Routledge Handbook on Spaces of Mental Health and Wellbeing

This handbook critically examines spaces of mental health and wellbeing across multiple, often intersecting, domains from green and blue spaces to lived and embodied spaces, creative spaces, work and home spaces, and institutional and post-institutional spaces.

The *Routledge Handbook on Spaces of Mental Health and Wellbeing* features 45 chapters from leading international scholars who collectively interrogate the spatial dimensions of mental health and wellbeing from conceptual and experiential viewpoints. The ways in which these theoretical developments prompt a re-thinking of mental health and wellbeing as concepts is also discussed before presenting some highlights from the handbook's five main sections – (1) green and blue spaces, (2) lived and embodied spaces, (3) creative spaces, (4) work and home spaces, and (5) institutional and post-institutional spaces. The key benefits of this book include a great appreciation of the complex networks and assemblages of mental health and wellbeing, the value of a geographical/ spatial approach to thinking about mental health, and the vast array of spaces and places that are implicated in human and posthuman notions of wellbeing.

This book will be of interest to students and scholars across the social sciences and the humanities as well as researchers and practitioners in the fields of psychology, psychiatry, social work, nursing, health geography, social and cultural geography, anthropology, mental health social studies, cultural theory, and architecture.

Candice P. Boyd is an artist-geographer and clinical psychologist. They are currently an honorary Principal Fellow in the School of Geography, Earth and Atmospheric Sciences at the University of Melbourne researching spaces of mental health and wellbeing, arts-based knowledge translation, and climate-related mental health issues. They are author of *Exhibiting Creative Geographies* (2023) and *Non-Representational Geographies of Therapeutic Art Making* (2017), co-author of *Emotion and the Contemporary Museum* (2020), and co-editor of *Non-Representational Theory and the Creative Arts* (2019).

Louise E. Boyle is a health geographer and Honorary Research Fellow in the School of Geographical and Earth Sciences at the University of Glasgow, Scotland. She completed an ESRC-funded PhD on *The Social and Anticipatory Geographies of Social Anxiety Disorder* (2019) and built on this research through an ESRC Post-Doctoral Research Fellowship (2020–2022). She is the author of *Anxious Geographies: Worlds of Social Anxiety* (Routledge, 2024).

Sarah L. Bell is a health geographer at the University of Exeter, whose work examines experiences of mental health, wellbeing, disability, and social inclusion in and with diverse forms of 'nature' – from parks, gardens, woodlands, coast, and countryside to the weather, seasons, and climate change (www.sensing-nature.com). Most recently, Sarah has been developing new collaborations to understand how the climate crisis – and prominent societal responses to it – is shaping the everyday lives and adaptive capacities of people with varied experiences and histories of disability (www.sensing-climate.com).

Ebba Högström is a professor in architecture at Umeå University. Her research interest is in social and experiential dimensions of architecture and the built environment. A specific interest is in geographies of welfare institutions and infrastructures of care. Currently, she is engaged in research projects addressing housing and living environments for vulnerable groups, i.e., people with mental ill-health and older people. Together with C Nord, she has edited the book *Caring Architecture: Institutions and Relational Practices* (2017).

Joshua Evans is an associate professor of human geography at the University of Alberta. He is a social geographer with interests in spaces of care, home, and work and their role in shaping the lived experiences of socially marginalized and vulnerable individuals, as well as spaces of policy development and implementation and their role in the creation of healthy, enabling, and equitable urban environments. His most recent research focuses on housing, homelessness, and urban justice.

Alak Paul is a health geographer at the University of Chittagong, Bangladesh. His research interest covers stigmatized diseases and public health. He focuses on everyday geographies of marginalized or vulnerable people in his research, especially how geographic space or place plays a role in reshaping the life of people or the environment. He is the author of *HIV/AIDS in Bangladesh: Stigmatized People, Policy and Place* (2020) and co-editor of *Geography in Bangladesh: Concepts Methods and Applications* (Routledge, 2019) and *The Palgrave Handbook of Social Fieldwork* (2023).

Ronan Foley is an associate professor in health geography and GIS at Maynooth University, Ireland, with expertise in therapeutic landscapes and geospatial planning within health and social care environments. His research focuses on relationships between water, health, and place, including two books and journal articles on holy wells, spas, social and cultural histories of swimming, and 'blue space'. He is an Editorial Board member of *Health & Place*, was Editor of *Irish Geography*, 2015–2022 and chairs the MU Healthy Campus Steering Group. He collaborates on water/health projects with colleagues in Ireland, UK, Spain, Germany, New Zealand, and Australia.

Routledge Handbook on Spaces of Mental Health and Wellbeing

Edited by Candice P. Boyd,
Louise E. Boyle, Sarah L. Bell,
Ebba Högström, Joshua Evans,
Alak Paul, and Ronan Foley

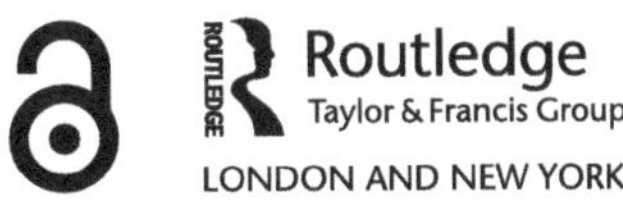

Designed cover image: © Getty Images

First published 2025
by Routledge
4 Park Square, Milton Park, Abingdon, Oxon OX14 4RN

and by Routledge
605 Third Avenue, New York, NY 10158

Routledge is an imprint of the Taylor & Francis Group, an informa business

British Library Cataloguing-in-Publication Data
A catalogue record for this book is available from the British Library

Library of Congress Cataloging-in-Publication Data
Names: Boyd, Candice P., 1970– editor.
Title: Routledge handbook on spaces of mental health and wellbeing /
edited by Candice P. Boyd, Louise E. Boyle, Sarah L. Bell, Ebba Högström,
Joshua Evans, Alak Paul, and Ronan Foley.
Other titles: Spaces of mental health and wellbeing
Description: Abingdon, Oxon; New York, NY: Routledge, 2025. |
Includes bibliographical references and index.
Identifiers: LCCN 2024030950 (print) | LCCN 2024030951 (ebook) |
ISBN 9781032385761 (hardback) | ISBN 9781032385815 (paperback) |
ISBN 9781003345725 (ebook)
Subjects: MESH: Mental Health | Environmental Health–methods | Environment Design | Nature
Classification: LCC RC454 .R68 2025 (print) | LCC RC454 (ebook) | NLM WM 31 |
DDC 616.89–dc23/eng/20240821
LC record available at https://lccn.loc.gov/2024030950
LC ebook record available at https://lccn.loc.gov/2024030951

ISBN: 9781032385761 (hbk)
ISBN: 9781032385815 (pbk)
ISBN: 9781003345725 (ebk)

DOI: 10.4324/9781003345725

Typeset in Sabon
by Newgen Publishing UK

Contents

Figures

Tables

Contributors

Joe Anderson received a PhD in Social Anthropology from the University of Edinburgh in 2020 and is now a research fellow on the *Suicide Cultures* project in the School of Health in Social Science at Edinburgh. Their research has focused on gun rights organisations in the United States and suicide in Scotland.

Kay Aranda is currently a Visiting Fellow in the School of Sport and Health Sciences at the University of Brighton. With a background in community and public health and theory informed qualitative research, she has published extensively in relation to health inequalities, gender and sexuality, and more recently on blue space and mental health, and sociomaterial practice theories, new materialisms and health equity.

Thomas Astell-Burt is the Professor of Cities and Planetary Health in the University of Sydney's School of Architecture, Design and Planning.

Gail E. Austen is a Postdoctoral Researcher at the Durrell Institute of Conservation and Ecology (DICE), University of Kent, UK. Her background is in conservation science, with a particular interest in species identification. Recently, her research has expanded across disciplines, and she is currently appreciating the opportunity to work on inter-disciplinary projects, addressing ecological and social aspects of biodiversity conservation, and working with non-academic partners.

Diti Bhattacharya is a Postdoctoral Research Fellow for an ARC Discovery Project with the Griffith Centre for Social and Cultural Research at Griffith University. She specialises in the study of South Asian diaspora in Australia. Her research expertise includes fitness cultures, sporting geographies, migration, heritage and mobilities. She is currently investigating the ways in which sporting practices and fitness cultures can be used as a social conduit through which marginalised communities experience a sense of belonging and community in Southeast Queensland. Trained as a human geographer, Diti specialises in posthuman critical feminist theories, non-representational theory and affect, and uses complex embodied practice-based research in her work.

Josephine Biglin is currently working as a lecturer in Social Psychology at the University of Salford and has previously worked as a lecturer in Sociology and Criminology. She was awarded her PhD from the University of Manchester in 2022. Her research centres around asylum, race, wellbeing, belonging and place. She is a qualitative researcher whose methodology is at the intersection of discursive approaches; sensory and embodied ways of knowing and arts-based participatory methods.

Shawn Bodden is Research Associate in Human Geography at the University of Glasgow. His research focuses on the geographies of community and social processes of shared experience.

Tore Dag Bøe is Professor of Mental Health Work in the Department of Psychosocial Health at the University of Agder, Norway. In his research, he is seeking to develop new forms of practice and new ways of understanding in the field of mental health, based on phenomenological, social, and ethical perspectives.

Candice P. Boyd is an artist-geographer and clinical psychologist. They are currently an honorary Principal Fellow in the School of Geography, Earth and Atmospheric Sciences at the University of Melbourne researching spaces of mental health and well-being, arts-based knowledge translation, and climate-related mental health issues. They are author of *Exhibiting Creative Geographies* (2023) and *Non-Representational Geographies of Therapeutic Art Making* (2017), co-author of *Emotion and the Contemporary Museum* (2020), and co-editor of *Non-Representational Theory and the Creative Arts* (2019).

Paul Callaghan is an Aboriginal man belonging to the land of the Worimi, coastal New South Wales, Australia. He uses his lived experience, cultural and community knowledge, experience and studies in commerce, and PhD in Creative Practice to advise organisations on how to implement strategic transformation initiatives that will increase the effectiveness of services targeting Aboriginal peoples. He is also a best-selling and award-winning author with his book *The Dreaming Path* providing insights on traditional Aboriginal ways of knowing, being and doing and how they can be used by all people to achieve improved wellbeing individually and globally.

Amy Chandler is Professor of the Sociology of Health and Illness. Her research centres qualitatively driven, sociologically informed studies of suicide, self-harm and mental illness in relation to social inequalities and injustice.

David A. G. Clarke lectures in Environmental Education at The University of Edinburgh, UK. He is a member of the University's Centre for Creative-Relational Inquiry (CCRI) and the Sustainability in Education Research Group (SIERG). His academic interests traverse education, creative inquiry, life experience and ethics in the Anthropocene.

Mary Coaten is a dance movement psychotherapist and practitioner/researcher working in the National Health Service in the UK where she delivers dance movement psychotherapy to groups in the acute adult mental health in-patient setting. Her special interest lies in how distress is expressed through the body, particularly in severe mental distress, and in embodied approaches to trauma. She completed her doctoral dissertation research in this area at the Institute of Medical Humanities, Durham University (2020). The research focused on the connection between movement patterns and the symbolic and metaphoric communications expressed during periods of acute mental distress. She is currently in Jungian Analytic training at the C.G. Jung Institute in Zurich.

Helen V. S. Cole is a senior researcher at the Barcelona Lab for Urban Environmental Justice and Sustainability (BCNUEJ) of the Institute of Environmental Science and Technology at the Autonomous University of Barcelona (ICTA-UAB). Her research explores whether, and how, healthier cities may also be made equitable, placing urban health interventions in the context of the broader urban social and political environments.

John Connell is Professor of Geography in the School of Geosciences at the University of Sydney. He has published widely on health in the island Pacific, including *The Global Health Care Chain. From the Pacific to the World* (2009), and on medical tourism.

Martin Dallimer is Professor of Environmental Change at the University of Leeds, UK. From April 2024, Martin will be based at Imperial College London. His research applies and integrates research techniques from across different disciplines to better understand, and provide solutions for, the sustainable management.

Charlie Dannreuther is a lecturer in European political economy at the University of Leeds in the School of Politics and International studies. Recent work inspired by collaborating in this team includes a piece on the pedagogy of "Feeling Political" in the desensitised environment of the University system, a piece on the political economy of whaling showing that capitalism kills and a new project exploring water infrastructure through changing ideals of the body.

Zoe G. Davies is Professor of Biodiversity Conservation at the Durrell Institute of Conservation and Ecology (DICE), University of Kent, UK. She is a landscape ecologist by training, but her research interests have expanded and increasingly cross traditional disciplinary boundaries. Nonetheless, the unifying theme throughout all of her work is that she uses empirical data to address questions of importance to conservation management and policy. She is particularly fascinated by understanding how biodiversity underpins human wellbeing.

Hannah Denton is a Counselling Psychologist working in Sussex Partnership Foundation Trust and a Visiting Fellow in the School of Sport and Health Sciences at the University of Brighton. Hannah has an interest in creative and mobile methodologies as a way to better understand the experience of outdoor swimming and how it relates to mental health and wellbeing. She has a number of publications in this area.

Nastaran Doroud is a Senior Lecturer in Occupational Therapy at School of Health Sciences, Swinburne University of Technology. She uses qualitative, participatory and photovoice research methodologies to explore how people with mental illness experience recovery and engage in meaningful activities. Nastaran's current projects include development and evaluation of a photovoice group intervention, recovery experiences for culturally diverse communities, and co-design of a university wellness program.

Kate E. W. Douglas is a PhD candidate in the School of Geography, Earth and Atmospheric Sciences at the University of Melbourne. Working within the theoretical and methodological bounds of cultural geography, her research examines the impact of creative recovery projects that emerged following the 2022 floods in the Northern Rivers of New South Wales, Australia.

Michelle Duffy is an Associate Professor of Human Geography at the School of Environmental and Life Sciences, University of Newcastle. Her research draws on participatory methodologies to explore how interactions between people and place contribute to notions of community and identity, and hence the processes of belonging and alienation. Current projects include the impact of disaster on community wellbeing;

festivals as spaces of social connection; and the role of sonic geographies and listening practices may play in reconnecting to our environments.

Christian Edwardes is an artist-researcher based in the UK. His work is centred around studio geographies and the geoaesthetics of artistic production, with a particular interest in artists' attachments to creative spaces and non-representational approaches to creative practising. He is Course Leader for BA Illustration at the Arts University Bournemouth and co-editor of *Non-Representational Theory and the Creative Arts* published in 2019.

Candela Sánchez-Rodilla Espeso is a Teaching Fellow in Counselling, Psychotherapy and Applied Social Science at the University of Edinburgh. She is currently a Co-Investigator for REALITIES, an AHRC-funded health disparities project. Her research interests and expertise fall within three areas: the concepts of place and space; phenomenological and embodied approaches to mental health; and space design and mobility.

Clifton Evers is a lecturer in Media and Cultural Studies at Newcastle University in the UK. He researches the intersections of men and masculinities, action and lifestyle sports, pollution, blue spaces, post-industrial placemaking, and just transitions. His research has been published widely in prestigious academic publications, as well as more public facing media such as TV and Radio. Clifton uses innovative participatory arts-based research methods (e.g., textile, perfumery, animation, performance art, film, photography, sound) and ethnography to conduct his studies. He is a curator of critically acclaimed arts-based research exhibitions.

Emma Farrell is a Chartered Psychologist and Senior Interdisciplinary Researcher in the School of Education, University College Dublin. With expertise in hermeneutic phenomenology, Emma's research focuses on understanding the lived experience of phenomena such as mental health, education and healthcare. She is author of 'Making Sense of Mental Health: A Practical Approach through Lived Experience' (2022). Her forthcoming book on supporting students with mental health difficulties in higher education will be published in 2025. Emma is a founding member of Jigsaw, Ireland's National Centre for Youth Mental Health; a former member of the Government Taskforce for Youth Mental Health, and a member of the Council of Gaisce, The President's Award. She is co-founder of thinkful.ie, an online platform that aims to empower conversations in philosophy and mental health.

Xiaoqi Feng is the Professor or Urban Health and Environment at the University of New South Wales' School of Population Health.

Fernando Ferrari is psychologist and professor at the University of Córdoba (Argentina) director of Ecos-Sud (France and Argentina) project and Director of Research in Secretaría de Ciencia y Técnica (UNC).

Jessica C. Fisher is a Conservation Social Scientist at the Durrell Institute of Conservation and Ecology, University of Kent, UK. While her background is in ecology, her research focuses on mixed methods approaches to social and environmental challenges, using techniques that cross traditional disciplinary boundaries.

Ellie Fossey is Professor and Head of Occupational Therapy at the School of Primary and Allied Health Care, Monash University. Her research focuses on understanding experiences of living with ongoing health conditions and addressing restrictions to participation in occupations of everyday life, primarily using collaborative and qualitative research approaches. Ellie's current projects include advancing recovery-oriented practices in mental health care, evaluation of a peer support enhanced vocational intervention, and consumer involvement and co-design in health professions education.

Jan Georg Friesinger is Associate Professor in the Department of Psychosocial Health at the University of Agder, Norway. His background is in sociology and his research focuses on materialities, public health, health geography, medical sociology, and community mental health.

Ann Fudge Schormans is an Associate Professor in the School of Social Work at McMaster University. Many years of social work practice with people living with disabilities, combined with ongoing activist work, informs her teaching and research. Employing inclusive, co-researcher methodologies and knowledge production, along with arts-informed methods, her research focuses on issues identified by people with disabilities as being important to their lives. Current projects include the parenting experiences and aspirations of people with intellectual disabilities; and friendships and social inclusion of youth with intellectual disabilities.

Marco Garrido-Cumbrera is a professor at the Department of Geography of the University of Seville and an international expert on urban health and environmental issues from a social and psychosocial perspective. Marco has completed university studies in Spain, Italy and France and has been a visiting professor at Maynooth University (Ireland), the Federal University of Rio de Janeiro (Brazil) and Columbia University (USA). He has participated in more than 50 research projects and co-authored more than 100 scientific publications in peer reviewed journals. He previously worked at the World Health Organization (WHO) in Geneva as project manager on different health atlases and currently leads the Health & Territory Research (HTR) team at the University of Seville on international projects measuring patient-reported outcomes, assessing the burden of mental disorders and work-related issues.

Hervé Guillemain is a historian at Le Mans University, France and member of TEMOS CNRS 9016. Specialised in the history of psychiatry, he is co-director of the French review *History, Medicine and Heath* and director of the DicoPolHiS project.

Andy Harrod is a senior teaching associate in human geography and PhD researcher in health and wellbeing geography in the Lancaster Environment Centre at Lancaster University. Andy is also a person-centred psychotherapist, with a particular interest in integrating person-centred theory with geographical place-based concepts. Andy's research focus on nature-based interventions and how participation influences participants' long-term wellbeing. Andy has specifically considered the agency of the facilitator(s) and participants in co-creating affective relational spaces as a significant influence on beneficial long-term changes to participants' wellbeing. Andy engages with creative qualitative methodologies and is interested in methods which can help diversify the range of voices involved in research.

Sophie-Bo Heinkel studied geography, ethnology and biology at the University of Bonn. After joining the Institute for Hygiene and Public Health, University Hospital Bonn, she conducted her doctoral research on the therapeutic effect of wetlands in Uganda. After graduation she took a postdoc position at the University of Cologne, running research projects in Asia focusing on disaster risk reduction. Sophie-Bo spent time researching and working in various African countries, including Uganda, Ethiopia and Burkina Faso. Next to her academic work, she offers trainings on intercultural communication.

Rebecca Helman is a Research Fellow on the University of Edinburgh's *Suicide Cultures: Reimagining Suicide Research* project. Rebecca's work explores the relationships between violence and various intersecting forms of inequality. She holds a PhD in Psychology from the University of South Africa.

Rachel Herron is a Professor in the Department of Geography and Environment at Brandon University, a Tier II CRC in Rural and Remote Mental Health, and founding Director of the Centre for Critical Studies of Rural Mental Health. Rachel works with researchers, students, and community partners to explore rural mental health, ageing, and care needs using a variety of qualitative methods. Her research examines safety in settings of care, social inclusion, and the diversity of experiences living with mental health problems.

Jesse Hodgetts is a Wangaaypuwan Ngiyampaa and Wiradjuri man of Western New South Wales, Australia. He is a lecturer in Aboriginal Studies at the Wollotuka Institute of The University of Newcastle. Jesse's experience as a songman and language practitioner supports Indigenous song making and language revitalisation through his Kinship ties and networks with other Indigenous cultural practitioners across the country. Jesse has recently completed a PhD in reawakening archived Ngiyampaa songs. His research focuses on First Nations Cultural revitalisation and the continuation of Indigenous Knowledge Systems and ways of being, particularly through the practice of Song, Language, and Kinship.

Ebba Högström is Professor in Architecture at Umeå University. Her research interest is in social and experiential dimensions of architecture and the built environment. A specific interest is in geographies of welfare institutions and infrastructures of care. Currently, she is engaged in research projects addressing housing and living environments for vulnerable groups, i.e., people with mental ill-health and older people. She has co-edited the book *Caring Architecture* (with C Nord).

Øyvind Hope is PhD candidate in Psycho-social Health at the Department of Psychosocial Health at the University of Agder, Norway. In his research, he is seeking to develop new forms of practice and new ways of understanding in the field of mental health, based on health geographical, social, and materialistic perspectives.

Sarah Huque is currently a Research Fellow on the *Suicide Cultures: Reimagining Suicide Research* project. Her research focuses on the intersection of social justice and public health, with an interest in methodological innovation. She holds a PhD in Geography from the University of St Andrews.

Sheena Hyland is Assistant Professor in Educational Development at University College Dublin. She holds a PhD from the UCD School of Philosophy on the phenomenological philosophy of Maurice Merleau-Ponty. Her research and teaching interests include phenomenology, the philosophy of education, and inclusion and equity in teaching and learning in higher education.

Katherine N. Irvine is a Senior Researcher in Environment, Wellbeing and Sustainable Behaviour at the James Hutton Institute, UK. She brings training in biology, conservation behaviour and environmental psychology, along with professional environmental education experience, to build bridges between disciplines and sectors at the nexus of the people-nature relationship. Incorporating theory, qualitative and quantitative methods, her transdisciplinary research evaluates the effectiveness of interventions to foster nature engagement and explores the contribution of biodiversity to multiple dimensions of well-being.

Robin Kearns is Professor of Geographer and Head of the School of Environment at the University of Auckland. He has published widely in the field of health geography and is an editor of the journal *Health and Place*. He is a coauthor of the Routledge book *Afterlives of the Psychiatric Asylum* (with G Moon and A. Joseph).

Juliana España Keller, PhD, is a Canadian, Swiss and British Sound and Performance Artist engaged in radical entanglements in soundpractices through speculative research that draws attention to quantum listening as a relational capacity and as a philosophical and temporal process. Her research framework of acoustic care and well-being through collective resonant ecologies is also entangled with human-non-human contact that engages in fluctuating sites with sensing subjects and tactile experimentation. She/Her is a sessional faculty member of Concordia University, Studio Arts Program in Montreal, Quebec, Canada. Juliana directs the International Creative Arts Residency 'Bajo el Olivo' in Malaga, Spain dedicated to artists and researchers who are looking for a private space to think, write and create during these exceptional times we are living on this planet. www.julianaespanakeller.com

Jonathan (Yotti) Kingsley is a Senior Lecturer in Health Promotion. Prior to moving into academia Jonathan worked in Aboriginal Community Controlled Health Organisations, government bodies, and NGOs across Australia in public health and community development. Jonathan views the natural environment as having the capacity to bridge health inequalities (the basis of his Honours, Masters, PhD and previous Visiting Academic position at Cambridge University). Dr Kingsley has published over 55 peer-reviewed papers (38 as first or last author) and received a number of grants to explore issues focused on the health benefits of urban agriculture and Aboriginal and Torres Strait Islander communities' connection to Country.

Thomas Kistemann studied geography, classical languages, educational psychology and medicine at the Universities of Aachen, Bonn and Gottingen. He is professor for Hygiene, Environmental Medicine and Medical Geography at the University of Bonn. At the Institute for Hygiene and Public Health, he is heading the GeoHealth Centre and the WHO Collaborating Centre for Health Promoting Water Management & Risk Communication. His research is focused on the water-health-nexus and the concept of therapeutic landscapes.

Hayden Lorimer is Chair of Human Geography at the University of Edinburgh. In his research and writing, he considers the geographical dimensions of place, landscape and practice, in the past, present and future.

Grace Lucas is a Senior Lecturer in Mental Health and Society in the School of Health and Psychological Sciences at City, University of London. Grace's research interests are interdisciplinary with a particular focus on embodied methodologies and bodywork practices for understanding, representing, and healing from mental distress. This interest was initially borne out of her lived experience of the eating disorder anorexia nervosa when she was a teenager. She is the author of *A Shape of My Own* (2006) / *Thin* (2007), a highly regarded memoir of anorexia and recovery.

Erin MacKenney has a background in education and close to 10 years of experience working in poverty reduction in the non-profit sector. Throughout her career she has developed a passion for developing and leading innovative projects to address her community's needs. This includes developing alternative educational programs for vulnerable youth and adults, building and implementing workplace training programs, and collaborating on a youth housing program. Erin believes in the importance of authentically engaging program participants in the work through the use of participatory action research and approaches program design through the lens of developmental evaluation. She believes that in order to solve our world's most complex issues, you must be bold, brave, and open to learning.

Judith Mair is an Associate Professor at the UQ Business School, University of Queensland, Australia. Judith's work aims to understand and enhance the positive impacts of tourism and events on the communities and societies which host them. She is working on a number of projects in fields including mega-event legacies, the future of events, the links between events and social connectivity and the potential impacts of climate change on the events sector.

Wendy Masterton is Lecturer in Criminology (specialising in substance use) at the University of Stirling. She is part of the Salvation Army Centre for Addiction Services and Research and the Scottish Centre for Crime and Justice Research. She holds a PhD in Sociology and Social Policy from University of Stirling, during which she developed a realist-informed intervention framework for greenspace programmes for improving mental health and supporting people with problem drug and alcohol use. Wendy's research interests include realist methods, substance use, harm reduction, mental health, health inequalities, and the health benefits of greenspace and greenspace interventions.

Gillean McDougall is a writer and editor based in Glasgow, Scotland. She worked in classical music and broadcasting before graduating with a MLitt with Distinction in Creative Writing from the University of Glasgow in 2017. Her PhD thesis (Doctor of Fine Arts) from the same university, the memoir 'A Year to Find My Father', was shortlisted for the *Mslexia* Memoir Prize in 2023. Gillean leads the archival creative projects *Honest Error*, *Writing the Asylum* and *the prescription* (on Charles Rennie Mackintosh, Gartnavel Royal Asylum and The Royal College of Physicians and Surgeons of Glasgow), and her first novel will be sent out to publishers in 2024.

Jamie Mcphie's work traverses Health, Environmental Humanities, and Experiential Education. He is a co-theme lead for one of the Learning, Education and Development Research Centre themes based at the University of Cumbria (UK). His research interests include therapeutic landscapes, environmental ethics, contemporary animisms, posthumanism and psychogeography. He recently authored the book *Mental Health and Wellbeing in the Anthropocene: A Posthuman Inquiry* (2019) and co-edited the book *New Materialisms and Environmental Education* (2023).

Cassandra Monette has a passion for blending art, research, and youth work together to create impact. She is dedicated to amplifying youth voice through arts-based storytelling and understands the influence narratives can have on identity and community membership. She currently holds a dual role as both the Youth Engagement and Research Specialist at the Teen Resource Centre, and directs the Youth Pillar at the HOME-RL research lab. She leads multiple participatory action research initiatives that strengthen partnerships between organisations and creates interdisciplinary teams to translate research data into social action.

Michael A. Navakatikyan is a Research Fellow in Statistics at the University of New South Wales' School of Population Health.

Ottar Ness is Professor at the Norwegian University of Science and Technology (NTNU) and Co-director of Nordic Research Center for Wellbeing and Social Sustainability (NTNU Welfare). He is also Adjunct Professor at University of Agder in Norway. His research focuses on transdisciplinary approaches to wellbeing, recovery, mental health, and citizenship.

Rebecca Olive is a Vice-Chancellor's Senior Research Fellow at RMIT University, Australia. With a background in cultural studies, gender studies, and anthropology, her recent work explores the role of recreational lifestyle sports and physical activities in human-ocean health and wellbeing with a particular interest in swimming, surfing and sailing. This work focuses on themes of human relationships to animals and pollution, as well as the politics of localism. You can read more about this work at www.movingoceans.com.

Deborah K. Padgett is a Professor at NYU Silver School of Social Work and an international expert on qualitative and mixed-methods research. Dr. Padgett's extensive research on unsheltered populations explores Housing First as a 'paradigm shifting' approach to addressing homelessness in the U.S. and abroad. Dr. Padgett has lectured widely on the topic across Europe as well as in Canada, India and Brasil. Padgett received the NYU Distinguished Teaching Award in 2012 and has been co-principal investigator on two R01 National Institute of Mental Health (NIMH) funded grants using qualitative methods to study the effects of Housing First. Since 2015, she has worked closely with The Banyan, an organization in Chennai, India that assists unhoused women with mental health issues.

Hester Parr is Chair of Human Geography at the University of Glasgow. In her research and writing, she considers the geographical dimensions of mental (ill) health and relationships to place.

Chris Philo is Professor of Geography at the University of Glasgow, Scotland. He is passionate about the value that a geographical perspective can bring to almost any academic inquiry. His specialist research is on the historical and social geographies of mental ill-health, psychiatric provisions and living with mental difference, and has also published widely on the history, theory, spirit, and purpose of his 'home' discipline.

Jesse Proudfoot is an Assistant Professor in the Department of Sociology at Durham University. His research is concerned with the relationship between socio-political forces such as racism and poverty and compulsive substance use, as well as critical theorisations of addiction and the politics of drug policy. Trained as a human geographer, he researches these issues through ethnographic fieldwork and life history interviews with people who use drugs in Canada, the United States, and UK. He has published in a variety of leading journals, including *Social Science and Medicine*; *Culture, Medicine and Psychiatry*; and *Progress in Human Geography*. He is currently co-investigator for the Discovery Research Platform for Medical Humanities, funded by the Wellcome Trust, alongside colleagues at Durham's Institute for Medical Humanities.

Virve Repo is Post-Doctoral Research Fellow in Social Sciences in Tampere University, Finland. With a background in human geography, she has specialised in carceral geography. Her studies have concentrated on spaces of care and control, such as nursing homes, psychiatric hospitals, and facilities of forensic psychiatric care. She also studies older individuals and their connections to space and surroundings from various viewpoints.

Thorben Peter Høj Simonsen is a Researcher at the Danish Center for Social Science Research (VIVE). Before coming to VIVE he was an Assistant Professor at the Department of Business IT at the IT University in Copenhagen, where he taught organisation theory. He gained his PhD at the Department of Organisation, Copenhagen Business School by investigating the spatial organisation of psychiatric practice, focusing specifically on the role of healing architecture. His research interests converge around problematics relating to space and place, welfare technologies, mental health, care, and digitalisation.

Elaine Stratford is Professor of Human Geography and Planning at the University of Tasmania. Her research is motivated by trying to understand the conditions in which people flourish in place, in their movements, in daily life, and over the life-course.

Alain Topor is Professor at the Department of Psychosocial Health at the University of Agder, Norway. He has previously worked as an "at home therapist" and family therapist in social services in Stockholm. As a psychologist, he actively participated in the closing of mental hospitals in Stockholm and in the development of alternative structures in the community. He then worked as head of Research and Development units. Together with colleagues from different countries he has explored recovery as a social, material, and relational process.

Margarita Triguero-Mas is an environmental health senior researcher at the Universitat Oberta de Catalunya (i.e. Open University of Catalonia, UOC) and at the Barcelona Institute of Global Health (ISGlobal). She is also an associated researcher at the Barcelona Lab for Urban Environmental Justice and Sustainability (BCNUEJ). Margarita's research focuses on how and why green and blue spaces benefit (or not) people's health, with a particular focus on health inequities and injustices.

Nadia Von Benzon is Lecturer in Human Geography at Lancaster University. She is a social geographer with particular interests in childhood, motherhood, disability, and nature. Recent publications include *Creative Methods in Human Geography* and *Birth in Unprecedented Times: Geographies of Risk in Birth Stories* (Routledge).

Belinda Wheaton is Professor in the School of Health at the University of Waikato Aotearoa New Zealand. Belinda is best known for her research on informal and lifestyle sport cultures, social inclusion and policy, which includes monographs *The Cultural*

Politics of Lifestyle Sports, Action Sports and the Olympic Games: Past, Present, Future (Wheaton & Thorpe, 2022). Belinda is Co-editor of The Palgrave Handbook of Feminism and Sport, Leisure and Physical Education and Managing Editor of *Annals of Leisure Research*. Belinda's recent research focuses on understanding Ocean-Human Relationships in coastal blue space leisure practices in Aotearoa, and how this contributes to wellbeing for communities and their environments.

Robert Wilton is a Professor in the School of Earth, Environment & Society at McMaster University. His research is concerned with the lived experiences of disabled people and the systemic barriers they face to social inclusion and participation. He has focused particular attention on people's experiences finding and keeping paid employment in both market and social economies; accessing and maintaining housing; and negotiating state welfare/disability benefits systems. Rob co-edited the books *Towards Enabling Geographies* and *Using Space* (Routledge).

Julia Woodhall-Melnik is an Associate Professor of Sociology at the University of New Brunswick in Saint John, co-director and founder of the Housing, Mobilization, and Engagement Research Lab (HOME-RL), and the Canada Research Chair in Resilient Communities. Her work focuses on housing justice, locational inequity, housing loss, climate and housing futures, and housing as a social determinant of physical and mental health. Julia is a community-based researcher, with expertise in mixed methods research. She is committed to incorporating the voices of people with lived experience of poverty and housing precarity into her research. Her work as the Principal Investigator at HOME-RL engages students, community members, and decision makers in research, and upholds values of social justice.

Emily Yue is PhD candidate on the Suicide Cultures research project and Research Fellow on Suicide in/as Politics at the University of Edinburgh. Her research centres on the intersections between 'mixed-race' and 'suicide/ality' in Britain.

Acknowledgements

We were delighted as contributors to the *Routledge Handbook of Health Geography* to be identified by one of its editors, Professor Gavin Andrews, as suitably qualified to put together a handbook on spaces of mental health and wellbeing. Being mostly early and mid-career researchers, it is an honour to be recognised by a senior colleague as key contributors to this exciting field of scholarship. We would like to thank him and commissioning editor at Routledge, Faye Leerink, for believing in us.

We are also grateful for the three rigorous reviews of our book proposal, which challenged us as an editorial team to extend our reach beyond our comfortable networks in the Global North. One of these reviewers, Professor Valorie Crooks (also an editor of the *Routledge Handbook of Health Geography*) introduced us to Dr Alak Paul who then joined the editorial team, and, as editors, we sought to include scholarship representative of the Global South and/or Indigenous geographies. Our efforts, however, fell well short of the fair balance we would had liked to have achieved. This is as much a reflection on the paucity of our own connections with Global South scholars as it is on the colonising nature of academic knowledge. Being pushed to make an effort by our reviewers, however, was very much appreciated.

We would like to individually thank partners, families, colleagues, and friends for their support of our efforts and for their continued mentorship, encouragement, understanding, and empathy. Projects such of these often 'bleed' into private time, impacting those around us as a result.

Our thanks to Prachi Priyanka, Editorial Assistant in Geography and Tourism at Routledge, for their invaluable support at the manuscript submission stage. Thanks also to the copyediting and design teams at Routledge who brought this book to publication. We would also like to acknowledge the support of our institutions, much of which is related to infrastructure rather than time.

Finally, we extend our deepest gratitude to all who authored chapters and recommended additional contributors to this handbook. Your dedication, expertise, and insightful contributions have been the backbone of this work. We acknowledge the precarious and unpaid nature of much of the labour that went into this endeavour from editors and contributors alike, especially those who are not in paid employment or who needed to take time out of their regular employment to prepare chapters. We recognise the substantial time and effort that each of you have devoted to ensuring the quality and depth of your chapters, which have enriched this publication immeasurably.

1 Introducing the *Routledge Handbook on Spaces of Mental Health and Wellbeing*

Candice P. Boyd, Louise E. Boyle, Ebba Högström,
Sarah L. Bell, Joshua Evans, Alak Paul, and Ronan Foley

In the context of a rapidly changing climate and global pandemic, our understandings of the geographies of mental health have never been more pertinent. These changes have far-reaching consequences for the material, social and affective relations that co-constitute people's everyday lives. This handbook, through the insights of its contributors, critically examines spaces of mental health and wellbeing across multiple, often intersecting, domains from green and blue spaces, lived and embodied spaces, creative spaces, spaces of work and home and institutional and post-institutional spaces. Incorporating contemporary and multi-disciplinary perspectives, contributors to this volume consider the social, emotional, and affective dimensions of treatment and recovery as well as the vernacular, everyday practices that create spaces for reflection and replenishment. In doing so, they also pay attention to experiences and practices that diminish wellbeing and our capacities for mental health, and how these are likewise embedded in place and space.

As a companion to the *Routledge Handbook of Health Geography*, the *Routledge Handbook on Spaces of Mental Health and Well-Being* adopts a relational framework for interrogating health-space connections, with a focus on mental health and wellbeing broadly conceived. As editors, however, we are acutely aware of wider debates across the social sciences and humanities about the value and validity of 'mental health' and 'wellbeing' as concepts. Although contributors to this volume problematise these terms to varying degrees (as we do as independent scholars), we have adopted a utilitarian, and somewhat mainstream, position as an editorial collective while simultaneously acknowledging that 'mental health' and 'wellbeing' have social and political implications that are far-reaching, complex, and sometimes harmful (see McGeachan & Philo, 2023). However, we are also cognisant of the fact that potential readers of this book will be unaware of these debates, instead approaching this book with an open curiosity about space-place relations and their relevance to mental health and wellbeing. With these readers in mind, we take mental health geography as our starting point for this introduction, providing a brief history of its trajectory before considering how current understandings within this field align with recent theoretical developments in health and human geography.

From mental health geography to 'geopsychiatry'?

Mental health geography emerged as a substantive subfield of human geography (Wolch & Philo, 2000) around the same time as health geography was transitioning from medical geography (Kearns & Moon, 2002). Acknowledged as having its origins in quantitative methods and spatial science (McGeachan & Philo, 2023), mental health geography

DOI: 10.4324/9781003345725-1

had a 'second wave' towards the end of the twentieth century, employing qualitative methods to better understand the experience of mental health and ill-health in different contexts and at different scales (Philo, 2005). Much of this early analysis was focused on institutional spaces (Philo, 1997) and spaces of the body (Parr, 1998) but later expanded to encompass the plethora of 'ad-hoc' facilities, therapeutic landscapes and spaces of community that play an integral role in shaping and defining the daily lives of individuals, particularly those transitioning out of institutional care and into the community (Knowles, 2000; Markström, Högström & Fjellfeldt, 2023; Parr & Philo, 2003; Davidson & Parr, 2007; Parr, 2008). This sustained attention to the lived geographies of institutionalised and deinstitutionalised communities (Parr, Philo and Burns, 2003, Högström, 2018) as well as to particular experiences and expressions of distress (Boyle, 2024; Davidson, 2003; Fjellfeldt, Högström and Markström, forthcoming; Nieuwenhuis and Knoll 2021) provide non-clinical, and specifically spatialised, insights into the taken-for-granted aspects of people's daily geographies.

Today, mental health geography is in its forecasted (Wolch & Philo, 2000), 'third' wave, where the advancement of affective and posthumanist perspectives across the social sciences and humanities have led to '… affirmative inquiries into the making of mentally healthy worlds' (McGeachan & Philo, 2023, p.1228) while still 'staying true' to its critical and humanist underpinnings (Andrews, 2018; Boyd, Parr & Philo, 2023). However, influences from psychiatric survivor critiques and voices and the emerging academic field of *Mad Studies*, have become more prominent which suggests that a 'fourth' wave of mental health geography might be approaching. Arising out of opposition to medicalised notions of mental health and wellbeing, mad studies is grounded in the people/survivor movement within anti-psychiatry and is strongly aligned to queer and crip theory (see Beresford & Russo, 2022; McRue, 2006) Developments within these fields have contributed to a contemporary re-thinking of mental health as well as highlighting a rich plethora of spaces for mental health and wellbeing, including spaces for mental health *care* other than the institutional spaces 'as we know them' .

At the heart of mental health geography is the established relationship between health and place, which in itself is based on an awareness of the unequal distribution of health and healthcare locally and across the globe (Brown, Andrews, Cummins, & Greenhough, 2017; Gatrell & Elliot, 2014). However, geographies of health and mental health do not simply regard 'place' in terms of 'location' but also conceptualise it in relational terms (Andrews, 2018). In contrast to the relatively fixed view of place as a 'point on a map', a relational view of place attends to the ways in which places are co-constructed 'in the moment' through 'a network of relations' which only temporarily come into being before dispersing and re-forming as a different set of relations. Thus, a relational view of health and mental health and their geographies is much more focused on the 'how' of health – i.e., its processes – than the 'where' (even though they to a great extent acknowledge the mutual influence between the 'how' and the 'where' as spatial processes become). Likewise, 'space' is not seen as a 'thing' or a 'container' in mental health geography but rather a 'product' of social forces which is similarly *in process* (see Crang & Thrift, 2000). The *Routledge Handbook on Spaces of Mental Health and Wellbeing* is replete with examples of relational ideas.

The relational view of mental health and wellbeing is not confined to the disciplinary boundaries of geography and resonates across the social sciences, humanities, the arts, architecture and what has become known as health and medical humanities. As De Leeuw et al. (2018) assert,

[t]raditional methods of both clinical and social science inquiry seek to neatly categorize and contain health and medical issues. Approaches used in the field of medical health humanities reject notions that what constitutes health and medicine has clear geographic or temporal boundaries ... [f]ormal explanations of health and disease might attempt to locate disease experiences within the confines of conventional spaces and places. More complex and creative understandings of health experiences (both personal and sociocultural) identify that health experiences unfurl and fold back, encompassing and linking together disparate geographies, positionalities, and subjectivities.

(p.289)

This style of thinking about health and medical issues has recently 'caught the eye' of researchers in psychiatry and psychology, with proposals to incorporate relational viewpoints into new interdisciplinary fields like 'geopsychiatry' (Castaldelli-Maria & Bhurga, 2022) and 'clinical geography' (Finlay & Rowles, 2021). Geographers, however, have warned against the slippage in concepts, or what is 'lost in translation', in these efforts (Rosenberg, 2021) as well as the neglect of decades of research in mental health geography and an appreciation of its disciplinary trajectory (Philo, Callard, McGeachan, & Parr, 2023). As editors, we would like to issue a similar caution to readers of the *Routledge Handbook on Spaces of Mental Health and Wellbeing* who might be approaching its contents from outside the social sciences and humanities, yet in many ways this is what this edited collection is for – a tribute to the power and relevance of geographical thought to contemporary understandings of mental health and wellbeing and a testament to mental health geography as a mature field of scholarship.

Re-thinking mental health and wellbeing

Wellbeing is a 'governing concept' in the field of health geography (Atkinson, 2017 and operationalised across wider academic and policy spaces for considering what constitutes a meaningful, fulfilling, and flourishing life. While approaches to, and conceptualisations of, wellbeing vary considerably across disciplinary spaces, the relationship between place and wellbeing is of fundamental concern in geographical research agendas (Fleuret and Atkinson, 2007; Kearns and Andrews, 2010; Atkinson, Fuller and Painter, 2012). As such, scholarship over the last two decades has centred on two key and, for the purposes of this summary, broad strands of research, namely: wellbeing agendas within wider neoliberal policy contexts (Atkinson and Joyce, 2011) and subjectively experienced wellbeing across a range of therapeutic landscapes, green and blue spaces, and embodied practices (Schwanen and Wang, 2014). In a geographical context, conceptualisations of wellbeing abound, but it is perhaps most commonly understood as '[a] holistic conception of positive human functioning ... extending beyond a physiological or biomedical notion of health to encompass the emotional, social, and in some cases, spiritual dimensions of what it means to be human' (Conradson 2012, p.16).

During what was widely lauded as the 'affective turn', human geography was one of several academic disciplines to contribute to, and draw upon, several developments in social theory and associated methodologies such as *actor network theory* (Latour, 2005; see McLeod, 2017 & Müller & Schurr, 2016), *assemblage theory* (Deleuze and Guattari, 1987; see Kanngieser, 2012 & Roberts, 2021), *new materialisms* (Barad, 2007; Braidotti, 2011; Manning, 2012; see Colls, 2012 & Whatmore, 2006), *ethico-aesthetics* (Guattari,

1992; see McCormack, 2002), *speculative realism* and *post-phenomenology* (Harman, 2010; Marion, 2002; Nancy, 1997; see Ash & Simpson, 2016), and *non-representational theory* (Thrift, 2007, Simpson, 2021; see Bissell, 2011, Boyd, 2017 & Dewsbury, 2003) – although many of these 'advancements' had their basis in phenomenological and process-oriented philosophies from a much earlier time (e.g., Merleau-Ponty, 1962; Spinoza, 2000; Whitehead, 1979). Regarding spaces of mental health and wellbeing, geographers informed by these theories emphasise how health, including mental health, emerges from embodied encounters between human and non-human entities (Andrews, 2020; Duff, 2014) in ways that are processual, eventful, pre-personal, and mobile (Andrews, Chen & Myers, 2014; Andrews & Duff, 2020).

The myriad of threats to human health posed by climate change have seen medicalised notions of Western health and wellbeing transform over the past decade (Adams, 2020). These new notions of health emphasise the interconnectedness of humans, animals, and ecosystems and the importance of understanding these links in responding to new health challenges (World Health Organisation, 2023). Such developments strongly align with new theoretical perspectives in human geography but also with Indigenous knowledges and lore (Elkington, 2023). As such, the call for Western scholars across the academy to develop a deeper knowledge and appreciation of Indigenous ways of knowing and being is stronger than ever (Jessen, Ban Claxton, & Darimont, 2021). Within geography, argu-ably a discipline already attuned to the 'more-than-human', there has been a developing interest in posthumanism (see Andrews & Rishworth, 2023;) both for its explana-tory power (Boyd, Parr, & Philo, 2023) and its methodological potential (Boyd, 2022; Williams, Patchett, Lapworth, Roberts, & Keating, 2019). Within these pages, we have several examples of the application of posthuman thinking to mental health (e.g., Keller, Chapter 25) as well as the importance of cultural practices and lore to Indigenous well-being (see Callaghan & Hodgetts, Chapter 23). The more-than-human approach also has connections to the concept of 'spatial agency'– or what spaces *do* – in both positive and negative sense. These 'doings' can act in contradictory as well as supportive ways to be both deliberately 'enabling', positive assemblages and ostensibly 'disabling', negative ones (Högström & Philo, 2023).

McPhie (2019) suggests, (see also Chapter 26 in this volume), that there is no such thing as mental health – mental health is *always* physical. Inherent in this view is a con-cept of relationality that is not 'inter' or between, but 'intra' or within. As such, health and place (or human and 'natural world') are not seen as separate entities in relation to one another but entangled and intertwined. As McPhie argues,

> [There] is not the naïve 'outside' that is proffered by binary bias as the healthful *nat-ural* world in opposition to an *artificial* sedentary 'inside' but an intra-relational out-side that is always already both inside and outside, natural and artificial, real and conceptual, physical and psychological. By this, I mean that psychological phenomena are necessarily physical; inside is also outside depending on your contextual and rela-tional situatedness; artificial is also always natural; and conceptual is also real, for how *on earth* could they not be?
>
> (emphasis in the original; 2019, pp.13–14)

Hayes-Conroy, Kinsey, and Hayes-Conroy (2022) take this further in their conceptu-alisation of the 'biosphere'. They similarly argue that binary thinking that divides the body and the mind is not helpful for understanding health and wellbeing. They instead call for non-dualistic, emergent, and plastic understandings of the body as 'contextually porous' – intra-affected within structural, discursive, and experiential domains of wellbeing in which the body is embedded (see Hayes-Conroy et al., 2022, p.5). Advancing twenty-first-century theorisations on [mental] health and wellbeing, they argue, necessitate non-hierarchical, non-binary, and intra-relational thinking across multiple locations at once. Centring a *new materialist* approach to health and wellbeing, their conceptualisation also attends to the dynamic 'matters' of body and environment while mapping out their 'interconnection with social processes, power, hierarchy, and/or discourse' (Hayes-Conroy et al., 2022, p.2; see also Bodden, Lorimer, & Parr, Chapter 16; Lucas Chapter 18; Chandler *et al.*, Chapter 19 this volume). This is particularly relevant to debates surrounding dominant narratives of 'mental' health, in which embodied experiences, expressions of distress and patterns of behaviour are recapitulated as individualised medical problems within diagnostic systems and not within systems of social injustice and oppression.

Posthuman and new materialist approaches to mental health and wellbeing recognise that 'rather than biological fact' [mental] health or embodied distress, 'is instead *mediated* by biological factors – expressed physiologically or behaviourally – and embodied by people situated in their relational and material worlds' (Boyle, 2024, p.4). Crucially, biology is resituated as biographical as the body is simultaneously lived and social (Hayes-Conroy et al. 2022) and features prominently as a site of on-going and collective sensing, meaning-making and identity processes. This further necessitates an embodied understanding of mental health and wellbeing as plural, 'embedded inextricably in relations of connectedness with others in space and the nature of these intersubjective experiences' (Harding and Mazzoli Smith, 2022, p.1). 'Biosociality' as a concept also emphasises that is the meaningful social relations formed through shared experiences of 'medicalised' conditions, that have the capacity to bridge into broader networks or 'biosolidarities' of community, advocacy, and activism (yley, 2021; Beresford & Russo, 2022; see also Bodden *et al.*, Chapter 16; Keller, Chapter 25 this volume), which are vital, not simply in terms of 'recovering from' but for living well with and through adverse health experiences and events (Power et al. 2019).

The book's structure and content

In many respects, the contents of this handbook reflect our expertise as editors and the networks we have cultivated based on our research interests. There are notable absences as a result. We are, however, pleased to be putting forward Global South and Indigenous perspectives across the book's different sections. At the same time, we acknowledge that these efforts don't go far enough in addressing the under-representation of the Global South and Indigenous scholarship in mental health geography or the academy at large. While a number of contributions are either influenced by or reflect upon authors' lived experiences, we acknowledge the limited contributions from queer, crip, critical race, or mad studies. In this regard, we would like to refer readers to key texts in these fields: *The Routledge International Handbook of Race, Culture and Mental Health* (Moody & Lee, 2023), *Exploring LGBT Spaces and Communities: Contrasting Identities, Belongings and Wellbeing* (Formby, 2017), *Crip Theory: Cultural Signs of Queerness and Disability*, and *The Routledge International Handbook of Mad Studies* (Beresford & Russo, 2022).

The Routledge Handbook on Spaces of Mental Health and Wellbeing comprises 44 chapters across five sections, including section introductions, authored by section editor(s). The first section, *Green and Blue Spaces*, is edited by health geographers Sarah Bell and Ronan Foley and is presented in two parts. Part A focuses on the potential held in green (land-based) spaces and blue (water-based) spaces for enhanced mental health and wellbeing. Part B, in contrast, comprises a range of critical reflections on the complexities of green/blue immersion, inequities in the access to green/blue spaces, and the notion of green/blue 'dosing'. The second section of the handbook, *Lived and Embodied Spaces*, is edited by health geographer Louise Boyle. This section offers insights into people's personal geographies across a range of experiences and expressions of distress that are typically framed by biomedical models of mental illness. The third section, *Creative Spaces*, is edited by artist-geographer and clinical psychologist, Candice Boyd. This section focuses on ways in which creative practices open up spaces which support (or sometimes diminish) mental health and wellbeing.

The fourth section of the *Routledge Handbook on Spaces of Mental Health and Wellbeing* is edited by human geographer Joshua Evans and health geographer Alak Paul. This section, titled *Spaces of Work and Home*, is concerned with housing and community-based recovery as well as place-based healing, employment, and care. The fifth and final section, titled *Institutional and Post-Institutional Spaces*, is edited by architect-geographer Ebba Högström. In this section, the present and past spaces of mental health care are in focus – all those 'other' spaces designed and organised for situations when mental health and wellbeing is weakened and when more-or-less organised care, support and/or treatment is considered needed (voluntarily or not). Bringing the edited collection to a close, this final section takes us 'full circle', reflecting on earlier mental health geographies while gesturing towards the future of alternative 'mad' place-making. It is our hope as editors that this book will be a useful resource for geography students and academics alike, and for those readers new to human geography, an exciting introduction to geographical thought.

References

Adams, M. (2020). *Anthropocene psychology: Being human in a more-than-human world.* New York: Routledge.

Andrews, G. (2018). Health and place. In T. Brown, G.J. Andrews, S. Cummins, B. Greenhough, D. Lewis and A. Power (Eds), *Health geographies: A critical introduction.* Oxford: Blackwell.

Andrews, G.J. (2020). *Non-representational theory & health: The health in life in space-time revealing.* New York: Routledge.

Andrews, G.J., & Duff, C. (2020). 'Whole onflow', the productive event: An articulation through health. *Social Science & Medicine, 265,* 113498.

Andrews, G.J., & Rishworth, A. (2023). New theoretical terrains in geographies of wellbeing: Key questions of the posthumanist turn. *Wellbeing, Space, and Society, 4,* 100130.

Andrews, G.J., Chen, S., & Myers, S. (2014). The 'taking place' of health and wellbeing: Towards non-representational theory. *Social Science & Medicine, 108,* 210–222.

Ash, J., & Simpson, P. (2016). Geography and post-phenomenology. *Progress in Human Geography, 40*(1), 48–66. https://doi.org/10.1177/0309132514544806

Atkinson, S. (2017). Health and Wellbeing. In D. Richardson, N. Castree, M. Goodchild, L. Weidong, A. Kobayashi, & R. Marston (Eds), *The international encyclopedia of geography: People, the earth, environment, and technology.* Hoboken, NJ: Wiley-Blackwell/AAG. https://doi.org/10.1002/9781118786352.wbieg0770

Atkinson, S., Fuller, S., & Painter, J. (2012). Wellbeing and place. In S. Atkinson, S. Fuller, & J. Painter (Eds.), *Wellbeing and Place* (pp. 1–14). London: Ashgate.

Atkinson, S., & Joyce, K. (2011). The place and practices of wellbeing in local governance. *Environment and Planning. C, Government and Policy*, 29(1), 133–148. https://doi.org/10.1068/c09200

Barad, K. (2007). *Meeting the university halfway: Quantum physics and the entanglement of matter and meaning*. Durham: Duke University Press.

Beresford, P. & Russo, J. (2022). *The Routledge International handbook of Mad studies*. New York: Routledge.

Bissell, D. (2011). Placing affective relations: Uncertain geographies of pain. In B. Anderson and P. Harrison (Eds), *Taking-place: Non-representational theories and geography*. London: Ashgate.

Boyd C.P, Parr H., Philo C. (2023). Climate anxiety as posthuman knowledge. *Wellbeing, Space & Society, 4,* 100120.

Boyd, C. P. (2022). Postqualitative geographies. *Geography Compass, 16*(10), e12661. https://doi.org/10.1111/gec3.12661

Boyd, C.P. (2017). *Non-representational geographies of therapeutic art making: Thinking through practice*. London: Palgrave.

Boyle, L.E. (2024). *Anxious geographies: Worlds of social anxiety*. London: Routledge.

Bradley, B. (2021). From biosociality to biosolidarity: The looping effects of finding and forming social networks for body-focused repetitive behaviours. *Anthropology & Medicine, 28*(4), 543–557 https://doi.org/10.1080/13648470.2020.1864807

Braidotti, R. (2011). *Nomadic theory: The portable Rosi Braidotti*. New York: Columbia University Press.

Brown, T., Andrews, G.J., Cummins, S., & Greenhough, B. (2017). *Health geographies: A critical introduction*. Oxford: Blackwell.

Castaldelli-Maia J. M., Bhugra D. (2022). What is geopsychiatry? *International Review of Psychiatry, 34*(1), 1–2

Colls, R. (2012). Feminism, bodily difference and non-representational geographies. *Transactions of the Institute of British Geographers, 37*(3), 430–445.

Conradson, D. (2012). Wellbeing: Reflections on geographical engagements. In S. Atkinson, S. Fuller, & J. Painter (Eds.), *Wellbeing and Place* (pp. 15–34). London: Ashgate

Crang, M., & Thrift, T. (2000). *Thinking space*. London: Routledge.

Davidson, J. (2003) *Phobic geographies: The phenomenology and spatiality of identity*. London: Routledge.

Davidson, J., & Parr, H. (2007). Anxious subjectivities and spaces of care: Therapeutic geographies of the UK National Phobics Society." In A. Williams (Ed), *Therapeutic landscapes* (pp. 95–110). Burlington, VT: Ashgate.

deLeeuw, S., Donovan, C., Schafenacker, N., Kearns, R., Neuwelt, P., Squier, S.M., McGeachan, C., Parr, H., Frank, A.W., Coyle, L.-A., Atkinson, S., El-Hadi, N., Shklanka, K., Shooner, C., Beljaars, D., & Anderson, J. (2018). Geographies of medical and health humanities: A cross-disciplinary conversation. *GeoHumanities, 4*(20), 285–334.

Deleuze, G. & Guattari, F. (1987). *A thousand plateaus: Capitalism and schizophrenia*. [Translated by Brian Massumi]. Minneapolis: University of Minnesota Press.

Dewsbury, J-D. (2003). Witnessing space: 'knowing without contemplation'. *Environment and Planning A: Economy and Space, 35*(11), 1907–1932. https://doi.org/10.1068/a3582.

Duff, C. (2014). *Assemblages of health: Deleuze's empiricism and the ethology of life*. New York: Springer.

Elkington, K. (2023). 'A'ole Pau Ka 'Ike I Ka Hālau Ho'okahi (knowledge is not restricted to one school of thought): Reflecting on the significance of Indigenous Knowledge in geography. *Society & Space*. Available at URL: www.societyandspace.org/articles/a-ole-pau-ka-ike-i-ka-halau-ho-okahi-knowledge-is-not-restricted-to-one-school-of-thought-reflecting-on-the-significance-of-indigenous-knowledge-in-geography

Finlay, J.M., & Rowles, G.D. (2021). Clinical geography: A proposal to embrace space, place and wellbeing through person-centred practice. *Wellbeing, Space and Society, 2,* 100035.

Fjellfeldt, M., Högström, E. & Markström, U. (forthcoming) *My place, your place, our place: A Photovoice study about spatial experiences among people with psychiatric disabilities.*

Fleuret, S., & Atkinson, S. (2007). Wellbeing, health and geography: A critical review and research agenda. *New Zealand Geographer, 63*(2), 106–118.

Formby, E. (2017). *Exploring LGBT spaces and communities: Contrasting identities, belongings and wellbeing.* New York: Routledge.

Gatrell, A.C., & Elliott, S.J. (2014). *Geographies of health: An introduction.* Oxford: Blackwell.

Guattari, F. (1992). *Chaosmosis: An ethico-aesthetic paradigm.* [Translated by Paul Bains and Julian Pefanis]. Bloomington: Indiana University Press.

Harding, S. and Mazzoli Smith, L. (2022). Freedom through constraint: Young women's embodiment, space and wellbeing during lockdown, *Wellbeing Space and Society, 3,* 1–7. https://doi.org/10.1016/j.wss.2022.100101

Harman, G. (2010). *Towards speculative realism.* London: Zero Books.

Hayes-Conroy, A., Kinsey, D., & Hayes-Conroy, J. (2022). Biosocial wellbeing: Conceptualizing relational and expansive well-bodies. *Wellbeing, Space and Society, 3,* 100105.

Högström, E. (2018) "It used to be here but moved somewhere else": Post-asylum spatialization – A new urban frontier? *Social & Cultural Geography, 19*(3), 314–335.

Högström, E. and Philo, C. (2023) 'Let there be light' or life in the dark? Vital geographies of mental healthcare. *Social Science & Medicine, 333,* 116137.

Jessen, T. D., Ban, N. C., Claxton, N. X., & Darimont, C. T. (2021). Contributions of Indigenous Knowledge to ecological and evolutionary understanding. *Frontiers in Ecology and the Environment, 20*(2), 93–101. https://doi.org/10.1002/fee.2435

Kanngieser, A., (2012). … And … and … and … The transversal politics of performative encounters. *Deleuze and Guattari Studies, 6*(2), 265–290.

Kearns, R. & Andrews, G.J. (2010). Geographies of wellbeing. In S. Smith, R. Pain, S. Marston & J.P. Jones (Eds), *Handbook of Social Geography.* London: SAGE.

Kearns, R., & Moon, G. (2002). From medical to health geography: Novelty, place and theory after a decade of change. *Progress in Human Geography, 26,* 605–625.

Knowles, C. (2000) Burger King, Dunkin' Donuts and community mental health care. *Health and Place, 6,* 213–224.

Latour, B. (2005). *Reassembling the social: An introduction to actor-network-theory / Bruno Latour.* Oxford: Oxford University Press.

Manning, E. (2012). *Relationscapes: Movement, art, philosophy.* Minneapolis: MIT Press.

Marion, J-L. (2002). *In excess: Studies of saturated phenomena.* New York: Fordham University Press.

Markström, U., Högström, E., & Fjellfeldt, M. (2023). Mental health supported accommodation services in a post-deinstitutionalised era. *Alter,* 39–56.

McCormack, D. (2002). A paper with an interest in rhythm. *Geoforum, 33*(4), 469–485.

McGeachan, C., & Philo, C. (2023). "Hanging around in their brokenness": On mental ill-health geography, asylums and camps, artworks and salvage. *Annals of the American Association of Geographers, 113*(5), 1224–1242.

McLeod, K. (2017). *Wellbeing machine: How health emerges from the assemblages of everyday life.* Durham: Carolina Academic Press.

McPhie, J. (2019). *Mental health and wellbeing in the Anthropocene: A posthuman inquiry.* Singapore: Palgrave.

McRue, R. (2006). *Crip theory: Cultural signs of queerness and disability.* New York: New York University Press.

Merleau-Ponty, M. (1962). *Phenomenology of perception.* [Translated by Colin Smith]. New York: Routledge.

Moody, R., & Lee, E. (2023). *The Routledge international handbook of race, culture and mental health.* New York: Routledge.

Müller, M., & Schurr, C. (2016). Assemblage thinking and actor-network theory: Conjunctions, disjunctions, cross-fertilisations. *Transactions of the Institute of British Geographers, 41*(3), 217–229. https://doi.org/10.1111/tran.12117.

Nancy, J.-L. (1997) *The sense of the world.* London: University of Minnesota Press.

Nieuwenhuis, M. and Knoll, E. (2021) Towards a geography of voice-hearing, Emotion. *Space and Society, 40,* 100812. https://doi.org/10.1016/j.emospa.2021.100812

Parr, H. (2008). *Mental health and social space.* Oxford: Blackwell.

Parr, H., (1998). Mental health, ethnography and the body. *Area, 30,* 28–37.

Parr, H., & Philo, C. (2003). Rural mental health and social geographies of caring. *Social & Cultural Geography, 4*(4), 471–488. https://doi.org/10.1080/1464936032000137911

Parr, H., Philo, C., and Burns, N. (2003) 'That awful place was home': Reflections on the contested meanings of Craig Dunain Asylum. *Scottish Geographical Journal,* 119(4), 341–360.

Philo C. (2005). The geography of mental health: An established field? *Current Opinion in Psychiatry, 18,* 585–591.

Philo, C. (1997). Across the water: Reviewing geographical studies of asylums and other mental health facilities. *Health and Place 3,* 73–89.

Philo, C., Callard, F., McGeachan, C., & Parr, H. (2023). Geopsychiatry and geography: A response. *International Journal of Social Psychiatry,* Online First. https://doi.org/10.1177/0020764023 1195289

Power, A., Bell, S.L., Kyle, R.G., and Andrews, G.J. (2019). Hopeful adaptation in health geographies: Seeking health and wellbeing in times of adversity. *Social Science and Medicine, 231,* 1–5.

Roberts, T. (2021). A constructivism of desire: Conceptualising the politics of assemblage with Deleuze and Guattari. *Area, 53*(4), 691–698. https://doi.org/10.1111/area.12735

Rosenberg, M.W. (2021). A commentary on clinical geography: A proposal to embrace space, place and wellbeing through person-centred practice. *Wellbeing, Space and Society, 2,* 100060.

Schwanen, T., & Wang, D. (2014). Well-Being, Context, and Everyday Activities in Space and Time. *Annals of the Association of American Geographers, 104*(4), 833–851. https://doi.org/ 10.1080/00045608.2014.912549

Simpson, P. (2021). *Non-representational theory.* New York: Routledge.

Spinoza, B. (2000). *Ethics.* [Translated by G.H.R. Parkinson]. Oxford: Oxford University Press.

Thrift, N. (2007). *Non-representational theory: Space, politics, affect.* New York: Routledge.

Whatmore, S. (2006). Materialist returns: Practising cultural geography in and for a more-than-human world. *Cultural Geographies, 13*(4), 600–609. https://doi.org/10.1191/1474474006c gj377oa

Whitehead, A.N. (1979). *Process and reality* (Corrected Edition). New York: Free Press.

Williams, N., Patchett, M., Lapworth, A., Roberts, T., & Keating, T. (2019). Practising posthumanism in geographical research. *Transactions of the Institute of British Geographers, 44*(4), 637–643. https://doi.org/10.1111/tran.12322

Wolch J., Philo C. (2000). From distributions of deviance to definitions of difference: Past and future mental health geographies. *Health & Place, 6,* 137–157.

World Health Organisation (WHO). (2023). One health fact sheet. Available from: www.who.int/ news-room/fact-sheets/detail/one-health

Section I
Green/blue spaces

2 Introduction to green/blue spaces

Sarah L. Bell and Ronan Foley

There is longstanding interest – across varied disciplines – in the potential for time spent with or near nonhuman nature to promote opportunities for mental health and wellbeing; from the extensive outdoor grounds of historic asylum environments (Eastoe, 2016) to contemporary forms of green and blue care, such as ecotherapy, horticultural therapy, animal assisted therapy, and green and blue 'prescriptions' (Steigen et al., 2016; Britton et al., 2020). Much of this work has focused on the role of so-called 'green' or 'blue' spaces in promoting mental health, from urban parks, community gardens, forests, woodland and countryside settings to a range of urban and rural freshwater and coastal sites. As discussed in a plethora of reviews in this area (e.g. Barakat and Yousufzai, 2020; Bray et al., 2022; Callaghan et al., 2021; Hermanski et al., 2022; Roberts et al., 2019; Zhang et al., 2021), this work ranges from population level studies examining associations between population mental health outcomes (such as low mood, anxiety, depression, PTSD) and presence of/proximity to neighbourhood green or blue spaces, to studies of specific blue or green care interventions, and in-depth qualitative work examining how and why green/blue experiences may contribute to or undermine a sense of mental health and wellbeing amongst particular groups and individuals.

Various mechanisms have been proposed for the positive outcomes observed, from the indirect mental health and wellbeing benefits of being physically or socially active in such environments (Masterton et al., 2020) to direct experiences of cognitive and relational restoration (Hartig et al., 2014; Hartig, 2021), flow (Csikszentmihalyi, 2002; Pitt, 2014), therapeutic accretion (Foley, 2017), awe and nostalgia (Severin et al., 2022), perspective – be it spatial or temporal (Bell et al., 2015; Conradson, 2005), or forging simple undemanding relationships with nonhuman others (Davidson and Smith, 2009). Yet, such benefits cannot be assumed or guaranteed, with concerns of 'environmental determinism' resulting in calls for more critical reflection on how green/blue spaces are theorised in connection with people's mental health and wellbeing (Rosenberg, 2017). The aim of this section is to interrogate the complexities of when, how and why people's mental health and wellbeing may unfold or indeed unravel through varied forms of green/ blue encounter. A number of cross-cutting themes recur across the section. We highlight three of these here.

The first theme relates to the affective and intimate ways in which green/blue encounters are sensed and made sense of, both individually and collectively. That <u>intimate sensing</u> is built around an embodied, emotional, and experiential engagement with the spaces around us and how these are lived by different bodies, human and

DOI: 10.4324/9781003345725-3

non-human, in different ways (Bell, Hickman & Houghton, 2023; Britton & Foley, 2020). Each sensory engagement is shaped by the specific setting, as noted by Astell-Burt et al.'s chapter on the complexity of biodiversity within green space, or in Evers' chapter on surfing within the unpromising blue space of a polluted ocean. That sensing is also a shared intimacy with others, as Biglin identifies within the context of refugees and other excluded groups, where a visible embodied presence matters. How exactly that intimate sensing is enacted and performed is a common theme across many of the chapters, such as Fisher et al.'s suggestion that perceptions of biodiversity can be directly linked to how they are sensed, while Harrod and Von Benzon show how a transformational experience is part and parcel of, and emergent from, nature-based interventions. In their chapters, Denton et al. and Wheaton and Olive each point to the value of therapeutic encounters that are explicitly immersive, with the body as a direct sensor in and from the water. This body sensor dimension is also noted by Evers in flagging up an important role for intimate sensing as a sentinel of environmental damage and an embodied pathway to care in and of place; something also identified by Heinkel and Kistemann in relation to biodiversity loss in the Global South and the negative affects of that loss, in terms of both place and livelihood.

The second theme concerns the <u>medicalisation</u> of people's green and blue space experiences, illustrated through the growing momentum to identify and 'prescribe' a healthy human 'dose' of 'nature'. As outlined in Garrido-Cumbrera's chapter, such 'doses' are understood in different ways, but typically consider duration of exposure, type of green/blue setting encountered, and the activities undertaken therein. Drawing on research focusing on the experiences of people with co-occurring mental health conditions and problem substance use, Masterton reflects on the value of realist approaches for developing context-specific green space interventions, alongside the challenges of sustaining such programmes in an unpredictable funding landscape. The importance of attending to context is demonstrated in Astell-Burt et al.'s chapter, which presents population-level findings from the Covid-19 pandemic that trouble the often taken-for-granted assumption that nature encounters can alleviate burnout. While there is promise in trying to 'prescribe' green/blue encounters that will best meet people's mental health needs, there are risks, too. For example, when such efforts fail to recognise the emergent, context-specific qualities of such experiences, or the legacy of long-term systematic exclusion from such encounters; a point taken up in Wheaton and Olive's chapter on surf therapy. As discussed in Harrod and Von Benzon's chapter on nature-based interventions, it's essential to empower people to find their own therapeutic 'dose' of nature in their own way and at their own pace. Although less discussed across the chapters, care is also needed in recognising the limits of the green/blue; that is, the perils of imposing individualised green/blue 'solutions' to mental distress rather than addressing the wider forms of structural and systemic violence that debilitate, harm and unravel people's mental health in the first place. The survivor-led movement of Mad Studies, for example, 'encourages appreciation of how we can be made mad by society and our circumstances within it', challenging the 'damaging dominance of prevailing medicalised individual models and the global psychiatric system' (Beresford, 2020, p. 1340).

Linked to the previous point, the third theme reflects the need to embed <u>social and environmental justice</u> within the growing momentum to connect people with nonhuman nature in the name of mental health and wellbeing. The challenges of social inequality are discussed in many of the section chapters, from inequalities in green/blue access (discussed in chapters by Kingsley, Denton et al., Wheaton and Olive, Masterton, Heinkel and Kistemann, and Biglin, for example) to the active displacement of multiply marginalised residents through the greening of urban environments in processes of green gentrification. Recognising such processes as preventable, Triguero-Mas and Cole's chapter calls for tangible measures to embed 'health in all policies' to ensure cities are 'sustainable, green, liveable, healthy and equitable'. The dominance of Global North scholars in the field of green/blue space, mental health and wellbeing – a dominance that is also reflected in the (im)balance of chapters in this section – is itself a form of injustice, that of epistemic injustice (Fricker, 2007). As indicated by Kingsley, and Wheaton and Olive, the widely critiqued tendency to view humans and nature as separate stems from narrow Western ideals and conceptions of what constitutes 'nature', 'health' and 'wellbeing'. In reducing nature to a 'resource' to be visited, owned, and extracted for human benefit (relating to health or otherwise), such ideals lack the richness of Indigenous perspectives that recognise people as *belonging to* and *of the land* (Panelli and Tipa, 2007; Panelli, 2008); relationships that emerge through lives that are deeply rooted in the land rather than relationships forged through periodic recreational excursions or visits to a pre-designated green/blue.

In summary, the section provides a rich and varied commentary on the ways that different types of natural spaces shape and trace mental health and wellbeing. Core themes such as equitable access, the dignity of risk, and care in and of place speak to the multiple immersive ways in which people's imbrication in green and blue spaces promote and protect mental health and wellbeing. Such themes are also evident in the varied settings and populations discussed elsewhere in the Handbook, though in the case of green and blue spaces, they can also be open, fluid and with less controllable or certain outcomes. That fluidity can be marked out in several ways, incorporating temporalities, shades, and traces. Parks, greenways, rivers, and lakes are often very different spaces, with highly varied mixes of human and nonhuman inhabitation, at night or across different seasons, so encounters never take shape in exactly the same way all the time or for all people, sometimes having anti-therapeutic dimensions (Li et al., 2019). While green and blue spaces are presented as representative colours, in reality there are many shades and palettes associated with such spaces, shaped by weather, climate, seasonality, run-off and other examples of human intervention, with further changes to unfold in the face of climate crisis. Such different palettes also reflect different shadings of effects and affects that shift based on the scale of spaces as well as the many different cohorts of human and nonhuman occupants. Finally, there are differences in terms of the social, cultural and affective relations and practices that act as a form of trace, that run within, but also across and through those differing green and blue spaces (Foley, 2019). There are omissions in the section, but these are always useful in identifying other research that is needed to trace mental health within green/blue space. These include more detailed work with children and young people, and people who identify as disabled, gender diverse and the increasingly fluid ways in which bodies are understood and made visible in public space. What is important to take forward, that each of the chapters discuss in different ways, are fuller understandings of relational connections between human and non-human bodies and ecologies, all of which document affective and experiential dimensions that emerge differently through the complexities of varied green and blue space encounters.

References

Barakat, C. and Yousufzai, S. (2020). Green space and mental health for vulnerable populations: A conceptual review of the evidence. *Journal of Military, Veteran and Family Health*, 6(S3), pp. 51–57.

Bell, SL., Hickman, C. and Houghton, F. (2023) From therapeutic landscape to therapeutic 'sensescape' experiences with nature? A scoping review. *Wellbeing, Space and Society*, 4, 100126. https://doi.org/10.1016/j.wss.2022.100126

Bell, S.L., Phoenix, C., Lovell, R. and Wheeler, B.W. (2015). Seeking everyday wellbeing: The coast as a therapeutic landscape. *Social Science and Medicine*, 142, pp. 56–67.

Beresford, P. (2020). 'Mad', Mad studies and advancing inclusive resistance. *Disability & Society*, 35(8), pp. 1337–1342.

Bray, I., Reece, R., Sinnett, D., Martin, F. and Hayward, R. (2022). Exploring the role of exposure to green and blue spaces in preventing anxiety and depression among young people aged 14-24 years living in urban settings: A systematic review and conceptual framework. *Environmental Research*, 214(4), 114081.

Britton, E., Foley, R. (2021). Sensing water: Uncovering health and well-being in the sea and surf. *Journal of Sport and Social Issues*, 45(1), pp. 60–87.

Britton, E., Kindermann, G., Domegan, C. and Carlin, C. (2020). Blue care: A systematic review of blue space interventions for health and wellbeing. *Health Promotion International*, 35(1), pp. 50–69.

Callaghan, A., McCombe, G., Harrold, A., McMeel, C., Mills, G., Moore-Cherry, N. and Cullen, W. (2021). The impact of green spaces on mental health in urban settings: A scoping review. *Journal of Mental Health*, 30(2), pp. 179–193.

Conradson, D. (2005). Landscape, care and the relational self: Therapeutic encounters in rural England. *Health and Place*, 11(4), pp. 337–348.

Csikszentmihalyi, M. (2002). *Flow*. London: Rider.

Davidson, J. and Smith, M. (2009). Autistic autobiographies and more-than-human emotional geographies. *Environment and Planning D: Society and Space*, 27, pp. 898–916.

Eastoe, S. (2016). 'Relieving gloomy and objectless lives'. The landscape of Caterham Imbecile Asylum. *Landscape Research*, 41(6), pp. 652–663.

Foley, R. (2017). Swimming as an accretive practice in healthy blue space. *Emotion, Space and Society*, 22, pp. 43–51.

Foley, R. (2019) Cartographies of Health: From Remote to Intimate Sensing. In Atkinson, S. and Hunt, R. (Eds.) *Geohumanities and Health*. (Global Perspectives on Health Geography). Cham, Springer Nature, pp. 261–277.

Fricker, M. (2007). *Epistemic injustice: Power and the ethics of knowing*. Oxford: Oxford University Press.

Hartig, T., Mitchell, R., de Vries, S., et al. (2014). Nature and health. *Annual Review of Public Health*, 35, pp. 207–228.

Hartig T. (2021). Restoration in Nature: Beyond the Conventional Narrative. In: Schutte A.R., Torquati J.C. and Stevens, J.R. (Eds.) *Nature and Psychology. Nebraska Symposium on Motivation*, Vol. 67. Springer, Cham. https://doi.org/10.1007/978-3-030-69020-5_5

Hermanski, A., McClelland, J., Pearce-Walker, J., Ruiz, J. and Verhougstraete, M. (2022). The effects of blue spaces on mental health and associated biomarkers. *International Journal of Mental Health*, 51(3), pp. 203–217.

Li, D., Zhai, Y., Xiao, Y., Newman, G. and Wang, D. (2019) Subtypes of park use and self-reported psychological benefits among older adults: A multilevel latent class analysis approach, *Landscape and Urban Planning*, 190, 103605.

Masterton, W., Carver, H., Parkes, T. and Park, K. (2020). Greenspace interventions for mental health in clinical and non-clinical populations: What works, for whom, and in what circumstances? *Health & Place*, 64, 102338.

Panelli, R. and Tipa, G. (2007). Placing well-being: A Māori case study of cultural and environmental specificity. *EcoHealth*, 4, 445–460.

Panelli, R. (2008). Social geographies: Encounters with Indigenous and more-than-White/Anglo geographies. *Progress in Human Geography*, 32(6), pp. 801–811.

Pitt, H. (2014). Therapeutic experiences of community gardens: Putting flow in its place. *Health and Place*, 27, pp. 84–91.

Roberts, H., van Lissa, C., Hagedoorn, P., Kellar, I. and Helbich, M. (2019). The effect of short-term exposure to the natural environment on depressive mood: A systematic review and meta-analysis. *Environmental Research*, 177, 108606.

Rosenberg, M. (2017). Health geography III: Old ideas, new ideas or new determinisms? *Progress in Human Geography*, 41(6), pp. 832–842.

Severin, M.I., Raes, F., Notebaert, E., Lambrecht, L., Everaert, G. and Buysse, A. (2022). A qualitative study on emotions experienced at the Coast and their influence on well-being. *Frontiers in Psychology*, 13, pp. 1–15. https://doi.org/10.3389/fpsyg.2022.902122

Steigen, A.M., Kogstad, R. and Hummelvoll, J.K. (2016). Green care services in the Nordic countries: An integrative literature review. *European Journal of Social Work*, 19(5), pp. 692–715.

Zhang, R., Zhang, C.-Q. and Rhodes, R.E. (2021). The pathways linking objectively-measured greenspace exposure and mental health: A systematic review of observational studies. *Environmental Research*, 198, 111233.

3 Greenspace programmes for mental health

Wendy Masterton

Introduction

The concept of nature being beneficial to health is not new, and it is now generally accepted that there are numerous biopsychosocial pathways by which this can happen (Markevych et al., 2017; Zhang, Zhang and Rhodes, 2021). Evidence of the link between greenspace and positive mental health is rapidly growing, and research has explored the relationship between greenspace and mental health in a myriad of domains (Reece et al., 2021; White et al., 2021). A study of approximately 19,000 people in England found that people who spent at least two hours in nature per week were consistently more likely to report higher levels of health and wellbeing, compared to people who spent less time in nature (White et al., 2019). Importantly, this pattern of a two-hour threshold was present for all included groups, including those with long-term illness or disability. This suggested that the results were not simply because people who visit nature are already a self-selected sample of healthier people.

Despite evidence that greenspace can improve health, exposure to greenspace may not be enough. In order to achieve desired mental health outcomes, research suggests that there must be a change in the physical greenspace environment alongside a planned intervention that will encourage people to use the space (Hunter et al., 2019). With this in mind, greenspace programmes are a type of targeted health intervention implemented in a variety of green settings like public parks, woodlands, wilderness, gardens, farms, and allotments (Fullam et al., 2021). A wide range of different activities may be used as part of these programmes such as: gardening; forest walks and forest bathing; wilderness or adventure programmes; forestry skills; nature-based mindfulness; conservation activities; and care farming, among others (Fullam et al., 2021; Garside et al., 2020). Previous systematic reviews of greenspace programmes for mental health have indicated success (Bowen & Neil, 2014; Cipriani et al, 2017; Genter et al., 2015), and from a mental health perspective, they have been cited as enabling the building of capacities in factors such as social cohesion and interaction, self-efficacy, and learning new skills (Fullam et al., 2021; Garside et al., 2020).

Despite increasing numbers of programmes that exist, there is still limited exploration of exactly why these programmes are effective for improving mental health, particularly for different population groups. Without knowing the components, processes, and influences within programmes, it is difficult to understand why they work, and how best to replicate and/or adapt them in ways that are appropriate to different contexts and population groups (Masterton et al., 2020). Additionally, an explanatory framework of programmes

DOI: 10.4324/9781003345725-4

is likely necessary to: facilitate partnership working; better raise awareness; increase confidence of greenspace programme services; and communicate outcomes to service users, their families, commissioners, and other bodies of mental health professionals (Garside et al., 2020). To address this gap, Masterton et al. (2020) conducted a realist review to synthesise the international evidence for greenspace programmes for mental health. The benefit of using a realist approach to evidence synthesis was that this methodology seeks to explore the causal mechanisms that explain why intervention outcomes occur (Pawson & Tilley, 1997). For these explanatory mechanisms to happen, they must be activated in the right contexts, and this relationship between the contexts, mechanisms, and outcomes is described as the 'programme theory' of why an intervention works (Pawson & Tilley, 1997). Programme theories provide greater insight into why interventions work and for whom. In their paper, Masterton and colleagues (2020) identified and refined seven programme theories to show why greenspace programmes appeared to improve poor mental health. These were: the feeling of escape and getting away from daily stressors; having space to reflect; increased physical activity; improved self-efficacy through learning new skills; feelings of purpose; improved relationships with staff/service providers; and increased shared experiences with peers. From these findings, the authors developed an initial intervention framework that aided understanding of how outcomes such as decreased stress, improved mood, improved self-esteem, and improved social cohesion occurred for clinical and non-clinical populations (Masterton et al., 2020).

Greenspace programmes and health inequalities

Notably, engagement with greenspace appears to be more beneficial for people with poor mental health compared to those with positive mental health (Rogerson et al., 2020). According to observational studies, time spent in greenspace also appears to be more beneficial to health for those from more socio-economically deprived areas compared to affluent areas (PHE, 2020). This evidence highlights that greenspace could be an asset in reducing existing health inequality. Indeed, as noted by Pearce, Mitchell and Shortt (2015), research frequently focuses solely on which characteristics of disadvantaged environments are harmful, how they are harmful, and who is most likely to be exposed to them. An alternate approach could be to explore why people stay well and what contributes to their health. If greenspace is shown to contribute positively to mental health, particularly for certain population groups, then increasing opportunities for engagement with greenspace, such as increased numbers of greenspace programmes, could play a role in reducing health inequalities and mitigating harm. One example might be exploring how greenspace could be used to support people with problem substance use (PSU). This type of substance use is associated with higher levels of risk and harm and with use that could be described as intensive or compulsive (Scottish Drugs Forum, 2020). Emerging evidence has suggested that greenspace programmes could be effective for this population group, who often experience high levels of physical and mental health inequality (Berry et al., 2021; Harper, Mott and Obee, 2019; Lehmann, Detweiler and Detweiler, 2018). Indeed, increased focus on how best to support people with PSU is timely since drug-related deaths are increasing globally (UNODC, 2022). From a UK-based perspective, in 2021, there were 4,859 drug-related deaths registered in England and Wales (ONS, 2022), and 1,330 drug-related deaths in Scotland (NRS, 2022).

Co-occurring mental health problems and PSU is often referred to as dual diagnosis, and it has been estimated that, in the UK, two thirds of the people who use drug services experience mental health problems (Scottish Government, 2022a). However, it has also been proposed that less than half of this group will engage with mental health services (Scottish Government, 2022a). Parallel, separate programmes provided for patients with dual diagnosis have been cited as ineffective (Alsuhaibani et al., 2021), and mental health and PSU services are currently fragmented in such a way that results in barriers to access for those who need support with both (Scottish Government, 2022a). Exploration of interventions which have the potential to provide holistic support for people with dual diagnosis is therefore essential. Unless they are based in an abstinence-focused setting such as a therapeutic community, greenspace programmes typically do not require people to be abstinent when taking part in programmes. This is an important consideration because one of the reasons that people can be denied appropriate mental health support and treatment is due to having to meet strict conditions such as a period of abstinence before accessing mental health services (Scottish Government, 2022a). Conversely, greenspace programmes can provide a 'no wrong door approach' for individuals with dual diagnosis meaning that they could support people regardless of their health needs. Although greenspace programmes for people experiencing dual diagnosis do exist, they are not currently supported by in-depth, theory-based frameworks which could aid implementation. Without this knowledge, programmes are less likely to be implemented successfully, stakeholder and service user buy-in is more difficult to ascertain, and continued funding is less likely to be secured. However, given the link between poor mental health and PSU, Masterton and colleagues suggested that their original framework (2020), specific to mental health support, could be transferable to programmes that support people with dual diagnosis through similar causal mechanisms.

Testing an intervention framework for greenspace programmes for dual diagnosis

Masterton et al. used qualitative interviews to explore whether the original framework (2020) could be transferable for use on greenspace programmes that support people with dual diagnosis (2022). To provide insight from a range of expertise, two different categories of participants were interviewed. The first category were staff that worked directly on greenspace programmes with people with dual diagnosis. Two staff worked on wilderness-based programmes, four staff worked on garden-based programmes, and two staff worked on conservation programmes. By interviewing staff from programmes that used different types of greenspace and where service users undertook different activities, this ensured the framework was tested for transferability across different greenspace programme types. The second category of participants interviewed were wider stakeholders whose work was linked to greenspace programmes for dual diagnosis support but did not work on the programmes themselves. Five stakeholders were academic researchers in the field, three stakeholders were National Health Service (NHS) practitioners who had previously been involved in supporting service users onto greenspace programmes, and one stakeholder worked in a managerial role within the third sector for an organisation specialising in providing greenspace programmes. No service users were included in the sample as, due to COVID-19, the majority of greenspace programmes were not operational/accepting visitors during the period of data collection. Further details on the sample, recruitment process, materials, and data analysis process can be found in the published manuscript (Masterton et al., 2022).

The research findings suggested that the original framework specific to mental health support was indeed transferable to programmes that supported people with dual diagnosis. Firstly, and perhaps unsurprisingly, programmes were described as successful because of the therapeutic effect of nature. Interviewees discussed how, as long as there was easy access to a planned programme, then mental wellbeing would be increased, and stress would be reduced. These outcomes were said to be as a result of service users 'getting away' from their day to day lives and stressors, experiencing reduced rumination, increased feelings of awe and increased connections to nature:

"Being able to get some distance and some perspective on your life is really, really good. [...] Looking at the mountains, looking at the trees, hearing the rivers, connecting with nature, with being outside. You are sort of separating from your own agenda and your own issues."

(Gerry (pseudonym), Staff)

Indeed, this concept of removal from daily stressors has previously been cited as important in greenspace programmes such as wilderness therapy for people with PSU (DeMille and Montgomery, 2016; Hoag, Massey and Roberts, 2014). Additionally, findings showed that greenspace provides physical space, but importantly, this space is non-clinical, in comparison to traditional treatment rooms which are also often located in buildings linked to statutory health services. This is potentially important given that mistrust of statutory health services is frequently reported by people with dual diagnosis (Paquette, Syvertsen and Pollini, 2018). Providing 'neutral' non-clinical space reportedly increases the likelihood of therapeutic conversations, as long as there is adequate time spent on the programme, because the greenspace allows service users to feel less 'boxed in', confined, and lectured to. One stakeholder explained:

"One of the things about natural environments as a setting for health promotion is that it's a sort of neutral space, a non-institutional space, which allows people to think about things differently, and have different types of conversations, than they would do in a therapist's room or a doctor's setting."

(Hayley, Stakeholder)

The findings also supported the original framework which indicated that greenspace programmes allow changes within the individual. Interviewees explained that increased physical activity was a benefit of engaging with greenspace. However, previous research has shown that provision of greenspace is not enough to change behaviour, and there must be structured programmes in place (Hunter et al., 2019). In line with this, interviewees discussed that when there are a variety of activities available, and programmes have the staff and equipment to support the activities, then service users will reportedly be more likely to enjoy the activities. It was this mechanism of enjoyment which was said to be crucial for increased engagement and, in turn, improved physical and mental health. Further, many interviewees discussed how the availability of trained facilitators to lead and support programmes, as well as the existence of supportive peers, was key for learning new skills. As service users developed skills, whether practical or psychological, these were said to be increasingly implemented in service users' lives outside the programme because of increased feelings of empowerment and confidence:

"The vehicle of going out and camping, walking, and putting up tents and chopping up sticks and making a fire and catching, whatever it might be, is just the vehicle.

> *Through that, what the person gets is an increased confidence [...] they find that they can do things, which then loops back on itself in a kind of "okay I'm good enough" sort of way."*
>
> (Ross, Stakeholder)

Relatedly, the structure and routine of the programmes was said to facilitate a sense of purpose and positive changes in self-identity. Interviewees discussed how service users would describe a sense of ownership around programme activities and see themselves as responsible for growing produce, tending plants, planning routes, or other central roles. This concept of positive changes in self-identity have previously been reported as key in aiding people with PSU to feel less characterised solely by their substance use (Webb et al., 2020). Interviewees also discussed how, when people struggle with their mental health and/or PSU, they often describe a sense of losing themselves and their interests. Greenspace programmes challenge this notion, as one staff member explained:

> *"Purpose is one of the big things. It's to give them some kind of "something" they see themselves as getting into, and it's fulfilling a need that they didn't have before."*
>
> (Malcolm, Staff)

As well as individual-level changes, programmes were described as improving social capital. One of the reasons why traditional treatment approaches have been described as unattractive for some people is that the doctor-patient mentality can still be seen in statutory health services, with therapy space designed and controlled by the therapist (Berger, 2006). Conversely, if an intervention has a 'doing with' and not 'doing for' culture, then these findings suggest that service users are more likely to buy into support because of increased communication, decreased power imbalance, feelings of trust and safety, and feelings of respect. Greenspace programmes may be particularly successful as generally the staff work alongside the service users doing the same activities. Indeed, a staff member discussed:

> *"If we stand on the side-lines and don't get involved, then there is not so much room for communication as you've still got that sort of official role that you are playing. But when you get your sleeves up and start getting involved with them, you start chatting about this, that, and the next thing, and then they suddenly feel a bit more comfortable."*
>
> (Alan, Staff)

As well as relationships with the staff/facilitators, improved relationships with peers were described as central to improved health outcomes. Improved peer relationships were said to be as a result of shared experiences while on the programme, as long as group dynamics and communication skills were supported by the staff since disagreements were said to be common. Through improved relationships and enhanced communication skills, interviewees explained how isolation can be reduced, and service users often report reduced feelings of stigma and judgement. This could be important, particularly for people with dual diagnosis, as there are high levels of stigma attached to both substance use and poor mental health (Scottish Government, 2022a). One staff member explained that service users report how they are once again *"part of the world, being seen, being heard, feeling like a person"* (Jess, Staff).

While these qualitative findings supported the original framework (Masterton et al., 2020), the data also added important refinements. Firstly, unsurprisingly, COVID-19 was discussed as impacting greenspace programme outcomes because services were unable to provide the same level of support. However, when the impact of COVID-19 on health interventions is lessened, this programme theory can be removed with no effect on the rest of the framework. Secondly, findings showed that programmes must have clear objectives and a multidisciplinary team approach consisting of the right expertise for service users to feel adequately supported and satisfied. As one stakeholder said:

"If there is a lack of support, and an expectation-delivery gap, that can have an independent effect in itself, never mind the effectiveness on the programme."

(Hayley, Stakeholder)

Indeed, previous research into community-based programmes has identified that people are much more likely to engage with a particular programme if it matches their expectations, and those with unrealistic expectations were least likely to maintain adherence (Husk et al., 2020).

The third refinement related to funding. Interviewees described having clear objectives and outcome measures for programmes as increasing the likelihood of stakeholder buy-in (such as funders, GPs, or social prescribers), and the likelihood of them believing programmes to be worthwhile. However, almost all interviewees spoke about how the funding landscape was unpredictable and remained one of the most significant barriers to programmes, regardless of the clarity of programme objectives and outcomes. This uncertainty around funding for mental health and substance use support, particularly within the third sector, has previously been well documented (Carver et al., 2020), and one interviewee explained:

"It is a huge barrier, not just the lack of quality funding, but it's just very short term [...] if you go to them and say we are running this programme for the next six weeks, they are not really that interested, because by the time they've actually spoken to people, and started to refer people into it, it's going to be gone again."

(Michael, Staff)

Finally, and in line with social-ecological models (Bronfenbrenner, 1979), the interview data highlighted the importance of acknowledging how micro-level influences could influence implementation and success. While these did not tie into programme theories, future work could explore how individual-level factors may mediate causal mechanisms and, in turn, affect outcome success. From the qualitative findings, Masterton et al. refined the original framework (2020), and it is presented below (Figure 3.1) as it appears in the published manuscript (2022).

Policy and practice implications

The potential of greenspace programmes in addressing several mental health policy and practice imperatives is clear. In Scotland, greenspace is central to the National Planning Framework 4 (Scottish Government, 2022b) which includes priorities such as improving access to quality greenspace for everyone to promote health and reduce inequalities. In the PHE Strategy 2020 to 2025 (2019), there is explicit discussion around how

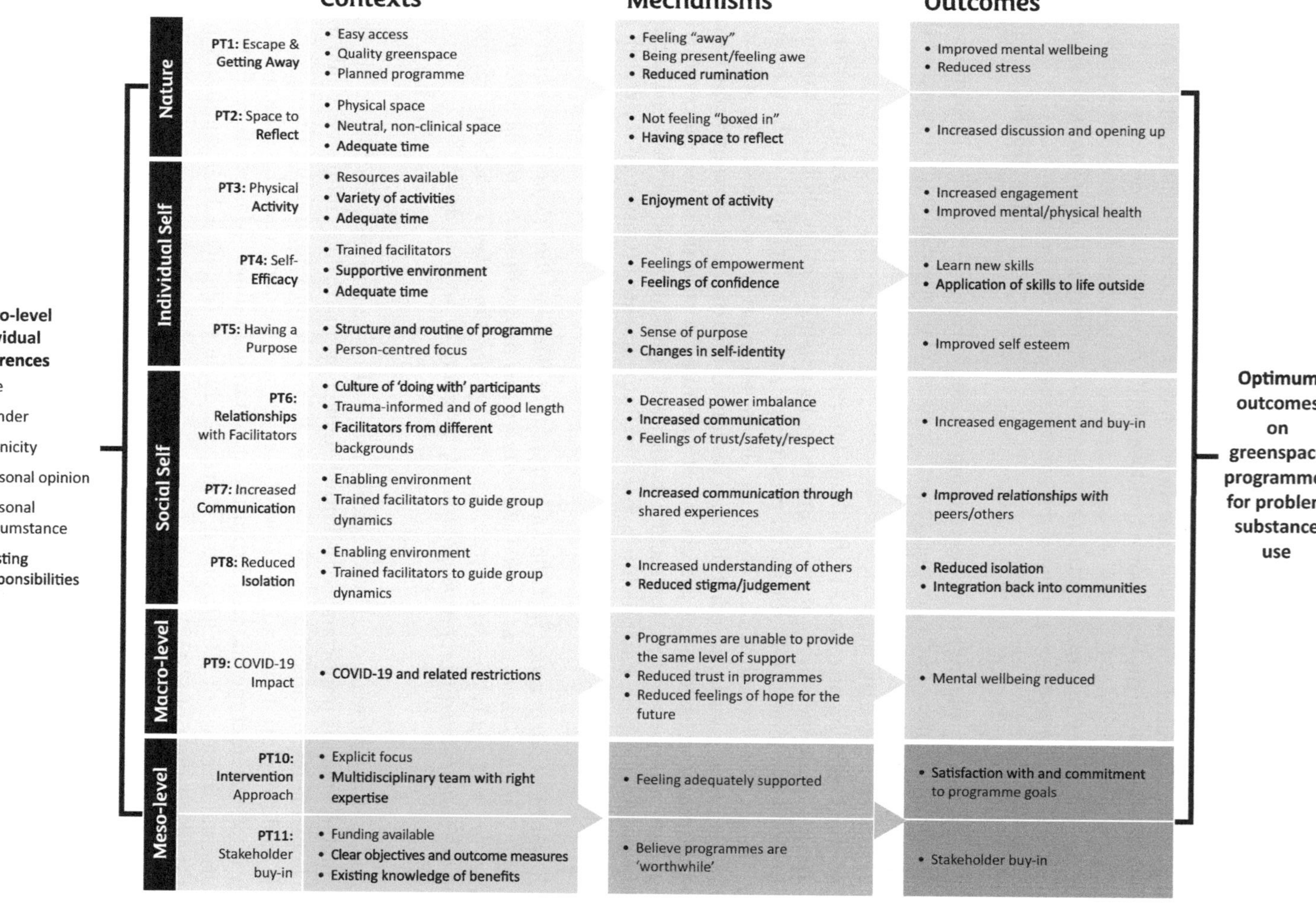

Figure 3.1 The proposed refined framework for greenspace programmes for people with dual diagnosis.

spatial planning for health is imperative, acknowledging the role that the environment has on mental health improvement. As well as development strategies, greenspace is also increasingly being integrated into health policy across regions of the UK through green prescribing, a type of social prescribing designed to improve physical and mental health and wellbeing through exposure to, and engagement with, nature (Fullam et al., 2021; McHale et al., 2020). As well as aligning with mental health strategy, greenspace programmes also connect with many of the recommendations and priorities provided in the UK Government's 10-year drug plan (UK Government, 2021) and the Drug Deaths Task Force (DDTF) final report (2022) such as: tackling stigma; delivering a holistic, 'no wrong door', public health approach; increased focus on engaging with those who do not currently access services; and more support and funding for community-based projects. Therefore, given the potential implications of greenspace programmes for the broader policy landscape, further research in this area is important.

It is essential to acknowledge that greenspace programmes are not a 'silver bullet' (Masterton et al., 2022). There are situations where greenspace programmes may be unsuitable for people, and circumstances where they will have very little effect. For example, people with dual diagnosis can experience wider vulnerabilities and face systemic challenges such as structural violence, insecure housing, and entrenched poverty that result in continuing inequalities, regardless of social interventions (Tyndall and Dodd, 2020). Therefore, the limitations of what greenspace programmes can provide must be made clear and should not be oversold. Going forward with future work, the voices of people with lived experience should be incorporated and central to framework refinement in order to truly show why programmes are successful, as well as why they may not work for some people and in some contexts. Future work must also consider how to better integrate multiple outcomes at an individual- and/or system-level and look to incorporate more quantitative outcome measures. For example, the use of validated psychometric assessment tools and/or physiological measures could allow a deeper understanding of how greenspace programmes can support diverse population groups that face mental health challenges (Masterton et al., 2022).

Conclusion

With rising levels of poor mental health and substance-related harm, there is increasing pressure on treatment and recovery services to deliver support to people with varying needs, while limiting costs (Scottish Government, 2022a). For people with dual diagnosis, the Scottish Government's Mental Health Strategy (2022a) acknowledges that many can "fall through the gaps" (p.30), because services are not joined up, and both the Scottish Government and UK Government agree that there is more effort needed to ensure that services provide both mental health and substance use support in a holistic way (2022a; 2021 respectively). Indeed, addressing mental health and substance use needs in a holistic and cost-effective way has the potential to lead to significant public health impact and improve population health, particularly among those already facing health and social inequalities. While greenspace programmes exist for marginalised groups, until this point there has been no framework showing why they are successful. Therefore, the findings of both the original and the tested/refined framework (Masterton et al. 2020; 2022) are not only theoretically novel, but have practical relevance for both policymakers, and those designing such interventions, by providing insight into how best to optimise, tailor, and implement future greenspace interventions.

References

Alsuhaibani, R., Smith, D.C., Lowrie, R., Aljhani, S. and Paudyal, V. (2021). Scope, quality and inclusivity of international clinical guidelines on mental health and substance abuse in relation to dual diagnosis, social and community outcomes: A systematic review. *BMC Psychiatry*, 21(1), pp. 1–23.

Berger, R. (2006). Beyond words: Nature-therapy in action. *Journal of Critical Psychology Counselling and Psychotherapy*, 6(4), p. 195.

Berry, M.S., Rung, J.M., Crawford, M.C., Yurasek, A.M., Ferreiro, A.V. and Almog, S. (2021). Using greenspace and nature exposure as an adjunctive treatment for opioid and substance use disorders: Preliminary evidence and potential mechanisms. *Behavioural Processes*, 186, 104344.

Bowen, D.J. and Neill, J.T. (2014). A meta-analysis of adventure therapy outcomes and moderators. *The Open Psychology Journal*, 6(1), pp. 28–53.

Bronfenbrenner, U. (1979). *The ecology of human development: Experiments by nature and design.* Harvard University Press.

Carver, H., Ring, N., Miler, J. and Parkes, T. (2020). What constitutes effective problematic substance use treatment from the perspective of people who are homeless? A systematic review and meta-ethnography. *Harm Reduction Journal*, 17(1), pp. 1–22.

Cipriani, J., Benz, A., Holmgren, A., Kinter, D., Mcgarry, J. and Rufino, G. (2017). A systematic review of the effects of horticultural therapy on persons with mental health conditions. *Occupational Therapy in Mental Health*, 33(1), pp. 47–69.

Demille, S.M. and Montgomery, M. (2016). Integrating narrative family therapy in an outdoor behavioral healthcare program: A case study. *Contemporary Family Therapy*, 38(1), pp. 3–13.

Drug Deaths Task Force. (2022). *Changing Lives – Final Report*. Available at: https://drugdeathstaskforce.scot/news-information/publications/reports/final-report/

Fullam, J., Hunt, H., Lovell, R., Husk, K., Byng, D.R., Bloomfield, D., Warber, S., Tarrant, M., Lloyd, J., Orr, N., Burns, L. and Garside, R. (2021). *A handbook for nature on prescription to promote mental health. Version 1.* University of Exeter. Available at: https://beyondgreenspace.net/green-social-prescribing-resources/nature-based-interventions-to-promote-health/ [Accessed October 2023]

Garside, R., Orr, N., Short, R., Lovell, B., Husk, K., Mceachan, R., Rashid, R. and Dickie, I. (2020). *Therapeutic nature: Nature-based social prescribing for diagnosed mental health conditions in the UK.* DEFRA. Available at: https://arc-swp.nihr.ac.uk/wp/wp-content/uploads/2021/06/15138_TherapeuticNature-Finalreport.pdf [Accessed October 2023]

Genter, C., Roberts, A., Richardson, J. and Sheaff, M. (2015). The contribution of allotment gardening to health and wellbeing: A systematic review of the literature. *The British Journal of Occupational Therapy*, 78(10), pp. 593–605.

Harper, N., Mott, A. and Obee, P. (2019). Client perspectives on wilderness therapy as a component of adolescent residential treatment for problematic substance use and mental health issues. *Children and Youth Services Review*, 105, 104450

Hoag, M.J., Massey, K.E. and Roberts, S.D. (2014). Dissecting the wilderness therapy client: Examining clinical trends, findings, and patterns. *Journal of Experiential Education*, 37(4), pp. 382–396.

Hunter, R.F., Cleland, C., Cleary, A., Droomers, M., Wheeler, B.W., Sinnett, D., Nieuwenhuijsen, M.J. and Braubach, M. (2019). Environmental, health, wellbeing, social and equity effects of urban green space interventions: A meta-narrative evidence synthesis. *Environment International*, 130, 104923.

Husk, K., Blockley, K., Lovell, R., Bethel, A., Lang, I., Byng, R. and Garside, R. (2020). What approaches to social prescribing work, for whom, and in what circumstances? A realist review. *Health and Social Care in the Community*, 28(2), pp. 309–324.

Lehmann, L.P., Detweiler, J.G. and Detweiler, M.B. (2018). Veterans in substance abuse treatment program self-initiate box gardening as a stress reducing therapeutic modality. *Complementary Therapies in Medicine,* 36, pp. 50–53.

Markevych, I., Schoierer, J., Hartig, T., Chudnovsky, A., Hystad, P., Dzhambov, A.M., De Vries, S., Triguero-Mas, M., Brauer, M., Nieuwenhuijsen, M.J., Lupp, G., Richardson, E.A., Astell-Burt, T., Dimitrova, D., Feng, X.Q., Sadeh, M., Standl, M., Heinrich, J. and Fuertes, E. (2017). Exploring pathways linking greenspace to health: Theoretical and methodological guidance. *Environmental Research,* 158, pp. 301–317.

Masterton, W., Carver, H., Parkes, T. and Park, K. (2020). Greenspace interventions for mental health in clinical and non-clinical populations: What works, for whom, and in what circumstances? *Health & Place,* 64, 102338.

Masterton, W., Parkes, T., Carver, H. and Park, K.J. (2022). Exploring how greenspace programmes might be effective in supporting people with problem substance use: A realist interview study. *BMC Public Health,* 22(1), pp. 1–19.

Mchale, S., Pearsons, A., Neubeck, L. and Hanson, C.L. (2020). Green health partnerships in scotland; Pathways for social prescribing and physical activity referral. *International Journal of Environmental Research and Public Health,* 17(18), pp. 1–13.

National Records of Scotland (NRS). (2022). *Drug-related deaths in Scotland in 2021.* National Records of Scotland. Available at: www.nrscotland.gov.uk/statistics-and-data/statistics/statistics-by-theme/vital-events/deaths/drug-related-deaths-in-scotland/2021 [Accessed October 2023]

Office for National Statistics (ONS). (2022). *Deaths related to drug poisoning in England and Wales: 2021 registrations.* Office for National Statistics. Available at: www.ons.gov.uk/peoplepopulationandcommunity/birthsdeathsandmarriages/deaths/bulletins/deathsrelatedtodrugpoisoninginenglandandwales/2021registrations [Accessed October 2023]

Paquette, C.E., Syvertsen, J.L. and Pollini, R.A. (2018). Stigma at every turn: Health services experiences among people who inject drugs. *International Journal of Drug Policy,* 57, pp. 104–110.

Pawson, R. & Tilley, N. (1997). *Realistic Evaluation.* London: SAGE.

Pearce, J., Mitchell, R. and Shortt, N. (2015). Place, space, and health inequalities. In: K.E. Smith, C., S.E. Hill, and Bambra, eds. *Health Inequalities: Critical Perspectives,* Oxford: Oxford University Press, pp. 192–205

Public Health England (PHE). (2020). *Improving access to greenspace – A new review for 2020.* Public Health England. Available at: https://assets.publishing.service.gov.uk/government/uploads/system/uploads/attachment_data/file/904439/Improving_access_to_greenspace_2020_review.pdf [Accessed October 2023]

Public Health England (PHE). (2019). *PHE strategy 2020 to 2025.* UK Government. Available at: www.gov.uk/government/publications/phe-strategy-2020-to-2025 [Accessed October 2023]

Reece, R., Bray, I., Sinnett, D., Hayward, R. and Martin, F. (2021). Exposure to green space and prevention of anxiety and depression among young people in urban settings: A global scoping review. *Journal of Public Mental Health,* 20(2), pp. 94–104

Rogerson, M., Wood, C., Pretty, J., Schoenmakers, P., Bloomfield, D. and Barton, J. (2020). Regular doses of nature: The efficacy of green exercise interventions for mental wellbeing. *International Journal of Environmental Research and Public Health,* 17(5), 1526.

Scottish Drugs Forum. (2020). *Moving beyond 'people-first' language. A glossary of contested terms in substance use.* Available at: www.sdf.org.uk/wp-content/uploads/2020/10/Moving-Beyond-People-First-Language.pdf [Accessed October 2023]

Scottish Government. (2022a). *Drug and alcohol services – co-occurring substance use and mental health concerns: literature and evidence review.* Scottish Government. Available at: www.gov.scot/publications/co-occurring-substance-use-mental-health-concerns-scotland-review-literature-evidence/ [Accessed October 2023]

Scottish Government. (2022b). *Scotland's Fourth National Planning Framework 4: revised draft.* Scottish Government. Available at: www.gov.scot/publications/national-planning-framework-4-revised-draft/ [Accessed October 2023]

Tyndall, M. and Dodd, Z. (2020). How structural violence, prohibition, and stigma have paralyzed North American responses to opioid overdose. *AMA Journal of Ethics,* 22 (8), pp. 723–728.

United Nations Office on Drugs and Crime (UNODC). (2022). *World Drug Report 2022.* United Nations. Available at: www.unodc.org/unodc/data-and-analysis/world-drug-report-2022.html [Accessed October 2023]

UK Government. (2021). *From harm to hope: A 10-year drugs plan to cut crime and save lives.* UK Government. Available at: www.gov.uk/government/publications/from-harm-to-hope-a-10-year-drugs-plan-to-cut-crime-and-save-lives?utm_medium=email&utm_campaign=govuk-notifications&utm_source=b26364cd-31a2-4cd5-87ca-f7795aee25e4&utm_content=immediately [Accessed October 2023]

Webb, L., Clayson, A., Duda-Mikulin, E. and Cox, N. (2020). 'I'm getting the balls to say no': Trajectories in long-term recovery from problem substance use. *Journal of Health Psychology,* 27(1), pp. 69–80.

White, M.P., Alcock, I., Grellier, J., Wheeler, B.W., Hartig, T., Warber, S.L., Bone, A., Depledge, M.H. and Fleming, L.E. (2019). Spending at least 120 minutes a week in nature is associated with good health and wellbeing. *Scientific Reports,* 9(1), pp. 1–11.

White, M.P., Elliott, L.R., Grellier, J., Economou, T., Bell, S., Bratman, G.N., Cirach, M., Gascon, M., Lima, M.L. and Lõhmus, M. (2021). Associations between green/blue spaces and mental health across 18 countries. *Scientific Reports,* 11(1), pp. 1–12.

Zhang, R., Zhang, C.-Q. and Rhodes, RE. (2021). The pathways linking objectively-measured greenspace exposure and mental health: A systematic review of observational studies. *Environmental Research,* 198, 111233.

4 Ten big picture actions for mainstreaming gardening into public and mental health policy and practice

Jonathan (Yotti) Kingsley

Introduction

I would like to pay my respects to Indigenous peoples and their Elders both past and present. Further, I want to acknowledge that Indigenous peoples' diverse connections to land, water, animals, and ancestry is ongoing, rich and has been built on tens of thousands of years of history that remains today

In the Australian context, where I write this chapter from, this acknowledgment to Country is an important and common practice to pay respect to our First Nations people that have a deep connection to these lands which are enmeshed in all elements of health and wellbeing (Thorpe et al., 2023). Therefore, before beginning this chapter, which focuses on connections to place through the act of gardening, I would like to acknowledge this historical and continual relationship that Indigenous people hold that allows us to be able to enjoy our garden spaces on planet earth today. I do not state this because it is common practice, nor a token platitude that I am required to say, but a recognition that this is central to the ideas I will put forward in the chapter on mainstreaming gardening in public and mental health.

In a recent collaborative paper that I wrote with Aboriginal and non-Indigenous scholars (Thorpe et al., 2023), the way we respectfully acknowledged this point was to position ourselves as authors regarding our background, how we came to write in the way we do and hold our perspectives/theoretical positions. In keeping with this process, I must acknowledge my background as a Jewish second-generation immigrant to Australia that has been an academic and has worked in non-government and government organisations to address health inequalities. The way I believe we can bridge these health inequalities is to engage and connect people with nature. Specifically, I explore how gardening and First Nations people's connection and caring for land impacts individual and population health and wellbeing.

This chapter is based on a keynote presentation I gave at the Australia Therapeutic Horticulture conference on November 1st, 2022, in front of approximately 100 delegates (for more information please see: https://tha.org.au/conference/). The presentation was titled "Ten big picture actions for therapeutic horticulture in Australia". The sections of this chapter are based on a similar structure and ideas I highlighted and proposed in the presentation. This was followed by a lively 30-minute conversation where delegates provided input into my ten suggested actions. I will also draw on my two decades of research into the public and mental health benefits of gardening and work in government and non-government organisations around health promotion and community

DOI: 10.4324/9781003345725-5

development. This will hopefully translate into a fruitful thought piece around integrating gardening into public health discourse at a global level.

The rationale for pushing this agenda forward is to address current structural issues commonly and currently faced around accessing garden spaces. These structural issues revolve around diminishing garden spaces in urban areas depriving segments of the population, based on for example socio-economic position and housing status, from enjoying this activity (e.g., Asl and Azadgar, 2022; Davoren et al., 2016; Gbedomon et al., 2015; Truong, Gray and Ward, 2022). To add to this complexity individuals come with their own gardening skills, ability and knowledge to these settings and capacity to upskill. Therefore, I believe actions are required to support more people in getting out and about and in their gardens for their mental and physical health.

The evidence-base surrounding gardening for our health and wellbeing

In the following section I will briefly share some of the literature focused on why gardening is important to human health and wellbeing. I will start at the larger scale exploring the health benefits of nature and associated theories of how this intersects with the act of gardening.

Nature, health and wellbeing

Nature has long been theorised as important to our physical and mental health and wellbeing. Nature is a broad term that is often applied too narrowly but I argue that to understand nature involves a "multi-layered and holistic relationship with our environments" (Kingsley & Lawson, 2015, p. 551). Theories explaining why connection, disconnection or destruction of nature is important to human existence and mental health include the well-known *Biophilia Hypothesis* (Wilson, 1984), *Attention Restoration Theory* (Kaplan & Kaplan, 1989), *Gaia* (Lovelock, 1979, 1991, 2009), *Deep Ecology* (Sessions, 1995; Simmons, 2006), and *Solastalgia* (Albrecht, 2005; Albrecht et al., 2007, 2008). Academics have been discussing the intersection between nature and physical and mental health for a longer period, with fields evolving on this topic since at least the mid-nineteenth century (Buse et al., 2018). Nonetheless, whenever discussing this intersection between nature and health I must again reiterate that Indigenous people have been practising these deep connections to land, nature, and place for tens of thousands of years (Burgess et al., 2009; Kingsley, Townsend and Henderson-Wilson, 2013; Kingsley et al., 2018; Thorpe et al., 2023). Further, I would like to quote a recent paper by Fletcher et al., (2021, p. 1) to flag a continuing issue around engagement in nature regarding it sometimes being considered a separate entity to human existence in ways that are reproduced by some of these popular human-nature relationship theories:

> [...] dominant... policy and public perceptions still fail to recognize that Indigenous and local peoples have long valued, used, and shaped "high-value" biodiverse landscapes. Moreover, the exclusion of people from many of these places under the guise of wilderness protection has degraded their ecological condition and is hastening the demise of a number of highly valued systems.

It is not surprising that public health evidence has been mounting on how connection and deeper engagement with nature impacts physical, social and mental health (Astell-Burt

& Feng, 2019; Astell-Burt et al., 2021, 2022a; Maller et al., 2006; Maas et al., 2009; Milligan, Gatrell & Bingley, 2004; Mitchell, Astell-Burt & Richardson, 2011; Richardson et al., 2012; Ulrich, 1983, 1984, 1986;). Some scholars go one step further, advocating and urging for mandated nature-based activities or nature prescriptions to improve population health (Astell-Burt et al., 2022b; Bratman et al., 2015; Fullam et al., 2021; Shanahan et al., 2016; Sia et al. 2020). These benefits go well beyond biomedical health and psychological wellbeing measures, with a recent systematic literature review highlighting that nature-based education for children reduces sedentary time, improves balance and increases risky play (Johnstone et al., 2022). However, some argue that a social and environmental justice lens needs to be applied to integrate these beneficial nature connections for human wellbeing appropriately (Kelly, Maller and Farahani, 2022). Access to garden spaces is but one example of environmental justice that is sometimes perceived differently within Indigenous communities (e.g., control of land/Country and stewardship) and 'settler' cultures (e.g., challenging the 'status quo') (Lambert, 2023).

Gardening as a sanctuary for our health and wellbeing

Gardening is one mechanism for connecting with nature and can come in many different forms such as community, allotment, guerrilla gardening to urban farming or agriculture that involves the production of "food, flowers, fibre, feed and herbs" on land and water (Kingsley et al., 2021, p. 2; Kingsley, In Press). Gardening throughout history has been a sanctuary for healing, relaxation, and therapy for our mental health (Kingsley, 2009; Marsh et al., 2021). Recent literature reviews have highlighted the significant health and wellbeing benefits of gardening (Dyg, Christensen and Peterson, 2020; Genter et al., 2015; Howarth et al., 2020; Soga, Gaston and Yamaura, 2017; Spano et al., 2020). Specifically, biomedical research indicates that gardening can reduce risks associated with cardiovascular disease, especially for older adults (Kingsley et al., 2022; Veldheer et al., In Press). Looking at psychological and mental health outcomes, Sia et al. (2020) found that participation in a therapeutic horticulture program directly improved cognitive function and reduced anxiety. Therefore, it is perhaps not surprising that urban agriculture has been identified as a potential nature-based solution to a range of environmental, social, health and economic challenges facing Australian cities (Kingsley et al., 2021).

Gardening is not just important in the Australian context but across the globe. This was particularly evident during the COVID-19 pandemic with researchers identifying the heightened health and wellbeing potential of this activity during this time (Corley et al., 2021; Theodorou et al., 2021. Scholars attributed this to the role of gardening in reducing stress, and increasing nature connectedness and resilience (Egerer et al., 2022; Sia et al., 2022; Wu et al., 2022). This led some public health researchers to advocate for greater opportunities and avenues for all populations to garden during times of high stress and crisis periods (Niala, 2020).

Ten big picture ideas for promoting gardening in public health

Although gardening is a popular leisure pursuit with a range of benefits, there is a disconnect when it comes to its application and promotion as a public and mental health intervention. Thus, the big question is how we could promote gardening into public health practice, policy, and discourse. This section highlights my ten big picture actions for doing so.

Action 1: *Integrating Indigenous concepts of land into gardening activities.*

Indigenous peoples worldwide have an intimate, holistic, complex, localised, and recip-rocal relationship to their 'Country' (as it is known in Australia), which includes elem-ents of the land, sea, waterways, sky, stars, and living and non-living entities (Thorpe et al., 2023). Country is more than something you see out there as a physical entity, it is a living system and tied to language, identity and customs incorporating the social, spir-itual, and cultural linkages of Indigenous peoples (Kingsley, Townsend and Henderson-Wilson, 2013; Lawson & Kingsley, 2020). If these concepts can be mainstreamed into government policy, organisational structures and society while promoting gardening, it is my belief that there will be better engagement in activities that promote nature con-nectedness. However, if this is not based on collaboration, listening to Indigenous voices and compensation for time and expertise that Indigenous knowledge holders share, this will not be effective (strategies to incorporate these elements are discussed in detail by Arabena and Kingsley, 2015).

Action 2: *We are all indigenous with a lower case 'i' to the universe.*

This action draws on Torres Strait Islander, Professor Kerry Arabena's, seminal book titled *Becoming Indigenous to the Universe*. Arebena (2015) explains that humans need to reconnect with the earth, to stop exploiting it and to engage in local knowledge systems to regain sustainability. To do this we must "remember the distinction between the use of capital 'I' Indigenous – referring to a member of the First Peoples of their respective countries – and a smaller 'i' indigenous – referring to a particular way of being in the Universe that validates us all as indigenous members of the Universe' (Arabena, 2015, p. 7). Arabena (2015, p. 57) explains that 'indigenous to the Universe' requires humans to look beyond the conventional narrative of belonging. There is a need to uncover the open, hybrid relationship that connects humans to different spaces, species, times and places. These relationships enhance the mutual presence that links humans and the Earth community". Arabena (2015) recommends that colonial language needs to change and be liberated, reflecting Indigenous holistic connections with nature that holds respect for diversity and equality beyond human gains. Thus, if we are to get serious about pro-moting gardening to benefit all humans and non-human systems then we need to engage in this discourse.

Action 3: *Creating a simple message of the physical and mental health benefits of gardening to a wider audience.*

Gardening is difficult to define because of the diversity of activities that it can involve (Kingsley, 2021), and the benefits are complex to transmit to a wider audience. Though any gardener understands these benefits intimately, it is yet to be transmitted across societies effectively. At the Australian Therapeutic Horticulture conference this was mentioned as the root problem in promoting and educating people in the therapeutic horticulture space. It caused debate because messaging around it needs to be defined more simply to a larger audience. This led me to consider a health communications textbook written by Lewis and Lewis (2015) that I use with my own undergraduate health promotion students. Lewis and Lewis (2015) recommended that to transmit a strong health message to the public you need one single, clear message, that is applied in partnership with all relevant stakeholders. The problem that came up in the conference is how do you simplify the numerous mental and physical health and wellbeing benefits of gardening into one clear concise message – this needs to be addressed if gardening as a public health intervention is to be accessible to more people.

Action 4: *A national course on social, therapeutic and health benefits of gardening.*

One suggestion I made at the conference, that raised some questions, was that a national certificate programme could be created that promotes and applies the health and wellbeing benefits of gardening. I recommended that to gain legitimacy across sectors it needed to be accredited and cut across allied health care, horticulture and social services. There was debate as to whether a certificate programme would be adequate to legitimise the field, with agreement that a university degree would increase the standard of practice in this space. There was support that this training needed to be run as a consortium across universities and disciplines like health, horticulture and social services to build its standing so that all students could access the best of each field when learning on related topics. There was also recognition that training programmes already existed in this space but to successfully promote this field an education programme should apply best practice and have a high standing at a national and global level. It should be flagged when mentioning university degrees that there are inequalities for some individuals accessing higher education so pathways into these degrees, like diplomas, may breakdown these barriers.

Action 5: *Intergenerational gardening programmes in every public school.*

There has been a growing recognition of the learning, educational and health benefits of bush kinder and gardening programmes throughout schooling (Campbell & Speldewinde, 2019, 2022; Lohr et al., 2020; Ohly et al., 2016). In addition, popular notions like nature deficit disorder explain that in modern society children often do not get enough play in nature which is thought to detrimentally impact their development (Louv, 2005). It is worth noting here that there have been various critiques of Louv's nature deficit disorder, for example that it requires a rethink to focus on psychological, interpersonal and culture factors that lead to children's disconnection from nature (Dickinson, 2013). Beyond this academic debate there seems to be much potential to incorporate gardening programmes into all schools that are tailored to their cultural needs. In applying this action, we should recognise that not all schools have access to garden spaces on their premises – to bridge this gap collaborations could be made with local allotment or community gardens to have long-term access to a suitable plot.

Action 6: *Mandate time out in gardens for people who are at risk, disadvantaged or marginalised in society.*

Initially this action had been for nursing home residents because of the impact of the COVID-19 pandemic on this population (Giri, Chenn and Romero-Ortuno, 2021). But through discussions at the conference, wider settings and populations were viewed as important. For instance, evidence substantiates the mental health and wellbeing benefits of gardening in settings like nursing homes (Magnussen, Alteren and Bondas, 2021), prisons (Brown, Bos and Brady, 2021), for people living with dementia (Lu et al., 2020;

Noone & Jenkins, 2018), people with neurological impairments (Lakhani et al., 2019), and autistic individuals (Scartazza et al., 2020). Full time carers were also identified as a group that may benefit from such experiences, as they are often overlooked within public and mental health interventions.

Like Action 5, if these garden interventions are to be effective and sustainable some rules need to be put in place, with the best interests of the gardeners themselves at the heart of the intervention. For example, there is a need to specify space parameters, resources and maintenance that abide by rules and regulations at a policy and organisation level of all and for all stakeholders involved. Interventions also need to prioritise the gardening skills, ability and knowledge of the participants themselves.

Actions 7, 8 and 9: *Combined actions that integrate gardening into the health care sector.*

These actions provide practical approaches to make gardening a public health intervention guided by health practitioners themselves. Recognising that health practitioners have competing priorities, this needs to be easily accessible and like Action 3 accompanied by simple but appropriate messaging.

Action 7: *Nature prescription advice and information integrated into medical/allied health textbooks.*

As previously mentioned, nature prescription has been identified as having many benefits (Kondo et al., 2020). Academic institutions, publishers and scholars have a responsibility to highlight the evidence on the potential benefits of nature/gardening and how to prescribe meaningful access to it in their core practice. All health textbooks should have sections on this that provide practical approaches as core business.

Action 8: *Develop a strategy for prescribing gardening in the health care sector.*

There are currently no global/universal prescription guidelines to implement gardening interventions in the health care sector. This needs to consider different forms of gardening, physical activity levels of diverse tasks (e.g., digging a trench compared with watering plants), and different physical and mental health and wellbeing benefits that will vary across age groups, cultures, genders, and settings. There has been initial work on this topic, for example, scholars have reviewed the different physical activity intensity levels of gardening practices (Gunn et al., 2002; Park, Lee and Son, 2011; Park et al., 2014) and some have looked at this within specific garden settings like allotment gardens (Hawkins et al., 2015). However, the exact details are lacking and therefore global guidelines that are specific and practical for different segments of the population and health conditions would assist health practitioners to embed gardening in their practices. This will be a difficult task based on different people's needs, priorities, abilities, and knowledge of gardens, on top of varied structural and organisational differences in the health care sector across the globe. However, the challenge also offers an opportunity to change the way we undertake public and mental health policy and programs in the future that are tailored to diverse needs with a focus on nature and equity.

Action 9: *Integrate therapy gardens into all hospital settings.*

Literature indicates the healing benefits of having nature and garden spaces in health care and hospital settings (George & Ethridge, 2023; Hartig & Marcus 2006; Weerasuriya, Henderson-Wilson and Townsend, 2019). These healing benefits include garden spaces acting as a place for reflection, destressing, and relaxing. Therefore it not surprising that recent evidence has linked increased amounts of weekly gardening opportunities with improved mental wellbeing and life satisfaction (Egerer et al., 2022; Fjaestad et al., 2023; Marsh et al., 2021). So for Action 9 I suggest increasing the value of integrating such spaces into all hospital settings in ways that are safe and therapeutic for staff and patients alike. Specifically, as Weerasuriya, Henderson-Wilson and Townsend (2019) found, having a hospital-based garden leads to enhanced control, choice, escapism, autonomy, privacy, social connections, and nature connectedness which in turn improves mental health.

Action 10: *Establishment of an accreditation body focused on the physical, mental and social health benefits of gardening.*

The final action I presented at the conference elicited mixed responses; accreditation for therapeutic horticulture to create a standard of practice that upholds ethics, integrity and the best outcomes for gardening as a public and mental health intervention. People working in hospital and health care settings mentioned how much this was needed to promote this activity but conversely other delegates mentioned how accreditation would take away the flexibility of gardening as an unstructured activity. Accreditation was also considered to add burdensome paperwork into the mix. Hence, while accreditation may be too burdensome, it seems important to explore the potential to create some sort of standard of practice that people working and undertaking gardening as a therapy can apply to ensure credibility and growth of this sector. This goes back full circle to **Action 1** in that if this is to be effective it is important to co-produce and integrate this with knowledge held by Indigenous and Traditional Owner groups.

Conclusion

I have put together these actions and a summary of the evidence in this chapter as a starting point for a discussion on where gardening as a public and mental health intervention could go in the future. I recognise these approaches will differ across countries, cultures, and populations. So now it is over to you to start pushing the agenda forward on the physical, mental, and social health benefits of gardens and adapting it into your health care settings based on the needs of your country, cultures, and different determinants of health impacting your communities. It's time to get our hands dirty to promote the potential of gardening for the mental health and wellbeing of all communities.

References

Albrecht, G. (2005). Solastalgia: A new concept in health and identity. *Philosophy, Activism and Nature (PAN)*, 3, pp. 41–55.

Albrecht, G., Higginbotham, N., Connor, L. & Freeman, S. (2008). Social and cultural perspectives on eco-health. In: K. Heggenhougen & S. Quah, eds, *International Encyclopaedia of Public Health* (vol. 6). San Diego: Academic Press.

Albrecht, G., Sartore, G.M., Connor, L., Higginbotham, N., Freeman, S., Kelly, B., Stain, H., Tonna, A. & Pollard, G. (2007). Solastalgia: The distress caused by environmental change. *Australasian Psychiatry*, 15(Suppl. 1), pp. S95–S98.

Arabena, K. (2015). *Becoming Indigenous to the Universe*. North Melbourne: Australian Scholarly Publishing.

Arabena, K. & Kingsley, J.Y. (2015). Climate change: Impact on country and Aboriginal and Torres Strait Islander culture. In: R. Walker & W. Mason, eds, *Climate Change Adaptation for Health and Social Services*. Canberra: CSIRO publishing.

Asl, S.R. & Azadgar, A. (2022). The spatial distribution of urban community gardens and their associated socio-economic status in Tehran, Iran. *Frontiers in Sustainable Food Systems*, 6, 949075.

Astell-Burt, T. & Feng, X. (2019). Association of urban green space with mental health and general health among adults in Australia. *JAMA Network Open*, 2(7), e198209.

Astell-Burt, T., Hartig, T., Eckermann, S., Nieuwenhuijsen, M., McMunn, A., Frumkin, H. & Feng, X. (2021). More green, less lonely? A longitudinal cohort study. *International Journal of Epidemiology*, 51(1), pp. 99–110.

Astell-Burt, T., Hartig, T., Putra, I.G.N.E., Walsan, R., Dendup, T. & Feng, X. (2022a). Green space and loneliness: A systematic review with theoretical and methodological guidance for future research. *Science of the Total Environment*, 847, 157521.

Astell-Burt, T., Pappas, E., Redfern, J. & Feng, X. (2022b). Nature prescriptions for community and planetary health: Unrealised potential to improve compliance and outcomes in physiotherapy. *Journal of Physiotherapy*, 68(3), pp. 151–152.

Bratman, G.N., Hamilton, J.P., Hahn, K.S., Daily, G.C. & Gross, J.J. (2015). Nature experience reduces rumination and subgenual prefrontal cortex activation. *Proceedings of the National Academy of Sciences (PNAS)*, 112(28), pp. 8567–8572.

Brown, G., Bos, E. & Brady, G. (2021). Building health and wellbeing in prison: Learning from the Master Gardener programme in a Midlands Prison. In: M. Maycock, R. Meek, & J Woodall, eds, *Issues and Innovations in Prison Health Research*. Palgrave Studies in Prisons and Penology. Cham, Switzerland: Palgrave Macmillan, Springer Nature.

Burgess, C.P., Johnston, F.H., Berry, H.L., McDonnell, J., Yibarbuk, D., Gunabarra, C., Mileran, A. & Bailie, R.S. (2009). Healthy country, healthy people: The relationship between Indigenous health status and "caring for country". *Medical Journal of Australia*, 190(10), pp. 567–572.

Buse, C.G., Oestreicher, J.S., Ellis, N.R., Patrick, R., Brisbois, B., Jenkins, A.P., McKellar, K., Kingsley, J., Gislason, M., Galway, L., McFarlane, R.A., Walker, J., Frumkin, H. & Parkes, M. (2018). Public health guide to field developments linking ecosystems, environments and health in the Anthropocene. *Journal of Epidemiology and Community Health*, 72(5), pp. 420–425.

Campbell, C. & Speldewinde, C. (2019). Bush kinder in Australia: A new learning 'place' and its effect on local policy. *Policy Futures in Education*, 17(4), pp. 541–559.

Campbell, C. & Speldewinde, C. (2022). Bush kinders in Australia: A creative place for outdoor STEM learning. In: K.J. Murcia, C. Campbell, M.M. Joubert & S. Wilson, eds, *Children's Creative Inquiry in STEM. Sociocultural Explorations of Science Education* (vol. 25). Cham, Switzerland: Springer Nature.

Corley, J., Okely, J.A., Taylor, A.M., Page, D., Welstead, M., Skarabela, B., Redmond, P., Cox, S.R. & Russ, T.C. (2021). Home garden use during COVID-19: Associations with physical and mental wellbeing in older adults. *Journal of Environmental Psychology*, 73, 101545.

Davoren, E., Siebert, S., Cilliers, S. & du Toit, M.J. (2016). Influence of socioeconomic status on design of Batswana home gardens and associated plant diversity patterns in northern South Africa. *Landscape Design and Urban Biodiversity*, 12, pp. 129–139.

Dickinson, E. (2013). The misdiagnosis: Rethinking "nature-deficit disorder". *Environmental Communications*, 7(3), pp. 315–335.

Dyg, P.M., Christensen, S. & Peterson, C.J. (2020). Community gardens and wellbeing amongst vulnerable populations: A thematic review. *Health Promotion International*, 35(4), pp. 790–803.

Egerer, M., Lin, B., Kingsley, J., Marsh, P., Diekmann, L. & Ossola, A. (2022) Gardening can relieve human stress and boost nature connection during the COVID-19 pandemic. *Urban Forestry & Urban Greening*, 68, 127483.

Fjaestad, S.L, Mackelprang, J.L, Sugiyama, T., Chandrabose, M., Owen, N., Turrell, G. & Kingsley, J. (2023) Associations of time spent gardening with mental wellbeing and life satisfaction in mid-to-late adulthood. *Journal of Environmental Psychology*, 87, 101993.

Fletcher, M.S, Hamilton, R., Dressler, W. & Palmer, L. (2021) Indigenous knowledge and the shackles of wilderness. *Proceedings of the National Academy of Sciences (PNAS)*, 118, e2022218118.

Fullam, J., Hunt, H., Lovell, R., Husk, K., Byng, R., Richard Byng, D.R., Bloomfield, D., Warber. S., Tarrant, M., Lloyd, J., Orr, N., Burns, L. and Garside, R. (2021). *A Handbook for Nature on Prescription to Promote Mental Health*. Farnham: Ashgate.

Gbedomon, R.C., Fandohan, A.B., Salako, V.K., Franck, A., Idohou, R., Kakaï, R.G. & Assogbadjo, A.E. (2015). Factors affecting home gardens ownership, diversity and structure: A case study from Benin. *Journal of Ethnobiology Ethnomedicine*, 11, p. 56.

Genter, C., Roberts, A., Richardson, J. & Sheaff, M. (2015) The contribution of allotment gardening to health and wellbeing: A systematic review of the literature. *British Journal of Occupational Therapy*, 78, pp. 593–605.

George, D.R. & Ethridge, A.E. (2023). Hospital-based community gardens as a strategic partner in addressing community health needs. *American Journal of Public Health*, 113(9), pp. 939–942.

Giri, S., Chenn, L.M. & Romero-Ortuno, R. (2021). Nursing homes during the COVID-19 pandemic: A scoping review of challenges and responses. *European Geriatric Medicine*, 12(6), pp. 1127–1136.

Gunn, S.M., Brooks, A.G., Withers, R.T., Gore, C.J., Owen, N., Booth, M.L. & Bauman, A.E. (2002). Determining energy expenditure during some household and garden tasks. *Medicine and Science in Sports and Exercise*, 34(5), pp. 895–902.

Hartig, T. & Marcus, C.C. (2006). Essay: Healing gardens—places for nature in health care. *The Lancet*, 368, pp. S36–S37.

Hawkins, J.L., Smith, A., Backx, K. & Clayton, D.A. (2015). Exercise intensities of gardening tasks within older adult allotment gardeners in Wales. *Journal of Aging and Physical Activity*, 23(2), pp. 161–168.

Howarth, M., Brettle, A., Hardman, M. & Maden, M. (2020). What is the evidence for the impact of gardens and gardening on health and well-being: A scoping review and evidence-based logic model to guide healthcare strategy decision making on the use of gardening approaches as a social prescription. *BMJ Open*, 10(7), e036923.

Johnstone, A., McCrorie, P., Cordovil, R., Fjørtoft, I., Livonen, S., Jidovtseff, B., Lopes, F., Reilly, J.J., Thomson, H., Wells, V. & Martin, A. (2022) Nature-based early childhood education and children's physical activity, sedentary behavior, motor competence, and other physical health outcomes: A mixed-methods systematic review. *Journal of Physical Activity and Health*, 19(6), pp. 456–472.

Kaplan, R. & Kaplan, S. (1989). *The experience of nature: A psychological perspective.* Sydney: Cambridge University Press.

Kelly, D., Maller, C. & Farahani, L.M. (2022). Wastelands to wetlands: Questioning wellbeing futures in urban greening. *Social and Cultural Geography*, 24(9), pp. 1576–1597.

Kingsley, J. (In Press). Nature and wellbeing. In: K. Dew & S. Donovan, eds, *Encyclopedia of Health Research in the Social Sciences*. Cheltenham: Edward Elgar Publishing.

Kingsley, J., Hadgraft, N., Owen, N., Sugiyama, T., Dunstan, D.W. & Chandrabose, M. (2022). Associations of vigorous gardening with cardiometabolic risk markers for middle-aged and older adults. *Journal of Aging and Physical Activity*, 30(3), pp. 466–472.

Kingsley, J., Egerer, M., Nuttman, S., Keniger, L., Pettitt, P., Frantzeskaki, N., Gray, T., Ossola, A., Lin, B., Bailey, A., Tracey, D., Barron, S. & Marsh, P. (2021). Urban agriculture as a nature-based solution to address socio-ecological challenges in Australian cities. *Urban Forestry & Urban Greening*, 60, 127059.

Kingsley, J. & Lawson, J. (2015). Finding a unified understanding of nature. *EcoHealth,* 12, pp. 551–552.

Kingsley, J., Townsend, M. & Henderson-Wilson, C. (2013) Exploring Aboriginal people's connection to Country to strengthen human–nature theoretical perspectives. In: M.K. Gislason, ed, *Ecological Health: Society, Ecology and Health.* Bingley: Emerald Group Publishing Limited.

Kingsley, J., Townsend, M. & Henderson-Wilson, C. (2009). Cultivating health and well-being: Members' perceptions of the health benefits of a Port Melbourne community garden. *Journal of Leisure Studies,* 28, pp. 207–219.

Kingsley, J., Munro-Harrison, E., Jenkins, A. & Thorpe, A. (2018). "Here we are part of a living culture": Understanding the cultural determinants of health in Aboriginal gathering places in Victoria, Australia. *Health & Place,* 54, pp. 210–220.

Kondo, M.C., Oyekanmi, K.O., Gibson, A., South, E.C., Bocarro, J. & Hipp, J.A. (2020). Nature prescriptions for health: A review of evidence and research opportunities. *International Journal of Environmental Research and Public Health,* 17(12), pp. 4213.

Lakhani, A., Norwood, M., Watling, D.P., Zeeman, H. & Kendall, E. (2019). Using the natural environment to address the psychosocial impact of neurological disability: A systematic review. *Health & Place,* 55, pp. 188–201.

Lambert, D. (2023). *Reframing the garden.* Available at: https://radicle.substack.com/p/reframing-the-garden?utm_source=post-email-title&publication_id=312977&post_id=117849027&isFreemail=true&utm_medium=email [Accessed 5th May, 2023].

Lawson, J. & Kingsley, J. (2020). The language of Australian human-ecological relationship: Identity, place and landscape. In: S.D Brunn & R. Kehrein, eds, *Landscape, Handbook of the Changing World Language Map.* Cham, Switzerland: Springer.

Lewis, B.S. & Lews, J.N. (2015). *Health communication: A media and cultural studies approach.* United Kingdom: Palgrave Macmillan.

Lohr, A.M., Krause, K.C., McClelland, D.J., Van Gorden, N., Gerald, L.B., Del Casino Jr, V., Wilkinson-Lee, A. & Carvajal, S.C. (2020). The impact of school gardens on youth social and emotional learning: A scoping review. *Journal of Adventure Education and Outdoor Learning,* 21(4), pp. 371–384.

Louv, R. (2005). *Last child in the woods: Saving our children from nature-deficit disorder,* New York: Algonquin Books.

Lovelock, J. (2009). *The vanishing face of Gaia: The final warning.* London: Allen Lane.

Lovelock, J.E. (1979). *Gaia: A new look at life on Earth.* Melbourne: Oxford University Press.

Lovelock, J. (1991). *Gaia: The practice science of planetary medicine.* Sydney: Allen & Unwin.

Lu, L-C., Lan, S-H., Hsieh, Y-P., Yen, Y-Y., Chen, J-C. & Lan, S-J. (2020). Horticultural therapy in patients with dementia: A systematic review and meta-analysis. *American Journal of Alzheimer's Disease & Other Dementias,* 35. https://doi.org/10.1177/1533317519883

Maas, J., Verheij, R., Vries, S., Spreeuwenberg, P., Schellevis, F.G. & Groenewegen, P. (2009). Morbidity is related to a green living environment. *Journal of Epidemiology & Community Health,* 63(12), pp. 967–973.

Magnussen, I-L., Alteren, J. & Bondas, T. (2021). "Human flourishing with dignity": A meta-ethnography of the meaning of gardens for elderly in nursing homes and residential care settings. *Global Qualitative Nursing Research,* 8, 1–17. https://doi.org/10.1177/23333936211035743

Maller, C., Townsend, M., Pryor, A., Brown, P. & St Leger, L. (2006). Healthy nature healthy people: 'Ccontact with nature' as an upstream health promotion intervention for populations. *Health Promotion International,* 21(1), pp. 45–54.

Marsh, P., Diekmann, L.O., Egerer, M., Lin, B., Ossola, A. & Kingsley, J. (2021). Where birds felt louder: The garden as a refuge during COVID-19. *Wellbeing, Space and Society,* 2, 100055.

Milligan, C., Gatrell, A. & Bingley, A. (2004). 'Cultivating health': Therapeutic landscapes and older people in northern England. *Social Science & Medicine,* 58, pp. 1781–1793.

Mitchell, R., Astell-Burt, T. & Richardson, E.A. (2011). A comparison of green spaces indicators for epidemiological research. *Journal of Epidemiology & Community Health,* 65(10), pp. 853–858.

Niala, J.C. (2020). Dig for vitality: UK urban allotments as a health-promoting response to COVID-19. *Cities & Health,* 5(S1), pp. S227–S231.

Noone, S. & Jenkins, N. (2018). Digging for dementia: Exploring the experience of community gardening from the perspectives of people with dementia. *Aging & Mental Health,* 22(7), pp. 881–888.

Ohly, H., Gentry, S., Wigglesworth, R., Bethel, A., Lovell, R. & Garside, R. (2016). A systematic review of the health and well-being impacts of school gardening: Synthesis of quantitative and qualitative evidence. *BMC Public Health,* 16, 286.

Park, S.A., Lee, K.S. & Son, K.C. (2011). Determining exercise intensities of gardening tasks as a physical activity using metabolic equivalents in older adults. *Hortscience,* 46(12), pp. 1706–1710.

Park, S.A., Lee A.Y., Lee, K.S. & Son, K.C. (2014) Gardening tasks performed by adults are moderate- to high-intensity physical activities. *Horttechnology,* 24(1), pp. 58–63.

Richardson, E.A., Mitchell, R., Hartig, T., de Vries, S., Astell-Burt, T. & Frumkin, H. (2012). Green cities and health: A question of scale? *Journal of Epidemiology & Community Health,* 66, pp. 160–165.

Scartazza, A., Mancini, M.L., Proietti, S., Moscatello, S., Mattioni, C., Costantini, F., Di Baccio, D., Villani, F. & Massacci, A. (2020). Caring local biodiversity in a healing garden: Therapeutic benefits in young subjects with autism. *Urban Forestry and Urban Greening,* 47, 126511.

Sessions, G. (1995). *Deep Ecology for the 21st century. Reading on the philosophy and practice of the new environmentalism.* London: Shambhala.

Shanahan, D., Bush, R., Gaston, K., Lin, B.B., Dean, J., Barber, E. & Fuller, R.A. (2016) Health benefits from nature experiences depend on dose. *Scientific Report,* 6, 28551.

Sia, A., Tam, W.W.S., Fogel, A., Kua, E.H., Khoo, K. & Ho, R.C.M. (2020). Nature-based activities improve the well-being of older adults. *Scientific Reports,* 10, 18178.

Sia, A., Tan, P.Y., Wong, J.C.M., Araib, S., Ang, W.F. & Er, K.B.H. (2022) The impact of gardening on mental resilience in times of stress: A case study during the COVID-19 pandemic in Singapore. *Urban Forestry and Urban Greening,* 68, 127448.

Simmons, I.G. (2006) Normative behaviour. In: N. Haenn & R.R. Wilk, eds, *The environment in anthropology: A reader in ecology, culture and sustainable living* (pp. 53–72). New York: New York University Press.

Soga, M., Gaston, K.J. & Yamaura, Y. (2017). Gardening is beneficial for health: A meta-analysis. *Preventive Medicine Reports,* 5, pp. 92–99.

Spano, G., D'Este, M., Giannico, V., Carrus, G., Elia, M., Lafortezza, R., Panno, A. & Sanesi, G. (2020). Are community gardening and horticultural interventions beneficial for psychosocial well-being? A meta-analysis. *International Journal of Environmental Research and Public Health,* 17(10), 3584.

Theodorou, A., Panno, A., Carrus, G., Carbone, G.A., Massullo, C. & Imperatori, C. (2021). Stay home, stay safe, stay green: The role of gardening activities on mental health during the Covid-19 home confinement. *Urban Forestry & Urban Greening,* 61, 127091.

Thorpe, A., Yashadhana, A., Biles, B., Munro-Harrison, E. & Kingsley, J. (2023). Indigenous health and connection to country. In: D. McQueen, ed, *Oxford Research Encyclopedia of Global Public Health.* New York: Oxford University Press.

Truong, S., Gray, T. & Ward, K.S. (2022). Enhancing urban nature and place-making in social housing through community gardening. *Urban Forestry Urban Greening,* 72, 127586.

Ulrich, R.S. (1983). Aesthetic and affective response to natural environment. In: I. Altman & J.F. Wohlwill, eds, *Behaviour and the natural environment.* New York: Plenum.

Ulrich, R.S. (1984). View through a window may influence recovery from surgery. *Science,* 224, pp. 420–421.

Ulrich, R.S. (1986). Human responses to vegetation and landscape. *Landscape and Urban Planning,* 13, pp. 29–44.

Veldheer, S., Tuan, W.-J., Al-Shaar, L., Wadsworth, M., Sinoway, L., Schmitz, K.H., Sciamanna, C. & Gao, X. (In Press). Gardening is associated with better cardiovascular health status among older adults in the United States: Analysis of the 2019 behavioral risk factor surveillance system survey. *Journal of the Academy of Nutrition and Dietetics*, 123(5), pp. 761–769.

Weerasuriya, R., Henderson-Wilson, C. and Townsend, M. (2019). A systematic review of access to green spaces in healthcare facilities. *Urban Forestry & Urban Greening*, 40, pp. 125–132.

Wilson, E.O. (1984). *Biophilia*. Cambridge: Harvard University Press.

Wu, C-F., Chou, L-W., Huang, H-C. & Tu, H-M. (2022). Perceived COVID-19-related stress drives home gardening intentions and improves human health in Taiwan. *Urban Forestry & Urban Greening*, 78, 127770.

5 What is the right dose of nature for mental health? Quantity, quality, distance, and exposure time

Marco Garrido-Cumbrera

Introduction

This chapter starts from the premise that, despite the evidence on the benefits of exposure to nature on mental health and emotional wellbeing, it is complex to identify an optimal 'healthy dose' of nature – in its different forms – for people with different health and wellbeing needs and priorities. To this end, we reflect on the role of different types of nature exposure in shaping wellbeing and mental health, including the importance of the proportion, size, and quality of urban green spaces, as well as the spatial distance from the residence. All this allows us to identify key aspects that should be considered when exploring the potential to include nature therapies as part of the support and improvement of mental health and emotional wellbeing.

Mental health conditions

Mental health conditions include common conditions such as depression or anxiety and severe mental illness such as bipolar disorder, Post-Traumatic Stress Disorder (PTSD), schizophrenia, obsessive-compulsive disorder and eating disorders, amongst others (World Health Organization, 2022). Mental health conditions affected more than 1 billion people globally in 2016 (Rehm & Shield, 2019), with neuropsychiatric conditions constituting five of the top ten biomedical causes of disability (Lopez & Murray, 1998). The prevalence of mental health conditions increased considerably during the COVID-19 pandemic (Winkler et al., 2020), affecting a higher proportion of children and women (Garrido-Cumbrera et al., 2023a; Pierce et al., 2020).

The aetiology of behavioural conditions can arise from biological, psychological, and social influences (Hamburg, 1970; Kinderman, 2005), although the causes appear to be multifactorial, which makes it difficult to establish associations between symptoms and outcomes (Kendler, 2005). Although most people believe that mental health conditions are caused solely by biological factors (Schomerus et al., 2006), their main aetiology stems from several biological, psychological, and social factors acting together (Kinderman, 2005). In addition, there are other factors to consider such as alcohol consumption (Regier et al., 1990), smoking (Cuijpers et al., 2007), use of other drugs such as opioids (Santo et al., 2022), sedentary lifestyles (Hoare et al., 2016), functional limitations (Buist-Bouwman et al., 2006), traumatic events (Bandelow et al., 2004), family economic hardship (Evans, 2018), financial crises (Belloni et al., 2016), and environmental aspects such as noise (Basner et al., 2014) or pollution (Ventriglio et al., 2021).

DOI: 10.4324/9781003345725-6

Similarly, there are pharmacological treatments – such as psychotropic medications – that, when prescribed by psychiatrists or general practitioners, can help control the symptoms of some mental illnesses (Frank et al., 2005). There are also cognitive behavioural therapies led by psychologists or therapists that focus on modifying distressing emotions, behaviours, and thoughts (Tolin, 2010). Relaxation techniques can help reduce stress and include meditation, deep breathing, visualization, or progressive muscle relaxation (Toussaint et al., 2021). Likewise, eating habits such as a balanced and healthy diet (Adan et al., 2019), healthy sleep (Liu et al., 2023), social factors such as stable relationships (Schön et al., 2009), emotional support from the family environment (Pernice-Duca, 2010) or a satisfactory job (Faragher et al., 2005) can contribute to maintaining good mental health.

Other determinants that may protect against the risk of mental distress include factors like social integration (Baumgartner & Susser, 2013), recreational or entertainment activities (Pondé & Santana, 2017) or environmental factors such as exposure to nature (Barton & Pretty, 2010; Bloomfield, 2017; Bratman et al., 2019; Vujcic et al., 2017). Among all these protective factors, contact with nature stands out for its benefits on the mental health and wellbeing of the population (Bratman et al., 2019; Mantler & Logan, 2015; McKinnon et al., 2016; Mitchell, 2013; Roe et al., 2013; Triguero-Mas et al., 2015). In addition to its low cost, exposure to urban green spaces has implications for the promotion of physical activity (Lee et al., 2015), social relations (Holtan et al., 2014) as well as supporting aspects of climate adaptation and environmental protection (Pitman et al., 2015).

Types of exposure to nature

Exposure to nature can be achieved directly by accessing and spending time in protected natural spaces (Buckley et al., 2019; Pullin et al., 2013), forests (Rosa et al., 2021), rural areas (Nicholson, 2008), urban green (Callaghan et al., 2021; Thompson et al., 2021) or blue spaces (Völker et al., 2018) and through enjoying other forms of greenery in cities (P. James et al., 2015). Nature exposure can also occur through indirect contact, such as views of greenery from home windows (Garrido-Cumbrera et al., 2023a) or through virtual reality (Szczepańska-Gieracha et al., 2021; Valtchanov et al., 2010), which does not require physical presence (Keniger et al., 2013). Direct contact with natural environments can be measured by number of visits to green (M. Van den Berg et al., 2016) or blue spaces (Poulsen et al., 2022), residential proximity/distance (Sturm, 2004) or percentage of greenness in a particular neighbourhood (Cottagiri et al., 2022).

Quantity, size, and quality of green spaces in neighbourhoods

Several studies have sought to understand how the quantity, size, and quality of green space in the neighbourhood may be linked to resident mental health and wellbeing. A study in Shanghai found that both the quantity of green space in the neighbourhood, measured as the proportion of green space in a given territory, and the quality of green space, measured by plant community structure and foliage habits, increased resident satisfaction (Ta et al., 2021). Residents are generally more satisfied living in greener neighbourhoods with more trees and shrubs (Kaplan, 1985; Kweon et al., 2010; White et al., 2013). A longitudinal study of Australian children identified associations between positive wellbeing in relation to greater amounts of greenness, specifically between 21%

and 40% of green space coverage (Feng & Astell-Burt, 2017). The Netherlands has set a standard for a minimum of 60 m² of green space per capita within a 500-metre radius around homes within healthy planning practice (Roo et al., 2011).

Likewise, having large green spaces can facilitate their use and, therefore, their potential health benefits. A Spanish study found a positive correlation between the size of green spaces and the frequency of walking, exercising, and relaxing (Rey Gozalo et al., 2019). However, the appropriate size of green spaces may vary from country to country, with a recommended size of >5 ha (Schipperijn, Stigsdotter, et al., 2010). Likewise, the quality of green spaces available in a neighbourhood is important for the mental health and wellbeing of the population, because even in places where there is a good amount of green space, if it is of low quality (i.e., unsafe), it may not be well used (Weimann et al., 2017). A study in the Perth metropolitan area (Australia) found that the quality of green space in a neighbourhood was more important than quantity for mental health (Francis et al., 2012). Another study of Public Open Spaces in Australia considered four domains (activities, environmental or aesthetic quality, services and safety), and found a relationship between accessibility to large and attractive spaces and their use for walking.

Another study in Spain evaluated the appreciation of eleven urban green space attributes including lighting, safety, cleanliness, walking routes, bike lanes, shaded areas, recreational areas, off-leash dog areas, children's playgrounds, drinking fountains, and pleasant views and found that older and more educated people, unemployed women, and single men were those who attributed the greatest importance to green spaces (Braçe et al., 2021).

How much residential distance to the nearest accessible green space?

The amount of green space within a given distance from residents' homes is one way of measuring accessibility to green space (Dzhambov et al., 2018). There is some evidence showing that proximity to parks and open spaces is associated with increased use and physical activity (Kaczynski & Henderson, 2007). Proximity to green space has been found to improve general psychological wellbeing (Annerstedt et al., 2012; Triguero-Mas et al., 2015), while frequency of use and walking distance have been positively associated for urban blue spaces (Völker et al., 2018).

In terms of accessibility and usage, an increase in distance to green space is linked with a decline in its use (Nielsen & Hansen, 2007), and proximity from residence to green spaces is related to health benefits (Ekkel & de Vries, 2017). It is important to consider the walking travel time or spatial distance, although there are different standards on what an acceptable distance is. The European Environment Agency (EEA) recommends that people should have access to green space within 15 minutes walking distance, roughly 900–1000m (Stanners & Bourdeau, 1995). Acceptable walking distance has also been separately defined as 1,500 metres from home (W. C. King et al., 2005) or as a 20-minute walk from home (W. C. King et al., 2003). According to a European study, all citizens in Brussels, Copenhagen, Glasgow, Gothenburg, Madrid, Milan, and Paris live within a 15-minute walk of urban green space, as well as the residents of many smaller cities (Stanners & Bourdeau, 1995). The 15-minute city represents a new possibility to reorganize the urban system so that green spaces can be made more accessible by walking (or wheeling) for all age groups (Allam et al., 2022).

Specifically in relation to health, the WHO Regional Office for Europe recommends living within walking distance of 300 metres for a green space of 0.5–1 ha (The WHO

Regional Office for Europe, 2016). A study in Los Angeles associated mental health and residential distance to parks of 400 meters (or ¼mile), which in turn corresponds to the US transit planning standard (Sturm & Cohen, 2014). For their part, different studies in Scandinavian countries have established a maximum distance of 300 metres from the home to an urban green space, as in the case of Denmark (Schipperijn, Ekholm, et al., 2010) and Sweden (Annerstedt et al., 2012).

How much exposure to nature does one need to benefit one's mental health?

Experiencing natural environments can be beneficial to health and wellbeing, but the duration of exposure time required to maximise the potential health benefits (Bell et al., 2019; Cox et al., 2017; Shanahan et al., 2016), including mental health specifically (Barton & Pretty, 2010; Hamer et al., 2009), has been lightly investigated to date. A study in Denver (USA) found that during the COVID-19 pandemic, spending more time in green space was significantly associated with lower depression and anxiety scores (Reid et al., 2022). A large cross-sectional population study demonstrated that visits to greenspace of 30 minutes per week could reduce depression prevalence in the general population by 7% (Shanahan et al., 2016). A study in England showed that spending at least 120 minutes a week in nature was associated with good health and wellbeing, regardless of whether the 120 minutes were achieved by one long visit or several short visits (White et al., 2019).

3-30-300 rule

The "3-30-300 rule" was proposed by Konijnendijk (2022) and could be useful for land use planning because of its simplicity and concreteness. It is based on three principles: residents should be able to see at least three trees from their homes (visibility); everyone should reside in a neighbourhood with at least 30% tree cover (quantity); and live within 300 meters of the nearest public green space (distance). However, other considerations such as exposure time or the quality of the nearest green space are yet to be included. In a study evaluating the association between compliance with the 3-30-300 rule and mental health in the city of Barcelona, it was observed that compliance with the complete rule was associated with better mental health, lower consumption of medication and fewer visits to a psychologist or psychiatrist, although it was significant only in the latter case (Nieuwenhuijsen et al., 2022).

Prescription of green and blue exposure to support mental health?

Nature prescription programmes are increasingly being adopted by health sectors as an adjunct to standard care to attend to health and social needs (Astell-Burt et al., 2023). But for healthcare professionals (HCPs) to include nature prescriptions in their work, it is important to understand how to identify appropriate 'doses' for such exposure to facilitate mental health benefits (Barton & Pretty, 2010; Hamer et al., 2009), which may vary according to the patient's health status, sociodemographic profile, and cultural context.

In 1998, the New Zealand Ministry of Health developed the "Green Prescription" programme with the aim of encouraging physical activity, with benefits in the treatment of depression (Hamlin et al., 2016; Patel et al., 2011). Around the same time in the US, the "Park Prescription" programme began to prescribe physical activity in parks to prevent and treat chronic illnesses and promote wellness (J. J. James et al., 2019). In

2015, there were more than 100 Park Prescription programmes in the US in which HCPs prescribed access to parks for patients to engage in physical activity in outdoor settings (Seltenrich, 2015). Currently, this Park Prescription programme allows physicians to issue prescriptions to enjoy the outdoors in thousands of parks across the US (Zarr et al., 2017). Park Prescription is a grassroots movement encouraging physicians to "prescribe" park visits to patients, with the aim of promoting a healthy lifestyle (James et al., 2019).

In Japan, forest bathing ('shinrin yoku') has been recommended to patients to support mental health and wellbeing since 1982 (initially in response to growing concerns about work-related burnout) (Antonelli et al., 2022). The Scottish National Health Service (NHS Scotland) launched the 'Nature Prescriptions' programme in Shetland from 2017 to help manage a range of conditions, including high blood pressure, anxiety, and depression (Bradley, 2021). Similarly, noteworthy is the UK's cross-government "Green social prescribing" project that began in 2020 to enable GPs to promote being active in nature to improve mental health and wellbeing (NHS, 2020). However, in most countries there is no nature prescription programme, nor are there consistent guidelines that would allow HCPs to include such prescriptions for their patients.

In general, studies suggest there is awareness and public support for nature-based social prescribing programmes. In this respect, for example, a national survey conducted by Astell-Burt and Feng during the COVID-19 pandemic found that 82% of Australian adults would be interested in receiving a nature prescription (Astell-Burt et al., 2023). About four billion people worldwide experienced periods of mandatory stay-at-home and business closure orders ("lockdowns") to reduce the spread of the COVID-19 pandemic from March 2020. From that point on, mental health conditions increased disproportionately, leading to concerns of a mental health crisis. While many people felt isolated, some populations suffered more than others, including homeless people, immigrants, and many people with disabilities who were particularly affected, as were young people and people (often women) with disproportionate caring responsibilities, among others (Garrido-Cumbrera et al., 2022; Garrido-Cumbrera, González-Marín et al., 2023; Garrido-Cumbrera, Rodriguez-Mateos et al., 2023). At the same time, many studies from around the world demonstrated the importance and increased use of urban nature during the COVID-19 pandemic to navigate the restrictions of the pandemic. At a time of increasing incidence and prevalence of mental health conditions – due in part to the consequences of the COVID-19 pandemic and lockdown – it is more necessary than ever to use all available means to protect and improve the mental health and wellbeing of the population. Park prescription is a low-cost intervention, easy-to-implement mode for HCPs, with benefits not only in mental health and wellbeing but in aspects such as the promotion of physical activity that could be explored and implemented with care, not only in high-income countries, but also in middle- and low-income countries.

Discussion

Opportunities for contact with nature in modern urban environments are not evenly distributed, with implications for who can experience the psychological and health benefits of nature (A. E. van den Berg et al., 2007). Exposure to nature can have beneficial effects for mental health and wellbeing and can be achieved directly by accessing and/or being exposed to a protected natural space (Pullin et al., 2013), a forest or enjoying a range of urban green or blue spaces (Gascon et al., 2018). Such exposures may also be available in more confined settings, for example through the view from home windows (Kaplan,

2001), indoor plants (Pérez-Urrestarazu et al., 2021), or even virtual reality (Valtchanov et al., 2010). An indication of potential nature contact can be gained through measures such as the number of number of visits to green (M. Van den Berg et al., 2016) or blue spaces (Poulsen et al., 2022), time spent in such settings (M. van den Berg et al., 2017), residential proximity (Orstad et al., 2020), or the percentage of greenery in a particular neighbourhood (Beyer et al., 2014; Van Herzele & de Vries, 2012).

Quantity, as measured by the percentage of green spaces in a neighbourhood or city, is one relevant aspect for comparative research, although it is also necessary to evaluate the quality of these green spaces by measuring the diversity of species or the attributes of green spaces as it too is important for the mental health and wellbeing of the population (Ta et al., 2021). Similarly, the proximity of homes to green spaces is important, and measures have been established ranging from 300 to 500 metres walking distance (Roo et al., 2011; The WHO Regional Office for Europe, 2016), which may be equivalent to a 10 to 15-minute walk; depending on age and mobility priorities and needs (T. L. King et al., 2012; Stanners & Bourdeau, 1995).

In addition, the duration of time spent in nature may play a role. Population-level studies have suggested that the beneficial effects of nature on health may appear through 120 minutes of exposure per week (White et al., 2019), although smaller durations, such as 30 minutes, have also been associated with a reduction in mental health disorders (Shanahan et al., 2016). Different doses may be appropriate for different groups and individuals, considering sociodemographic characteristics (such as age, gender, disability, sexuality, race, ethnicity, income), existing mental health conditions, as well as key qualities of green or blue spaces and other environmental characteristics such as temperature, shade, lighting or safety (Braçe et al., 2021). The social contexts of a visit may also be important (e.g. alone, with children, with another adult or with the dog) (Garrido-Cumbrera et al., 2020).

Despite growing interest in the potential to prescribe nature, there are important limitations to consider in the implementation of park prescription initiatives (Hamlin et al., 2016; Patel et al., 2011). Most of the evidence of how nature exposure is associated with improvements in mental health and wellbeing comes from cross-sectional studies that cannot prove *causal* relationships between types of exposure and mental health improvements; more longitudinal studies are needed to deepen understanding of those causal relationships. In addition, there is great heterogeneity with respect to the measures used to assess nature exposure. A scoping review found that measures of green space were often vague and varied across the included studies, making accurate comparisons difficult (Callaghan et al., 2021). There is variability in measures of mental health (diagnosed by a physician, through validated scales or self-reported), types of exposure to nature (direct, through windows or virtual) (Pullin et al., 2013; Garrido-Cumbrera et al., 2023a; Szczepańska-Gieracha et al., 2021), number of green spaces in the neighbourhood (Weimann et al., 2017), or distance to green spaces from home (Annerstedt et al., 2012). In addition, there are important differences between types of green spaces (urban green spaces, forests, protected areas), between urban and rural areas (Callaghan et al., 2021; Nicholson, 2008), between geographic areas or between green spaces versus blue spaces (Völker et al., 2018). Such heterogeneity makes it difficult to establish solid and robust scientific evidence to support nature exposure as an effective mental health intervention in clinical practice, particularly when trying to tailor such exposure to the specific needs and priorities of different people (Aerts et al., 2022; Astell-Burt et al., 2023; Müller-Riemenschneider et al., 2020). Personalized medicine is increasingly used in many areas of clinical practice, with the aim of providing personalized, individualized, and patient-tailored care (Hayes et al., 2014). As with approaches to the management of other health conditions, nature or green social prescribing programmes should be personalized (NHS, 2020), considering sociodemographic characteristics (i.e., gender, age, race, ethnicity, income, marital status), health conditions, (physical or mental), disability status, alongside other personal and socio-cultural and historical factors.

Conclusions

This chapter has presented several ways to measure the impacts of nature on mental health and wellbeing, including distance, quantity, quality, and exposure time. Establishing the most appropriate distance, quantity, quality, and time spent in the natural environment – both to protect us and to improve our mental health and wellbeing – will contribute to generating solid evidence and practical guidelines that will enable HCPs to prescribe contact with nature to patients. Fuller evidence on the percentage of green spaces in a neighbourhood or city, as well as their characteristics and quality, and the minimum exposure time per week, will be necessary to support mental health/wellbeing benefits for different individuals and groups. This knowledge will allow progress in the establishment of appropriate green social prescribing programmes, especially in countries where they have not been implemented, as well as their consolidation where they already exist (such as New Zealand, the United States, Japan, or the United Kingdom). If the aim is to improve the health and wellbeing of the population, it is necessary to integrate public health principles into urban planning in all types of neighbourhoods and communities. In a planet increasingly threatened by climate breakdown, environmental issues affecting cities and their effects on mental health and wellbeing must be put on the agenda as a matter of urgency.

References

Adan, R. A. H., van der Beek, E. M., Buitelaar, J. K., Cryan, J. F., Hebebrand, J., Higgs, S., Schellekens, H., & Dickson, S. L. (2019). Nutritional psychiatry: Towards improving mental health by what you eat. *European Neuropsychopharmacology*, 29(12), pp. 1321–1332. https://doi.org/10.1016/J.EURONEURO.2019.10.011

Aerts, R., Vanlessen, N., Dujardin, S., Nemery, B., Van Nieuwenhuyse, A., Bauwelinck, M., Casas, L., Demoury, C., Plusquin, M., & Nawrot, T. S. (2022). Residential green space and mental health-related prescription medication sales: An ecological study in Belgium. *Environmental Research*, 211, 113056. https://doi.org/10.1016/j.envres.2022.113056

Allam, Z., Nieuwenhuijsen, M., Chabaud, D., & Moreno, C. (2022). The 15-minute city offers a new framework for sustainability, liveability, and health. *The Lancet Planetary Health*, 6(3), pp. e181–e183.

Annerstedt, M., Östergren, P. O., Björk, J., Grahn, P., Skärbäck, E., & Währborg, P. (2012). Green qualities in the neighbourhood and mental health – Results from a longitudinal cohort study in Southern Sweden. *BMC Public Health*, 12(1). https://doi.org/10.1186/1471-2458-12-337

Antonelli, M., Donelli, D., Carlone, L., Maggini, V., Firenzuoli, F., & Bedeschi, E. (2022). Effects of forest bathing (shinrin-yoku) on individual well-being: An umbrella review. *International Journal of Environmental Health Research*, 32(8), pp. 1842–1867. https://doi.org/10.1080/09603123.2021.1919293

Astell-Burt, T., Hipp, J. A., Gatersleben, B., Adlakha, D., Marselle, M., Olcoń, K., Pappas, E., Kondo, M., Booth, G., Bacon, S., Lem, M., Francois, M., Halcomb, E., Moxham, L., Davidson,

P., & Feng, X. (2023). Need and interest in nature prescriptions to protect cardiovascular and mental health: A nationally-representative study with insights for future randomised trials. *Heart Lung and Circulation*, 32(1), pp. 114–123. https://doi.org/10.1016/j.hlc.2022.11.008

Bandelow, B., Torrente, A. C., Wedekind, D., Broocks, A., Hajak, G., & Rüther, E. (2004). Early traumatic life events, parental rearing styles, family history of mental disorders, and birth risk factors in patients with social anxiety disorder. *European Archives of Psychiatry and Clinical Neuroscience*, 254(6), pp. 397–405. https://doi.org/10.1007/S00406-004-0521-2/METRICS

Barton, J., & Pretty, J. (2010). What is the best dose of nature and green exercise for improving mental health- A multi-study analysis. *Environmental Science and Technology*, 44(10), pp. 3947–3955. https://doi.org/10.1021/ES903183R

Basner, M., Babisch, W., Davis, A., Brink, M., Clark, C., Janssen, S., & Stansfeld, S. (2014). Auditory and non-auditory effects of noise on health. *Lancet*, 383(9925), pp. 1325–1332. https://doi.org/10.1016/S0140-6736(13)61613-X

Baumgartner, J. N., & Susser, E. (2013). Social integration in global mental health: What is it and how can it be measured? *Epidemiology and Psychiatric Sciences*, 22(1), pp. 29–37. https://doi.org/10.1017/S2045796012000303

Bell, S. L., Leyshon, C., Foley, R., & Kearns, R. A. (2019). The "healthy dose" of nature: A cautionary tale. *Geography Compass*, 13(1), e12415. https://doi.org/10.1111/GEC3.12415

Belloni, M., Meschi, E., & Pasini, G. (2016). The effect on mental health of retiring during the economic crisis. *Health Economics*, 25, pp. 126–140. https://doi.org/10.1002/hec.3377

Beyer, K. M. M., Kaltenbach, A., Szabo, A., Bogar, S., Javier Nieto, F., & Malecki, K. M. (2014). Exposure to neighborhood green space and mental health: Evidence from the survey of the health of Wisconsin. *International Journal of Environmental Research and Public Health*, 11(3), pp. 3453–3472. https://doi.org/10.3390/IJERPH110303453

Bloomfield, D. (2017). What makes nature-based interventions for mental health successful? *BJPsych. International*, 14(4), pp. 82–85. https://doi.org/10.1192/S2056474000002063

Braçe, O., Garrido-Cumbrera, M., & Correa-Fernández, J. (2021). Gender differences in the perceptions of green spaces characteristics. *Social Science Quarterly*, 102(6), pp. 2640–2648. https://doi.org/10.1111/ssqu.13074

Bratman, G. N., Anderson, C. B., Berman, M. G., Cochran, B., de Vries, S., Flanders, J., Folke, C., Frumkin, H., Gross, J. J., Hartig, T., Kahn, P. H., Kuo, M., Lawler, J. J., Levin, P. S., Lindahl, T., Meyer-Lindenberg, A., Mitchell, R., Ouyang, Z., Roe, J., … Daily, G. C. (2019). Nature and mental health: An ecosystem service perspective. *Science Advances*, 5(7), eaax0903. https://doi.org/10.1126/SCIADV.AAX0903

Buckley, R., Brough, P., Hague, L. et al. (2019). Economic value of protected areas via visitor mental health. *Nature Communications 10*, 5005 . https://doi.org/10.1038/s41467-019-12631-6

Buist-Bouwman, M. A., De Graaf, R., Vollebergh, W. A. M., Alonso, J., Bruffaerts, R., Ormel, J., Angermeyer, M., Bernert, S., Brugha, T. S., De Girolamo, G., Demyttenaere, K., Gasquet, I., Haro, J. M., Katz, S. J., Kessler, R. C., Kovess, V., Lépine, J. P., Polidori, G., & Vilagut, G. (2006). Functional disability of mental disorders and comparison with physical disorders: A study among the general population of six European countries. *Acta Psychiatrica Scandinavica*, 113(6), pp. 492–500. https://doi.org/10.1111/j.1600-0447.2005.00684.x

Callaghan, A., McCombe, G., Harrold, A., McMeel, C., Mills, G., Moore-Cherry, N., & Cullen, W. (2021). The impact of green spaces on mental health in urban settings: A scoping review. *Journal of Mental Health*, 30(2), pp. 179–193. https://doi.org/10.1080/09638237.2020.1755027

Cottagiri, S. A., Villeneuve, P. J., Raina, P., Griffith, L. E., Rainham, D., Dales, R., Peters, C. E., Ross, N. A., & Crouse, D. L. (2022). Increased urban greenness associated with improved mental health among middle-aged and older adults of the Canadian Longitudinal Study on Aging (CLSA). *Environmental Research*, 206, 112587. https://doi.org/10.1016/J.ENVRES.2021.112587

Cox, D. T. C., Shanahan, D. F., Hudson, H. L., Fuller, R. A., Anderson, K., Hancock, S., & Gaston, K. J. (2017). Doses of nearby nature simultaneously associated with multiple health benefits. *International Journal of Environmental Research and Public Health*, 14(2). https://doi.org/10.3390/IJERPH14020172

Cuijpers, P., Smit, F., Ten Have, M., & De Graaf, R. (2007). Smoking is associated with first-ever incidence of mental disorders: A prospective population-based study. *Addiction*, 102(8), pp. 1303–1309. https://doi.org/10.1111/J.1360-0443.2007.01885.X

Dzhambov, A., Hartig, T., Markevych, I., Tilov, B., & Dimitrova, D. (2018). Urban residential greenspace and mental health in youth: Different approaches to testing multiple pathways yield different conclusions. *Environmental Research*, 160, pp. 47–59. https://doi.org/10.1016/j.envres.2017.09.015

Ekkel, E. D., & de Vries, S. (2017). Nearby green space and human health: Evaluating accessibility metrics. *Landscape and Urban Planning*, 157, pp. 214–220. https://doi.org/10.1016/j.landurbplan.2016.06.00

Evans, K. (2018). Treating financial difficulty – The missing link in mental health care? *Journal of Mental Health*, 27(6), pp. 487–489. https://doi.org/10.1080/09638237.2018.1520972

Faragher, E. B., Cass, M., & Cooper, C. L. (2005). The relationship between job satisfaction and health: A meta-analysis. *Occupational and Environmental Medicine*, 62(2), pp. 105–112. https://doi.org/10.1136/OEM.2002.006734

Feng, X., & Astell-Burt, T. (2017). Residential green space quantity and quality and child well-being: A longitudinal study. *American Journal of Preventive Medicine*, 53(5), pp. 616–624. https://doi.org/10.1016/J.AMEPRE.2017.06.035

Francis, J., Wood, L. J., Knuiman, M., & Giles-Corti, B. (2012). Quality or quantity? Exploring the relationship between public open space attributes and mental health in Perth, Western Australia. *Social Science and Medicine*, 74(10), pp. 1570–1577. https://doi.org/10.1016/j.socscimed.2012.01.032

Frank, R. G., Conti, R. M., & Goldman, H. H. (2005). Mental health policy and psychotropic drugs. *The Milbank Quarterly*, 83(2), pp. 271–298. https://doi.org/10.1111/J.1468-0009.2005.00347.X

Garrido-Cumbrera, M., Braçe, O., Suárez-Cáceres, G., & Correa-Fernández, J. (2020). Does having children or a dog influence visits to urban green spaces? *Landscape Research*, 45(8), pp. 1018–1031. https://doi.org/10.1080/01426397.2020.1808966

Garrido-Cumbrera, M., Foley, R., Correa-Fernández, J., González-Marín, A., Braçe, O., & Hewlett, D. (2022). The importance for wellbeing of having views of nature from and in the home during the COVID-19 pandemic. Results from the GreenCOVID study. *Journal of Environmental Psychology*, 83. https://doi.org/10.1016/j.jenvp.2022.101864

Garrido-Cumbrera, M., González-Marín, A., Correa-Fernández, J., Braçe, O., & Foley, R. (2023a). Can views and contact with nature at home help Combat anxiety and depression during the Pandemic? Results of the Green COVID study. *Brain and Behavior*, 13, e2875. https://doi.org/10.1002/brb3.2875

Garrido-Cumbrera, M., Rodriguez-Mateos, J. C., & López-Lara, E. (2023b). Impact of the COVID-19 Pandemic on People with Disabilities and Inequalities. In L. Bertelmann, M. Kempf, M. F. Reichstein, A. Rohrmann, & L. Wissenbach (Eds.), *Planning and Development of Social Services for Persons with Disabilities*, pp. 249–258. Siegen, Germany: University of Siegen.

Gascon, M., Sánchez-Benavides, G., Dadvand, P., Martínez, D., Gramunt, N., Gotsens, X., Cirach, M., Vert, C., Molinuevo, J. L., Crous-Bou, M., & Nieuwenhuijsen, M. (2018). Long-term exposure to residential green and blue spaces and anxiety and depression in adults: A cross-sectional study. *Environmental Research*, 162, pp. 231–239. https://doi.org/10.1016/J.ENVRES.2018.01.012

Hamburg, D. A. (1970). *Psychiatry as a Behavioral Science. The Behavioral and Social Sciences Survey*. Englewood Cliffs, NJ: Prentice Hall.

Hamer, M., Stamatakis, E., & Steptoe, A. (2009). Dose-response relationship between physical activity and mental health: The Scottish Health Survey. *British Journal of Sports Medicine*, 43(14), pp. 1111–1114. https://doi.org/10.1136/BJSM.2008.046243

Hamlin, M. J., Yule, E., Elliot, C. A., Stoner, L., & Kathiravel, Y. (2016). Long-term effectiveness of the New Zealand Green prescription primary health care exercise initiative. *Public Health, 140,* pp. 102–108. https://doi.org/10.1016/J.PUHE.2016.07.014

Hayes, D. F., Markus, H. S., Leslie, R. D., & Topol, E. J. (2014). Personalized medicine: Risk prediction, targeted therapies and mobile health technology. *BMC Medicine, 12*(1), pp. 1–8. https://doi.org/10.1186/1741-7015-12-37/FIGURES/4

Hoare, E., Milton, K., Foster, C., & Allender, S. (2016). The associations between sedentary behaviour and mental health among adolescents: A systematic review. *International Journal of Behavioral Nutrition and Physical Activity, 13*(1). https://doi.org/10.1186/s12966-016-0432-4

Holtan, M. T., Dieterlen, S. L., & Sullivan, W. C. (2014). Social life under cover: Tree canopy and social capital in Baltimore. *Maryland Environ Behavior, 47*(5), pp. 502–525. https://doi.org/10.1177/0013916513518064

James, J. J., Christiana, R. W., & Battista, R. A. (2019). A historical and critical analysis of park prescriptions. *Journal of Leisure Research, 50*(4), pp. 311–329. https://doi.org/10.1080/00222 216.2019.1617647

James, P., Banay, R. F., Hart, J. E., & Laden, F. (2015). A review of the health benefits of greenness. *Current Epidemiology Reports, 2*(2), pp. 131–142. https://doi.org/10.1007/S40471-015-0043-7

Kaczynski, A. T., & Henderson, K. A. (2007). Environmental correlates of physical activity: A review of evidence about parks and recreation. *Leisure Sciences, 29*(4), pp. 315–354. https://doi.org/10.1080/01490400701394865

Kaplan, R. (1985). Nature at the doorstep – residential satisfaction and the nearby environment. *Journal of Architectural & Planning Research, 2*(2), pp. 115–127.

Kaplan, R. (2001). The nature of the view from home. *Environment and Behavior, 33*(4), pp. 507–542. https://doi.org/10.1177/00139160121973115

Kendler, K. S. (2005). 'A gene for ...': the nature of gene action in psychiatric disorders. *American Journal of Psychiatry, 162*(7), pp. 1243–1252. https://doi.org/10.1176/appi.ajp.162.7.1243

Keniger, L. E., Gaston, K. J., Irvine, K. N., & Fuller, R. A. (2013). What are the benefits of interacting with nature? *International Journal of Environmental Research and Public Health, 10*(3), pp. 913–935. https://doi.org/10.3390/IJERPH10030913

Kinderman, P. (2005). A psychological model of mental disorder. *Harvard Review of Psychiatry, 13*(4), pp. 206–217. https://doi.org/10.1080/10673220500243349

King, T. L., Thornton, L. E., Bentley, R. J., & Kavanagh, A. M. (2012). Does Parkland influence walking? The relationship between area of parkland and walking trips in Melbourne, Australia. *International Journal of Behavioral Nutrition and Physical Activity, 9.* https://doi.org/10.1186/ 1479-5868-9-115

King, W. C., Belle, S. H., Brach, J. S., Simkin-Silverman, L. R., Soska, T., & Kriska, A. M. (2005). Objective measures of neighborhood environment and physical activity in older women. *American Journal of Preventive Medicine, 28*(5), pp. 461–469. https://doi.org/10.1016/J.AME PRE.2005.02.001

King, W. C., Brach, J. S., Belle, S., Killingsworth, R., Fenton, M., & Kriska, A. M. (2003). The relationship between convenience of destinations and walking levels in older women. *American Journal of Health Promotion: AJHP, 18*(1), pp. 74–82. https://doi.org/10.4278/ 0890-1171-18.1.74

Konijnendijk, C. C. (2022). Evidence-based guidelines for greener, healthier, more resilient neighbourhoods: Introducing the 3–30–300 rule. *Journal of Forestry Research, 1,* pp. 1–10. https://doi.org/10.1007/S11676-022-01523-Z/FIGURES/1

Kweon, B. S., Ellis, C. D., Leiva, P. I., & Rogers, G. O. (2010). Landscape components, land use, and neighborhood satisfaction. *Environment and Planning B: Planning and Design, 37*(3), pp. 500–517. https://doi.org/10.1068/B35059

Lee, A. C. K., Jordan, H. C., & Horsley, J. (2015). Value of urban green spaces in promoting healthy living and wellbeing: Prospects for planning. *Risk Management and Healthcare Policy, 8,* pp. 131–137. https://doi.org/10.2147/RMHP.S61654

Liu, M., Ye, Z., Wu, Q., Yang, S., Zhang, Y., Zhou, C., He, P., Zhang, Y., & Qin, X. (2023). Healthy sleep, mental health, genetic susceptibility, and risk of irritable bowel syndrome. *Journal of Affective Disorders, 331*, pp. 25–32. https://doi.org/10.1016/J.JAD.2023.03.033

Lopez, A. D., & Murray, C. C. J. L. (1998). The global burden of disease, 1990–2020. *Nature Medicine, 4*(11), pp. 1241–1243. https://doi.org/10.1038/3218

Mantler, A., & Logan, A. C. (2015). Natural environments and mental health. *Advances in Integrative Medicine, 2*(1), pp. 5–12. https://doi.org/10.1016/J.AIMED.2015.03.002

McKinnon, M. C., Cheng, S. H., Dupre, S., Edmond, J., Garside, R., Glew, L., Holland, M. B., Levine, E., Masuda, Y. J., Miller, D. C., Oliveira, I., Revenaz, J., Roe, D., Shamer, S., Wilkie, D., Wongbusarakum, S., & Woodhouse, E. (2016). What are the effects of nature conservation on human well-being? A systematic map of empirical evidence from developing countries. *Environmental Evidence, 5*(1). https://doi.org/10.1186/S13750-016-0058-7

Mitchell, R. (2013). Is physical activity in natural environments better for mental health than physical activity in other environments? *Social Science & Medicine, 91*, pp. 130–134. https://doi.org/10.1016/J.SOCSCIMED.2012.04.012

Müller-Riemenschneider, F., Petrunoff, N., Yao, J., Ng, A., Sia, A., Ramiah, A., Wong, M., Han, J., Tai, B. C., & Uijtdewilligen, L. (2020). Effectiveness of prescribing physical activity in parks to improve health and wellbeing-the park prescription randomized controlled trial. *International Journal of Behavioral Nutrition and Physical Activity, 17*(1). https://doi.org/10.1186/S12966-020-00941-8

NHS. (2020). *NHS England Green social prescribing.* www.england.nhs.uk/personalisedcare/social-prescribing/green-social-prescribing/

Nicholson, L. A. (2008). Rural mental health. *Advances in Psychiatric Treatment, 14*(4), pp. 302–311. https://doi.org/10.1192/APT.BP.107.005009

Nielsen, T. S., & Hansen, K. B. (2007). Do green areas affect health? Results from a Danish survey on the use of green areas and health indicators. *Health & Place, 13*(4), pp. 839–850. https://doi.org/10.1016/J.HEALTHPLACE.2007.02.001

Nieuwenhuijsen, M. J., Dadvand, P., Márquez, S., Bartoll, X., Barboza, E. P., Cirach, M., Borrell, C., & Zijlema, W. L. (2022). The evaluation of the 3-30-300 green space rule and mental health. *Environmental Research, 215*, p. 114387. https://doi.org/10.1016/J.ENVRES.2022.114387

Orstad, S. L., Szuhany, K., Tamura, K., Thorpe, L. E., & Jay, M. (2020). Park proximity and use for physical activity among urban residents: Associations with mental health. *International Journal of Environmental Research and Public Health, 17*(13), pp. 1–13. https://doi.org/10.3390/ijerph17134885

Patel, A., Schofield, G. M., Kolt, G. S., & Keogh, J. W. L. (2011). General practitioners' views and experiences of counselling for physical activity through the New Zealand green prescription program. *BMC Family Practice, 12*(1), pp. 1–8. https://doi.org/10.1186/1471-2296-12-119/TABLES/2

Pérez-Urrestarazu, L., Kaltsidi, M. P., Nektarios, P. A., Markakis, G., Loges, V., Perini, K., & Fernández-Cañero, R. (2021). Particularities of having plants at home during the confinement due to the COVID-19 pandemic. *Urban Forestry & Urban Greening, 59*, 126919. https://doi.org/10.1016/J.UFUG.2020.126919

Pernice-Duca, F. (2010). Family network support and mental health recovery. *Journal of Marital and Family Therapy, 36*(1), pp. 13–27. https://doi.org/10.1111/J.1752-0606.2009.00182.X

Pierce, M., Hope, H., Ford, T., Hatch, S., Hotopf, M., John, A., Kontopantelis, E., Webb, R., Wessely, S., McManus, S., & Abel, K. M. (2020). Mental health before and during the COVID-19 pandemic: A longitudinal probability sample survey of the UK population. *The Lancet Psychiatry, 7*(10), pp. 883–892. https://doi.org/10.1016/s2215-0366(20)30308-4

Pitman, S. D., Daniels, C. B., & Ely, M. E. (2015). Green infrastructure as life support: Urban nature and climate change. *Transactions of the Royal Society of South Australia, 139*(1), pp. 97–112. https://doi.org/10.1080/03721426.2015.1035219

Pondé, M. P., & Santana, V. S. (2017). Participation in leisure activities: Is it a protective factor for women's mental health? *Journal of Leisure Research*, 32(4), pp. 457–472. https://doi.org/10.1080/00222216.2000.11949927

Poulsen, M. N., Nordberg, C. M., Fiedler, A., DeWalle, J., Mercer, D., & Schwartz, B. S. (2022). Factors associated with visiting freshwater blue space: The role of restoration and relations with mental health and well-being. *Landscape and Urban Planning*, 217. https://doi.org/10.1016/j.landurbplan.2021.104282

Pullin, A. S., Bangpan, M., Dalrymple, S., Dickson, K., Haddaway, N. R., Healey, J. R., Hauari, H., Hockley, N., Jones, J. P. G., Knight, T., Vigurs, C., & Oliver, S. (2013). Human well-being impacts of terrestrial protected areas. *Environmental Evidence*, 2(1). https://doi.org/10.1186/2047-2382-2-19

Regier, D. A., Farmer, M. E., Rae, D. S., Locke, B. Z., Keith, S. J., Judd, L. L., & Goodwin, F. K. (1990). Comorbidity of mental disorders with alcohol and other drug abuse: Results from the Epidemiologic Catchment Area (ECA) study. *JAMA*, 264(19), pp. 2511–2518. https://doi.org/10.1001/JAMA.1990.03450190043026

Rehm, J., & Shield, K. D. (2019). Global burden of disease and the impact of mental and addictive disorders. *Current Psychiatry Reports*, 21(2), pp. 1–7. https://doi.org/10.1007/S11920-019-0997-0/METRICS

Reid, C. E., Rieves, E. S., & Carlson, K. (2022). Perceptions of green space usage, abundance, and quality of green space were associated with better mental health during the COVID-19 pandemic among residents of Denver. *PloS One*, 17(3), e0263779. https://doi.org/10.1371/journal.pone.0263779

Rey Gozalo, G., Barrigón Morillas, J. M., & Montes González, D. (2019). Perceptions and use of urban green spaces on the basis of size. *Urban Forestry & Urban Greening*, 46, 126470. https://doi.org/10.1016/J.UFUG.2019.126470

Roe, J. J., Ward Thompson, C., Aspinall, P. A., Brewer, M. J., Duff, E. I., Miller, D., Mitchell, R., & Clow, A. (2013). Green space and stress: Evidence from cortisol measures in deprived urban communities. *International Journal of Environmental Research and Public Health*, 10(9), pp. 4086–4103. https://doi.org/10.3390/IJERPH10094086

Roo, M., Kuypers, V., & Lenzholzer, S. (2011). *The green city guidelines: techniques for a healthy liveable city*. https://library.wur.nl/WebQuery/wurpubs/410448

Rosa, C. D., Larson, L. R., Collado, S., & Profice, C. C. (2021). Forest therapy can prevent and treat depression: Evidence from meta-analyses. *Urban Forestry and Urban Greening*, 57, 126943. https://doi.org/10.1016/J.UFUG.2020.126943

Bradley, E. (2021). *Nature Prescriptions: Supporting the health of people and nature*. A report on the outcomes of an urban pilot of Nature Prescriptions in Edinburgh. The Royal Society for the Protection of Birds (RSPB): Edinburgh, UK. p. 59. Available at: https://base-prod.rspb-prod.magnolia-platform.com/dam/jcr:1eb5f06d-adb0-4517-8168-70a08fcf4d98/Edinburgh-pilot-final-report.pdf

Santo, T., Campbell, G., Gisev, N., Martino-Burke, D., Wilson, J., Colledge-Frisby, S., Clark, B., Tran, L. T., & Degenhardt, L. (2022). Prevalence of mental disorders among people with opioid use disorder: A systematic review and meta-analysis. *Drug and Alcohol Dependence*, 238, 109551. https://doi.org/10.1016/J.DRUGALCDEP.2022.109551

Schipperijn, J., Ekholm, O., Stigsdotter, U. K., Toftager, M., Bentsen, P., Kamper-Jørgensen, F., & Randrup, T. B. (2010). Factors influencing the use of green space: Results from a Danish national representative survey. *Landscape and Urban Planning*, 95(3), pp. 130–137. https://doi.org/10.1016/j.landurbplan.2009.12.010

Schipperijn, J., Stigsdotter, U. K., Randrup, T. B., & Troelsen, J. (2010). Influences on the use of urban green space – A case study in Odense, Denmark. *Urban Forestry and Urban Greening*, 9(1), pp. 25–32. https://doi.org/10.1016/J.UFUG.2009.09.002

Schomerus, G., Matschinger, H., & Angermeyer, M. C. (2006). Public beliefs about the causes of mental disorders revisited. *Psychiatry Research*, 144(2–3), pp. 233–236. https://doi.org/10.1016/J.PSYCHRES.2006.05.002

Schön, U. K., Denhov, A., & Topor, A. (2009). Social relationships as a decisive factor in recovering from severe mental illness. *International Journal of Social Psychiatry, 55*(4), pp. 336–347. https://doi.org/10.1177/0020764008093686

Seltenrich, N. (2015). Just what the doctor ordered: Using parks to improve children's health. *Environmental Health Perspectives, 123*(10), A254. https://doi.org/10.1289/EHP.123-A254

Shanahan, D. F., Bush, R., Gaston, K. J., Lin, B. B., Dean, J., Barber, E., & Fuller, R. A. (2016). Health benefits from nature experiences depend on dose. *Scientific Reports, 6.* https://doi.org/10.1038/SREP28551

Stanners, D., & Bourdeau, P. (1995). The urban environment. In *Europe's Environment: The Dobris Assessment*, pp. 261–296. Luxembourg: Office for Official Publications of the European Communities.

Sturm, R. (2004). The economics of physical activity: Societal trends and rationales for interventions. *American Journal of Preventive Medicine, 27*(Suppl. 3), pp. 126–135. https://doi.org/10.1016/j.amepre.2004.06.013.

Sturm, R., & Cohen, D. (2014). Proximity to urban parks and mental health. *Journal of Mental Health Policy and Economics, 17*(1), p. 19. /pmc/articles/PMC4049158/

Szczepańska-Gieracha, J., Cieślik, B., Serweta, A., & Klajs, K. (2021). Virtual therapeutic garden: A promising method supporting the treatment of depressive symptoms in late-life: A randomized pilot study. *Journal of Clinical Medicine, 10*(9), 1942. https://doi.org/10.3390/JCM10091942

Ta, N., Li, H., Zhu, Q., & Wu, J. (2021). Contributions of the quantity and quality of neighborhood green space to residential satisfaction in suburban Shanghai. *Urban Forestry & Urban Greening, 64*, 127293. https://doi.org/10.1016/J.UFUG.2021.127293

The WHO Regional Office for Europe. (2016). *Urban green spaces and health. Technical report World health Organization Copenhagen: WHO regional office for Europe.* https://apps.who.int/iris/handle/10665/345751

Thompson, D.A., Fry, R., Watkins, A., Mizen, A., Akbari, A., Garrett, J., Geary, R., Lovell, R., Lyons, R., Nieuwenhuijsen, M., Rowney, F., Stratton, G., Wheeler, B., White, M., White, J., Williams, S., Rodgers, S. (2021). Exposure to green-blue spaces and mental health: a retrospective e-cohort study in Wales. *The Lancet, 398*, S85. 10.1016/S0140-6736(21)02628-3.

Tolin, D. F. (2010). Is cognitive–behavioral therapy more effective than other therapies? A meta-analytic review. *Clinical Psychology Review, 30*(6), pp. 710–720. https://doi.org/10.1016/J.CPR.2010.05.003

Toussaint, L., Nguyen, Q. A., Roettger, C., Dixon, K., Offenbächer, M., Kohls, N., Hirsch, J., & Sirois, F. (2021). Effectiveness of progressive muscle relaxation, deep breathing, and guided imagery in promoting psychological and physiological states of relaxation. *Evidence-Based Complementary and Alternative Medicine: ECAM, 2021*(1). https://doi.org/10.1155/2021/5924040

Triguero-Mas, M., Dadvand, P., Cirach, M., Martínez, D., Medina, A., Mompart, A., Basagaña, X., Gražulevičiene, R., & Nieuwenhuijsen, M. J. (2015). Natural outdoor environments and mental and physical health: Relationships and mechanisms. *Environment International, 77*, pp. 35–41. https://doi.org/10.1016/j.envint.2015.01.012

Valtchanov, D., Barton, K. R., & Ellard, C. (2010). Restorative effects of virtual nature settings. *Cyberpsychol Behaviour Society Networks, 13*(5), pp. 503–512. https://doi.org/10.1089/cyber.2009.0308

van den Berg, A. E., Hartig, T., & Staats, H. (2007). Preference for nature in urbanized societies: Stress, restoration, and the pursuit of sustainability. *Journal of Social Issues, 63*(1), pp. 79–96. https://doi.org/10.1111/J.1540-4560.2007.00497.X

van den Berg, M., van Poppel, M., Smith, G., Triguero-Mas, M., Andrusaityte, S., van Kamp, I., van Mechelen, W., Gidlow, C., Gražulevičiene, R., Nieuwenhuijsen, M. J., Kruize, H., & Maas, J. (2017). Does time spent on visits to green space mediate the associations between the level of residential greenness and mental health? *Urban Forestry & Urban Greening, 25*, pp. 94–102. https://doi.org/10.1016/J.UFUG.2017.04.010

Van den Berg, M., Van Poppel, M., Van Kamp, I., Andrusaityte, S., Balseviciene, B., Cirach, M., Danileviciute, A., Ellis, N., Hurst, G., Masterson, D., Smith, G., Triguero-Mas, M.,

Uzdanaviciute, I., Wit, P. de, Van Mechelen, W., Gidlow, C., Grazuleviciene, R., Nieuwenhuijsen, M. J., Kruize, H., & Maas, J. (2016). Visiting green space is associated with mental health and vitality: A cross-sectional study in four European cities. *Health & Place, 38*, pp. 8–15. https://doi.org/10.1016/J.HEALTHPLACE.2016.01.003

Van Herzele, A., & de Vries, S. (2012). Linking green space to health: A comparative study of two urban neighbourhoods in Ghent, Belgium. *Population and Environment, 34*(2), pp. 171–193. https://doi.org/10.1007/s11111-011-0153-1

Ventriglio, A., Bellomo, A., Di Gioia, I., Di Sabatino, D., Favale, D., De Berardis, D., & Cianconi, P. (2021). Environmental pollution and mental health: A narrative review of literature. *CNS Spectrums, 26*(1), pp. 51–61. https://doi.org/10.1017/S1092852920001303

Völker, S., Heiler, A., Pollmann, T., Claßen, T., Hornberg, C., & Kistemann, T. (2018). Do perceived walking distance to and use of urban blue spaces affect self-reported physical and mental health? *Urban Forestry & Urban Greening, 29*, pp. 1–9. https://doi.org/10.1016/J.UFUG.2017.10.014

Vujcic, M., Tomicevic-Dubljevic, J., Grbic, M., Lecic-Tosevski, D., Vukovic, O., & Toskovic, O. (2017). Nature based solution for improving mental health and well-being in urban areas. *Environmental Research, 158*, pp. 385–392. https://doi.org/10.1016/J.ENVRES.2017.06.030

Weimann, H., Rylander, L., van den Bosch, M. A., Albin, M., Skärbäck, E., Grahn, P., & Björk, J. (2017). Perception of safety is a prerequisite for the association between neighbourhood green qualities and physical activity: Results from a cross-sectional study in Sweden. *Health and Place, 45*, pp. 124–130. https://doi.org/10.1016/j.healthplace.2017.03.011

White, M. P., Alcock, I., Grellier, J., Wheeler, B. W., Hartig, T., Warber, S. L., Bone, A., Depledge, M. H., & Fleming, L. E. (2019). Spending at least 120 minutes a week in nature is associated with good health and wellbeing. *Scientific Reports, 9*(1). https://doi.org/10.1038/s41598-019-44097-3

White, M. P., Alcock, I., Wheeler, B. W., & Depledge, M. H. (2013). Would you be happier living in a greener urban area? A fixed-effects analysis of panel data. *24*(6), pp. 920–928. https://doi.org/10.1177/0956797612464659

Winkler, P., Formanek, T., Mlada, K., Kagstrom, A., Mohrova, Z., Mohr, P., & Csemy, L. (2020). Increase in prevalence of current mental disorders in the context of COVID-19: Analysis of repeated nationwide cross-sectional surveys. *Epidemiology and Psychiatric Sciences, 29*, e173. https://doi.org/10.1017/S2045796020000888

World Health Organization. (2022). *Mental disorders.* www.who.int/news-room/fact-sheets/detail/mental-disorders

Zarr, R., Cottrell, L., & Merrill, C. (2017). Park prescription (DC Park Rx): A new strategy to combat chronic disease in children. *Journal of Physical Activity and Health, 14*(1), pp. 1–2. https://doi.org/10.1123/JPAH.2017-0021

6 Nature contact and burnout

Thomas Astell-Burt, Michael Navakatikyan, and Xiaoqi Feng

Introduction

Among the many things revealed (and potentially aggravated) by institutional responses to the COVID-19 pandemic has been the widespread issue of work-related burnout (Parandeh et al., 2022). *"[E]xhaustion because of excessing demands on energy, strength, or resources"* was how Freudenberger described burnout in 1975 (p.73). Prior to this, there had been a history of denial and unwillingness to discuss burnout that, to some extent, continues to this day (e.g. over reputational fears; Maslach, 2017). Maslach (2001) considered burnout as characterised by any number of the following experiences: (1) excessive workload demands that feel insurmountable; (2) insufficient control over resources to accomplish work; (3) an absence of appreciation for work done well (e.g. social approval, financial rewards); (4) a felt deprivation of meaningful support and community spirit at work; (5) perceived inequity in the workplace, such as disparities in pay for the same work; and (6) a conflict between institutional and personal values and aspirations. Therefore, clear resonances are evident between how burnout has been understood thus far and a legion of research on social determinants of health that, among a constellation of risk factors, strongly identifies control over one's life and full social participation as fundamental human needs (Marmot, 2006).

Although chronically stressful demands in other life domains have led some researchers to suggest that unemployed people can feel burnout (Bianchi et al., 2014), it has long been studied as a work-specific phenomenon. For example, a range of evidence reviews report high levels of burnout in nurses (Dall'Ora et al., 2020), surgeons (Galaiya et al., 2020), mental health professionals (O'Connor et al., 2018), and school teachers (García-Carmona et al., 2019). The World Health Organization (WHO) includes burnout in the 11th Revision of the International Classification of Diseases (ICD-11). Rather than a disease, the WHO classifies burnout as an occupational syndrome characterised by feelings of energy depletion or exhaustion, increased mental distance to one's occupation, and reduced feelings of professional efficacy (World Health Organization, 2019). In other words, burnout is still widely linked to chronic and unresolved workplace stress; separate to but concomitant with evidence of psychosocial stressors experienced in other life domains such as housing and food insecurity, relationships, caring, and discrimination (World Health Organization, 2008).

There is some debate as to the extent of overlap between burnout and depression, given their concomitance and shared precipitants (Sen, 2022). However, like depression, it is challenging to over-estimate the full impact of burnout on society and economy.

DOI: 10.4324/9781003345725-7

Many attempts to do this are not only specific to certain sectors, but also to professional specialities and cultural contexts. For instance, before the aforementioned global pandemic, burnout had been estimated to cost at least US $4.6 billion in physician turnout and reduced clinical hours per year in the United States (or $7600 per employed physician per year; Han et al., 2019). It means we have shed light on only a very narrow sliver of the total worldwide economic impact of burnout. This, along with the reticence to discuss it, may also help to explain the lack of successful attempts to prevent or alleviate burnout, with the failure to reduce its onset or provide sustained relief having serious consequences for the individuals directly affected. For example, epidemiological studies from the early 1990s reported individuals experiencing burnout had elevated cardiovascular disease risk (Melamed et al., 1992; Appels and Schouten, 1991). Other studies have subsequently pointed to a wide range of other physical, psychological and occupational harms that can eventuate from uninterrupted burnout (Salvagioni et al., 2017). It can also negatively affect people who interact with those who are experiencing burnout, such as the increased potential for medical errors (Menon et al., 2020; Al-Ghunaim et al., 2022; Crijns et al., 2020), diminished patient quality of care (Dall'Ora et al., 2020), and reduced academic achievement and motivation for learning in students (Madigan and Kim, 2021).

Another factor in the challenge to identify scalable, effective solutions is that burnout – like loneliness – has been studied mostly in social, clinical, and organisational psychology (Maslach, 2017). Among many major contributions, researchers in these fields of psychology have helped to identify harms that burnout can result in and also cultivated the 'areas-of-work-life' conceptual model, which emphasises burnout as the outcome of unfavourable interactions between an individual and their occupation, instead of it being exclusively of one or the other (Leiter and Maslach, 1999). But despite the context-specific understanding of burnout predominating, contextual or environmental interventions have been ignored in favour of individual-level treatment-oriented initiatives (even though it is not a disease) that lack robust evidence of efficacy (Maslach, 2017).

Perhaps there is a role for increasing contact with nature to help remedy, maybe even lower the risk of burnout from manifesting? There is certainly some plausibility to harnessing nature as a potential solution, given evidence of green space (and, to some extent, blue space) supporting health and wellbeing through capacity restoring and strengthening domain pathways (Markevych et al., 2017; Hartig et al., 2014). It is suggested that the practice of *shinrin yoku* – or 'forest bathing' – promoted by the Japanese government in the 1980s was driven by concerns about an overworked labour force; various randomised trials in Japan and South Korea report that *shinrin yoku* interventions can have mental and physical health benefits (Chun et al., 2017; Lee et al., 2011, 2018; Shin et al., 2012). Studies of healing gardens and therapeutic landscapes point to psychological, spiritual, and emotional benefits of nature contact (Adevi and Mårtensson, 2013; Corazon et al., 2012; Gonzalez et al., 2010; Hartig and Marcus, 2006). Accordingly, the restorative qualities of contact with nature may play a potent role in alleviating and preventing burnout from occurring through diversionary experiences, momentary and sustained, that afford rest of the neurocognitive mechanism and renewal of capacities depleted through adaptation to chronic stressors that precipitate burnout. As such, we hypothesise that individuals with more contact with nature will have a lower risk of experiencing burnout, whether that be through reducing onset or providing timely relief.

Moreover, recent theoretical developments in this rapidly expanding literature have elaborated on the role of personal, relational, and collective experiences with nature (Hartig, 2021). They have also extended research to loneliness (Astell-Burt et al., 2022a), a close bedfellow of work-related burnout (Seppala and King, 2017) for which there is rapidly emerging evidence of benefit from nature contact (e.g. Astell-Burt et al., 2022a, 2022c; Hammoud et al., 2021; Maas et al., 2009). This advancement extended the domain pathways conceptual model by highlighting the importance of congruent interactions between green spaces and places, individual characteristics, and the co-occurrence of other relevant contextual factors, including the presence of other people (Astell-Burt et al., 2022a; Feng and Astell-Burt, 2023). In other words, one can feel lonely – and burned out – if the contexts to which they are exposed are absent of the things that nourish and fulfil their health, social and personal needs, or in which there are harmful things present (e.g., sources of structural discrimination). But also, the degree of benefit one might accrue from contact with nature may be contingent upon other circumstances that are present i.e., there may be greater restorative potential for people exposed to sources of chronic stress that precipitate burnout. Accordingly, we hypothesise that those individuals who are in occupations that have excess demands and offer individuals low levels of control, security, and imbalance between effort and reward (i.e., low 'job quality'), will have higher risks of burnout, but also greater potential to benefit from contact with nature as a result.

We assessed both hypotheses in a national longitudinal cohort study conducted during the COVID-19 pandemic in Australia with multiple measures of nature contact. This marked an unusual and especially stressful period for many individuals directly affected by protracted lockdowns, spatial restrictions, social isolation, and economic turbulence (Kramer and Kramer, 2020; Penninx et al., 2022; Rahimi-Ardabili et al., 2022). Increased contact with natural environments and felt mental, social, and physical health benefits have been reported in Australia (Astell-Burt and Feng, 2021; Feng and Astell-Burt, 2022) and elsewhere (Labib et al., 2022), though declines have also been reported for some groups by other researchers e.g., in the UK (Burnett et al., 2021). Although increasing burnout has been reported in this period, such as in health professionals (Galanis et al., 2021, Ghahramani et al., 2021, Macaron et al., 2023), the potential benefits of contact with nature for preventing and alleviating burnout have not been investigated in these or general populations (Middleton and Astell-Burt, 2023), making our study especially relevant and timely.

Methods

Data

Baseline and follow-up surveys were conducted on the nationally representative Life in Australia™ panel run by the Social Research Centre. Participants were aged 18 years or older and were the sole respondents from the homes in which they lived. Participants were living across all states and territories of Australia and provided a $10 incentive as either a gift card, direct payment, or a donation to charity. All surveys were conducted in English language only, facilitated by trained interviewers. The baseline survey was conducted between October 12 and 26 2020, which was when Australia had mostly relaxed COVID-19 stay-at-home orders and people were again permitted to travel and visit nature spaces with limited restrictions, except for people living in Melbourne who were coming to the end of a 3-month lockdown period that was no longer in place during the follow-up survey. The follow-up was conducted between February 15 and March 1, 2021, predominantly online (95%). Participants who were uncomfortable with an online survey were afforded the option to complete it via a telephone. A total of 3,043 (78.8% response) of baseline surveys were completed, among whom 2,743 also completed the follow-up survey. Geographical data was missing for 326 participants, and they were omitted from the sample. The focus on job-related burnout meant our sample was then restricted to 1,258 participants in employment. The University of Wollongong HREC granted ethical approval for this study (2020/343).

Outcomes

Burn-out was measured at both time-points using a question from the stress-related Exhaustion Disorder (s-ED) scale (Glise et al., 2010): *"Do you currently feel, and have felt for more than 2 weeks, physically and/or mentally exhausted? (yes/no)"* This single-item response was selected for its brevity, specificity of duration and time-period, and encapsulation of both mental and/or physical exhaustion. It is not strictly a direct measure of burnout in the way that has been done previously, for example, with the more widely used Maslach Burnout Inventory (MBI). However, the MBI is a commercially distributed scale and overly long for inclusion in a general survey, consisting of 22 items for three subscales (emotional exhaustion, depersonalisation, and professional accomplishment). So we acknowledge that the single-item measure used only focuses on the exhaustion component, though researchers have suggested that this (along with depersonalisation) is most relevant, with a lack of professional accomplishment being both a precipitant or symptom, rather than a characteristic of burnout (Lawrence et al., 2022). Further work has involved creating new burnout scales, such as the Copenhagen Burnout Inventory (CBI) that is free to use, but similarly long (19 items). As the CBI conceptualises the severity of psychological and physical exhaustion and fatigue as the core characteristics of burnout, we reasoned that the abovementioned single item used was a feasible starting point ahead of more detailed study.

Two outcomes were derived. First, onset of burnout was identified in those participants who indicated negatively (i.e., favourably) at baseline, but for whom there was a positive (i.e., unfavourable) response at follow-up. Second, relief from burnout was identified in the converse sense, with a negative response at baseline and a positive one at follow-up. Accordingly, this meant splitting the sample into two, contingent upon burnout at baseline.

Contact with nature

We considered both subjective and objective measures of nature contact, as follows:

- Total green space, tree canopy, open grass and shrub, and park availability within 400m, 800m, and 1600m buffers: Data on total green space, tree canopy and open grass and shrub were extracted from the Geovision raster (Pitney Bowes Ltd) for 2016, a high-resolution 2-m surface cover with tree canopy, open grass and shrub included as pre-defined categories. Total green space was the aggregate of all three subtypes. Tree canopy includes all trees, both within parks and along streets, deciduous and evergreen. Open grass and shrub included all low-lying vegetation regardless of whether it was publicly available (e.g., parks and reserves) or in private ownership (e.g., back gardens, school sports grounds). Grass and shrub are underestimated as that which lies beneath tree canopy was not measurable. Park availability was measured for the same buffer sizes using Mesh Block land-use data developed by the Australian Bureau of Statistics. Mesh Blocks are the smallest geographical boundary set in Australia, comprising 30-60 dwellings where populated; those classified as parkland mostly have zero population counts. Parkland includes parks, nature reserves and sports grounds, and can also include other facilities that may not always be publicly accessible, such as golf courses, but does not include private gardens or farmland. These variables (n= 12) were classified into quintiles.

- Time spent in green or blue space in the last week at baseline: This was measured subjectively using the question *"Approximately how many hours did you spend in green spaces and/or blue spaces (e.g., park, reserve, woodland, beach) in total over the last 7 days?"* Responses were classified as none, up to 1-2 hours, 3-4, 4-9, 10 or more.
- Time to reach the nearest green or blue space at baseline: This was also measured subjectively using the question *"How long would it take for you to walk to the nearest green space and/or blue space from your home?"* Responses were classified as 0-4 minutes, 5-9, 10-14, 15-19, 20 or above. This measure was preferred to an objective option given prior research indicating poor correlation between park access variables measured subjectively and objectively (Macintyre et al., 2008), and it is how an individual feels about access that determines visitation of a natural space, rather than how far it is calculated to be.

Job quality

A job quality scale that permits insights into work-related stressors used in the Household Income and Labour Dynamics in Australia (HILDA) survey was replicated in our survey at baseline. This scale has three subscales pertaining to job demands and complexity (three items), job control (three items), and perceived job security (three items). These scales and their aggregation reflect many of the commonly cited precipitants of burnout such as time pressure, excessive complexity and other high psychosocial demands (low levels of job control and autonomy). Participants were required to respond to the following statements with a 5-point Likert scale (strongly disagree to strongly agree):

a) My job is more stressful than I had ever imagined
b) I fear that the amount of stress in my job will make me physically ill
c) I get paid fairly for the things I do in my job
d) I have a secure future in my job
e) The company/organisation I work for will still be in business five years from now
f) I worry about the future of my job
g) My job is complex and difficult
h) My job often requires me to learn new skills
i) I use many of my skills and abilities in my current job
j) I have a lot of freedom to decide how I do my own work
k) I have a lot of say about what happens on my job
l) I have a lot of freedom to decide when I do my work

All items were re-coded in the same direction and the three scales were summed to give an overall job quality scale; wherein higher scores were more favourable. This approach is aligned with that used in previous studies reporting that higher scores on this job quality scale are associated with better mental and physical health (Butterworth et al., 2011, Welsh et al., 2016). As our purpose was to examine whether those with lower job quality and therefore at higher risk of burnout were more likely to benefit from a potentially protective effect of nature contact, we focused on the overall job quality scale only.

Confounders

We took into consideration a range of factors at baseline that are known to be associated with mental health and may also influence the degree of nature contact an individual might have. These included sex and age group, a broad indication of whether people were born in English-speaking or non-English-speaking countries if outside of Australia, whether they were married or with a partner, their highest level of educational qualification, and the annual combined income of the household in which they were resident. We also took into account the level of socioeconomic disadvantage within the neighbourhood of residence, measured using the Socio-Economic Index For Areas (SEIFA) scale, developed from multiple Census variables by the Australian Bureau of Statistics. Finally, we did not take into account differences in labour market status as the sample was already restricted to those who were in employment.

Statistical analysis

We used crosstabulations and percentages to describe the two samples. These samples were weighted for national representativeness, with weights developed by the Social Research Centre taking into account location, age group, gender, annual household income, citizenship status, language(s) spoken other than English, country of birth, Aboriginal or Torres Strait Islander status, number of adults and children in the household, employment status, marital status, highest education, television viewing and internet browsing habits, smoking and drinking status, general health, life satisfaction, early adopter status, caregiving, disability status, volunteer status, concession card status, and telephony status. Multilevel logistic regressions were used to define the odds of onset of, or relief from, burnout in separate models. The clustering of participants at level 1 within cities and regional areas as level 2 (i.e., random intercept) was accounted for using Markov Chain Monte Carlo (MCMC) estimation, with a burn-in period of 30,000 iterations and another 300,000 for the full model. All models were fitted in MLwIN (Browne, 2005; Rasbash et al., 2000).

Results

A total of 689 participants did not experience burnout at baseline, among whom 29.3% experienced an onset of burnout at follow-up (Table A6.1). Onset of burnout was higher among females (32.4%) than males (26.8%), much higher among younger adults (50.9% among 18–24-year-olds) compared to older age groups, lower among those with higher education or income, and lower for those born in Australia or predominantly English-speaking countries. There was little difference in onset of burnout by couple status, but there was very clear evidence of higher onset among those in the lowest job quality quintile and the highest (43.5%, compared with 24.7%). Onset was also higher in more socioeconomically disadvantaged areas. Patterns of burnout onset were less pronounced with respect to the objectively measured green space variables (Table A6.2). There was some indication of higher onset with lower duration of contact and longer journey time. Multilevel models for each of the objectively measured green space variables measured with 400m buffers (Table A6.3) confirmed the absence of association indicated by the descriptive summaries. Higher job quality was, as expected, strongly associated with lower odds of burnout onset. Most other covariates did not reach statistical significance.

Relief was felt by 27.1% of 569 participants identified as experiencing burnout at baseline (Table A6.4). Relief tended to be higher among males than females (31.4% compared with 23.0%), higher in couples or those born in Australia, higher among those with more education, incomes or in socioeconomically advantaged areas, and higher with better job quality. There was little consistent evidence of a pattern between relief from burnout and any of the nature contact variables (Table A6.5). This was confirmed for those objectively measured green space variables within 400m (Table A6.6). Females had 31% lower odds of experiencing relief from burnout than males, whereas those with better job quality had higher odds of finding relief. Assessment of objectively measured green space variables within 800m and 1600m also yielded null associations for both outcomes (Tables A6.7 and A6.8). Neither onset nor relief outcomes were associated with time spent in nature (Table A6.9). Only onset of burnout was associated with journey time to green or blue space (Table A6.10). Two-way interaction terms between each of the nature contact variables with the job quality variable were all not statistically significant, indicating no evidence of effect modification i.e., all indicators of nature contact were consistently not associated with either burnout outcome, regardless of the level of job quality (results not shown in tables).

Discussion

Surprisingly, given the wealth of evidence for restorative benefits of nature contact, the main finding from this study of working adults has been the apparent absence of evidence for it as an effective remedy or preventive measure for work-related burnout. This result was consistent whether participants were at a greater risk of burnout or not, as defined by lower levels of job quality.

These results align with a small number of recent studies. A cross-sectional study in Sweden found no statistically significant associations between a measure of burnout and objectively measured green space variables after adjustment for confounding variables and regardless of whether the population investigated were in gainful employment or not (Klein et al., 2022). A non-randomised controlled evaluation of a walk and talk intervention in a natural setting set in The Netherlands gave some indication of potential benefit overall, though the rate of improvement in level of burnout for the intervention group was not statistically significantly different to that of a passive control group (van den Berg and Beute, 2021). Finally, a randomised trial with waitlist control of healthcare workers in Mexico reported no evidence of a *shinrin yoku* (forest bathing) intervention impacting burnout, though the authors suggest the trial may have been underpowered (Kavanaugh et al., 2022). Currently, it appears that there is limited evidence to suggest that investing in nature contact is an effective way to address the major challenge of burnout.

Our study adds to this small but rapidly emerging literature in a number of ways. First, this is a nationally representative longitudinal study permitting assessment of both onset and relief of burnout. This permits inferences that have greater resonance for urban planners supporting entire populations of working adults, in comparison with those studies that focus on specific groups (e.g., healthcare workers). Second, it offers a more comprehensive examination of contrasting nature contact measures than has previously been attempted in the few studies conducted so far on burnout; consistently null results across different objectively measured green space types across contrasting buffer sizes complement the null results from the subjective measures of contact duration and journey time. The literature on nature and health more generally is replete with studies that use only limited broadscale measures of nature contact (e.g. normalised difference vegetation index, 'NDVI') from which it is impossible to discern how much of what type of green space is most important for a particular outcome, and equally if not more importantly, whether people actually have meaningful contact with it (and if not, why e.g., lacks certain qualities; Astell-Burt and Feng, 2022; Nguyen et al., 2021). The combination of objective and subjective measures of nature contact is therefore an important strength of the study.

Third, it is also the only study of those highlighted above that incorporated a measure of job quality to account for underlying variations in burnout risk within the population. Evidently, some occupations are more demanding and restrictive than others and it is how each person feels individually about their job circumstances, rather than whether they have one or not, that is key to understanding burnout in an occupational context. Finally, caregiving responsibilities, home schooling and other demands placed on many individuals during the COVID-19 period are likely to have aggravated levels of burnout (Aznar et al., 2021; Dellafiore et al., 2022; Muldrew et al., 2022), and perhaps especially in those with low job quality; it may be that associations between burnout and contact with nature during this period are limited to more specific groups of individuals than we have examined in the current study.

That said, there remain ample opportunities for future research before we close the chapter on nature-based solutions for burnout. It is important to note that our study examined job quality as an overall indicator of underlying risk, but it may well be that specific aspects of job quality are more potent determinants of burnout than others; separate analyses are warranted in future work. Second, follow-up of our sample was over the course of four months and maybe a longer duration between survey waves might reveal something different, if the putative mechanisms take longer to have an impact. Third, the single-item measure of burnout as a binary indicator may mask more subtle changes in the degree of burnout experienced; there may be smaller improvements than the current measure can detect. Further dedicated surveys on this topic with more space to include a long-form burnout question-set would be useful to investigate this further. The CBI's context-specific utility may make it ideal in this regard and might be complemented by new measures of nature contact around workplace locations, were that level of geographical precision to become available.

Fourth, the context in which this study was conducted was during the COVID-19 pandemic, with major socioeconomic upheaval and transition to working from home ongoing, albeit to varying degrees in different sectors and geographically. Participants in Melbourne were coming to the end of a long and protracted lockdown, whereas those in Sydney – a city of comparable size and population – were much less restricted by comparison. Our work has already shown that people in Melbourne benefited much more from contact with nature than their counterparts in Sydney during this period, in terms of physical activity, social connection, and feelings of respite and solace (Astell-Burt and

Feng, 2021). These benefits were also far stronger among those who were able to visit higher quality green and blue spaces (Feng and Astell-Burt, 2022). So, it may be that potential benefits of nature contact for preventing and alleviating burnout are contingent upon the qualities in those natural settings and the broader contextual circumstances at play, including whether people are permitted to work from home and to what extent that influences job quality. For instance, it may be that for people who work from offices or other on-site facilities, the quantity and quality of nearby-workplace greenery available may be relatively more important because of duration of time spent there (provided they have sufficient job control to visit it), as compared with a person who works mostly from home and would stand to benefit more from visiting natural settings where they live. A critical caveat here is control in other aspects of one's life; people working from home may be able to harness their discretionary time spent not commuting for more contact with nature, provided they have access to it. But the selection of work from home outside of pandemic-related mandate is likely to be highly entwined with other factors, such as looking after dependent family members, which may mean the time not commuting is not in fact discretionary. Proximity to nature, therefore, does not necessarily translate into use or benefit and much more research on the ongoing bifurcation of labour into those able or unable to work from home will need to be sensitive to this and other common complexities that result in contingent effects.

Finally, with only one randomised trial (Kavanaugh et al., 2022) conducted thus far, there is a clear need to develop and test interventions that enable and empower people with or at high risk of burnout to spend more time in nature, to examine whether this helps to improve their situations. Current evidence is not sufficient to provide any guidance to employers on how to harness nature for reducing employee burnout, but it could improve quickly. The absence of association in well-controlled observational studies does not necessarily mean there is no benefit. With prior evidence suggesting that nature based interventions (including 'nature prescriptions') could lead to meaningful increases in physical activity and reductions in depression, anxiety, and blood pressure (Nguyen et al., 2023), these would be valuable results for people experiencing burnout even if the intervention does not achieve its primary outcome. Our recent work has indicated strong interest among Australian adults in nature prescriptions (Astell-Burt et al., 2023) amid demonstrable application among health professionals in some countries (e.g., Canada; Astell-Burt et al., 2022b; Sherman et al., 2021). Co-design of nature-based interventions with employers and employees is essential to ensure buy-in from key stakeholders and the potential for rapid translation at scale is built-in so everyone who could benefit does so. It may even be that the process of engaging in the co-design and trialling of nature-based solutions by employer's signals to employees (especially if they themselves are engaged in the process of co-design) an intent to improve job quality and reduce burnout as a part of their commitments to sustainability and community.

In conclusion, the findings from the current study indicate that nature contact may not be singularly sufficient to prevent or alleviate burnout in working adults. Companies and organisations interested in reducing burnout must take direct action to protect employee wellbeing, such as by strengthening job and career security, reducing exposure to stressful (and toxic) workplace environments, and prioritising autonomy and on-task control. Still, there is huge potential for health, societal and environmental co-benefits through trialling a nature-based approach to addressing burnout and improving psychological wellbeing in employees as an adjunct to the aforementioned actions that must be taken. Building the evidence will require collaborations involving researchers from many disciplines and methods to reveal the impacts of 'greening' places, including neighbourhoods and workplaces, as well interventions designed to enable and empower people to spend more time in nature for purposes of preventing and alleviating burnout. This adds up to a significant program of work still to be done and it may be a key opportunity for new multisectoral research partnerships.

References

Adevi, A. A. & Mårtensson, F. (2013). Stress rehabilitation through garden therapy: The garden as a place in the recovery from stress. *Urban Forestry & Urban Greening*, 12, pp. 230–237.

Al-Ghunaim, T., Johnson, J., Biyani, C. S. & O'Connor, D. B. (2022). How UK surgeons experience burnout and the link between burnout and patient care: A qualitative investigation. *Scottish Medical Journal*, 67, pp. 197–206.

Appels, A. & Schouten, E. (1991). Burnout as a risk factor for coronary heart disease. *Behavioral Medicine*, 17, pp. 53–59.

Astell-Burt, T. & Feng, X. (2021). Time for 'green' during COVID-19? Inequities in green and blue space access, visitation and felt benefits. *International Journal of Environmental Research and Public Health*, 18, 2757.

Astell-Burt, T. & Feng, X. (2022). Paths through the woods. *International Journal of Epidemiology*, 51, pp. 1–5.

Astell-Burt, T., Hartig, T., Putra, I. G. N. E., Walsan, R., Dendup, T. & Feng, X. (2022a). Green space and loneliness: A systematic review with theoretical and methodological guidance for future research. *Science of the Total Environment*, 847, 157521.

Astell-Burt, T., Hipp, A., Gatersleben, B., Adlakha, D., Marselle, M., Olcoń, K., Pappas, E., Kondo, M., Booth, G. L., Bacon, S., Lem, M., Francois, M., Halcomb, E., Moxham, L., Davidson, P. M. & Feng, X. (2023). Need and interest in nature prescriptions to protect cardiovascular and mental health: A nationally-representative study with insights for future randomised trials. *Heart, Lung & Circulation*, 32, pp. 114–123.

Astell-Burt, T., Pappas, E., Redfern, J. & Feng, X. (2022b). Nature prescriptions for community and planetary health: Unrealised potential to improve compliance and outcomes in physiotherapy. *Journal of Physiotherapy*, 68(3), pp. 151–152.

Astell-Burt, T., Walsan, R., Davis, W. & Feng, X. (2022c). What types of green space disrupt a lonelygenic environment? A cohort study. *Social Psychiatry and Psychiatric Epidemiology*, 58(5), pp. 745–755.

Aznar, A., Sowden, P., Bayless, S., Ross, K., Warhurst, A. & Pachi, D. (2021). Home-schooling during COVID-19 lockdown: Effects of coping style, home space, and everyday creativity on stress and home-schooling outcomes. *Couple and Family Psychology: Research and Practice*, 10, 294.

Bianchi, R., Truchot, D., Laurent, E., Brisson, R. & Schonfeld, I. S. (2014). Is burnout solely job-related? A critical comment. *Scandinavian Journal of Psychology*, 55, pp. 357–361.

Browne, W. J. (2005). *MCMC estimation in MLwiN: Version 2.0*, Bristol, Centre for Multilevel Modelling, University of Bristol.

Burnett, H., Olsen, J. R., Nicholls, N. & Mitchell, R. (2021). Change in time spent visiting and experiences of green space following restrictions on movement during the COVID-19 pandemic: A nationally representative cross-sectional study of UK adults. *BMJ Open*, 11, e044067.

Butterworth, P., Leach, L. S., Rodgers, B., Broom, D. H., Olesen, S. C. & Strazdins, L. (2011). Psychosocial job adversity and health in Australia: Analysis of data from the HILDA Survey. *Australian and New Zealand Journal of Public Health*, 35, pp. 564–571.

Chun, M. H., Chang, M. C. & Lee, S.-J. (2017). The effects of forest therapy on depression and anxiety in patients with chronic stroke. *International Journal of Neuroscience*, 127, pp. 199–203.

Corazon, S. S., Stigsdotter, U. K., Moeller, M. S. & Rasmussen, S. M. (2012). Nature as therapist: Integrating permaculture with mindfulness- and acceptance-based therapy in the Danish healing forest garden Nacadia. *European Journal of Psychotherapy and Counselling*, 14, pp. 335–347.

Crijns, T. J., Kortlever, J. T., Guitton, T. G., Ring, D. & Barron, G. C. (2020). Symptoms of burnout among surgeons are correlated with a higher incidence of perceived medical errors. *HSS Journal®*, 16, pp. 305–310.

Dall'Ora, C., Ball, J., Reinius, M. & Griffiths, P. (2020). Burnout in nursing: A theoretical review. *Human Resources for Health*, 18, pp. 1–17.

Dellafiore, F., Arrigoni, C., Nania, T., Caruso, R., Baroni, I., Vangone, I., Russo, S. & Barello, S. (2022). The impact of COVID-19 pandemic on family caregivers' mental health: A rapid systematic review of the current evidence. *Acta Bio Medica: Atenei Parmensis*, 93, pp. 1–12.

Feng, X. & Astell-Burt, T. (2022). Perceived qualities, visitation and felt benefits of preferred nature spaces during the COVID-19 Pandemic in Australia: A nationally-representative cross-sectional study of 2940 adults. *Land*, 11, 904.

Feng, X. & Astell-Burt, T. (2023). Lonelygenic environments: A call for research on multilevel determinants of loneliness. *The Lancet Planetary Health*, 6, pp. E933–E934.

Freudenberger, H. J. (1975). The staff burn-out syndrome in alternative institutions. *Psychotherapy: Theory, Research & Practice*, 12, p. 73.

Galaiya, R., Kinross, J. & Arulampalam, T. (2020). Factors associated with burnout syndrome in surgeons: A systematic review. *The Annals of The Royal College of Surgeons of England*, 102, pp. 401–407.

Galanis, P., Vraka, I., Fragkou, D., Bilali, A. & Kaitelidou, D. (2021). Nurses' burnout and associated risk factors during the COVID-19 pandemic: A systematic review and meta-analysis. *Journal of Advanced Nursing*, 77, pp. 3286–3302.

García-Carmona, M., Marín, M. D. & Aguayo, R. (2019). Burnout syndrome in secondary school teachers: A systematic review and meta-analysis. *Social Psychology of Education*, 22, pp. 189–208.

Ghahramani, S., Lankarani, K. B., Yousefi, M., Heydari, K., Shahabi, S. & Azmand, S. (2021). A systematic review and meta-analysis of burnout among healthcare workers during COVID-19. *Frontiers in Psychiatry*, 12, 758849.

Glise, K., Hadzibajramovic, E., Jonsdottir, I. H. & Ahlborg, G. (2010). Self-reported exhaustion: A possible indicator of reduced work ability and increased risk of sickness absence among human service workers. *International Archives of Occupational and Environmental Health*, 83, pp. 511–520.

Gonzalez, M. T., Hartig, T., Patil, G. G., Martinsen, E. W. & Kirkevold, M. (2010). Therapeutic horticulture in clinical depression: A prospective study of active components. *Journal of Advanced Nursing*, 66, pp. 2002–2013.

Hammoud, R., Tognin, S., Bakolis, I., Ivanova, D., Fitzpatrick, N., Burgess, L., Smythe, M., Gibbons, J., Davidson, N. & Mechelli, A. (2021). Lonely in a crowd: Investigating the association between overcrowding and loneliness using smartphone technologies. *Scientific Reports*, 11, pp. 1–11.

Han, S., Shanafelt, T. D., Sinsky, C. A., Awad, K. M., Dyrbye, L. N., Fiscus, L. C., Trockel, M. & Goh, J. (2019). Estimating the attributable cost of physician burnout in the United States. *Annals of Internal Medicine*, 170, pp. 784–790.

Hartig, T. (2021). Restoration in nature: Beyond the conventional narrative. *In:* Schutte, A. R., Torquati, J. & Stevens, J. R. (eds.) *Nature and psychology: Biological, cognitive, developmental, and social pathways to well-being (Proceedings of the 67th Annual Nebraska Symposium on Motivation)*. Cham, Switzerland: Springer Nature.

Hartig, T. & Marcus, C. C. (2006). Essay: Healing gardens—places for nature in health care. *The Lancet*, 368, pp. S36–S37.

Hartig, T., Mitchell, R., De Vries, S. & Frumkin, H. (2014). Nature and health. *Annual Review of Public Health*, 35, pp. 207–228.

Kavanaugh, J., Hardison, M. E., Rogers, H. H., White, C. & Gross, J. (2022). Assessing the impact of a Shinrin-Yoku (Forest Bathing) intervention on physician/healthcare professional burnout: A randomized, controlled trial. *International Journal of Environmental Research and Public Health,* 19, 14505.

Klein, Y., Lindfors, P., Osika, W., Magnusson Hanson, L. L. & Stenfors, C. U. (2022). Residential greenspace is associated with lower levels of depressive and burnout symptoms, and higher levels of life satisfaction: A nationwide population-based study in Sweden. *International Journal of Environmental Research and Public Health,* 19, 5668.

Kramer, A. & Kramer, K. Z. (2020). The potential impact of the Covid-19 pandemic on occupational status, work from home, and occupational mobility. *Journal of Vocational Behavior,* 119, 103442.

Labib, S., Browning, M. H., Rigolon, A., Helbich, M. & James, P. (2022). Nature's contributions in coping with a pandemic in the 21st century: A narrative review of evidence during COVID-19. *Science of The Total Environment,* 833, 155095.

Lawrence, J. A., Davis, B. A., Corbette, T., Hill, E. V., Williams, D. R. & Reede, J. Y. (2022). Racial/ethnic differences in burnout: A systematic review. *Journal of Racial and Ethnic Health Disparities,* 9, pp. 257–269.

Lee, J., Miyazaki, Y., Park, B. J., Tsunetsugu, Y., Ohira, T. & Kagawa, T. (2011). Effect of forest bathing on physiological and psychological responses in young Japanese male subjects. *Public Health,* 125, pp. 93–100.

Lee, K. J., Hur, J., Yang, K.-S., Lee, M.-K. & Lee, S.-J. (2018). Acute biophysical responses and psychological effects of different types of forests in patients with metabolic syndrome. *Environment and Behavior,* 50, pp. 298–323.

Leiter, M. P. & Maslach, C. (1999). Six areas of worklife: A model of the organizational context of burnout. *Journal of Health and Human Services Administration,* 21(4), pp. 472–489.

Maas, J., Van Dillen, S. M. E., Verheij, R. A. & Groenewegen, P. P. (2009). Social contacts as a possible mechanism behind the relation between green space and health. *Health & Place,* 15, pp. 586–595.

Macaron, M. M., Segun-Omosehin, O. A., Matar, R., Beran, A., Nakanishi, H., Than, C. A. & Abulseoud, O. (2023). A systematic review and meta analysis on burnout in physicians during the COVID-19 pandemic: A hidden healthcare crisis. *Frontiers in Psychiatry,* 13, 1071397.

Macintyre, S., Macdonald, L. & Ellaway, A. (2008). Lack of agreement between measured and self-reported distance from public green parks in Glasgow, Scotland. *International Journal of Behavioral Nutrition and Physical Activity,* 5, 26.

Madigan, D. J. & Kim, L. E. (2021). Does teacher burnout affect students? A systematic review of its association with academic achievement and student-reported outcomes. *International Journal of Educational Research,* 105, 101714.

Markevych, I., Schoierer, J., Hartig, T., Chudnovsky, A., De Vries, S., Triguero-Mas, M., Brauer, M., Dzhambov, A., Dadvand, P., Nieuwenhuijsen, M. J., Lupp, G., Richardson, E. A., Astell-Burt, T., Hystad, P., Dimitrova, D., Feng, X., Sadeh, M., Standl, M., Heinrich, J. & Fuertes, E. (2017). Exploring pathways linking greenspace to health: Theoretical and methodological guidance. *Environmental Research,* 158, pp. 301–317.

Marmot, M. G. (2006). Status syndrome. *JAMA: The Journal of the American Medical Association,* 295, pp. 1304–1307.

Maslach, C. (2017). Finding solutions to the problem of burnout. *Consulting Psychology Journal: Practice and Research,* 69, p. 143.

Maslach, C., Schaufeli, W. B. & Leiter, M. P. (2001). Job burnout. *Annual Review of Psychology,* 52, pp. 397–422.

Melamed, S., Kushnir, T. & Shirom, A. (1992). Burnout and risk factors for cardiovascular diseases. *Behavioral Medicine,* 18, pp. 53–60.

Menon, N. K., Shanafelt, T. D., Sinsky, C. A., Linzer, M., Carlasare, L., Brady, K. J., Stillman, M. J. & Trockel, M. T. (2020). Association of physician burnout with suicidal ideation and medical errors. *JAMA Network Open,* 3, e2028780.

Middleton, R. & Astell-Burt, T. (2023). Nurses and nature; Does green space make a difference? *Journal of Clinical Nursing*, 32, pp. 4214–4216. https://doi.org/10.1111/jocn.16697.

Muldrew, D. H., Fee, A. & Coates, V. (2022). Impact of the COVID-19 pandemic on family carers in the community: A scoping review. *Health & Social Care in the Community*, 30, pp. 1275–1285.

Nguyen, P.-Y., Astell-Burt, T., Rahimi-Ardabili, H. & Feng, X. (2021). Green space quality and health: A systematic freview. *International Journal of Environmental Research and Public Health*, 18, 11028.

Nguyen, P.-Y., Astell-Burt, T., Rahimi-Ardabili, H. & Feng, X. (2023). Effect of nature prescriptions on cardiometabolic and mental health, and physical activity: A systematic review. *The Lancet Planetary Health*, 7, pp. e313–328.

O'Connor, K., Neff, D. M. & Pitman, S. (2018). Burnout in mental health professionals: A systematic review and meta-analysis of prevalence and determinants. *European Psychiatry*, 53, pp. 74–99.

Parandeh, A., Ashtari, S., Rahimi-Bashar, F., Gohari-Moghadam, K. & Vahedian-Azimi, A. (2022). Prevalence of burnout among health care workers during coronavirus disease (COVID-19) pandemic: A systematic review and meta-analysis. *Professional Psychology: Research and Practice* 53(6), pp. 564–573.

Penninx, B. W., Benros, M. E., Klein, R. S. & Vinkers, C. H. (2022). How COVID-19 shaped mental health: From infection to pandemic effects. *Nature Medicine*, 28, pp. 2027–2037.

Rahimi-Ardabili, H., Feng, X., Nguyen, P.-Y. & Astell-Burt, T. (2022). Have deaths of despair risen during the COVID-19 Pandemic? A systematic review. *International Journal of Environmental Research and Public Health*, 19, 12835.

Rasbash, J., Browne, W., Goldstein, H., Yang, M., Plewis, I., Healy, M., Woodhouse, G., Draper, D., Langford, I. & Lewis, T. (2000). *A user's guide to MLwiN*, London, Institute of Education.

Salvagioni, D. A. J., Melanda, F. N., Mesas, A. E., González, A. D., Gabani, F. L. & Andrade, S. M. D. (2017). Physical, psychological and occupational consequences of job burnout: A systematic review of prospective studies. *PloS One*, 12, e0185781.

Sen, S. (2022). Is it burnout or depression? Expanding efforts to improve physician well-being. *New England Journal of Medicine*, 387, pp. 1629–1630.

Seppala, E. & King, M. (2017). Burnout at work isn't just about exhaustion. It's also about loneliness. *Harvard Business Review*, 29, pp. 2–4.

Sherman, J. D., Mcgain, F., Lem, M., Mortimer, F., Jonas, W. B. & Macneill, A. J. (2021). Net zero healthcare: A call for clinician action. *BMJ*, 374, pp. 1–6.

Shin, W. S., Shin, C. S. & Yeoun, P. S. (2012). The influence of forest therapy camp on depression in alcoholics. *Environmental Health and Preventive Medicine*, 17, pp. 73–76.

Van Den Berg, A. E. & Beute, F. (2021). Walk it off! The effectiveness of walk and talk coaching in nature for individuals with burnout-and stress-related complaints. *Journal of Environmental Psychology*, 76, 101641.

Welsh, J., Strazdins, L., Charlesworth, S., Kulik, C. T. & Butterworth, P. (2016). Health or harm? A cohort study of the importance of job quality in extended workforce participation by older adults. *BMC Public Health*, 16, pp. 1–14.

World Health Organization. (2008). *Closing the gap in a generation: Health equity through action on the social determinants of health. Final report of the Commission of Social Determinants of Health*, Geneva, World Health Organization.

World Health Organization. (2019). *Burn-out an "occupational phenomenon": International Classification of Diseases* [Online]. Available: www.who.int/news/item/28-05-2019-burn-out-an-occupational-phenomenon-international-classification-of-diseases [Accessed].

Appendices

Table A6.1 Descriptive statistics for burnout onset – demographics and socioeconomics

Variable	Items	Onset of burnout	
		Total (no burnout at baseline)	% Onset of burnout
Full sample		689	29.3
Gender	Male	368	26.8
	Female	321	32.4
Age group	18-24y	58	50.9
	25-34y	153	32.3
	35-44y	150	36.2
	45-54y	151	25.0
	55-64y	136	20.2
	65y +	41	10.1
Geography	Greater Sydney	156	27.0
	Rest of NSW	69	30.2
	Greater Melbourne	121	23.5
	Rest of Vic.	43	36.5
	Greater Brisbane	69	33.2
	Rest of Qld	71	19.4
	Greater Adelaide	45	40.8
	Greater Perth	81	35.1
	Other	33.0	39.4
Education	School	195	33.3
	Diploma	246	28.1
	University	239	28.2
	Missing	10	15.2
Income (AUD)	0-29K	24	33.2
	30-69K	132	32.0
	70-100K	139	24.3
	100K +	367	29.1
	Missing	27	43.6
Couple status	In a couple	528	29.0
	Not in a couple	161	30.9
Country of birth	Australia	434	28.6
	Other English-speaking country	107	28.1
	Other non-English-speaking country	148	32.6
Overall job quality (quintiles)	1 (score 12 to 33, lower quality)	83	43.5
	2 (score 34 to 36)	109	34.1
	3 (score 37 to 39)	172	24.2
	4 (score 40 to 42)	150	29.5
	5 (score 43 to 60, higher quality)	174	24.7
Area-level disadvantage (quintiles)	1 (low disadvantage)	146	19.7
	2	173	34.2
	3	137	29.4
	4	129	35.7
	5 (high disadvantage)	103	27.2

Table A6.2 Descriptive statistics for burnout onset and nature contact variables

Variable	Items	Onset of burnout	
		Total (no burnout at baseline)	% Onset of burnout
Full sample		689	29.3
Total green space < 400m (quintiles)	1 (0 to 12.3%)	135	31.8
	2 (12.3 to 22.6%)	141	27.4
	3 (22.6 to 33.4%)	161	31.4
	4 (33.4 to 52%)	120	24.1
	5 (52 to 100%)	131	31.5
Total green space < 800m (quintiles)	1 (0 to 14.7%)	139	28.1
	2 (14.7 to 26.8%)	145	32.5
	3 (26.8 to 38.6%)	159	30.9
	4 (38.6 to 58%)	115	22.9
	5 (58 to 100%)	131	31.3
Total green space < 1600m (quintiles)	1 (0 to 17.7%)	145	30.3
	2 (17.8 to 30.8%)	150	30.4
	3 (30.8 to 42.2%)	142	30.2
	4 (42.3 to 61.1%)	132	25.5
	5 (61.1 to 100%)	120	30.5
Tree canopy < 400m (quintiles)	1 (0 to 0%)	131	26.4
	2 (0 to 4.8%)	114	21.7
	3 (4.8 to 11.8%)	164	40.5
	4 (11.8 to 23.2%)	158	26.2
	5 (23.2 to 100%)	123	28.9
Tree canopy < 800m (quintiles)	1 (0 to 1.0%)	125	25.0
	2 (1.0 to 7.1%)	124	30.3
	3 (7.1 to 13.9%)	163	31.6
	4 (13.9 to 25.7%)	155	29.0
	5 (25.8 to 100%)	122	30.6
Tree canopy < 1600m (quintiles)	1 (0 to 2.5%)	125	22.7
	2 (2.5 to 8.8%)	131	39.0
	3 (8.8 to 15.9%)	169	27.3
	4 (15.9 to 28.3%)	141	29.7
	5 (28.4 to 100%)	123	28.5
Grass and shrub < 400m (quintiles)	1 (0 to 5.5%)	125	26.6
	2 (5.5 to 10.9%)	151	34.3
	3 (10.9 to 18%)	165	26.3
	4 (18 to 29.2%)	126	33.4
	5 (29.3 to 100%)	123	26.2
Grass and shrub < 800m (quintiles)	1 (0 to 6.8%)	131	32.1
	2 (6.8 to 12.4%)	151	28.6
	3 (12.5 to 19.9%)	146	29.8
	4 (19.9 to 33.3%)	141	25.4
	5 (33.4 to 100%)	120	31.7
Grass and shrub < 1600m (quintiles)	1 (0 to 8.6%)	144	35.8
	2 (8.6 to 13.9%)	133	20.8
	3 (13.9 to 21.5%)	154	31.1
	4 (21.5 to 35.3%)	129	30.8
	5 (35.3 to 100%)	129	27.6

(*Continued*)

Table A6.2 (Continued)

Variable	Items	Onset of burnout	
		Total (no burnout at baseline)	% Onset of burnout
Parks < 400m (quintiles)	1 (0 to 0%)	138	25.4
	2 (0 to 4.9%)	143	32.5
	3 (4.9 to 10.6%)	143	35.7
	4 (10.6 to 19.3%)	158	28.1
	5 (19.3 to 100%)	107	23.9
Parks < 800m (quintiles)	1 (0 to 3.1%)	148	26.9
	2 (3.1 to 7.3%)	144	30.0
	3 (7.3 to 13.3%)	152	30.0
	4 (13.3 to 22.4%)	139	33.0
	5 (22.4 to 100%)	106	26.5
Parks < 1600m (quintiles)	1 (0 to 6.0%)	154	30.5
	2 (6.0 to 10.8%)	141	29.1
	3 (10.8 to 15.9%)	158	29.4
	4 (15.9 to 24.6%)	123	33.0
	5 (24.6 to 100%)	113	24.3
Time spent in green/blue spent per week (hours)	None	114	34.6
	1-2	209	21.0
	3-4	150	37.8
	5-9	125	32.3
	10 or more	91	24.4
Time to reach preferred green/blue space (minutes)	0-4	220	23.9
	5-9	227	32.0
	10-14	109	18.7
	15-19	55	30.9
	20 or above	78	51.3

Table A6.3 Models for availability of nature space within 400m and onset of burnout

Model	Outcome: Onset of burnout			
	1	*2*	*3*	*4*
	Odds Ratio (95% Credible Interval)			
Total green space < 400m	0.99 (0.92, 1.07)			
Tree canopy < 400m		0.98 (0.87, 1.09)		
Grass and shrub < 400m			1.01 (0.91, 1.11)	
Parks < 400m				1.01 (0.86, 1.17)
Gender (ref=Male)				
Female	1.20 (0.84, 1.74)	1.21 (0.84, 1.76)	1.21 (0.83, 1.75)	1.20 (0.83, 1.74)
Age group (ref=18-24y)				
25-34y	0.71 (0.24, 2.11)	0.68 (0.23, 2.10)	0.71 (0.23, 2.18)	0.71 (0.24, 2.13)
35-44y	0.71 (0.24, 2.05)	0.69 (0.24, 2.04)	0.71 (0.24, 2.14)	0.71 (0.25, 2.08)
45-54y	0.42 (0.14, 1.24)	0.41 (0.14, 1.22)	0.42 (0.14, 1.26)	0.42 (0.15, 1.23)
55-64y	0.45 (0.16, 1.29)	0.44 (0.15, 1.29)	0.44 (0.15, 1.34)	0.45 (0.16, 1.30)
65y +				
Education (ref=School)				
Diploma	1.24 (0.70, 2.21)	1.25 (0.71, 2.20)	1.24 (0.70, 2.20)	1.24 (0.71, 2.20)
University	0.98 (0.59, 1.66)	0.99 (0.59, 1.66)	0.98 (0.59, 1.66)	0.98 (0.59, 1.65)
Missing	0.97 (0.11, 6.06)	0.98 (0.12, 6.14)	0.98 (0.11, 6.13)	0.98 (0.11, 6.07)
Income (AUD, ref=0-29K)				
30-69K	0.71 (0.26, 2.09)	0.72 (0.26, 2.05)	0.73 (0.26, 2.05)	0.70 (0.25, 2.00)
70-100K	0.47 (0.16, 1.39)	0.47 (0.16, 1.38)	0.47 (0.16, 1.37)	0.46 (0.16, 1.35)
100K +	0.62 (0.23, 1.74)	0.62 (0.23, 1.72)	0.63 (0.23, 1.72)	0.61 (0.23, 1.69)
Missing	0.95 (0.25, 3.53)	0.95 (0.26, 3.48)	0.96 (0.26, 3.48)	0.93 (0.25, 3.41)
Couple status (ref=in a couple)				
Not in a couple	1.24 (0.79, 1.91)	1.24 (0.80, 1.91)	1.24 (0.80, 1.93)	1.24 (0.80, 1.91)
Country of birth (ref=Australia)				
Other English-speaking country	1.01 (0.56, 1.76)	1.00 (0.56, 1.75)	1.01 (0.56, 1.78)	1.01 (0.56, 1.76)
Other non-English-speaking country	1.19 (0.72, 1.93)	1.19 (0.72, 1.94)	1.19 (0.72, 1.95)	1.19 (0.72, 1.93)
Overall job quality	0.95 (0.91, 0.98) x	0.95 (0.91, 0.98) x	0.95 (0.91, 0.98) x	0.94 (0.91, 0.98) x

(Continued)

Table A6.3 (Continued)

Model	Outcome: Onset of burnout			
	1	2	3	4
	Odds Ratio (95% Credible Interval)			
Area-level disadvantage (quintiles, ref=1)				
2	1.49 (0.86, 2.60)	1.48 (0.85, 2.58)	1.49 (0.86, 2.59)	1.50 (0.86, 2.63)
3	1.39 (0.78, 2.50)	1.38 (0.77, 2.48)	1.40 (0.78, 2.49)	1.40 (0.78, 2.50)
4	2.13 (1.18, 3.87) +	2.10 (1.16, 3.80) +	2.13 (1.18, 3.83) +	2.15 (1.19, 3.90) +
5 (most disadvantaged)	1.13 (0.59, 2.14)	1.12 (0.59, 2.11)	1.13 (0.59, 2.14)	1.14 (0.60, 2.15)
RANDOM PART	Variance (95% Credible interval)			
Geography	0.031 (0.001, 0.186)	0.033 (0.001, 0.198)	0.035 (0.001, 0.217)	0.032 (0.001, 0.197)
N Geographical areas	14	14	14	14
N Individuals	689	689	689	689

Note: * P≤0.001, x P≤0.01, + P≤0.05 | MCMC procedure using MLwiN with 30000-300000 burn-in and sample iterations. | Random intercept was associated with capital areas and the rest of states and territories in Australia. | Green space variables show a coefficient related to 10% change. | Overall job quality coefficient is related to a change per 1 unit.

Table A6.4 Descriptive statistics for burnout relief – demographics and socioeconomics

Variable	Items	Relief from burnout	
		Total (burnout at baseline)	*% Relief from burnout*
Full sample		569	27.1
Gender	Male	266	31.4
	Female	303	23.0
Age group	18-24y	74	22.3
	25-34y	144	24.5
	35-44y	168	29.2
	45-54y	111	26.8
	55-64y	62	31.6
	65y +	9	30.0
Geography	Greater Sydney	120	27.6
	Rest of NSW	64	22.5
	Greater Melbourne	131	31.1
	Rest of Vic.	47	25.4
	Greater Brisbane	52	13.5
	Rest of Qld	46	19.9
	Greater Adelaide	30	40.4
	Greater Perth	52	35.5
	Other	27	22.2
Education	School	126	25.0
	Diploma	243	22.5
	University	194	34.1
	Missing	7	14.0
Income (AUD)	0-29K	27	22.4
	30-69K	135	17.7
	70-100K	122	26.5
	100K +	260	31.8
	Missing	25	32.6
Couple status	In a couple	432	27.5
	Not in a couple	137	24.9
Country of birth	Australia	395	25.9
	Other English-speaking country	60	30.2
	Other non-English-speaking country	113	28.8
Overall job quality (quintiles)	1 (score 12 to 33, lower quality)	165	21.3
	2 (score 34 to 36)	132	30.3
	3 (score 37 to 39)	111	27.1
	4 (score 40 to 42)	92	24.7
	5 (score 43 to 60, higher quality)	69	36.4
Area-level disadvantage (quintiles)	1 (low disadvantage)	136	30.5
	2	115	33.3
	3	119	19.1
	4	110	23.7
	5 (high disadvantage)	90	27.6

Table A6.5 Descriptive statistics for burnout relief and nature contact variables

Variable	Items	Relief from burnout	
		Total (burnout at baseline)	*% Relief from burnout*
Full sample		569	27.1
Total green space < 400m (quintiles)	1 (0 to 12.3%)	129	23.5
	2 (12.3 to 22.6%)	139	26.3
	3 (22.6 to 33.4%)	105	29.0
	4 (33.4 to 52%)	117	30.2
	5 (52 to 100%)	79	25.7
Total green space < 800m (quintiles)	1 (0 to 14.7%)	124	27.1
	2 (14.7 to 26.8%)	137	26.9
	3 (26.8 to 38.6%)	113	29.1
	4 (38.6 to 58%)	112	24.1
	5 (58 to 100%)	83	27.5
Total green space < 1600m (quintiles)	1 (0 to 17.7%)	119	25.8
	2 (17.8 to 30.8%)	132	29.5
	3 (30.8 to 42.2%)	109	26.0
	4 (42.3 to 61.1%)	123	28.5
	5 (61.1 to 100%)	86	23.4
Tree canopy < 400m (quintiles)	1 (0 to 0%)	156	29.2
	2 (0 to 4.8%)	92	24.2
	3 (4.8 to 11.8%)	123	25.7
	4 (11.8 to 23.2%)	101	21.8
	5 (23.2 to 100%)	97	32.7
Tree canopy < 800m (quintiles)	1 (0 to 1.0%)	149	29.0
	2 (1.0 to 7.1%)	103	24.7
	3 (7.1 to 13.9%)	114	28.6
	4 (13.9 to 25.7%)	107	20.0
	5 (25.8 to 100%)	97	31.5
Tree canopy < 1600m (quintiles)	1 (0 to 2.5%)	143	23.1
	2 (2.5 to 8.8%)	109	36.3
	3 (8.8 to 15.9%)	114	26.1
	4 (15.9 to 28.3%)	107	20.4
	5 (28.4 to 100%)	96	30.2
Grass and shrub < 400m (quintiles)	1 (0 to 5.5%)	108	25.3
	2 (5.5 to 10.9%)	134	30.3
	3 (10.9 to 18%)	125	21.6
	4 (18 to 29.2%)	109	34.6
	5 (29.3 to 100%)	93	22.1
Grass and shrub < 800m (quintiles)	1 (0 to 6.8%)	107	29.2
	2 (6.8 to 12.4%)	134	21.4
	3 (12.5 to 19.9%)	123	31.4
	4 (19.9 to 33.3%)	110	31.6
	5 (33.4 to 100%)	96	20.9
Grass and shrub < 1600m (quintiles)	1 (0 to 8.6%)	101	25.0
	2 (8.6 to 13.9%)	127	22.5
	3 (13.9 to 21.5%)	128	32.4
	4 (21.5 to 35.3%)	110	32.9
	5 (35.3 to 100%)	103	21.0

Table A6.5 (Continued)

Variable	Items	Total (burnout at baseline)	% Relief from burnout
		Relief from burnout	
Parks < 400m (quintiles)	1 (0 to 0%)	110	28.1
	2 (0 to 4.9%)	113	37.1
	3 (4.9 to 10.6%)	125	23.9
	4 (10.6 to 19.3%)	116	15.4
	5 (19.3 to 100%)	105	31.0
Parks < 800m (quintiles)	1 (0 to 3.1%)	114	26.7
	2 (3.1 to 7.3%)	121	30.0
	3 (7.3 to 13.3%)	117	30.1
	4 (13.3 to 22.4%)	119	21.5
	5 (22.4 to 100%)	98	26.2
Parks < 1600m (quintiles)	1 (0 to 6.0%)	108	20.3
	2 (6.0 to 10.8%)	107	33.6
	3 (10.8 to 15.9%)	122	26.4
	4 (15.9 to 24.6%)	120	30.9
	5 (24.6 to 100%)	111	23.2
Time spent in green/blue spent per week (hours)	None	124	21.7
	1-2	170	35.0
	3-4	128	25.4
	5-9	95	22.3
	10 or more	51	24.9
Time to reach preferred green/blue space (minutes)	0-4	173	24.8
	5-9	177	37.6
	10-14	103	23.7
	15-19	51	14.1
	20 or above	65	18.5

Table A6.6 Availability of nature space within 400m and relief from burnout

Model	Outcome: Relief from burnout			
	1	2	3	4
	Odds Ratio (95% Credible Interval)			
Total green space < 400m	1.03 (0.95, 1.13)			
Tree canopy < 400m		1.12 (0.99, 1.28)		
Grass and shrub < 400m			0.96 (0.84, 1.08)	
Parks < 400m				1.00 (0.83, 1.20)
Gender (ref=Male)				
Female	0.69 (0.46, 1.04)	0.68 (0.45, 1.03)	0.70 (0.46, 1.06)	0.70 (0.46, 1.05)
Age group (ref=18-24y)				
25-34y	1.06 (0.38, 3.21)	1.06 (0.38, 3.11)	1.09 (0.39, 3.27)	1.07 (0.39, 3.13)
35-44y	1.30 (0.48, 3.87)	1.32 (0.49, 3.82)	1.37 (0.50, 4.01)	1.32 (0.49, 3.75)
45-54y	1.63 (0.59, 4.88)	1.60 (0.59, 4.72)	1.71 (0.61, 5.01)	1.65 (0.61, 4.74)
55-64y	1.33 (0.47, 4.03)	1.34 (0.48, 4.02)	1.45 (0.51, 4.37)	1.38 (0.50, 4.01)
65y +	1.51 (0.35, 6.51)	1.44 (0.33, 6.22)	1.65 (0.38, 7.01)	1.58 (0.38, 6.51)
Education (ref=School)				
Diploma	0.95 (0.50, 1.81)	0.93 (0.49, 1.78)	0.94 (0.50, 1.79)	0.94 (0.50, 1.78)
University	1.17 (0.64, 2.18)	1.15 (0.63, 2.15)	1.15 (0.63, 2.14)	1.15 (0.63, 2.13)
Missing	0.16 (0.01, 1.71)	0.16 (0.01, 1.73)	0.16 (0.01, 1.70)	0.16 (0.01, 1.71)
Income (AUD, ref=0-29K)				
30-69K	0.50 (0.19, 1.38)	0.51 (0.19, 1.40)	0.53 (0.20, 1.46)	0.51 (0.19, 1.39)
70-100K	0.65 (0.24, 1.79)	0.67 (0.25, 1.86)	0.68 (0.25, 1.90)	0.66 (0.25, 1.78)
100K +	0.83 (0.32, 2.22)	0.86 (0.33, 2.31)	0.87 (0.34, 2.37)	0.84 (0.33, 2.22)
Missing	1.17 (0.32, 4.19)	1.12 (0.29, 4.15)	1.19 (0.32, 4.39)	1.17 (0.32, 4.26)

Couple status (ref=in a couple)				
Not in a couple	1.07 (0.67, 1.71)	1.11 (0.68, 1.78)	1.04 (0.65, 1.66)	1.05 (0.66, 1.67)
Country of birth (ref=Australia)				
Other English-speaking country	0.96 (0.47, 1.88)	0.93 (0.46, 1.84)	0.92 (0.45, 1.81)	0.94 (0.47, 1.85)
Other non-English-speaking country	1.27 (0.72, 2.22)	1.29 (0.73, 2.27)	1.22 (0.70, 2.13)	1.24 (0.70, 2.18)
Overall job quality	1.07 (1.03, 1.11) x	1.07 (1.03, 1.11) x	1.07 (1.03, 1.11) *	1.07 (1.03, 1.11) *
Area-level disadvantage (quintiles, ref=1)				
2	1.13 (0.64, 2.02)	1.18 (0.66, 2.11)	1.14 (0.64, 2.03)	1.12 (0.63, 2.01)
3	0.72 (0.37, 1.38)	0.77 (0.40, 1.47)	0.71 (0.37, 1.34)	0.71 (0.37, 1.33)
4	0.80 (0.41, 1.52)	0.85 (0.44, 1.64)	0.81 (0.42, 1.54)	0.79 (0.41, 1.52)
5 (most disadvantaged)	1.69 (0.88, 3.24)	1.81 (0.93, 3.51)	1.66 (0.87, 3.18)	1.64 (0.86, 3.13)
RANDOM PART	Variance (95% Credible interval)			
Geography	0.067 (0.001, 0.390)	0.105 (0.001, 0.575)	0.064 (0.001, 0.388)	0.066 (0.001, 0.392)
N Geographical areas	14	14	14	14
N Individuals	569	569	569	569

Note: * P≤0.001, x P≤0.01, + P≤0.05 | MCMC procedure using MLwiN with 30000-300000 burn-in and sample iterations. | Random intercept was associated with capital areas and the rest of states and territories in Australia. | Green space variables show a coefficient related to 10% change. | Overall job quality coefficient is related to a change per 1 unit.

Table A6.7 Availability of nature space within 800m and 1600m and onset of burnout

% green space measured within	Onset of burnout	
	<800m	<1600m
	Odds Ratio (95% Credible Interval)	
Total green space	0.99 (0.91, 1.07)	0.97 (0.90, 1.05)
Tree canopy	1.00 (0.89, 1.11)	0.98 (0.88, 1.09)
Grass and shrub	0.98 (0.88, 1.08)	0.97 (0.87, 1.08)
Parks	1.12 (0.97, 1.29)	1.00 (0.87, 1.15)

Note: * P≤0.001, x P≤0.01, + P≤0.05 | MCMC procedure using MLwiN with 30000-300000 burn-in and sample iterations. | Random intercept was associated with capital areas and the rest of states and territories in Australia. | Green space variables show a coefficient related to 10% change. | Models are fitted with all covariates, including job quality index.

Table A6.8 Availability of nature space within 800m and 1600m and relief from burnout

% green space measured within	Relief from burnout	
	<800m	<1600m
	Odds Ratio (95% Credible Interval)	
Total green space	1.05 (0.96, 1.15)	1.04 (0.95, 1.15)
Tree canopy	1.12 (0.99, 1.27)	1.06 (0.94, 1.20)
Grass and shrub	0.98 (0.87, 1.10)	1.01 (0.89, 1.13)
Parks	1.10 (0.94, 1.29)	1.09 (0.93, 1.28)

Note: * P≤0.001, x P≤0.01, + P≤0.05 | MCMC procedure using MLwiN with 30000-300000 burn-in and sample iterations. | Random intercept was associated with capital areas and the rest of states and territories in Australia. | Green space variables show a coefficient related to 10% change. | Models are fitted with all covariates, including job quality index.

Table A6.9 Time in nature space for both outcomes

	Onset of burnout	Relief from burnout
	Odds Ratio (95% Credible Interval)	
Time spent in nature per week (hours)		
Ref=None		
1-2 hrs	0.65 (0.36, 1.18)	1.73 (0.95, 3.22)
3-4 hrs	0.63 (0.33, 1.20)	1.67 (0.85, 3.28)
5-9 hrs	1.05 (0.56, 1.99)	1.28 (0.63, 2.61)
10 hrs or more	0.68 (0.34, 1.38)	1.34 (0.60, 2.93)

Note: * P≤0.001, x P≤0.01, + P≤0.05 | MCMC procedure using MLwiN with 30000-300000 burn-in and sample iterations. | Random intercept was associated with capital areas and the rest of states and territories in Australia. | Green space variables show a coefficient related to 10% change. | Models are fitted with all covariates, including job quality index.

Table A6.10 Distance to nature space for both outcomes

	Onset of burnout	Relief from burnout
	Odds Ratio (95% Credible Interval)	
Time to nature (minutes)		
Ref=0-4 mins		
5-9 mins	1.42 (0.89, 2.26)	1.46 (0.88, 2.44)
10-14 mins	0.58 (0.31, 1.08)	1.15 (0.65, 2.04)
15-19 mins	1.39 (0.66, 2.85)	0.84 (0.38, 1.80)
20 mins or more	2.13 (1.13, 3.99) +	0.94 (0.42, 2.04)

Note: * P≤0.001, x P≤0.01, + P≤0.05 | MCMC procedure using MLwiN with 30000-300000 burn-in and sample iterations. | Random intercept was associated with capital areas and the rest of states and territories in Australia. | Green space variables show a coefficient related to 10% change. | Models are fitted with all covariates, including job quality index.

7 Biodiversity for health and wellbeing

Jessica C. Fisher, Gail E. Austen, Katherine N. Irvine, Martin Dallimer, and Zoe G. Davies

Green and blue space characteristics

It is now widely accepted across research, policy and practice that nature, in both 'green' (e.g. parks, gardens, forests) and 'blue' spaces (e.g. canals, rivers, coastlines), can benefit human health and wellbeing. For instance, higher remote-sensed satellite measurements of 'greenness' (e.g. Normalised Difference Vegetation Index [NDVI]) in residential areas are associated with lower anti-depressant prescription rates (Gascon et al., 2015), lower odds of depression (Tomita et al., 2017), and lower healthcare costs (Van Den Eeden et al., 2022). Likewise, people living closer to the coast report better general health (Hooyberg et al., 2020), and those with more blue space visibility report less psychological distress (Nutsford et al., 2016).

Despite these promising findings, such approaches tend to assume that green/blue spaces are homogeneous entities, rarely examining what features within the spaces are actually responsible for underpinning human health and wellbeing (Eigenbrod et al., 2010; Irvine et al., 2023). For instance, the presence of vegetation, butterflies and water can offer multisensory engagement opportunities which elicit wellbeing (Gobster et al., 2023), and seasonal changes in trees and flowering plants can stimulate joy (Paraskevopoulou et al., 2018).

The value different people place on particular green/blue space features also varies between individuals. In Sweden, the sound of birdsong and rustling leaves in urban greenery led to greater feelings of calmness for women and the elderly, than for men and younger participants (Hedblom et al., 2017). Similarly, in the UK, individuals who had sight, smell, and hearing impairments indicated lower scores on a scale measuring the physical, cognitive, emotional, social, and spiritual wellbeing benefits associated with biodiversity in a woodland setting (Irvine et al., 2023). People's background and social experiences can also influence their perceptions of safety when confronted with different structures and densities of vegetation in urban green spaces (Gargiulo et al., 2020; Jansson et al., 2013).

Indeed, how individuals perceive biodiversity is a critical factor in whether or not, and the extent to which, they derive benefits from that experience (Pett et al., 2016). Seminal work from researchers exposing the interlinkages between biodiversity and human wellbeing examined actual species richness of plants, butterflies and birds, as well as measures of perceived species richness for these taxonomic groups. They found that positive perceptions, rather than objective measurements, were related to improved wellbeing (Dallimer et al., 2012; Fuller et al., 2007). This work revealed a 'people-biodiversity

DOI: 10.4324/9781003345725-8

paradox', whereby people express a preference for greater levels of biodiversity, but have a limited ability to accurately perceive the biodiversity that exists around them (Pett et al., 2016).

In this chapter, we explore the multifaceted and complex ways in which biodiversity influences people's health and wellbeing. We begin by discussing the multiple theories and frameworks designed to map out biodiversity-human wellbeing relationships, and then examine the existing empirical evidence. Finally, we outline how the evidence may inform policy and practice, in terms of both biodiversity conservation and public health.

Biodiversity-human wellbeing theories and mechanisms

A range of theories and conceptual frameworks have been used to help define and unpack the intricacies and peculiarities of biodiversity-human wellbeing relationships. Until recently, most have considered nature rather than biodiversity *per se*.

Psychoevolutionary theory, also known as stress-reduction theory, postulates that upon entering a natural environment, an individual experiences an initial positive emotive reaction. In turn, this influences their behavioural response and cognitive appraisal, which leads to additional emotional and physiological responses (Ulrich et al., 1991). More biodiverse environments are associated with enhanced mood, arousal and reduced physiological stress indicators (Cracknell et al., 2017; Wolf et al., 2017).

Attention restoration theory stipulates that spending time in natural environments restores a person's ability to concentrate and focus attention, thereby improving their memory, information processing and problem-solving capabilities (Kaplan and Kaplan, 1989). Certain experiential qualities facilitate this process, including fascination (interesting stimuli attract attention), coherence (how stimuli are arranged), compatibility (whether individuals can carry out purposes freely) and being away (distance from tasks that demand attention). Biodiversity is associated with enhancements in each of these qualities (Marselle et al., 2016).

The biophilia hypothesis proposes that people have evolved an inherent emotional affiliation with nature (Fromm, 1964; Kellert and Wilson, 1993). Consequently, we are predisposed to exhibit certain responses to biodiversity (e.g. fear of snakes) and, for example, it is thought to be why people prefer more complex birdsong rather than that of a single species singing (Hedblom et al., 2014). The concept of biophilia, which also partially underpins elements of psychoevolutionary theory (i.e. positive emotive reactions are relics of human evolution in natural environments) (Ulrich et al., 1991), is criticised for the fact that: (i) human species have always lived in natural environments, so there would have been no selection pressure for this mechanism to evolve; and (ii) most research is on student populations in developed countries, thus limiting the applicability of such theories elsewhere (Joye and de Block, 2011; Joye and van den Berg, 2011). As an extension of biophilia, topophilia implies that people's relationships with the natural environment stem from cultural learning, though place attachment, in combination with natural selection (Beery et al., 2015; Tuan, 1974).

Ecosystem services are a construct to explain how biodiversity provides benefits and disbenefits to human wellbeing, originally grouped into four broad categories: provisioning, regulating, supporting and cultural services (Millenium Ecosystem Assessment, 2005). The cultural ecosystem service benefits provided by biodiversity are considerable, including contributing to the formation of people's identities (e.g. sense of place), enabling

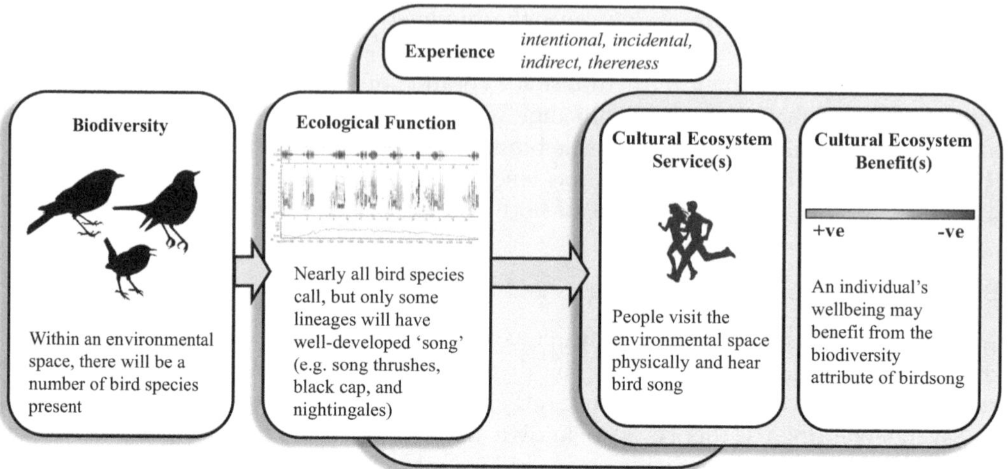

Figure 7.1 Conceptual framework for how biodiversity can underpin human wellbeing through cultural ecosystem services, using birds as an example.

experiences (e.g. feelings of escape) and equipping capabilities (e.g. knowledge) (see Fish et al., 2016). Far less is understood about the role of biodiversity for cultural ecosystem services, compared with provisioning or regulating services (Brockerhoff et al., 2017; Garrett et al., 2023). The mechanism through which biodiversity attributes could elicit human wellbeing through cultural ecosystem services is proposed in Figure 7.1.

In this example, birds produce birdsong, which has an ecological function (e.g. mating strategies; Friis et al., 2022). Additionally, birdsong can provide an ecosystem service benefit when experienced by people (Ratcliffe et al., 2013). This experience could be intentional (e.g. a person visits a park to listen to the birds), incidental (e.g. a person goes to a park for a run and happens to hear birds), indirect (e.g. a person hears birds singing on television) or 'thereness' (e.g. a person benefits from conceiving and imagining birds singing outdoors) (Kaplan, 2010; Keniger et al., 2013).

The outcomes for different individuals can vary. Nature-health theories have been used to underpin frameworks that illustrate how biodiversity affects human health and wellbeing (e.g. risk of depression, allergies, perceived overall health) through a series of mediators. The mediating processes by which biodiversity elicits wellbeing responses can be both positive and negative, including reducing harm (e.g. providing medicine), causing harm (e.g. infectious diseases), restoring capacities (e.g. reducing stress) and building capacities (e.g. transcendent experiences) (Marselle et al., 2021). Outcomes can also link to past experiences or phobias (Pett et al., 2016), and not everyone will experience the species in the same way. For instance, people's attitudes toward biodiversity are also informed by social norms, personal identities and other factors specific to the cultural context (Gatersleben et al., 2014).

A parallel field of research contests that the relationship between biodiversity and human wellbeing is mediated by people's 'nature connection', which is how separate or connected a person feels with/from nature (e.g. Richardson et al., 2016). Many psychological scales have been developed to capture affective, cognitive and experiential constructs such as 'nature-relatedness', 'connectedness to nature' and 'inclusion with nature' (Nisbet et al., 2009; Richardson et al., 2019; Schultz, 2002). While there is some suggestion that restoring or increasing human connection with nature could improve pro-environmental attitudes and behaviour, as well as enhancing health and wellbeing (Alcock et al., 2020; Liu et al., 2022), the definitions and theoretical underpinning of these constructs (i.e. what is nature; what is a connection) remain ambiguous. Asserting that people and nature are distinct reinforces a disassociation between the two (Fletcher, 2017). Indeed, in many cultural contexts there is no distinction between people and nature, and therefore the idea of (re)connecting does not apply (Fletcher, 2017).

Researchers have called for better recognition of people's relationships with, and responsibilities for, biodiversity. Rather than the dichotomous notion of instrumental values (nature for human's sake) and intrinsic values (nature for nature's sake), the concept of 'relational values' (e.g. preferences, principles, social norms) encompasses people-nature relationships from an individual and social perspective (Chan et al., 2016). This approach incorporates better representation of how nature is valued across cultures, leading to more inclusive and better informed policy and practice (Chan et al., 2016). In response to calls for greater recognition of the diverse perspectives and worldviews underpinning how people relate to biodiversity for their wellbeing, the Intergovernmental Science-Policy Platform on Biodiversity and Ecosystem Services (IPBES) was established to provide policy-relevant knowledge by harnessing expertise from different scientific disciplines and knowledge communities (IPBES, 2019).

The broad definition of ecosystem services (Millenium Ecosystem Assessment, 2003) considers links to many aspects of human wellbeing but is predominantly informed by ecology and economics (Díaz et al., 2018). Concerned with sustainable development and conservation, IPBES has reframed ecosystem services as 'nature's contributions to people', with the aim of better integrating the relationships between biodiversity, ecosystem services and human wellbeing into decision-making (Pascual et al., 2017). This reframing recognises the role of culture in people-nature relationships and highlights the importance of indigenous and local knowledge in understanding these contributions (Díaz et al., 2018).

Empirical evidence linking biodiversity to health and wellbeing

Urban green spaces (i.e. parks) are the principal focus of existing empirical evidence linking biodiversity to human health and wellbeing. However, other types of ecosystems have been examined, including mountains (Dorwart et al., 2010), woodlands (Austen et al., 2021; Austen et al., 2022) and wetlands (Maund et al., 2019). Evidence regarding 'blue spaces' (rivers, lakes, coastline) is accruing (White et al., 2020) and, although only a handful have explored the role of biodiversity *per se*, such experiences are found to improve people's wellbeing (Bell et al., 2017; Fisher et al., 2021a; White et al., 2017).

The evidence-base for biodiversity-human wellbeing relationships is growing across continents. In Hong Kong, for instance, a survey found older adults had better mental wellbeing when they had a view of blue space from their homes, and were more likely to visit urban blue space if they believed that they would encounter wildlife (Garrett et al., 2019). Nonetheless, most of the empirical research originates from middle- and high-income countries, thus limiting the interpretation of this evidence to diverse populations elsewhere. This geographical skew has been repeatedly underlined in reviews of the literature on nature exposure and health and wellbeing (Barragan-Jason et al., 2023).

Understanding this diversity is critical, if we are to identify what constitutes a health-promoting, or 'salutogenic' environment from a biodiversity perspective, and for whom.

Across green and blue spaces, the research examining biodiversity-human wellbeing relationships is predominantly quantitative, harnessing a diverse range of sampling methodologies, including population-scale cross-sectional approaches (e.g. Methorst et al., 2021b), app-based momentary experience sampling (e.g. Bakolis et al., 2018) and *in situ* questionnaires with passers-by combined with ecological surveys (e.g. Dallimer et al., 2012). Qualitative, participatory and creative research approaches are increasingly being used, providing in-depth insight into the mechanisms through which biodiversity is experienced as beneficial to people (e.g. Austen et al., 2023; Gobster et al., 2023). Better-tailored information about what works for whom could be gathered through participatory mapping exercises (e.g. Klain and Chan, 2012), or by incorporating members of the community as co-researchers (e.g. Fisher et al., 2021c).

Existing biodiversity-human wellbeing studies have generally been limited to certain taxonomic groups (e.g. flowering plants, Hoyle et al., 2018; birds, White et al., 2023), and focused predominantly on species richness and abundance as metrics of biodiversity (e.g. Cox et al., 2017; Methorst et al., 2021a). For example, higher bird species richness has been positively associated with mental health in Germany (Methorst et al., 2021a), higher life satisfaction across 26 countries in Europe (Methorst et al., 2021b), and greater psychological wellbeing in England (Southon et al., 2017). A study in Costa Rica identified 20 traits from 199 bird species that elicited cultural ecosystem service benefits (e.g. aesthetic traits were important for birdwatching) and disbenefits (e.g. carnivorous raptors preying on farm animals), although they did not investigate wellbeing as an outcome (Echeverri et al., 2020).

Trees make a considerable contribution to people's health. Higher tree density in Leipzig, Germany, has been associated with lower anti-depressant prescription rates (Marselle et al., 2020). In the UK, trees and forests provide approximately £202 million per annum in mental health benefits to people, based on the avoided costs of living with and treating mental health difficulties, as well as costs to employers for sick-days (Forest Research, 2021). In urban green spaces of Kathmandu, Nepal, Nawrath et al. (2022) found that specific tree species, such as the socially and spiritually significant sacred fig (*Ficus religiosa*), contributed to relieving the burden of mental ill-health burden for low-income residents.

Specific species, and their sounds, smells and morphology, are beginning to be explored in relation to human wellbeing. For instance, Zhang et al. (2023) documented specific psychological effects from blue-coloured flowers, which elicited relaxation and stress reduction. By contrast, flowers that were orange, yellow or red stimulated uplifting emotions. In urban green spaces in Guyana, natural sounds like birdsong were associated with greater enjoyment and higher perceived restorativeness when compared with anthropogenic noises such as traffic (Fisher et al., 2021b). In turn, this enhanced positive emotions. In rural USA, Ferraro et al. (2020) played birdsong through hidden speakers along a walking trail and demonstrated better psychological restoration of hikers, mediated by people's perceptions of the bird species richness around them.

Biodiversity encounters are multisensory, and personal preferences can be expressed via different senses, for example vision (e.g. colour determining psychological effects; Zhang et al., 2023), smell (e.g. woodland smells affecting biopsychosocial-spiritual wellbeing; Bentley and Fisher et al., 2022) and touch (curiosity of how plants feel; Austen et al., 2021). As well as the range of species' attributes, and the mechanisms by which people experience them, human health and wellbeing is influenced by both experiences and memories, individual and collective. Austen et al. (2021) found that despite using woodlands as a study system, people's preferences for biodiversity attributes were influenced by 'everyday' encounters, through short-term (e.g. in the garden/park, walking to work) and longer-term memories (e.g. tree climbing and playing conkers in childhood). Cultural influences (e.g. literature, games, popular media) and memories linked to particular people and places were also prominent (Austen et al. 2023). Such memories do not have to be first-person experiences, as likes and dislikes can be influenced by narratives from other people (e.g. 'Grandad's favourite bird'; Austen et al., 2021), popular media (e.g. bats and zoonoses; Cerri et al., 2022) and representation in literature (e.g. children's stories; Burke and Copenhaver, 2004). In this respect, mistaken ideas or misidentification of species can lead to negative associations (Austen et al., 2021; Soga et al., 2023). This mechanism of cultural influence on negative perceptions of biodiversity was illustrated by Fisher et al. (2021a) in Georgetown, Guyana, where folklore about the West Indian manatee (*Trichechus manatus*) and species of marine fish, as well as mistaken ideas about the presence of venomous snakes, evoked fear and discomfort amongst participants.

Securing biodiversity and human wellbeing

Implications for biodiversity conservation

Biodiversity conservation is reliant on intact habitats (Chase et al., 2020), yet anthropogenic pressures are reducing the extent and quality of habitats, driving biodiversity loss and constraining ecosystem functioning (Williams et al., 2020). Ecological degradation and climate change are both ubiquitous, rapidly accelerating and threatening human quality of life, with the impacts recognised as emergencies by scientists and policymakers alike (Ripple et al., 2021; Roe, 2019). Such challenges are interdependent, and global strategies to mitigate their impacts should be treated as such (Dinerstein et al., 2020). Consequently, a series of international initiatives have been devised and implemented. The United Nations (UN) have established the Decade on Ecosystem Restoration, aiming to stop, reverse and prevent ecosystem degradation to halt biodiversity declines, combat climate change and relieve poverty (United Nations, 2021). Likewise, the Global Biodiversity Framework is an intergovernmental agreement which aims to conserve 30% of land and sea areas across the world by 2030 (CBD, 2022).

Demonstrating where spaces containing biodiversity have benefits for human health and wellbeing could be a powerful tool to justify conservation to decision-makers. At one end of the spectrum, spaces managed primarily for biodiversity, could be highlighted as a public health resource (Davies et al., 2019). In Europe, ancient woodlands support high levels of biodiversity and species unique to old-growth forest (Dean et al., 2020; Woodland Trust, 2009). Simultaneously, ancient woodlands are linked to improved wellbeing for visitors, through multisensory experiences of biodiversity attributes like 'earthy' smells (Bentley and Fisher et al., 2022). Protected areas, many of which were designated historically for human recreation, are now an integral component of global conservation policies (Hanson et al., 2020). They also, however, improve mental health of visitors, at an estimated value of $6 trillion per annum in quality-adjusted life years (Buckley et al.,

2019). For instance, visitors to a protected area in Australia, acquired both physical and social wellbeing benefits (Wolf and Wohlfart, 2014). At the other end of the spectrum, are spaces managed primarily for people, but which could also provide important habitat for biodiversity. Urban allotments, for example, provide resources for pollinating insects (Baldock, 2020) and are associated with improved physical, psychological, and social wellbeing benefits (Genter et al., 2015).

Conservation gains could also be made through people, whereby positive experiences with biodiversity could stimulate concern and willingness to protect it. When retrofitting or designing new green and blue spaces, it is important to capture the heterogeneity in people's biodiversity preferences to ensure that initiatives are inclusive and socially just in the benefits they deliver (Cole et al., 2017; Erbaugh et al., 2020). Indeed, any conservation strategies that are implemented in landscapes where people live and work must engender public support and stewardship to ensure their long-term success (e.g. Austen et al., 2023; Coleman et al., 2021). Green/blue spaces can also be designed as heterogeneous in themselves, adopting zoning approaches to meet a greater variety of needs for people, as well as biodiversity.

Implications for public health

Mounting pressure on public health care systems has fuelled the growth of non-medical, low-cost social prescribing, now implemented in countries across the world (Morse et al., 2022). Activities that involve interactions with biodiversity, termed 'green' or 'nature-based' social prescribing, may benefit human health and wellbeing through two main avenues: (i) as a treatment to help recover from ill-health (e.g. provision of hospital gardens); and (ii) as a preventative measure (e.g. enhancing residential neighbourhood planting regimes) (Shanahan et al., 2019). Significant cost-savings are likely when scaled across entire populations. For instance, the UK Department of Health has estimated that exposure to biodiversity could save the National Health Service £2.1 billion per annum (Department for Environment Food and Rural Affairs, 2011). Promoting nature-based social prescribing initiatives has knock-on benefits to biodiversity through creating new, and enhancing existing, natural habitats.

At present, nature-based public health interventions do not currently consider biodiversity in all its complexity. For instance, trees significantly reduce urban heat islands (Iungman et al., 2023), benefit mental health (Marselle et al., 2020) and provide opportunities for nutritional supplements and poverty alleviation (Hunte et al., 2019). Yet, they are also a significant source of pollen-related allergies and asthma, and contradictory information about tree pollen allergenicity is offered by different land-use planning guidance (Sousa-Silva et al., 2021) with potentially significant implications for tree-planting and public health (Sousa-Silva et al., 2020).

The benefits of biodiversity for human health and wellbeing are not universal. Research has demonstrated, for instance, that the health gains associated with exposure to biodiversity are greater amongst socio-economically deprived communities (Clitherow et al., 2019; Mitchell and Popham, 2008). Such deprivation is often connected to a higher prevalence of non-communicable disease and less access to natural spaces (Mitchell and Popham, 2008). For women, biodiversity that is not maintained or offers dark hiding spaces could be perceived as dangerous, thus prohibiting health benefits (Gargiulo et al., 2020). Importantly, as people move throughout their life course, their circumstances and priorities will shift (Bell et al., 2019), as will their relational values with biodiversity.

For example, someone navigating the onset of visual impairment might initially be overwhelmed by feelings of uncertainty about how to interact with biodiversity in ways that do not rely primarily on sight, despite being able to recall positive experiences (Bell and Foley, 2021).

Conclusion

While nature's benefits to human health and wellbeing are well known, the role of biodiversity specifically is far more complex than often assumed. People's relationships with biodiversity are highly variable, related to past experiences, memories, beliefs and other factors. Although the existing evidence is geographically skewed, a multitude of theories and frameworks are proliferating from both within and between academic disciplines to conceptualise how humans can derive health and wellbeing benefits through biodiversity exposure. Rigorous systematic assessments of sustainable land-use planning initiatives and nature-based public health interventions are required, with careful consideration of the biodiversity, to supply synergistic benefits for both people and nature.

Acknowledgements

This work was funded by the European Research Council (ERC) through the Horizon 2020 Research and Innovation Programme (Consolidator Grant no. 726104). K.N.I. was also supported by Scottish Government Rural and Environment Science and Analytical Services Division, Strategic Research Programmes 2022–2027 (JHI-C6-1: Reciprocal Care for Nature and Wellbeing; JHI-D4-1: People and Nature).

References

Alcock, I., White, M.P., Pahl, S., Duarte-Davidson, R., Fleming, L.E. (2020). Associations between pro-environmental behaviour and neighbourhood nature, nature visit frequency and nature appreciation: Evidence from a nationally representative survey in England. *Environment International* 136, 105441. https://doi.org/10.1016/j.envint.2019.105441

Austen, G.E., Dallimer, M., Irvine, K.N., Fisher, J.C., Fish, R.D., Davies, Z.G. (2022. The diversity of people's relationships with biodiversity should inform forest restoration and creation. *Conservation Letters* 16(1), e12930. https://doi.org/10.1111/conl.12930

Austen, G.E., Dallimer, M., Irvine, K.N., Maund, P.R., Fish, R.D., Davies, Z.G. (2021). Exploring shared public perspectives on biodiversity attributes. *People and Nature* 3, pp. 901–913. https://doi.org/10.1002/pan3.10237

Bakolis, I., Hammoud, R., Smythe, M., Gibbons, J., Davidson, N., Tognin, S., Mechelli, A. (2018). Urban mind: Using smartphone technologies to investigate the impact of nature on mental wellbeing in real time. *BioScience* 68, pp. 134–145. https://doi.org/10.1093/biosci/bix149

Baldock, K.C. (2020). Opportunities and threats for pollinator conservation in global towns and cities. *Current Opinion in Insect Science* 38, pp. 63–71. https://doi.org/10.1016/j.cois.2020.01.006

Barragan-Jason, G., Loreau, M., de Mazancourt, C., Singer, M.C., Parmesan, C. (2023). Psychological and physical connections with nature improve both human well-being and nature conservation: A systematic review of meta-analyses. *Biological Conservation* 277, 109842. https://doi.org/10.1016/j.biocon.2022.109842

Beery, T.H., Jönsson, K.I., Elmberg, J. (2015). From environmental connectedness to sustainable futures: Topophilia and human affiliation with nature. *Sustainability* 7, pp. 8837–8854. https://doi.org/10.3390/su7078837

88 *Jessica C. Fisher et al.*

Bell, S.L., Foley, R. (2021). A(nother) time for nature? Situating non-human nature experiences within the emotional transitions of sight loss. *Social Science and Medicine* 276, 113867. https://doi.org/10.1016/j.socscimed.2021.113867

Bell, S.L., Leyshon, C., Foley, R., Kearns, R.A. (2019). The "healthy dose" of nature: A cautionary tale. *Geography Compass* 13, pp. 1–14. https://doi.org/10.1111/gec3.12415

Bell, S.L., Weston, M.A., Lovell, R., Wheeler, B.W. (2017). Everyday green space and experienced well-being: The significance of wildlife encounters. *Landscape Research* 43, pp. 8–19. https://doi.org/10.1080/01426397.2016.1267721

Bentley, P.R., Fisher, J.C., Dallimer, M., Fish, R.D., Austen, G.E., Irvine, K.N., Davies, Z.G. (2022). Nature, smells, and human wellbeing. *Ambio* 52(1), pp. 1–14. https://doi.org/10.1007/s13280-022-01760-w

Brockerhoff, E.G., Barbaro, L., Castagneyrol, B., Forrester, D.I., Gardiner, B., González-Olabarria, J.R., Lyver, P.O., Meurisse, N., Oxbrough, A., Taki, H., Thompson, I.D., van der Plas, F., Jactel, H. (2017V. Forest biodiversity, ecosystem functioning and the provision of ecosystem services. *Biodiversity Conservation* 26, pp. 3005–3035. https://doi.org/10.1007/s10531-017-1453-2

Buckley, R., Brough, P., Hague, L., Chauvenet, A., Fleming, C., Roche, E., Sofija, E., Harris, N. (2019). Economic value of protected areas via visitor mental health. *Nature Communications* 10, 5005. https://doi.org/10.1038/s41467-019-12631-6

Burke, C.L., Copenhaver, J.G. (2004). Animals as people in children's literature. *Language Arts* 81(3), pp. 205–213.

CBD. (2022). *Kunming-Montreal Global biodiversity framework* (Draft decision submitted by the President No. CBD/COP/15/L.25). UN Environment Programme, Montréal, Canada. https://doi.org/10.5281/ZENODO.3831673

Cerri, J., Mori, E., Ancillotto, L., Russo, D., Bertolino, S. (2022). COVID-19, media coverage of bats and related Web searches: A turning point for bat conservation? *Mammal Review* 52, pp. 16–25. https://doi.org/10.1111/mam.12261

Chan, K.M.A., Balvanera, P., Benessaiah, K., Chapman, M., Díaz, S., Gómez-Baggethun, E., Gould, R., Hannahs, N., Jax, K., Klain, S., Luck, G.W., Martín-López, B., Muraca, B., Norton, B., Ott, K., Pascual, U., Satterfield, T., Tadaki, M., Taggart, J., Turner, N. (2016). Why protect nature? Rethinking values and the environment. *Proceedings of the National Academy of Sciences of the United States of America* 113, pp. 1462–1465. https://doi.org/10.1073/pnas.1525002113

Chase, J. M., Blowes, S. A., Knight, T. M., Gerstner, K., & May, F. (2020). Ecosystem decay exacerbates biodiversity loss with habitat loss. Nature, 584(7820), pp. 238–243.

Clitherow, T., Garrett, J.K., White, M.P., Wheeler, B.W., Fleming, L.E. (2019). Coastal proximity and mental health among urban populations in England: The moderating effect of household income. *Health and Place*, 59, 102200. https://doi.org/10.1016/j.healthplace.2019.102200

Cole, H.V.S., Garcia Lamarca, M., Connolly, J.J.T., Anguelovski, I. (2017). Are green cities healthy and equitable? Unpacking the relationship between health, green space and gentrification. *Journal of Epidemiology Community Health* 71(11), pp. 1118–1121. https://doi.org/10.1136/jech-2017-209201

Coleman, E.A., Schultz, B., Ramprasad, V., Fischer, H., Rana, P., Filippi, A.M., Güneralp, B., Ma, A., Rodriguez Solorzano, C., Guleria, V., Rana, R., Fleischman, F. (2021). Limited effects of tree planting on forest canopy cover and rural livelihoods in Northern India. *Nature Sustainability* 4, pp. 997–1004. https://doi.org/10.1038/s41893-021-00761-z

Cox, D.T.C., Shanahan, D.F., Hudson, H.L., Plummer, K.E., Siriwardena, G.M., Fuller, R.A., Anderson, K., Hancock, S., Gaston, K.J. (2017). Doses of neighborhood nature: The benefits for mental health of living with nature. *BioScience* 67, pp. 147–155. https://doi.org/10.1093/biosci/biw173

Cracknell, D., White, M.P., Pahl, S., Depledge, M.H. (2017). A preliminary investigation into the restorative potential of public aquaria exhibits: A UK student-based study. *Landscape Research* 42, pp. 18–32. https://doi.org/10.1080/01426397.2016.1243236

Dallimer, M., Irvine, K.N., Skinner, A.M.J., Davies, Z.G., Rouquette, J.R., Maltby, L.M., Warren, P.H., Armsworth, P.R., Gaston, K.J. (2012). Biodiversity and the feel-good factor: Understanding associations between self-reported human well-being and species richness. *BioScience* 62, pp. 47–55. https://doi.org/10.1525/bio.2012.62.1.9

Davies, Z.G., Dallimer, M., Fisher, J.C., Fuller, R.A. (2019). Biodiversity and Health: Implications for Conservation, in: Marselle, M., Stadler, J., Korn, H., Irvine, K.N., Bonn, A. (eds.), *Biodiversity and Health in the Face of Climate Change*. Springer, Cham, Switzerland, pp. 283–294.

Dean, C., Kirkpatrick, J.B., Doyle, R.B., Osborn, J., Fitzgerald, N.B., Roxburgh, S.H. (2020). The overlooked soil carbon under large, old trees. *Geoderma* 376, 114541. https://doi.org/10.1016/j.geoderma.2020.114541

Department for Environment Food and Rural Affairs. (2011). *The Natural Choice: Securing the value of nature*. DEFRA, UK Government.

Díaz, S., Pascual, U., Stenseke, M., Martín-López, B., Watson, R.T., Molnár, Z., Hill, R., Chan, K.M.A., Baste, I.A., Brauman, K.A., Polasky, S., Church, A., Lonsdale, M., Larigauderie, A., Leadley, P.W., van Oudenhoven, A.P.E., van der Plaat, F., Schröter, M., Lavorel, S., Aumeeruddy-Thomas, Y., Bukvareva, E., Davies, K., Demissew, S., Erpul, G., Failler, P., Guerra, C.A., Hewitt, C.L., Keune, H., Lindley, S., Shirayama, Y. (2018). Assessing nature's contributions to people. *Science* 359, pp. 270–272. https://doi.org/10.1126/science.aap8826

Dinerstein, E., Joshi, A.R., Vynne, C., Lee, A.T.L., Pharand-Deschênes, F., França, M., Fernando, S., Birch, T., Burkart, K., Asner, G.P., Olson, D. (2020). A "Global safety net" to reverse biodiversity loss and stabilize Earth's climate. *Science Advances* 6, eabb2824. https://doi.org/10.1126/sciadv.abb2824

Dorwart, C.E., Moore, R.L., Leung, Y.F. (2010). Visitors' perceptions of a trail environment and effects on experiences: A model for nature-based recreation experiences. *Leisure Sciences* 32, pp. 33–54. https://doi.org/10.1080/01490400903430863

Echeverri, A., Karp, D.S., Naidoo, R., Tobias, J.A., Zhao, J., Chan, K.M.A. (2020). Can avian functional traits predict cultural ecosystem services? *People and Nature* 2, pp. 138–151. https://doi.org/10.1002/pan3.10058

Eigenbrod, F., Armsworth, P.R., Anderson, B.J., Heinemeyer, A., Gillings, S., Roy, D.B., Thomas, C.D., Gaston, K.J. (2010). The impact of proxy-based methods on mapping the distribution of ecosystem services. *Journal of Applied Ecology* 47, pp. 377–385. https://doi.org/10.1111/j.1365-2664.2010.01777.x

Erbaugh, J.T., Pradhan, N., Adams, J., Oldekop, J.A., Agrawal, A., Brockington, D., Pritchard, R., Chhatre, A. (2020). Global forest restoration and the importance of prioritizing local communities. *Nature Ecology and Evolution* 4, pp. 1472–1476. https://doi.org/10.1038/s41559-020-01282-2

Ferraro, D.M., Miller, Z.D., Ferguson, L.A., Taff, B.D., Barber, J.R., Newman, P., Francis, C.D. (2020). The phantom chorus: Birdsong boosts human well-being in protected areas. *Proceedings of the Royal Society B: Biological Sciences* 287, 20201811. https://doi.org/10.1098/rspb.2020.1811

Fish, R.D., Church, A., Winter, M. (2016). Conceptualising cultural ecosystem services: A novel framework for research and critical engagement. *Ecosystem Services* 21, pp. 208–217. https://doi.org/10.1016/j.ecoser.2016.09.002

Fisher, J.C., Bicknell, J.E., Irvine, K.N., Hayes, W.M., Fernandes, D., Mistry, J., Davies, Z.G. (2021a). Bird diversity and psychological wellbeing: A comparison of green and coastal blue space in a neotropical city. *Science of the Total Environment* 793, 148653. https://doi.org/10.1016/j.scitotenv.2021.148653

Fisher, J.C., Irvine, K.N., Bicknell, J.E., Hayes, W.M., Fernandes, D., Mistry, J., Davies, Z.G. (2021b). Perceived biodiversity, sound, naturalness and safety enhance the restorative quality and wellbeing benefits of green and blue space in a neotropical city. *Science of the Total Environment* 755, 143095. https://doi.org/10.1016/j.scitotenv.2020.143095

Fisher, J.C., Mistry, J., Pierre, M.A., Yang, H., Harris, A., Hunte, N., Fernandes, D., Bicknell, J.E., Davies, Z.G. (2021c). Using participatory video to share people's experiences of neotropical urban green and blue spaces with decision-makers. *Geographical Journal* 187, pp. 346–360. https://doi.org/10.1111/geoj.12406

Fletcher, R. (2017). Connection with nature is an oxymoron: A political ecology of "nature-deficit disorder". *The Journal of Environmental Education* 48, pp. 226–233. https://doi.org/10.1080/00958964.2016.1139534

Forest Research. (2021). *Valuing the mental health benefits of woodlands, Valuing the mental health benefits of woodlands*. Forest Research, Edinburgh.

Friis, J.I., Sabino, J., Santos, P., Dabelsteen, T., Cardoso, G.C. (2022). Ecological adaptation and birdsong: How body and bill sizes affect passerine sound frequencies. *Behavioral Ecology* 33, pp. 798–806. https://doi.org/10.1093/beheco/arac042

Fromm, E. (1964). *The heart of man*. Harper and Row Publishers, London.

Fuller, R.A., Irvine, K.N., Devine-Wright, P., Warren, P.H., Gaston, K.J. (2007). Psychological benefits of greenspace increase with biodiversity. *Biology Letters* 3, pp. 390–394. https://doi.org/10.1098/rsbl.2007.0149

Gargiulo, I., Garcia, X., Benages-Albert, M., Martinez, J., Pfeffer, K., Vall-Casas, P. (2020). Women's safety perception assessment in an urban stream corridor: Developing a safety map based on qualitative GIS. *Landscape and Urban Planning* 198, 103779. https://doi.org/10.1016/j.landurbplan.2020.103779

Garrett, J.K., White, M.P., Elliott, L.R., Grellier, J., Bell, S., Bratman, G.N., Economou, T., Gascon, M., Lõhmus, M., Nieuwenhuijsen, M., Ojala, A., Roiko, A., van den Bosch, M., Ward Thompson, C., Fleming, L.E. (2023). Applying an ecosystem services framework on nature and mental health to recreational blue space visits across 18 countries. *Science Report* 13, 2209. https://doi.org/10.1038/s41598-023-28544-w

Garrett, J.K., White, M.P., Huang, J., Ng, S., Hui, Z., Leung, C., Tse, L.A., Fung, F., Elliott, L.R., Depledge, M.H., Wong, M.C.S. (2019). Urban blue space and health and wellbeing in Hong Kong: Results from a survey of older adults. *Health and Place* 55, pp. 100–110. https://doi.org/10.1016/j.healthplace.2018.11.003

Gascon, M., Triguero-Mas, M., Martínez, D., Dadvand, P., Forns, J., Plasència, A., Nieuwenhuijsen, M.J. (2015.) Mental health benefits of long-term exposure to residential green and blue spaces: A systematic review. *International Journal of Environmental Research Public Health* 12, pp. 4354–4379. https://doi.org/10.3390/ijerph120404354

Gatersleben, B., Murtagh, N., Abrahamse, W. (2014). Values, identity and pro-environmental behaviour. *Contemporary Social Science* 9, pp. 374–392. https://doi.org/10.1080/21582041.2012.682086

Genter, C., Roberts, A., Richardson, J., Sheaff, M. (2015). The contribution of allotment gardening to health and wellbeing: A systematic review of the literature. *British Journal of Occupational Therapy* 78, pp. 593–605. https://doi.org/10.1177/0308022615599408

Gobster, P.H., Kruger, L.E., Schultz, C.L., Henderson, J.R. (2023). Key characteristics of forest therapy trails: A guided, integrative approach. *Forests* 14, 186. https://doi.org/10.3390/f14020186

Hanson, J.O., Rhodes, J.R., Butchart, S.H.M., Buchanan, G.M., Rondinini, C., Ficetola, G.F., Fuller, R.A. (2020). Global conservation of species' niches. *Nature* 580, pp. 232–234. https://doi.org/10.1038/s41586-020-2138-7

Hedblom, M., Heyman, E., Antonsson, H., Gunnarsson, B. (2014). Bird song diversity influences young people's appreciation of urban landscapes. *Urban Forestry and Urban Greening* 13, pp. 469–474. https://doi.org/10.1016/j.ufug.2014.04.002

Hedblom, M., Knez, I., Sang, A.O., Gunnarsson, B. (2017). Evaluation of natural sounds in urban greenery: Potential impact for urban nature preservation. *Royal Society Open Science* 4(2), 170037. https://doi.org/10.1098/rsos.170037

Hooyberg, A., Roose, H., Grellier, J., Elliott, L.R., Lonneville, B., White, M.P., Michels, N., Henauw, S.D., Vandegehuchte, M., Everaert, G. (2020). General health and residential proximity to the coast in Belgium: Results from a cross-sectional health survey. *Environmental Research*, 184, 109225. https://doi.org/10.1016/j.envres.2020.109225

Hoyle, H., Norton, B., Dunnett, N., Richards, J.P., Russell, J.M., Warren, P. (2018). Plant species or flower colour diversity? Identifying the drivers of public and invertebrate response to designed annual meadows. *Landscape and Urban Planning* 180, pp. 103–113. https://doi.org/10.1016/J.LANDURBPLAN.2018.08.017

Hunte, N., Roopsind, A., Ansari, A.A., Trevor Caughlin, T. (2019). Colonial history impacts urban tree species distribution in a tropical city. *Urban Forestry and Urban Greening* 41, pp. 313–322. https://doi.org/10.1016/j.ufug.2019.04.010

IPBES. (2019). *Global assessment report on biodiversity and ecosystem services of the Intergovernmental Science-Policy Platform on Biodiversity and Ecosystem Services.* IPBES Secretariat, Bonn, Germany. https://doi.org/10.5281/zenodo.3831673

Irvine, K.N., Fisher, J.C., Bentley, P.R., Nawrath, M., Dallimer, M., Austen, G.E., Fish, R., Davies, Z.G. (2023). BIO-WELL: The development and validation of a human wellbeing scale that measures responses to biodiversity. *Journal of Environmental Psychology* 85, 101921. https://doi.org/10.1016/j.jenvp.2022.101921

Iungman, T., Cirach, M., Marando, F., Barboza, E.P., Khomenko, S., Masselot, P., Quijal-Zamorano, M., Mueller, N., Gasparrini, A., Urquiza, J., Heris, M., Thondoo, M., Nieuwenhuijsen, M. (2023). Cooling cities through urban green infrastructure: A health impact assessment of European cities. *The Lancet* 401(10376), pp. 577–589. https://doi.org/10.1016/S0140-6736(22)02585-5

Jansson, M., Fors, H., Lindgren, T., & Wiström, B. (2013). Perceived personal safety in relation to urban woodland vegetation–A review. *Urban Forestry & Urban Greening*, 12(2), pp. 127–133.

Joye, Y., de Block, A. (2011). "Nature and I are two": A critical examination of the biophilia hypothesis. *Environmental Values* 20, pp. 189–215. https://doi.org/10.3197/096327111X12997574391724

Joye, Y., van den Berg, A. (2011). Is love for green in our genes? A critical analysis of evolutionary assumptions in restorative environments research. *Urban Forestry and Urban Greening* 10, pp. 261–268. https://doi.org/10.1016/j.ufug.2011.07.004

Kaplan, R. (2010). Intrinsic and aesthetic values of urban nature: A psychological perspective, in: Douglas, I., Goode, D., Houck, M.C. and Maddox, D. (eds.), *The Routledge Handbook of Urban Ecology.* Routledge, Farnham, pp. 385–393.

Kaplan, R., Kaplan, S. (1989). *The experience of nature: A psychological perspective.* Cambridge University Press, Cambridge, UK.

Kellert, Stephen R., Wilson, E.O. (1993). *The Biophilia Hypothesis.* Island Press, Washington, DC.

Keniger, L.E., Gaston, K.J., Irvine, K.N., Fuller, R.A. (2013). What are the benefits of interacting with nature? *International Journal of Environmental Research and Public Health* 10, pp. 913–935. https://doi.org/10.3390/ijerph10030913

Klain, S.C., Chan, K.M.A. (2012. Navigating coastal values: Participatory mapping of ecosystem services for spatial planning. *Ecological Economics* 82, pp. 104–113. https://doi.org/10.1016/j.ecolecon.2012.07.008

Liu, Y., Cleary, A., Fielding, K.S., Murray, Z., Roiko, A. (2022). Nature connection, pro-environmental behaviours and wellbeing: Understanding the mediating role of nature contact. *Landscape and Urban Planning* 228, 104550. https://doi.org/10.1016/j.landurbplan.2022.104550

Marselle, M.R., Bowler, D.E., Watzema, J., Eichenberg, D., Kirsten, T., Bonn, A. (2020). Urban street tree biodiversity and antidepressant prescriptions. *Science Report* 10, 22445. https://doi.org/10.1038/s41598-020-79924-5

Marselle, M.R., Hartig, T., Cox, D.T.C., de Bell, S., Knapp, S., Lindley, S., Triguero-Mas, M., Böhning-Gaese, K., Braubach, M., Cook, P.A., de Vries, S., Heintz-Buschart, A., Hofmann, M., Irvine, K.N., Kabisch, N., Kolek, F., Kraemer, R., Markevych, I., Martens, D., Müller, R., Nieuwenhuijsen, M., Potts, J.M., Stadler, J., Walton, S., Warber, S.L., Bonn, A. (2021). Pathways linking biodiversity to human health: A conceptual framework. *Environment International* 150, 106420. https://doi.org/10.1016/j.envint.2021.106420

Marselle, M.R., Irvine, K.N., Lorenzo-Arribas, A., Warber, S.L. (2016). Does perceived restorativeness mediate the effects of perceived biodiversity and perceived naturalness on emotional well-being following group walks in nature? *Journal of Environmental Psychology* 46, pp. 217–232. https://doi.org/10.1016/j.jenvp.2016.04.008

Maund, P.R., Irvine, K.N., Reeves, J., Strong, E., Cromie, R., Dallimer, M., Davies, Z.G. (2019). Wetlands for wellbeing: Piloting a nature-based health intervention for the management of anxiety and depression. *International Journal of Environmental Research and Public Health* 16(22), 4413. https://doi.org/10.3390/ijerph16224413

Methorst, J., Bonn, A., Marselle, M.R., Böhning-Gaese, K., Rehdanz, K. (2021a). Species richness is positively related to mental health – A study for Germany. *Landscape and Urban Planning* 211, 104084. https://doi.org/10.1016/j.landurbplan.2021.104084

Methorst, J., Rehdanz, K., Mueller, T., Hansjürgens, B., Bonn, A., Böhning-Gaese, K. (2021b). The importance of species diversity for human well-being in Europe. *Ecological Economics* 181, 106917. https://doi.org/10.1016/j.ecolecon.2020.106917

Millenium Ecosystem Assessment (2003). Ecosystems and human well-being: A framework for assessment. www.millenniumassessment.org/documents/document.48.aspx.pdf

Mitchell, R.J., Popham, F. (2008). Effect of exposure to natural environment on health inequalities: An observational population study. *The Lancet* 372, pp. 1655–1660.

Morse, D.F., Sandhu, S., Mulligan, K., Tierney, S., Polley, M., Chiva Giurca, B., Slade, S., Dias, S., Mahtani, K.R., Wells, L., Wang, H., Zhao, B., De Figueiredo, C.E.M., Meijs, J.J., Nam, H.K., Lee, K.H., Wallace, C., Elliott, M., Mendive, J.M., Robinson, D., Palo, M., Herrmann, W., Østergaard Nielsen, R., Husk, K. (2022). Global developments in social prescribing. *BMJ Global Health* 7, e008524. https://doi.org/10.1136/bmjgh-2022-008524

Nawrath, M., Elsey, H., Dallimer, M. (2022). Why cultural ecosystem services matter most: Exploring the pathways linking greenspaces and mental health in a low-income country. *Science of the Total Environment* 806, 150551. https://doi.org/10.1016/j.scitotenv.2021.150551

Nisbet, E.K., Zelenski, J.M., Murphy, S.A. (2009). The nature relatedness scale – Linking individuals' connection with nature to environmental concern and behavior. *Environment and Behavior* 27, pp. 1–26. https://doi.org/10.1177/0013916506295574

Nutsford, D., Pearson, A.L., Kingham, S., Reitsma, F. (2016). Residential exposure to visible blue space (but not green space) associated with lower psychological distress in a capital city. *Health and Place* 39, pp. 70–78. https://doi.org/10.1016/j.healthplace.2016.03.002

Paraskevopoulou, A.T., Kamperi, E., Demiris, N., Economou, M., Theleritis, C., Kitsonas, M., Papageorgiou, C. (2018). The impact of seasonal colour change in planting on patients with psychotic disorders using biosensors. *Urban Forestry and Urban Greening* 36, pp. 50–56. https://doi.org/10.1016/j.ufug.2018.09.006

Pascual, U., Balvanera, P., Díaz, S., Pataki, G., Roth, E., Stenseke, M., Watson, R.T., Dessane, E.B., Islar, M., Kelemen, E. and Maris, V. (2017). Valuing nature's contributions to people: the IPBES approach. *Current Opinion in Environmental Sustainability*, 26, pp. 7–16.

Pett, T.J., Shwartz, A., Irvine, K.N., Dallimer, M., Davies, Z.G. (2016). Unpacking the people–biodiversity paradox: A conceptual framework. *BioScience* 66(7), pp. 576–583. https://doi.org/10.1093/biosci/biw036

Ratcliffe, E., Gatersleben, B., Sowden, P.T. (2013). Bird sounds and their contributions to perceived attention restoration and stress recovery. *Journal of Environmental Psychology* 36, pp. 221–228. https://doi.org/10.1016/j.jenvp.2013.08.004

Richardson, M., Cormack, A., McRobert, L., Underhill, R. (2016). 30 days wild: Development and evaluation of a large-scale nature engagement campaign to improve well-being. *PLoS ONE* 11, pp. 1–13. https://doi.org/10.1371/journal.pone.0149777

Richardson, M., Hunt, A., Hinds, J., Bragg, R., Fido, D., Petronzi, D., Barbett, L., Clitherow, T., White, M. (2019). A measure of nature connectedness for children and adults: Validation, performance, and insights. *Sustainability* 11, pp. 1–16. https://doi.org/10.3390/SU11123250

Ripple, W.J., Wolf, C., Newsome, T.M., Gregg, J.W., Lenton, T.M., Palomo, I., Eikelboom, J.A.J., Law, B.E., Huq, S., Duffy, P.B., Rockström, J. (2021). World scientists' warning of a climate emergency 2021. *BioScience* 71, pp. 894–898. https://doi.org/10.1093/biosci/biab079

Roe, D. (2019). Biodiversity loss — More than an environmental emergency. *The Lancet Planetary Health* 3, pp. e287–e289. https://doi.org/10.1016/S2542-5196(19)30113-5

Schultz, P.W. (2002). *Inclusion with nature: The psychology of human-nature relations*, in: *Psychology of Sustainable Development*. Springer, Boston, MA.

Shanahan, D.F., Astell–Burt, T., Barber, E.A., Brymer, E., Cox, D.T.C., Dean, J., Depledge, M., Fuller, R.A., Hartig, T., Irvine, K.N., Jones, A., Kikillus, H., Lovell, R., Mitchell, R.J., Niemelä, J., Nieuwenhuijsen, M., Pretty, J., Townsend, M., van Heezik, Y., Warber, S., Gaston, K.J. (2019). Nature-based interventions for improving health and wellbeing: The purpose, the people and the outcomes. *Sports* 7, 141. https://doi.org/10.3390/sports7060141

Soga, M., Gaston, K.J., Fukano, Y., Evans, M.J. (2023). The vicious cycle of biophobia. *Trends in Ecology & Evolution* 38(6), pp. 512–520. https://doi.org/10.1016/j.tree.2022.12.012

Sousa-Silva, R., Smargiassi, A., Kneeshaw, D., Dupras, J., Zinszer, K., Paquette, A. (2021). Strong variations in urban allergenicity riskscapes due to poor knowledge of tree pollen allergenic potential. *Science Report* 11, 10196. https://doi.org/10.1038/s41598-021-89353-7

Sousa-Silva, R., Smargiassi, A., Paquette, A., Kaiser, D., Kneeshaw, D. (2020). Exactly what do we know about tree pollen allergenicity? *The Lancet Respiratory Medicine* 8, e10. https://doi.org/10.1016/S2213-2600(19)30472-2

Southon, G.E., Jorgensen, A., Dunnett, N., Hoyle, H., Evans, K.L. (2017). Biodiverse perennial meadows have aesthetic value and increase residents' perceptions of site quality in urban greenspace. *Landscape and Urban Planning* 158, pp. 105–118. https://doi.org/10.1016/j.landurbplan.2016.08.003

Tomita, A., Vandormael, A.M., Cuadros, D., Di Minin, E., Heikinheimo, V., Tanser, F., Slotow, R., Burns, J.K. (2017). Green environment and incident depression in South Africa: A geospatial analysis and mental health implications in a resource-limited setting. *The Lancet Planetary Health* 1, pp. e152–e162. https://doi.org/10.1016/S2542-5196(17)30063-3

Tuan, Y.-F. (1974). *Topophilia: A study of environmental perceptions, attitudes and values.* Prentice Hall, Englewood Cliffs, NJ.

Ulrich, R.S., Simons, R.F., Losito, B.D., Fiorito, E., Miles, M.A., Zelson, M. (1991). Stress recovery during exposure to natural and urban environments. *Journal of Environmental Psychology* 11, pp. 201–230.

United Nations. (2021). *Becoming #GenerationRestoration. Ecosystem restoration for people, nature and climate* (No. ISBN 978-92-807-3864-3). United Nations Environment Programme, Nairobi, Kenya.

Van Den Eeden, S.K., H.E.M. Browning, M., Becker, D.A., Shan, J., Alexeeff, S.E., Thomas Ray, G., Quesenberry, C.P., Kuo, M. (2022). Association between residential green cover and direct healthcare costs in Northern California: An individual level analysis of 5 million persons. *Environment International* 163, 107174. https://doi.org/10.1016/j.envint.2022.107174

White, M.E., Hamlin, I., Butler, C.W., Richardson, M. (2023). The Joy of birds: The effect of rating for joy or counting garden bird species on wellbeing, anxiety, and nature connection. *Urban Ecosystem* 26(3), pp. 755–765. https://doi.org/10.1007/s11252-023-01334-y

White, M.P., Elliott, L.R., Gascón, M., Roberts, B., Fleming, L.E. (2020). Blue space, health and well-being: A narrative overview and synthesis of potential benefits. *Environmental Research* 191, 110169. https://doi.org/10.1016/j.envres.2020.110169

White, M.P., Weeks, A., Hooper, T., Bleakley, L., Cracknell, D., Lovell, R., Jefferson, R.L. (2017). Marine wildlife as an important component of coastal visits: The role of perceived biodiversity and species behaviour. *Marine Policy* 78, pp. 80–89. https://doi.org/10.1016/j.marpol.2017.01.005

Williams, A., & de Vries, F. T. (2020). Plant root exudation under drought: implications for ecosystem functioning. *New Phytologist*, 225(5), pp. 1899–1905.

Wolf, I.D., Wohlfart, T. (2014). Walking, hiking and running in parks: A multidisciplinary assessment of health and well-being benefits. *Landscape and Urban Planning* 130, pp. 89–103. https://doi.org/10.1016/j.landurbplan.2014.06.006

Wolf, L.J., zu Ermgassen, S., Balmford, A., White, M.P., Weinstein, N. (2017). Is variety the spice of life? An experimental investigation into the effects of species richness on self-reported mental well-being. *PloS One* 12, e0170225. https://doi.org/10.1371/journal.pone.0170225

Woodland Trust. (2009). *Ancient tree guide 6: The special wildlife of trees* (Practical Guidance). Woodland Trust, UK.

Zhang, L., Dempsey, N., Cameron, R. (2023). Flowers – Sunshine for the soul! How does floral colour influence preference, feelings of relaxation and positive up-lift? *Urban Forestry and* Urban Greening 79, 127795. https://doi.org/10.1016/j.ufug.2022.127795

8 The affective quality of blue spaces
The case study of a wetland in Wakiso District, Uganda

Sophie-Bo Heinkel and Thomas Kistemann

Introduction

Wetlands supply freshwater, improve water quality, support primary industries, provide food and storm water mitigation, act as a carbon sink, provide habitat for biodiversity and threatened species, provide recreational and touristic opportunities to communities, and are often of particular significance amongst Indigenous peoples. Globally, wetlands are ecosystems that many people depend on, since wetlands support resident livelihoods (WHO, 2005) including the provision of key resources such as water and food. Wetlands are landscapes characterised by a unique assemblage of plants and animals.

Wetlands are an important sub-category of blue spaces, though freshwater spaces in general, have not been discussed extensively in the literature (De Bell et al., 2017). Through the health lens, blue spaces have been defined as 'health-enabling places and spaces, where water is at the centre of a range of environments with identifiable potential for the promotion of human wellbeing' (Foley & Kistemann, 2015, p. 158). Wetlands create opportunities for an intense type of blue therapeutic landscape experience, as they are markedly rich in colours, shapes, and borders (Lengen, 2015). Wetlands are also areas of high biodiversity, which has been linked to human wellbeing in the context of urban green spaces (Fuller et al., 2007; Kaplan & Kaplan, 1989; Ulrich, 1983). Interest in the lived experiences of health within blue spaces is increasing, but the understanding of how this process occurs remains rather limited (Foley et al., 2020).

There are particular gaps in understanding how blue spaces are perceived by varied communities in the Global South, and how different cultural, spatial and affective responses to freshwater blue spaces can support both general and mental health. The main body of literature concerning the links between blue spaces and health is informed by research conducted within European countries, Australia and New Zealand. Here, blue spaces are thought to support health through enabling leisure and a range of physical and social activities (Brückner et al., 2022). These topics have received far less attention in research conducted in African countries, so far (Cilliers et al., 2013). In such contexts, more attention has been given to the role of blue spaces, especially wetlands, as an increasingly sparse environmental resource, with scarcity often leading to conflict (Heinkel, 2018).

In this chapter, we initially outline different theoretical approaches used to understand perceptions of blue space landscapes. Thereafter, methods are presented to assess people's emotional and affective responses to a case study wetland in the Wakiso District, Uganda. To understand and interpret the results, it is important to consider the political, cultural,

DOI: 10.4324/9781003345725-9

and environmental setting of the wetland. We discuss how local residents perceive the wetland and highlight the positive and negative emotions evoked by this specific landscape. Finally, we note limitations of our study and draw some conclusions.

Perceiving landscapes

Embodiment, intersubjectivity, physical activity, and symbolism have been proposed as dimensions which may cast light on how and why blue spaces matter for health and wellbeing (Foley & Kistemann, 2015). Feminist geography, in particular, has highlighted the role of the physical body in the relationship between people and places, critiquing the Cartesian separation of body and mind (Longhurst, 1997). Sensory engagements within one's surroundings have been considered, as well as the individual's consciousness of living in a body (Kazig, 2013; Thrift, 1999). The idea of embodiment is relevant in the analysis of human-environment-relationships, since it means the sense of being localised with sensory and emotional feelings within one's physical body (Lea, 2008; Wylie, 2006). Landscapes are perceived and embodied (Kazig, 2013) as physical, material entities that are nonetheless interpreted in various ways, shaped by individual experiences, alongside diverse cultural and societal meanings (Hinchliffe, 2002; Wylie, 2006). This understanding of landscapes recognises the subjectivity of landscapes as perceived entities (Claßen, 2016; Ipsen, 2006).

Landscape is a product of individual everyday lives and activities in a landscape. This includes activities with the landscape's non-human materials as well as human interactions (Rose, 2002). Wylie (2006) defines landscape as an emerging relationship between narratives, visual aesthetics, and sensibilities predicated on cultural-historical patterns as well as materialities of immanent topographies. Geographies dealing with landscapes have revealed emotional dimensions of landscape perception and experience (Wylie, 2006). A landscape is not only what observers see, but also what they feel about these elements, and so correspondingly a construct of both materialism and sensibilities (Wylie, 2006), which is expressed in narratives with immanent topographies. The interaction of human beings with a landscape generates a sense of coherence (Antonovsky, 1987), with the individuals' manner of acting providing insights into the representation of landscape in their minds. Thus, a landscape's change is considered as a dynamic process also in human mental representations. Assessing this dialectic of tectonics and semiotics of a landscape requires a view beyond the discipline of geography to neighbouring disciplines.

Our study therefore draws on methodologies developed within environmental psychology. Environmental psychology has explored the intuitive and spontaneous change in emotional state, e.g. from pleasantness to unpleasantness, in response to the aesthetic appearance of natural environments (Russell & Pratt, 1980; Ulrich, 1983). Russell's (1980) circumplex model visualises these core affects, which are "neurophysiological state[s] consciously accessible as the simplest raw (nonreflective) feelings evident in moods and emotions" (Russell, 2003, p. 148). In our study, wetland-directed attributed affects were investigated. An attributed affect is an object-directed change of emotional states due to a prior event or exposure to a place; it is a change in a neurophysiological state in moods and emotions and builds to the initial point of an emotional reaction, such as facial and emotional oral expressions. In addition to the affective quality of wetlands, their mentally supportive character merits emphasis, in particular with regard to reciprocal concepts of people and places (Brandenburg & Carroll, 1995; Low & Altman 1992). This is not a trivial point, since mental wellbeing is perceived intuitively (Horwitz & Finlayson, 2011) and its supportive environments such as health-promoting landscapes are often taken for granted.

Study area and method

Wetland residents in Uganda have lives and livelihoods interconnected with the wetland and can be seen as part of the ecosystem. At least 10% of the Ugandan population, constituting more than 2.7 million people, is dependent on wetlands by direct or subsistence employment (Republic of Uganda, 2014). Uganda has an annual population growth of 3.2% (data.worldbank.org); thus, the pressure of producing food is still increasing. Further, the extent of unused wetlands is decreasing while encroachment is permanently increasing. Current news coverage highlights the Ugandan government's action against encroachers and evictions (Heinkel, 2014). This reflects the sensitivity surrounding matters of land property and key resources, which wetlands provide, as conflict-raising topics between the government and subsistence farmers.

The Ugandan National Regulations, No.3/2000 (National Environmental Act, Sec 107 Cap 153) place wetlands under protection and provide clear rules at different scales regarding the conditions under which these ecosystems may be used. The document allows the traditional use of wetlands in terms of: (a) harvesting of papyrus, medicinal plants, trees and reeds; (b) any cultivation where the cultivated area is not more than 25% of the total area of the wetland; (c) fishing using traps, spears and baskets or other methods than weirs; (d) collection of water for domestic use; and (e) hunting under the rule of the provisions of the Wildlife Act. The reality, however, looks different: already in 2009, highly impacted wetlands are apparent widely across Uganda.

The wetland in Wakiso District, Uganda is an inland valley, which is seasonally flooded (Figure 8.1). Within the investigated basin, green dominates in numerous shades, of various grasses and papyrus reed, bushes and palm trees. From the ridge of the upper wetland, there is a broad view of plants, fields and houses between the trees and vegetation. In the dry season, the dusty roads contribute with red and brownish colours to that impression, while some types of grasses in the upper areas dry out. During the rainy season, the green is more saturated and the dusty roads tend to be more brown than red and are covered by puddles filled with brown water (Figure 8.2). In the central area of the wetland, the acoustic background of cicadas and birds stands out. Within the lower wetlands, there is hardly any sound from machines or humans, besides the voices of some field workers or subsistence farmers. On hot days, the change of the air temperature from very hot and dusty in the upper land to fresh and less dusty in the central green area is apparent. Many colourful birds, small monkeys and various insects have their habitats in the whole basin, while chameleons and snakes live in the lower areas between the papyrus reed, palm trees and bamboo. Moreover, the Crested Crane, both a subspecies of the grey-crowned crane and the national bird of Uganda, settles down in flocks within this wetland.

Wetland users, who had their residence in the case study communities for this study, were invited to participate in group interviews by the local councils. The group interviews were carried out in three local communities. One community was located in a rural and very remote area (I). Two of the three communities were located in urban fringe areas.

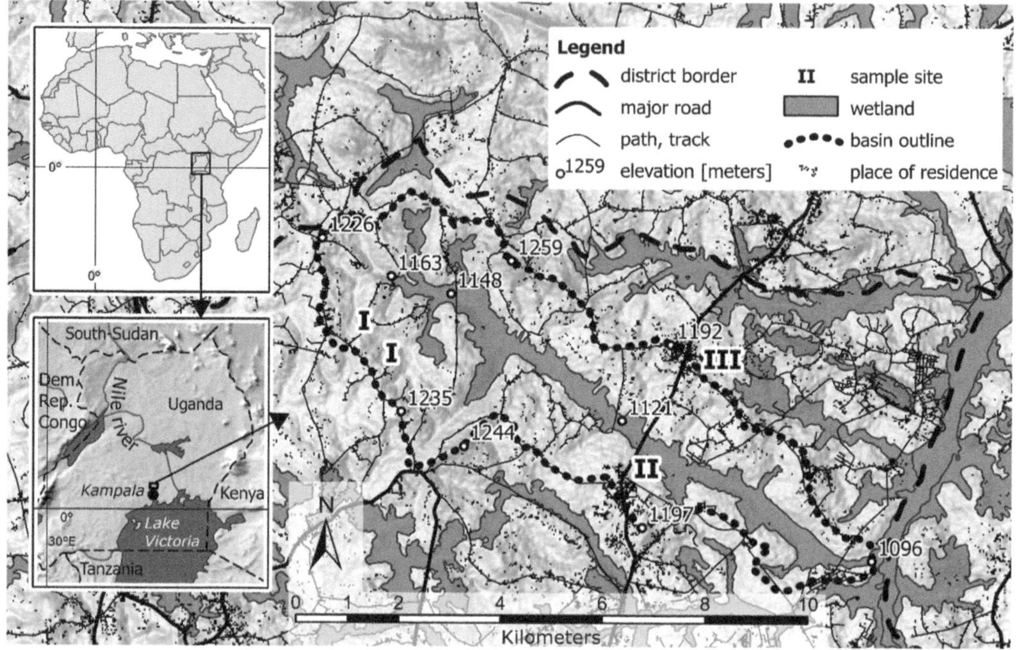

Figure 8.1 Map of the research area and data collection spots.

The land properties of one community of the urban fringe area were under the purview of a national research institute (II), thus this land was managed with a top-down mentality. Subsistence farmers of the other investigated areas of jurisdictions experienced fewer restrictions (III).

Group interviews with six to ten men and six to ten women were conducted in each community. The interviews were held in English with simultaneous translation to the local language, Luganda. Participatory Rapid Appraisal Methods (Chambers, 1994) were used. The process was audio recorded. A transcript of each audio recording was devised and translated by a neutral translator with expertise in the local language, Luganda, into English. The study was ethically approved by the ethical committees of the Medical Faculties of the University of Bonn (Nr. 248/14) and the Makerere University of Kampala (#REC REF 2016-053). After receiving accessible information on the project and the researchers in Luganda, each participant was asked for their informed consent in participating in the study.

A free listing about the wetland and the place of residence was used to examine the participants' cognitive and emotional associations with the landscape. This was done by asking the question: "What comes into your mind, when I say they word 'wetland'[1]"? The immediate verbal expressions of the participants were audio recorded and transcribed. During the interviews, the interviewees were not aware of the assessment

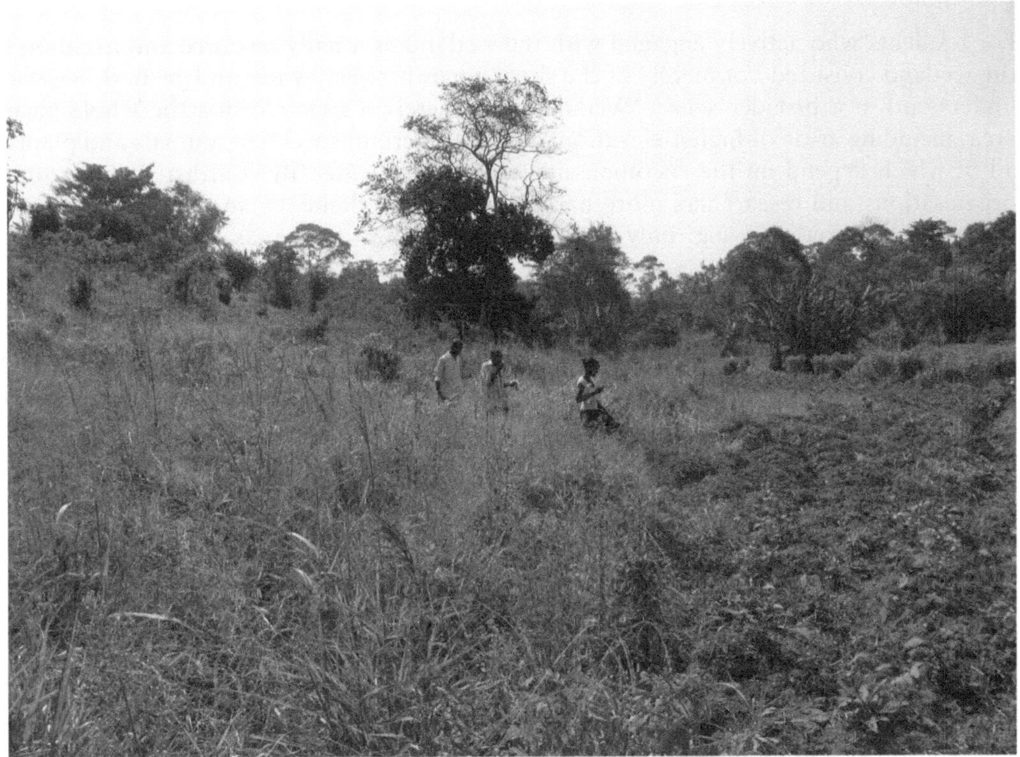

Figure 8.2 View into the wetland from Research area I.

of their emotional expressions. The results were surprising, since the pure association of the wetland elicited a number of emotional affects amongst the respondents (Russell and Pratt, 1980). For example: *"I see water flowing down a valley. The valley is surrounded by hills. As the water flows down the valley it is surrounded by shrubs. I also see sandy soil, clay soil, muddy soil as well as papyrus reeds since I have a passion for mats. That is what I see. May God bless you!"*

These verbal expressions of attributed affects were further coded and classified. A code could be any spoken emotional expression about or association with the wetland, whether negative or positive, e.g. (A) *"when I think about the wetland I never imagine myself building anything since I cannot protect myself effectively from the much water. I want to build a house as far away as possible [...]"* or (B) *"I pride myself a lot in the swamps simply because of the presence of water. Since water is life, as we all know"*.

Within the six group interviews, 54 separate emotional expressions were identified. All evaluative expressions and descriptions about the wetland were selected and screened for emotional expressions. These were assigned to states of pleasure or displeasure and the state of arousal, then translated into specific emotions (Russell & Lanius, 1984). The code families were categorised into feelings arising from Russell's core affect model (Russell, 1980; 2003).

Results and discussion

For residents who actively engaged with the wetland as a daily resource and livelihood, the wetland consisted not merely of the shore zones between water and ground, but was understood in a broader sense. 'Wetland' was merely a synonym for the whole basin area, including areas of higher elevation, as well as certain species of animals and plants, all of which depend on the encompassing resource of water. By contrast, international organisations and researchers more narrowly define wetlands by specific technical and scientific characteristics, e.g. only the swampy areas of a valley as the 'wetland areas' drawn in Figure 8.1.

The wetland was psychologically represented in the minds of its residents and people who felt emotionally attached to it. For the interviewees, the wetland is a unique place endowed with meanings and values (Tuan, 1977). The imagination of the wetland evoked varied affects in people, including both positive and negative emotions. In the rural community, positive expressions predominated, while in one of the communities of the urban fringe, negative feelings about the wetland predominated (Figure 8.3).

The wetland generated pleasure through both its appearance and the provision of resources such as water (Figure 8.4). The green colour and the various types of grasses were recognised. People mentioned the important function of this landscape in terms of temperature regulation during hot days. This made residents proud of "their" wetland since they see it as "essential to humanity". Thinking of the wetland as an intact ecosystem inspired the participants' creativity. By simple association to the local expression for wetland, they immediately imagined a detailed picture of the landscape in their minds. Additionally, often a whole range of business ideas and opportunities based on materials generated by the ecosystem came up.

Words like "passion" indicated a high appreciation and deep commitment to the landscape. Additionally, there was an association of the wetland with spirit and God. Others

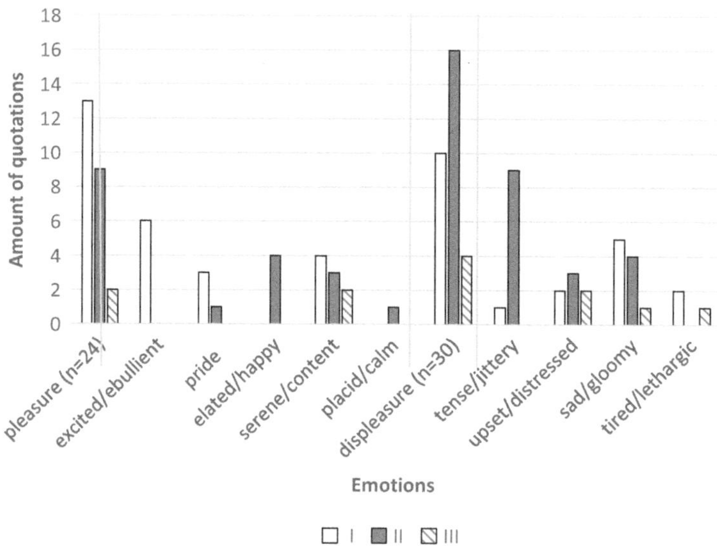

Figure 8.3 Wetland-attributed feelings of pleasure (1) and displeasure (2).

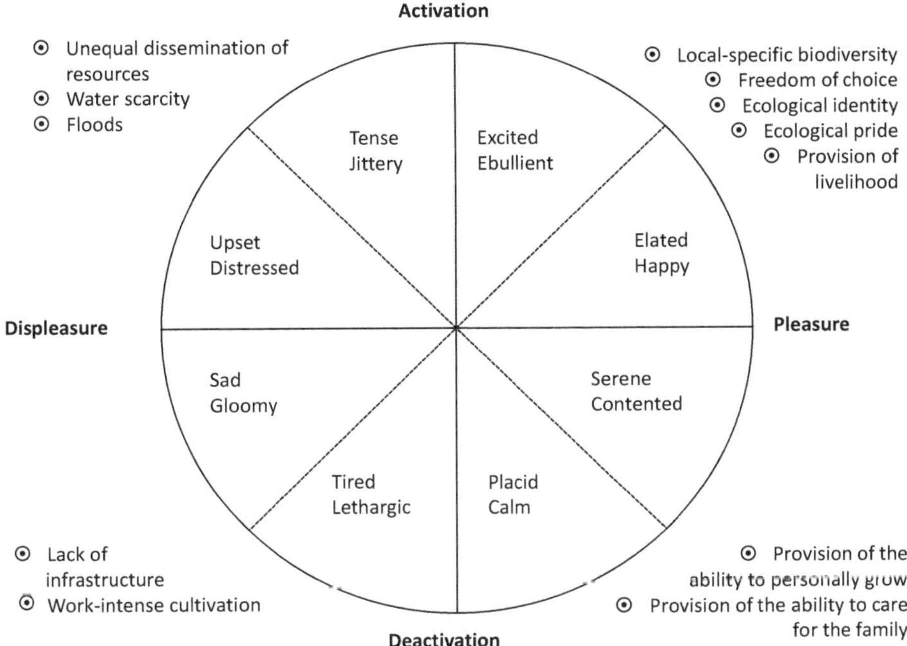

Figure 8.4 Affects provoked by aspects related to wetland embedded into Russell's (1980) circumplex model.

used the term "pride" when they talked about the large variety of products as well as the self-fulfilment they received from the wetland. Happiness was related to the freedom to farm and autonomy to produce the products of their choice. The opportunity to grow crops in the wetland strongly supported farmers' wellbeing. The wetland was seen to provide support in the face of droughts and food scarcity; the subsistence farmers' protection against disaster if the natural circumstances on the mainland change in a way to threaten their families. The wetland was associated with support in terms of food security, financial wellbeing, as well as a means by which to achieve goals and to obtain a better life. The wetland comprised a specific composition of plants unique to its ecosystem. The provision of material, such as papyrus reed and tree leaves, played an important role in the perception of the wetland as an activity and social space (Völker & Kistemann, 2015). The residents of the rural areas gathered materials from the wetland from which they produced craftworks, such as mats. Many women sat together, chatting and creating products out of the material. Such activity fosters social coherence (Antonovsky, 1996) as well as a sense of belonging to the wetland (Relph, 1976). By living in towns and more urbanised areas, residents had fewer possibilities to participate in the socialising and joint production of handicrafts. This influenced the perception of the wetlands as an activity space and may explain local differences in perceptions and mental representations of the wetlands.

Activities happening in or being closely related to the wetland trigger appreciation for the ecosystem and landscape. Especially in the remote areas, many people articulated pride when they talked about the wetland. Pride is a secondary emotion of love and happiness (Edelstein & Shaver, 2007), which presupposes an internal evaluation (Russell, 2003) of the wetland. Pride was apparent when farmers talked about the wetland as their property and the role of the wetland for supporting financial wellbeing, a source of freedom of choice and opportunities (Smith et al., 2013) and ensuring opportunities for personal growth (Ryff & Keyes, 1995). Notably, farmers and business people relied on wetland products and services. Moreover, the local specific biodiversity was seen as something to be proud of, with the feeling of taking pride in the ecosystem representing a conscious positive identification with the wetland. Thus, "ecological pride" is a consciously felt appreciation for a landscape. The key items in the core affect model revealed that positive emotions are also related to low activity levels and a level of low mobilization. In regions where the degradation of the wetland was not visible yet, and the livelihood-providing ecosystem services were still fully functioning, people were satisfied by the provision of ecosystem services and did not feel the need to be proactive in preserving their source of livelihood.

Negative feelings were associated with the exhausting, long journeys to water sources and the general hard work of cultivation in the wetland. Additionally, the lack of infrastructure and the lack of improved farming techniques caused tiredness and lethargy. When wetland resources were unavailable or inaccessible, people felt helpless: *"At the moment, most of our swamps dried up a long time ago. They no longer have water. We do need assistance."* Distress emerges when water is not available and food becomes scarce. With accelerating climate change, periods of water scarcity will become more frequent, thus there are risks that people will experience greater distress within the near future, potentially including climate anxiety (Dodds, 2021; Ogunbode et al., 2022, 2023; Whitmarsh et al., 2022) as well as solastalgia; a place-based distress due to environmental change and loss of belonging (Albrecht, 2005; Askland & Bunn, 2018; Tschakert et al., 2013). On the other hand, people also expressed concern about the overabundance of water during the rainy season.

The scarcity of land for purchase was another source of tension; it posed a threat of hunger and poverty to the farmers, as subsistence farmers usually have no reserves or savings. Such people had a high risk of losing their whole means of existence due to environmental shifts and damage to the wetland or eviction. These conditions caused feelings of fear and despair. More pressing negative affects had their origins mostly in social hierarchies and social pressures. The insecurity of land availability affected the farmers' economic wellbeing and their ability to plan their future. Even as to the immediate future, the existence of the residents was insecure. Under such conditions, the risk of "learning" helplessness (Maier & Seligman, 1976) appeared in relation to the unpredictability of shifts in the social space. Changes in the social fabric and hierarchical construction of place are sources of tension. Mental health issues, such as stress in relation to the wetlands, can develop in the context of land-use conflicts, e.g. political restrictions. People living in densely-populated areas expressed a sense of displeasure and perceived injustice in terms of the social rules and land ownership in the wetland.

The highly restricted access to key resources, land and water, and the comparison of participants' own lives with those of others generated feelings of injustice and anger: *"[...] there are quarters, they have the restriction, but others they have not"*. The missing of "homeland", and unfulfilled wishes and dreams made people sad. Many people, especially in the "restricted" community, experienced feelings of anger and injustice when they talked about the wetland in terms of the distribution of land properties *"[...] I need the wetlands in this area, according to what I do to cultivate some crops. [...] To buy food is now becoming an expensive thing. So, for my wellbeing, I need to work somewhere, where I can at least cultivate something instead of going for everything to the shops [...].*" This was a source of tension, despair and fear for people since they experienced the landscape as being *"monopolised by institutions and rich people"*.

Limitations

This study was designed by a German researcher in the frame of their PhD research project. Before conducting the study onsite, all questions and activities were discussed and critically reworked with the local research assistant, who identified herself as Baganda (Baganda is the local ethnic majority in the research area). The first contact with the participants was made through the local councillors in respect to the local hierarchies and societal structures. The research team took care to exclude colonial behaviour and demonstration of power during the research. However, during the group interviews, cultural differences between the Bagandan participants, the German researcher and even the highly educated and intercultural experienced Baganda research assistant in expressing anger or happiness or any other feeling by body language could not be overcome. In this context, it is not clear how much information was lost by the transcription of the Bagandan interpreter and the translation into English. The cultural bias posed a challenge and might have hampered the gathering of better and clearer information on the feelings and expressions provoked by the wetland, and the culturally appropriate interpretation of participant responses. Even though the research team was culturally sensitive and self-reflective, it cannot be ruled out that study participants might have felt intimidated by a perceived power gradient between themselves and the researchers. Further studies on the emotional expressions would need longer-term processes of in-depth research co-design, implementation and analysis with a local research team, who speak the same language, as well as use the same body language, and share similar points of cultural reference as the participants.

The group discussions took place in regular assembly areas of the villages, which were located in the immediate vicinity, partly in sight of the wetland. Drawing on the work of Andrews, Chen and Myers (2014), it was assumed that imaginations of the wetland landscapes would have a similar effect as being physically *in* the landscape. However, alternative verbal and non-verbal embodied responses may have been elicited through conducting the interviews directly in situ within the wetland, perhaps on a 1:1 basis rather than in group situations. It might be the case, that only the most intense, present or culturally shared emotions evoked by the wetlands were captured.

Conclusions

Blue spaces can support a range of specific sensory experiences, e.g. they have a cooling effect during hot days, provide borders for orientation, etc. This study highlights how blue spaces, specifically the sub-category of wetlands, can have a highly affective quality, triggering both positive and negative emotions. Wetlands as provisional ecosystems foster emotional bonding with and within these landscapes, eliciting detailed and multi-faceted mental representations amongst people who experience this emotional bonding. As unique and livelihood-providing landscapes, wetlands are places of identification with high potential to support mental wellbeing. In this respect, their aesthetic appearance is important for cultural identity and for the development of a sense of place (Jorgensen & Stedman, 2001; Lengen & Kistemann, 2012; Relph, 1976; Shamai, 1991; Tuan, 1977). Sense of place reflects the emotional attachment of people to places (DeMiglio

& Williams, 2008, p. 16). This includes emotional affects provoked by the place itself as well as the cognitive evaluation of the place. Furthermore, intact wetlands play a crucial role in the promotion of resident health. Wetlands support personal growth, freedom of choice, autonomy and financial security amongst those who depend on wetland ecosystem services. The emotional supportive character of blue spaces needs more attention concerning environmental protection activities, including key questions concerning the maintenance of the crucial life and livelihood supportive ecosystem functions of wetlands. Due to the difficulties in providing evidence on the supportive character of blue spaces on mental wellbeing, environmental scientists highlight that there is a need to embed more social science in the topic of protecting wetlands (McInnes et al., 2016).

The method used here to identify the range of emotions elicited through imagining a specific wetland of local importance is innovative and provides promising progress. Firstly, it highlights that sustainable ecosystem management and the effective protection of wetlands in the Global South needs the meaningful involvement of wetland residents, in this instance subsistence farmers, in environmental planning. Secondly, it also shows that people become more aware of the emotionally supportive functions of blue spaces when resources diminish or dry up and ecosystems are obviously degrading. Framing blue spaces, where environmental and social meanings meet, as health-enabling resources provides a strong, but still underestimated argument for the need for sustainable water body management (Foley & Kistemann, 2015). The wetland case, a thus far overlooked but nonetheless constitutive part of the blue world, is important in further promoting the healthy blue space agenda.

Acknowledgements

This research was carried out in the frame of the joint research project "GlobE – Wetlands in East Africa: Reconciling future food production with environmental protection" funded by the German Federal Ministry of Education and Research (Funding Code: 031A250D). Our special thanks go to Joan Kresser for her invaluable support in terms of data collection and translation into the local language. Additionally, we thank Christoph Höser for providing the maps. We thank also Dr Noeline Nakasujja (Head of Department of Psychatry at Makerere University, Uganda) and Isaac Kakande and also the local councillors of our data sampling areas for their support in data collection and all participants of the study.

Note

1 In Luganda, there are two expressions for "wetland", which are partly used synonymously. Both words, "Lutobazi" and "Kyseni", were named in this context.

References

Albrecht, G. (2005). "Solastalgia". A new concept in health and identity. *Philosophy Activism Nature*, 3, pp. 41–55.
Andrews, G. J., Chen, S., & Myers, S. (2014). The 'taking place' of health and wellbeing: Towards non-representational theory. *Social Science & Medicine*, 108, pp. 210–222. https://doi.org/10.1016/j.socscimed.2014.02.037

Antonovsky, A. (1987). *Unraveling the mystery of health: How people manage stress and stay well* (1st ed.) San Francisco: Jossey-Bass.

Antonovsky, A. (1996). The salutogenic model as a theory to guide health promotion. *Health Promotion International*, 11(1), pp. 11–18. https://doi.org/10.1093/heapro/11.1.11

Askland, H. H., & Bunn, M. (2018). Lived experiences of environmental change: Solastalgia, power and place. *Emotion, Space and Society*, 27, pp. 16–22. https://doi.org/10.1016/j.emospa.2018.02.003

Brandenburg, A. M., & Carroll, M. S. (1995). Your place or mine?: The effect of place creation on environmental values and landscape meanings. *Society & Natural Resources*, 8(5), pp. 381–398. https://doi.org/10.1080/08941929509380931

Brückner, A., Falkenberg, T., Heinzel, C., & Kistemann, T. (2022). The regeneration of urban blue spaces: A public health intervention? Reviewing the evidence. *Frontiers in Public Health*, 9, 782101. https://doi.org/10.3389/fpubh.2021.782101

Chambers, R. (1994). Participatory Rural Appraisal (PRA): Challenges, potentials and paradigm. *World Development*, 22(10), pp. 1437–1454.

Cilliers, S., Cilliers, J., Lubbe, R., & Siebert, S. (2013). Ecosystem services of urban green spaces in African countries—Perspectives and challenges. *Urban Ecosystems*, 16(4), pp. 681–702. https://doi.org/10.1007/s11252-012-0254-3

Claßen, T. (2016). Landschaft. In: U. Gebhard & T. Kistemann, eds., *Landschaft, Identität und Gesundheit*. Wiesbaden: Springer Fachmedien. https://doi.org/10.1007/978-3-531-19723-4_3

De Bell, S., Graham, H., Jarvis, S., & White, P. (2017). The importance of nature in mediating social and psychological benefits associated with visits to freshwater blue space. *Landscape and Urban Planning*, 167, pp. 118–127. https://doi.org/10.1016/j.landurbplan.2017.06.003

DeMiglio, L., & Williams, A. (2008). A sense of place, A sense of well-being. In: J. Eyles & A. Williams, eds., *Sense of Place, Health and Quality of Life*. Abingdon: Routledge.

Dodds, J. (2021). The psychology of climate anxiety. *BJPSYCH Bulletin*, 45(4), pp. 222–226. https://doi.org/10.1192/bjb.2021.18

Edelstein, R. S., & Shaver, P. R. (2007). A cross-cultural examination of lexical studies of self-conscious emotions. In: J.L. Tracy, R.W. Robins, & J.P. Tangney, eds., *The Self-Conscious Emotions: Theory and Research*. New York: The Guildford Press.

Foley, R., Kearns, R. A., Kistemann, T., & Wheeler, B. (eds.) (2020). Introduction. In: *Blue Space, Health and Wellbeing: Hydrophilia Unbounded*. Abingdon: Routledge Taylor & Francis Group.

Foley, R., & Kistemann, T. (2015). Blue space geographies: Enabling health in place. *Health and Place*, 35, pp. 157–165. https://doi.org/10.1016/j.healthplace.2015.07.003

Fuller, R. A., Irvine, K. N., Devine-Wright, P., Warren, P. H., & Gaston, K. J. (2007). Psychological benefits of greenspace increase with biodiversity. *Biology Letters*, 3(4), pp. 390–394.

Heinkel, S.-B. (2018). *Therapeutic Effects of Wetlands on Mental Well-Being. The Concept of Therapeutic Landscapes Applied to an Ecosystem in Uganda*. PhD Thesis, Rheinische Friedrich-Wilhelms-Universität Bonn. https://bonndoc.ulb.uni-bonn.de/xmlui/handle/20.500.11811/7588

Heinkel, S.-B. (2014). Wetlands in Uganda – Ecosystems under pressure A newspaper review from Uganda. *WHOCC Newsletter Water & Risk*, 23, pp. 7–9.

Hinchliffe, S. (2002). Inhabiting—Landscapes and natures. In: K. Anderson, M. Domosh, S. Pile, & N. Thrift, eds., *Handbook of Cultural Geography*. London, UK: SAGE Publications. https://doi.org/10.4135/9781848608252

Horwitz, P., & Finlayson, M. (2011). Wetlands as settings for human health: Incorporating ecosystem services and health impact assessment into water resource management. *BioScience*, 61(9), pp. 678–688. https://doi.org/10.1525/bio.2011.61.9.6

Ipsen, D. (2006). *Ort und Landschaft*. Wiesbaden: VS, Verlag für Sozialwissenschaften.

Jorgensen, B. S., & Stedman, R. C. (2001). Sense of place as an attitude: Lakeshore owners attitudes toward their properties. *Journal of Environmental Psychology*, 21(3), pp. 233–248. https://doi.org/10.1006/jevp.2001.0226

Kaplan, R., & Kaplan, S. (1989). *The experience of nature: A psychological perspective.* Cambridge: Cambridge University Press. https://doi.org/10.1037/030621

Kazig, R. (2013). Landschaft mit allen Sinnen-Zum Wert des Atmosphärenbegriffs für die Landschaftsforschung. In: O. Kühne & D. Bruns, eds., *Landschaften: Theorie, Praxis und internationale Bezüge.* Barcelona: Oceano.

Lea, J. (2008). Retreating to nature: Rethinking 'therapeutic landscapes'. *Area,* 40(1), pp. 90–98. https://doi.org/10.1111/j.1475-4762.2008.00789.x

Lengen, C. (2015). The effects of colours, shapes and boundaries of landscapes on perception, emotion and mentalising processes promoting health and well-being. *Health & Place,* 35, pp. 166–177. http://dx.doi.org/10.1016/j.healthplace.2015.05.016

Lengen, C., & Kistemann, T. (2012). Sense of place and place identity: Review of neuroscientific evidence. *Health & Place,* 18(5), pp. 1162–1171. https://doi.org/10.1016/j.healthplace.2012.01.012

Longhurst, R. (1997). (Dis)embodied geographies. *Progress in Human Geography,* 21(4), pp. 486–501. https://doi.org/10.1191/030913297668704177

Low, S.M. & Altman, I. (1992). Place attachment: A conceptual Inquiry. In: I. Altman, S.M. Low, eds., *Place Attachment. Human Behavior and Environment,* 12. Boston, US: Springer. https://doi.org/10.1007/978-1-4684-8753-4_1.

Maier, S. F., & Seligman, M. E. (1976). Learned helplessness: Theory and evidence. *Journal of Experimental Psychology: General,* 105(1), pp. 3–46. https://doi.org/10.1037/0096-3445.105.1.3

McInnes, R., Smith, G., Greaves, J., Watson, D., Wood, N., & Everard, M. (2016). Multicriteria decision analysis for the evaluation of water quality improvement and ecosystem service provision. *Water and Environment Journal,* 30(3–4), pp. 298–309. https://doi.org/10.1111/wej.12195

Ogunbode, C. A., Doran, R., Hanss, D., Ojala, M., Salmela-Aro, K., Van Den Broek, K. L., Bhullar, N., Aquino, S. D., Marot, T., Schermer, J. A., Wlodarczyk, A., Lu, S., Jiang, F., Maran, D. A., Yadav, R., Ardi, R., Chegeni, R., Ghanbarian, E., Zand, S., … Karasu, M. (2022). Climate anxiety, wellbeing and pro-environmental action: Correlates of negative emotional responses to climate change in 32 countries. *Journal of Environmental Psychology,* 84, 101887. https://doi.org/10.1016/j.jenvp.2022.101887

Ogunbode, C. A., Pallesen, S., Böhm, G., Doran, R., Bhullar, N., Aquino, S., Marot, T., Schermer, J. A., Wlodarczyk, A., Lu, S., Jiang, F., Salmela-Aro, K., Hanss, D., Maran, D. A., Ardi, R., Chegeni, R., Tahir, H., Ghanbarian, E., Park, J., … Lomas, M. J. (2023). Negative emotions about climate change are related to insomnia symptoms and mental health: Cross-sectional evidence from 25 countries. *Current Psychology,* 42(2), pp. 845–854. https://doi.org/10.1007/s12144-021-01385-4

Relph, E. (1976). *Place and placelessness.* London: Pion.

Republic of Uganda, Ministry of Water and Environment, Climate Change Department (2014). Uganda Second National Communication to the United Nations Framework Convention on Climate Change. Kampala, p. 11.

Rose, M. (2002). Landscape and labyrinths. *Geoforum,* 33(4), pp. 455–467. http://dx.doi.org/10.1016/S0016-7185(02)00030-1

Russell, J. (1980). A circumplex model of affect. *Journal of Personality and Social Psychology,* 39(6), pp. 1161–1178. https://doi.org/10.1037/h0077714

Russell, J. (2003). Core affect and the psychological construction of emotion. *Psychological Review,* 110(1), pp. 145–172. https://doi.org/10.1037/0033-295X.110.1.145

Russell, J., & Lanius, U. F. (1984). Adaptation level and the affective appraisal of environments. *Journal of Environmental Psychology,* 4(2), pp. 119–135. https://doi.org/10.1016/S0272-4944(84)80029-8

Russell, J., & Pratt, G. (1980). A description of the affective quality attributed to environments. *Journal of Personality and Social Psychology,* 38(2), pp. 311–322.

Ryff, C. D., & Keyes, C. L. M. (1995). The structure of psychological well-being revisited. *Journal of Personality and Social Psychology,* 69(4), pp. 719–727. https://doi.org/10.1037/0022-3514.69.4.719

Shamai, S. (1991). Sense of place: An empirical measurement. *Geoforum*, 22(3), pp. 347–358. https://doi.org/10.1016/0016-7185(91)90017-K

Smith, L. M., Case, J. L., Smith, H. M., Harwell, L. C., & Summers, J. K. (2013). Relating ecoystem services to domains of human well-being: Foundation for a U.S. index. *Ecological Indicators*, 28(0), pp. 79–90. https://doi.org/10.1016/j.ecolind.2012.02.032

Thrift, N. (1999). Steps to an ecology of place. In: D. B. Massey, J. Allen, & P. Sarre, eds., *Human Geography Today*. Cambridge: Polity Press.

Tschakert, P., Van Oort, B., St. Clair, A. L., & LaMadrid, A. (2013). Inequality and transformation analyses: A complementary lens for addressing vulnerability to climate change. *Climate and Development*, 5(4), pp. 340–350. https://doi.org/10.1080/17565529.2013.828583

Tuan, Y.-F. (1977). *Space and place: The perspective of experience*. 8th ed. Minneapolis: University of Minnesota Press.

Ulrich, R. S. (1983). Aesthetic and affective response to natural environment. In: I. Altman & J. F. Wohlwill, eds., *Behavior and the Natural Environment*. New York and London: Plenum Press. https://doi.org/10.1007/978-1-4613-3539-9_4

Völker, S., & Kistemann, T. (2015). Developing the urban blue: Comparative health responses to blue and green urban open spaces in Germany. *Health & Place*, 35, pp. 196–205. http://dx.doi.org/10.1016/j.healthplace.2014.10.015

Whitmarsh, L., Player, L., Jiongco, A., James, M., Williams, M., Marks, E., & Kennedy-Williams, P. (2022). Climate anxiety: What predicts it and how is it related to climate action? *Journal of Environmental Psychology*, 83, 101866. https://doi.org/10.1016/j.jenvp.2022.101866

WHO (2005). Ecosystems and human well-being: health synthesis: A report of the Millennium Ecosystem Assessment. Geneva: World Health Organization.

Wylie, J. (2006). Depths and folds: On landscape and the gazing subject. *Environment and Planning D: Society and Space*, 24(4), pp. 519–535. https://doi.org/10.1068/d380t

9 Untangling nature-based interventions' influences on participants' mental wellbeing

Critiquing 'nature on prescription'

Andy Harrod and Nadia von Benzon

Introduction

Nature-based interventions involve facilitated engagement with nature to benefit human health. These interventions, typically including agricultural and/or gardening activities, have occurred since Ancient Greece (Gallis, 2013), within hospitals, prisons, and asylums, providing routine, meaningful work, and reflective spaces in support of people's mental and physical recovery (Sempik, Hine and Wilcox, 2010). Since the 1970s, people with mental ill health have been treated through community care initiatives (Killaspy, 2006). This includes occupational therapists' use of established gardening and farming practices to provide opportunities for vulnerable people within communities to engage with nature for their wellbeing. This led to the development of social and therapeutic horticulture (Sempik and Bragg, 2013). The range of nature-based interventions has since expanded to include environmental conservation, care-farming, green and blue exercise, adventure activities, and ecotherapy.

Community-based support is increasingly being provided through social prescribing; an approach which recognises that human health is influenced by a range of economic, environmental, and social factors (NHS England, 2020). Social prescribing seeks to support people in taking greater care of their health, as well as reduce pressure on the UK National Health Service (NHS) through non-clinical sources of psychosocial support and activities within the local community, based on personal interests. The prescribing of nature-based interventions is a growing area of social prescribing (Robinson et al., 2020) informed by an evidence-base linking nature exposure and engagement to improved emotional regulation and processing for both children and adults (e.g., Keniger et al., 2013; Mughal et al., 2022). Nature-based interventions integrate nature through facilitated, structured and regular activities to co-create active therapeutic processes (Bragg and Atkins, 2016; Sempik, Hine and Wilcox, 2010). As such, nature-based interventions aim to improve participants' wellbeing by providing defined programmes for individuals with a specific need and/or health promotion projects for the general population (Van den Berg, 2017).

Three core components have been identified as characterising nature-based interventions, including: nature; meaningful activity; and social interaction (Bragg and Atkins, 2016). Activities are deemed meaningful when they provide opportunities for participants to develop skills (e.g., caring for animals, habitat creation), improve mobility and/or fitness (e.g., horticultural, adventure), and/or mindfully engage with nature.

DOI: 10.4324/9781003345725-10

Through these types of activities, participants have reported feeling valued, developing connections with nature and people, enhancing their emotional regulation, and nurturing their sense of self (Conlon et al., 2018; Rotheram, McGarrol and Watkins, 2017). Participating in the activities as part of a group supports engagement with a diverse range of people, which can improve social skills and promote a sense of belonging (Biglin, 2020; O'Brien, 2018). Herein, nature is viewed as the connecting characteristic, which is engaged with through the environmental settings and where the meaningful activities and the social interactions take place.

Whilst there is a wealth of research highlighting the efficacy of nature-based interventions in supporting short-term changes to wellbeing, there are limited follow-up studies, so there is uncertainty regarding the sustainability of benefits. This leads to uncertainty regarding how nature-based interventions work to create both short and long-term shifts in participants' wellbeing. Existing theories primarily focus on peoples' immediate experience, rather than ongoing effects after and outside the therapeutic event. We will consider these uncertainties and the future of nature-based interventions research by firstly providing a review of the literature. We follow by exploring how nature-based interventions have been theorised. Thirdly, we consider the 'black boxes' of nature-based interventions; for this we recommend engaging with psychological theories regarding therapeutic processes to understand how participation influences wellbeing over time. We conclude with our reflections on the field, including implications for research, policy, and practice.

Nature-based interventions: Recognising an assemblage of activities, natural and social influences

Nature-based interventions are complex assemblages where several human and other-than-human actants come together, which can influence participants' experiences and their mental wellbeing. Studies have tended to report on the beneficial impacts to mental wellbeing at the time, relating these impacts to the core components of nature, meaningful activity, and social interaction (e.g., Harris, 2017; Pálsdóttir et al., 2018). Whilst there has been recognition that 'safe spaces' are co-created through the combination of the actants present at nature-based interventions, researchers often report their findings in relation to specific core components (e.g., Howarth, Lawler and Da Silva, 2021; Sudmann, 2018). As such we critically discuss the aspects separately to highlight their role in co-creating therapeutic experiences, rather than in combination as would be experienced in practice.

We begin with nature, where the contact with nature either at the environmental setting or through the involvement of specific animals is regarded as the connecting characteristic between different types of nature-based interventions (Gallis, 2013). Studies suggest a range of nature-full settings – from allotments (Biglin, 2020) to wetlands (Maund et al., 2019) – can contribute to improvements in participants' emotional wellbeing. The opportunity for participants to immerse themselves in nature-focused environments outside their everyday experience – and contrasting to their previous experience of clinical settings (Cacciatore, Gorman and Thieleman, 2020) – is reported as an important factor in enabling change, particularly where environments provide disconnection from technology, and moments of awe and reflection (Conlon et al., 2018). For example, Fernee et al.'s (2019) research involving 16-18-year-olds with a mental health diagnosis, at a wilderness therapy intervention in Norway, demonstrated that participants were empowered to change via entering into an unknown and challenging wilderness environment. Within this environment, participants reported improvements in their mood and wellbeing. Participants also reported reduced feelings of stress and pressures when actively moving through or by being in the wilderness.

Fostering safe and supportive environments for nature-based interventions is also important. Pálsdóttir et al. (2018) explore the factors involved in providing a supportive environment at the Alnarp rehabilitation garden in Sweden. Participants with a stress-related illness attended the garden for a 12-week rehabilitation programme involving group therapy. An important aspect was the provision of refuge with vegetation; participants felt safe where hedges and planting provided shelter, but these spaces needed to also provide a view of the garden and escape routes, in case other participants came too close. In these locations, also noted as being serene and rich in species, participants felt able to release and be with their emotions. Adevi and Lieberg (2012) propose, based on their research with caregivers at Alnarp, that participants' sensory impression of their chosen spaces supports their healing process as aspects of the space 'receive' their current mood. These interactions with specific spaces provide participants with an uncomplicated relationship, which develops into a place attachment providing meaning and positively impacting their stress recovery process. Collins, Avey and Lekkas (2016) similarly note the importance of safe places where people with mental health problems can relate to others on their own terms and find spaces that are private and calm. Such places can be considered to offer 'affective sanctuary' through providing a contained calming space that offers opportunities for supportive encounters with other people, as well as for personal reflection (Butterfield and Martin, 2016).

Environmental settings are also multi-sensory, influencing how individuals perceive, relate, and make sense of them (Bell, Hickman and Houghton, 2023). Gorman (2017a) considers smell at care farms, reporting how the different smells of wood helped engage participants in a wood carving exercise. Smells also influenced participants' preferences regarding where to work and socialise, choosing to be away from particularly strong smells: for some participants, the smells of the farm were overwhelmingly off-putting, preventing engagement altogether. Meanwhile, Cérwen, Pedersen and Pálsdóttir (2016) at a rehabilitation garden, found sounds of nature were reported by participants as having a soothing effect and stimulated memories of past enjoyable activities and important others. These natural sounds were often referred to as quiet and silent by participants despite the presence of noise.

Animals have been considered a key source of social connection. For example, Gorman's (2017b; 2017c) study of care farms describes how participants felt welcomed by the animals, forming emotional bonds with them, and feeling as if the animals remembered them through their repeated visits, creating a sense of belonging. This promoted acts of nurturing, development of familiar and secure spaces, and facilitated social interaction with fellow participants. Additionally, the animals broke down barriers between participants and visitors to the site, where the participants could show their knowledge and skills through telling the stories of the animals. Meanwhile, Cacciatore, Gorman and Thieleman (2020a) found that being amongst animals provided participants with spaces of reflection, emotional regulation, and connection. For some, animals formed the entry-point to accessing the care farm, as understanding the farm as a site of sanctuary for rescued animals helped to position the farm as a site of safety for participants. However, the presence of animals may not always be conducive to a therapeutic encounter, for example, when phobias shape someone's engagement (Gorman, 2017b).

In addition to working with animals, nature-based intervention activities can be as varied as woodland crafts (O'Brien, 2018), gardening (Milligan, Gatrell and Bingley, 2004), and group exercise (Paddon, 2020). These activities provide a regular structure, which Pitt (2014) found to create a sense of flow and relax the body. Activities can also support participants' wellbeing by providing opportunities to learn new skills and through being trusted to practise this new learning in a working environment. For example, Rotheram, McGarrol and Watkins (2017) found that participants with a learning disability at a care farm experienced improved emotional wellbeing through developing confidence and a sense of purpose by realising their abilities and being given responsibility.

O'Brien (2018) reports the role of facilitators in shaping activities to suit participants as an important factor in engaging participants. The attitude and behaviours of facilitators influences the space the activities take place in: through non-judgmental, flexible, supportive and encouraging approaches, a safe and inclusive space is created, where participants are supported at their pace to try new experiences (Crowther, 2019; O'Brien, 2018). Kogstad et al. (2014) highlight the importance of the facilitator in enabling changes in participants' understanding of their self, their confidence, and the development of skills allowing them to return to school or employment. However, facilitation can also negatively affect how participants engage with nature. For example, von Benzon (2017) reports how facilitators' perception of the vulnerability of learning disabled young people within natural spaces limited their independence.

Engagement with fellow participants over shared experiences can create a sense of community. Sudmann's (2018) research at a care farm, which included equine-assisted therapy for drug users, reports the significance of participants learning to ride together and sharing their riding experiences with others. An inclusive community, fostered as much through mundane conversation as riding, enabled participants to return after a relapse. Meanwhile, Rotheram, McGarrol and Watkins' (2017) study found participants with a learning disability at a care farm made new friendships, providing supportive and meaningful interactions, and producing a space of inclusion. These friendships were an important factor in continuing attendance. Harris (2017) saw friendships extending outside the researched intervention, with participants meeting up with one another away from the site.

As we have shown, a broad evidence base has been developed regarding the efficiency of nature-based interventions for maintaining and enhancing participants' short-term mental wellbeing. This evidence base provides justification for including a range of nature-based prescriptions to support and improve people's mental health (Mughal et al., 2022). However, social prescribing can shift responsibility onto the facilitators of interventions to be sufficiently skilled in providing therapeutic environments and the participants to self-manage their health (Calderón-Larrañaga et al., 2022). Yet, the majority of research studies have neglected to explore critically the role of these two key actants. This includes exploring the role of the individual and relational qualities involved in providing affective facilitation, and understanding participants' encounters as situated within their biography. This is alongside limited follow-up studies to understand how participants' wellbeing is maintained and enhanced beyond the nature-based intervention across the life course. The shortage of research in these areas has implications for how, how long, and to whom, different nature-based interventions are prescribed.

Nature-based interventions: Theorising facilitated health-place interactions

Researchers of nature-based interventions have applied several theoretical frameworks to understand how nature-based interventions work to co-create beneficial therapeutic experiences for participants. Two dominant approaches are Attention Restoration Theory (ART), which propose natural environments as spaces of cognitive restoration (Kaplan and Kaplan, 1989) and therapeutic landscapes that consider the social, cultural, symbolic, and environmental facets to people's therapeutic engagements with places (Gesler, 1992). ART has commonly been used by researchers as a framework to explain people's beneficial experiences at nature-based interventions, for example, during green exercise, at gardens, and in forest therapy (Han, 2021; Pálsdóttir et al., 2018; Sonntag-Ostrom et al., 2015). In ART, the improvements in participants' mental wellbeing due to being active in natural environments are attributed to participants' contact with nature rather than how participants shape a place through their embodied engagements with the activities and the space (Pitt, 2014). Similar criticisms might be levied at Wilson's (1984) biophilia hypothesis, which proposes humans have an innate emotional affiliation with other species, natural landscapes/habitats due to evolving adaptive responses within these environments during human evolution. This assumed universal relationship underpins the concept of 'a dose of nature' – that engaging with nature is unequivocally good for people's health, especially at a particular intensity, duration, and frequency. However, these suggestions are based on research which standardises people and their practices. This standardisation risks excluding the variety of ways people embody, relate to, and conceptualise nature, as certain types of interactions with nature are normalised (Bell et al., 2019).

By contrast, Gesler (1992) proposed therapeutic landscapes as a concept to examine the interactions between the environmental, social, and symbolic aspects of a place in promoting healing. Since then, therapeutic landscapes have become a popular concept to explore the interactions that occur at nature-based interventions, including: care farms (Gorman, 2017a; Kaley, Hatton and Milligan, 2019); gardens (Howarth, Lawler and Da Silva, 2021; Milligan, Gatrell and Bingley, 2004); therapeutic camping programmes (Dunkley, 2009); and walking groups (Paddon, 2020). Gesler's initial focus on places that had a reputation for healing, particularly extraordinary places and events – including national parks (Palka, 1999) and pilgrimages (Gesler, 1996) – led to critiques of the concept. Critiques also included Gesler's focus on short-term experiences rather than how connection to place supports long-term health and wellbeing (English, Wilson and Keller-Olaman, 2008). Also critiqued was the idea that through the presence of particular phenomena, certain places can be framed as intrinsically therapeutic, equating presence within these places as sufficient for therapeutic benefits (Conradson, 2005). The concern here centres on the identification of places with certain attributes as automatically supportive of wellbeing. This idea was effectively critiqued by Milligan and Bingley's (2007) research regarding young people and woodlands. The authors demonstrated that natural spaces are not always therapeutic, as environmental experience is mediated by a person's past experience and by their understanding of cultural representations of that place. Thus, the benefits of a particular place or environment are not universal, but rather a product of the way in which the space is perceived and engaged with by each person (Conradson, 2005).

In addition to the value of past experience and cultural representation, Dunkley's (2009) study of youths at a therapeutic camping programme foregrounds activities as formative for individual relationships to place, as well as their understanding and view of their self. Dunkley (2009) proposed 'taskscapes', where meaning occurs through participants' engagement with place-based activities. Here the meaning ascribed to the place is influenced by the timing and quality of the engagement, and so is subject to ongoing negotiation. The dynamism of meaning-making within natural places and how this influences a sense of self is supported by von Benzon's (2018) research with learning disabled young people, exploring their perceptions and experiences of nature. Von Benzon (2018) reports that through 'doing', the young people engaged with different environmental settings to develop free play, involving their imagination, the environmental setting, and their social context to co-produce environmental affordances that provide opportunities to engage. The provision of these opportunities occurs through multiple relational factors, which assemble an encounter, whereby the therapeutic value is co-produced between the participant and the social interaction, activities, and environment. This emphasis on relational understandings is a strength of therapeutic landscapes and supports researchers' engagement with a vast range of individual place-based practices in understanding the co-creation of personal affective encounters. The use of mixed methodologies can support researchers to work with marginalised communities, producing rich data that can help explain why and how places become therapeutic for different people at different times (Bell et al., 2018; Foley 2020).

By contrast, the 'dose of nature' concept risks embedding a reductionist approach to nature-health encounters (Bell et al., 2019), whereby nature is engaged with for a fixed duration on a set number of occasions and with specific activity types and intensity to deliver the required health benefits (Barton and Pretty, 2010; Shanahan et al., 2015). The concept of a dose of nature is viewed as providing a cost-effective tool in improving people's wellbeing and as a therapy with no apparent side effects. However, defining an appropriate dose of nature is challenging due to the range of influences on a person's nature preferences, including: cultural (perception of nature, exercise preferences); socio-economic (access to and availability of natural spaces); and individual (age, gender, health, ethnicity) (Shanahan et al., 2015). Relational dynamics in the more-than-human encounters between humans and nature – including how nature is conceptualised, embodied, and experienced – are central to wellbeing outcomes. Nevertheless, the concept is still pursued as a means to provide public recommendations regarding the benefits of engaging with nature, whilst simplifying the complexities of such engagements (Shanahan et al., 2015).

Black boxes: Long-term wellbeing and therapeutic processes

As we have shown, there has been a focus on the short-term impacts of participating in nature-based interventions on recovery and respite, rather than considering them as spaces of transformation with longer-term influences on participants' wellbeing. However, the limited follow-up studies conducted have found that positive wellbeing changes occurring during nature-based interventions can continue post attendance. In wilderness therapy, Roberts et al. (2017) found that the improvements in mental wellbeing (reduced anxiety, depression, and stress) for the young adult participants were maintained 18 months later. One-year follow-ups of participants attending rehabilitation gardens also report that the positive changes, which occurred during the nature-based intervention, were sustained a year later. These included: reductions in GP visits and long-term sick leave (Corazon et al., 2018); reductions in stress; improved social interactions; increased contact with nature and creative activities (Pálsdóttir, Grahn and Persson, 2014); and overall improved psychological wellbeing and decreased burnout (Stigsdotter et al., 2018).

This focus on the short-term has also meant that whilst the affective characteristics of nature-based interventions have been described and attributed to improvements in participants' wellbeing, less attention has been turned to how nature-based interventions co-create these beneficial effects. To consider both aspects, we recommend engaging with psychological theories regarding therapeutic processes to understand the therapeutic processes involved at nature-based interventions and how these can go beyond in-the-moment respite and recovery to co-create transformational experiences. A recent follow-up study by Fernee et al. (2021) concerning wilderness therapy, suggests a supportive psychosocial environment, alongside time spent in nature, may facilitate shifts in participants' awareness and acceptance of their selves and situations, promoting their agency and exportation of self towards fulfilling their potential. To identify long-term effects of nature-based interventions requires understanding how wellbeing is co-created as a relational and sensory process, and why specific kinds of relating shape long-term influences on a person's wellbeing. As such, future research needs to incorporate two key actants of nature-based interventions that are largely missing from the literature: facilitators and participants. Fernee et al.'s (2021) study does consider the role of participants in co-creating their experiences and in maintaining and enhancing the benefits to their mental wellbeing 12 months later. The authors report that participants experienced improved mood, emotional regulation, and increased social interactions, as well as being able to adapt nature-based strategies to manage stress. Fernee et al. (2021) propose this is due to participants developing greater autonomy and agency, which occurs due to improvements in their self-awareness and acceptance of self. The follow-up interviews suggest most of the participants have continued this self-growth and have been able to sustain the alternative narratives they had developed. This suggests that the participants have both engaged with a supportive psychosocial environment at the wilderness therapy and been supported to continue their own personal growth as they define it.

How people are related to influences the therapeutic effect of a place and the potential for this influence to continue into a person's daily life. Kaley, Hatton and Milligan's (2019) research on the influence of the care farm experience on participants' daily lives reports that fixed boundaries between the care farm and participants' everyday lives – for example, where the care farm was viewed as a retreat from challenging circumstances – reduced the flow of wellbeing gains beyond the care farm itself. Kaley, Hatton and Milligan (2019) argue that a person's wider socio-environmental networks need to be considered when exploring the therapeutic potential of nature-based interventions. This relates to Harper et al.'s (2007) proposal, based on their study of wilderness therapy, that to maintain positive mental health and behavioural outcomes requires supportive transitions and aftercare, as well as the involvement of the family. The authors identified this as requiring further research.

To further understand the process of transformative change, one valuable source of explanation may lie in Carl Rogers' (1951; 1957) conceptualisations of the person and the therapeutic relationship, which informs person-centred psychotherapy. Harrod, Von Benzon and Limmer (2023) highlight the importance of the relational dynamics involving the facilitators and participants at nature-based interventions in co-creating long-term changes in participants' sense of self, actions, and emotional regulation. These are key actants who have been largely missing from the literature. The authors draw on person-centred psychotherapy as an explanation for these changes. This work suggests that the relational environments a person is part of can facilitate a person to develop trust in their own feelings and thoughts or to defer to others and become reliant on looking for validation from others, at the expense of relying on their own judgement (Sanders, 2007). In supportive environments, people develop a sense of security in their own choices based on their perception of the world, helping them to flourish (Mearns and Cooper, 2018). However, in unsupportive environments people become estranged from their own appraisals of their experience, denying and distorting them to fit the judgements of others (Sanders, 2007). This leads to psychological distress. Whilst an incongruent identity may become fixed, it is possible for it to loosen and for shifts to occur towards a more authentic sense of self, within unthreatening relationships. Rogers (1957) proposed these co-created therapeutic relationships are experienced by the client as authentic, empathic, and non-judgemental, whereby the client experiences a sense of safety and a way of relating that does not reject them but accepts them for who they are (Mearns and Cooper, 2018). The role of non-judgemental and empathic encounters has been recognised as important in the formation of affective sanctuaries (Parry and Glover, 2010) – Rogers' theory provides an explanation for why these encounters are effective. Through drawing on person-centred psychotherapy to understand nature-based interventions, Harrod, Von Benzon and Limmer (2023) bring to the fore the agency of facilitators and participants in understanding how therapeutic encounters occur and a depth of understanding to how relationships facilitate or hinder a person's wellbeing.

To understand the long-term effects of participating at nature-based interventions requires researching how wellbeing is co-created as a relational and sensory process and why specific kinds of relating support and develop a person's wellbeing. This requires consideration of participants as situated in their on-going biography and the influence of wider socio-environmental relations on supporting or hindering participants' long-term wellbeing. This relates to Bell et al.'s (2014) call to consider the role of individual and relational agency in understanding how people relate to and engage with green spaces for their wellbeing, within the context of their everyday lives. Consequently, we propose a shift from focusing on the core components of nature, activities, and social interaction and their role in providing short-term beneficial influences on participants' mental wellbeing, to exploring the varied ways people relate to one another and the influence of these on a person's ongoing maintenance and enhancement of their mental health.

Reflections

In this chapter we have outlined the state of research concerning nature-based interventions and their influence on participants' mental health. We have highlighted a developing evidence-base regarding the role of the core components of nature, activities, and social interaction in co-creating short-term benefits to participants' mental wellbeing. Due to the complexity of nature-based interventions we have also recognised the importance of therapeutic landscapes as a helpful concept for exploring the relations between people, the environmental, cultural, and symbolic aspects of a place in promoting a sense of being well. However, there are still unanswered questions regarding how participating at nature-based interventions influences participants' wellbeing at the time, as well as how long-term wellbeing is co-created through the participation. Future research that incorporates two key actants of nature-based interventions: facilitators and participants, is required to explore the role of relational dynamics in the co-creation of enabling places and how beneficial effects that are co-created at interventions are supported or hindered by wider socio-environment networks.

Creative research approaches may be useful in gaining such insights in future work. Creative methods may: facilitate the sharing and expression of experiences that are sensitive or may not be easily verbalised (Bagnoli, 2009); encourage a range of communication, enabling 'quiet' voices to be heard (Trell and Van Hoven, 2010); and challenge power relations by being creative together (Hawkins, 2019). For example, life mapping supports participants to explore in-depth their lifecourse, situating significant influences within their biographies (Worth, 2011). Meanwhile, poetry can enable participants to connect to their emotions and imagination in response to research questions (Bishop and Willis, 2014). Such approaches could help diversify the people involved in nature-based interventions research and enrich researchers' understanding of what it means to different people to become well and the salient aspects of these complex assemblages. Continuing to develop our understanding of how nature-based interventions work and influence wellbeing over time will enhance theoretical conceptualisations of enabling people-place encounters, while also supporting practices and policies that shape nature-based interventions, for example, developing pedagogies and training for facilitators. With the increasing drive to construct a specific 'healthy dose of nature', it is important to recognise that nature-based interventions appear to work best when they empower participants to find their own dose at their own pace.

References

Adevi, A. A. & Lieberg, M. (2012). Stress rehabilitation through garden therapy: A caregiver perspective on factors considered most essential to the recovery process. *Urban Forestry & Urban Greening*, 11(1), pp. 51–58.

Bagnoli, A. (2009). Beyond the standard interview: The use of graphic elicitation and arts-based methods. *Qualitative Research*, 9(5), pp. 547–570.

Barton, J. & Pretty, J. (2010). What is the best dose of nature and green exercise for improving mental health? A multi-study analysis. *Environmental Science & Technology*, 44(10), pp. 3947–3955.

Bell, S. L., Foley, R., Houghton, F., Maddrell, A. & Williams, A. M. (2018). From therapeutic landscapes to healthy spaces, places and practices: A scoping review. *Social Science & Medicine*, 196, pp. 123–130.

Bell, S. L., Hickman, C. & Houghton, F. (2023). From therapeutic landscape to therapeutic 'sensescape' experiences with nature? A scoping review. *Wellbeing, Space and Society*, 4, 100126.

Bell, S. L., Leyshon, C., Foley, R. & Kearns, R. A. (2019). The "healthy dose" of nature: A cautionary tale. *Geography Compass*, 13(1), e12415.

Bell, S. L., Phoenix, C., Lovell, R. & Wheeler, B. W. (2014). Green space, health and wellbeing: Making space for individual agency. *Health Place*, 30, pp. 287–292.

Biglin, J. (2020). Embodied and sensory experiences of therapeutic space: Refugee place-making within an urban allotment. *Health & Place*, 62, 102309.

Bishop, E. & Willis, K. (2014). 'Hope is that fiery feeling': Using poetry as data to explore the meanings of hope for young people. *Forum, Qualitative Social Research*, 15(1).

Bragg, R. & Atkins, G. (2016). *A review of nature-based interventions for mental health care (NECR204)*. Natural England.

Butterfield, A. & Martin, D. (2016). Affective sanctuaries: Understanding Maggie's as therapeutic landscapes. *Landscape Research*, 41(6), pp. 695–706.

Cacciatore, J., Gorman, R. & Thieleman, K. (2020). Evaluating care farming as a means to care for those in trauma and grief. *Health & Place*, 62, 102281.

Calderón-Larrañaga, S., Greenhalgh, T., Finer, S. & Clinch, M. (2022). What does the literature mean by social prescribing? A critical review using discourse analysis. *Sociology of Health and Illness*, 44(4-5), pp. 848–868.

Cérwen, G., Pedersen, E. & Pálsdóttir, A. M. (2016). The role of soundscape in nature-based rehabilitation: A patient perspective. *International Journal of Environmental Research and Public Health*, 13(12), 1229.

Collins, J., Avey, S. & Lekkas, P. (2016). Lost landscapes of healing: The decline of therapeutic mental health landscapes. *Landscape Research*, 41(6), pp. 664–677.

Conlon, C. M., Wilson, C. E., Gaffney, P. & Stoker, M. (2018). Wilderness therapy intervention with adolescents: Exploring the process of change. *Journal of Adventure Education and Outdoor Learning*, 18(4), pp. 353–366.

Conradson, D. (2005). Landscape, care and the relational self: Therapeutic encounters in rural England. *Health and Place*, 11(4), pp. 337–348.

Corazon, S. S., Nyed, P. K., Sidenius, U., Poulsen, D. V. & Stigsdotter, U. K. (2018). A long-term follow-up of the efficacy of nature-based therapy for adults suffering from stress-related illnesses on levels of healthcare consumption and sick-leave absence: A randomized controlled trial. *International Journal of Environmental Research and Public Health*, 15(1), 137.

Crowther, R. (2019). *Wellbeing and Self-Transformation in Natural Landscapes*. Switzerland: Palgrave Macmillan.

Dunkley, C. M. (2009). A therapeutic taskscape: Theorizing place-making, discipline and care at a camp for troubled youth. *Health & Place*, 15(1), pp. 88–96.

English, J., Wilson, K. & Keller-Olaman, S. (2008). Health, healing and recovery: Therapeutic landscapes and the everyday lives of breast cancer survivors. *Social Science and Medicine*, 67(1), pp. 68–78.

Fernee, C. R., Gabrielsen, L. E., Andersen, A. J. W. & Mesel, T. (2021). Emerging stories of self: Long-term outcomes of wilderness therapy in Norway. *Journal of adventure education and outdoor learning*, 21(1), pp. 67–81.

Fernee, C. R., Mesel, T., Andersen, A. J. W. & Gabrielsen, L. E. (2019). Therapy the natural way: A realist exploration of the wilderness therapy treatment process in adolescent mental health care in Norway. *Qualitative Health Research*, 29(9), pp. 1358–1377.

Foley, R. (2020). Therapeutic Landscapes. In: A. Kobayashi, ed., *International Encyclopedia of Human Geography*. 2nd Edition. Oxford: Elsevier.

Gallis, C. (2013). What is Green Care? Introduction, History, and Origins. In: C. Gallis, C., ed., *Green Care: For Human Therapy, Social Innovation, Rural Economy, and Education*. New York: Nova Science.

Gesler, W. (1996). Lourdes: healing in a place of pilgrimage. *Health & Place*, 2(2), pp. 95–105.

Gesler, W. M. (1992). Therapeutic landscapes: Medical issues in light of the new cultural geography. *Social Science & Medicine*, 34(7), pp. 735–746.

Gorman, R. (2017a). Smelling therapeutic landscapes: Embodied encounters within spaces of care farming. *Health & Place*, 47, pp. 22–28.

Gorman, R. (2017b). Therapeutic landscapes and non-human animals: The roles and contested positions of animals within care farming assemblages. *Social & Cultural Geography*, 18(3), pp. 315–335.

Gorman, R. (2017c). Thinking critically about health and human-animal relations: Therapeutic affect within spaces of care farming. *Social Science & Medicine*, 231, pp. 6–12.

Han, K.-T. (2021). Effects of three levels of green exercise, physical and social environments, personality traits, physical activity, and engagement with nature on emotions and attention. *Sustainability (Basel, Switzerland)*, 13(5), 2686.

Harper, N. J., Russell, K. C., Cooley, R. & Cupples, J. (2007). Catherine Freer wilderness therapy expeditions: An exploratory case study of adolescent wilderness therapy, family functioning, and the maintenance of change. *Child & Youth Care Forum*, 36(2-3), pp. 111–129.

Harris, H. (2017). The social dimensions of therapeutic horticulture. *Health & Social Care in the Community*, 25(4), pp. 1328–1336.

Harrod, A., Von Benzon, N. & Limmer, M. (2023). 'It's probably more about the people': For a person-centred approach to understanding benefits of nature-based interventions. *Area* 00, pp. 1–9. https://doi.org/10.1111/area.12867.

Hawkins, H. (2019). Geography's creative (re)turn: Toward a critical framework. *Progress in Human Geography*, 43(6), pp. 963–984.

Howarth, M., Lawler, C. & Da Silva, A. (2021). Creating a transformative space for change: A qualitative evaluation of the RHS Wellbeing Programme for people with long term conditions. *Health & Place*, 71, 102654.

Kaley, A., Hatton, C. & Milligan, C. (2019). Therapeutic spaces of care farming: Transformative or ameliorating? *Social Science & Medicine*, 227, pp. 10–20.

Kaplan, R. & Kaplan, S. (1989). *The experience of nature: A psychological perspective*. Cambridge, New York: Cambridge University Press.

Keniger, L. E., Gaston, K. J., Irvine, K. N. & Fuller, R. A. (2013). What are the benefits of interacting with nature? *International Journal of Environmental Research and Public Health*, 10(3), pp. 913–935.

Killaspy, H. (2006). From the asylum to community care: Learning from experience. *British Medical Bulletin*, 79-80(1), pp. 245–258.

Kogstad, R. E., Agdal, R. & Hopfenbeck, M. S. (2014). Narratives of natural recovery: Youth experience of social inclusion through green care. *International Journal of Environmental Research and Public Health*, 11(6), pp. 6052–6068.

Maund, P. R., Irvine, K. N., Reeves, J., Strong, E., Cromie, R., Dallimer, M. & Davies, Z. G. (2019). Wetlands for wellbeing: Piloting a nature-based health intervention for the management of anxiety and depression. *International Journal of Environmental Research and Public Health*, 16(22), 4413.

Mearns, D. & Cooper, M. (2018). *Working at relational depth in counselling and psychotherapy*. 2nd Edition. UK: Sage Publications.

Milligan, C. & Bingley, A. (2007). Restorative places or scary spaces? The impact of woodland on the mental well-being of young adults. *Health and Place*, 13(4), pp. 799–811.

Milligan, C., Gatrell, A. & Bingley, A. (2004). 'Cultivating health': Therapeutic landscapes and older people in northern England. *Social Science & Medicine*, 58(9), pp. 1781–1793.

Mughal, R., Seers, H., Polley, M., Sabey, A. & Chatterjee, H. J. (2022). *How the natural environment can support health and wellbeing through social prescribing*. England: National Academy for Social Prescribing.

NHS England. (2020). *Social prescribing and community-based support: Summary guide*. England: NHS England.

O'Brien, L. (2018). Engaging with and shaping nature: A nature-based intervention for those with mental health and behavioural problems at the Westonbirt Arboretum in England. *International Journal of Environmental Research and Public Health*, 15(10), 2214.

Paddon, L. I. (2020). Therapeutic or detrimental mobilities? Walking groups for older adults. *Health and Place*, 63, 102346.

Palka, E. (1999). Accessible Wilderness as a Therapeutic Landscape: Experiencing the Nature of Denali National Park, Alaska. In: A. Williams, ed., *Therapeutic Landscapes: the Dynamic Between Place and wellness*. America: University Press of America.

Parry, D. C., & Glover, T. D. (2010). Dignity, hope, and transcendence: Gilda's Club as complementary care for cancer survivors. *Journal of Leisure Research*, 42, pp. 347–364.

Pitt, H. (2014) Therapeutic experiences of community gardens: Putting flow in its place. *Health and Place*, 27, pp. 84–91.

Pálsdóttir, A. M., Grahn, P. & Persson, D. (2014). Changes in experienced value of everyday occupations after nature-based vocational rehabilitation. *Scandinavian Journal of Occupational Therapy*, 21(1), pp. 58–68.

Pálsdóttir, A. M., Stigsdotter, U. K., Persson, D., Thorpert, P. & Grahn, P. (2018). The qualities of natural environments that support the rehabilitation process of individuals with stress-related mental disorder in nature-based rehabilitation. *Urban Forestry & Urban Greening, 29*, pp. 312–321.

Roberts, S. D., Stroud, D., Hoag, M. J. & Massey, K. E. (2017). Outdoor behavioral health care: A longitudinal assessment of young adult outcomes. *Journal of Counseling and Development, 95*(1), pp. 45–55.

Robinson, J. M., Jorgensen, A., Cameron, R. & Brindley, P. (2020). Let nature be thy medicine: A socioecological exploration of green prescribing in the UK. *International Journal of Environmental Research and Public Health, 17*(10), 3460.

Rogers, C. R. (1951). *Client-centered therapy: Its current practice, implications and theory.* London: Constable.

Rogers, C. R. (1957). The necessary and sufficient conditions of therapeutic personality change. *Journal of Consulting Psychology, 21*(2), pp. 95–103.

Rotheram, S., McGarrol, S. & Watkins, F. (2017). Care farms as a space of wellbeing for people with a learning disability in the United Kingdom. *Health and Place, 48*, pp. 123–131.

Sanders, P. (2007). Introduction to the Theory of Person-Centred Therapy. In: Cooper, M., O'Hara, M., Schmid, P. F. & Whyatt, G. (eds.) *The Handbook of Person-Centred Psychotherapy and Counselling.* Great Britain: Palgrave Macmillan.

Sempik, J. & Bragg, R. (2013). Green Care: Origins and Activities. In: C. Gallis, ed., *Green Care: For Human Therapy, Social innovation, Rural Economy, and Education.* New York: Nova Science Publishers.

Sempik, J., Hine, R. & Wilcox, D. (2010). *Green Care: A Conceptual Framework.* A report of the Working Group on the Health Benefits of Green Care, COST Action 866, Green Care in Agriculture. Loughborough: Centre for Child and Family Research.

Shanahan, D. F., Fuller, R. A., Bush, R., Lin, B. B. & Gaston, K. J. (2015). The health benefits of urban nature. How much do we need? *BioScience, 65*(5), pp. 476–485.

Sonntag-Ostrom, E., Stenlund, T., Nordin, M., Lundell, Y., Ahlgren, C., Fjellman-Wiklund, A., Jarvholm, L. S. & Dolling, A. (2015). "Nature's effect on my mind" – Patients' qualitative experiences of a forest-based rehabilitation programme. *Urban Forestry & Urban Greening, 14*(3), pp. 607–614.

Stigsdotter, U. K., Corazon, S. S., Sidenius, U., Nyed, P. K., Larsen, H. B. & Fjorback, L. O. (2018). Efficacy of nature-based therapy for individuals with stress-related illnesses: Randomised controlled trial. *British Journal of Psychiatry, 213*(1), pp. 404–411.

Sudmann, T. T. (2018). Communitas and Friluftsliv: Equine-facilitated activities for drug users. *Community Development Journal, 53*(3), pp. 556–573.

Trell, E.-M. & Van Hoven, B. (2010). Making sense of place: Exploring creative and active research methods with young people. *Fennia, 188*(1), pp. 91–104.

Van Den Berg, A. E. (2017). From green space to green prescriptions: Challenges and opportunities for research and practice. *Frontiers in Psychology, 8*, pp. 1–4.

Von Benzon, N. (2017). Unruly children in unbounded spaces: School-based nature experiences for urban learning disabled young people in Greater Manchester, UK. *Journal of Rural Studies, 51*, pp. 240–250.

Von Benzon, N. (2018). Discussing Nature, 'Doing' Nature: For an emancipatory approach to conceptualizing young people's access to outdoor green space. *Geoforum, 93*, pp. 79–86.

Wilson, E. O. (1984). *Biophilia: The human bond with other species.* Cambridge, USA: Harvard University Press.

Worth, N. (2011). Evaluating life maps as a versatile method for lifecourse geographies: Life maps as a method for lifecourse geographies. *Area, 43*(4), pp. 405–412.

10 Seeking asylum, 'therapeutic landscapes', agency and lived citizenship

Josephine Biglin

Introduction

The concept, therapeutic landscapes, refers to where 'physical and built environments, social conditions and human perceptions combine to produce an atmosphere which is conducive of healing' (Gesler, 1996, p. 96). Since the term's inception, the therapeutic landscapes concept has gained momentum as a key framework to explore the links between health and place. Initially, the term was used to explore the literal relationship between health and place, by focusing on places with extraordinary healing potential, for example, hot springs (Gesler, 1998). However, the potential therapeutic value of encounters with everyday space was soon identified. Green and blue spaces dominate much of the therapeutic landscape's literature. The benefits of interactions within local parks, community green and grow spaces, and spending time in or near forests, rivers, lakes and the sea have all been documented as potentially beneficial for wellbeing, in many cases amongst people experiencing specific physical and/or mental health challenges (Bell et al., 2018).

Place philosophy has demonstrated that places are not fixed sites but rather place is an 'event' (Cresswell, 2004, p. 39); places not only *are* but they *happen* through the day-to-day experiences of those who create them (Casey, 1997). Thus, whilst therapeutic spaces were initially treated as possessing inherently therapeutic qualities, evidence suggests that places may be therapeutic for some, but stress inducing for others (see for example, Milligan and Bingley, 2007; Milligan et al. 2004) leading to an understanding of the fundamental relational aspect of the concept. A therapeutic experience within place is never guaranteed because places do not hold inherent qualities, but wellbeing experiences happen through interactions with place whether that be sociocultural, material, affective or sensuous, or a complex combination of all of these. There is limited literature on asylum seekers and refugees' experiences of therapeutic landscapes. However, the literature that does exist finds places of worship and green spaces, such as local parks and allotments, to be key sites in creating anchors in new places; reducing social isolation and generating a sense of community and belonging, all of which improve wellbeing (see Agyekum and Newbold, 2016; Biglin, 2020; 2021a; Ermansons et al., 2023; Rishbeth et al., 2019; Sampson and Gifford, 2010).

Although it is established that therapeutic landscapes are produced by the people who engage with these spaces, there has been minimal discussion and observation of asylum seekers and refugees' production of therapeutic space relying on a form of agency that evades dominant representations of asylum seekers as agentless. For asylum seekers, agency has been linked to alternative forms of citizenship (see for example, Biglin,

DOI: 10.4324/9781003345725-11

2022; Erel et al., 2018; O'Neill, 2018). Citizenship is often understood as relating to formal rights and duties, however, alternative readings of citizenship explore the wider sociological meanings, encompassing participation and belonging as it is experienced and enacted within real-life everyday contexts (Lister, 2007; Isin, 2008; Erel, 2013; Kallio et al., 2020). This chapter brings together an exploration of therapeutic landscape experiences amongst refugee and asylum seekers with theories of lived citizenship (Lister, 2007).

The chapter is structured as follows: initially there is a brief outline of the social context asylum seekers find themselves in whilst in the UK and how this impacts on wellbeing. This is followed by the details of the research that informs the chapter. Then I will explore the links between therapeutic landscapes and theories of lived citizenship before finally turning to the question of where this leaves the therapeutic landscapes concept to conclude the chapter.

The wellbeing of asylum seekers in the UK: A hostile and racist environment

Refugees and people seeking asylum have higher rates of mental ill health than the general population, including anxiety, PTSD, psychosis and depression (Blackmore et al., 2020; Turrini et al., 2017). Pre-migration trauma of forced dispossession of land, war and climate disaster have a profound impact on mental wellbeing (Keller et al., 2017; WHO, 2021). Most people who experience forced displacement remain internally displaced or in neighbouring countries, however, many choose to make long and dangerous journeys to Europe and the UK. These, often traumatic, journeys can exacerbate existing mental health problems and contribute to new ones (Carlson and Sonne, 2018; WHO, 2021).

Experiences within postmigration contexts can further compromise mental health and wellbeing. In the UK and much of the West, securing and controlling borders have become a defining feature of contemporary states (Squires, 2009). A rise in nationalistic rhetoric across the globe in recent years means that those considered the 'anti-citizen' (migrants, racially, ethnically, religiously and sexually minoritised groups) are viewed as a threat to those who can claim an 'authentic' belonging to the nation state ('citizens') (May et al., 2020). Thus, citizenship, as an official category, is highly restrictive and selective, and life is made very difficult for those subject to immigration control.

Although hostility towards immigration predates this, the Immigration and Asylum Act 1999 was a turning point in the UK, as a number of asylum policies were introduced that increased 'restrictions, control and experimentation with various means of detention, dispersal and deterrence' (Darling, 2011, p. 264). This includes the introduction of the dispersal policy which involves the placement of asylum seekers on a no-choice basis into accommodation within designated 'dispersal areas' of the UK, which since 2012 has been contracted to private companies. In addition, the policy limits asylum seekers' access to welfare and the labour market. Hirschler (2021, p. 142) has explored the harmful physical and psychological impacts of living in privatised asylum dispersal accommodation and finds that poor housing quality with 'high levels of disrepair and unhygienic conditions' were identified as sources of anxiety and concern relating to physical and mental wellbeing. Evidence suggests that within dispersal systems people are forced to live with a chronic sense of fear, exclusion, powerlessness, insecurity, temporariness, and a highly controlled sense of liminality (O'Reilly, 2019). Darling (2022, p. 2–3) has powerfully argued that the dispersal policy represents a form of 'slow violence' that produces and sustains suffering and social abjection.

In 2012, what is commonly termed the Hostile Environment was introduced, signifying a new wave of discrimination against refugees and asylum seekers and those racialised as non-white. As both a medium and outcome of a range of policies implemented through the Immigration Acts 2014 and 2016, the Hostile Environment is encompassing of an attitude of unwelcomeness and suspicion of racialised migrants (Liberty, 2018). Those who can be identified as foreign, largely through non-whiteness, are assumed to be unlawful and must prove their status. Being forced to recount traumatic experiences to prove worthiness of protection has been shown to cause immense psychological harm (Good, 2011). The Refugee Council (2022) reports that people seeking asylum in the UK suffer from acute anxiety due to the complexity of the asylum process. The Hostile Environment is also characterised by a continued defunding of essential migrant services and increasing eligibility conditions for support that is available. Resources continue to be directed towards enforcement, detention and removal, as opposed to funding already strained asylum casework teams and other forms of welfare and care resources (Darling, 2016; Liberty, 2018), leaving vulnerable migrants with little access to support.

Debates over immigration and national identity continue to dominate politics, particularly the 'stop the boats' agenda of the current Conservative government, which plans to deport people to offshore detention centres and determine asylum cases based on entry route. Thus, continuing to expose vulnerable people to suffering. Moreover, asylum seekers and refugees have higher rates of destitution and thus are increasingly exposed to the ongoing cost of living crisis (Scottish Refugee Council, 2022).

Immigration and asylum policy has dire consequences for the mental and physical wellbeing of asylum seekers and refugees through pushing people to the margins of the margins (O'Neill, 2018), and exposing them to suffering. This section has provided a brief overview of the socio-political context that refugees and people seeking asylum in the UK might be seeking therapeutic respite from. The following section outlines the research that informs this chapter.

Research context: therapeutic landscapes for asylum seekers and refugees

This chapter draws on two projects conducted with asylum seekers and refugees in the UK. The first is an ethnography, carried out in 2017, of an urban allotment ran by a charitable organisation as an enrichment activity for refugees and people seeking asylum. The project used Sarah Pink's (2015) sensory and embodied ethnographic approaches to carry out research exploring participants' wellbeing within the allotment. Sensory ethnography as laid out by Pink (2015) involves incorporating the following three principles into the ethnographic observation: the serendipitous sensory learning of being there; the ethnographer as a sensory apprentice and joining others in embodied experiences, as well as probing sensory and embodied experiences within the interview (more details on this study can be found in Biglin, 2020). The second study is a photovoice project carried out in 2019 where over forty people who were currently seeking asylum or had refugee status took part. Photovoice is a creative participatory methodology developed by Wang and Burris (1997) where participants use photography to explore and represent their experiences of a research topic and then engage in group dialogue sessions. Participants used photography to represent their experiences of place, belonging and citizenship in the Greater Manchester area (more details on this study can be found in Biglin, 2021a; 2021b; 2022).

The findings from these two studies suggest that through participants' place-making activities they were seeking out and shaping therapeutic landscape experiences within a range of green and public urban spaces. These activities had the potential to improve wellbeing through tackling social isolation; transnational and local belonging; friendship and solidarity; and symbolic expressions of hope and justice. The following subsections evidence this and provide some examples.

Growing practices and produce from 'home': transnational belonging

All the participants in the allotment came from an agrarian background, such that attending the allotment was a way to engage in familiar activities. As well as the physical act of gardening, the food grown was found to be a key link between past and present selves (Biglin, 2020), illustrated in the following example:

> I saw the plant, the same plant was from my country, the plant was the same colour [...] I said my god look at that! Here in the allotment, it is most like home, the corn, the potato, apples, you know we have more types of apples in Africa, we have a really small one, but still I like to see an apple because it's just like the things we have back home.
>
> (Fred, quoted in Biglin, 2020)

Participants in the photovoice project also highlighted the significance of finding produce from former countries:

> And you find food from home, like the green veggies they sell, it's not like normal spinach that you get here, it's from home, and they also have this maize flour that we have at home and some other vegetables like the white sweet potato, those types of

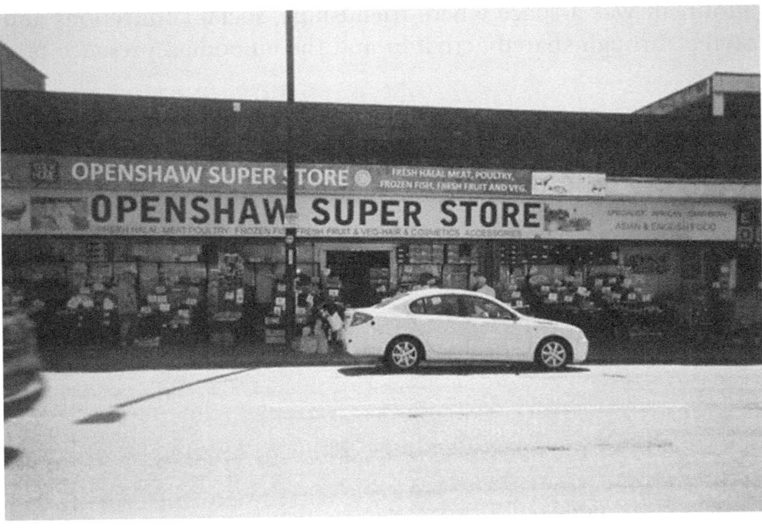

Figure 10.1 Photograph of a superstore taken by Gabrielle.

things. Even the way they cut the meats is like back home. It was a life saver for me. Because I have felt so alone but eating something familiar is so important.

(Gabrielle)

The participants demonstrated the joy and significance of finding or growing produce that is similar to what would be grown/eaten in their former countries. It was evident that familiar food had the potential to generate a sense of place and home when in new surroundings. A feeling of home is important to wellbeing, as Gabrielle highlighted, it reduces feelings of aloneness (see also Boccagni, 2017). Moreover, Biglin (2020) argues this to be a form of 'sensory nostalgia', that can create a healthy sense of continuity of the self, where positive perceptions of the past can foster a sense of meaning in the present. Furthermore, Oyangen (2009) has discussed the gustatory identity of immigrants and explains that putting something into our body is a potentially anxiety provoking activity. Cultural food system rules help to relieve this anxiety. A food system regulates how and what we eat. Allotment tending and cultural supermarkets gave the participants a way to make eating food in a new place familiar. The food norms and values of their former countries appeared to stay with them through symbolic reminders and transplantation of traditional growing, preparing and eating practices. Thus, growing food or finding food from former countries was a way in which transnational membership and belonging was sustained.

Green space: embodied presence and symbolism

Solace was sought in green space for several reasons. Some participants used plants to tell cathartic stories of displacement and replacement (see Biglin, 2020) and symbolism of hope for alternative futures was found within nature.

This is hope, a growing seedling, is a similarity with hopes. It can symbolise that I have hope for my future.

(Duaa, quoted in Biglin, 2022)

Furthermore, the allotment was a space where friendships, social connections and solidarity could be fostered through shared activities and the embodied presence of others (Biglin, 2020).

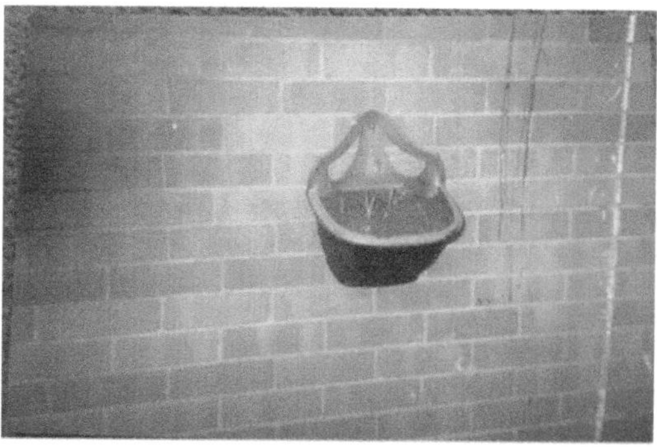

Figure 10.2 Photograph of a seedling taken by Duaa (Biglin, 2022).

I don't always like to talk, I can just do my watering, but it doesn't matter if I'm not talking to anyone, just being here with everyone means that I am not alone.

(Aster, quoted in Biglin, 2020)

There are all different languages here, we can't all speak the same language, and not everyone can speak English that well, so like I said we don't need to be talking all the time we can just be here.

(Solomon, quoted in Biglin, 2020)

These opportunities tackled social isolation and loneliness, which are common amongst asylum seekers and refugees (Lim, 2022). Green spaces, such as the allotment or local parks, were places where participants felt they were distracted from stress as they were moved to a more positive affective state, either through physical activity or simply through the fresh air offered. The following photograph shows this:

This park relaxes me like every time I was stressing, I would wake up in my accommodation and feel like I can't breathe, like everything is overwhelming me, I would go to this park and walk round, and it calms me. [...] It feels like the air is different here.

(Gabrielle, quoted in Biglin, 2021a)

The busyness of urban green spaces such as Piccadilly Gardens, a public green space in the centre of Manchester, was also highlighted as being important in reducing stress and social isolation.

Here I like because shopping, buses, café. When I am here, so busy all the time, all the people, all stresses are gone.

(Aleena)

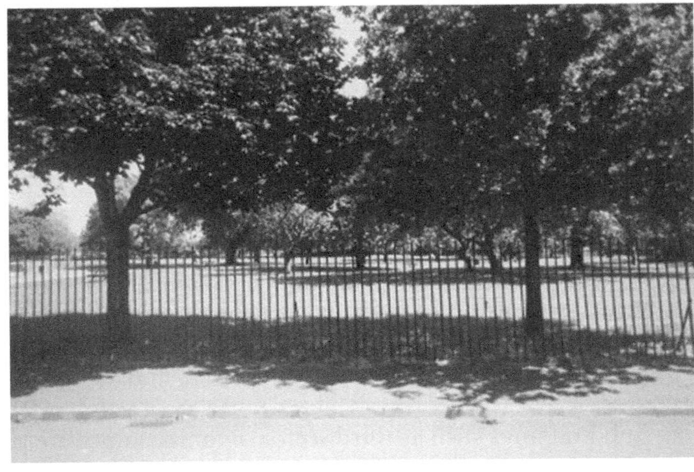

Figure 10.3 Photograph of a park taken by Gabrielle (Biglin, 2021a).

Yes, it is a place that can distract you from problems just for a while.

(Duaa)

(both quoted in Biglin, 2021a)

But Piccadilly Gardens was more than just a place to reduce stress. The environment there meant it was a hive of community activity that participants felt they could be a part of:

Piccadilly and open spaces like that, everyone is the same, we're just there to relax, we are there to enjoy the weather when it is like this, also it is entertaining. [...] And it is free, you can sit and relax on the grass, there is always music. And you know people are always friendly. I like Piccadilly, the water, the kids are playing, you can almost like forget where you are, and all of your problems, you can enjoy what is in front of you.

(Gabrielle, quoted in Biglin, 2021a)

In these examples participants highlight the ways in which engagement in urban green and public space has the potential to improve wellbeing through the symbolism that can be found within nature, but also where these spaces provide opportunities for social engagements and participation in the local community. Strang and Quinn (2019) have argued isolation undermines wellbeing as it results in a lack of emotional support and can create difficulties in accessing health services. Thus, these engagements with place that tackle isolation are key mitigators of poor wellbeing, as are community hub buildings, outlined in the following section.

Community hubs: identity and solidarity

There were also non-green spaces that were important for wellbeing such as libraries, third sector organisations and the church. The participants tended to find these places to be important sources of respite from exclusionary spaces such as immigration sign in centres, the job centre or the domestic space, and therefore have been theorised as 'third places' (see Biglin, 2021a). It is important to note, however, that this is not always the case as these places can be hierarchical and exclusionary for some individuals and groups. The following photograph is of Manchester Central Library:

In the house there can be no peace, I look after everybody, and I can be stressed by that too much sometimes. And you know I am refugee, and it is hard I have to go job centre and sign and do many things, but in the library, I am student and that's it.

(Hamza)

Here Hamza describes the way being in the library is a way to escape the stresses of home life and drop the refugee label in favour of being a student. Thus, the library, as a community hub, appears to be a safe space for identity forming, learning and self-expression. This reflects Brewster's (2014) argument that, for people with mental health challenges, the library is simultaneously familiar and welcoming, comforting and calming, and empowering.

Furthermore, community hub buildings such as third sector organisations were places that fostered a sense of local community, belonging and solidarity with others. For example, Adam discussed the third sector organisation he visited:

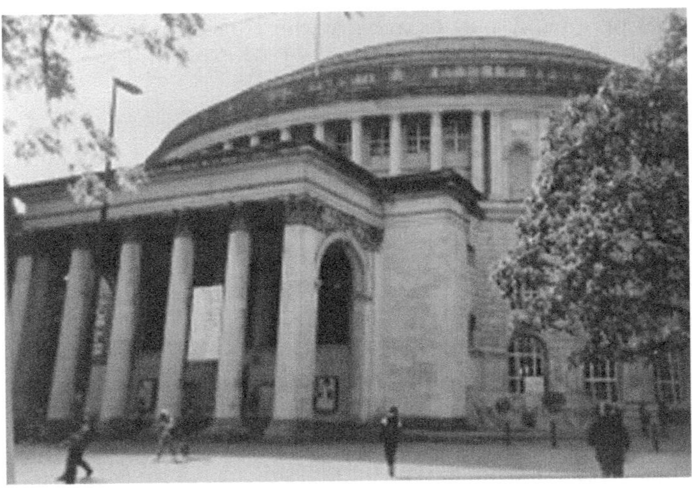

Figure 10.4 Photograph of the library taken by Hamza (Biglin, 2022).

You know here we make food, and it means something like this place is so friendly. Here you can see people from all other communities, and you can get a lot of different type of support here. I have spent a lot of time in this place. It is community with other people here, relationships with other communities. So, it is meaningful.

(Adam)

Here Adam highlights the importance of friendship and a local sense of belonging, to the community, but also different communities that come together within one place to offer support and solidarity.

In this section I have documented an array of different place-making activities that participants in the two studies were engaging in, and the varying ways in which they create therapeutic landscape experiences (Biglin, 2020; 2021a). What is key amongst all participants' interactions with place is the participants' agency in seeking out and shaping these spaces as therapeutic. This is discussed in the following section.

'Therapeutic landscapes', agency and lived citizenship

It is well established in the therapeutic landscapes literature that places do not hold inherent qualities, but rather are produced and sought out through the place-making activities of those seeking the therapeutic encounter (Biglin, 2020; Sampson and Gifford, 2010). As the excerpts detailed above show, a therapeutic experience within place is enabled by a complex assemblage of sociocultural-material-affective-sensuous experience. Crucially, Bell et al. (2014) have pointed out, on the topic of green space use and wellbeing, that we cannot assume people will always use green space for wellbeing purposes. In fact, we must consider more subtle aspects of individual agency in use patterns and well-being effects. People seek out and engage with place for wellbeing in relation to shifting life circumstances and personal identities; past place experiences; social relationships and adaptive agency, whereby people shift their actions and interactions with place to generate the best possible wellbeing outcomes (Bell et al., 2014). Thus, the production of therapeutic landscapes relies on agentic participation within space by those seeking the therapeutic encounter. I argue that for asylum seekers and refugees, this agency can be understood through the lens of lived citizenship.

Citizenship, as an official category, is mainly understood to represent formal rights and duties, and is highly selective, restrictive and racialised. Under official definitions of citizenship, refugees and asylum seekers will always be considered the 'Other'. However, official definitions of citizenship tend to ignore the participation in domestic, informal and private spaces that is often engaged in by women and marginalised groups (Lister, 2007; 2008). Therefore, alternative readings of citizenship highlight where those excluded from formal citizenship processes enact and perform citizenship regardless of status. These enactments might be understood through the lived citizenship concept (Lister, 2007). Drawing on critical and feminist studies, lived citizenship, as an analytical lens, places at the centre of inquiry the embodied performance of citizenship and how people negotiate rights, responsibilities, identities and belonging within everyday life (Lister 2007) – irrespective of formal citizenship status (Kallio et al., 2020).

Lived citizenship is about the everyday. The 'everyday' has been described by Pink (2015, p. 143) as 'at the centre of human existence, the essence of who we are and our location in the world'. Thus, the everyday is key in understanding how the state infiltrates and mediates people's intimate spaces and seemingly mundane aspects of daily life. Within everyday life people seeking asylum and refugees are, through discourse and policy, racialised, marginalised, and exposed to suffering. Lived citizenship centres human agency, and the ways in which people engage in civic practice. Thus, the lived citizenship concept allows us to view citizenship as an act that encompasses participation and belonging as it is experienced and enacted within real-life everyday contexts (see for example, Isin, 2008).

The links between lived citizenship and maintaining wellbeing have been made by scholars. For example, Müller (2021) has explored the ways in which Eritrean diaspora communities, that lack formal citizenship, in Nairobi, Addis Ababa and Khartoum dealt with the COVID-19 pandemic. It was found that participants 'secure their livelihoods and wellbeing through behaving like citizens' and engaging in 'everyday humanitarianism' (Müller, 2022, p. 21). Here everyday humanitarianism is used to mean aiming to alleviate suffering within everyday lives outside of traditional structures of humanitarian action (Müller, 2022; Richey, 2018). For example, where mutual support and solidarity was drawn from informal networks of peer-to-peer or local community or faith-based groups. O'Neill (2018) has also made the links between wellbeing and citizenship in her work with women asylum seekers, exploring their journeys and search for asylum. Themes discussed included: the importance of women's story telling capacities; self-determination and agency in the search for freedom; the barriers they face and overcome, and the relational sense of transnational belonging occasionally expressed as solidarity. In their search for freedom and alleviation from suffering, the women engage in lived citizenship practices – going to the park, the library or community café. These were places where the women felt a sense of freedom, community and belonging and had a positive impact on their overall wellbeing. The women also discussed the significance of friendship and solidarity in maintaining wellbeing whilst waiting for asylum.

Elsewhere I have argued that place-making by asylum seekers and refugees is linked to alternative citizenships because it is an everyday practice that relies on agency. It claims the right to space and constitutes their active and present membership of the local community. In so doing, it disrupts the categories of citizen/Other (Biglin, 2022). In the discussion of participants' production of therapeutic landscapes, evidenced in this chapter, we see that participants are key actors in mitigating the harmful effects of asylum policies through various place-making practices. The research discussed in this chapter demonstrates that the participants' place-making in green and public urban space is largely about seeking wellbeing through negotiating forms of transnational belonging; determination for asylum and justice, at times articulated through plants and nature to symbolise hope; places where they build friendships and solidarity with others; and identities beyond the asylum seeker/refugee label. It is these various practices of participation and belonging that *produce* therapeutic landscape experiences, rather than therapeutic landscapes being a stage on which people perform. Refugees and asylum seekers are often represented as passive and agentless which is why I argue that we should view interactions with place, that actively seek out and shape wellbeing opportunities, as a form of agency that counteracts this representation. This agency and engagement in everyday participation and belonging within place, which sustains a sense of wellbeing, against a backdrop of forced suffering, constitutes a form of lived citizenship.

Conclusion: Where does this leave the therapeutic landscapes concept for asylum seekers and refugees?

Since its inception the therapeutic landscapes concept has been applied in many different contexts and with different social groups to explore the links between health and place. However, within existing literature there lacks a deeper understanding of the links between therapeutic landscapes and theories of lived citizenship, which this chapter has examined. I have argued that for asylum seekers and refugees, opportunities to create therapeutic landscapes are part of lived citizenship. Through various forms of participation, and belonging, asylum seekers and refugees behave like 'citizens' in search of wellbeing and alleviation from suffering.

When using the therapeutic landscapes concept, it is important to consider to what extent these 'therapeutic' encounters that we discuss are a deep source of transformation or a temporary source of respite (Kaley et al., 2019). I would argue that the term 'therapeutic' may not be entirely appropriate in the current context as the political project that participants seek respite from cannot be 'cured' by urban green and public space. This links to a wider discussion of the limits of community provision in relation to long term effectiveness of efforts to 'welcome' migrants, as 'welcome' does very little to change the fundamental precariousness of many migrants' situations (see for example Bagelman, 2013, 2016; Darling, 2017). Some scholars argue that movements seeking to welcome migrants (for example, the City of Sanctuary movement) may depoliticise the harm caused by asylum policies by aiming to make the wait for an asylum claim productive, rather than actually addressing and contesting the forced suffering imposed by the state (Bagelman, 2013). Similarly, on the topic of therapeutic landscapes amongst refugees and asylum seekers, highlighting that people are able to mitigate their suffering may depoliticise that suffering through failing to challenge the politics that produce that suffering in the first place.

However, what is key in the research discussed here is that power does not sit solely within these places to offer welcome and belonging to participants; power is within the participants to seek out, construct and shape place to meet their needs and offer a range of wellbeing opportunities. Through their relational encounters with place participants were active in creating and (re)producing these spaces into places that could potentially improve their wellbeing through forms of embodied presence and social engagement; transnational and local belonging; friendship and solidarity; and symbolic expressions of hope and justice. Therefore, production of therapeutic landscapes by asylum seekers and refugees can be understood through the lens of lived citizenship. It is an active process that evades forced suffering and disrupts the binary notion of 'citizen' and 'Other'.

To conclude then, therapeutic landscapes for refugees and asylum seekers are about more than just improving wellbeing, they are about the way everyday acts of participation and belonging can 'operate as an arena for the contestation and transformation of […] often oppressive modalities of citizenship' (Dickinson et al., 2008, p. 105).

Acknowledgements

Figures 10.2 and 10.4 were published in Biglin, J. (2022). 'Photovoice as an unfamiliar act of citizenship: Everyday belonging, place-making and political subjectivity' *Citizenship Studies*, 26(3), pp. 263–286.
Figure 10.3 was published in Biglin, J. (2021a). 'Photovoice accounts of third places: Refugee and asylum seeker populations' experiences of therapeutic space.' *Health and Place*, 71, pp. 102663

References

Agyekum, B. and Newbold, B. K. (2016). 'Religion/spirituality, therapeutic landscape and migrant mental well-being amongst African migrants to Canada.' *Mental Health, Religion and Culture*, 19(7), pp. 674–685.

Bagelman, J. (2013). 'Sanctuary: A politics of ease?' *Alternatives: Global, Local, Political*, 38(1), pp. 49–62.

Bagelman, J. (2016). *Sanctuary City: A Suspended State*. London: Palgrave Macmillan.

Bell, S., Phoenix, C., Lovell, R. and Wheeler, B. (2014). 'Green space, health and wellbeing: Making space for individual agency.' *Health and Place*, 30, pp. 287–292.

Bell, S. L., Foley, R., Houghton, F., Maddrell, A. and Williams, A. M. (2018). 'From therapeutic landscapes to health spaces, places and practices: A scoping review.' *Social Science and Medicine*, 196, pp. 123–130.

Biglin, J. (2022). 'Photovoice as an unfamiliar act of citizenship: Everyday belonging, place-making and political subjectivity' *Citizenship Studies*, 26(3), pp. 263–286.

Biglin, J. (2021a). 'Photovoice accounts of third places: Refugee and asylum seeker populations' experiences of therapeutic space.' *Health and Place*, 71, 102663

Biglin, J. (2021b). 'Photovoice accounts of borders and home: Asylum seeker and refugee perspectives' *Borderlands*, 20(2), pp. 91–123.

Biglin, J. (2020). 'Embodied and sensory experiences of therapeutic space: Refugee place-making within an urban allotment.' *Health and Place*, 62, 102309

Blackmore, R., Boyle, J. A., Fazel, M., Ranasinha, S., Gray, K. M, Fitzgerald G, Misso, M. and Gibson-Helm, M. (2020). 'The prevalence of mental illness in refugees and asylum seekers: A systematic review and meta-analysis.' *PLOS MEDICINE*, DOI: 10.1371/journal.pmed.1003337

Boccagni, P. (2017). *Migration and the Search for Home*. New York: Palgrave/ Springer Nature.

Brewster, L. (2014). 'The public library as therapeutic landscape: A qualitative case study.' *Health and Place*, 26, pp. 94–99.

Carlson, J and Sonne, C. (2018). 'Mental Health, Pre-Migratory Trauma and Post-migratory Stressors Among Adult Refugees.' Morina, N and Nickerson, A. (eds.) *Mental Health of Refugee and Conflict-Affected Populations*, Switzerland: Springer, pp. 15–35.

Casey, E. S. (1997). *The Fate of Place: A Philosophical History*. California: University of California Press.

Cresswell, T. (2004). *Place: An Introduction*. Oxford: Wiley-Blackwell.

Darling, J. (2011). 'Domopolitics, governmentality and the regulation of asylum accommodation.' *Political Geography*, 30(5), pp. 263–271.

Darling, J. (2016). Asylum in austere times: Instability, privatization and experimentation within the UK asylum dispersal system. *Journal of Refugee Studies*, 29(4), pp. 484–505.

Darling, J. (2017). 'Forced migration and the city: Irregularity, informality, and the politics of presence.' *Progress in Human Geography*, 41(2) 178–198.

Darling, J. (2022). *Systems of Suffering: Dispersal and the Denial of Asylum*. London: Pluto Press.

Dickinson, J., Andrucki, J., Rawlins, E., Hale, D. and Cook, V. (2008). 'Introduction: Geographies of everyday citizenship.' *ACME: An International E-Journal for Critical Geographies*, 7(2), pp. 100–112.

Erel, U. (2013). 'Kurdish migrant mothers in London enacting citizenship.' *Citizenship Studies*, 17(8), pp. 970–984.

Erel, U., T. Reynolds, and Kaptani, E. (2018). 'Migrant mothers' creative interventions in racialized citizenship.' *Ethnic and Racial Studies*, 41(1), pp. 55–72.

Ermansons, G., Kienzler, H., Asif, Z. and Schofield, P. (2023). 'Refugee mental health and the role of place in the Global North countries: A scoping review.' *Health and Place*, 79, 102964.

Gesler, W. M. (1996). 'Lourdes: healing in a place of pilgrimage.' *Health and Place*, 2(2), pp. 95–105.

Gesler, W. (1998). 'Bath's Reputation as a Healing Place.' In Kearns, R., Gesler, W. (eds.) *Putting Health into Place*. Syracuse, NY: Syracuse University Press, pp. 17–36.

Good, A. (2011). 'Tales of suffering: Asylum narratives in the refugee determination process.' *West Cost Line*, 68, pp. 80–89.

Hirschler, S. (2021). *Hostile Homes: Violence, Harm and the Marketisation of UK Asylum Housing*. Cham: Palgrave Macmillan.

Isin, E. (2008). 'Theorising Acts of Citizenship.' In *Acts of Citizenship*, Isin, E. and Nielsen, G. M. (eds.) London, NY: Palgrave Macmillan, pp. 15–43.

Kaley, A., Hatton, C. and Milligan, C. (2019). 'Therapeutic spaces of care farming: Transformative or Ameliorating?' *Social Science Medicine*, DOI: 10.1016/j.socscimed.2018.05.011.

Kallio, K. P., Wood, B. E. and Häkli, J. (2020). 'Lived citizenship: Conceptualising an emerging field.' *Citizenship Studies*, 24, p. 6, DOI: 10.1080/13621025.2020.1739227

Keller, A., Joscelyne, A., Granski, M. and Rosenfeld, B. (2017). 'Pre-migration trauma exposure and mental health functioning among Central American Migrants arriving at the US Border.' *PLOS ONE*, DOI: 10.1371/journal.pone.0168692

Liberty. (2018). *A Guide to the Hostile Environment*. London: Liberty. Available at: www.liberty humanrights.org.uk/wp-content/uploads/2020/02/Hostile-Environment-Guide---update-May-2019_0.pdf (Accessed on 14th August 2021).

Lim, M., Van Hulst, A., Pisanu, S. and Merry, L. (2022). 'Social isolation, loneliness and health: A descriptive study of the experiences of migrant mothers with young children (0-5 Years Old) at La Maison Bleue.' *Frontiers in Global Women's Health*, 3, 823632

Lister, R. (2007). 'Inclusive citizenship: Realising the potential.' *Citizenship Studies*, 11(1), pp. 49–61.

Lister, R. (2008). 'Unpacking Children's Citizenship.' In Invernizzi, A. and Williams, J. (eds.) *Children and Citizenship*. London: Sage, pp. 9–19.

May, V., Byrne, B., Holmes, H. and Takhar, S. (2020). 'Introduction: Nationalism's futures.' *Sociology*, 54(6), pp. 1055–1071.

Milligan, C. and Bingley, A. (2007). 'Restorative places or scary spaces? The impact of woodland on the mental well-being of young adults.' *Health and Place* 13(4), pp. 799–811.

Milligan, C., Gatrell, T. and Bingley, A. (2004). 'Cultivating health: Therapeutic landscapes and older people in northern England.' *Social Science and Medicine,* 58(9), pp. 1781–1793.

Müller, T. (2022). 'Covid-19 and urban migrants in the Horn of Africa: Lived citizenship and everyday humanitarianism.' *IDS Bulletin,* 53(2), pp. 11–27.

O'Neill, M. (2018). 'Walking, well-being and community: Racialized mothers building cultural citizenship using participatory arts and participatory action research.' *Ethical and Racial Studies,* 41(1), pp. 73–97.

O'Reilly, Z. (2019). 'Living liminality: Everyday experiences of asylum seekers in the "Direct provision" system in Ireland.' *Gender, Place and Culture,* 25(6), pp. 821–842.

Oyangen, K. (2009) 'The gastrodynamics of displacement: Place-making and gustatory identity in the immigrants' midwest'. *Journal of Interdisciplinary History,* 39(3), pp. 323–348.

Pink, S. (2015). *Sensory Ethnography.* 2nd ed. London: Sage.

Refugee Council. (2022). Mental health support for refugees and asylum seekers. Online. Available: www.refugeecouncil.org.uk/our-work/mental-health-support-for-refugees-and-asylum-seekers/ (Accessed on 4th Feb 2023).

Richey, L. A. (2018). 'Conceptualizing "Everyday humanitarianism": Ethics, affects, and practices of contemporary global helping. *New Political Science* 40(4), pp. 625–639.

Rishbeth, C., Blachnicka-Ciacek, D. and Darling, J. (2019). 'Participation and wellbeing in urban greenspace: "curating sociability" for refugees and asylum seekers.' *Geoforum,* 106, pp. 125–134.

Sampson, R. and Gifford, S. (2010). 'Place-making, settlement and well-being: The therapeutic landscapes of recently arrived youth with refugee backgrounds.' *Health & Place,* 16(1), pp. 116–131.

Scottish Refugee Council. (2022). Cost of Living Crisis: Asylum seekers need more support. Online. Available: https://scottishrefugeecouncil.org.uk/our-calls-for-increases-to-asylum-support/ (Accessed on 4th Feb 2023).

Squire, V. (2009). *The Exclusionary Politics of Asylum.* Basingstoke: Palgrave Macmillan.

Strang, A. and Quinn, N. (2019). 'Integration or isolation? Refugees' social connections and well-being.' *Journal of Refugee Studies,* 34(1), pp. 328–353.

Turrini, G., Purgato, M., Ballette, F., Nosè, M., Ostuzzi, G. and Barbu, C. (2017). 'Common mental disorders in asylum seekers and refugees: Umbrella review of prevalence and intervention studies.' *International Journal of Mental Health,* 11(51), pp. 1–14.

Wang, C. and Burris, M. A. (1997). 'Photovoice: Concept, methodology, and use for participatory needs assessment.' *Health Education and Behaviour,* 24(3), pp. 369–387.

WHO. (2021). 'Mental health and forced displacement.' Online. Available: www.who.int/newsroom/fact-sheets/detail/mental-health-and-forced-displacement Accessed on 5th February 2023.

11 Green gentrification and its impacts on mental health

Unveiling the evidence on sociocultural and physical exclusion linked to green and blue spaces

Margarita Triguero-Mas and Helen V. S. Cole

Introduction

In this chapter, we aim to present the existing scientific evidence on the potential links between green gentrification and people's mental health. To accomplish this goal, we start by defining gentrification and green gentrification, then we move onto detailing the prevalence of green gentrification within and between municipalities, before exploring the nexus between green gentrification and mental health. We finish this chapter with a discussion of potential next steps and future directions in research, and draw together our conclusions on green gentrification's (mental) health impacts.

Conceptualising gentrification and green gentrification

Socioeconomical and racial segregation by neighbourhood is evident in cities around the world. For example, in the USA, historical discriminatory housing policies and practices have created segregated neighbourhoods where mostly Black and Latinx residents live with limited access to services (such as healthy foods and good-quality schools), concentrated poverty and high crime rates (Krieger, 2014; Bailey *et al.*, 2017). All these inequitably distributed conditions have been linked to poor health (Collins and Williams, 1999; Dai, 2010; Kershaw, Albrecht and Carnethon, 2013; Williams, Sternthal and Wright, 2009). These neighbourhoods, marked by socioeconomic and racial segregation, face the risk of gentrification if they experience an influx of capital, particularly when they are desirable to more socially privileged residents due to, for example, their central location or historical architecture. Definitions of social privilege (and underprivilege) exhibit variability across diverse contexts, yet they can be broadly characterised as having financial, political and sociocultural power (or lacking this power in the case of underprivileged residents). This is due to the interplay of intersectional factors, such as classism and racism, which promote privileged residents to have economic opportunities or empower them to have a political voice (while underprivileged residents are excluded from these opportunities). Privileged residents generally include majority ethnic and racial groups, and upper-class individuals (e.g. highly educated, wealthy, white populations).

Gentrification was first coined by Ruth Glass in 1964 to describe the process of middle-class residents moving to working-class London neighbourhoods and displacing long-term working-class residents. In its original definition, gentrification was also characterised by stables, cottages and Victorian houses becoming elegant expensive residences and the transformation of the neighbourhood social environment (Brown-Saracino, 2010).

DOI: 10.4324/9781003345725-12

Nowadays, we can define gentrification as the social, economic, cultural and physical transformation of a place, including the change in its amenities, that indicate a shift towards a more privileged population capable of purchasing newly developed or upgraded, higher-priced residences, simultaneously fostering novel cultural and consumption patterns (Brown-Saracino, 2010; Lees, Shin and López-Morales, 2015; Smith, 1982, 1996). Gentrification leads to sociocultural exclusion as the population shifts towards a more privileged one. It may lead to the physical displacement of long-term – often underprivileged – residents due to their inability to afford the increasing housing and living expenses which, in turn, may exacerbate existing residential socioeconomic and racial segregation (Musterd *et al.*, 2017). Research shows that gentrification is linked to worse mental health (i.e. sleep deprivation, higher anxiety, stress and depression) and to worse physical health (i.e. more respiratory diseases and preterm births) for under-privileged residents (Bhavsar, Kumar and Richman, 2020; Jelks, Jennings and Rigolon, 2021; Mehdipanah et al., 2018; Schnake-Mahl et al., 2020; Tulier et al., 2019). Research about the relationship between gentrification and health has grown over the past decade but mostly focuses on gentrification itself as the exposure of interest and on general physical health rather than mental health (for some examples of studies exploring the links between gentrification and mental health, see Smith, Lehning and Kim, 2018; Tran et al., 2020). Also, debates remain about the best methods of measurement for gentrification in quantitative studies.

In gentrification processes, usually multiple drivers – such as an influx of retail or residential investments, tourism, and influx of wealthy student populations, or the introduction or improvement of greenspaces, and others – overlap. However, depending on the setting, any one of the different drivers may be more prominent in the gentrification process. Accordingly, the most impactful driver can be used to characterise the type of gentrification (e.g. retail gentrification, tourism gentrification, studentification, green gentrification). These drivers – and associated neighbourhood changes in general – have an effect on health, with outcomes that can be paradoxical (Cole, Mehdipanah, et al., 2021). For example, shops selling organic or other healthy food could suggest that the neighbourhood design is more conducive to the better health and wellbeing of its inhabitants. But underprivileged residents may not be able to afford or feel welcomed in these amenities, so these gentrification drivers may – indeed – increase health inequities.

Cities across the globe are progressively creating and restoring green and blue spaces. These interventions aim to tackle a wide range of socio-environmental and health challenges such as adapting for and mitigating the effects of climate change and protecting citizens' mental health (Kabisch et al., 2017). However, there is also an increasing body of evidence indicating that these interventions may entice new investment, consequently elevating the risk of gentrification for these areas – a process known as green gentrification. Green gentrification, also known as environmental or eco-gentrification, refers to the physical and socio-cultural exclusion and displacement of underprivileged residents originated from environmental planning strategies and the incorporation of new environmental amenities (Dooling, 2009; Gould and Lewis, 2017). Green and/or blue space interventions spur or hasten gentrification through tangible and discursive processes. On one hand, green/blue spaces lead to higher land and property values, while also giving rise to urban green grabbing practices (where developers appropriate from the social and financial benefits stemming from new or projected green/blue spaces) (Czembrowski and Kronenberg, 2016; García-Lamarca et al., 2022; Safransky, 2014). On the other hand, green/blue interventions are articulated around a green/nature narrative that serves to (re-)brand cities (known as urban green boosterism), ultimately generating commodified environmental amenities (Garcia-Lamarca et al., 2019; Triguero-Mas et al., 2021). Accordingly, the process of green gentrification might compromise the positive effects of green/blue interventions and – instead of contributing to just and sustainable neighbourhoods (Agyeman et al., 2016) – green gentrification might lead to the emergence of novel social and environmental injustices. Apart from displacement, green gentrification is linked to environmental privilege. Privileged residents may – as usual – be the key actors in producing the accepted and branded environmental knowledge and discourse that shape the placement, accessibility and features of green/blue spaces (Anguelovski, 2016; Rigolon and Németh, 2018). Consequently, green/blue spaces may become GreenLULUs (Locally Unwanted Land Uses) (Anguelovski, 2016) or disruptive green landscapes (Triguero-Mas et al., 2021) for underprivileged residents.

The spread of green gentrification

Exposure to green space plays a vital role in enhancing human physical and mental health (Frumkin et al., 2017), while concurrently providing an array of ecosystem services, including mitigating climate change and decreasing air and noise pollution, among others (Derkzen, van Teeffelen and Verburg, 2015; Vargas-Hernández, Pallagst and Zdunek-Wielgołaska, 2018). Nonetheless, to effectively implement green/blue interventions capable of tackling health and socio-environmental challenges while avoiding the forementioned adverse impacts of gentrification, it is crucial to have a clear understanding of the prevalence of green gentrification, the circumstances in which it emerges, and the scale of its effects (Pearsall and Eller, 2020). Cases of green gentrification have been well-documented in various urban settings, especially in connection with flagship projects, such as interventions in the US (e.g. the BeltLine in Atlanta or the High Line Park in New York City), in Europe (e.g. the Noorderpark in Amsterdam or the Lene-Voigt Park in Germany) and also in East Asia (e.g. the Gyeongui Line Forest Park or Cheonggyecheon Stream Restoration Project in South Korea) (Anguelovski and Connolly, 2021; Black and Richards, 2020; Haase et al., 2017; Immergluck and Balan, 2018; Kwon et al., 2017; Loughran, 2014; Sandberg, 2014; Weber et al., 2017).

However, much of the literature to date has been dominated by qualitative case study analyses of a specific city and/or of a particular neighbourhood (Anguelovski and Connolly, 2021; Curran and Hamilton, 2012; Loughran, 2014). The few quantitative studies on green gentrification that exist show mixed findings, with most of the studies focusing on a specific context (usually US) and time period, finding that greening is linked to gentrification. In contrast, studies exploring a diversity of contexts and/or time periods report that, for some cities and time periods, associations may be null or even negative (Anguelovski et al., 2018, 2022; Chen et al., 2021; Connolly, 2019; Conway et al., 2010; Donovan et al., 2021; Du and Zhang, 2020; Irwin, 2002; Kim and Wu, 2022; Kwon et al., 2017; Maantay and Maroko, 2018; Pearsall and Eller, 2020; Rigolon and Németh, 2020; Shokry, Connolly and Anguelovski, 2020; Schinasi et al., 2021).

Additionally, a limited number of the quantitative studies that try to better understand green gentrification examine the diversity of urban greenspace in terms of size, vegetation coverage, biodiversity, facilities, protection status, or other socioenvironmental features (all of these are factors that have important implications for the potential of these spaces as health or socioecological interventions). An increasing number of scientific studies indicate that extensive urban greening projects like the 606 rails-to-trails project in Chicago or the BeltLine in Atlanta may instigate environmental gentrification given that they may be intentionally planned – at least in part – with the aim of increasing property values (Black and Richards, 2020; Chen et al., 2021; Immergluck and Balan, 2018; Kwon et al., 2017; Loughran, 2014). Nevertheless, the findings from one study encompassing ten major and medium-size cities in the US revealed no significant impact of park size on gentrification (Rigolon and Németh, 2020). In parallel, it is hypothesized that smaller greenspaces are elements of a 'just green enough' urban planning design which may deliver environmental and health benefits without spurring gentrification (Chen et al., 2021; Wolch, Byrne and Newell, 2014)). To delve further, distinct greenspace attributes are related to different greenspaces typologies (e.g. parks, allotments or nature preserves) (Smith et al., 2017). These diverse greenspace types may, subsequently, result in distinct gentrification patterns driven by their distinct uses and levels of appreciation amongst residents (Amorim Maia et al., 2020). Very little research (mainly US-based) has examined the relationships between property prices and green space typologies (Czembrowski and Kronenberg, 2016; Donovan et al., 2021; Lutzenhiser and Netusil, 2001). Despite this, researchers have emphasized that exploring how greenspace typologies are associated with green gentrification is important (Pearsall and Eller, 2020; Stuhlmacher, Kim and Kim, 2022). There is scarce but slowly growing evidence that the associations between gentrification and greenspaces may differ by greenspace type (with other factors such as distance to the city centre also being linked to gentrification) (Chen et al., 2021; Czembrowski and Kronenberg, 2016; Kim and Wu, 2022; Kwon et al., 2017; Lutzenhiser and Netusil, 2001; Maantay and Maroko, 2018; Rigolon and Németh, 2020; Triguero-Mas et al., 2022).

Regarding parks, the most comprehensive research conducted so far, which included 28 cities in Europe and North America and a diversity of green space types (i.e., parks, gardens, nature preserves, recreational spaces and greenways), found that parks were the greenspace type more consistently positively associated with gentrification, especially in the US settings – apart from historically Black disinvested postindustrial cities with significant amounts of vacant land (Triguero-Mas et al., 2022). Similarly, one study focusing on five contiguous districts of Barcelona city showed that new urban parks were linked to gentrification in their vicinity, while neighbourhoods characterised by aging housing units that are challenging to renovate were not (Anguelovski et al., 2018). Nevertheless, Rigolon and Németh did not reveal any relationship between the size of new parks (apart from other characteristics) and gentrification in their aggregated analysis of data from ten large and medium-sized US cities (Rigolon and Németh, 2020). Together, all this evidence indicates that parks may be the type of greenspace most employed in green branding (Garcia-Lamarca et al., 2019) and, consequently, also strongly linked to green gentrification processes. People may be willing to pay higher prices to live near to parks because residents may use parks more than other spaces, as parks offer a diversity of recreational options and a feeling of familiarity, as they usually have a "normative" aesthetic (Amorim Maia et al., 2020; Chan, Peters and Marafa, 2015). For instance, features such as elaborate landscapes, meticulously designed gardens, and fences (which might make spaces feel safer) may aesthetically appeal to gentrifiers and real estate developers, making parks more attractive for investment (Chen et al., 2021).

The evidence on the relationship between gentrification and other types of greenspace is more heterogeneous, which may indicate that greenspaces that are not parks have a diversity of roles in gentrification processes, probably due to their different functionalities, aesthetics and access characteristics, which create different use patterns. A study by Rigolon and Németh focusing on US cities reported that census tracts with centroids located within a half mile of greenways had over 200% increased odds of gentrification compared to census tracts located farther away from greenways (Rigolon and Németh, 2020). Likewise, the presence of gardens has been found to be linked to increased gentrification in Brooklyn, New York (Maantay and Maroko, 2018) and in St. Louis, Missouri (Braswell, 2018). Meanwhile, another recent study in New York City showed that greenspaces not designed for the practise of high-level physical activity and which were natural (non-manicured, wild) were linked to gentrification processes (Kim and Wu, 2022). However, a more extensive study including Canadian, US and European cities showed negative associations between newly designated nature preserves and gentrification, and mixed results for new gardens, recreational spaces and greenways (Triguero-Mas et al., 2022).

Apart from considering the heterogeneity of greenspace socio-environmental characteristics when studying green gentrification, context differences may be relevant too. Several studies show different patterns between North American and European cities (Anguelovski et al., 2022; Triguero-Mas et al., 2022) which may be attributed to distinct policy and planning realities, as European cities typically having a greater and more robust array of anti-displacement tools and equitable greening practices (Oscilowicz et al., 2022) compared to their counterparts in the US cities.

Green gentrification and mental health

Multiple studies illustrate the links between exposure to green space and good mental health although scholars are still working to improve how to assess green space exposure, and to understand the pathways that would explain these associations (Frumkin et al., 2017). Moreover, research that considers the relationship between green/blue spaces, gentrification and health is nascent, yet much needed in order to parse out the interplay between these interconnected factors. This research is based on studies exploring the associations between greenspace exposure and health outcomes, and explores how green gentrification processes (as described above) may impact who benefits from greenspaces, and the potential role of gentrification on the associations between exposure to greenspace and inequalities (Cole et al., 2017). Studying the health effects of green gentrification is one way to contextualize the effects of greenspace exposures within a broader socio-political urban context.

The few studies that have explored this topic so far indicate that green gentrification negatively impacts underprivileged residents (Jelks, Jennings and Rigolon, 2021). For instance, in a study investigating the interplay between green/blue space, gentrification, and health among New York City residents, the authors found that only residents with high education and income living in gentrifying neighbourhoods experienced health benefits from greenspaces (Cole et al., 2019). Meanwhile those living in non-gentrifying neighbourhoods or those with less education or income in gentrifying neighbourhoods showed no health benefit from greenspaces. A similar study conducted in Barcelona and focusing on mental health reported that only residents of gentrifiable census tracts who were exposed to greenways had lower odds of reporting poor mental health (in that case, depression/anxiety), with no differences by socioeconomic status (Zayas-Costa et al., 2021). These studies, however, looked only at existing greenspaces, and therefore did not include a measure of green gentrification itself.

A research study specifically focusing on green gentrification and based on over 100 qualitative interviews from five cities in Canada, the United States and Western Europe, revealed that when green/blue spaces were newly built or improved in neighbourhoods that were also gentrifying, these spaces were perceived as non-therapeutic by underprivileged neighbourhood residents (Triguero-Mas et al., 2021), instead of being perceived as healthy spaces – or as spaces promoting opportunities for "therapeutic landscape" experiences (Atuoye et al., 2019; Bell et al., 2018; Conradson, 2005; Finlay, 2018). That is, the study found that underprivileged neighbourhood residents were not physically or emotionally engaged with these spaces. Gentrification was perceived to affect all dimensions of green/blue spaces as (non-) therapeutic landscapes: relational (such as the ineffectiveness of green/blue spaces to counteract other factors detrimental to health); spiritual-symbolic-cultural (such as not feeling welcomed and feeling socially controlled in green/blue spaces, with conflicts experienced between users, and also green/blue spaces being used for city branding and housing marketing); social (such as the hindrance of some social contacts); and environmental-material-physical (such as decreased accessibility due to privatization of access routes, environmental harms remaining unmitigated in green/blue spaces and residential displacement from the neighbourhood) (Triguero-Mas et al., 2021).

This body of recent research diverges from a large body of scholarly work that – without considering aspects such as gentrification processes – suggests that the health of socially underprivileged groups may benefit more than privileged groups from contact with green/blue spaces close to their residence (Kabisch et al., 2017; Mitchell et al., 2015; Pearce et al., 2018; Triguero-Mas et al., 2017). The differences between these previous findings focusing on green/blue spaces and health and the findings of those studies also including gentrification, could be explained by the fact that extremely underprivileged individuals are usually forced to move from re-naturalised neighbourhoods to areas with fewer green/blue spaces, while some less underprivileged individuals may be able to stay in environmentally improved (and gentrifying) neighbourhoods.

As a whole, the findings in this area pose fundamental questions about cities' capacity to integrate green/blue interventions with sustainability, greening, healthy liveable environments and equity (Anguelovski et al., 2020; Gould and Lewis, 2017) or if underprivileged neighbourhood residents can only have the right to the unhealthy deprived (ungreen) city (O'Neill et al., 2023). However, the available evidence on the associations between mental health and green gentrification remains scarce. It is of paramount importance to delve deeper into the magnitude of health inequities in gentrifying neighbourhoods with newly created green/blue spaces along with the intricate connections among various health determinants (i.e. personal, social, cultural, economic, environmental, political and other contextual factors that influence individual health), with a particular focus on contextual factors (Frumkin et al., 2017) like gentrification.

Next steps and future directions

There are many recent advances from related lines of research which could lead to robust studies on the relationship between green gentrification and mental health. For example, researchers studying the health effects of greenspace exposures have compared and contrasted the many methods for conceptualising and measuring exposures (Vilcins et al., 2022) which could be used in future studies in this field. Recent studies of gentrification and health have begun to incorporate longitudinal measures (Agbai, 2021), which would allow researchers to better determine the timeframe during which the mental health impacts of green gentrification may develop. There are also many sources of (often publicly) accessible spatial, health and demographic data which are representative of the populations of cities (such as the annual health survey of New York City, or the 500 cities dataset from the US Centers for Disease Control and Prevention, both of which present data on the health of city residents which is tied to spatial indicators such as zip codes or census tracts); national censuses which often include the sociodemographic data necessary to approximate a quantitative measure of gentrification; and many sources of green spatial data such as those used in the studies described throughout.

In addition, the power of qualitative methods to contribute to our understanding of how and under which circumstances green gentrification may affect mental health should not be underestimated. Qualitative methods have proven their potential in this field through several past studies, as they complement broad quantitative findings by uncovering mechanisms. This has been demonstrated previously with the disruptive green landscapes concept (Triguero-Mas et al., 2021). They can also assist researchers to disentangle such effects amidst complex social and environmental contexts (Cole, Anguelovski, et al., 2021). Finally, attention to mental health is growing in public health research, along with advances in measuring and conceptualising mental health conditions among populations or sub-populations. Future research in the field would benefit from transdisciplinary approaches, including methods and approaches used by public health (environmental and equity), urban planning and green/blue spaces experts, among others.

Conclusions

In this chapter, we have presented how certain urban processes – such as green gentrification – may impact the potential (mental) health benefits derived from well-established health determinants such as green/blue spaces. Based on the knowledge we have so far, it is essential that all stakeholders (including scientists, policy makers and planners) embrace that green/blue spaces can be perceived, conceptualised and experienced as healthy or not, according to different lived experiences and neighbourhood processes (including gentrification). Green/blue spaces are landscapes linked to gradients of well-being, gradients that may differ by sociodemographic groups as people experience green/blue spaces at different moments in time, and might not always experience them as a 'healthy' resource. As such, green/blue spaces might act as therapeutic or non-therapeutic, disruptive landscapes. Despite the best intentions of those who design and implement new greenspace projects, these nuances and potential for unintended consequences (such as the potential for exacerbating health inequalities if protections are not put in place), need to be considered.

At the same time as producing more and higher quality research that examines relationships between green gentrification and mental health, it is essential to raise awareness of social and power dynamics that, through hegemony and resistance, may legitimate particular discourses about green/blue spaces and potentially even overshadow empirical evidence. Moreover, we should understand and claim clearly that the harmful impacts of gentrification on green/blue space-health relationships are preventable. There is a need to find political solutions and to secure resources for people who struggle with certain health determinants and outcomes and we should all make efforts in that direction. Especially, policy makers and planners should be mindful of all these challenges and needs, and integrate innovative approaches to overcome these limitations, especially within green/blue space planning and the development of healthy cities. Tangible measures are needed to protect the right to (high-quality) housing for underprivileged residents and to embed "health in all policies". In pursuit of this goal, supporting community-based interventions and implementing policies that address gentrification and those that promote green/blue spaces – similar to the ones undertaken by Nantes, Vienna, and Portland – could be of paramount importance (Oscilowicz et al., 2022). Only through such actions will cities become sustainable, green, liveable, healthy and equitable. In summary, given the environmental and health benefits offered by urban green/blue spaces, cities should continue their efforts to enhance access to these spaces while at the same time implementing anti-displacement and inclusive green policies.

References

Agbai, C.O. (2021). Shifting neighborhoods, shifting health: A longitudinal analysis of gentrification and health in Los Angeles County. *Social Science Research*, 100, 102603.

Agyeman, J., Schlosberg, D., Craven, L. and Matthews, C. (2016). Trends and directions in environmental justice: From inequity to everyday life, community, and just sustainabilities. *Annual Review of Environment and Resources*, 41(1), pp. 321–340.

Amorim Maia, A.T., Calcagni, F., Connolly, J.J.T., Anguelovski, I. and Langemeyer, J. (2020). Hidden drivers of social injustice: Uncovering unequal cultural ecosystem services behind green gentrification. *Environmental Science & Policy*, 112, pp. 254–263.

Anguelovski, I. (2016). From toxic sites to parks as (Green) LULUs? New challenges of inequity, privilege, gentrification, and exclusion for urban environmental justice. *Journal of Planning Literature*, 31(1), pp. 23–36.

Anguelovski, I., Connolly, J.J.T., Masip, L. and Pearsall, H. (2018). Assessing green gentrification in historically disenfranchised neighborhoods: A longitudinal and spatial analysis of Barcelona. *Urban Geography*, 39(3), pp. 458–491.

Anguelovski, I., Brand, A.L., Connolly, J.J.T., Corbera, E., Kotsila, P., Steil, J., García-Lamarca, M., Triguero-Mas, M., Cole, H., Baró, F., Langemeyer, J., Pérez del Pulgar, C., Shokry, G., Sekulova, F. and Ramos, L.A. (2020). Expanding the boundaries of justice in urban greening scholarship: Toward an emancipatory, antisubordination, intersectional, and relational approach. *Annals of the American Association of Geographers*, 110(6), pp. 1743–1769 .

Anguelovski, I., Connolly, J.J.T., Cole, H., García-Lamarca, M., Triguero-Mas, M., Baró, F., Martin, N., Conesa, D., Shokry, G., Pérez del Pulgar, C., Ramos, L.A., Matheney, A., Gallez, E., Oscilowicz, E., López-Máñez, J., Sarzo, B., Beltrán, M.A., and Minaya, J.M. (2022). Green gentrification in European and North American cities. *Nature Communications*, 13(1), 3816.

Anguelovski, I. and Connolly, J.J. (eds) (2021). *The Green City and Social Injustice: 21 Tales from North America and Europe*. Abingdon, Oxon: New York, NY: Routledge (Routledge equity, justice and the sustainable city series).

Atuoye, K.N., Luginaah, I., Hambati, H. and Campbell, G. (2019). Politics, economics, how about our health? Impacts of large-scale land acquisitions on therapeutic spaces and wellbeing in coastal Tanzania. *Social Science & Medicine*, 220, pp. 283–291.

Bailey, Z.D., Krieger, N., Agénor, M., Graves, J., Linos, N. and Bassett, M.T. (2017). Structural racism and health inequities in the USA: Evidence and interventions. *The Lancet*, 389(10077), pp. 1453–1463.

Bell, S.L., Foley, R., Houghton, F., Maddrell, A., and Williams, A.M. (2018) From therapeutic landscapes to healthy spaces, places and practices: A scoping review. *Social Science & Medicine*, 196, pp. 123–130.

Bhavsar, N.A., Kumar, M. and Richman, L. (2020). Defining gentrification for epidemiologic research: A systematic review. *PLOS ONE*, 15(5), e0233361.

Black, K.J. and Richards, M. (2020). Eco-gentrification and who benefits from urban green amenities: NYC's high Line. *Landscape and Urban Planning*, 204, 103900.

Braswell, T.H. (2018). Fresh food, new faces: Community gardening as ecological gentrification in St. Louis, Missouri. *Agriculture and Human Values*, 35(4), pp. 809–822. Available at: https://doi.org/10.1007/s10460-018-9875-3.

Brown-Saracino, J. (2010). *The Gentrification Debates. A Reader*. New York, USA: Routledge.

Chan, C.S., Peters, M. and Marafa, L.M. (2015). Public parks in city branding: Perceptions of visitors vis-à-vis residents in Hong Kong, *Urban Forestry and Urban Greening*, 14(4), pp. 1157–1165.

Chen, Y., Xu, Z., Byrne, J., Xu, T., Wang, S. and Wu, J. (2021). Can smaller parks limit green gentrification? Insights from Hangzhou, China. *Urban Forestry & Urban Greening*, 59, 127009.

Cole, H.V.S., García-Lamarca, M.G., Connolly, J.J.T. and Anguelovski, I. (2017). Are green cities healthy and equitable? Unpacking the relationship between health, green space and gentrification. *Journal of Epidemiology and Community Health*, 71(11), pp. 1118–1121.

Cole, H.V.S., Triguero-Mas, M., Connolly, J.J.T. and Anguelovski, I. (2019). Determining the health benefits of green space: Does gentrification matter? *Health & Place*, 57, pp. 1–11.

Cole, H.V.S., Anguelovski, I., Connolly, J.J.T., García-Lamarca, M., Pérez del Pulgar, C., Shokry, G. and Triguero-Mas, M. (2021). Adapting the environmental risk transition theory for urban health inequities: An observational study examining complex environmental riskscapes in seven neighborhoods in Global North cities. *Social Science & Medicine*, 277, 113907.

Cole, H.V.S., Mehdipanah, R., Gullón, P. and Triguero-Mas, M. (2021). Breaking down and building up: Gentrification, its drivers, and urban health inequality. *Current Environmental Health Reports*, 8, pp. 157–166.

Collins, C.A. and Williams, D.R. (1999). Segregation and mortality: The deadly effects of racism? *Sociological Forum*, 14, pp. 496–523.

Connolly, J.J.T. (2019). From Jacobs to the Just City: A foundation for challenging the green planning orthodoxy. *Cities*, 91, pp. 64–70.

Conradson, D. (2005). Landscape, care and the relational self: Therapeutic encounters in rural England. *Health & Place*, 11(4), pp. 337–348.

Conway, D., Li, C.Q., Wolch, J., Kahle, C. and Jerrett, M. (2010). A spatial autocorrelation approach for examining the effects of urban greenspace on residential property values. *The Journal of Real Estate Finance and Economics*, 41(2), pp. 150–169.

Curran, W. and Hamilton, T. (2012). Just green enough: Contesting environmental gentrification in Greenpoint, Brooklyn. *Local Environment*, 17(9), pp. 1027–1042.

Czembrowski, P. and Kronenberg, J. (2016). Hedonic pricing and different urban green space types and sizes: Insights into the discussion on valuing ecosystem services. *Landscape and Urban Planning*, 146, pp. 11–19.

Dai, D. (2010). Black residential segregation, disparities in spatial access to health care facilities, and late-stage breast cancer diagnosis in metropolitan Detroit. *Health & Place*, 16(5), pp. 1038–1052.

Derkzen, M.L., van Teeffelen, A.J.A. and Verburg, P.H. (2015). REVIEW: Quantifying urban ecosystem services based on high-resolution data of urban green space: An assessment for Rotterdam, the Netherlands. *Journal of Applied Ecology*, 52(4), pp. 1020–1032.

Donovan, G.H., Prestemon, J.P., Butry, D.T., Kaminski, A.R., and Monleon, V.J. (2021). The politics of urban trees: Tree planting is associated with gentrification in Portland, Oregon. *Forest Policy and Economics*, 124, 102387.

Dooling, S. (2009). Ecological gentrification: A research agenda exploring justice in the City. *International Journal of Urban and Regional Research*, 33(3), pp. 621–639.

Du, M. and Zhang, X. (2020). Urban greening: A new paradox of economic or social sustainability? *Land Use Policy*, 92, 104487.

Finlay, J.M. (2018). "Walk like a penguin": Older Minnesotans' experiences of (non)therapeutic white space. *Social Science & Medicine*, 198, pp. 77–84.

Frumkin, H., Bratman, G.N., Breslow, S.J., Cochran, B., Kahn Jr, P.H., Lawler, J.J., Levin, P.S., Tandon, P.S., Varanasi, U., Wolf, K.L. and Wood, S.A. (2017). Nature contact and human health: A research agenda. *Environmental Health Perspectives*, 125(7), 075001.

García-Lamarca, M., Anguelovski, I., Cole, H., Connolly, J.J.T., Argüelles, L., Baró, F., Loveless, S., Péres Del Pulgar Frowein, C. and Shokry, G. (2019). Urban green boosterism and city affordability: For whom is the "branded" green city? *Urban Studies*, 58(1), pp. 90–112.

García-Lamarca, M., Anguelovski, I., Cole, H.V.S., Connolly, J.J.T., Péres Del Pulgar, C., Shokry, G. and Triguero-Mas, M. (2022) Urban green grabbing: Residential real estate developers discourse and practice in gentrifying Global North neighborhoods. *Geoforum*, 128, pp. 1–10.

Gould, K.A. and Lewis, T.L. (2017). *Green Gentrification: Urban Sustainability and the Struggle for Environmental Justice*. London and New York: Routledge, Taylor & Francis Group.

Haase, D., Kabisch, S., Haase, A., Andersson, E., Banzhaf, E., Baró, F., Brenck, M., Fischer, L.K., Frantzeskaki, N., Kabisch, N., Krellenberg, K., Kremer, P., Kronenberg, J., Larondelle, N., Mathey, J., Pauleit, S., Ring, I., Rink, D., Schwarz, N. and Wolff, M. (2017) Greening cities – To be socially inclusive? About the alleged paradox of society and ecology in cities. *Habitat International*, 64, pp. 41–48.

Immergluck, D. and Balan, T. (2018). Sustainable for whom? Green urban development, environmental gentrification, and the Atlanta Beltline. *Urban Geography*, 39(4), pp. 546–562.

Irwin, E.G. (2002). The effects of open space on residential property values. *Land Economics*, 78(4), pp. 465–480.

Jelks, N.O., Jennings, V. and Rigolon, A. (2021). Green gentrification and health: A scoping review. *International Journal of Environmental Research and Public Health*, 18(3), 907.

Kabisch, N., Korn, H., Stadler, J. and Bonn, A. (eds) (2017). *Nature-Based Solutions to Climate Change Adaptation in Urban Areas: Linkages between Science, Policy and Practice*. Cham, Switzerland: Springer International Publishing (Theory and Practice of Urban Sustainability Transitions).

Kershaw, K.N., Albrecht, S.S. and Carnethon, M.R. (2013). Racial and ethnic residential segregation, the neighborhood socioeconomic environment, and obesity among blacks and mexican americans. *American Journal of Epidemiology*, 177(4), pp. 299–309.

Kim, S.K. and Wu, L. (2022). Do the characteristics of new green space contribute to gentrification? *Urban Studies*, 59(2), pp. 360–380.

Krieger, N. (2014). Discrimination and health inequities. In: L.F. Berkman, I. Kawachi, and M.M. Glymour, eds, *Social Epidemiology*. 2nd edition. Oxford: Oxford University Press.

Kwon, Y., Joo, S., Han, S. and Park, C. (2017). Mapping the distribution pattern of gentrification near Urban Parks in the case of Gyeongui Line Forest Park, Seoul, Korea. *Sustainability*, 9(2), 231.

Lees, L., Shin, H.B. and López-Morales, E. (eds) (2015). *Global Gentrifications: Uneven Development and Displacement*. Bristol, UK Chicago, IL: Policy Press.

Loughran, K. (2014). Parks for profit: The high line, growth machines, and the uneven development of urban public spaces. *City & Community*, 13(1), pp. 49–68.

Lutzenhiser, M. and Netusil, N.R. (2001). The effect of open spaces on a home's sale price. *Contemporary Economic Policy*, 19(3), pp. 291–298.

Maantay, J. and Maroko, A. (2018). Brownfields to greenfields: Environmental justice versus environmental sentrification. *International Journal of Environmental Research and Public Health*, 15(10), 2233.

Mehdipanah, R., Marra, G., Melis, G. and Gelormino, E. (2018). Urban renewal, gentrification and health equity: A realist perspective. *European Journal of Public Health*, 28(2), pp. 243–248.

Mitchell, R.J., Richardson, E.A., Shortt, N.K. and Pearce, J.R. (2015) Neighborhood environments and socioeconomic inequalities in mental well-being. *American Journal of Preventive Medicine*, 49(1), pp. 80–84.

Musterd, S., Marcińczak, S., van Ham, M. and Tammaru, T. (2017). Socioeconomic segregation in European capital cities. Increasing separation between poor and rich. *Urban Geography*, 38(7), pp. 1062–1083.

O'Neill, E., Cole, H.V.S., García-Lamarca, M., Anguelovski, I., Gullón, P. and Triguero-Mas, M. (2023). The right to the unhealthy deprived city: An exploration into the impacts of state-led redevelopment projects on the determinants of mental health. *Social Science & Medicine*, 318, 115634.

Oscilowicz, E., Anguelovski, I., Triguero-Mas, M., García-Lamarca, M., Baró, F. and Cole, H.V.S. (2022). Green justice through policy and practice: A call for further research into tools that foster healthy green cities for all. *Cities & Health*, 6, pp. 878–893.

Pearce, J., Cherrie, M., Shortt, N., Deary, I. and Ward Thompson, C. (2018). Life course of place: A longitudinal study of mental health and place. *Transactions of the Institute of British Geographers*, 43(4), pp. 555–572.

Pearsall, H. and Eller, J.K. (2020). Locating the green space paradox: A study of gentrification and public green space accessibility in Philadelphia, Pennsylvania. *Landscape and Urban Planning*, 195, 103708.

Rigolon, A. and Németh, J. (2018). Privately owned parks in New Urbanist communities: A study of environmental privilege, equity, and inclusion. *Journal of Urban Affairs*, 40(4), pp. 543–559.

Rigolon, A. and Németh, J. (2020). Green gentrification or "just green enough": Do park location, size and function affect whether a place gentrifies or not? *Urban Studies*, 57(2), pp. 402–420.

Safransky, S. (2014). Greening the urban frontier: Race, property, and resettlement in Detroit. *Geoforum*, 56, pp. 237–248.

Sandberg, L.A. (2014) Environmental gentrification in a post-industrial landscape: The case of the Limhamn quarry, Malmö, Sweden. *Local Environment*, 19(10), pp. 1068–1085.

Schinasi, L.H., Cole, H.V.S., Hirsch, J.A., Hamra, G.B., Gullon, P., Bayer, F., Melly, S.J., Neckerman, K.M., Clougherty, J.E. and Lovasi, G.S. (2021). Associations between greenspace and gentrification-related Sociodemographic and housing cost changes in major metropolitan areas across the United States. *International Journal of Environmental Research and Public Health*, 18(6), 3315.

Schnake-Mahl, A.S., Jahn, J.L., Subramanian, S.V., Waters, M.C. and Arcaya, M. (2020) Gentrification, neighborhood change, and population health: A systematic review. *Journal of Urban Health*, 97(1), pp. 1–25.

Shokry, G., Connolly, J.J. and Anguelovski, I. (2020). Understanding climate gentrification and shifting landscapes of protection and vulnerability in green resilient Philadelphia. *Urban Climate*, 31, 100539.

Smith, G., Cirach, M., Swart, W., Dėdelė, A., Gidlow, C., van Kempen, E., Kruize, H., Gražulevičienė, R. and Nieuwenhuijsen, M.J. (2017) Characterisation of the natural environment: Quantitative indicators across Europe. *International Journal of Health Geographics*, 16, 16.

Smith, N. (1982). Gentrification and uneven development. *Economic Geography*, 58(2), pp. 139–155.

Smith, N. (1996). *The New Urban Frontier: Gentrification and the Revanchist City*. London and New York: Routledge.

Smith, R.J., Lehning, A.J. and Kim, K. (2018). Aging in place in gentrifying neighborhoods: Implications for physical and mental health. *The Gerontologist*, 58(1), pp. 26–35.

Stuhlmacher, M., Kim, Y. and Kim, J.E. (2022). The role of green space in Chicago's gentrification. *Urban Forestry and Urban Greening*, 71, 127569.

Tran, L.D., Rice, T.H., Ong, P.M., Banerjee, S., Liou, J. and Ponce, N.A. (2020). Impact of gentrification on adult mental health. *Health Services Research*, 55(3), pp. 432–444.

Triguero-Mas, M., Donaire-Gonzalez, D., Seto, E., Valentín, A., Martínez, D., Smith, G., Hurst, G., Carrasco-Turigas, G., Masterson, D., van den Berg, M., Ambròs, A., Martínez-Íñiguez, T., Dedele, A., Ellis, N., Grazulevicius, T., Voorsmit, M., Cirach, M., Cirac-Claveras, J., Swart, W., Clasquin, E. and Niuewenhuijsen, M.J. (2017). Natural outdoor environments and mental health: Stress as a possible mechanism. *Environmental Research*, 159, pp. 629–638.

Triguero-Mas, M., Anguelovski, I., García-Lamarca, M., Argüelles, L., Pérez-del-Pulgar, C., Shokry, G., Connolly, J.J.T. and Cole, H.V.S. (2021). Natural outdoor environments' health effects in gentrifying neighborhoods: Disruptive green landscapes for underprivileged neighborhood residents. *Social Science & Medicine*, 279, 113964.

Triguero-Mas, M., Anguelovski, I., Connolly, J.J.T., Martin, N., Matheney, A., Cole, H.V.S., Pérez-del-Pulgar, C., García-Lamarca, M., Shokry, G., Argüelles, L., Conesa, D., Gallez, E., Sarzo, B., Angel Beltrán, M., López Máñez, J., Martínez-Minaya, J., Oscilowicz, E., Arcaya, M.C. and Baró, F. (2022). Exploring green gentrification in 28 global North cities: The role of urban parks and other types of greenspaces. *Environmental Research Letters*, 17(10), 104035.

Tulier, M.E., Reid, C., Mujahid, M.S. and Allen, A.M. (2019). "Clear action requires clear thinking": A systematic review of gentrification and health research in the United States. *Health & Place*, 59, 102173.

Vargas-Hernández, J.G., Pallagst, K. and Zdunek-Wielgołaska, J. (2018). Urban green spaces as a component of an ecosystem. In: J. Marques, ed, *Handbook of Engaged Sustainability*. Switzerland, Cham: Springer International Publishing.

Vilcins, D., Sly, P.D., Scarth, P. and Mavoa, S. (2022). Green space in health research: An overview of common indicators of greenness. *Reviews on Environmental Health*, 39(2), pp. 221–231. https://doi.org/10.1515/reveh-2022-0083.

Weber, S., Boley, B.B., Palardy, N. and Johnson Gaither, C. (2017). The impact of urban greenways on residential concerns: Findings from the Atlanta BeltLine Trail. *Landscape and Urban Planning*, 167, pp. 147–156.

Williams, D.R., Sternthal, M. and Wright, R.J. (2009). Social determinants: Taking the social context of asthma seriously. *Pediatrics*, 123(Supplement_3), pp. S174–S184.

Wolch, J.R., Byrne, J. and Newell, J.P. (2014). Urban green space, public health, and environmental justice: The challenge of making cities "just green enough". *Landscape and Urban Planning*, 125, pp. 234–244.

Zayas-Costa, M., Cole, H.V.S., Anguelovski, I., Connolly, J.J.T., Bartoll, X. and Triguero-Mas, M. (2021). Mental health outcomes in Barcelona: The interplay between gentrification and greenspace. *International Journal of Environmental Research and Public Health*, 18(17), 9314. Available at: https://doi.org/10.3390/ijerph18179314.

12 How do we understand the impact of immersion in blue space on mental health and wellbeing?

Hannah Denton, Charlie Dannreuther, and Kay Aranda

Splashing about! Introduction

The pleasures of outdoor water-based activities, particularly cold-water swimming, are no longer the secret of a few enthusiasts. Now mainstream, the experience of immersion in blue space, and the potential impact on mental health and wellbeing, is increasingly a focus of researchers (Foley et al., 2019). Blue space, which can include all visible outdoor surface water (White et al., 2016), is thought to have unique qualities that can positively impact those who visit (Gascon, 2017). Much of the research into the benefits of outdoor exercise on mental health and wellbeing has focused on land-based activities (Cumming, 2017), with less exploration of the specific experience of activity while submerged in water. In this chapter we share our developing understandings of the impacts of outdoor aquatic immersion on mental health and wellbeing. In doing so, we reflect on what research methods have been used across this work to date, and what different methods tell us about the experience of submerging our bodies in watery worlds.

Muddy water? Clarifying terminologies

Researchers interested in immersion in blue space approach the topic from within different research paradigms and with a multitude of methodologies in geography, physiology, health care, psychology and sociology, amongst others. This range of perspectives adds richness but also confusion, as the same terms are used and understood differently. In this chapter we will focus on research that investigates activities that take place in outdoor blue space, requiring full immersion, including swimming, surfing, diving. We have, however, included some studies that do not make a distinction between activities that take place largely on the water, for example kayaking, windsurfing, stand-up paddle-boarding. The blue spaces considered include all bodies of water where these activities can take place including the sea, reservoirs, lakes, lochs, rivers, harbours, canals and lidos.

Reflecting the complexity of the experiences that they are endeavouring to illuminate, what comprises mental health and wellbeing are understood in a myriad of different ways. The term wellbeing has been used interchangeably with happiness, life satisfaction, quality of life, personal growth and self-care (Evers and Phoenix, 2022). The background of the researcher leading a study often determines the methodologies that are favoured and therefore the insights gained. Qualitative researchers recognise wellbeing and mental health as multi-faceted and fluid, developing conceptual understandings

DOI: 10.4324/9781003345725-13

that are unique and individual. Quantitative researchers favour standardised measures so that comparisons can be made. Geographers exploring the ways in which certain environments can contribute to a sense of healing have highlighted the importance of dynamic, multisensory relationships with place (Atkinson and Scott, 2015). Experiences of landscape are understood as an assemblage (Anderson, 2012), comprised of more-than-human materiality, affects and experience in a particular timespace (lisahunter and Stoodley, 2021). There is often an associated feeling of belonging or 'home' and the opportunity to express one's self identity in and with place (Eyles and Williams, 2008) that may develop through repeated encounters over time (Jellard and Bell, 2021).

Awash with ideas! Developing qualitative methods.

The vast majority of research into immersion in blue space has relied on qualitative methods to explore and gain depth of insight into the experience (McNamara et al., 2020. Many researchers have collected data after the event using semi-structured interviews, free text questionnaires and diaries (Burlingham, 2022; Jellard and Bell, 2021; McDougall et al., 2022; Thompson and Wilkie, 2021). Others have explored using a variety of mobile or agile, in-situ, multisensory and emplaced methods to get as close to the experience as possible (Bates and Moles, 2022; Denton et al., 2021; lisahunter and Stoodley, 2021). This has, in part, been made possible by developments in technology such as the easy use of video cameras in the water which enable in-the-moment interviewing and recording. There have also been developments in research techniques whereby different creative methods are combined. This includes autoethnographic approaches that grapple with the overlap and interplay between researcher and participant. lisahunter and Stoodley argue that 'new theory-methods are required to facilitate understanding of this constantly fluctuating, watery, multi-dimensional, and under conceptualised assemblage of more-than-human (human, nature, technology) experience and relationships' (2021, p. 89). However, methodological approaches where researchers are both observer and participant are not without issues (Smith, 2021) so, whilst the use of mobile methods gets closer to the experience, there is a recognition that the recording of the experience also impacts on the experience. Furthermore, both blue space and human wellbeing may be undermined by the presence of technology (lisahunter and Stoodley, 2021, p. 101).

Reflecting the immersive quality of being in the water, and the exploration of mobile and in-situ methods, blue-space researchers are querying the distinction between human and non-human worlds. This interest in creative, novel and innovative spaces to map immersion follows the call for post-qualitative inquiry. Using this philosophical and theory-driven approach would be to move beyond conventional qualitative research to focus on the differential flows, energies, affect and desires inherent to the emergent phenomena of immersion (Fox and Powell, 2021; Lather, 2016; St Pierre, 2015, 2023). A diversification and experimentation within a complex ecology of inventing and innovating practices (St Pierre, 2023) is needed in order to more fully understand practices, potentials or capacities for action, interaction, feelings and desire produced in and through these networks or assemblages. These are assemblages developing in unpredictable and unequal ways, creating networks of habitual and non-habitual connections that future, more ontologically focused, empirical research would seek to analyse and understand (Fox and Powell, 2021).

Diving in! What have we learned about immersion?

Regular participants in immersing activities tend to prevail in the literature, with details of their experience used to discern what draws people to engage in these sports. Common themes of how this might be beneficial for mental health and wellbeing suggest that being submerged in water may offer an encounter unlike any other activity. Participants and researchers often report an experience of 'mindfulness', of being present in the moment that, rather than requiring effort to achieve, is impossible to avoid. Although slightly dependent on the activity, the kind of blue space and the season, there are common factors that force the participant to *'be present'* (McDougall et al., 2022). Aspects of being in outdoor blue space which are compelling and claim attention include the sensations associated with being submerged in cold water (Tipton et al., 2017), the changing conditions noticed through the embodied sensory experience (Britton and Foley, 2021; Thompson and Wilkie, 2021), the requirement to focus on breathing (Straughan, 2012), and a 'unique nature engagement that is distinct to that experienced during other activities and forms of exercise' (McDougall et al., p11). This focus on what is happening in the moment, along with the altered perspective of being in a watery world, enables a feeling of escape from the demands of everyday life (Denton and Aranda, 2020). This includes not only moving from a 'terrestrial place to a watery place, but also moving from the "head" and into the body' (Britton and Foley, 2021, p11). This experience of escape can provide respite from traumatic memories (Caddick et al., 2015). The surf zone can be experienced as a liminal space that dislocates people from their everyday lives (Anderson, 2013, p956). The calmness, serenity and equanimity that this elicits (Thompson and Wilkie, 2021) is a fundamental part of the experience. These moments were captured by lisahunter and Stoodley (2021) in 'subconscious rituals' that included stroking the surface of the water, staring out to the horizon, and humming a song.

Another core aspect of the experience, which although overlapping, is almost a contrast, is the feeling of exhilaration. Alongside calmness, there can be excitement, challenge, fear and elation (Denton and Aranda, 2020). The degree to which this is a part of the experience is somewhat dependent on the activity and the body of water. The sea, and to a lesser extent rivers, are wild and unpredictable. Fast moving and powerful water, in the form of strong currents and waves, provide challenging conditions that need to be navigated. A participant in this activity may develop skills, strength and fitness that enable greater challenges to be safely achieved however, the water always 'commands your respect and a constant state of vigilance' (Thompson and Wilkie, 2021, p. 9). Limits may change over time (Foley, 2018), with both experienced and 'new' swimmers becoming overwhelmed by emotions and feelings of anxiety 'when experiencing a sudden sensory stimulation, body sensation, or new movements in an unpredictable and ever-changing fluid environment of the sea' (Britton and Foley, 2021, p. 14). However, a part of the enjoyment is turning a potentially risky practice into an enabling one (Britton and Foley, 2021). However, not all outdoor blue spaces offer the same level of challenge. Lochs and lakes can offer a more peaceful environment, with boundaries that are visible, eliciting descriptions of the pleasures of the *'breaking glass'* moment when the surface is totally still (McDougall et al., 2022, p10). These differ from swimming pools which are, in comparison, more controlled and therefore safer. Indoor pools are often described as being important for fitness and accuracy of measurement (Ward, 2016) but can be experienced as 'chlorinated, sanitised, regulated and bounded' (Olive, 2023). In contrast, swimmers in outdoor blue space describe a sense of being able to move more freely, enjoying the sensation of being 'free to experience the water in diverse and inclusive ways' (Bates and Moles, 2022).

Approaching the impact of immersion from a different perspective, some researchers have investigated the changes in the physiology of the body in response to cold water. A significant proportion of this research has involved submerging research participants in tanks so conditions can be controlled and where equipment for measuring changes is easily accessible. This research has added to the understanding of what might be happening in the body when different hormones are released as the body adjusts to this different environment. This research has indicated that when fully submerged in cold water, both the sympathetic and the parasympathetic nervous systems are stimulated, perhaps reflecting the combination of both the sense of calm and the 'high' that are often reported (e.g. Hirvonen et al., 2002; Tipton et al., 2017). Researching these changes outside the laboratory has proved challenging, however, as the unruly nature of the environments under investigation do not lend themselves easily to precise scientific measuring of the bodies within them (Burlingham et al., 2022). Accurate measurements of physical tests are easier when captured in the context of experiments conducted in controlled environments that are typically indoors (Collier et al., 2015; Smolander et al., 2004).

Social wetworking? Immersion and community

Social and community-related qualities of experience are also regularly described in research exploring immersion in blue space (Caddick et al., 2015; lisahunter and Stoodley, 2021; McDougall et al., 2022). Whether this involves engaging in the activity together, helping each other and passing on knowledge (Thompson and Wilkie, 2021), or a post-swim chat with coffee and cake (Costello et al., 2019), the connection with others is often a key aspect of the experience. Although 'wild swimming' might be seen as a solitary pursuit where people retreat and connect with nature, the social interactions are often fundamental to engagement with blue space (Gould et al., 2021). People describe a closeness with their blue space buddies, sometimes relying on them for motivation, encouragement and occasionally safety, yet appreciate that conversation is often 'undemanding' (Bell et al., 2015) with a focus on the experience of being immersed rather than more stressful details of wider life. As such, people can come to feel included, whatever their background or current situation is, as long as they are a participant in the activity (Denton and Aranda, 2020). There are also reports of blue space communities stretching beyond the blue space, being there for each other when engaging in the activity is not possible (Costello et al., 2019), with vital connections being made as a result of being in and around water (Bates and Moles, 2022).

Bodies that otherwise might feel excluded, 'overlooked or problematised' can find a welcoming place in the water (Throsby, 2013, p. 103), with the 'unhealthy land body' transformed into a 'healthy sea-body' (Foley, 2015, p. 224). Bodies that might feel judged or limited in other exercise spaces can find room to move outside of the gaze of others once in the water. Measuring distances and times is fruitless when the water is moving, discouraging comparison either with others or with one's own performances on different days; whilst for some this is a barrier, for others it provides a release from expectation. As the water holds the body buoyant, it allows people to engage in exercise when land-based activities might be impossible (Tanaka, 2009), providing opportunities for 'healthy aging' (Costello et al., 2019). Participants also report using coastal and immersive activities to negotiate challenging life transitions or injury (Jellard and Bell, 2021; McDougall et al., 2022) as a result of benefits to both physical and mental health. Outdoor swimming can challenge established narratives of what constitutes a 'good body', widening it to include strong, acclimatised, insulated bodies (Bates and Moles, 2022, p6).

Frozen out? Unequal access to blue space

As the number of people engaging in activities within blue space increases, a less rosy picture of the experience is however also developing; one that is more challenging and fragmented, and in which many groups are excluded. While experienced by some as a freer space away from the gaze of others, worries about body size and the tight clothing required for water sports are reported as a barrier (Doughty, 2019) and may impact on people's ability to connect with the experience as a result of feeling self-conscious (McDougall et al., 2022). There can be differences in the ways that people enjoy the water, ranging from expert surfers and endurance swimmers who push the boundaries, to the lone swimmers, the wetsuit wearers and those who swim in 'skins', the head-up breaststrokers, the front crawlers, the dippers and bobbers who derive their pleasure purely from the immersive experience of being in the water, and triathletes who embrace technologies of wetsuits and Garmins to shave off the seconds; each having a different swimming experience (Bates and Moles, 2022). There can also be tensions between the blue space 'locals' or 'old timers' and the visitors or 'new adopters' (Olive, 2015). While there can be friction between and judgement towards each other, different groups may learn to co-exist as they coalesce and settle into their different forms of blue space engagement and 'negotiate a path between caring for a place and feeling a sense of place-based entitlement' (Olive, 2015 p. 507).

As well as relatively benign politics of water use, where there might be tensions and conflicts, but everyone still has access, there are groups that continue to be excluded. The coast is not a place of freedom for everyone (Britton et al., 2018) as 'place is experienced differently by different people' (Foley, 2015, p. 218). Blue space activities 'are shaped and constrained by a range of social, cultural, historical and geographical factors' (Britton et al., 2018, p. 147–148). Green and blue spaces can be racialised (Byrne and Wolch, 2009) and at the seaside 'racialised bodies' have been 'constructed as corporeal markers of undesirability and non-belonging' (Burdsey, 2013, p. 98). Young people from lower income backgrounds can feel socially and culturally excluded as a result of the social norms around water sports and surfing (Hignett et al., 2018). Lakes and swimming pools often require payment and internet access to book a visit and so 'the correct cultural and economic capital' is needed to access the water (Bates and Moles, 2022, p. 4). Although these facilities may provide safety cover as well as provide information about swimming safely, such regulations serve to control access, 'privileging certain bodies and granting the right to swim to only particular groups, at particular times' (Bates and Moles, 2022, p. 4). The ability to swim varies with people from black and minoritised ethnicities and individuals from lower income backgrounds less likely to have had opportunities to learn and feel comfortable in the water. Statistics from a number of different national contexts show that white people are less likely to drown than people of minoritised ethnicities (Giles et al., 2010) and that access to swimming pools is a barrier for lower socio-economic groups to become competent swimmers in many Western contexts (Giles et al., 2010; Wiltse, 2007). Both positive and negative associations with water can be passed through the generations (Britton, 2019). The exclusionary forces in outdoor blue spaces, including the 'process of othering' and the role of socio-political narratives in shaping their use, has led to concerns that these 'therapeutic landscape experiences' can become a 'privilege' of dominant groups within society (Bell et al., 2019; Conradson, 2014). Understanding how blue spaces can prompt trauma, fear and disengagement, as well as health and wellbeing, therefore warrants further attention (lisahunter and Stoodley, 2021, p. 106).

Slippery when wet! Can immersion in blue space be a therapeutic intervention?

Practitioners of blue space activities describe the positive emotions they experience as a result of being immersed in water (Burlingham et al., 2022; McDougall et al., 2022). These positive emotions can extend beyond the swim, throughout the day and even longer term (Massey et al., 2022). They can also link back to childhood memories, at times resulting in childlike behaviours whilst in the water (Foley, 2017). The reliable positive feeling associated with being immersed means it is often seen by participants as being like a drug or medicine for mental health (Costello et al., 2019; Charlier and Chaineux, 2009). The habitual practice of outdoor swimming is also understood as resulting in a heightened resilience, accreted over time, that enables swimmers to tolerate physically and mentally challenging circumstances (Foley, 2017). McDougall et al. (2022) described a participant who reported that her resilience was in part generated by knowing she would be able to go into the water again in the future. Conversely, there are adverse health and wellbeing impacts if regular participants are unable to swim (Foley, 2015). Veterans with PTSD emphasised the need to go surfing regularly to gain respite from symptoms (Caddick et al., 2015). Restrictions to immersing in blue space were imposed during the initial phase of the Covid 19 pandemic, when the RNLI and Surfing England released guidelines warning against entering the sea. Participants interviewed by Jellard and Bell (2021, p. 4) described a 'real longing for the ocean', and that immersing in water is 'not just important but necessary'. Whilst some visited the sea, and exercised alongside the water, this more distant encounter did not have the same impact as the intensive haptic sensory experience of aquatic immersion.

With the recognition that immersion in blue space might have a positive impact on mental health and wellbeing, practitioners have explored whether it can be used as an intervention for people who are struggling with mental health. There are increasing numbers of 'surf therapy' wellbeing initiatives that enable people to benefit from the 'all-encompassing sensory nature of being in the ocean' (Wheaton et al., 2020, p. 86). Devine-Wright and Godfrey (2015, 2018) found consistent and sustained improvements in the mental health and physical wellbeing of the vulnerable young people that participated in their six-week surf therapy groups. They suggested this was as a result of the sensory, social and inclusive qualities of the program. In a study exploring the impact of an outdoor swimming course for people with depression and anxiety, Burlingham et al. (2022) found significant reductions in participant scores on standardised measures undertaken pre versus post the swim course. The lower scores were maintained at follow up three months later. A parallel qualitative analysis indicated that confronting challenges, becoming a community and appreciating the moment were key to participants enjoying immediate positive changes in mood, improved mental and physical health and an increased motivation to swim. Britton et al. (2018) undertook a systematic review exploring the impact of blue space 'blue care' interventions and concluded that, although there were limited studies in the area, overall blue care can have direct benefit for health, especially mental health and psycho-social wellbeing.

Concerns have been raised, however, about how consistently these interventions can be offered. Navigating the risks of being immersed in blue space can be an important aspect resulting in positive benefits (Britton et al., 2020; Devine-Wright and Godfrey, 2015, 2018), but there is still little research about whether all outdoor water-based instructors have the capacity to support these interventions (Juster-Horsfield and Bell, 2022). Juster-Horsfield and Bell (2022, p. 141) suggest the need for a 'blue care skillset' that includes recognising potential risks, ensuring participants are fully informed of the risks, being responsive to individual need and understanding when to support participants to take risks that match their ability. The potential for participants to be excluded as a result of resourcing has also been identified, whether that is because they are not able to sustain the financial commitment or because programme funding is ad hoc or short term (James et al., 2019). Finally, there is a danger that using blue space for health interventions might medicalise activities that people engage in for pleasure (Juster-Horsfield and Bell, 2022).

Quantitative methods are generally the mainstay for health research, with the randomised controlled trial (RCT) considered the gold standard in determining the efficacy of an intervention and therefore key to developing the evidence base required for public funding. However, there are limited numbers of quantitative studies within blue space, perhaps reflecting the challenges in using such research methodologies in blue care contexts. By design, quantitative studies reduce experience to component and measurable parts to determine changes. There is a requirement for order and precision so that studies can be generalised and replicable. However, most outdoor blue space is untamed and somewhat unpredictable. Of the 33 studies included in the blue care review undertaken by Britton et al. (2018), 13 explored the impact of immersion in blue space and only 7 of those were quantitative. As well as noting a lack of structured quantitative studies in this area, Britton et al. identified no RCTs. However, they also questioned how feasible it would be to employ this methodology with the difficulties of blinding participants to an intervention arm, the ethics of allocating participants to a control arm, and the financial uncertainty of the organisations delivering the interventions. There are also challenges with choosing appropriate measures, as participants might feel uncomfortable being evaluated by questionnaires that are overly clinical or problem-focused (Britton et al., 2018), that are not designed to meet the particular needs of a target population and place (Linton et al, 2016) or fail to reflect the complexities of how wellbeing takes shape for different people, including indigenous understandings and experiences of wellbeing (Ritchie et al, 2014). Despite the importance of assessing the impact of immersion in blue space, and the continued expectation to use RCTs in developing the evidence base necessary for blue space interventions to be widely offered to populations who might benefit, there are many challenges.

Wading through sh**! Immersion and pollution

Extending beyond the human-centric focus, researchers have also attended to the more-than-human aspects of the environment. It has been pointed out that not all outdoor water is blue (Foley et al. 2019; Pitt, 2018) but includes green-blue (Finlay et al., 2015), the grey-blue of water in urban spaces (Völker and Kistemann, 2015), brown (Pitt, 2018), and even the white of winter landscapes (Finlay, 2018). Regardless of colour, it is important to recognise which are 'health-enabling places and spaces', where the water in these environments has 'identifiable potential for the promotion of human-wellbeing' (Foley and Kistemann, 2015, p. 158). Water pollution can be a health hazard for water users, even when beaches appear to be clean (Evers, 2019; Wheaton, 2007). Water quality, and the associated health risks of exposure to polluted waters, are a particular concern (Leonard et al., 2018). The development of the safer seas app, and the information provided by the environmental charity, Surfers Against Sewage, has highlighted the extent to which raw sewage is being discharged into waterways (Brown, 2021). While regular blue space users were largely aware of this to varying degrees (Evers, 2019), and might avoid blue space immersion following significant rainfall or reports of sewage outflows, this app has brought this knowledge into the mainstream. The greater awareness of potential threats causes dilemmas for water users, with some rethinking their immersive practices (BBC, 2021) and others continuing regardless (Evers, 2019). Those that continue report efforts to ignore the potential threats, feeling that to dwell on them would compromise the potential for enhanced mental health and wellbeing (Evers and Phoenix, 2022). There is also an emerging recognition of the importance of the weather (Bell et al. 2019), and how this can shape the sensory experience of aquatic encounters. Although not yet widely researched, the health impacts of regular blue space immersion may lead to a greater eco-awareness and concern, encouraging people to recognise our entanglement with the more-than-human world (Britton, 2019).

Land Ahoy? Grounding blue space research: concluding remarks

Water research is transdisciplinary and offers opportunities for more participatory and agnostic ways of producing knowledge (Krueger et al., 2016). Through the use of creative qualitative methodologies, an understanding of the in-the-moment experience of being in water outdoors is emerging. As well as the pleasures and benefits of immersing in watery worlds, an awareness of some of the challenges faced by water users is also developing. In addition to polluted waters, resulting in additional risks to immersion, it is becoming clear that there are significant inequalities in access with some members of the population much less likely to be able to enjoy aquatic activities. As a result of the reported positive impact on mental health, 'blue-care' water-based activities are being explored as a possible therapeutic intervention to benefit mental health. However, a randomised control trial, the mainstay of medical and health research, is yet to be undertaken. Perhaps reflecting the unruly and unpredictable environment of outdoor water, quantitative methods, requiring controlled conditions and precise measurement, are proving elusive. These methods may resist recognising so-called water 'cures', much as they did in the nineteenth century (Adams, 2015). Epistemologies that can reflect entangled relationships with nature, community and self may be more relevant in understanding immersion in blue space, elucidating meaning in water bodies (Strang, 2005) in ways that transcend the abyssal divide between spiritual and scientific meanings of water (Hayashi et al., 2021). These insights urge us to reframe human/nonhuman nature relationships, for example around principles of kinship, to accommodate ontologies of thinking-feeling and to acknowledge a pluriverse of world views and epistemologies (Escobar, 2019; Boelens et al., 2016, 2022). The challenges of categorising, understanding, measuring and abstracting seem to be greater in water. However, conversely, these challenges may offer new insights into all contemporary research attempting to understand the human experience.

References

Adams, J.M., (2016). Healing with water: English spas and the water cure, 1840–1960. In *Healing with water*. Manchester University Press.

Anderson, J. (2012). Relational places: The surfed wave as assemblage and convergence. *Environment and Planning D: Society and Space*, 30(4), pp.570–587.

Anderson, J. (2013). Cathedrals of the surf zone: Regulating access to a space of spirituality. *Social & Cultural Geography*, 14(8), pp.954–972.

Atkinson, S. and Scott, K. (2015). Stable and destabilised states of subjective well-being: Dance and movement as catalysts of transition. *Social & Cultural Geography*, 16(1), pp.75–94.

Bates, C. and Moles, K. (2022). Immersive encounters: Video, swimming and wellbeing. *Visual Studies*, 38(1), pp.69–80.

Bates, C. and Moles, K. (2022). Bobbing in the park: Wild swimming, conviviality and belonging. *Leisure Studies*, pp.1–13.

BBC. (2021). St Ives: Open Water Swimmers Quitting over River Sewage Risk. British Broadcasting Commission, 29 October 2021. Available online: www.bbc.co.uk/news/uk-england-cambridgesh ire-59082896.

Bell, S.L., Leyshon, C. and Phoenix, C. (2019). Negotiating nature's weather worlds in the con-text of life with sight impairment. *Transactions of the Institute of British Geographers*, 44(2), pp.270–283.

Bell, S.L., Phoenix, C., Lovell, R. and Wheeler, B.W. (2015). Seeking everyday wellbeing: The coast as a therapeutic landscape. *Social Science & Medicine*, 142, pp.56–67.

Boelens, R., Hoogesteger, J., Swyngedouw, E., Vos, J. and Wester, P. (2016). Hydrosocial terri-tories: A political ecology perspective. *Water International*, 41(1), pp.1–14.

Boelens, R., Escobar, A., Bakker, K., Hommes, L., Swyngedouw, E., Hogenboom, B., Huijbens, E.H., Jackson, S., Vos, J., Harris, L.M. and Joy, K.J. (2022). Riverhood: political ecologies of socionature commoning and translocal struggles for water justice 50 (3). *Journal of Peasant Studies*, 50(3), pp.1–32.

Britton, E. and Foley, R. (2021). Sensing water: Uncovering health and well-being in the sea and surf. *Journal of Sport and Social Issues*, 45(1), pp.60–87.

Britton, E., Kindermann, G., Domegan, C. and Carlin, C. (2020). Blue care: A systematic review of blue space interventions for health and wellbeing. *Health Promotion International*, 35(1), pp.50–69.

Britton, E. (2018). 'Be like water': Reflections on strategies developing cross-cultural programmes for women, surfing and social good. In *The Palgrave Handbook of Feminism and Sport, Leisure and Physical Education* Mansfield, L., Caudwell, J., Wheaton, B., Watson, B. (Eds.) (pp.793–807). Palgrave Macmillan. https://doi.org/10.1057/978-1-137-53318-0_50

Britton, E., Olive, R. and Wheaton, B. (2018). Surfers and leisure: 'Freedom' to surf? Contested spaces on the coast. In *Living with the Sea* Brown, M., Peters, K. (Eds.) (pp.147–166). Routledge.

Britton, E. (2019). Dúchas: Being and belonging on the borderlands of surfing, senses and self. In *Blue Space, Health and Wellbeing* Foley, R., Kearns, R., Kistemann, T., Wheeler, B.W. (Eds.) (pp.95–116). Routledge.

Burdsey, D. (2013). 'The foreignness is still quite visible in this town': Multiculture, marginality and prejudice at the English seaside. *Patterns of Prejudice*, 47(2), pp.95–116.

Burlingham, A., Denton, H., Massey, H., Vides, N. and Harper, C.M. (2022). Sea swimming as a novel intervention for depression and anxiety-A feasibility study exploring engagement and acceptability. *Mental Health and Physical Activity*, 23, 100472.

Brown, D. Sewage Discharged into Rivers 400,000 Times in 2020. British Broadcasting Commission, 31 March 2021. Available online: www.bbc.co.uk/news/science-environment-56590219 (accessed on 13 December 2021).

Byrne, J. and Wolch, J. (2009). Nature, race, and parks: Past research and future directions for geographic research. *Progress in Human Geography*, 33(6), pp.743–765.

Caddick, N., Smith, B. and Phoenix, C. (2015). The effects of surfing and the natural environment on the well-being of combat veterans. *Qualitative Health Research*, 25(1), pp.76–86.

Charlier, R.H. and Chaineux, M.C.P. (2009). The healing sea: A sustainable coastal ocean resource: Thalassotherapy. *Journal of Coastal Research*, 25(4), pp.838–856.

Collier, N., Massey, H.C., Lomax, M., Harper, M. and Tipton, M.J. (2015, December). Cold water swimming and upper respiratory tract infections. *Extreme Physiology & Medicine*, 4(1), pp.1–2.

Conradson, D. (2014). Health and well-being. In: *Introducing Human Geographies*, 3rd Edition Cloke, P., Crang, P., Goodwin, M. (Eds.) (pp.599–612). Routledge.

Costello, L., McDermott, M.L., Patel, P. and Dare, J. (2019). 'A lot better than medicine'-Self-organised ocean swimming groups as facilitators for healthy ageing. *Health & Place*, 60, 102212.

Cumming, I. (2017). *The health & wellbeing benefits of swimming*. Swim England's Swimming and Health Commission.

Denton, H. and Aranda, K. (2020). The wellbeing benefits of sea swimming. Is it time to revisit the sea cure? *Qualitative Research in Sport, Exercise and Health*, 12(5), pp.647–663.

Denton, H., Dannreuther, C. and Aranda, K. (2021). Researching at sea: Exploring the 'swim-along' interview method. *Health & Place*, 67, 102466.

Devine-Wright, H. and Godfrey, C. (2018. Surf therapy: The long-term impact. *An Independent Longitudinal Evaluation of the Impact of the Wave Project on Vulnerable Young People 2013-2017*, [viewed 5-7-2024 @ www.waveproject.co.uk/wp-content/uploads/2018/05/Wave-Project-Evaluation-2018.pdf]

Devine-Wright, H. and Godfrey, C. (2015). From Positive Outcomes to Lasting Impact. In *An Independent Evaluation of the Wave Project's Impact on Vulnerable Young People over 3 Years from 2013-2015*. Exeter: Wave Project. [viewed 5-7-2024 @ for The Wave Project available at www.waveproject.co.uk]

Doughty, K. (2019). From water as curative agent to enabling waterscapes: Diverse experiences of the 'therapeutic blue'. In *Blue Space, Health and Wellbeing* Foley, R., Kearns, R., Kistemann, T., Wheeler, B.W. (Eds.) (pp.77–94). Routledge.

Escobar, A. (2019). Territorial Struggles and the Ontological Dimension of the Epistemologies of the South. In *Knowledges Born in the Struggle: Constructing the Epistemologies of the Global South*. de Sousa Santos, B., Menenses, M. (Eds.) (pp.11–32). Routledge.

Evers, C.W. (2019). Polluted leisure. *Leisure Sciences*, 41(5), pp.423–440.

Evers, C. and Phoenix, C. (2022). Relationships between recreation and pollution when striving for wellbeing in blue spaces. *International Journal of Environmental Research and Public Health*, 19(7), 4170.

Eyles, J. and Williams, A. eds. (2008). *Sense of place, health and quality of life*. Ashgate Publishing.

Finlay, J.M., 2018. 'Walk like a penguin': Older Minnesotans' experiences of (non) therapeutic white space. *Social Science & Medicine*, 198, pp.77–84.

Finlay, J., Franke, T., McKay, H. and Sims-Gould, J. (2015). Therapeutic landscapes and well-being in later life: Impacts of blue and green spaces for older adults. *Health & Place*, 34, pp.97–106.

Foley, R. (2017). Swimming as an accretive practice in healthy blue space. *Emotion, Space and Society*, 22, pp.43–51.

Foley, R., Kearns, R., Kistemann, T. and Wheeler, B. (2019). *Blue space, health and wellbeing*. Hydrophilia Unbounded, Routledge, London. https://doi.org/10.4324/9780815359159.

Foley, R. (2018). Mapping a blue trace: An intermittent swimming life. In *Water, Creativity and Meaning* Roberts, L., Phillips, K. (Eds.) (pp.86–102). Routledge.

Foley, R. (2015). Swimming in Ireland: Immersions in therapeutic blue space. *Health & Place*, 35, pp.218–225.

Foley, R. and Kistemann, T. (2015). Blue space geographies: Enabling health in place. *Health & Place*, 35, pp.157–165.

Fox, N.J. and Powell, K., (2021). Non-human matter, health disparities and a thousand tiny dis/advantages. *Sociology of Health & Illness*, 43(3), pp.779–795.

Gascon, M., Zijlema, W., Vert, C., White, M.P. and Nieuwenhuijsen, M.J. (2017). Outdoor blue spaces, human health and well-being: A systematic review of quantitative studies. *International Journal of Hygiene and Environmental Health*, 220(8), pp.1207–1221.

Giles, A.R., Castleden, H. and Baker, A.C. (2010). "We listen to our Elders. You live longer that way": Examining aquatic risk communication and water safety practices in Canada's North. *Health & place*, 16(1), pp.1–9.

Gould, S., McLachlan, F. and McDonald, B. (2021). Swimming with the Bicheno "Coffee Club": The textured world of wild swimming. *Journal of Sport and Social Issues*, 45(1), pp.39–59.

Hayashi, Y., Christie, M., Gaillard, J.C., Banks, E.W., Batelaan, O. and Ellis, J. (2021). A transdisciplinary engagement with Australian Aboriginal water and the hydrology of a small bedrock island. *Hydrological Sciences Journal*, 66(13), pp.1845–1856.

Hignett, A., White, M.P., Pahl, S., Jenkin, R. and Froy, M.L. (2018). Evaluation of a surfing programme designed to increase personal well-being and connectedness to the natural environment among 'at risk' young people. *Journal of Adventure Education and Outdoor Learning*, 18(1), pp.53–69.

Hirvonen, J., Lindeman, S., Joukamaa, M. and Huttunen, P. (2002). Plasma catecholamines, serotonin and their metabolites and beta-endorphin of winter swimmers during one winter. Possible correlations to psychological traits. *International Journal of Circumpolar Health*, 61(4), pp.363–372.

James, J.J., Christiana, R.W. and Battista, R.A. (2019). A historical and critical analysis of park prescriptions. *Journal of Leisure Research*, 50(4), pp.311–329.

Jellard, S. and Bell, S.L. (2021). A fragmented sense of home: Reconfiguring therapeutic coastal encounters in Covid-19 times. *Emotion, Space and Society*, 40, 100818.

Juster-Horsfield, H.H. and Bell, S.L. (2022). Supporting 'blue care 'through outdoor water-based activities: Practitioner perspectives. *Qualitative Research in Sport, Exercise and Health*, 14(1), pp.137–150.

Krueger, T., Maynard, C., Carr, G., Bruns, A., Mueller, E.N. and Lane, S., (2016). A transdisciplinary account of water research. *Wiley Interdisciplinary Reviews: Water*, 3(3), pp.369–389.

Lather, P. (2016). Top Ten+ List: (Re) thinking ontology in (Post) qualitative research. *Cultural Studies? Critical Methodologies*, 16(2), pp.125–131.

Leonard, A.F., Singer, A., Ukoumunne, O.C., Gaze, W.H. and Garside, R. (2018). Is it safe to go back into the water? A systematic review and meta-analysis of the risk of acquiring infections from recreational exposure to seawater. *International Journal of Epidemiology*, 47(2), pp.572–586

Linton, M.J., Dieppe, P. and Medina-Lara, A. (2016). Review of 99 self-report measures for assessing well-being in adults: Exploring dimensions of well-being and developments over time. *BMJ Open*, 6(7), e010641

Lisahunter and Stoodley, L. (2021). Bluespace, senses, wellbeing, and surfing: Prototype cyborg theory-methods. *Journal of Sport and Social Issues*, 45(1), pp.88–112.

Massey, H., Gorczynski, P., Harper, C.M., Sansom, L., McEwan, K., Yankouskaya, A. and Denton, H. (2022). Perceived impact of outdoor swimming on health: Web-based survey. *Interactive Journal of Medical Research*, 11(1), e25589.

McDougall, C.W., Foley, R., Hanley, N., Quilliam, R.S. and Oliver, D.M. (2022). Freshwater wild swimming, health and well-being: Understanding the importance of place and risk. *Sustainability*, 14(10), 6364.

McNamara, M., Murphy, A., Dowler, F. and Foley, R. (2020). Blue spaces as resources for health and wellbeing: Survey comparisons of indoor and outdoor settings from Ireland. *Revista de Estudios Andaluces*, 39, pp.8–22.

Olive, R. (2015). Surfing, localism, place-based pedagogies and ecological sensibilities in Australia. In B. Humberstone, H. Prince, and K. A. Henderson (eds) *Routledge International Handbook of Outdoor Studies* (pp.501–510). Routledge.

Olive, R. (2023). How to swim without water: Swimming as an ecological sensibility. In *Living with water* Bates, C., Moles, K. (Eds.) (pp.235–253). Manchester University Press.

Pitt, H. (2018). Muddying the waters: What urban waterways reveal about bluespaces and well-being. *Geoforum*, 92, pp.161–170.

Ritchie, S.D., Wabano, M.J., Russell, K., Enosse, L. and Young, N.L. (2014). Promoting resilience and wellbeing through an outdoor intervention designed for Aboriginal adolescents. *Rural and Remote Health*, 14(1), pp.83–101.

St Pierre, E.A. (2015). Practices for the "new" in new empiricisms, new materialisms, and post qualitative research. In N. K. Denzin and M. D. Giardina (eds) *Qualitative Inquiry and the Politics of Research* (pp.75–95). Routledge.

St. Pierre, E.A. (2023). Poststructuralism and post qualitative inquiry: What can and must be thought. *Qualitative Inquiry*, 29(1), pp.20–32.

Smith, T.S. (2021). Therapeutic taskscapes and craft geography: Cultivating well-being and atmospheres of recovery in the workshop. *Social & Cultural Geography*, 22(2), pp.151–169.

Smolander, J., Mikkelsson, M., Oksa, J., Westerlund, T., Leppäluoto, J. and Huttunen, P. (2004). Thermal sensation and comfort in women exposed repeatedly to whole-body cryotherapy and winter swimming in ice-cold water. *Physiology & Behavior*, 82(4), pp.691–695.

Strang, V. (2005). Common senses: Water, sensory experience and the generation of meaning. *Journal of Material Culture*, 10(1), pp.92–120.

Straughan, E.R. (2012). Touched by water: The body in scuba diving. *Emotion, Space and Society*, 5(1), pp.19–26.

Tanaka, H. (2009). Swimming exercise: Impact of aquatic exercise on cardiovascular health. *Sports Medicine*, 39, pp.377–387.

Thompson, N. and Wilkie, S. (2021). 'I'm just lost in the world': The impact of blue exercise on participant well-being. *Qualitative Research in Sport, Exercise and Health*, 13(4), pp.624–638.

Throsby, K. (2013). 'If I go in like a cranky sea lion, I come out like a smiling dolphin': Marathon swimming and the unexpected pleasures of being a body in water. *Feminist Review*, 103(1), pp.5–22.

Tipton, M.J., Collier, N., Massey, H., Corbett, J. and Harper, M. (2017). Cold water immersion: Kill or cure? *Experimental Physiology*, 102(11), pp.1335–1355.

Ward, M. (2016). Swimming in a contained space: Understanding the experience of indoor lap swimmers. *Health & Place*, 46, pp.315–321.

Wheaton, B. (2007). Identity, politics, and the beach: Environmental activism in surfers against sewage. *Leisure Studies*, 26(3), pp.279–302.

Wheaton, B., Waiti, J., Cosgriff, M. and Burrows, L. (2020). Coastal blue space and wellbeing research: Looking beyond western tides. *Leisure Studies*, 39(1), pp.83–95.

White, R., Abraham, C., Smith, J.R., White, M. and Staiger, P.K. (2016). Recovery under sail: Rehabilitation clients' experience of a sail training voyage. *Addiction Research & Theory*, 24(5), pp.355–365.

Wiltse, J. (2007). *Contested waters: A social history of swimming pools in America*. University of North Carolina Press.

Völker, S. and Kistemann, T. (2015). Developing the urban blue: Comparative health responses to blue and green urban open spaces in Germany. *Health & Place*, 35, pp.196–205.

13 Lifestyle sports, blue space and mental health
Examining the case of surf therapy

Belinda Wheaton and Rebecca Olive

Introduction

An increasingly vibrant body of multidisciplinary research shows that sport and leisure activities, from playing on shorelines to physical activities on and in water, are central to how people's relationships with blue spaces are forged (Bell et al., 2015). This research 'recognises that our relationships to water can shape our identities, sense of belonging and place, and influence our physical, emotional and spiritual wellbeing' (Olive & Wheaton, 2021, p.4). In this chapter, we focus on recreational "lifestyle sports" (Wheaton, 2004, 2013), such as surfing, swimming, paddling, and sailing, which are practised in and on blue spaces including oceans, rivers, reservoirs, pools, and harbours. Lifestyle sport participation and experiences are wide-ranging, from those of people who swim or paddle as one of many different blue space recreation activities, to avid and committed enthusiasts and professional 'athletes'. Many lifestyle sports have informal and individualistic cultures without explicit rules, regulations, spatial boundaries, or institutional settings. However, for some participants, engagement is more formalised and involves structured, organised sporting competitions, clubs or programmes. In this chapter we build on our previous research on blue spaces, sport, health and wellbeing to discuss how lifestyle sports are important for understanding how we experience and access blue spaces, from everyday encounters to local micro-adventures and international tourism, and how these practices impact participants' mental health and wellbeing (Olive & Wheaton, 2021). As we discuss below, nature-based therapy interventions involving activities such as surfing and swimming, are one of the emerging ways in which informal lifestyle sports activities are being adapted into programmes to enrich people's lives.

Rather than consider the capacities of a range of sports and blue spaces, our commentary focuses on surfing. In particular, we consider participants' relationships to the complex interactions they have in the sites of engagement, i.e. coasts and oceans, and how these impact health and wellbeing for recreational lifestyle sport participants. First, we provide a brief overview of the multidisciplinary literature exploring blue spaces, physical recreation, and health and wellbeing, highlighting key research approaches and foci. We highlight the value of place-based approaches that focus on different blue spaces, and the need to consider both the barriers and inequalities in access to blue spaces, as well as the benefits. Then we discuss the rapidly expanding "surf therapy" movement that has stemmed from growing interest in the therapeutic, immersive capacities of sport and physical activities in blue spaces. We provide an overview of research and evaluations of the potential of surf therapy programmes for fostering physical, mental, social, and

DOI: 10.4324/9781003345725-14

spiritual health and wellbeing. In assessing these claims about surf therapy interventions, we argue that while they have many benefits, they also present challenges that limit their potential as a tool for promoting mental health, which are largely unaccounted for in the literature. In the final section of the chapter, we focus on health and wellbeing inequalities, reflecting on the ways informal lifestyle sport participation/surf therapy can reproduce existing inequalities and injustices, including in health and wellbeing. In this, our aim is not to dismiss the important role that many therapy programmes can and do provide, but to recognise the complexity of blue space lifestyle sports as therapeutic beyond time-constrained and funding-reliant organised programmes and interventions.

Blue spaces, health and wellbeing

Over recent decades, a body of research across the humanities and social sciences has focused on the role of blue spaces in shaping human health and wellbeing (Foley et al., 2019; Olive & Wheaton, 2021). As White et al. (2020) illustrate in a synthesis of this research, diverse methodologies have been adopted across the field, including both quantitative (e.g. epidemiological studies, field and laboratory experiments, visitor surveys) and in-depth qualitative research (e.g. interviews and in situ fieldwork). Themes and approaches have often been developed using questions and findings from green space literature, such as considerations of if, how, and why 'time spent with nature can contribute to human health and well-being' (Frumkin et al., 2017, quoted in Bell et al., 2019, p.1). While a detailed overview of this field of research is beyond our scope here, we draw attention to key productive shifts. First, the move from a pathogenic focus on health risks and problems to more salutogenic approaches. Second, from positivistic understandings of individual health and wellbeing towards approaches that conceptualise health and wellbeing as subjective, transpersonal, contextual, relational, and situated. And third, research contributions, especially from health geographers, who have increased the field's focus on the spatial determinants of health and the forms of individual and social interactions that influence wellbeing (c.f. Kearns & Gesler, 1998; Kearns & Moon, 2002). Underpinning each of these shifts are wider ontological understandings of "health", "wellbeing" and "nature" among researchers and participants.

Bio/health scientists have historically maintained a pathogenic focus on health risks and problems. Blue space environments pose a wide range of threats to human health and wellbeing such as drowning, water-borne diseases and flooding, pollution, and microplastics, which are 'generally far better articulated and documented than the benefits' (White et al., 2020, p.2). More salutogenic approaches focus on factors that support health and wellbeing, such as the 'affective, life-enhancing, and health-enabling' qualities of water (Foley et al., 2019, p.2) and the sense of perspective and vulnerability that immersive, multispecies encounters can bring (Olive, 2022). The shift to a more salutogenic lens reflects social models that 'emphasise the promotion and protection of health and wellbeing rather than the causes of illness' and locate 'individual experience within social contexts' (Philips & Evans, 2015, p. 2342). These insights have become embedded in health geographies, where the disciplinary focus has 'shifted away from illness and disease towards a focus on the place-based facilitation of health' (Smith & Reid, 2018, p. 811). This approach has become more broadly accepted. For example, the UN World Health Organization constitution states that 'health is a state of complete physical, mental and social well-being and not merely the absence of disease or infirmity' (WHO, 2023). These changes in approach have meant that in contemporary health research, mental health is understood to be more than just the absence of mental disorders, illness or impairment; recognising that it is connected to factors including social structures, physical movement, and the health of the places we live, work and play in.

Alongside changing conceptions of 'health', the term 'wellbeing' has become prevalent within policy and research (Phillips, Evans & Muirhead, 2015). Yet, despite an increasingly large and multi-disciplinary literature on wellbeing, an ongoing lack of clarity and consensus on what wellbeing is, and how to measure it, continues to present challenges for research, policy and community understandings (Atkinson & Joyce, 2011). Psychological models emphasising subjective wellbeing and individual happiness, initially dominated particularly in wellbeing policies. However, extensive critiques have been made about these approaches. The focus on individual rather than social wellbeing masks the importance of social inequalities and fails to recognise how wellbeing cuts 'across the personal, social, and material world' (Mansfield, Daykin & Kay, 2020, p.1). Recent reconceptualisations, including within the fields of health and cultural geographies, have presented wellbeing as subjective, transpersonal, contextual, relational, and situated, with increased focus on the complex interactions across physical, mental, emotional, spiritual, societal and environmental domains (Bell et al., 2019; Fleuret & Atkinson, 2007). These understandings have become increasingly influential in sociocultural research on blue space, sport, leisure, health, and wellbeing (Evers & Phoenix, 2022; Moles, 2021; Olive & Wheaton, 2021).

While changing social conceptions of health and wellbeing have contributed significant developments in the field, shifting from instrumental conceptions of the spaces themselves has been less universal. However, binary and universalised understandings of "nature" – such as those within policy imperatives seeking to show the economic value of "nature" for human health – have been problematised. For example, in questioning the health policy shift towards "nature prescriptions" for health, Bell et al. (2019) argue that standardised 'dose-response frameworks' tend to conceptualise nature in universal ways and fail to recognise the different ways in which cultures and communities understand, perceive and experience nature. Instead, they suggest, experiences of health and wellbeing 'emerge through dynamic, more-than-human relations' and connections (Bell et al. 2019, p. 1). Exemplifying this point, a number of researchers have offered in depth examples of such human/non-human relations, including with animals (Olive, 2022), materialities (e.g. rocks, sand, waves) (Booth, 2019), weather (Phoenix, Bell & Wheeler, 2021-2022), as well as culture and ancestors (Stronach & Adair, 2020; Waiti & Awatere, 2019). This work highlights that through 'multispecies and non-human encounters, nature-based sports and physical activities allow us to *feel* the illusion of human/nature separation' (Olive, 2022, p. 3, italics original).

These shifts align with popular interest in the potential role of nature in supporting 'therapeutic landscape' experiences (Gesler, 1992). The idea that encounters with landscapes may be culturally, emotionally, and spiritually therapeutic (Philips, Evans and Muirhead, 2015) has been widely used to illustrate how blue space experiences connect to a range of physical, cognitive, emotional, spiritual, economic, and sociocultural processes (Bell et al., 2018; Foley, 2015; 2017). As we highlight elsewhere, the significance of sport, leisure, and physical cultures to how we access and experience blue spaces has given rise to a growing emphasis on the role of blue spaces in human wellbeing (Olive & Wheaton, 2021). For example, Bell et al.'s (2015) research exploring local leisure-based coastal interactions in England illustrates these interconnected dimensions in people's encounters on, by, and in the sea. They identify four overlapping "therapeutic experience" dimensions in participants' coastal leisure interactions, namely, 'symbolic, achieving, immersive, and social' (2015, p. 58).

While simply living by the coast can have benefits (Ballesteros-Olza, Gracia-de-Rentería, Pérez-Zabaleta, 2020) it is suggested that ocean immersion activities such as swimming and surfing have unique effects on promoting physical, mental, emotional, and spiritual wellbeing for individuals (Foley et al., 2019). Surfing and open water swimming are two sport and leisure activities that have garnered research attention across different sites, geographies, climates, communities, and demographics, including sex/gender, ethnicity, age, war veterans and newcomers (see for example, Burlingham et al., 2022; Caddick, Smith and Phoenix, 2015; Olive, 2019; Wheaton, 2017). Adopting qualitative methodologies – from in-depth interviews and participant observations to 'in situ' mobile methods such as swim-alongs – this research shows how people obtain skills and knowledge, develop a sense of collective identity and belonging, and experience spirituality and connection to nature (Denton & Aranda, 2019; lisahunter & Stoodley, 2021). Furthermore, in-line with socio-ecological models of health and more-than-human scholarship, such research has revealed the interconnectedness of people, places, ecologies, and multispecies entities (Olive, 2022). Individuals who regularly swim in open waters report experiencing increased connection to place and the 'natural environment' (Foley, 2015; 2017; Moles, 2021). Surfers can develop an ethic of care, and responsibility for local environments, contributing to the ongoing management, safeguarding, and restoration of place (Evers & Phoenix, 2022; Olive, 2015; Wheaton, 2007; 2020).

More recently, there has been growing recognition that blue spaces can also be sites of exclusion and inequity; how different 'subjects and bodies access and experience blue spaces' impacts who can use blue spaces, and 'how they can be used' (Olive & Wheaton 2021, p. 8). White, non-disabled, coastal dwelling, middle class people are the most dominant group represented in existing research. Yet, for many outside this group, intersecting factors relating to geography, race and ethnicity, sex/gender, class, and dis/ability (see e.g. Darcy et al., 2022) have significant, and complex impacts. For example, a recent Surfing and Diversity report by Wave Wahines, a girls' surf organisation in the UK, highlighted the prohibitive costs of equipment and travel, geographical distances, a lack of public transport, and the White and male-dominated cultures associated with surfing as significant barriers (Curtis, 2023). Such barriers could amplify a sense of exclusion and lead to worse mental health outcomes for people. Given the clear health and wellbeing benefits that can come from sport and leisure in blue spaces, the exclusionary impacts of these various barriers and tensions are significant. To explore these issues further, in the following section we focus on surf therapy programmes, and explore the various ways in which surfing is used to promote mental health and wellbeing amongst diverse groups.

Surf therapy

Policy imperatives seeking to show the value of "nature" for health and wellbeing, particularly as a form of health prescription, have proliferated over the past decades. As Bell et al. (2019, p. 10) discuss, these tend to be driven by economic and quantitative measures, hence many researchers have focused on identifying a 'healthy dose' of nature that is the 'ideal' level of 'exposure to a specific type of nature at a specified frequency and duration'. In some countries, doctors are able to prescribe nature to individuals; sport and physical activity programmes are a key way in which dosing is promoted, including walking, running, open water or 'wild' swimming, and surfing. Focused on programmes in blue spaces, Britton et al. (2020, p. 60) conducted a systematic review of 'blue space interventions' (BSI) that emphasised a 'therapeutic approach'. BSI are defined as 'pre-designed activities or programmes (typically physical) in a natural water setting, targeting individuals to manage illness, promote or restore health and/or wellbeing for that group' (2020, p. 51). Britton et al.'s review highlighted that the main purpose of these interventions, was 'health promotion, restoration and awareness', using or learning 'from nature to improve health or manage illness' (Britton et al., 2020, p. 51). They also identified thirty-two different BSIs, including surfing, sailing, swimming, kayaking, scuba-diving, drag boat racing, and beach activities. While lakes and rivers appeared, seas and beaches were the most prevalent settings for interventions, and surfing the most frequent activity, representing 11 of the 32 included BSIs.

As a 'therapeutic', physically active blue space 'dose', surf therapy programmes have been rapidly expanding in popularity. The health and wellbeing possibilities of surf therapy are so widely accepted that in 2017, the International Surf Therapy Organization (ISTO) [https://intlsurftherapy.org/] was founded as a collective of international surf therapy programmes and researchers who advocate for the benefits of surf therapy and to collaborate on research and best practices (Sarkisian et al., 2020). Surf therapy has also garnered increasing multi-disciplinary academic interest over the past decade including across psychology, therapy, public health, and sport development (see e.g., Marshall et al., 2019; Godfrey et al., 2015; Drake et al., 2021). For example, a special issue of *The Global Journal of Community Psychology Practice* (Sarkisian et al., 2020) focuses on surf therapy. It features eight different surf therapy programmes delivered in six countries across Europe, the USA, Australia, and South Africa. The editors of this special issue (Sarkisian et al., 2020) identify health promotion rather than various forms of symptom reduction as the general goal across these therapy programmes (see also Britton et al., 2020). As they argue, their focus is on 'the promotion of wellbeing and involve the measurement of hope, wellbeing, or positive affect' (Sarkisian et al., 2020 p. 3).

Most Surf Therapy programmes include an element of surf instruction typically focused on absolute beginners, along with health and wellbeing-related mentorship and therapy activities (e.g. talking circles, psychoeducation). Britton et al. (2020) suggest the 'ocean therapy' approach adopted by many programmes is informed by "nature-based therapy" (NBT) emerging from occupational therapy, whereby 'participation in meaningful activities within the natural environment is both part of the therapeutic process and a desired outcome' (Rogers et al., 2014 cited in Britton et al., 2020, p. 60). Similarly, Sarkisian et al. (2020) observed that programmes represented in their special issue tend to adopt four key community psychology practice competencies in the delivery of surf therapy, namely; empowerment, mentorship, community inclusion and partnership, and health promotion. However, the "dosage" (i.e. session frequency, duration and programme length), structure, programming and the targeted populations vary considerably (Sarkisian et al., 2020), and as Britton et al. (2020) note, in some cases, the therapeutic addition is minimal.

Across this growing body of research, evidence is offered to suggest that surf therapy can have 'direct benefit for health, especially mental health and psycho-social wellbeing' (Britton et al., 2020, p. 50; Benninger et al., 2020; Sarkisian et al., 2020). However, several caveats are important to note. First, the research and evaluation methodologies differ widely (see Benninger et al., 2020). Quantitative approaches range from randomised control trials to statistical evaluations using self-reported psychometric measures, and commonly used self-reported wellbeing indicators capturing dimensions of self-esteem, self-efficacy, social confidence, resilience, stress, and mood (Britton et al., 2020). Qualitative inductive research (e.g. life history interviews, focus group discussions, participant observation, field notes, including adopting grounded theory) has become more prevalent (e.g. Gibbs et al., 2022; Marshall et al., 2023; Podavkova & Dolejs, 2022), as have mixed methods (e.g. McKenzie et al., 2021). However, as Benninger et al.'s (2020) scoping review shows, observational pre-test/post-test and case studies are the more commonly adopted research designs. They highlight 'significant variability in the measures utilized, and inconsistency in the way the same constructs (i.e. trauma, physical fitness) were measured across studies' (p. 7).

Much of this research has centred on programme evaluation that measures changes in participants over the course of an intervention, not the processes of implementing a programme (Britton et al., 2020; Sarkisian et al., 2020). Such an approach to evaluation is not able to explain whether any reported changes are due to the surf therapy, or other factors (Sarkisian et al., 2020). Furthermore, the evaluations of these programmes are often instigated by the need to show evidence of success to achieve further funding and support. Therefore, better understanding of the different approaches and their impacts is required for assessing the potential impact of surf therapy programmes for mental health and wellbeing benefits (Britton et al., 2020). We agree with Bell et al. (2019) who argue that a focus on social practices, rather than 'dose-response frameworks', is important to reveal how 'different materialities become meaningful amongst people with different forms of embodied knowledges, skills and competencies' (p.8).

The targeted populations in the programmes are also diverse. Benninger et al.'s (2020) scoping review reports that therapeutic benefits were reported for populations including vulnerable youth, autistic youth and people with disabilities (e.g. military service members, military veterans including those with PTSD, young adult cancer survivors, and adults in recovery from addiction). While these studies all suggest that mental health, especially psycho-social wellbeing, can be improved through surfing, given the diversity of participants, and the specific issues creating challenges to mental health amongst these populations, generalisations are problematic (see also Benninger et al., 2020).

Additionally, there is great variety in 'doses' and structures across the interventions themselves. The duration of interventions reviewed by Britton et al. (2020) ranged from one day to six months, and in Sarkisian et al. (2020) from one day, to three years. While short-term benefits were reported, few studies considered the longer-term effects, particularly whether health outcomes were sustained (Britton et al. 2020, p. 61). One study that has collected data on outcomes beyond the programme found that the benefits participants reported during the programme were no longer being experienced 6-weeks after the programme (Olive et al., 2023). Limitations related to a lack of critique about realistic long- term benefits are perhaps unsurprising as many surf therapy projects are delivered by charitable organisations and constrained by short-term funding models.

Nonetheless, the research data suggests significant mental, emotional, and spiritual wellbeing benefits of participation in surf therapy programmes. For example, Caddick, Smith and Phoenix's (2015) research on surf therapy for combat veterans with post-traumatic stress disorder (PTSD) highlighted the significance of "escape" from everyday difficulties. "Respite" emerged to describe the way surfing allowed participants to 'just leave all that away somewhere on the beach' (2015, p. 69). The authors highlight that ocean environments are both fun and unpredictable, and the all-encompassing sensory nature of being in ocean waves was central to the effectiveness of respite. These findings were reflected in the experiences of populations of at-risk youth, for whom the immersive, multisensory and physically demanding nature of surfing was also highlighted (Hignett et al., 2018).

> participants must focus attention on each moment while learning to ride a wave. The focus of mind and body required by the ocean environment simultaneously brings respite, a break from trauma symptoms, or from being stigmatized due to being part of a disenfranchised group.
>
> (Walter et al., 2020, p. 1)

As Hignett et al. (2018) explain, surfing can provoke strong positive emotions and "stoke" experiences, which for some troubled youth lessen their more routine strong emotions of anger and frustration. The affective and sensory nature of surfing immersion, and its wellbeing benefits have been widely discussed in surfing research (see lisahunter & Stoodley, 2021). To some extent many of the recorded benefits in surf therapy mirror wider literatures on surfing participation and wellbeing, such as spirituality (Anderson, 2013), personal empowerment, and a sense of connection to people, places and oceanic environments (e.g. lisahunter & Stoodley, 2021; Olive, 2015).

Our own research in surfing development programmes in Aotearoa New Zealand and Australia, several of which were providing mental health-related surfing-based interventions, also highlighted many of the mental and spiritual benefits other surf therapy researchers have documented, including freedom or respite, a sense of personal empowerment, and social and place-based connectiveness (Wheaton, Roy and Olive, 2017). However, we also found a tendency for providers, all of whom were surfers themselves, to romanticise the activity and its benefits. We argued that surf therapy providers often perceive surfing as being 'unique in its capacity for personal experience and development, and communion with nature' (2017, p. 2). They therefore tended to promote an almost "evangelical belief" in the 'power of surfing to reform, protect or heal those who participate in it, and for them to be able to transcend all boundaries and constraints' (Wheaton, Roy and Olive, 2017, p. 2). Often this belief stemmed from having experienced 'personal awakening through surfing' in their own lives (p. 7). Our interviews also showed that surfing therapy interventions presented unique challenges. Geographic accessibility is a significant factor; surfing, like other coastal blue space activities is limited to those with proximity to the coast. Our interviewees cited cost as a key factor in the sustainability of programmes, including of transport, specialised equipment, and qualified staff. The unpredictable ocean and weather conditions that can hamper ocean-based activities also had significant implications, particularly in relation to safety regulations.

Furthermore, surfing is a largely informal recreation/sport, with its own cultural ethos and practices, and specific barriers or challenges for participation. Surfing clubs and organisations are often based on high performance or social competition rather than participation or learning. Participants not interested in competitions need at least basic surf literacies (from assessing where and when to surf, to buying suitable equipment), skills, and aptitudes to be able to self-organise their recreation safely on their own or with like-minded others. This informality has implications for the sustainability of mental health outcomes beyond formal surf therapy, as participants often do not have access to adequate support or equipment following their structured programme (see also Curtis, 2023). Surfing spaces may offer outcomes such as social connectedness, and a supportive, non-judgmental safe environment, but these are certainly not guaranteed for a 'newcomer' recreational surfer. Indeed, the politics of surfing cultures can be hostile to newcomers and less skilled surfers in ways that might contribute to mental health stress (Olive, 2019). Facilitating pathways to independent surfing access might be key in assuring the long-term mental health and wellbeing benefits of surfing.

Bluespaces and health and wellbeing inequities and injustices

Clearly, the momentum for surf therapy programmes is growing. At ISTO's third conference in November 2019, contributing member surf therapy organisations had grown from eight to more than sixty in three years (Walter et al., 2020). Research is beginning to include more diverse populations and geographic locales, such as Sierra Leone and post-conflict Liberia (Marshall et al. 2020). The latter, taking a more traditional sport-for-development approach, has an explicit focus on mental health and wellbeing to support young people in post-conflict and post-epidemic contexts. Research in Aotearoa New Zealand suggests that surf therapy can have particular value for Indigenous and First Nations youth as a space to connect with cultural knowledges and practices in relation to being in the sea and to a sense of wellbeing in significant ways (Leonard, Tairi and Blampied, 2022; Waiti & Awatere, 2019; Wheaton, Roy and Olive, 2017). However, like many sport-for-development projects, Western-centric goals and models of health often dominate. For example, the ISTO are committed in their belief that surf therapy has the potential to be 'a standard form of healthcare' (Walter et al., 2020, p. 9). However, to develop the evidence base that will support health funding agencies to include surf therapy as a standard form of healthcare means adopting a pathologised framework of health and wellbeing such as the 'optimal dose of surf therapy programs' (Walter et al., 2020, p .7).

Certainly, a compelling body of research suggests surf therapy contributes to mental and spiritual health and wellbeing. Nonetheless, we remain cautious about overstating the significance of this evidence. As Benninger et al., (2020, p. 11) also conclude, 'Overall, there is a lack of generalizability of the research results, due to small sample sizes, lack of control groups, biases potentially skewing data collection, confounding factors, lack of validated standardized measures, and significant variability in surf conditions.' Furthermore, as Bell et al. (2019, p. 2) argue, prescribing health interventions across populations and contexts in universal ways can be 'illusionary and potentially exclusionary'. Such approaches fail to recognise people's 'unique and relational embodied practices' (2019, p. 10), and how diverse cultures and communities understand, perceive and experience "nature", "health" and "wellbeing" in ways that may not align with dominant Western cultural understandings and representations. Surf therapy programmes may be understood as extractive if not accompanied by approaches that care for the health and wellbeing of places in return, as well as the social and cultural politics of the places in which they are carried out (Olive, 2023).

Associated with this is the assumption that oceans are always good for our health and wellbeing. As Surfers Against Sewage activism in the UK has long shown, in some geographical contexts people are cautioned against entering the sea due to detrimental effects caused, for example, by pollution (Evers & Phoenix, 2022; Wheaton, 2007). Furthermore, although in many countries in the global North, the beach is understood symbolically and materially as a place for leisure and pleasure, this is not the case for all (e.g. Booth, 2019; Phoenix, Bell and Hollenbeck, 2021). Oceanic spaces have identity politics and histories, and demographic, cultural, socio-political, and geographic factors can impact the access of particular cultural/ethnic/gendered individuals and bodies (Wheaton et al., 2020). As Olive's research illustrates, the ongoing male-dominated cultural politics in surfing continues to be experienced as a barrier for many women (Olive, 2019). Unsurprisingly, many surf therapy interventions appear to target men or teenage boys, while research on women's experiences in surf therapy remains limited (see Glassman et al., 2021). Wheaton, Roy and Olive's (2017) research found some providers were aware of the particular challenges for women in surfing spaces, which drove them to focus their surfing programmes on girls and women (see also, Curtis, 2023).

In conclusion, with growing government and health promotion interest and funding in the capacity of surf therapy to contribute to better mental health and wellbeing of diverse groups, 'more rigorous forms of research and evaluation methods' are crucial in providing a 'compelling evidence base to support surf therapy funding' (Sarkisian et al., 2020, p. 3). Alongside this, better understanding of which populations can benefit from surf therapy and why is needed; and to challenge existing surf therapy programmes to account for the knowledges and assumptions that underpin the programmes, to increase the diversity of people who can participate, and establish long term visions for how participants can continue to surf after the programme. Perhaps rather than tying them to organised programmes, providers should enable participants to integrate surfing into their lives on their own terms. Such work will require more interdisciplinary collaborations and qualitative methods to meaningfully engage with and ensure the best outcomes for the complexities of lived wellbeing experiences of diverse surf therapy participants.

References

Anderson, J. (2013). Cathedrals of the surf zone: Regulating access to a space of spirituality. *Social & Cultural Geography*, 14(8), pp. 954–972.

Atkinson, S., & Joyce, K.E. (2011). The place and practices of well-being in local governance. *Environment and Planning C: Government and Policy*, 29(1), pp. 133–148. https://doi.org/10.1068/c09200

Ballesteros-Olza, M., Gracia-de-Rentería, P., & Pérez-Zabaleta, A. (2020). Effects on general health associated with beach proximity in Barcelona (Spain). *Health Promotion International*, 35(6), pp. 1406–1414.

Bell, S.L., Leyshon, C., Foley, R., & Kearns, R.A. (2019). The "healthy dose" of nature: A cautionary tale. *Geography Compass*, 13(1), e12415.

Bell, S.L., Foley, R., Houghton, F., Maddrell, A., & Williams, A.M. (2018). From therapeutic landscapes to healthy spaces, places and practices: A scoping review. *Social Science & Medicine*, 196, pp. 123–130.

Bell, S.L., Phoenix, C., Lovell, R., & Wheeler, B.W. (2015). Seeking everyday wellbeing: The coast as a therapeutic landscape. *Social Science & Medicine*, 142, pp. 56–67.

Benninger, E., Curtis, C., Sarkisian, G.V., Rogers, C.M., Bender, K. and Comer, M. (2020). Surf therapy: A scoping review of the qualitative and quantitative evidence. *Global Journal of Community Psychology Practice*, 11(2), pp. 1–26.

Booth, D. (2019). Physical culture and the making and preservation of Bondi Beach. *The International Journal of the History of Sport*, 36(6), pp. 570–591.

Britton, E., Kindermann, G., Domegan, C., & Carlin, C. (2020). Blue care: A systematic review of blue space interventions for health and wellbeing. *Health Promotion International*, 35(1), pp. 50–69.

Burlingham, A., Denton, H., Massey, H., Vides, N., & Harper, C.M. (2022). Sea swimming as a novel intervention for depression and anxiety – A feasibility study exploring engagement and acceptability. *Mental Health and Physical Activity*, 23, 100472. https://doi.org/https://doi.org/10.1016/j.mhpa.2022.100472

Caddick, N., Smith, B. & Phoenix, C. (2015). The effects of surfing and the natural environment on the w-being of Combat Veterans. *Qualitative Health Research*, 25, pp. 76–86.

Curtis, Y. (2023). *Surfing & Diversity*. Report for Wave Wahines CIC. Available at: https://img1.wsimg.com/blobby/go/7e2a9826-cf4c-47ff-96f8-0897309718dd/Surfing%20for%20Diversity%202022%20Report.pdf [Accessed 6 March 2023]

Darcy, S., Maxwell, H., Edwards, M., & Almond, B. (2022). Disability inclusion in beach precincts: beach for all abilities – A community development approach through a social relational model of disability lens. *Sport Management Review*, 26(1), pp. 1–23. https://doi.org/10.1080/14413523.2022.2059998

Denton, H., & Aranda, K. (2020). The wellbeing benefits of sea swimming. Is it time to revisit the sea cure? *Qualitative Research in Sport, Exercise and Health*, 12(5), pp. 647–663. https://doi.org/10.1080/2159676X.2019.1649714

Evers, C., & Phoenix, C. (2022). Relationships between recreation and pollution when striving for wellbeing in blue spaces. *International Journal of Environmental Research and Public Health*, 19(7), 4170.

Fleuret, S., & Atkinson, S. (2007). Wellbeing, health and geography: A critical review and research agenda. *New Zealand Geographer*, 63(2), pp. 106–118. https://doi.org/https://doi.org/10.1111/j.1745-7939.2007.00093.x

Foley, R. (2017). Swimming as an accretive practice in healthy blue space. *Emotion, Space and Society*, 22, pp. 43–51. https://doi.org/https://doi.org/10.1016/j.emospa.2016.12.001

Foley, R. (2015). Swimming in Ireland: Immersions in therapeutic blue space. *Health & Place*, 35, pp. 218–225. www.sciencedirect.com/science/article/pii/S1755458615300591

Foley, R., Kearns, R., Kistemann, T., & Wheeler, B. (2019). *Blue Space, Health and Wellbeing: Hydrophilia Unbounded*. Abingdon: Routledge.

Frumkin, H., Bratman, G.N., Breslow, S.J., Cochran, B., Kahn, P.H. Jr., Lawler, J.J., Levin, P.S., Tandon, P.S., Varanasi, U., Wolf, K.L. and Wood, S.A. (2017). Nature contact and human health: A research agenda. *Environmental Health Perspectives*, 125(7), 075001. https://doi.org/10.1289/EHP1663

Gesler, W.M. (1992). Therapeutic landscapes: Medical issues in light of the new cultural geography. *Social Science & Medicine*, 34(7), pp. 735–746. https://doi.org/https://doi.org/10.1016/0277-9536(92)90360-3

Gibbs, K., Wilkie, L., Jarman, J., Barker-Smith, A., Kemp, A.H., & Fisher, Z. (2022). Riding the wave into wellbeing: A qualitative evaluation of surf therapy for individuals living with acquired brain injury. *Plos One*, 17(4), 0266388.

Glassman, L.H., Otis, N.P., Michalewicz-Kragh, B., & Walter, K.H. (2021). Gender differences in psychological outcomes following surf therapy sessions among US service members. *International Journal of Environmental Research and Public Health*, 18(9), 4634.

Godfrey, C., Devine-Wright, H., & Taylor, J. (2015). The positive impact of structured surfing courses on the wellbeing of vulnerable young people. *Community Practitioner*, 88(1), pp. 26–29.

Hignett, A., White, M.P., Pahl, S., Jenkin, R., & Froy, M.L. (2018). Evaluation of a surfing programme designed to increase personal well-being and connectedness to the natural environment among 'at risk' young people. *Journal of Adventure Education and Outdoor Learning*, 18(1), pp. 53–69.

Kearns, R.A., & Gesler, W.M. (1998). *Putting Health into Place: Landscape, Identity, and Wellbeing*. New York: Syracuse University Press.

Kearns R.A., Moon, G. (2002) From medical to health geography: Novelty, place and theory after a decade of change. *Progress in Human Geography*, 26, pp. 605–625

Leonard, A., Tairi, T., & Blampied, N.M. (2022). Tai Wātea/Waves of freedom: An evaluation of a surf therapy programme for improving psychosocial functioning in young men at high risk of adverse life outcomes. *Journal of Adventure Education and Outdoor Learning*, 24(1), pp. 1–21. https://doi.org/10.1080/14729679.2022.2153370.

lisahunter, & Stoodley, L. (2021). Bluespace, senses, wellbeing, and surfing: Prototype cyborg theory-methods. *Journal of Sport and Social Issues*, 45(1), 88–112. https://doi.org/10.1177/0193723520928593

Mansfield, L., Daykin, N., & Kay, T. (2020). Leisure and wellbeing. *Leisure Studies*, 39(1), pp. 1–10. https://doi.org/10.1080/02614367.2020.1713195

Marshall, J., Kelly, P., & Niven, A. (2019). "When I go there, I feel like *i* can be myself." Exploring programme theory within the wave project surf therapy intervention. *International Journal of Environmental Research and Public Health*, 16(12), 2159.

Marshall, J., Kamuskay, S., Samai, M.M., Marah, I., Tonkara, F., Conteh, J., Keita, S., Jalloh, O., Missalie, M., Bangura, M., Messeh-Leone, O., Leone, M., Ferrier, B., & Martindale, R. (2021). A mixed methods exploration of surf therapy piloted for youth well-being in post-conflict Sierra Leone. *International Journal of Environmental Research and Public Health*, 18(12), 6267.

Marshall, J., Ferrier, B., Ward, P.B., & Martindale, R. (2020). "I feel happy when I surf because it takes stress from my mind": An initial exploration of program theory within waves for change surf therapy in Post-Conflict Liberia. *Journal of Sport for Development*, 9(1), pp. 1–17.

Marshall, J., Ferrier, B., Martindale, R., & Ward, P.B. (2023). A grounded theory exploration of programme theory within Waves of Wellness surf therapy intervention. *Psychology & Health*, 1–23. https://doi.org/10.1080/08870446.2023.2214590

McKenzie, R.J., Chambers, T.P., Nicholson-Perry, K., Pilgrim, J., & Ward, P.B. (2021). "Feels good to get wet": The unique affordances of surf therapy among Australian Youth. *Frontiers in Psychology*, 12, 721238.

Moles, K. (2021). The social world of outdoor swimming: Cultural practices, shared meanings, and bodily encounters. *Journal of Sport and Social Issues*, 45(1), pp. 20–38.

Olive, L., Dober, M., Mazza, C., Turner, A., Mohebbi, M., Berk, M., & Telford, R. (2023). Surf therapy for improving child and adolescent mental health: A pilot randomised control trial. *Psychology of Sport and Exercise*, 65, 102349.

Olive, R. (2019). The trouble with newcomers: Women, localism and the politics of surfing. *Journal of Australian Studies*, 43(1), pp. 39–54. https://doi.org/10.1080/14443058.2019.1574861

Olive, R. (2023). How to swim without water: Swimming as an ecological sensibility. In: C. Bates and K. Moles, eds., *Living with Water: Everyday Encounters and Liquid Connections* (pp. 235–253). Manchester: Manchester University Press.

Olive, R. (2022). Swimming and surfing in ocean ecologies: Encounter and vulnerability in nature-based sport and physical activity. *Leisure Studies*, 42(5), pp. 679–692. DOI: 10.1080/02614367.2022.2149842

Olive, R. (2015). Surfing, localism, place-based pedagogies, and ecological sensibilities in Australia. In: B. Humberstone, H. Prince and K.A. Henderson, eds., *Routledge International Handbook of Outdoor Studies* (pp. 501–510). Abingdon, Oxon, UK: Routledge.

Olive, R., & Wheaton, B. (2021). Understanding blue spaces: Sport, bodies, wellbeing, and the sea. *Journal of Sport and Social Issues*, 45(1), pp. 3–19.

Phillips, R., Evans, B., & Muirhead, S. (2015). Curiosity, place and wellbeing: Encouraging place-specific curiosity as a 'way to wellbeing'. *Environment and Planning A: Economy and Space*, 47(11), pp. 2339–2354. doi:10.1177/0308518X15599290

Phoenix, C. Bell, S.L., & Wheeler, B., (2021-2022) *Weathered Lives*. Available at: www.durham.ac.uk/research/institutes-and-centres/medical-humanities/our-research/projects/weathered-lives/ [Accessed 23 March 2023].

Phoenix, C., Bell, S.L., & Hollenbeck, J. (2021). Segregation and the sea: Toward a critical understanding of race and coastal blue space in greater Miami. *Journal of Sport and Social Issues*, 45(2), pp. 115–137.

Podavkova, T., & Dolejs, M. (2022). Surf therapy—Qualitative analysis: Organization and structure of surf programs and requirements, demands and expectations of personal staff. *International Journal of Environmental Research and Public Health*, 19(4), 2299.

Rogers, C. M., Mallinson, T., Peppers, D. (2014). High-intensity sports for post traumatic stress disorder and depression: Feasibility study of Ocean Therapy with veterans of Operation Enduring Freedom and Operation Iraqi Freedom. *American Journal of Occupational Therapy*, 68, pp. 395–404.

Sarkisian, G.V., Walter, K.H., Martinez, G., & Ward, P.B. (2020). Introduction to the special issue on surf therapy around the Globe. *Global Journal of Community Psychology Practice*, 11, pp. 1–10.

Smith, T.S.J. & Reid, L. (2018). Which 'being' in wellbeing? Ontology, wellness and the geographies of happiness. *Progress in Human Geography*, 42(6), pp. 807–829. https://doi.org/10.1177/0309132517717100

Stronach, M., & Adair, D. (2020). Swimming for their lives: Palawa women of Lutruwita (Van Diemen's Land). *Sporting Traditions*, 37(2), pp. 47–70.

Waiti, J.T.A., & Awatere, S. (2019). Kaihekengaru: Māori Surfers' and a sense of place. *Journal of Coastal Research*, 87(sp1), pp. 35–43. https://doi.org/10.2112/SI87-004.1

Walter, K.H., Sarkisian, G.V., Martínez, G., & Ward, P.B. (2020). Surf therapy practice, research, and coalition building: Future directions. *Global Journal of Community Psychology Practice*, 11(2), pp. 1–11.

Wheaton, B. (Ed.). (2004). *Understanding Lifestyle Sports: Consumption, Identity and Difference*. Routledge.

Wheaton, B. (2013). *The Cultural Politics of Lifestyle Sport*. Routledge.

Wheaton, B., Roy, G., & Olive, R. (2017). Exploring critical alternatives for youth development through lifestyle sport: Surfing and community development in Aotearoa/New Zealand. *Sustainability*, 9(12), 2298.

Wheaton, B., Waiti, J., Cosgriff, M., & Burrows, L. (2020). Coastal blue space and wellbeing research: Looking beyond western tides. *Leisure Studies*, 39(1), pp. 83–95.

Wheaton, B. (2020). Surfing and Environmental Sustainability. In: B. Wilson & B. Millington, eds., *Sport and the Environment* (pp. 157–178). Bingley: Emerald Publishing Limited.

Wheaton, B. (2017). Surfing through the life-course: Silver surfers' negotiation of ageing. *Annals of Leisure Research*, 20(1), pp. 96–116. https://doi.org/10.1080/11745398.2016.1167610

Wheaton, B. (2007). Identity, politics, and the beach: Environmental activism in Surfers Against Sewage. *Leisure Studies*, 26(3), pp. 279–302.

White, M.P., Elliott, L.R., Gascon, M., Roberts, B., & Fleming, L.E. (2020). Blue space, health and well-being: A narrative overview and synthesis of potential benefits. *Environmental Research*, 191, 110169.

World Health Organization (WHO). (2023). *Health and Wellbeing. The Global Health Observatory*. Available at: www.who.int/data/gho/data/major-themes/health-and-well-being [Accessed 2 March 2023].

14 Intoxicated

Men, mental health, wellbeing, and pollution in blue spaces

Clifton Evers

Introduction

I regularly visit an environmentally damaged man-made promontory called South Gare, on the heavily industrialised Northeast coast of England. It is about two miles in length, created in the 1880s from waste slag (a by-product of a bygone booming iron and steel industry). The region has a 200-year heavy industrial history (e.g., shipbuilding, manufacturing, chemical). South Gare is polluted. The air pollution is, at times, some of England's worst. Untreated sewage release into the North Sea here is regular. The river is being dredged (2022–ongoing) to further develop the industrial port. There have been mass die offs of hundreds of thousands of crabs and lobster because, arguably, the dredging stirred up previously settled industrial chemicals (BBC News, 2022). I, along with others from the community, go to South Gare for blue space nature-based recreation – for example, beachcombing, swimming, walking, fishing, and surfing – to seek out joy and associated mental health and wellbeing benefits.

In this chapter, I use art-based autoethnography to explore a few gendered ways in which some men negotiate pollution as they strive for mental health and wellbeing in a blue space that is part of a compounding socio-ecological crisis. The study proceeds from Hannah Pitt's (2018) argument for the importance of more relational perspectives of blue space and any salutogenic claims. Salutogenesis, a term introduced by Aaron Antonovsky in his book "Health, Stress and Coping" in 1979 and elaborated upon in subsequent works, refers to the salutogenic model of health. This model proposes that life experiences contribute to an individual's sense of coherence, or how understandable, manageable, and meaningful they perceive their life to be. I argue that pollution shapes men's experiences of nature-based recreation in blue spaces and subsequently how they strive for and experience mental health and wellbeing through such. By 'blue spaces' I am referring to "all visible outdoor, natural surface waters with potential to improve human health and wellbeing" (Britton et al., 2018, p. 2).

Initially, I offer an indicative outline of the literature on the links between blue spaces, outdoor recreation, and mental health and wellbeing, before briefly explaining what I mean by mental health/wellbeing and masculinities. Following this, I discuss my arts-based autoethnographic approach to the research. Next, I present a study of South Gare, with a focus on the nature-based recreation of surfing and men. Finally, I contemplate what my analysis reveals about how some men in the UK are dealing with contamination while striving for mental health and wellbeing in blue spaces. So far, there is a lack of scholarly studies that directly investigate how sports and physical activity affect people

DOI: 10.4324/9781003345725-15

and groups as they strive for salutogenic benefits as they live through disasters, including being on the fence-line of deindustrialisation, resource extraction, and economic downturn (Cherrington and Black, 2023).

When I go surfing my goal is to feel 'stoked' – a deeply embodied mixed sensibility of joy, pleasure, and satisfaction. I experience salutogenesis. Researchers are focusing on the positive therapeutic (Bell et al., 2018), healing benefits and mental health advantages of being in or near water in blue spaces (Foley et al., 2019; Foley and Kistemann, 2015). Access to blue spaces is also being advocated for public health policies linked to mental health and wellbeing, including the potential 'prescription' of blue space activities (Grellier et al., 2017; Juster-Horsfield and Bell, 2022).

There is evidence that participating in physical activities and sport in blue spaces can improve wellbeing and health, for example through sensory experiences of being in and near water (Britton and Foley, 2021; Olive and Wheaton, 2021). Going surfing can also be therapeutic. For example, helping participants to recover from trauma and illness, cultivate autonomy and a sense of belonging, manage fear and anxiety, nurture resilience, mend self-esteem, and build resilience (for example, see Benninger et al., 2020; Caddick, Smith, and Phoenix, 2015; Clapham et al., 2014; Godfrey et al., 2015; Marshall et al., 2019).

It is important to also be aware of factors that diminish any therapeutic health and wellbeing benefits of nature-based recreation and the 'prescribing' of nature-based activities more widely. Sport and physical activity cultures as well as blue spaces are contested when it comes to access, cultural norms and values, vulnerabilities, risks, and ability. For instance, proximity, race, gender, ethnicity, religion, disability, socio-economics, urban/rural considerations, age, built environment, (e.g., signage), subcultural capital, hazardous animals (e.g. sharks, mosquitoes, jellyfish), drowning, and pollution can erode the potential for mental health and wellbeing benefits of blue spaces for different people in different ways (Duff, 2011; Evers and Phoenix, 2022; Gibbs and Warren, 2015; Olive, 2022; Pitt, 2018).

I comprehend mental health and wellbeing as relational and multiscalar. Mental health and wellbeing are products of qualitative evaluations of shifting biological, emotional, economic, psychological, sociological, cultural, spiritual, and environmental relationships that multiply or reduce a person's capacities to act in the world (Atkinson, 2013; Liamputtong et al., 2012; Mackenzie and Hodge, 2020). Here, following the work of Rebecca Olive and Belinda Wheaton (2021) on physical activity and sport in blue spaces, I focus on a subjective dimension of evaluation of whether capacities are multiplied and enriched (or not) when determining wellbeing and mental health. I am especially intrigued by the notion that people's emotions are "prime arbiters of value" when it comes to such matters (Testoni et al., 2018, p. 816). In fact, as noted by de Boise and Hearn (2017), there is an urgent need for studies of men's everyday emotional lives to understand how men experience and evaluate their mental health and wellbeing (River and Flood, 2021).

The way men perceive mental health and ask for help, either from institutions or people close to them, or suffer in silence, is shaped by masculinity (Sharp et al., 2023). The relationships between men, mental health, wellbeing, and masculinities are also relational and multiscalar (Connell, 2005; Sharp et al., 2023). Throughout history, different settings and spaces have played a role in shaping norms of masculinity, whether they be institutional, cultural, sporting, social, or domestic. However, individuals also actively participate in the development of their own masculine identities within these contexts

(Evers, 2009; Waling, 2020). Leisure activities, for instance, can foster a shared feeling of joy among men and create a space for intimate discussions on sensitive environmental issues. Despite this, men often use humour to avoid any potential erotic interpretations of these intimate moments, with humour becoming an integral aspect of their masculine identity (Evers and Green, 2020). Pollution, which has not been commonly accounted for in discussions on masculinities, is now a potent factor influencing and multiplying these masculine arrangements. Pollution can both create and hinder opportunities for intimacy among men, with humour often employed as a coping mechanism in such situations.

Methodology

The methodology I have been using for my research (2016–ongoing) is an arts-based autoethnography. Autoethnography is an approach to ethnography that involves using the subjective as an entry point into studying wider relational socio-cultural-environmental arrangements. Carefully analysing contextual subjective experiences of relationships between bodies, emotions, artefacts, activities, non-humans, culture, society, and environments can help researchers better know what is happening and how. It can also illuminate how power is operating in ways that produce unjust circumstances and/or damage to people's mental health and wellbeing as well as to nonhumans and the environment (Probyn, 2016). Inspired by feminist researchers, I emphasise researching through my body and emotions (Blakely, 2007). It is an approach at odds with normative research about masculinities which tends to write about emotions and bodies rather than with them. My autoethnography is not wholly human though. Given mental health and wellbeing are relational, I also account for how the researcher and research occur as part of more-than-human, more-than-textual, multisensual worlds (Lorimer, 2010).

I keep reflexive fieldnotes, as well as using an audio-recorder to speak into, record ambient sounds, and to informally interview other users of blue spaces. A wider ethnography is also underway. During this chapter I enter into discussion with some of this ethnography to establish multiple points of validity. I also film and photograph experiences and settings both on land and in the sea to later analyse fleeting action and sensory impressions that happen in-situ (Evers, 2016; lisahunter and Stoodley, 2021).

As part of the auto-ethnography I am using arts-based research methods (ABR) to craft data and analyse it. Patricia Leavy (2017) defines ABR as a transdisciplinary approach to knowledge-building that utilises the tenets of the creative arts in research contexts. The aim is not to pin down meaning at the end of fieldwork but to allow it to evolve from the middle through hesitations, shifting sensibilities, noticing something new, and altered orientations while making 'aha moments!' I treat data as constructed and performative, rather than found 'out there' (Riddett-Moore and Siegesmund, 2012). As I arrive at realisations, I produce themes for analysis in dialogue with a desk review of materials e.g., media, academic studies, the fieldwork documentation.

Intoxicated

I've been living on the Northeast coast of England for eight years, arriving in 2015. I grew up in Australia as white and working class. I am a very experienced surfer. My experiences of the relationship between blue spaces, mental health/wellbeing, and nature-based recreation are privileged. It has been rare not to feel stoked, although I have had to negotiate violence e.g., territorialism, codes of masculinised respect, and homophobia.

I rarely had to deal directly with pollution. I lived according to what Alexander and O'Hare (2020) call "technologies of (un)knowing", by which they mean with an infrastructure that distracts from waste, rubbish, and pollution to depoliticise them. Further, I was not a member of a "fence-line community" most exposed to the violent effects of resource extraction, economic decline, deindustrialisation, and pollution (Taylor, 2014). My stoke came at the expense of fence-line communities and their health, mental health, and wellbeing somewhere "over there".

Since arriving in England, I have focused my nature-based physical activity and sport in nearby blue spaces, such as the promontory, which are fence-line. I see, taste, smell, hear, and feel pollution in the sea foam, the anthropogenic geology layers replete with mining waste, the water-borne illnesses and infections I commonly experience, the apocalyptic dead shellfish masses washed up on the beach, and the official names of some places I surf within (e.g., blast beach, chemical beach) that sit alongside unofficial surf names (e.g., 'shitpipe', 'oilies'). My body and cultural knowledge are going through a process of familiarization with what Lora Wainwright (2021) calls "toxic nature", whereby pollution becomes an all-pervading part of the natural environment affecting its appearance, how it functions, as well as how inhabitants look, feel, act, and know.

As a newcomer my initial reaction to the promontory was one of awe. The sheer scale of industry and pollution for me was previously unimaginable. I experienced an initial aesthetic thrill because of a "post-industrial sublime" (Gormley, 2007, p. 5). For example, surfing in the glow of the lights of the chemical plant while the last rays of sun turned massive rusted and broken industrial infrastructure golden. That post-industrial sublime enhanced my mental health and sense of wellbeing. Pollution and its infrastructure, ironically, may benefit how nature-based physical activity and sport benefit mental health and wellbeing. What I was doing was engaging in "ruin porn", which trades in sensationalised imagery that obscures the historical and structural history and impacts of pollution (Strangleman, 2013).

Early on, my place-attachment with South Gare was weak. Place attachment is a combination of emotional, social, cultural, physical, and spiritual links between people and their environment, along with the corresponding history and social and technical systems such as businesses, institutions, and infrastructure that are part of daily life (Manzo and Devine-Wright, 2021). This attachment to a place may range from weak to strong, and people may feel either disconnected or deeply attached to the places they live, have lived, or will live in (bid). As my attachment to this place has evolved, the relationships between the physical activity/sport, wellbeing, mental health, blue space, pollution, and masculinity have changed.

I learned more about the history of the promontory and fence-line community and in my own small way begin to become part of it. Striving for wellbeing and mental health through nature-based recreation with this blue space involves negotiating longstanding fence-line community poverty and health/wellbeing inequalities because of deindustrialisation and government austerity policies (Office of National Statistics, 2021). There is a stigma that the local fence-line community is "contaminated". Mind you, the community are much further along in their journey through toxic nature. For example, local surfers have always been amid "tangible brutality" that is "plain to see" both in the water and on land (Davies, 2022, p. 13). Experiences of ecological collapse and the everyday living of such is unevenly distributed and consequently takes different forms due to environmental justice differences produced by structural socio-cultural processes of gender, class, ethnicity, religion, sexuality, disability, caste, age, nationality, and location (Taylor, 2014;

Sultana, 2022). Many academics view environmental justice as referring to issues such as unequal distribution, lack of acknowledgment, disempowerment and exclusion, as well as broader negative effects on the fundamental necessities, capacities, and operations of both individuals and communities (Schlosberg, 2009).

While I was capturing photographic and video footage at the promontory, some of the long-term, resident surfers (all men) were intrigued by the images that blended surfing, heavy industry, and pollution. They homed in on the multi-generational pride attached to the industries that had previously given the region economic success. Their pride was linked to an industrial/breadwinner interpretation of masculinity (Hultman and Pulé, 2018). However, to strive for this proud industrial/breadwinner interpretation of masculinity they and their community had to persist in spite of health risks from pollution, which still influences their wellbeing and mental health today. The discussion segues into one about how some men in this region now regularly experience depression due to the region's ailing economy and the concomitant lack of opportunity to gain a sense of self-worth through work, as well as legacy health problems due to pollution. Surfing helps them escape negative thoughts, yet not always because it is, again, plain to see all around them even when riding waves. According to the Office of National Statistics (2021), the suicide rate of men in this area is one of the highest in the UK. Nature-based recreation can be beneficial to men's mental health, but benefits are mitigated by "slow violence" (Nixon, 2011). Pollution's effects can be insidious, since they may not be immediately visible and can accumulate over time, affecting multiple generations (Ibid).

At the promontory, I make collages to examine a contrived ignorance theme I have produced. I have the privilege of being able to detach myself from the history of poverty and pollution and deprivation of the fence-line community. I have also had a lifetime of training in a masculine identity orientated by a masculine logic of domination and dualistic thinking framing of the world: man-woman, culture-nature, mind-body, reason-emotion (Plumwood, 1993). I have learned to understand myself as apart from nature rather than as a part of nature (MacGregor & Seymour, 2017; Plumwood, 1993; Sikka, 2019). The term White m(A)nthropocene has been coined to draw attention to the perpetuation of environmental and social harm through a white masculine framework (Di Chiro, 2017; Plumwood, 1993). As a result, men are over-represented in areas such as carbon emissions, damaging ecological footprints, climate denialism, and lower perceptions of risk about geoengineering 'solutions' to environmental crises. Furthermore, men tend to have strong relationships with fossil fuels, both intellectually and emotionally, conceptually and physically (Alaimo, 2016; Brough et al., 2016; Daggett, 2018; Hultman & Pulé, 2018; Macgregor & Seymour, 2017; Twine, 2021). Although there are men who are working towards improving their relationship with the environment through initiatives such as environmental stewardship, sustainable agriculture, and renewable energy, many of them still attempt to control and dominate nature.

Arrangements of masculinity, men, and the environment are not so straightforward for those I surf and research with. I can "switch off" when surfing to enhance wellbeing and mental health benefits, however for them toxic nature has for too long been in their skin, blood, and bones. They don't feel apart from pollution but rather a part of pollution. My contrived ignorance is a way of avoiding confronting the pollution and its consequences. It is a psychological defence mechanism for my wellbeing and mental health. However, as my place-attachment grows and my body also becomes intoxicated, an eco-anxiety appears more and more in my collages and complicates my upbringing. It is juxtaposed with stoke. Eco-anxiety typically encompasses feelings of anxiety and distress related to ecological crises. However, it is also associated with a range of other emotions, including grief, guilt, anger, and despair, as well as feelings of expectation, motivation, and hope (Pihkala, 2020).

Emotions are intimately entangled with mental health, wellbeing, and living with pollution, and more widely climate change (Verlie, 2021; Wang, 2020). The emotional state of eco-anxiety encompasses more than just anxiousness, but a broad range of emotions such as guilt, fear, despair, dread, sadness, anxiety, and anger (Coffey et al., 2021). Eco-anxiety can be de-motivating, as well as relate to perceptions of lower wellbeing and poor mental health (Stanley et al., 2021). Sometimes, eco-anxiety may prompt eco-anger (Ibid). It is suggested that the latter is more likely to lead to pro-environmental behaviour, and for some people that activism may benefit mental health and wellbeing (Stanley et al., 2021).

While I experience de-motivation and through privilege mobilise a contrived ignorance, at other times the eco-anxiety has prompted anger. With a little bit of encouragement from some men I surf with, I have joined activist groups and protests led by the fishing and surfing communities who are seeking a moratorium on dredging of the river until a proper environmental assessment is in place (Craigie, 2022). However, at the town meetings and protests I attend I become overwhelmed by the magnitude of the environmental issues we face. The eco-anxiety takes over because of what appear to be never-ending troubles. I find myself using my privileged emotional and financial resources to contrive ignorance and for a while 'turn way' from the challenges to help manage my eco-anxiety. Different cohorts of people experience eco-anxiety differently due to socio-cultural histories and expectations, including those filtered through gender (Coffey et al., 2021). The men I associate with tend not to acknowledge or express their eco-anxiety because of a regional normative masculine expectation that they should be strong and stoic (Nayak, 2006). This norm makes it difficult for them to seek formal help for eco-anxiety.

One way the men I surf with seek help and help others regarding eco-anxiety is through an informal pollution pedagogy, an accretive more-than-human know-how developed and shared while immersed in toxic geographies. This pollution pedagogy involves learning and sharing how to recognise different pollution and how to mitigate harms through everyday cultural practices. For example, washing off with fresh water after surfing, not surfing after heavy rainfall, drinking coca cola to kill bugs in the stomach after surfing, regularly spitting out seawater, and knowing where to paddle out to avoid injury on toxic infrastructure. The pollution pedagogy can lessen the purchase pollution has on the men's mental health, health, and wellbeing.

Informed by a pollution pedagogy I prepare and act a performance art piece, performed in Newcastle and Paris. I recreate a specific experience. During one surf session after heavy rain the water turned orange while a group of newcomers and I were surfing. We assumed the colour came from local clay run-off. Neil – a local – saw us surfing and waited for us to finish. With a concerned furrowed brow, Neil asked: "what the hell are you lot doing out there? That water is full of stuff from the mine today." Until 31 December 1999, mine operators could abandon a mine without notifying anyone and disregard any responsibility for allowing contaminated water to enter waterways. Abandoned metal mines continue to be responsible for high levels of cadmium, zinc, arsenic, lead and copper found in estuaries, streams, rivers. Local surfers know that while you must wait for the tide, swell, wind, and other elements to coalesce favourably for good waves to occur, it is also necessary to evaluate pollution level via the colour of the water. A pollution pedagogy involves a contaminated mode of attention, an 'oddkin' conversation, to strive for mental health and wellbeing (see Haraway, 2016). I thanked Neil and have subsequently become great friends with him as he has continued the pollution pedagogy. He contributed to the performance art. When men share expertise via the pollution pedagogy it can foster social bonds and is how they demonstrate care for the physical and mental health of others. The pollution pedagogy creates informal opportunities to connect that can enhance mental health and wellbeing for both the teacher and student in damaged blue spaces.

Men utilize leisure activities to construct and affirm their identity and sense of belonging, according to Blackshaw (2003). Through leisure activities, men also acquire knowledge about the world and express their masculine identities, which can be shaped by factors such as age, race, and sexuality (Evers, 2019; Johnson & Cousineau, 2018; Pringle et al., 2011). However, the impact of pollution and environmental challenges on men's leisure experiences and related masculine identities has been largely overlooked, despite the common encounters with toxic chemicals, plastics, bacteria, sewage, and radiation during activities.

Conclusion

During my visits and ABR, I have discovered how some men use recreation in a toxic geography to improve their mental health and wellbeing, in addition to how pollution erodes or contains any improvements. This is a gender-specific process, which involves mediation of masculine standards as one engages in place-making while gaining knowledge of its materials, creatures, atmosphere, histories, and social-cultural issues. As my own place-attachment grew, I experienced eco-anxiety. I have learned that men experience eco-anxiety in relation to societal expectations about gender as well as in relation to a masculine logic of domination and dualism. To manage this eco-anxiety, some men mobilise an informal pollution pedagogy. By sharing knowledge about pollution hazards and how to mitigate them, men can foster social bonds and demonstrate care, not only for their own physical and mental health but also that of others.

Pollution erodes wellbeing and mental health during nature-based recreation in blue spaces. Controversially, it may be perceived as also improving some men's mental health and wellbeing. Pollution is now ecological, and that arrangement complicates any positive nature-human relationship achieved through immersion in blue spaces. As Jane Bennett (2004, p. 365) writes, when something is called "ecological" it is to acknowledge a "necessary implication in a network of relations, to mark its persistent tendency to enter into a working system" that is "more or less mobile, more or less transient, more or less conflictual". Relationships between blue spaces, mental health, and wellbeing cannot be untangled from pollution and gender.

References

Alaimo, S. (2016) *Exposed: Environmental politics and pleasure in posthuman times.* Minneapolis: University of Minnesota Press.

Alexander, C. and O'Hare, P. (2020) 'Waste and its disguises: Technologies of (un)knowing', *Ethnos* [online]. Available at www.tandfonline.com/doi/full/10.1080/00141844.2020.1796734

Atkinson, S. (2013) 'Beyond components of wellbeing the effects of relational and situated assemblage', *Topoi*, 32, pp. 137–1440.

BBC News. (2022) 'Crab death: Academic calls for Teesside freeport dredging to be paused', 25 October [online]. Available at www.bbc.co.uk/news/uk-england-tees-63392210

Bell, S.L., Foley, R., Houghton, F., Maddrell, A. and Williams, A.M. (2018) 'From therapeutic landscapes to healthy spaces, places and practices: A scoping review', *Social Science & Medicine*, 196, pp. 123–130.

Bennett, J. (2004) 'The force of things: Steps toward an ecology of matter', *Political Theory*, 32(3), pp. 347–372.

Benninger, E., Curtis, C., Sarkisian, G. V., Rogers, C. M., Bender, K. and Comer, M. (2020) 'Surf therapy: A scoping review of the qualitative and quantitative research evidence', *Global Journal of Community Psychology Practice*, 11, pp. 1–26.

Blakely, K. (2007) 'Reflections on the role of emotion in feminist research', *International Journal of Qualitative Methods*, 6(2), pp. 59–68.

Britton, E., Kindermann, G., Domegan, C. and Carlin, C. (2018) 'Blue care: A systematic review of blue space interventions for health and wellbeing', *Health Promotion International*, 103, pp. 1–20.

Britton, E. and Foley, R. (2021) 'Sensing water: Uncovering health and well-being in the sea and surf', *Journal of Sport and Social Issues*, 45(1), pp. 60–87.

Brough, A. R., Wilkie, J. E. B., Ma, J., Isaac, M. S. and Gal, D. (2016) 'Is eco-friendly unmanly? The green-feminine stereotype and its effect on sustainable consumption', *Journal of Consumer Research*, 43(4), pp. 567–582.

Caddick, N., Smith, B. and Phoenix, C. (2015) 'The effects of surfing and the natural environment on the wellbeing of combat veterans', *Qualitative Health Research*, 25, pp. 76–86.

Cherrington, J. and Black, J. (2023) *Sport and physical activity in catastrophic environments*. London: Routledge.

Clapham, E., Armitano, C., Lamont, L. and Audette, J. (2014) 'The ocean as a unique therapeutic environment: Developing a surfing program', *Journal of Physical Education, Recreation and Dance*, 85(4), pp. 8–14.

Coffey, Y., Bhullar, N., Durkin, J., Islam, M.S. and Usher, K. (2021) 'Understanding eco-anxiety: A systematic scoping review of current literature and identified knowledge gaps', *The Journal of Climate Change and Health*, 3, 100047.

Connell R. W. (2005) *Masculinities*. London: Polity.

Craigie, E. (2022) 'Teesworks to resume dredging in March 2023 amid fishing concern', *The Northern Echo*, 3 December [online]. Available at www.thenorthernecho.co.uk/news/23167614.teesworks-resume-dredging-march-2023-amid-fishing-concern/

Davies, T. (2022) 'Slow violence and toxic geographies: 'Out of sight' to whom?', *Environment and Planning C: Politics and Space*, 40(2), pp. 409–427.

Daggett, C. (2018) 'Petro-masculinity: Fossil fuels and authoritarian desire', *Millennium*, 47(1), pp. 25–44.

de Boise, S. and Hearn, J. (2017) 'Are men getting more emotional? Critical sociological perspectives on men, masculinities and emotions', *The Sociological Review*, 65(4), pp. 779–796.

Di Chiro, G. (2017) 'Welcome to the white (M)Anthropocene? A feminist-environmentalist critique' in MacGregor, S. (ed.) *Routledge handbook of gender and environment*. London: Routledge, pp. 487–505.

Duff, C. (2011) Networks, resources and agencies: On the character and production of enabling places. *Health & Place*, 17, pp. 149–156.

Evers, C. (2009) '"The point': Surfing, geography and a sensual life of men and masculinity on the Gold Coast, Australia', *Social & Cultural Geography*, 10(8), pp. 893–908.

Evers, C. (2016) 'Researching action sport with a GoPro™ camera: an embodied and emotional mobile video tale of the sea, masculinity, and men-who-Surf'. In Wellard, I. (ed.) *Researching embodied sport: exploring movement cultures*. London: Routledge, pp. 145–162.

Evers, C. (2019) 'Polluted leisure', *Leisure Sciences*, 41(5), pp. 423–440.

Evers, C. and Phoenix, C. (2022) 'Relationships between recreation and pollution when striving for wellbeing in blue spaces', *International Journal of Environmental Research and Public Health*, 19(7), 4170.

Foley, R., Kearns, R., Kistemann, T. and Wheeler, B. (eds.) (2019) *Blue space, health and wellbeing: hydrophilia unbounded*. Abingdon: Routledge.

Foley, R. and Kistemann, T. (2015) 'Blue space geographies: enabling health in place', *Health Place*, 35, pp. 157–165.

Gibbs L. and Warren A. (2015) 'Transforming shark hazard policy: learning from ocean-users and shark encounter in Western Australia', *Marine Policy*, 58, pp. 116–124.

Godfrey, C., Devine-Wright, H. and Taylor, J. (2015) 'The positive impact of structured surfing courses on the wellbeing of vulnerable young people', *Community Practice*, 88, pp. 26–29.

Gormley, A. (2007). The post-industrial sublime. *Modern Times*, 56, pp. 5–6.

Green, K. and Evers, C. (2020) Intimacy on the mats and in the surf. *Contexts*, 19(2), pp. 10–15.

Grellier, J., White, M.P., Albin, M., et al. (2017) 'BlueHealth: a study programme protocol for mapping and quantifying the potential benefits to public health and well-being from Europe's blue spaces', *BMJ Open*, 7, e016188. Available at https://bmjopen.bmj.com/content/7/6/e016188

Haraway, D. J. (2016) *Staying with the trouble: making kin in the chthulucene*. Durham: Duke University Press.

Hultman, M. and Pulé, P.M. (2018) *Ecological masculinities: theoretical foundations and practical guidance*. London: Routledge.

Johnson, C. W. and Cousineau, L. S. (2018) 'Manning up and manning on: masculinities, hegemonic masculinity, and leisure studies' in Parry, D. (Ed.) *Feminisms in leisure studies: advancing a fourth wave*. London: Routledge, pp. 127–148.

Juster-Horsfield, H.H. and Bell, S.L. (2022) 'Supporting 'blue care' through outdoor water-based activities: practitioner perspectives', *Qualitative Research in Sport, Exercise and Health*, 14(1), pp. 137–150.

Leavy, P. (2017) *Research design: quantitative, qualitative, mixed methods, arts-based, and community-based participatory research approaches*. New York: The Guilford Press.

Liamputtong P., Fanany R. and Verrinder G. (2012) *Health, illness and wellbeing: perspectives and social determinants*. Oxford: Oxford University Press.

lisahunter. and Stoodley, L. (2021) 'Bluespace, senses, wellbeing, and surfing: prototype cyborg theory-methods', *Journal of Sport & Social Issues*, 45(1), pp. 88–112.

Lora-Wainwright, A. (2021) *Resigned activism: living with pollution in rural China*. Massachusetts: MIT Press.

Lorimer, J. (2010) 'Moving image methodologies for more-than-human geographies', *Cultural Geographies*, 17(2), pp. 237–258.

Marshall, J., Kelly, P. and Niven, A. (2019) '"When I go there, I feel like I can be myself." exploring programme theory within the wave project surf therapy intervention', *International Journal of Environmental Research and Public Health*, 16, pp. 2159–2176.

Mackenzie, S.H. and Hodge, K. (2020) 'Adventure recreation and subjective well-being: a conceptual framework', *Leisure Studies*, 39(1), pp. 26–40.

Manzo, L. and Devine-Wright, P. (2021) *Place attachment: advances in theory, methods and applications*. London: Routledge.

MacGregor, S. and Seymour, N. (eds.) (2017). 'Men and nature: hegemonic masculinities and environmental change', *Rachel Carson Centre Perspectives*, 4 [online]. Available at www.environmentandsociety.org/perspectives/2017/4/men-and-nature-hegemonic-masculinities-and-environmental-change

Nayak, A. (2006) 'Displaced masculinities: chavs, youth and class in the post-industrial city', *Sociology*, 40(5), pp. 813–831.

Nixon, R. (2011) *Slow violence and the environmentalism of the poor*. Cambridge: Harvard University Press.

Office of National Statistics. (2021) *Redcar & Cleveland: local statistics* [online]. Available at www.redcar-cleveland.gov.uk/about-the-council/local-statistics

Olive, R. (2022) 'Swimming and surfing in ocean ecologies: encounter and vulnerability in nature-based sport and physical activity', *Leisure Studies*, 42(5), 679–692. Available at www.tandfonline.com/doi/full/10.1080/02614367.2022.2149842

Olive, R. and Wheaton, B. (2021) 'Understanding blue spaces: sport, bodies, wellbeing, and the sea', *Journal of Sport and Social Issues*, 45(1), pp. 3–19.

Pihkala, P. (2020) 'Eco-anxiety and environmental education', *Sustainability*, 12(23), 10149.

Pitt, H. (2018) 'Muddying the waters: what urban waterways reveal about bluespaces and wellbeing', *Geoforum*, 92, pp. 161–170.

Plumwood, V. (1993) *Feminism and the mastery of nature*. London: Routledge.

Pringle, R., Kay, T. and Jenkins, J. M. (2011) 'Masculinities, gender relations and leisure studies: are we there yet?', *Annals of Leisure Research*, 14(2-3), pp. 107–119.

Probyn, E. (2016) *Eating the ocean*. Durham: Duke University Press.

Riddett-Moore, K. and Siegesmund, R. (2012) Arts-based research: data are constructed, not found. In Klein, S. R. (Ed.) *Action research methods*. Palgrave Macmillan: New York, pp. 105–132.

River, J. and Flood, M. (2021) 'Masculinities, emotions and men's suicide', *Sociology of Health and Illness*, 43(4), pp. 910–927.

Schlosberg, D. (2009) *Defining environmental justice: theories, movements, and nature*. Cary: Oxford University Press.

Sharp,. P., Oliffe, J. L., Bottorff, J. L., Rice, S. M., Schulenkorf, N. and Caperchione, C. M. (2023) Connecting Australian masculinities and culture to mental health: men's perspectives and experiences. *Men and Masculinities*, 26(1), pp. 112–133. Available at https://journals.sagepub.com/doi/10.1177/1097184X221149985

Sikka, T. (2019) *Climate technology, gender, and justice: the standpoint of the vulnerable*. Berlin: Springer-Verlag.

Stanley, S.K., Hogg, T.L., Leviston, Z. and Walker, I. (2021) 'From anger to action: differential impacts of eco-anxiety, eco-depression, and eco-anger on climate action and wellbeing', *The Journal of Climate Change and Health*, 1, 100003.

Strangleman, T. (2013) "Smokestack nostalgia," "ruin porn" or working-class obituary: the role and meaning of deindustrial representation', *International Labour and Working-Class History*, 84, pp. 23–37.

Sultana, F. (2022). 'The unbearable heaviness of climate coloniality', *Political Geography*, 99, 102638.

Taylor, D. (2014) *Toxic communities: environmental racism, industrial pollution, and residential mobility*. New York: NYU Press.

Testoni, S., Mansfield, L. and Dolan, P. (2018) 'Defining and measuring subjective wellbeing for sport policy', *International Journal of Sport Policy and Politics*, 10(4), pp. 815–827.

Twine, R. (2021) 'Masculinity, nature, ecofeminism, and the "Anthropo"cene" in Pulé, P.M. and Hultman M. (eds.) *Men, masculinities, and earth*. Cham: Palgrave Macmillan, pp. 117–134.

Verlie, B. (2021) *Learning to live with climate change: from anxiety to transformation*. London: Taylor & Francis.

Waling, A. (2020). *White masculinity in contemporary Australia: the good ol' aussie bloke*. London: Routledge.

Wang, L. (2020) Impacts of environmental pollution behaviors on mental health emotions and relevant countermeasures. *Revista Argentina de clínica psicológica*, 29(1), pp. 701–707

Section II

Lived and embodied spaces

15 Introduction to lived and embodied spaces

Louise E. Boyle

Introduction

This section draws together geographical contributions, alongside contributions from the wider social sciences with a 'geographical sensibility' towards health and place, to consider the lived and embodied spaces of mental health, wellbeing and 'recovery'. The chapters in this section reflect a decades-long history of geographical research, which has sought to develop through qualitative inquiry, social and spatial understandings of various embodied 'conditions', practices and patterns of behaviour that are framed, to varying degrees, under biomedical models of mental illness. Collectively, they reflect scholarly endeavours in the geographies of mental health that aim to bring "more sharply into view the faces and voices of people with mental health problems and the community geographies that they occupy and embody" (Parr, 2008, pp. 11–12). Engaging relational and embodied conceptualisations of distress, the chapters offer insights into personal geographies across a range of experiences and expressions of distress, including seasonal affective disorder (SAD), panic, psychosis, anorexia nervosa (AN) and suicide and self-harm. Methodologically, this section reflects a range of approaches, from traditional interview and ethnographic methods (Bodden, Lorimer and Parr, Chapter 16; Chandler *et al.*, Chapter 20; Farrell and Hyland, Chapter 21), to more creative and embodied approaches that include walking and arts-based interviews (Sánchez-Rodilla Espeso, Chapter 16) and body-orientated practices such as dance movement therapy (DMP) (Coaten, Chapter 19) and yoga (Lucas, Chapter 18). Collectively, the accounts documented throughout are nourished by experiential and reflective accounts from authors and research participants alike, providing a rich and varied commentary on the ways that experiences of distress are lived, embodied and emplaced.

As in other parts of this volume, a number of cross-cutting themes emerged both between chapters in this section and across other sections of this book. Four of these are outlined here. As a number of contributors note, lived experience research on their respective topics and contexts is scarce. The first theme relates to the **experiential insights** offered by these accounts, which contribute to a legacy of spatially-informed research on specific 'conditions' including agoraphobia, compulsions and compulsive 'disorders', neurodiversity, social anxiety, specific phobias, suicide and voice-hearing (Parr, 1999; Davidson, 2003, 2005; Segrott and Doel, 2004; Stevenson, 2016; Nieuwenhuis and Knoll, 2021; Beljaars, 2022; Kenna, 2022; Boyle, 2024). Crucially, the collective insights offered in the following chapters, enable a critical and relational reframing of mental health that challenges and nuances deep-rooted individualised and medicalised accounts of embodied distress centring spatial, temporal and embodied dynamics throughout.

DOI: 10.4324/9781003345725-17

Bodden *et al.* conceptualise seasonal affective disorder as an "environmental illness", one that is contingent with the environmental conditions and relations associated with changing seasonality and winter light. Sánchez-Rodilla Espeso's contribution reconceptualises panic 'disorder' as "a disruption of the relational structures" between self and body, self and others and self and space. Similar, self -world relations are explored by Lucas reflecting on her own experiences of healing from anorexia nervosa. Disrupting individualised models of AN, alongside internalised conceptualisations of embodiment prominent in brain sciences, the embodiment of anorexia is reframed as dynamic and relational, as "learnt and inhabited from the outside in". Drawing from research with those who have attempted or been bereaved by suicide, Chandler *et al.* consider suicide as an "embodied social practice". Rather than an isolated event, it is one resolutely shaped by and embedded within the social contexts in which it takes place. Overall, the chapters take a more nuanced and even ambivalent approach to the diagnostic labels assigned to various experiences and bodily practices explored throughout this section, in ways that acknowledge that diagnostic process and practice "are temporally and spatially complex, and have effects at different scales" (Callard, 2014, p. 526). Pertinent here, is Farrell and Hyland's exploration of students' experiences of distress. They examine the 'force' of the university in shaping students' experiences of distress and how their experiences are validated and alienated by structures and resources designed to support them.

The second theme is concerned, perhaps unsurprisingly, with the **relations between health, place and space**. Chapters both implicitly and explicitly examine the role of place and space, or more accurately, 'place-assemblages' (Fox and Powell, 2023), and their capacities for supporting, or indeed, diminishing health and wellbeing. Contributors explore various spaces, each interconnected with the spaces and themes explored across the other sections of this book, ranging from spaces of the body, home, local communities, public spaces, rural and urban locales, built and natural environments and institutional spaces. Chandler et al. offer critical reflections on 'sites of suicide' arguing that the narrow focus on 'locations of concern', more commonly referred to as 'suicide hotspots', in suicide prevention and intervention policy fails to adequately address the wider affective, social, cultural and economic factors that may explain why suicides occur in these locations. They focus on three sites, bridges, forests and homes in urban and rural areas of Scotland, as potential sites of suicide. Coaten describes the therapeutic process and practice involved in Dance Movement Psychotherapy, which she delivers for people experiencing psychosis in in-patient mental health care settings. She centres her discussion around the creation of a 'temenos', a safe and therapeutic space or container, that enables the profound disembodiment experienced during psychosis to be 'worked through'. Temenos becomes a metaphor that helps to conceptualise the physical, relational and embodied spaces of the therapeutic encounter and the emotional and affective atmospheres that emerge within it. However, the therapeutic temenos is always juxtaposed by the clinical and 'sterile' landscape and realities of the ward beyond. Sánchez-Rodilla Espeso argues that the relational disruption experienced during panic "fragments" everyday places, dividing them into a "patchwork of 'safe' and 'phobic' spaces", affecting how people relate to and move through them. Similar geographies are evident in the lives of people with social anxiety, wherein taken-for-granted routines and mobilities are "continuously written, unwritten and rewritten" as they navigate encounters with others in their everyday social and spatial worlds (Boyle, 2019).

The third theme challenges notions of **self as separated from environment**. Recent endeavours have been concerned with the wider social, cultural, political and structural drivers and contexts that incite and exacerbate trauma and distress such as austerity (Lowe and DeVerteuil, 2020a), forced mobility and displacement (Lowe and DeVerteuil, 2020b; Ehrkamp, Loyd and Secor, 2022) the COVID-19 pandemic (Boyle, Parr and Philo, 2021) and climate change (Boyd, Parr and Philo, 2023). Experiences are interrogated alongside wider social, political and cultural traumas and environmental exposures that shape and, in some cases, dominate people's everyday lives. On an environmental level, reduced exposure to sunlight is realised through the body in experiences of SAD as people become slow and lethargic and "weighed down by wintertime" (Bodden et al.). In a time when nature-based interventions are promoted for their capacity to facilitate and improve well-being (see also *Blue and Green Spaces* for critical reflections), they offer unique insights into environmental conditions that *incite* rather than alleviate feelings of despair and isolation. Farrell and Hyland argue that the historical context alongside the "structures and requirements" of the university cannot but shape students experiences of distress along "positivist lines". The 'affective force' of the university plays an integral role in shaping students' understandings of distress and by extension, understandings of self. Lucas notes that AN is inevitably bound up in discourses of bodily objectification and social and cultural pressures about the body, but that many bodies are also excluded from existing research so a complete picture of embodiment in this context cannot be realised. While Chandler *et al.* argue that suicide and suicide attempts do not occur in a vacuum. They address a range of factors that incite suicide and suicide attempts, including wholly insufficient intervention practices that prioritise physical, rather than emotional safety and point to wider policies and politics of austerity, poverty and forced evictions as "social drivers of misery, distress and self-inflicted death" that fuel hostile, and for some, unliveable conditions.

The final theme relates to **help-seeking practices, living and coping with, and/or 'recovery'**. First, Chandler *et al.* draw critical attention to the consequences that arise when there is a sustained lack of resources, opportunities, support, care and dignity for individuals residing in marginalised and deprived communities. They point to long-standing failures within local services' response to suicide and misguided suicide prevention practices and interventions. It bears mentioning that individualised models of mental health, further exacerbated by recovery narratives that privilege neoliberal discourses of responsible individualism, significantly reduce the possibilities for living well with or enacting possibly recoveries (Woods, Hart and Spandler, 2022). Yet, the geographies discussed here do offer insights into how bodies and experiences can be rescripted and embedded within wider narratives of community and social and environmental justice. As part of their programme of research, Bodden *et al.* ran participant workshops, fostering "dialogic spaces", where people with SAD could come together, build community and create "imaginative and transformative potentials for collective and shared wellbeing", ones that can bridge into wider "biosolidarities" of community and advocacy. Two chapters also outline the therapeutic potentials of body-orientated practices: Lucas integrates yoga as a form of "embodied healing" for AN; while Coaten, explores the therapeutic and integrative capacities of the moving body for those experiencing psychosis. DMP priorities the exploration and expression of unconscious feelings and emotional states through movement. For Lucas, healing from AN is intricately linked to issues of social justice. She advocates for bodies that 'take up' space in order to challenge and resist powerful social, cultural and moralising discourses about the body and anorexia more broadly.

In summary, *Lived and Embodied Spaces* offers critical and pertinent insights into the personal geographies of experience and the complex, often hidden social geographies, that comprise them. Bodies tell stories; they are integral sites of meaning-making and identity. Therefore, the focus on embodiment concerns how personal, social, and physical environments are embedded in, expressed by, and mediated through bodies and biology, but are never simply reducible to them. The contributions in this section highlight the importance of attending to dynamic 'matters' of body, affectivity and environment whilst simultaneously mapping the interconnections between the body, health and wellbeing and wider "with social processes, power, hierarchy, and/or discourse" (Hayes-Conroy, Kinsey and Hayes-Conroy, 2022, p. 2).

References

Beljaars, D.N.M. (2022) *Compulsive Body Spaces.* Milton, United Kingdom: Taylor & Francis Group.

Boyd, C., Parr, H. and Philo, C. (2023) 'Climate anxiety as posthuman knowledge', *Wellbeing, Space and Society*, 4, 100120. Available at: https://doi.org/10.1016/j.wss.2022.100120.

Boyle, L.E. (2019) 'The (un)habitual geographies of Social Anxiety Disorder', *Social Science & Medicine*, 231, pp. 31–37. Available at: https://doi.org/10.1016/j.socscimed.2018.03.002.

Boyle, L.E., Parr, H. and Philo, C. (2021) 'Mental ill-health and anxious pandemic geographies', in G.J. Andrews et al. (eds) *COVID-19 and Similar Futures: Pandemic Geographies.* Cham: Springer International Publishing (Global Perspectives on Health Geography), pp. 365–372. Available at: https://doi.org/10.1007/978-3-030-70179-6_48.

Boyle, L.E. (2024) *Anxious Geographies: Worlds of Social Anxiety.* London: Routledge.

Callard, F. (2014) 'Psychiatric diagnosis: The indispensability of ambivalence', *Journal of Medical Ethics*, 40(8), pp. 526–530. Available at: https://doi.org/10.1136/medethics-2013-101763.

Davidson, J. (2003) *Phobic Geographies: The Phenomenology and Spatiality of Identity.* London: Routledge. Available at: https://doi.org/10.4324/9781315246864.

Davidson, J. (2005) 'Contesting stigma and contested emotions: Personal experience and public perception of specific phobias', *Social Science & Medicine*, 61(10), pp. 2155–2164. Available at: https://doi.org/10.1016/j.socscimed.2005.04.030.

Ehrkamp, P., Loyd, J.M. and Secor, A.J. (2022) 'Trauma as displacement: Observations from refugee resettlement', *Annals of the American Association of Geographers*, 112(3), pp. 715–722. Available at: https://doi.org/10.1080/24694452.2021.1956296.

Fox, N.J. and Powell, K. (2023) 'Place, health and dis/advantage: A sociomaterial analysis', *Health: An Interdisciplinary Journal for the Social Study of Health, Illness and Medicine*, 27(2), pp. 226–243. Available at: https://doi.org/10.1177/13634593211014925.

Hayes-Conroy, A., Kinsey, D. and Hayes-Conroy, J. (2022) 'Biosocial wellbeing: Conceptualizing relational and expansive well-bodies', *Wellbeing, Space and Society*, 3, 100105. Available at: https://doi.org/10.1016/j.wss.2022.100105.

Kenna, T. (2022) 'Cities of neurodiversity: New directions for an urban geography of neurodiversity', *Area*, 54(4), pp. 646–654. Available at: https://doi.org/10.1111/area.12803.

Lowe, J. and DeVerteuil, G. (2020a) 'Austerity Britain, poverty management and the missing geographies of mental health', *Health & Place*, 64, 102358. Available at: https://doi.org/10.1016/j.healthplace.2020.102358.

Lowe, J. and DeVerteuil, G. (2020b) 'Power, powerlessness and the politics of mobility: Reconsidering mental health geographies', *Social Science & Medicine*, 252, 112918. Available at: https://doi.org/10.1016/j.socscimed.2020.112918.

Nieuwenhuis, M. and Knoll, E. (2021) 'Towards a geography of voice-hearing', *Emotion, Space and Society*, 40, 100812. Available at: https://doi.org/10.1016/j.emospa.2021.100812.

Parr, H. (1999) 'Delusional geographies: The experiential worlds of people during madness/illness', *Environment and Planning D: Society and Space*, 17(6), pp. 673–690. Available at: https://doi.org/10.1068/d170673.

Parr, H. (2008) *Mental Health and Social Space: Towards Inclusionary Geographies?* London: Wiley Books.

Segrott, J. and Doel, M.A. (2004) 'Disturbing geography: Obsessive-compulsive disorder as spatial practice', *Social & Cultural Geography*, 5(4), pp. 597–614. Available at: https://doi.org/10.1080/1464936042000317721.

Stevenson, O. (2016) 'Suicidal journeys: Attempted suicide as geographies of intended death', *Social & Cultural Geography*, 17(2), pp. 189–206. Available at: https://doi.org/10.1080/14649365.2015.1118152.

Woods, A., Hart, A. and Spandler, H. (2022) 'The recovery narrative: Politics and possibilities of a genre', *Culture, Medicine, and Psychiatry*, 46(2), pp. 221–247. Available at: https://doi.org/10.1007/s11013-019-09623-y.

16 Feeling SAD

Embodied geographies of seasonal affective disorder

Shawn Bodden, Hayden Lorimer, and Hester Parr

Introduction

Presently, there is wide-ranging public commentary and plentiful academic writing on the relationship between climate change and mental health, as part of a critical analysis of the impact of the Anthropocene (Albrecht, 2007; Boyd et al, 2022; Ojala et al, 2021; Romanello et al, 2021). Across the spectrum of interdisciplinary research, there is increasing attention to psychological, behavioural and psychosocial relations with changing natures, as a way to understand the diffuse mental health risks and 'affective discomfort' (Adams, 2016, p. 131) of climate change. We situate this chapter in conversation with these new genres of literature, particularly those which seek to create agendas for 'psychosocial research' in dialogue with ecological crisis (ibid, p 238; and see Boyd et al, 2022). However, our attention below is not so much on an unprecedented unravelling of human-nature relations in crisis-led scenarios, but on *already existing* complexities bound up with seasonal natures and light and mental health, and ones that exist for around 3 in every 100 people according to the UK's Royal College of Psychiatrists. In what follows, we explore *Seasonal Affective Disorder* (SAD) with a distinct concern that this condition is likely to become much more commonplace within a context of climatically disrupted seasonal rhythms: it may well represent an expanding (if globally diverse) geography of mental health that might become much more commonplace for all (if still differentiated and tied to local cultural and natural contexts) in an era of protracted climate change.

Geographers have a long history of researching mental ill-health, but they have curiously neglected how illness is tied to questions of seasonality, climate, weather and light. Wolch and Philo (2000) highlighted three 'waves' of geographical studies of mental health and ill-health, reflective of major genres of geographical thought in the later-twentieth century, but in each there is little-to-no engagement with questions of seasons and climate. This chapter addresses the mental ill-health dimensions of SAD in ways that directly comment on nature relations and embodied experience. In doing so we seek to insert SAD into a disciplinary engagement with geographies of mental (ill) health and reflect on some aspects of this diagnostic category's particular modern history. SAD's history is interesting because of its debated and evolving status (Bodden et al., in press) and how it ties into climate related mental health literatures in which the changing world relates to changing mental health conditions. Given that mental health related embodied relations are often experienced in isolation, we also comment on the hopeful potential of *biosociality* (a dialogic space where people with shared conditions come together to

DOI: 10.4324/9781003345725-18

form social networks, (after Bradley, 2020 and see Parr et al, forthcoming) to disrupt and change SAD sensibilities. In conclusion, we return to questions of mental health and future seasonal climate change.

There is little social science and humanities-led research to date on SAD, and so our own contribution is distinctive in this regard. As such, we engage with neglected voices of people with SAD – ones collected as part of a 'Living with SAD' research project based in Scotland, UK – and here we particularly focus on the *embodied* experience of winter-light in ways that communicate sensorial and affective relations. Our informants were individuals who self-identify as experiencing symptoms of SAD (only some of which will have a diagnosed disorder and who receive treatment). The study was deliberately situated in West of Scotland health board areas which overlap with a climatic region renowned for extended winter gloom as the result of latitude, high precipitation, overcast conditions and low seasonal light levels. Our survey recruited 350 people, in addition, 5 people opted to undertake 6-week time-space diaries; 15 individuals took part in biographical interviews and 20 people were recruited for a practice-led 'Wintering Well' workshop programme for people with SAD which took place over 2022–2023. We draw on the range of material collected as part of these research-led engagements to elaborate the embodied geographies of feeling SAD.

Seasonal Affective Disorder: a brief history

SAD is an 'environmental illness' of recent invention and remains one with an uncertain, disputed status. SAD was first recognised as a mental health condition in 1987 in the *Diagnostic and Statistical Manual-III-R* of the American Psychiatric Association. By 2013 the condition was no longer afforded a discrete entry in DSM-5's diagnostic criteria, instead being recognised as a sub-type of major depression or low mood with seasonal patterns (and see Callard's 2014 critique of the DSM). The UK National Health Service states 'the exact cause of SAD is not well understood' and that 'SAD can be difficult to diagnose' (NHS, 2022). The online entry lists the symptomology of SAD as 'winter depression', persistent low mood, a loss of pleasure in everyday life, and feelings of lethargy or despair that can affect normal functioning. While causes of SAD are not entirely understood, as noted, it is obviously contingent on environmental conditions and relations, with a particular link to seasonal changes in the levels of natural light. The lack of sunlight in wintertime is understood to impact the physiological production of the hormones melatonin and serotonin which are themselves known to be associated with feelings of depression and sleepiness (Rosenthal 2009; Lambert G, Reid C, Kaye D, *et al*, 2002). The body's internal clock – its circadian rhythm – is also affected by lowered light conditions and reduced exposure to sunlight, technically determined as a reading of the level of environmental illumination by the unit-measure *lux* (Geddes, 2019), perceptible most notably during shorter autumn and winter days. People experiencing SAD symptoms during wintertime are less inclined to spend periods of time exposed to natural light outdoors, which can compound their situation. It is unclear why some people experience SAD and some do not, although Targum and Rosenthal (2008) suggest geographic location and genetic disposition have a role, while Fonte and Coutinho (2021) suggest the significance of co-morbidity with other psychiatric conditions. Our purpose in this chapter is not to debate these possibilities, but instead to communicate more about the embodied experience of SAD, drawing on cultural-geographical research with light-affected people who have self-identified as suffering from wintertime low-mood and

SAD. This task is important as, unlike many other mental health conditions, there is no longer any national advocacy or charitable organisation to provide insight into SAD lives or cultivate biosociality for those experiencing it.

Embodying SAD

What I have noticed is that you know, when it's autumn time I start to have thoughts of 'ugh … Here we go again. My thoughts are going to 'clocks will be changing in two weeks'. So, I'm very aware of when that is. In years gone by my mood has changed, it has become a bit lower. And my activity has just basically become zero.

(Sharon, Research interview)

Many people affected by SAD describe feelings of heaviness and sluggishness, not just as a lack of energy, but as a feeling of being weighed down by wintertime changes and lack of light. Sometimes this comes on slowly, as part of an Autumnal sensibility, as described by Sharon, above, while at other times it can be a sudden or distinct embodied realisation that the season is upon them, as these research interview excerpts reveal:

My body slows down, there isn't enough light in the day to achieve everything. It feels dark so much of the time.

(Lorna)

I feel sluggish, like I'm fighting my body; trying to make it do the things that are good for it, like exercise.

(Derek)

Wading through sludge – everything is hard work.

(Shashi)

Low mood sets in, like a blanket covering you, creeping up slowly, then covering your whole body and soul.

(Jim)

While individual experiences with SAD frequently identify specific aspects of the winter that influence and trigger these changes, they can commonly blame *themselves* for not being able to cope like others do with seasonal changes – while some also report receiving similar comments from family and GPs. One particularly notable experience is a sense of embodied estrangement during the winter season, as though their own bodies have gone 'out of control' or are at winter's mercy. This involves a sense of lethargy and an impulse to 'hibernate' until these bodily changes pass:

Grey days, lonely days and the damp creeps slowly up my legs as the day progresses.

(Pam)

November through to April, I am more prone to headaches. I have joint pain which increases with the damp and cold, which then makes me more irritable. I know this is

happening and it upsets me pushing my feelings of depression and hopelessness more
to the forefront.

(Peter)

I find it oppressive, and it feels like the sky is very heavy on my head, almost pushing
it down.

(Maureen)

These embodied relationships with low winter light focus on the weight of the world,
experienced as a heaviness and creeping pain that brings slowness. These sensations are
often coupled with feelings of frustration, irritation, guilt, anger and sadness.

Feeling SAD with others: failing to organise

In the UK, SAD has had a complex social life which can be told through a short history of community-making: one culminating in dissolution and fragmentation rather
than biosocial coalescence. The Seasonal Affective Disorder Association (hereafter
SADA) was a UK-based voluntary organisation, established with the stated intention of
helping people of all ages affected by SAD. SADA existed between 1986 and 2017, held
registered charity status, and operated as a patient-led organisation. Initially, it attracted
plenty of press and media interest, including radio programmes, partly prompted by
the work of prominent academic and clinician Norman Rosenthal (2012), author of
Winter Blues: Everything You Need to Know to Beat Seasonal Affective Disorder. The
account we offer here draws on oral testimonies presented in 2013 at a 'witness seminar' (Overy and Tansey, 2014, organised by University of London's History of Modern
Biomedicine Research Group, funded by The Wellcome Trust), along with material from
recent communications and formal interviews with former SADA committee members as
part of data-gathering activity on lived experiences of SAD.
While serving as SADA's chairperson, Betty described the situation at hand:

Hundreds of SAD sufferers treat themselves, guided by information gleaned from the
media and us. Their stories are often untold and the experience of this very specific
form of depression goes unexplored.

Some difficulties SADA faced were ordinary operational ones; not least because it
remained largely low-tech during the digital transition. Perhaps the key issue identified, however, was the challenge in maintaining credibility among clinicians. Over time,
the initial spike of interest that SADA had attracted from medical professionals drifted
and dwindled. Meanwhile, biological and psychological inquiries and scientific funding
gravitated towards circadian rhythm research, a field where the particular seasonality of
SAD experience became a little lost:

We revamped and produced a new handbook we wrote lots and lots of articles and we
sort of co-opted a few scientists to write occasional articles ... but we were a charity
run by volunteers and we were up against charities, who were real charities with sal-
aried workers, and they could ... pay for fancy websites ... and SAD had kind of gone
off the agenda, if you like, [since] we had no support really from experts.

(Betty, research interview)

When SADA members put themselves in public view, the media did respond, raising public awareness of the condition, although this coverage would sometimes prompt negative reactions, including disbelief that sufferers were depressed by winter or the weather – with the significance of light perhaps subsumed within the UK's peculiarly 'meteorological culture' (Veale et al, 2014):

> I mean we're absolutely obsessed with the weather in the UK aren't we? We get quite a lot of different kinds of weather, so I do think that there's a lot of it to do with our weather patterns that play into it. We've also got that sort of British stoicism that we 'just grin and bear it'. I got splashed across the Daily Mail – I'd been used as a case study – but I just got so much abuse … from people telling me to stop being pathetic. You know it's hard when you're trying to be open and honest about something. We still have … an attitude of "just get on with it" and especially when it's something to do with life. I mean SAD sounds [pulls face] – the acronym doesn't help!
>
> (Shona, research interview)

The legitimacy and validity of embodied SAD experience was subject to scrutiny (Lobello, 2017, Young, 2017), some scepticism, and a changed status in *DSM-5* (2013), as simply a subset of major depression rather than a stand-alone condition.

Feeling SAD with others: disconnections

In our research with those experiencing negative winter feelings and affect, the reduced light of winter contributes to and compounds on the reduced social and physical activity of the season. Many encounter what can seem like a shrunken version of the world, in which winter disrupts or constrains local services, public transport and social life more generally. Participants in our survey described reducing their own activities and ambitions as a response to the increased difficulty of life in winter:

> The darkness reduces social contact especially as older folk aren't keen to drive.
>
> (Hugo)

> My energy tends to be lower in the winter so it takes more effort to make plans, or I reduce my aims.
>
> (Allie)

This reduction of activity during winter can be a source of frustration, guilt and disappointment; with our UK-wide survey showing over 95% of 350 participants spending less time outdoors, with reduced wintertime life and light a particularly widespread challenge (Bodden et al, 2022):

> In December at the height of winter and it's cloudy the light has gone by 4pm, so any walking, cycling or normal outdoor activities are greatly reduced or gone, making it a long night if you are alone.
>
> (Bea)

> I can be more difficult to be with when I am down, I reduce when I see people in case it affects our relationship.
>
> (Beth)

I don't want to see friends; I don't want to go out. Don't want to join in in things I just want to almost completely hibernate …

(Riya)

Seasonal changes in light levels are reported to result in less social, less mobile and less varied lives during the winter season: for those facing extreme winter affect, the season is 'life limiting'. Moreover, those activities that do continue often feel less fulfilling and more exhausting. The feeling of a reduced wintertime life includes decreased activity, but also a lowered sense of the quality and value of their day-to-day life. Participants describe being outside as generally more negative in winter, feeling a need to hurry back home, a desire to avoid the darkness, and an inability to stand still for an extended period of time due to the weather. When participants reduce their winter activity it is not a straight-forwardly deliberate choice: recognising these changes in their behaviour, participants report feeling 'like someone else' or as though they are 'avoiding life':

I feel I'm half the person I know I am. I feel as if I'm in a cocoon waiting for the better weather. Just button down until it's over then I can re-emerge as the real me.

(Kayla)

Only 23.6% (n=82) of our survey participants indicated that they had previously sought out or connected with others who experienced winter affect and lowered winter mood; a small number of participants described making connections through social media groups and online forums, mental health groups and cafes, and counselling. Only one participant specifically mentioned the Seasonal Affective Disorder Association (SADA). More frequently, participants described occasions when the topic came up during casual conversations, sometimes with regards to their own personal experience but often focusing on winter more generally. Some participants observed that the 'general moaning' about the weather could worsen their mood: 'Lots of moaning about the weather, everyone seems more fed up and unhappy, less tolerance of each other.' This contributed to worries that their own problems could be dismissed as 'just moaning' and so sharing these experiences can be inhibited by worries about stigma or misunderstanding:

When I worked in an office with no natural light a clerk brought a light box in and the managers were very scathing and dismissive and concerned about the fact it was using their electricity.

(Sue)

A slightly larger number of participants, just over 28.4% (n=99) indicated that they had spoken about their experiences of winter affect with their GP or another medical pro-fessional. Experiences were varied, including both highly positive and highly negative encounters with medical practitioners, which could shade and influence future efforts to find help: 'They laughed and said it [SAD] doesn't exist.' In these conversations, the diffi-culty of disentangling experiences of winter affect from other mental and physical health conditions — particularly depression — posed a particular problem for getting help, with SAD often treated as a lesser or secondary concern: 'They said because I was already diagnosed with depression that they wouldn't put it in my notes.' Participants who did receive support recounted a range of recommended courses of action, including CBT, vitamin D, therapeutic lightboxes, anti-depressants, meditation, regular walks outside and advice to 'try to keep positive'. Participants' feelings about the usefulness of this advice varied. As with relationships with friends and family, participants commented positively about those GPs who were 'understanding' and 'supportive' even in the absence of definitive treatment options.

Biosocial human geographies

Having acknowledged some of the challenges previously faced by the UK's fragmented SAD 'community' in maintaining momentum and gaining recognition in clinical communities and health services, as well as the isolating experience of individuals, we are interested in identifying alternative models for 'biosocial solidarity'. In Bradley's (2021) work on body-focused repetitive behaviours (BFRB), experiences that are rare, unrecognised and isolating, biosocial validation is more likely to occur from similar others rather than from medical diagnosis (although the latter is welcomed by some). In discussing BFRB, Bradley (2021, p.10) notes how many forms of biosociality are processual and uncertain: 'biosociality is complex, and the different interpretations, expectations and practices of coming together with shared experiences of illness are deeply nuanced'. We have drawn inspiration from such work in how we have organised and pursued outreach and knowledge-exchange opportunities building on our research within the 'Living with SAD' project.

The programme of research for 'Living with SAD' included a workshop series which took place across the autumn and winter of 2022–23, co-designed with artist-poet Alec Finlay and CBT-experts Living Life to the Full (https://llttf.com/).[1] The workshops comprised seven Glasgow-based events with 20 SAD-affected participants. Our approach in the workshops was to create a creative and supportive 'biosocial space' where participants could be invited to experiment out-of-doors with creative activities, generating dialogue regarding things seen, heard, written, and felt while experiencing and working to counter feelings of wintertime lowered mood. The workshops encouraged new kinds of curiosity about weather-and-light worlds and were based on practice-led and artistic activity involving outdoor work and indoor conversation, including activities like 'sky framing', 'letter writing' and a 'collective poetic manifesto'. Although there is much more that can be said about the workshops, our focus here is on the changing experience of community and 'biosocial solidarity' over the course of the whole workshop series. At each event we asked participants what aspect of our joint work had made them re-think their SAD experience and how they might anticipate embodying winter differently in future. For some this involved a new feeling of *being together* and thus a changing experience of their own condition. One participant recorded that they had been rethinking *'openness and readiness'* for SAD times, while another noted *'feel[ing] less like an over dramatic kid for struggling'*. In the workshop series, environmental experience, so central to SAD, was *shared*, enabling conceptual shifts for the group regarding the nature of their condition and, hence, what they could do about it: *'It's not 'the dark', it's the light!'*. Here, shared thinking has offered the beginnings of new ways for one person to shift their understanding of the fundamental problem causing their feelings of seasonal depression. Instead of focussing on battling (or suffering) through the dark, their focus turns to finding what light *is* available and what they *can do* with that light. Another participant's comment echoes the importance of this shift in perspective: *'maybe need to change what I/we frame'* (See Figure 16.1).

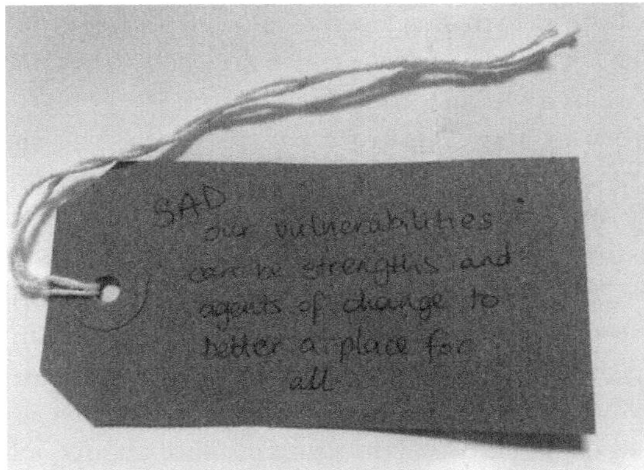

Figure 16.1 Expressions of biosocial hope in the *Wintering Well* programme, 2022–2023 (author photograph).

What does this amount to in biosocial terms? As we write, our SAD winter workshop series has come to a close, but there is an emergent sense of community around the experience of seasonal depression. That much is clear:

> There is power in community. You don't have to endure and overcome SAD alone
>
> (Evaluation, Workshop 3)

> The comfort of listening to one another and recognising parts of yourself …
>
> (Evaluation, Workshop 3)

> Knowing more about how SAD affects me can help me help others in my community
>
> (Evaluation, Workshop 6)

Members of our workshop group are continuing to meet independently in their own local version of a SAD community: holding informal social get-togethers over the summer months and creating an itinerary of wintertime activities. We venture that its short-term continuation already shows that the workshops enable a creative and generative form of relationship, starting new trajectories for learning how to live better in winter – a specific expression of biosolidarity. The challenges of being together when feeling SAD are already emphasised, and our workshops have asked participants to reimagine their winter lives by reinhabiting their local environment and everyday lives in new ways, to light up the dark of SAD. This experience not only outlines the potential for living differently – and biosocially – with seasonality but underscores the importance of working with and learning from those most affected by the challenges brought on by seasonal change.

Conclusions: SAD lessons for cultural geographies of mental health

It is important to consider that embodied relations with place and nature do not always feature nurturing and restorative modes. In writing about SAD, we have illuminated the uncomfortable affects of winter and months of low light. In doing so, we have attended to an embodied condition which has been neglected in geographies of mental health, but one that also holds lessons for future times and new configurations of psychosocial natures, and it is to this area we turn to in conclusion.

The uncertain history of the diagnostic category of SAD, the fractured history of SADA, and the lack of community for those who experience the condition tell us that interventions in 'environmental' mental health problems are tricky. Here, embodied relations that seem distinct yet distinctively connected to seasons of low light and winter social life are experienced as isolating, even stigmatising. Although our own research project seeks to disrupt these associations and find new creative pathways to SAD biosociality, there are difficult messages here for other forms of environmental illness, particularly ones that might arrive with ongoing climate change.

In the emergent field of literature connecting climate change and mental health, there is a focus on emotional states like dread, hopelessness, anxiety, and grief as well as some attention (but less so) on depression. Some attention is also paid to ways in which these states may be associated with new forms of engagement with climate action from small personal changes to larger scale collective forms of action (Ojala et al, 2021). It is notable that 'talking' and 'meaning-making' with others helps to engender feelings of 'adaptive control', from psychological perspectives, especially when dealing with 'macro worries' like climate change (Ojala et al., 2021). Such generalisations are contextualised by observations that 'distressing emotions may also be dependent on place and cultural identity as well as living and working relationships related to the natural world' (Cunsolo and Ellis, 2018, p. 279). Our own research with people living with SAD suggests that nature-relations that induce mental ill health are isolating experiences which are not well understood, but that opportunities to talk and share are meaningful for adapting the SAD-self to projections or imaginaries of future winter life. In this regard we confirm and complement emerging research in this field, but also suggest new ways in which we might manage this phenomenon. Those living with SAD are already expert at managing changing seasons of light and have an acute sense of what it is to suffer shifts in weather and atmospheric conditions and temperature. This seasonal expertise has arguably been a negative individual experience, held in suspicion by others, especially in the Global North, where, for the time being, everyday life can still be disassociated from direct climate change damage. While we wish to resist making crass and too-easy connections to research with other peoples in other places, especially indigenous peoples who have suffered profound and on-going mental health consequences of climate-changed relations with their environments for many decades (Middleton et al., 2020), we also believe there are points for greater connection and opportunities for expanded environmental solidarities. We might imagine these as ones existing between people with SAD experience in the Global North and those who experience a range of 'intangible' mental health affects in indigenous communities around the world connected to changing relations with environments and places (ibid). As Middleton et al (2020) have argued, it is only recently that global institutions have begun to recognise these affects and conditions as part of a global social and economic recognition of 'loss and damage'. In summing up their article, these authors (ibid, p.13) argue:

> In recognizing the highly interconnected and potentially pervasive mental health challenges Indigenous Peoples will face, there exist important opportunities for global research efforts to engage Indigenous Peoples on this topic, while building upon existing

causal understandings to better plan and prepare for the mental health implications of rapid climatic change

Given such calls to engage, and the realities to which they are connected, it may not seem so implausible to imagine that future cultural geographies of mental health might seek to actively connect people with SAD, and SAD stories, with others experiencing climate-related mental health challenges in other parts of the world in order to think through the more radical potentials of global biosocial community making.

Acknowledgements

'Living with SAD' is an ESRC funded research project: number ES/V002473/1. This chapter is written with thanks to the Wintering Well Collective, and our partners artist-poet Alec Finlay and Living Life to the Full.

Note

1 Living Life to the Full is a leading provider of online CBT-based resources for people experiencing diverse mental health challenges, building on the 'Five Areas' approach developed by Chris Williams.

References

Adams, Matthew. (2016). *Ecological crisis, sustainability and the psychosocial subject: Beyond behaviour change*. Palgrave Macmillan. https://doi.org/10.1057/978-1-137-35160-9

Albrecht, G. (2007). Solastalgia: the distress caused by environmental change. *Australas Psychiatry*, *15*, pp. 95–98.

Bodden, S., Finlay, A., Lorimer, H., Parr, H. and Williams, C. (2022). Winter worries: understanding experiences of seasonal affective disorder in the UK through the 2022 'Big SAD survey'Interim project report. https://eprints.gla.ac.uk/292974/

Bodden, S., Lorimer, H., Parr, H. and Williams, C. (in press) SAD geographies: making light matter *Progress in Human Geography*.

Boyd, C. *et al* (2022). Climate anxiety as posthuman knowledge. *Wellbeing, Space and Society, 4*, ISSN 2666-5581.

Bradley, B. (2021). From biosociality to biosolidarity: the looping effects of finding and forming social networks for body-focused repetitive behaviours. *Anthropology & Medicine, 28*(4), pp. 543–557. doi: 10.1080/13648470.2020.1864807

Callard F. (2014). Psychiatric diagnosis: the indispensability of ambivalence. *Journal of Medical Ethics, 40*, pp. 526–530.

Cunsolo A, Ellis N.R. 2018. Ecological grief as a mental health response to climate change-related loss. *Nature Climate Change, 8*(4), pp. 275–281.

Fonte A. and Coutinho B. (2021). Seasonal sensitivity and psychiatric morbidity: study about seasonal affective disorder. *BMC Psychiatry, 21*(1), p. 317. doi: 10.1186/s12888-021-03313-z

Geddes, L. (2019). *Chasing the Sun*. London: Wellcome Collection.

Lambert, G.W., Reid, C., Kaye, D.M., Jennings, G.L. and Esler, M.D. (2002). Effect of sunlight and season on serotonin turnover in the brain. *Lancet, 360*(9348), pp. 1840–1842. doi: 10.1016/s0140-6736(02)11737-5. PMID: 12480364.

LoBello, S.G. (2017). The validity of major depression with seasonal pattern: reply to young (2017). *Clinical Psychological Science, 5*(4), pp. 755–757. Available at: https://doi.org/10.1177/2167702617702420.

NHS. (2022). Seasonal affective disorder (SAD). *NHS inform*. Online: www.nhsinform.scot/illnes ses-and-conditions/mental-health/seasonal-affective-disorder-sad/

Middleton, J., Cunsolo, A., Jones-Bitton, A., Wright, C.J. and Harper, S.L., 2020. Indigenous mental health in a changing climate: a systematic scoping review of the global literature. *Environmental Research Letters*, 15(5), 053001.

Ojala, M., Cunsolo, A., Ogunbode, C.A. and Middleton, J. (2021). Anxiety, worry, and grief in a time of environmental and climate crisis: a narrative review. *Annual Review of Environment and Resources*, 46, pp. 35–58.

Overy, C. and Tansey, E. M. (2014). The recent history of Seasonal Affective Disorder (SAD): the transcript of a Witness Seminar held by the History of Biomedicine Research Group. Queen Mary, University of London, on 10 December 2013. Witness Seminar https://wellcomecollect ion.org/works/qqz94jmg

Parr, H., Bodden, S. and Lorimer, H. (submitted, forthcoming). In a positive light? Experiencing Seasonal Affective Disorder (SAD) and the promise of biosolidarity. *Social and Cultural Geography*, 1–19. https://doi.org/10.1080/14649365.2024.2347873

Romanello, M., McGushin, A., Di Napoli, C., Drummond, P., Hughes, N., Jamart, L., Kennard, H., Lampard, P., Rodriguez, B.S., Arnell, N. and Ayeb-Karlsson, S., 2021. The 2021 report of the Lancet Countdown on health and climate change: code red for a healthy future. *The Lancet*, 398(10311), pp. 1619–1662.

Rosenthal, N (2009). Issues for DSM-V: seasonal affective disorder and seasonality. *American Journal of Psychiatry*. doi: 10.1176/appi.ajp.2009.09020188

Rosenthal, N. (2012). *Winter Blues: Everything You Need to Know to Beat Seasonal Affective Disorder*. 4th ed. The Guildford Press.

Targum S.D. and Rosenthal, N. (2008). Seasonal affective disorder. *Psychiatry (Edgmont)*, 5(5), pp. 31–33. PMID: 19727250; PMCID: PMC2686645.

Veale, L., Endfield, G. and Naylor, S. (2014). Knowing weather in place: the Helm Wind of Cross Fell. *Journal of Historical Geography*, 45, p. 25.

Wolch, J.R. & Philo, C. (2000). From distributions of deviance to definitions of difference: past and future mental health geographies. *Health Place*, 6, pp. 137–157.

Young, M.A. (2017). Does seasonal affective disorder exist? A Commentary on Traffanstedt, Mehta, and LoBello (2016). *Clinical Psychological Science*, 5(4). https://doi.org/10.1177/21677 02616689086

17 Geographies of panic

Towards a relational conceptualisation of panic 'disorder'

Candela Sánchez-Rodilla Espeso

Introduction

The phenomenon and experience of panic was not conceptualised as a 'mental disorder' until the publication of the 3rd Diagnostic and Statistical Manual of Mental Disorders (DSM-III) in 1980 (Nardi and Freire, 2016). Prior to this, panic was described largely as a cardiovascular illness and was based around research during war time (Angst, 1998). It was not until Klein's (1988, 1994 work that the positivist onto-epistemology of the psychological and physiological symptoms of panic were brought together and culminated in the creation of 'panic disorder' as a clinical entity.

Since then, panic disorder[1] (defined with or without agoraphobia[2]) has largely been understood and treated within biomedical and psychological science models of mental illness. These models *locate* panic in the individual. In other words, panic disorder is understood as a set of physiological symptoms (e.g. palpitations, trembling, shaking) and the misinterpretation of these (e.g. fear of going 'crazy', fear of dying), which then lead people to engage in maladaptive behaviours (e.g. avoidance behaviours). All of these are seen as symptoms of a malfunction *in* and *of* the person through which the body becomes objectified and medicalised as the source of illness and the site for treatment.

On the other hand, a small sub-field of medical and health geographies, mental health geography investigates the worlds of institutionalisation, deinstitutionalisation, community care, and everyday life of people with mental health issues (Wolch and Philo, 2000; McGeachan and Philo, 2017). Since the 1990s, mental health geographers have focused on the emotional, experiential and situated elements of mental health issues, not normally available within the clinical models of ill-health and a positivistic onto-epistemology (Kearns, 1993; Kearns and Moon, 2002; Parr, 2002; McGeachan and Philo, 2017). The more recent 'third wave' of mental health geographies (see Wolch and Philo, 2000) draws from feminist, phenomenological, post-colonial, post-humanist and psychotherapeutic approaches. This has provided the theoretical basis to offer a) alternatives to the dominant reductive conceptualisations of mental ill-health, and b) critical scrutiny of medical ideas, practices and spaces.

It is within this academic landscape that a small number of geographers and critical theorists have investigated the phenomenon of agoraphobia (Bankey, 2002, 2004; Davidson, 2002, 2003; Callard, 2006, 2016; Trigg, 2013b, 2013a, 2016, 2018). Relationality, space, place and embodiment feature as important themes in their investigations. In this chapter, I build on this work and offer a relational, and necessarily embodied, conceptualisation of panic. I hope that by moving towards a deeply situated,

DOI: 10.4324/9781003345725-19

contextualised and embodied understanding of panic that recovery approaches will also attend and embrace the ways in which anxious bodies produce phobic materialities and vice versa.

Panic as the disruption of relational structures

To construct a relational conceptualisation of panic, I draw from the findings of a qualitative study on the experiences of, and 'recovering' journeys from, panic (Sánchez-Rodilla Espeso, 2021; 2022). The qualitative material produced in this study consists of semi-structured interviews, 'go-along' interviews and drawing methods undertaken with four research participants. Theresa, Anna, Raul and Grant. The semi-structured interview explored each participant's history of panica alongside how they make sense of and experience panic. This initial interview was followed by an invitation to use drawing materials (specifically, a selection of charcoal, graphite sticks, pencils, coloured pencils, coloured markers and gouache) to explore what their experience of panic meant to each of them. Finally, the 'go-along' interviews involved walking around and through a place that the participant had previously had an anxious relationship with – and very often avoided due to fear of panicking while in it. The findings are discussed here to highlight that panic is constituted by three relational elements: self and the body, between the self and others, between the self and space. The experience of panic disrupts the relational elements through which space becomes fragmented into, as I have argued elsewhere, a patchwork of safe and phobic places (Sánchez-Rodilla Espeso, 2021, 2022).

The self and the body: Embodiment, ontological security, and mobility

The experience of panic is commonly associated, in both popular culture and in biomedical accounts, to the onset of panic attacks. Panic attacks are deeply embodied. While exploring the body is key to understanding the experience of panic, biomedical and psychological science accounts present the body as a set of discrete physical symptoms that give an 'objective' picture of what a panic attack 'is' (e.g. palpitations, sweating, trembling and so on). In this section, I explore the relationship between the self and the body in panic beyond this set of physiological symptoms.

In order to explore the role that the 'panicking body' has in reconceptualising panic as a relational entity, let us consider the body in space, and how it allows us to experience ourselves as unified and mobile individuals. First, when we are not anxious, we can move from one place to another, or from one area of the room to another while retaining full agency of our movements and without questioning this movement (Trigg, 2018). That is, we can move through space as whole, secure beings whose 'ontological security' is intact. Ontological security is a concept developed by Laing (1959) within the field of existential psychoanalysis, which refers to the existential sense of safety required to live 'normally'. According to Laing (1959), to live our lives normally, our everyday experience is not riddled by questions about our own existence. Therefore, we must have a sense of stability and safety *in ourselves* in such a way that we take for granted our sense of self.

The second aspect to our mobility is our experience of space as a continuous and homogeneous fabric. That is not to say that space is 'all the same' but, rather, that we take for granted the existence of a continuous spatial fabric that is available to us through movement. Malpas's (2012ab; 2017; 2018) conceptualisation of relational space and place is particularly helpful here. Malpas (2012b) encourages us to think of space and place in terms of three key concepts: boundedness, opennesss and appearance. A place becomes 'a place' not as a fixed point or area on a map, but rather as something that *appears* as *bounded* in the *openness* of space. This appearance is further conceptualised in terms of salience and withdrawal:

> The structure of place is such that it draws towards its centre — towards the *there,* the *here,* the *this,* that is salient within it — but as it draws in towards, so place envelops and surrounds, but in a way that also itself draws away, withdraws.
>
> (Malpas, 2012a, p. 237)

This tension between the salience and withdrawal of place yields the boundaries of place, thus *producing* a place. When we are not anxious, our experience of space is as a continued *openness* comprised by areas of spatial *salience* that make up what we recognise as distinctive places. And yet, the spatial fabric that connects all of these remains intact.

In anxiety, both of these are disrupted (Boyle, 2019). The disruption of the intersubjective and spatial elements is accompanied by the experience of panic attacks. Panic attacks, as embodied anxiety, undermine our sense of selfhood and our ability to move through space as ontologically secure selves. The accounts of panic discussed throughout this chapter, illustrate how, for each participant, panic is experienced and embodied differently. For example, Theresa's panic travels all the way through her spine causing a tightening of her throat, resulting in feelings of nausea and unsteady legs. For Raul, the very notion of losing control over his own body is so deeply terrifying that he manages to keep panic attacks invisible, but even then continues to experience "breathing problems". These embodied aspects of panic result in both participants' inability to relate to themselves as whole and 'secure' beings. The body becomes, not only the expression of panic, but the very 'object' of it. In other words, in panic, the body becomes 'it', a thing almost divorced from themselves that "starts dysfunctioning" (Theresa), takes on a mind of its own and behaves in ways that they do not want it to and have no control over. Trigg (2018) discusses this in his exploration of agoraphobia in which he draws on the phenomenological works of Merleau-Ponty to argue that the body can appear at times as *thinglike.* The experience of being disconnected from the body is one of the ways in which anxious and phobic bodies disrupt our sense of whole integral selves.

The possibility that the body might start 'dysfunctioning' when encountering certain places or certain situations leads to the disruption of space as a continuous fabric, one in which a person can move freely and safely. This second way in which the embodiment of panic disrupts mobility contributes to embodied spatial fragmentation (see Trigg, 2018). This involves the experience of space as fragmented; with some places becoming phobic (to be avoided) and others safe.

The self and 'Others': The breakdown of intersubjectivity

Alongside disruptions in their sense of self and mobility, panic also disrupts participant's sense of belonging among others. During the drawing interviews, I asked participants to draw what panic felt like for them. Theresa drew the following image:

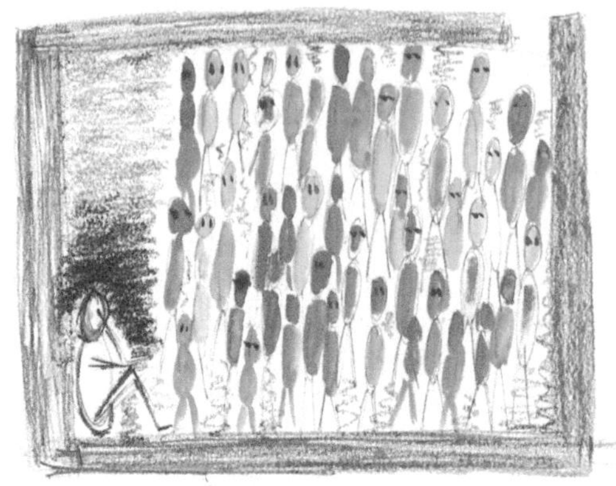

Figure 17.1 Theresa's drawing of 'panic' (Authors photograph).

For Theresa, panic is being in a space where a) escaping will be difficult and b) there is a feeling of deep existential separation from 'the crowd'. Theresa explained this in more detail through her use of colour with each colour giving emphasis and meaning to different elements of what she experiences and embodies during panic. The yellow section (in the top right hand corner) symbolises a potential exit and represents what she feels when she is able to leave a phobic place as "any bright colours would mean joy to me, so the yellow, yeah… a bit of sunlight, a bit of sun light, a bit of, you know, something… yeah…" (Theresa). She uses black (for herself, the 'cloudy' area around her and between people, and the borders of the room) to symbolise *where* panic is for her. The panic is not only in her but also in the room, in the walls and the space is within the room, and particularly in the cloud surrounding her head. Thus, the experience of panic depicted here is explicitly spatial. Panic is not just about what goes on inside but it develops *in relation* to the space that she has drawn, where she imagines herself to be. Crucially, panic takes place at the intersections between the self, the body and the material arrangements (including other selves and other bodies) that make-up a 'phobic place'. Finally, she notes that red is "really the aggression, like I find… you know, so many people being present here like it's really aggressives in my face, it's there, you know, and I can't not see them" (Theresa). Red (depicts 'the crowd') emphasises the intersubjectivity of panic as other people are not just in the background but rather constitutive of that experience. In Theresa's case, this intersubjective element of panic has two separate parts. Others are experienced both as other bodies, that restrict her ability to move through space, as well as through the perceived 'gaze of the other'. I discuss each of these in turn.

Theresa describes how panic disrupts her ability (or lack thereof) to navigate the mass of bodies illustrated in her drawing:

Yeah… so this kind of… physical and… you can't go through, you can't escape easily, you would have to physically move people to actually get out […] then… you know, I'm gonna have to move people physically to get to the door [she laughs slighty as she says this]. […] And then all these people are all the same colour because they are all the same, just a mass of people, like they can't really… I don't differentiate [between] them, you know, they can't be different colours or different shapes cos they are just a mass of people that are just in the way.

The people in the space become a mass of bodies that obstruct her movement to the point that she feels she will have to move them to get out of that room. Theresa drew them using the same colour and shape to emphasise that she does not perceive them as separate individuals who may relate to Theresa (and Theresa to them) on an individual basis. This illustrates how Theresa's panic is one in which her ability to relate to and differentiate individual others breaks down; instead, a solid boundary emerges between her and the mass of others she is sharing space with. Here I would like to introduce two concepts from Heidegger's (1962) discussion of anxiety that are particularly useful for thinking through Theresa's account and for considering the role of 'other people' in the experience of panic. These are the 'Others' and 'modes of encounter'.

The Others is an existential term. Heidegger does not refer to Others as a collection of individuals that a person is always part of by being in proximity (spatially) with other people. Others refers to the 'whole' to which one belongs and from which oneself cannot be – ontologically – separated, with the exception being that in an anxious mood the 'self' anxiety estranged (or 'individualised', in Heidegger's terms) from the Others. In order to understand what he means by this, it is important to understand the concept of 'modes of encounter'. According to Heidegger, a reflexive and self-conscious subject[3] encounters entities in the world in three different ways, through: readiness-to-hand; presence-at-hand; and unreadiness-to-hand. In this discussion I focus specifically on 'readiness' and 'unreadiness'.

We encounter most entities as 'equipment', meaning that we have no conscious experience of them existing as independent objects. In other words, according to Heidegger, my experience of entities that I encounter in my everyday life is always mediated by the set of actions in which I become familiarised with them. Therefore, my familiarisation and making sense of, say, a pen as an entity always takes place within a particular context in which I use the pen. This is what Heidegger calls readiness-to-hand. Unreadiness-to-hand is the mode of existing of entities that we experience when an activity or an action is disturbed by a broken or a malfunctioning piece of equipment. Thus, these entities are not 'phenomenologically transparent' to us, that is to say that the means through which people understand and become familiar with these entities is no longer straightforward. This ability to make sense of an entity does not take place in the performance of an activity, but in the disruption of such an activity. Now, Heidegger argues that all ready-to-hand entities that we encounter in our everyday (for example, the keyboard in which I am typing now, or my notebook, or my cup of tea), we encounter them as existing always in essential reference to Others (for example, the person who made the keyboard, the person who dispatched it to the shop where I bought it, the shop assistant who sold it to me, and so on). This is also the case for entities that are encountered as unready-to-hand. This is the reason why Heidegger defines the Others as a collective whole in which the 'I' is always embedded in.

In anxiety, however, the self is separated and estranged from the Others. As in the case of Theresa where she cannot relate to the people in the room as individuals, all of them comprising a societal whole to which she belongs. Instead, and suddenly, the bodies of others become an entangled mesh, undifferentiated and blocking her way out and a way to safety. This way of relating to 'Others-as-bodies' through the experience of disruption (or, to use Heidegger's terms in an unready-to-hand mode) contributes to the feeling of not being able to escape or to move. Crucially, the experience of Others-as-bodies by disruption is produced relationally; it is not an inherent property of the Others, as much as it is not an intrinsic property of Theresa's perception of other people. Others are viewed/experienced/perceived only as disrupting bodies. In other words, Theresa's relationship to Others becomes problematic and disruptive specifically and *only* when Theresa is panicking and feels an urgent need to escape to a place of relative safety.

This boundary that emerges between Theresa and the Others is partly related to, and fuelled by, the second intersubjective element of Theresa's panic. In addition to obstructing Theresa's movement and ability to escape this phobic place, this mass of red people depicted in her drawing are also 'watchful people':

> It's just like… those people will be… psych- [interrupts herself]… you know, aware if I start dysfunctioning as a human, fainting, puking… […] yeah, so… red really for the aggression… uhm… the fact that those people are not just… they have eyes cos, you know, they can definitely see me fainting, puking, whatever… which has never happened, and the dark really, yeah, cos you can't avoid it, it's there, it's clouding your judgement, your vision, your anything […]

The gaze of others is deeply embedded in Theresa's experience of panic as it separates and individualises Theresa from them. This aspect of panic is discussed by both Trigg (2018) and Davidson (2003) in their investigations of agoraphobia. Davidson (2003) draws from Sartre and Goffman to argue that agoraphobia sufferers become hypersensitive to the gaze of others. This look of the others highlights both their self-consciousness and the ways in which their bodies are not able to comply with specific place-embodiments.

Theresa, too, becomes aware of her own body panicking and experiences place differently from other people. This produces what Theresa calls "physical loneliness":

> [Y]ou feel really… you know… in your head you can't be part of this, like you are really… it's too hard to pretend to be part of this, you, you know, you will be… uhm… … …yeah, you will be… …unable to behave like the rest of the people that are around basically, behaving in a certain way, soo… and then… …yeah, the very kind of feeling of… it's not something that anybody else can experience with you, so it's physically, physical loneliness.
>
> (Theresa)

Thus, to be in a place involves also taking in a particular way of perceiving the world and taking in a particular way of behaving in order to be a successful social agent of that specific place (see Foucault, 1984; Giddens, 1991). While at the same time, an individual being in a place and exerting the necessary and appropriate body performances for that place, contributes to the constitution of that very place. Thus, encounters, actions and affectivities that tangle bodies and places produce both a sense of place and a sense of identification and acceptance in that place. In turn, this produces what Seamon (1980) calls 'place ballets', the interaction of individual bodily routines rooted in a specific place that produces meaning and attachment to that place. In anxiety, the panicking body does not conform to these specific ways of behaving (e.g. patiently waiting in a queue or being in an enclosed busy place calmly and mindlessly). The panicking body draws attention from others and this 'gaze' further separates Theresa from the crowd.

The self and space: The world becomes uncanny

Finally, the third element that panic disrupts is the relationship between the self and space. This is, of course, related to the discussions I have presented already, but it is nevertheless useful to pay special attention to what panic *does* to space and how panicking bodies sense and make sense of the world differently.

During our interview, Theresa recalled that her first panic attack took place in the canteen of her university. After this, the particular spatial aspects of that place took on a phobic meaning, to the point that these spatialities become part of what it means to panic for Theresa. The canteen was a loud, busy with a lot of noise and a lot of movement and since her initial panic attack, "*[...] loud, busy spaces with a lot of noise equals a panic attack, type of thing*". As such, other places that share similar qualities, such as cinemas and music venues become phobic places too.

During our 'go-along' interviews, Theresa spoke of the cinema as a similarly phobic space:

> [...] loads of people, loads of noise, loads of movement, loads of different lights and kind of information" and when she was feeling anxious all of these sensory elements would become "louder, brighter, and lighter. [...] Eh... but like... you know, everything used to be like really amplified and really... just louder.

This space provoked an intense sensory overload that could end in the outburst of a panic attack. Theresa also spoke of the density of information and the density of space as attributes of phobic places. She remarked that the area below the mezzanine inside the cinema hall, where the ceiling is lower and the overhead lights are closer to one's body, is an even more difficult area to be in. She mentioned similar aspects in relation to music venues:

> The... the physical volume of the... place is something that I find really important [...] Yeah... so... I find it... a lot easier to hang out in clubs with higher ceiling... than things like... on the ground.

Consequently, the relationship that Theresa forms with the specific materialities of the canteen, the cinema, and music venues is transformed and takes on an aggressive and threatening sense. As she stated: "I would feel like really...ergh, I don't know... attacked by the environment". And in this, the world does indeed become an uncanny and unfamiliar place.

The production of phobic places involves, not only, thinking about the boundaries that define specific places but how these places are sensed and made sense of as increasingly hostile spaces. Exploring these aspects allows us to start understanding how anxious bodies perceive space differently and how this in turn leads to the production of phobic places.

Spatial fragmentation and the production of phobic places

Participants spoke of a variety of phobic places that they have avoided or still avoid (at the time of our interviews) because their experience of panic is tightly bound to the spatialities of those places. Theresa spoke of cinemas, pubs, clubs and music venues. Raul spoke of some cinemas, airplanes, and buses. Anna spoke of her family home and her current office. While, Grant spoke of schools, colleges, universities, and narrow streets. I have discussed how panic disrupts how participants relate to their body and mobility through space; the way in which they relate to Others; and the way in which they sense the world and feel familiarity in it. The question is: how do these disruptions lead to specific places becoming phobic?

Earlier in this chapter I introduced relational conceptualisations of space and place through Malpas' work (2012a, 2012b, 2017, 2018). The concept Boundaries[4] are key to understanding place relationally and is particularly useful for thinking about the emergence of phobic places. What makes a place *that* place? Or, in other words, with all the meaning that this entails, what makes, for instance, your house *your home*?

The boundaries of places are produced by the tension between the *salience* of place, and the *withdrawal* of place. The salience of place is everything that makes a place, that draws towards its centre whereas the withdrawal of place is everything that stands in contrast, or that pulls away from such a place. These notions are purposefully vague, they reflect the way in which place is, "always bounded, yet it is also always open and dynamic" (Malpas, 2012a, p. 236). Furthermore, acknowledging this complexity enables us to imagine place as emerging within *many* different sets of relational structures, and importantly, how these are experienced (Gendlin, 1997; Duff, 2011). To go back to the example of a house; what makes that house *your home* is the particular affective, material, cultural, generational and relational elements that have become *salient* in the relationship between you and the particular building that you have now come to see *your home*.

Phobic places emerge in much the same way, although through disruption. Phobic places emerge, not due to the elements that become salient in the relationship between a person and that phobic place. Instead, the *salience* of a phobic place emerges as a *disruption* of the three relational elements discussed throughout: between the self and the body; between the self and Others; and between the self and space. The *withdrawal* of phobic places is everything that allows for that disruption to diminish and for the individual to begin to restore their sense of safety.

The boundaries of the phobic places do not necessarily match the physical boundaries of those places. These boundaries are subjective and make up the kind of spatial fragmentation that each panic sufferer experiences. Yet, this does not mean that these boundaries are any less 'hard'. Crossing these boundaries can be extremely challenging because it involves being confronted by the disruption of the three elements that I discuss earlier in this chapter. For Anna, for example, the walk to her office is a difficult space to be. The first part of her walk is usually not as challenging. In the walk, there is a road crossing where, once she crosses, she will be able to see her office. This crossing is particularly significant for Anna and her experience of boundaries because she might either turn and walk back home *before* crossing it or decide to cross it and continue on.

The boundaries of phobic places are constantly redrawn and managed on a daily basis, as Boyle (2019) discusses in her investigation of social anxiety. Moreover, they change throughout processes of recovery. While, for example, the anxiety may be focused around, say, a restaurant (as it was for Theresa) it may be that the boundaries of that phobic place extend for a large enough radius around it so that she would not be able to go anywhere where the restaurant is visible. Only when she felt able to manage her anxiety, the boundaries of that phobic place would reduce and she would feel able to go by the street where the restaurant was, as long as she was not actually walking inside of it. This is also the case for Anna, when on a 'bad day' leaving the house to go to the office is already problematic; and on 'good days' the boundaries of the office-phobic-place change. And Raul, for whom airplanes as phobic places extended to include the airport and the bus that would take him to the airport. As he became less anxious about airplanes the boundaries of those as a phobic place also changed; and he was able to manage entering the airport, even if not the airplane.

Concluding thoughts

This chapter develops a relational and spatial conceptualisation of panic. In doing so, it highlights the significance of thinking geographically about mental health and aims to demonstrate what a phenomenological – and geographically informed – analysis of mental health can offer future debates – both clinically and within mental health geographies. Understanding the relationship between the context in which panic attacks emerges, how people make sense of them, and the embodiment of panic in itself is not something to be weeded out in order to find the objective elements that make up panic disorder. Instead, paying attention to the embodiment of panic and how it affects one's sense of ontological security and mobility is crucial to understanding panic as an ongoing disruption between self, space, and others.

Panic attacks, rather than being decontextualised and unexpected, emerge at the intersections between selves and space. They disrupt our sense of self and render us ontologically insecure disrupting how people move through the world. Being in or near phobic places can trigger these panic symptoms leading to the avoidance of such places. Conversely, experiencing panic in a specific location can contribute to the perception of that place as phobic. The real issue is not the embodied symptoms themselves, as clinical accounts of panic have tended to assume, but the threat that these symptoms experienced in particular places pose to our ontological security and mobility.

As demonstrated in this chapter, investigating panic relationally shifts our 'investigative gaze' away from what might be wrong inside the individual, to the bodily, spatial and intersubjective aspects of anxiety, as well as the role of prior experiences of panic. This shift is important, because it produces a departure from the conceptual assumptions that current models of illness rest upon. It also presents opportunities for more nuanced approaches to recovery that pay careful attention to the relationships between the individual and space.

Notes

1 In this chapter I refer to panic disorder when speaking about a biomedical understanding of this mental health issue, and I refer to panic when I speak of the whole experience of panic phenomenologically. I refer to panic attacks when speaking about individual panic surges that an individual may experience. I make this distinction because discussing mental health and mental ill-health necessarily come with terminological issues (Wolch and Philo, 2000). Terms such as mental disability or mental disorder bring with them issues around 1) negativity (something that the person is lacking) and 2) essentialist views of the individual which can be problematic (implying that this disorder is an essential and core element of the identity of the person who experiences such a mental health issue). Terms such as mental illness imply a medical

understanding of the individual and of mental health issues, from which this chapter wants to depart. In light of this, I refer to people with mental health issues when speaking about individuals who are affected by mental ill-health.

2 Panic disorder and agoraphobia have historically been defined along the same continuum (Cassano *et al.*, 1998). In the third edition of the DSM, agoraphobia appears as a separate disorder from panic disorder, which can be diagnosed with or without the presence of panic attacks (American Psychiatric Association, 1980). Subsequent research into the relationship between panic and agoraphobia in the 1980s led to panic disorder being understood as the precursor of agoraphobia (Garvey and Tuason, 1984; Noyes *et al.*, 1986). Noyes et al (1986) for example argue that agoraphobia is a more severe form of panic disorder. Consequently, in the fourth edition of the DSM, panic disorder appears as a disorder diagnosed either with or without agoraphobia (American Psychiatric Association, 1994). The notion that agoraphobia is a secondary manifestation of panic disorder still existed until 2013 with the publication of the most recent version of the DSM (American Psychiatric Association, 2013).

3 Note that Heidegger's discussion here surrounds his concept of Dasein, rather than a subject. Dasein is a concept that emerges from Heidegger's (1962) exploration into the metaphysical question of being. Dasein is the particular type of existing realised by human beings. The reason why Heidegger makes this particular distinction - between the mode of existing done by human beings alone and the rest of entities in the world - is twofold. First, according to Heidegger (1962), human beings are conscious of themselves as 'beings'; and second, they are also able to reflect upon what it means to be. However, for simplicity and due to the short scope of this Chapter, I am referring here to 'reflexive self-conscious subject' instead.

4 I am aware the notion of boundaries is a particularly contested theme within relational conceptualisations of space and place. Massey (2005, p. 152) argues that one issue of thinking of place as being bounded is that it "can so easily be yet another way of constructing a counter position between 'us' and 'them'". This way of thinking about boundaries has been taken up by most human geographers who have embraced post-structuralist notions of openness and fluidity (Cresswell, 2004), with Nigel Thrift (2008) arguing that there is no such thing as a boundary. Yet, I contest this view on two grounds. First, if we do conceptualise place as relational; and emerging within relational structures we must recognise that the very concept of boundary is what establishes the possibility of the concept of relationality in the first instance. Boundaries and boundedness are necessary for thinking of space. They are also necessary for thinking of the emergence of places within the relational field of space, as well as the elements within a particular place. Second, I agree with Massey (2005) that thinking of boundaries involves thinking of an 'us' and 'them'; but this is precisely the way in which the participants of this study all speak of places and people within places. Thus, it does not seem useful to simply negate the existence of boundaries altogether. Instead, relational conceptualisations of space and place does not mean that we must forgo discussions about boundaries. Instead, they allow us to re-imagine boundaries more creatively. In the same way place is fluid and constantly evolving, so are boundaries. And this, in turn, is a useful framework to explore phobic places; the way in which they appear, but also how their boundaries are constantly redefined and managed.

References

American Psychiatric Association. (1980) *Diagnostic and statistical manual of mental disorders (DSM-III)*. Arlington: American Psychiatric Publishing.

American Psychiatric Association. (1994) *Diagnostic and statistical manual of mental disorders (DSM-IV)*. Arlington: American Psychiatric Publishing.

American Psychiatric Association. (2013) *Diagnostic and statistical manual of mental disorders: DSM-5*. 5th edn. Arlington, VA: American Psychiatric Publishing.

Angst, J. (1998) 'Panic disorder: History and epidemiology', *European Psychiatry*, 13, pp. 51s–55s. Available at: https://doi.org/10.1016/S0924-9338(98)80014-X.

Bankey, R. (2002) 'Embodying Agoraphobia: Rethinking Geographies of Women's Fear', in Bondi et al. (ed.) *Subjectivities, Knowledges and Feminist Geographies*. Oxford: Rowman & Littlefield.

Bankey, R. (2004) 'The agoraphobic condition', *Cultural Geographies*, 11(3), pp. 347–355.

Boyle, L.E. (2019) 'The (un) habitual geographies of Social Anxiety Disorder', *Social Science & Medicine*, 231, pp. 31–37.

Callard, F. (2006) '"The sensation of infinite vastness"; or, the emergence of agoraphobia in the late 19th century', *Environment and Planning D: Society and Space*, 24(6), pp. 873–889.

Callard, F. (2016) 'The intimate geographies of panic disorder: Parsing anxiety through psycho-pharmacological dissection', *Osiris*, 31(1), pp. 203–226.

Cassano, G.B. *et al.* (1998) 'The panic-agoraphobic spectrum: Rationale, assessment, and clinical usefulness', *CNS Spectrums*, 3(4), pp. 35–48. Available at: https://doi.org/10.1017/S109285290 0005848.

Cresswell, T. (2004) 'Defining Place', in *Place: A Short Introduction*. Malden, MA: Blackwell Ltd, 12.

Davidson, J. (2002) 'All in the Mind?: Women, Agoraphobia, and the Subject of Self-Help', in Bondi et al. (ed.) *Subjectivities, Knowledges and Feminist Geographies*. Oxford: Rowman & Littlefield.

Davidson, J. (2003) *Phobic geographies: The phenomenology and spatiality of identity*. Aldershot: Ashgate Publishing.

Duff, C. (2011) 'Networks, resources and agencies: On the character and production of enabling places', *Health & Place*, 17, pp. 149–156.

Foucault, M. (1984) 'Docile bodies', *The Foucault Reader*, pp. 179–187.

Garvey, M.J. and Tuason, V. (1984) 'The relationship of panic disorder to agoraphobia', *Comprehensive Psychiatry*, 25(5), pp. 529–531.

Gendlin, E.T. (1997) *Experiencing and the creation of meaning: A philosophical and psychological approach to the subjective*. Evanston: Northwestern University Press.

Giddens, A. (1991) *Modernity and self-identity*. Cambridge: Polity Press.

Heidegger, M. (1962) *Being and time*. Translated by J. Macquarrie and E. Robinson. Oxford: Blackwell.

Kearns, R. and Moon, G. (2002) 'From medical to health geography: Novelty, place and theory after a decade of change', *Progress in Human Geography*, 26(5), pp. 605–625.

Kearns, R.A. (1993) 'Place and health: Towards a reformed medical geography', *The Professional Geographer*, 45(2), pp. 139–147.

Klein, D.F. (1988) 'The cause and treatment of agoraphobia-reply', *Archives of General Psychiatry*, 45(4), pp. 389–392.

Klein, D.F. (1994) 'Testing the suffocation false alarm theory of panic disorder', *Anxiety*, 1(1), pp. 1–7.

Laing, R.D. (1959) *The divided self: An existential study into sanity and madness*. 1990th edn. London: Penguin Books.

Malpas, J. (2012a) *Heidegger and the thinking of place: Explorations in the topology of being*. Minneapolis: MIT Press.

Malpas, J. (2012b) 'Putting space in place: Philosophical topography and relational geography', *Environment and Planning D: Society and Space*, 30(2), pp. 226–242.

Malpas, J. (2017) 'Thinking topographically. Place, space, and geography', *Il Cannocchiale: Rivista di Studi Filosofici*, XLII, pp. 1–2.

Malpas, J. (2018) *Place and experience: A philosophical topography*. New York: Routledge.

Massey, D. (2005) *For space*. New York: Sage.

McGeachan, C. and Philo, C. (2017) Occupying space: mental health geography and global directions. In: White, R. G., Jain, S., Orr, D. M.R. and Read, U. M. (eds.) The Palgrave Handbook of Sociocultural Perspectives on Global Mental Health. Series: Palgrave handbooks. Palgrave Macmillan: London, pp. 31-50. ISBN 9781137395092 (doi: 10.1057/978-1-137-39510-8_2)

Nardi, A.E., Freire, R.C.R. (2016). The Panic Disorder Concept: A Historical Perspective. In: Nardi, A., Freire, R. (eds) Panic Disorder. Springer, Cham. https://doi.org/10.1007/978-3-319-12538-1_1

Noyes, R. *et al.* (1986) 'Relationship between panic disorder and agoraphobia: A family study', *Archives of General Psychiatry*, 43(3), pp. 227–232.

Parr, H. (2002) 'Medical geography: Diagnosing the body in medical and health geography, 1999-2000', *Progress in Human Geography*, 26(2), pp. 240–251.

Sánchez-Rodilla Espeso, C. (2021) 'Therapeutic relationships to landscapes: The role of place in panic and panic recovery', *PhD Thesis, The University of Edinburgh* [Preprint].

Sánchez-Rodilla Espeso, C. (2022) 'From safe places to therapeutic landscapes: The role of the home in panic disorder recovery', *Wellbeing, Space and Society*, 3, 100108. Available at: https://doi.org/10.1016/j.wss.2022.100108.

Seamon, D. (1980) Body-subject, time space routines, and place-ballets. In: Buttimer, A., and Seamon, D. (eds.) *The Human Experience of Space and Place*. London: Routledge.

Thrift, N. (2008) *Non-representational theory: Space, politics, affect*. New York: Routledge.

Trigg, D. (2013a) 'Bodily moods and unhomely environments: The hermeneutics of agoraphobia and the Spirit of place', *Interpreting Nature: The Emerging Field of Environmental Hermeneutics*, pp. 160–177.

Trigg, D. (2013b) 'The body of the other: Intercorporeality and the phenomenology of agoraphobia', *Continental Philosophy Review*, 46(3), pp. 413–429.

Trigg, D. (2016) *Topophobia: A phenomenology of anxiety*. London: Bloomsbury Publishing.

Trigg, D. (2018) 'Situated anxiety: A Phenomenology of Agoraphobia', in *Situatedness and Place*. Springer, pp. 187–201.

Wheeler, M. (2020) 'Martin Heidegger', in E.N. Zalta (ed.) *The Stanford Encyclopedia of Philosophy*. Fall 2020. Metaphysics Research Lab, Stanford University. Available at: https://plato.stanford.edu/archives/fall2020/entries/heidegger/.

Wolch, J. and Philo, C. (2000) 'From distributions of deviance to definitions of difference: Past and future mental health geographies', *Health & Place*, 6, pp. 137–157.

18 Taking up space
Anorexia nervosa and embodied healing

Grace Lucas

Anorexia nervosa: minds and bodies

Anorexia nervosa (AN) is an eating disorder (ED) that is defined by restriction of energy intake, low body weight, fear of gaining weight, and a disturbed experience of body weight or shape (American Psychiatric Association, 2013). It mainly affects young women and evidence suggests its incidence is increasing in younger people under the age of 15 (van Eeden, van Hoeken and Hoek, 2021). Relapse rates are high and the overall prognosis is poor (Khalsa et al., 2017). AN has the highest mortality rate of any psychiatric illness (Morris and Twaddle, 2007). Eating disorders are defined as mental disorders, although the physical manifestation of AN makes it profoundly bodily in nature. Psychiatric approaches to treatment tend to focus on this body problem in relation to physical symptoms such as low Body Mass Index (BMI) through cognitive behavioural means and thereby work therapeutically from the head down (NICE, 2017).

In recent years, increasing research interest has been paid to the role of bodily experiences in understanding the development and maintenance of AN. Whilst distorted body image has long been considered a core symptom of AN and has been targeted in treatment, the concept of embodiment, which focuses on the body as the centre of experiencing the world, more helpfully considers the broader sense of how it feels and what it means to be and have a body (Burychka, Miragall & Baños, 2021; Cook-Cottone, 2020; McBride and Kwee 2018; Gaete and Fuchs 2016). As Perey and Cook-Cottone (2020) explain, a sense of embodiment can be both positive – leading to a sense of mind-body connection – or can be experienced negatively as a disruption to the sense of having and being a body. In the context of ED, measures of embodiment have been designed to assess these varied experiences including the 'Experience of Embodiment Scale' (Piran, 2019) and 'Identity and Eating Disorders Questionnaire' (Stanghellini et al., 2012). Indeed, from this perspective, AN has been conceived as a possible disturbance or 'conflict' of embodiment (Fuchs, 2020). However, the concept of embodiment is differently articulated and understood across disciplinary spaces, leading to varied conclusions about how this embodied problem might be best addressed and treated.

Conceptualising anorexia nervosa: meanings of embodiment

Studies on embodiment in brain sciences have analysed potentially significant features of inner body perception in AN relating to distortions in how the body is perceived versus its 'true' physical form. From this perspective, the embodied problem is an internal one. In

DOI: 10.4324/9781003345725-20

a systematic review, Malighetti *et al.* (2022) found 'deficits' in interoception (perceptions of sensations in the body) (Price and Hooven, 2018) – and proprioception (perception of where the body is in terms of its location and movement) (Taylor, 2009) – in people with AN. In a study by Beckmann *et al.,* (2021), people with AN rotated their shoulders to fit through a space that they (mis)perceived was too narrow for them, suggesting 'distortion' in body schema (which controls automatic actions and body posture in space). In this way, AN may relate to a problem of how inner body space is felt from within and how outer space is negotiated. As a result interventions are suggested that focus on these 'faulty' perceptions and body representations (Malighetti et al. 2022; Engel and Keizer, 2017). Virtual reality interventions, working with virtual space, for example, have been proposed as possible ways of helping people with AN address these distortions (Riva, Malighetti and Serino, 2021). Whilst mending perception through virtual means might be useful to feel and sense the body differently in a controlled space, the real world is not so controllable.

Although these neuroscientific approaches provide insight into processes that might lead to people with AN reporting difficulty in bodily connection, they do so from a largely internalised understanding of what embodiment means. The medical model of ED situates them as related to the individual's wrong perception of their body – a flawed connection – often treated by cognitively addressing the problem. However, when considered through a broader biopsychosocial lens (Frank, 2016), this individualised approach leaves the 'social' aspect of ED largely unaddressed. Indeed, when individual body perception and sensation is overlaid with sociocultural ideals of a desirable body object, it can be argued that a person with AN *'perceives all too well'* how their body should look (Threadcraft, 2015, p.220) and how they should treat it. It makes sense that a person might judge or evaluate their body critically because of the influence of a proliferation of images of body ideals through social media, which do not always reflect reality (Vandenbosch, Fardouly, Tiggemann, 2022). Arguably, perception becomes more distorted after layers of online filters and edits have been added to photos and 'reality' turns out to be an increasingly malleable concept. Furthermore, body size, shape and appearance are physically changeable with increased exposure and availability of physical modifications via cosmetics procedures (Cook and Dwyer, 2017). With fast changing standards and expectations, it is easy to overestimate or misperceive the problem of our bodies. Perception of size and space is not an abstract concept separately circling inside the brain but one that is defined, learned and remade from embodied experiences of living in the world. The more the body is an object to be changed and adapted, monitored and controlled, the less a person might feel that they 'are' their body. AN is not only an issue with misreading an outside image of the body, its weight or shape but is entangled with, and more deeply experienced within a sense of self. In AN, where the body's fundamental needs are overwritten and the focus is driven to restricting intake and reducing the body's size, the anorexic body powerfully and problematically enacts societal ideals of mind-over-matter body objectification (Threadcraft, 2015). A disturbance of embodiment is one that is learnt, remade and inhabited from the outside in.

Research about AN in the context of social and cultural pressures around the body (Underwood, 2013) has grown from feminist roots and has typically focused on young, white, middle-class women (Franko et al., 2007). Feminist perspectives have been invaluable in analysing AN beyond the internalised, individualised model to illustrate the power of patriarchal and capitalist contexts and their damaging influence on women's bodies and minds. However, broader social inequities in ED more generally risk highlighting the need to understand the ED experiences of racialized groups, those identifying as LGBTQ+, and people of lower socioeconomic status. Many voices are currently excluded from spaces of ED research and thus evidence about prevalence and impact can only be partial (Burnette et al., 2022). A more nuanced approach to the meanings and manifestations of embodiment is required. Eating disorders are bound up with personal distress but also bring to the fore the social and structural conditions that have laid the foundations for that distress (Eli, 2018). If we understand that embodiment is about how people experience the world around them, and how the world gets under the skin, then ED also relates to how bodies are marginalised, discriminated against or stigmatised by the social worlds and contexts in which they grow, develop and live (Piran & Teall, 2012). If a person experiences trauma, stigma or discrimination, these may disrupt feelings of embodiment. In response to adverse events it may feel safer to escape bodily sensation and disconnect from it entirely. The streets on which we walk teach us a lesson about how we are perceived and we quickly learn, adapt and manoeuvre in relation to those spaces. Our bodies are shaped by our environments. Embodiment is not only a feeling from within that stops at the surface of the skin. Bodily freedom (or lack of it) is bound up with layers of power and privilege and an intersectional lens is needed to unpack this (Burke et al., 2020).

Healing from anorexia – layers of space

In a similar way to understanding how (dis)embodiment and (mis)perception of the body might lead to the development of AN, these concepts are also helpful in relation to healing from AN. This healing can be thought of as different engagements with 'layers of space'.

The first layer helps us attend to the idea of internal space – a renegotiation with how the body feels from within. Finding 'positive embodiment' has been put forward as a possible protective factor for ED as well as a healing mechanism (Piran, 2016). In a thesis on the role of embodied affective experience in recovery from AN, Beyer (2016) writes how a person recovering from AN can move from resenting or reviling their body to having a positive embodied experience, connected to their body, and feeling freed as a result. Although cognitive behavioural therapy is the recommended treatment, there are therapeutic approaches (such as body oriented psychotherapy, yoga, body awareness therapy and dance movement therapy) that are specifically body-oriented and take a 'bottom-up approach'; working with people's emotions, body perceptions, and self-awareness (van de Kamp et al., 2019). It makes sense that if the problem relates to proprioception or interoception difficulties, then physically exploring these bodily experiences and sensations might be helpful therapeutically. I have written about my own experiences of healing from AN based on a non-verbal sensory enquiry (Lucas, 2022). I practiced yoga and became a yoga teacher because I began to notice a changed relationship with my body through meditative movement and focused physical attention. I realised how much feeling there was in my body space and breath and, through movement, I was able to feel space open up. Through this practice I was able to access a different form of engagement with my body – no longer felt as an object but instead expressing the very fibres of my 'self'. Through feeling the sensations of the body – whether that be through tapping, shaking, twisting, balancing, stretching, pressing and making contact with the skin or breathing into its different parts – over time, there can come a realisation that the self is not entirely located in the head. More explicitly then, the concept of 'positive embodiment' can provide a bridge to understanding that selfhood is as somatic as it is cerebral.

For people with AN, who may have experienced a radical disconnection between self and body in attempts to diminish and shrink the physical body (and may not remember any other way of being) the experience of selfhood as emerging from the body can be profound – a flooding of sensation into the limbs, a radical recentring of feeling in the chest or stomach (Doyle, 2023). This may be temporarily experienced in a movement class, for example, and once this feeling of 'subjective immersion' is ignited (Piran and Neumark-Sztainer, 2020) it can be practiced, with new pathways to experiences laid down, as emotions are explored through bodily sensations via 'bodily resonance' (Fuchs & Koch, 2014).

Off the mat, or away from the therapeutic environment, as the body moves through the world, healing needs to be cultivated further. Healing the relationship with the embodied self goes beyond addressing unhelpful thoughts; it might involve noticing and recognising the way a person has been made to feel in the spaces and places they inhabit, the patterns they have adopted to feel safe, and the way these experiences have changed, altered or disturbed their body sense. It might involve reflection on how experiences are felt in sensations on the skin and in the nervous system; seeking to understand how the body reacts, contracts, tightens or tenses up in different situations, listening to them, feeling them and working through them, rather than cutting them off.

Embodied healing may start with resolving feelings within the inner space and sensation within the body but it also requires re-negotiating a relationship with the spaces we inhabit from the outside in. Viewed through a social justice and health equity lens, positive embodiment may be about making a challenge to the spaces of the world that the body is made to fit into. Chrisler and Johnston-Robeldo (2018) write that, for women, the experience of positive embodiment comes with social empowerment and freedom. Indeed, healing from AN can be conceptualised as 'taking up space'; having enough self-value and worth to allow one's body to inhabit the world, rather than apologetically trying to shrink oneself. In some ways, this is a metaphorical engagement with the idea of taking up space – a belief that one is good enough or worthy enough, a feeling that a person has the right to belong. In other ways, taking up space is experienced physically through (perhaps) being bigger, feeling fuller and heavier and allowing oneself to sink into the body and its feeling, rather than float around in the head, trying to control the body from above. Of course, this is arguably easier for some bodies than others, given the power of weight stigma (Tomiyama *et al.*, 2018) and moral discourse around eating habits (Lucas, Olander & Salmon 2023).

In time, and as recovery progresses, it becomes clearer that AN at its deep roots has little to do with an image or picture of a body, this is only a surface projection of a deeper embodied problem. AN is a defence against a world that is unfair and unequal and which suggests success and power can be gained through controlling and managing the body, through becoming smaller. Initially, in the experience of AN, the more the body conforms to this control, the more power is felt – for a while (Lucas, 2007; Ngo, 2019). Anorexia, so paradoxically, in its self-destruction, appears to provide a layer of protection; a layer of space between body, self and world – a way of backing out of the world and not having to confront difficult feelings that surface in that engagement. Healing from AN involves reforming a relationship with layers of space. It is about finding a renewed relationship with internal space through being able to adjust to the feelings in the body and sitting with any uncomfortable sensations that arise. It involves learning how to inhabit the body again – practicising how the body moves in space, feeling its lines and edges and resonance in the world around. Second, it is about tuning into broader, powerful discourse, recognising the narratives that seek to objectify the body, and resisting them. It involves thinking through the body, rather than controlling the body top-down. It is about feeling your way through, and deciding to take up space when the world loudly tells you not to do so.

References

American Psychiatric Association. (2013) *Diagnostic and statistical manual of mental disorders* (5th ed.). Washington, DC: American Psychiatric Association.

Beckmann, N., Baumann, P., Herpertz, S., Trojan, J., & Diers, M. (2021) 'How the unconscious mind controls body movements: Body schema distortion in anorexia nervosa,' *International Journal of Eating Disorders*, 54, 578– 586.

Beyer, C.D. (2016) 'Seeking the body electric: The role of embodied affective experience in the process of recovery from anorexia nervosa' (Thesis). Trinity Western University.

Burke, N.L., Schaefer, L.M., Hazzard, V.M., & Rodgers, R.F. (2020) 'Where identities converge: The importance of intersectionality in eating disorders research', *International Journal of Eating Disorders*, 53, 1605–1609.

Burnette, C.B., Luzier, J.L., Weisenmuller, C.M., & Boutté, R.L. (2022) 'A systematic review of sociodemographic reporting and representation in eating disorder psychotherapy treatment trials in the United States', *International Journal of Eating Disorders*, 55(4), 423–454.

Burychka, D., Miragall, M., & Baños, R.M. (2021) 'Towards a comprehensive understanding of body image: Integrating positive body image, embodiment and self-compassion', *Psychologica Belgica*, 61(1), 248–261.

Chrisler, J.C., & Johnston-Robledo, I. (2018) 'Woman's embodied self: An introduction', in J.C. Chrisler & I. Johnston-Robledo (Eds.) *Woman's embodied self: Feminist perspectives on identity and image*. Arlington: American Psychological Association (pp. 3–14).

Cook-Cottone, C.P. (2020) *Embodiment and the treatment of eating disorders: The body as a resource in recovery*. New York: W. W. Norton.

Cook, P.S., Dwyer, A. (2017) 'No longer raising eyebrows: The contexts and domestication of Botox as a mundane medical and cultural artefact', *Journal of Consumer Culture*, 17(3), 887–909. https://doi.org/10.1177/1469540516634414

Doyle, G. (2023) *How to Follow the Wisdom of Your Body with Dr. Hillary McBride* [podcast] We Can Do Hard Things with Glennon Doyle. Available at: http://wecandohardthingspodcast.com/ [Accessed 03.06.23]

Eli, K. (2018) 'Striving for liminality: Eating disorders and social suffering', *Transcultural Psychiatry*, 55(4), 475–494.

Engel, M.M., & Keizer, A. (2017) 'Body representation disturbances in visual perception and affordance perception persist in eating disorder patients after completing treatment', *Scientific Reports*, 7, 16184. Available at: https://doi.org/10.1038/s41598-017-16362-w

Frank, G.K. (2016) 'The perfect storm – A bio-psycho-social risk model for developing and maintaining eating disorders', *Frontiers in Behavioral Neuroscience*, 10(10), 44. Available at: https://doi.org/10.3389/fnbeh.2016.00044

Franko, D.L., Becker, A.E., Thomas, J.J., & Herzog, D.B. (2007) 'Cross-ethnic differences in eating disorder symptoms and related distress', *International Journal of Eating Disorders*, 40(2), 156–164.

Fuchs T. (2020) 'The disappearing body: Anorexia as a conflict of embodiment', *Eating and Weight Disorders*, 27(1), 109–117.

Fuchs, T., Koch, S.C. (2014) 'Embodied affectivity: On moving and being moved', *Frontiers in Psychology*, 6(5), 508. Available at: https://doi.org/10.3389/fpsyg.2014.00508

Gaete, M.I. & Fuchs, T. (2016) 'From body image to emotional bodily experience in eating disorders', *Journal of Phenomenological Psychology*, 47, 17–40.

Khalsa, S.S., Portnoff, L.C., McCurdy-McKinnon, D., & Feusner, J.D. (2017) 'What happens after treatment? A systematic review of relapse, remission, and recovery in anorexia nervosa', *Journal of Eating Disorders*, 14(5), 20. Available at: https://doi.org/10.1186/s40337-017-0145-3

Lucas, G. (2007) *Thin*. London: Penguin.

Lucas, G., Olander, E.K., & Salmon, D. (2023) 'Bodies of concern? A qualitative exploration of eating, moving and embodiment in young mothers', *Health*, 27(4), 607–624. doi:10.1177/13634593211060760

Lucas, G. (2022) 'Moving matters: Living in the body after anorexia', In I. Parker, M. Hopfenbeck, J. Downs, H. Lewis, N. Schnackenberg (Eds.) *The practical handbook of eating difficulties: A comprehensive guide from professional and personal perspectives.* Shoreham-by-Sea: Pavillion Press (pp. 331–338).

Malighetti, C., Sansoni, M., Gaudio, S., Matamala-Gomez, M., Di Lernia, D., Serino, S. and Riva, G., (2022) 'From virtual reality to regenerative virtual therapy: Some insights from a systematic review exploring inner body perception in Anorexia and Bulimia Nervosa', *Journal of Clinical Medicine*, 11(23), 7134. Available at: https://doi.org/10.3390/jcm11237134

McBride, H.L., Kwee, J.L. (2018) *Embodiment and eating disorders. Theory, research, prevention and treatment.* London: Routledge.

Morris, J. & Twaddle, S. (2007) 'Anorexia nervosa', *BMJ*, 334(7599), 894–898.

Ngo, N.T. (2019) 'What historical ideals of women's shapes teach us about women's self perception and body decisions today', *AMA Journal of Ethics*, 21(10), E879–E901. Available at: https://doi.org/10.1001/amajethics.2019.879

NICE. (2017) *Eating disorders: Recognition and treatment, NICE guideline [NG69].* Available at: www.nice.org.uk/guidance/ng69

Perey, I. & Cook-Cottone, C. (2020) 'Eating disorders, embodiment, and yoga: A conceptual overview', *Eating Disorders*, 28,4, 315–329.

Piran, N. (2016), 'Embodied possibilities and disruptions: The emergence of the Experience of Embodiment construct from qualitative studies with girls and women', *Body Image*, 18, 43–60.

Piran, N. (2019). 'The experience of embodiment construct: Reflecting the quality of embodied lives', In T.L. Tylka & N. Piran (Eds.) *Handbook of positive body image and embodiment.* Oxford: Oxford University Press, pp. 11–21.

Piran, N., & Neumark-Sztainer, D. (2020). 'Yoga and the experience of embodiment: A discussion of possible links', *Eating Disorders*, 28(4), 330–348

Piran, N., & Teall, T. (2012). The developmental theory of embodiment. In G. McVey, M.P. Levine, N. Piran, & H.B. Ferguson (Eds.) *Preventing eating-related and weight-related disorders: Collaborative research, advocacy, and policy change* Waterloo, ON: Wilfred Laurier Press (pp. 171–199).

Price, C.J., & Hooven, C. (2018) 'Interoceptive awareness skills for emotion regulation: Theory and approach of mindful Awareness in Body-Oriented Therapy (MABT)', *Frontiers in Psychology*, 28(9), 798. Available at: https://doi.org/10.3389/fpsyg.2018.00798

Riva, G., Malighetti, C., & Serino, S. (2021) 'Virtual reality in the treatment of eating disorders', *Clinical Psychology and Psychotherapy*, 28(3), 477–488.

Stanghellini, G., Castellini, G., Brogna, P., Faravelli, C., & Ricca, V. (2012) 'Identity and eating disorders (IDEA): A questionnaire evaluating identity and embodiment in eating disorder patients', *Psychopathology*, 45(3), 147–158.

Taylor, J.L. (2009) 'Proprioception' in L.R. Squire *Encyclopedia of Neuroscience*. Cambridge, MA: Academic Press, pp, 1143–1149.

Threadcraft, S. (2015) 'Embodiment' in L. Disch and M. Hawkesworth (Eds) *The Oxford Handbook of Feminist Theory*. Oxford: Oxford University Press. pp. 207–226.

Tomiyama, A., Carr, D., Granberg, E. *et al.* (2018) 'How and why weight stigma drives the obesity 'epidemic' and harms health', *BMC Medicine*, 16, 123.

Underwood, M. (2013) 'Body as choice or body as compulsion: An experiential perspective on body–self relations and the boundary between normal and pathological', *Health Sociology Review*, 22(4), 377–388.

Vandenbosch, L., Fardouly, J. Tiggemann, M. (2022) 'Social media and body image: Recent trends and future directions', *Current Opinion in Psychology*, 45, 101289. https://doi.org/10.1016/j.copsyc.2021.12.002.

van de Kamp, M.M., Scheffers, M., Hatzmann, J., Emck, C., Cuijpers, P., and Beek, P.J. (2019) 'Body- and movement-oriented interventions for posttraumatic stress disorder: A systematic review and meta-analysis', *Journal of Traumatic Stress*, 32(6), 967–976.

van Eeden, AE., van Hoeken, D., and Hoek, HW. (2021) 'Incidence, prevalence and mortality of anorexia nervosa and bulimia nervosa', *Current Opinion in Psychiatry*, 34(6), 515–524.

19 Dance movement psychotherapy in acute adult psychiatry

Space, time and affective atmospheres in the ward landscape

Mary Coaten

Dance movement psychotherapy and psychosis

For the past 15 years I have delivered Dance Movement Psychotherapy (DMP) to individuals and groups within acute adult in-patient National Health Service (NHS) mental health settings in the UK, specifically those experiencing psychosis. DMP is defined by the Association for Dance Movement Psychotherapy UK as a therapeutic practice that:

> recognises body movement as an implicit and expressive instrument of communication and expression. DMP is a relational process in which client(s) and therapist engage creatively using body movement and dance, as well as verbal and non-verbal reflection.
>
> (ADMPUK, 2023)

As a dance movement psychotherapist, my focus lies in the therapeutic and integrative potential of the moving body, particularly for individuals navigating severe distress and trauma. In experiences of psychosis, there is a disruption in the foundational sense of self, evident in the breakdown of implicit bodily functions and the disintegration of daily life routines (Fuchs and Schlimme, 2009, Fuchs, 2015). The lived experience of psychosis is also marked by "core existential themes" that "permeate self-world boundaries" and lead to a pervasive sense of detachment and overwhelming feeling of unreality (Fusar-Poli et al, 2022). Kean argues that this results in a "dissolved", "disorientated" and "disembodied" self through which a person is unable to "comfortably relate to the world or [their] inner self" (2009, p. 1035). Describing her own experiences, Kean (2009, p. 1034) writes:

> Despite the "usual" voices, alien thoughts and paranoia, what scared me the most was a sense that I had lost myself, a constant feeling that my 'self' no longer belonged to me. [...] Everything I experience is through a dense fog, created by my own mind, yet it also resides outside my mind. I feel that my real self has left me, seeping through the fog toward a separate reality, which engulfs and dissolves this self. This has nothing to do with the suspicious thoughts or voices; it is purely a distorted state of being. The clinical symptoms come and go, but this nothingness of the self is permanently there.

In my research (Coaten, 2020; 2021; 2022), I explore the therapeutic and integrative capacities of DMP for navigating the intricate and often complex life-worlds of psychosis.

DOI: 10.4324/9781003345725-21

By engaging with improvised movement and creative expression, DMP seeks to address profound existential concerns, like those described above, by fostering a process of self-discovery and integration that goes beyond traditional clinical symptom management. Building upon this foundation, I outline four mechanisms of embodied and existential disruption that manifest during periods of psychosis and how DMP can be implemented therapeutically to address these issues through creative and improvisational movements. These are summarised as follows:

1) **Altered experience of time:** DMP engages individuals in movement and dance, focusing on pacing, timing and spatial awareness in the presence of others to foster a sense of rhythmic connection.
2) **Interpersonal and intersubjective difficulties:** Through movement and dance, DMP helps to develop social connection and cohesion utilising rhythm and interactional synchrony ('attunement') to address interpersonal and intersubjective challenges.
3) **Disruption of predictive mechanisms:** DMP targets balance, proprioception and motor co-ordination to improve an individual's sense of space and time.
4) **Prevalence of delusions and hallucinations:** DMP embraces symbolic and metaphorical expressions of delusions and hallucinations, incorporating them into dance and artistic expression.

DMP engages with these challenges both verbally and non-verbally, employing embodied movement alongside artistic and creative expression to foster empathetic and therapeutic relationships with one's self and others. The practice is designed to tap into unconscious material through imitation, imagination, symbolism and metaphor. An integral aspect of the approach is the emphasis on reflection, creativity and movement narratives.

In this chapter, I discuss my role as a dance movement psychotherapist within the distinctive environment of acute adult in-patient mental health settings. I discuss the components of this therapeutic practice, encompassing improvisation, movement, dance and symbolic representation. These elements are analysed in connection with geographical and psychotherapeutic literatures exploring dynamics of moving bodies, affective atmospheres and emotions. Throughout, I offer a reflection on the DMP session, contemplating these elements in relation to Jung's (2002) concept of "Temenos". This examination provides insights into the therapeutic capacities of DMP, offering a nuanced understanding of how the practice contributes to the over well-being and the 'transformative' experiences of individuals in mental health settings.

The "temenos"

In this chapter, I consider the dynamic space and practice of DMP through the Jungian concept of "temenos", defined as a sacred precinct or 'container' in which psychological integration and transformation of the body and psyche can occur (Noack, 2003). Jung (1975) recognised that the body, through its physiological responses, gestures, postures and movements, serves as a vehicle for unconscious expression and self-discovery, most notably through processes of 'active imagination'.[1] A temenos can be considered an "alchemical space" (Di Rezze, 2020) in which symbolic language and "archetypal" imagery, crucial for understanding the personal and collective unconscious can be tapped into and worked through. During a session, individuals will express themselves through symbolic movement using props and artistic expression. Participants often express trauma, distress and dissociative states through 'mytho-poetic' images including religious references to god, heaven and hell, as well as aliens, outer space, ghosts, acid house 'smileys' and pregnancy (Coaten, 2022). These images constitute part of what Jung calls the "archetypal experience",[2] a subjective and transformative experience that includes both images (representations) and affects (Chodorow, 1991). A temenos provides a 'contained' space in which to draw out and explore unconscious material through creative and imaginative processes.

While considered a 'container', it is important to note that within this therapeutic space, "to contain the affect is not to suppress or deny it [nor] to get rid of it through a cathartic purge [but] to feel deeply what is in us, bear witness to the terrible discomfort, and find a way to express it" (Chodorow, 1991, p. 37). Temenos comes to represent what Bondi argues lies "[a]t the heart of psychotherapy", that is, "the idea of holding open a space for processes of symbolisation into which people come to make new 'sense' of themselves, their lives and their interpersonal relationships" (2005, p.444). This holds particular relevance as I, in the role of therapist, strive to establish a secure and supportive environment for individuals to engage in movement expression while fostering a space "within which unconscious fantasies and conscious dilemmas can be safely dealt with" (Chodorow, 1991, p. 7). Therefore, temenos intends to capture the aesthetics of embodied and therapeutic practice that emerge within the DMP session, which subsequently works to "spatialise the self, the other and the endless possible worlds that unfold in this open-ended relational process" (Nieuwenhuis and Knoll, 2021, p. 2).

The practice of DMP

DMP operates on the fundamental premise of mind-body interconnections with changes in one sphere having a concomitant effect on the other (Acolin, 2016). It also posits that (un)conscious feelings and emotions are externalised and find expression through movement and dance (Hayes, 2013). In my therapeutic practice I must not only remain attentive to and trust my own "embodied knowing" but work towards a "co-creative knowing" with clients (Allegranti, 2011). I observe shifts in physical sensations and tensions in my body as well as changes in breathing, speed, postures and gestures articulated by those participating in the session. I am attuned to the movements and atmospheres expressed during the session, actively seeking what Atmodiwirjo (2014) refers to as "affordances" – the opportunities and potentials for movement, expression, and interaction that unfold within the therapeutic space.

This approach enables me to embrace moments for creative expression through the use of improvisation, metaphors, and movement. Rather than seeking 'to know', I cultivate a mindset of curiosity and openness during the session and attune myself to the often creative, sometimes chaotic, nature of the session. This may involve navigating through moments of confusion or fear and, at times, simply being present without predetermined expectations. I pay close attention to subtle, fragments of movements – a twist here, a lift of the shoulders there, a jump, an intentional move forwards or a deliberate retreat backwards. I promote clients' self-inquiry, fostering heightened self-reflection, connection, and understanding, which have been identified as key factors in therapeutic change (Meekums, 2002). The inclusion of artistic elements, like music, props, and visual arts enhances creative expression These foundational elements of the practice are now discussed.

Dance improvisation

Dance improvisation is a foundational aspect of the practice, emerging from an individual's inner impulses, feelings and thoughts. It serves as a powerful and generative tool for self-expression, exploration and therapeutic communication, allowing for unconscious or pre-reflective content to be perceived or find expression through movement (McCormack, 2008). Improvisation is an ongoing flow emerging from the "ever-changing kinetic world of possibilities", one which requires no separation between the acts of thinking and doing (Sheets-Johnstone, 1999, p. 30). In dance improvisation, the therapist may opt to explore specific themes, emotions or associations that arise within the client's movement expressions. This process facilitates the transition of unconscious elements into conscious awareness within a secure and contained therapeutic environment. The content that emerges is then shaped into tangible form through words, images or movement metaphors, which may unveil aspects previously unknown to the individual. Images and movements are frequently inspired by the music, lyrics and the ongoing movements happening around them.

Movement metaphors

Movement metaphors are also central to the praxis (Mcckums 2002). Whether embodied in a movement, phrase, motif or posture, these metaphors serve as unique forms of non-verbal communication between the client and therapist. Movements such as the level and direction of movement, flowing or restrained movement, gestures and shapes, patterns and mirroring, and synchrony can represent or convey deeper psychological and emotional states. Movement and the body are embedded in many metaphorical expressions in the English language, for example: "going out on a limb", "elbow room", "jumping out of one's skin", or "falling to pieces". Props, including scarves, cloth, stretchy elastic and various objects such as garden canes, are also incorporated into movement and have a "catalytic" function (McCormack 2003, p.498), sparking imaginative, symbolic and affective interactions and enhancing the relational aspects of the therapeutic process. In this context, movement metaphors also allow individuals to embody and externalise their inner experiences, transforming abstract or complex emotional experiences into more tangible and accessible forms for exploration. Metaphors may be personal carrying meaning from personal histories and experience or be 'archetypal' deeply embedded in collective and cultural consciousness (Samaritter, 2009).

Moving together

Kean (2009, p. 1035) notes that when "the very elementary basis of self-experience is disrupted, communicating to, and participating with, others will automatically seem secondary, even insignificant". Thus, participation in a group setting promotes social cohesion and collective group responses to the material being explored. Dancing together creates an intersubjective and socially oriented space where clients engage in their own expressive movements alongside those of who they are dancing with. I aim to develop a therapeutic relationship through "the empathic reflection of expression movement qualities", also called 'mirroring', where I imitate the movements and expressions of clients, while group interaction and cohesion is supported "through rhythmic group synchrony" (Meekums et al. 2015, p. 6). Here, props serve as 'bridges' for initiating movement, promoting connection and setting boundaries with and between clients. For instance, a simple act like two people holding opposite ends of a long piece of cloth, creates a connection albeit at a distance. This also aids in building rapport and trust between myself and the client while creating a sense of safety and autonomy for them.

A dance movement therapy session

Entering the ward

The creative and vibrant work done in therapeutic sessions stands in stark contrast to the clinical, often bleak, atmosphere of the ward. When I enter the ward, I pass through a 'double door airlock system', a security measure that requires one door to be completely closed before the second door can be opened. Within this secure and enclosed zone, cut off from the rest of the ward and the outside world, there is an immediate sense of being somewhere very different, characterised by sense of emptiness that is heightened by the temporary suspension in this restricted vacuum. Inside the wards, uniformed staff move swiftly through the corridors, attending to daily tasks such as issuing medications. As I walk along the corridor to the rooms where I hold my sessions, I see people sitting on the window-seats huddled together and some individuals sitting alone. Adjacent to the main corridor are individual pods where the bedrooms are located, each featuring seating areas with soft furnishings. In these spaces, several individuals sit alone, gazing out of the windows. Overall, the ward is not set up for interaction which, as one person describes, contributes to the "mind-numbing boredom of the ward" (Coaten, 2020, p. 120). This lack of life and vitality echoes Högström and Philo's concerns about what is offered and, crucially, lost in the design of 'modern' Western mental healthcare spaces, where spaces are often "too clinical, too sterile, even too empty, perhaps detrimental to mental and physical health" (2023, p.8). DMP has the capacity to restore what they describe as the " 'vital' –lively, affectively-charged, embodied, emplaced – dimensions of health and healthcare" (ibid. 2023, p. 2).[3]

The in-patient unit consists of two wards, one designated for men and the other for women, both with a capacity of 22 beds. Patients within the age range of 18-65 are admitted for various reasons, including drug-induced psychosis, suicide attempts, and 'depressive' episodes, 'manic' episodes and 'psychotic' episodes. Admissions can be voluntarily or on section[4] under the Mental Health Act (MHA, 2007). The length of stay on the ward varies, ranging from a short duration to several months, contingent on factors such as the duration of symptoms and considerations related to social and housing issues.

DMP sessions take place at the same time and place each week, which helps provide a sense of regularity and stability in an already fluctuating environment. Spanning from one hour to an hour and a half, the sessions adopt an open format, allowing clients to join or leave at their discretion. This flexibility means attendance can fluctuate with anywhere between one and ten participants in attendance. Some individuals are regulars, others may drop in sporadically or attend only once. They may stay for part of or attend the whole session. The crucial aspect is that I regularly maintain the space, even in sessions with minimal or no participants. Regularity is a key aspect of temenos.

Separate sessions are run for men and women. The men's session takes place in the dining room of the men's ward. It is a bright room with tables and a sink with no taps – a safety precaution in case someone pulls them off the wall and uses them in a threatening way. Information notices hang on the wall behind plastic screens. The windows look out onto the central courtyard and carpark. In the women's ward the session takes place in the activity room, which is immediately adjacent to the nursing office. The windows are constructed with slits that only open enough for you to slide your hand through, akin to a fortified castle. The view from the men's room is of a beautiful silver birch tree in the car park area and a view to the hills around the town. The view from the women's ward is onto the central enclosed internal garden where service users sit and chat.

I rush to set up the session, pushing tables back to clear a space on the floor. I lay out props and art materials and turn on the music to inject a more vibrant and life-affirming energy to the bleak atmosphere of this space. I also set up a single camera in a fixed position, used in my research to capture group participation and movement.[5] In order to channel a sense of openness to others, I take off my badge and shoes and leave the door open throughout the session. The music spills into the corridor, signalling the start of the session and serves as an invitation to encourage clients to come in.

Some clients burst energetically into the room while others linger tentatively at the threshold, as if waiting for the right moment to cross. I dim the lights, to signal a moment of inner reflection as the session commences. During the session, the moving bodies respond dynamically to the interplay of music, lyrics, props and lighting, collectively forming an 'other' space distinct from the surrounding ward.

Altered sense of time and space

During acute episodes of severe distress, individuals experience disruptions in their perception and experience of both time and space. Temporal alterations encompass distortions in the typical flow and progression of time. Such distortions can manifest as a feeling that time is either 'accelerating', stretched out or prolonged, or 'decelerating', where events unfold at a slower pace (Stanghellini et. al., 2016). These altered time experiences are closely intertwined with disturbances in a person's "core sense of self", that is, the foundational framework shaping how individuals perceive and navigate the world and maintain a sense of cohesion and continuity within it (Fusar-Poli et al., 2022). This not only impacts how individuals relate to themselves but also results in an "intersubjective desynchronisation" affecting their interactions with others and the world around them (Vogels et al., 2019). In this context, the sense of containment created by the temenos and the atmosphere cultivated within the DMP session plays a role in addressing this lack of, "temporal continuity underlying conscious awareness" (ibid. p 1). Utilising movement and body-focused interventions within the temenos can enhance bodily awareness, which help foster a more grounded sense of self and time.

This heightened self-awareness can lead to movement that appears slowed down akin to feeling as if events around you are unfolding in slow motion, impacting interactions and communication with others. When approaching someone who is experiencing the world in this way, this understandably impacts our interaction which is mediated through our moving bodies. Clients might exhibit an increase in acceleration, engaging in fast forward or rushing movements breaking with the 'rhythmic group synchrony' and introducing a sense of imbalance to the interaction. In response, DMP addresses these issues through a combination of techniques including pacing, timing, spatial awareness and interactional synchrony. The rhythmic elements of the music, coupled with the therapist's movement, collectively contribute to mitigating experiences of de-animation and de-temporalisation.

Martin,[6] a disc jockey who likes 1980s and 1990s music, enters the room. He loves to dance and move across the room in undulating motions, his movements are predominantly ascending and descending, in simple terms moving up and down in the vertical plane. Martin appears restless, struggling to keep his legs still and expresses a desire to dance with me. As we dance he comments that my dancing is "good … especially for your age" – (he is in his mid-40s and I am 55.)

I observe as he jumps up and dances very energetically and I match his movements, creating a movement dialogue that establishes a "kinaesthetic intersubjectivity" (Payne and Samaritter, 2013) – an awareness of and shared connection through gesture, movement or theme. This interpersonal relatedness is particularly crucial for those who may otherwise feel isolated from themselves and others.

Following his high energy dance, Martin sits quietly and draws a 'smiley acid house image', emphasising its importance as a symbol of his disc jockey status. While the "smiley face" image has its cultural origins in the 1960s, its significance has changed "like a constantly mutating virus: from early 70s fad to late-80s acid house culture from millennial txt [sic] option to serial killer signature to ubiquitous emoticon." (Savage, 2009, n.p.). The smiley face holds personal significance for Martin, reflecting his passions, interests and perhaps memories associated with electronic dance music and sub-cultures.

Then, Daniel enters the room, exuding life and energy. Lupton (2017) notes that "affective atmospheres can be understood as an assemblage of affects […] that is constantly changing as new actors enter and leave spaces". Daniel's entrance brings something quite different into the atmosphere of the group, notably a sense of fun and mischief. He playfully enhances Martin's smiley face with a spaceship and makes it more 'psychedelic', sparking discussions about aliens, outer space and the ability to become younger by traversing space faster than the speed of light. This metaphorical expression hints at the potential to transcend, swiftly moving away or beyond certain aspects of their experience.

The sense of fun and play enriched by active imagination flourishes as Daniel and Martin collaborate on the images and dance. I find this scene very funny and cannot help but burst into laughter. Daniel grabs the image from Martin, bringing it towards the camera set up in the room. Daniel creates a light-hearted moment by dancing around with the image and playfully zooming in and out from the camera. The entire group joins in, incorporating the 'smiley' image into their collective dance. Placing it over their faces, they each move in close to and then pull away from the camera, accompanied by laughter, running and jumping. They ask me to dance with it and then they go behind the camera to have a look. It makes me feel as if they want me to 'try on' what they are feeling. I notice that this makes me feel like a part of the group and they get a chance to look at me and the group in action, literally through a 'different lens', demonstrating the link between images, movement and group sociality. Notably, this 'smiley' face symbol became central to the group, expressing their emotions symbolically through chaos and anti-establishment. It serves as a non-verbal expression of understanding and solidarity between the group members. The 'smiley' image becomes a shared expression, providing a means of communication when verbal expression is challenging. Individual needs, feelings and desires find expression through the symbol, initiating a collective response from the group.

Symbols, metaphors and the imaginal landscape

Symbolism in DMP serves as a channel through which an individual can revisit, act out and re-experience personal challenges on a symbolic level. There is a sense of social cohesion and solidarity created through the use of rhythm and symbol, which in DMP we understand as a "synchronistic" organising principle "that has the power to transform" (Lewis, 1993 cited in Sandel et al.1993, p. 166). As feelings are expressed in a shared rhythm, a heightened sense of confidence, strength and security emerges. The change seems to occur when the person is ready to allow him or herself to experience the action in their body. Chaiklin and Schmais (1986, p.78) emphasise the use of "symbolic body action to communicate emotions and ideas" as well as giving expression to the complexity and depth of feelings that cannot be put into words. In other words, expressing that which can only be communicated, in that moment, through symbolic body action.

Symbols in general can have personal and collective significance for those in the session. Here, the 'smiley' face takes on multiple meanings as both a 'feel-good' symbol from the 1960s and a somewhat anarchic and anti-establishment one from the 1980s. Created by Martin as a personal symbol through which he expressed joy, positivity and a connection to the music as well as his personal connection to the social phenomenon of the sub-culture movement, it evolved into a potent collective symbol that the group wanted me to 'try on'. The link between the movement and the symbolic and metaphoric is evident in the group adoption of Martin's symbol and their shared and collective movements around it. Ultimately, the 'smiley' becomes the group emblem for the session illustrating a collective response through a "thematic [and] imaginal improvisation" (Lewis, 1993 cited in Sandel et al., 1993 p. 167).

Post-session landscape

As we near the end of the session, the tempo of the music gradually slows, gently guiding the group towards a sense of closure. During this concluding phase, I engage in reflective dialogue with those who remain, exploring any topic brought to mind, such as their reflections on the images, the music or their movement throughout the session. I often reflect back to the group what I have noticed, for example, how the atmosphere changed throughout the session. Others will reflect on the images, metaphors or symbols and others may cry as they discuss what brought them to the session. Some laugh and talk about family, friends or the ward atmosphere.

The atmosphere shifts from one of high and expressive energy to one of quiet and meditative stillness, signalled also by the change in sounds and qualities of the movement. There is a sense of being more grounded and less chaotic. I notice these changes in myself and in others. There is a sense of coming into the body and a connectedness with each other, plus a respect for the depth and intensity of what has taken place, all of which feel like participants are making new 'sense' of themselves. I signal the end of this reflective period and say that I will come again next week at the same time. Participants thank me and begin to leave the room. As I put my shoes on and start to pack up, gathering the art materials, props and the music, some linger while others leave quickly.

When I finish, I carry all my things in a bag and go out into the curved corridor of the ward. Sometimes people sit together on the windowsill afterwards and seem to be different, more alive with a sense of togetherness. Occasionally the corridor is deserted as if they have hurried back into their rooms. In these moments, the ward landscape still seems bleak and the contrast between it and the sessional space even more stark. Walking towards the exit, I often sing, carrying the sessions vibrant and therapeutic atmosphere through the ward.

Stepping back out into the ward corridor, I begin the long walk towards the exit door. As I pass, those huddled on the windowsill thank me for coming, I say "see you next week", but that is not what someone wants to hear, as no one wants to be on the ward next week, so I quickly change it to, "I'll be here next week". Sometimes someone is hovering at the door hoping to leave and I have to wait until they have moved away from the door before I can exit, or others are waiting to go out to the garden or out of the hospital to smoke. I pass through into the airlock between the security doors again and wait to leave the ward. Once again, it feels empty, lacking the vibrancy and creativity of the DMP atmosphere created within the ward.

Conclusion

The practice of DMP places strong emphasis on embodiment, recognising the body as a primary vehicle for self-expression and integration by drawing attention to the role of bodily sensations, expressions and movements in the therapeutic process. The temenos serves as an intentional space or container that holds and honours the embodied experiences of individuals engaging in movement and expression. It provides a secure environment for the holistic integration of body and mind, which encourages individuals to fully embody their experiences and facilitate a deeper connection with (un)conscious memories, emotions and others in the therapeutic space. In this chapter I have captured the often lively nature of the DMP session, the embodied experiences of time and space and the affective atmospheres that emerge within and through the therapeutic space and practice. This is all set against, often in stark contrast to, the ostensibly mundane spaces of acute adult in-patient mental health care settings.

I have also described this change from dining-room or activity room to temenos with reference to specific elements, that is, the creation of a 'container' which takes place consistently at the same time, same day, with myself attending and being creatively alert to these opportunities to connect with whoever enters the space. I use music with rhythms and lyrics which individuals can connect with, evoking strong feelings both individually and collectively. I also use scarves and cloth as props which can take on a symbolic function. I provide art materials for image-making, and crucially I leave the door open both physically and metaphorically, to create an entrance, a 'way-in' for those that care to cross that threshold. This space and the interplay of these elements offer the opportunity for the individual to move from a sense of fragmentation towards integration and social cohesiveness.

Clearly, the inter-disciplinarity between geographical research into the spaces of moving bodies and DMP, offer insights that can help recovery in mental health by transforming spaces. Geographers are interested in space in terms of affective atmospheres, affordances and the moving body, as is dance movement psychotherapy. I have endeavoured to highlight this inter-disciplinarity and what and how it can add to aiding recovery in mental health in-patient settings. Both disciplines offer the potential for further combined research in this field.

Notes

1 Active imagination in Jung's analytic method is "a method of assimilating unconscious content (dreams, fantasies, etc.) through some form of self-expression [...] to give voice to sides of the personality that are normally not heard, thereby establishing a line of communication between consciousness and the unconscious" (Sharp, 1991, n.p.).
2 Archetypes serve as basic building blocks of the collective unconscious and play a crucial role on shaping individual and collective psyches. They often manifest as "archetypal images" in various

forms, motifs and symbols, influencing how individuals perceive themselves and the world around them. Sharp (1991, n.p.) notes that they are the "basic content of religions, mythologies, legends and fairy tales." Jung (1959) argued that exploring and understanding archetypes can lead to greater self-awareness and comprehension of the human psyche. Analysing dreams, myths and personal symbols through the lens of archetypes can help individuals recognise patterns, overcome challenges and integrate different aspects of their personalities.

3 While not the specific focus of this chapter, there is a wealth of geographical literature exploring the "spatial stories" of modern mental healthcare environments often with comparison and contrast to older asylum landscapes examining the positive and negatives memories and feelings of nostalgia provoked by such spaces and also the 'usability' and relational aspects of common and shared spaces on wards (Woods et al. 2015; Högström and Philo, 2023).

4 Sectioning is a serious legal intervention and refers to the process of being involuntarily admitted to a psychiatric hospital for assessment and treatment. This is typically done when there is a concern for the person's safety and wellbeing and/or they are unable or unwilling to seek help voluntarily.

5 The camera was set up to capture the movement patterns using the Kestenberg Movement Profile – a system for observing and analysing movement and non-verbal behaviours (Loman and Merriman, 1996). The footage was analysed by myself at the end of the fieldwork period. Participants did not voice any concerns about the camera and informed consent was received from them to record the sessions for research purposes. It was explained in detail in the participant information leaflet and consent obtained to record participants. However, I'm not sure if there were others who would like to have taken part but did not because of the camera. The camera was only explicitly referred to when it was used by some of the participants in a playful way. I had thought the presence of the camera could be problematic around issues of surveillance but in fact my sense is that it acted as a witness and enhanced feelings of 'being seen' in a positive and inclusive way.

6 All participants have been assigned pseudonyms.

References

Acolin, J. (2016) The Mind–Body Connection in Dance/Movement Therapy: Theory and Empirical Support, *American Journal of Dance Therapy*, Vol. 38, pp. 311–333.

Allegranti, B. (2011) Ethics and Body Politics: Interdisciplinary Possibilities for Embodied Psychotherapeutic Practice and Research, *British Journal of Guidance & Counselling*, Vol. 39(5), pp. 487–500.

Association of Dance Movement Psychotherapy UK. (2023) Available at: https://admp.org.uk/what-is-dance-movement-psychotherapy/ Accessed: 29/09/2023

Atmodiwirjo, P. (2014) Space Affordances, Adaptive Responses and Sensory Integration by Autistic Children, *International Journal of Design*, Vol. 8(3), pp. 35–47.

Bondi, L. (2005) Making Connections and Thinking through emotions: Between Geography and Psychotherapy, *Transactions of the Institute of British Geographers, Wiley on behalf of the Royal Geographical Society, New Series*, Vol. 30(4), pp. 433–448.

Chaiklin, S. and Schmais, C. (1986) The Chace Approach to Dance Movement Therapy, in Bernstein, P. ed. *Eight Theoretical Approaches in Dance-Movement Therapy*, Kendall/Hunt, Dubuque, USA.

Chodorow, J. (1991) *Dance therapy and depth psychology: The moving imagination*, Routledge, London, New York.

Coaten, M. (2020) Dance Movement Psychotherapy (DMP) in acute adult psychiatry: A mixed methods study, Unpublished PhD Thesis, Durham University, UK.

Coaten, M. (2021) Dance Movement Psychotherapy and Voice Hearing: Looking Outward and Inward, in Parker, P. Schnackenberg, J., and Hopfenbeck, M. (eds.) *The Practical Handbook of Hearing Voices*, PCCS Books, Monmouth UK.

Coaten, M (2022) Voice-Hearing and Lived Space, in Woods, A., Alderson-Day, B., and Fernyhough, C. (eds.) *Voices in Psychosis: Interdisciplinary Perspectives*, pp. 161–168, Oxford, Oxford Unversity Press:

Di Rezze, G. (2020) Creating Temenos in the Classroom: Relational Encounter and the Subtle Alchemy of Transformation, *Canadian Journal for the Study of Adult Education*, Vol. 32(2), pp. 37–48.

Fuchs, T. (2015) The Intersubjectivity of Delusions, *World Psychiatry*, Vol. 14(2), p. 178.

Fuchs, T. and J. Schlimme. (2009) Embodiment and Psychopathology: A Phenomenological Perspective, *Current Opinion Psychiatry*, Vol. 22(6), pp. 570–575.

Fusar-Poli, P., Estradé, A., and Stanghellini, G., et al. (2022) The Lived Experience of Psychosis: A Bottom-Up Review Co-Written by Experts by Experiences and Academics, *World Psychiatry*, Vol. 21(2), pp. 168–188. doi: 10.1002/wps.20959

Hayes, J. (2013) *Soul and Spirit in Dance Movement Psychotherapy: A Transpersonal Approach*, Jessica Kingsley Publishers, London and Philadelphia.

Högström, E. and Philo, C. (2023) Let There Be Light' or Life in the Dark? Vital Geographies of Mental Healthcare, *Social Science Medicine*, Vol. 33, pp. 1–10. DOI: 10.1016/j.socscimed.2023.116137

Jung, C. (1959) Archetypes of the Collective Unconscious, In *The Archetypes and the Collective Unconscious* (Vol. 9). Part 1. Translated by R.F.C Hull. Routledge & Kegan Paul, London.

Jung, C. (1975/1916) The Transcendent Function, In *Collected Works*, Vol. 8, pp. 67–91. Princeton: Princeton University Press,.

Jung, C. (2002/1974) Dreams, Hull, R. (trans.), Routledge Classics, London and New York.

Kean, C. (2009) Silencing the Self: Schizophrenia as a Self-disturbance, *Schizophr Bulletin*, Vol. 35(6), pp. 1034–1036.

Loman, S. and Merman, H. (1996) The KMP: A tool for dance/movement therapy, *American Journal of Dance Therapy*, Vol. 18, pp. 29–52. https://doi.org/10.1007/BF02360220

Lupton, D. (2017). How does health feel? Towards research on the affective atmospheres of digital health. *Digital Health*, Vol. 3. doi:10.1177/2055207617701276

McCormack, D. (2003) An Event of Geographical Ethics in Spaces of Affect, *Transactions of the Institute of British Geographers*, Vol 28(4), pp. 488–507. https://doi.org/10.1111/j.0020-2754.2003.00106.x

McCormack, D. (2008) Geographies for Moving Bodies: Thinking, Dancing, Spaces, *Geography Compass*, Vol. 2(6), pp. 1822–1835.

Meekums, B. (2002) *Dance Movement Psychotherapy, A Creative Psychotherapeutic Approach*, Sage, London.

Meekums, B., Karkou, V., and Nelson, E. A. (2015) Dance Movement Therapy for Depression. *The Cochrane Database of Systematic Reviews*, Vol. 2, pp. 1–50. https://doi.org/10.1002/14651858.CD009895.pub2

Mental Health Act (MHA) 1983. Amended by the Mental Health Act 2007 [online] Revised (2007) Available at: www.legislation.gov.uk/ukpga/1983/20/contents Accessed: 29/03/2023

Nieuwenhuis, M. and Knoll, E. (2021) Towards a geography of voice-hearing, Emotion, *Space and Society*, Vol. 40. https://doi.org/10.1016/j.emospa.2021.100812

Noack, A. (2003) On a Jungian Approach to Dance Movement Therapy, in Payne, H. (ed.), *Dance Movement Therapy: Theory and Practice*, pp. 182–201, Routledge, London.

Payne, H. and Samaritter, R. (2013) Kinaesthetic Intersubjectivity: A Dance Informed Contribution to Self-Other Relatedness and Shared Experience in Nonverbal Psychotherapy with an Example from Autism, *Arts in Psychotherapy*, Vol. 40(1), pp. 143–150.

Samaritter, R. (2009) The use of metaphors in dance movement therapy, *Body, Movement and Dance in Psychotherapy*, Vol. 4(1), pp. 33–43.

Sandel, S., Chaiklin, S., and S. Lohn, (1993) *Foundations of Dance/Movement Therapy: The Life and Work of Marian Chace, American Dance Therapy Association*. The Marian Chace Memorial Fund, Columbia, Maryland.

Savage, J. (2009) A design for life – Smiley face design history. The Guardian [Online] www.theg
uardian.com/artanddesign/2009/feb/21/smiley-face-design-history The Primacy of Movement.

Sharp, S. (1991) *Jung Lexicon: A Primer of Terms and Concepts.* Inner City Books. Available
at: https://jungpage.org/learn/jung-lexicon#active Accessed: 01/02/2024

Sheets-Johnstone, M. (1999) *The Primacy of Movement,* John Benjamins Publishing
Company, USA.

Stanghellini, G., *et al.* (2016) The Psychopathology of Lived Time: Abnormal Timing Experience
in Persons with Achizophrenia, *Bulletin,* Vol. 42 (1), pp. 45–55.

Wood, V.J., Gesler, W., Curtis, S.E., Spencer, I.H., Close, H.J., Mason, J., and Reilly, J.G.
(2015) 'Therapeutic Landscapes' and the Importance of Nostalgia, Solastalgia, Salvage and
Abandonment for Psychiatric Hospital Design, *Health and Place,* Vol. 33, pp. 83–89.

Vogel, D. et al. (2019) Disturbed Time Experience During and After Psychosis, *Schizophrenia
Research: Cognition, Science Direct,* Vol. 17, 10036. https://doi.org/10.1016/j.scog.2019.10036

20 Embodiment and space in understandings of suicide and self-harm

Amy Chandler, Sarah Huque, Rebecca Helman, Joe Anderson, and Emily Yue

Introduction

> … literature on suicide severs self-destruction from time, space, and place.
>
> (Balayannis and Cook, 2016, p. 530)

As Balayannis and Cook (2015) have argued, while suicide and self-harm are inherently embodied and emplaced, these elements are rarely visible in much published suicide research. Instead, research tends to focus on these practices in isolation from the material and environmental contexts in which they occur, and in which they are given meaning. A key exception to this, where 'space' and 'place' do become present, is via a focus on 'locations of concern' or 'hotspots' (Linskens et al., 2022; Pirkis et al., 2015). Though there is debate about the terminology (Owens, 2016), these are public places, understood locally (sometimes nationally) as a site of suicide, attracting concern and action in an attempt to reduce the possibility of suicide in these places. Many suicide prevention strategies include identification and intervention into particular 'hotspots' (Oaten, Jordan, Chandler, & Marzetti, 2022; Platt & Niederkrotenthaler, 2020).

Conversely, another arena where 'space' and 'place' are present in suicide prevention – though not often foregrounded in policies themselves – is the contrasting 'place of safety'. In the UK, transporting those at risk of suicide to a 'place of safety' is often a key feature of suicide prevention practices, and closely tied to the use of mental health legislation, particularly Section 136 of the 1983 Mental Health Act. However, such 'places of safety' can be sites of contestation. Local areas often lack appropriate places for people in distress, especially when the place of distress is at 'home'. This results in the inappropriate use of police cells, psychiatric hospitalisation, or busy Accident and Emergency departments (Bendelow, Warrington, Jones, & Markham, 2019).

Self-harm and suicide are both inherently bodily and embodied practices. They are shaped by the intimate and broader contexts in which they occur, or are imagined in, interacting with and informed by space and place. Despite this, another absence can be noted in much research on self-harm and suicide. As well as neglecting place and space, the bodies of those who harm or kill themselves are also often missing from scholarly analysis (Jaworski, 2014). In contrast, our own work approaches self-harm and suicide as embodied social practices (Chandler, 2016, 2019), and seeks – like Jaworski – to avoid 'forgetting' that these are practices that intimately involve bodies, and that bodies are always located: socially, culturally and materially. This builds also on work by Stevenson, which similarly sought to make "suicidal bodies matter" (2016, p. 165).

DOI: 10.4324/9781003345725-22

In this chapter, we introduce and develop the concept of 'suicidescapes' to illustrate how working with the notion of embodied space can help to productively trouble some of the taken for granted practices of suicide prevention. In particular, we use the concept to pay attention to how both 'locations of concern' and 'places of safety' are produced in this work. To do so, we draw from an ongoing ethnographic and interview-based interdisciplinary study of suicide in Scotland. Our work identifies challenges and limitations of addressing 'locations of concern' within attempts to prevent suicide. Alongside this, our research points to the role of less 'spectacular' sites where suicide, and suicidality, are shaped. Indeed, a key concern with a focus on public suicides is that the vast majority of deaths by suicide occur within private homes. Considering 'home' as a rather different 'location of concern' provides further ways in which an engagement with embodied space may help us to think differently about suicide, and suicide prevention.

Our ongoing research engages with suicide using multiple methods, including embedded ethnographic research with a number of communities, spending time with people affected by suicide and/or engaged in suicide prevention work. Alongside this, we are holding qualitative interviews with people who have attempted or been bereaved by suicide, and those who work with people affected by suicide. The locations in which we are working are in Scotland, UK, and reflect a range of settings – urban and rural, socioeconomically privileged, and disadvantaged. Aside from the country in which we are working, all other names of places and people are pseudonymised. Our fieldwork is focused on three broad geographical areas of Scotland, with Authors JA, RH and SH each working intensively with communities and organisations within these areas.

Locations of concern and places of safety as suicidescapes

Space and place are rarely explicitly highlighted in studies of suicide, but they are certainly present through some of the core practices advocated by suicide prevention researchers. Locations of concern refer to places in a locality that are understood to be "specific, accessible and usually public sites" (Cox et al., 2013 p. 1) and have a 'reputation' for being a place where suicides often occur. Designing interventions that target such places is advocated in many suicide prevention strategies and recommendations (Owens, Lloyd-Tomlins, Emmens, & Aitken, 2009). Such interventions might include physical measures, such as barriers on bridges or high buildings; the installation of help-phones, with posters detailing numbers of crisis lines; or facilitating regular surveillance – either via CCTV cameras, or urban design approaches that encourage more regular footfall (Beautrais, 2007; Platt & Niederkrotenthaler, 2020). Coming under the broader category of 'restricting access to means', a substantial number of studies have sought to explore the extent to which these interventions can reduce deaths a) at a particular site; and b) in an area overall (Pirkis et al., 2015).

As with much suicide research (Abrutyn & Mueller, 2019; Marsh, 2020; White, Marsh, Kral, & Morris, 2016), the focus of these intervention studies tends to be on measurement, using quantitative methodologies (Sueki, 2021). As Stevenson (2016) has underlined, such approaches leave absent and under-explored the associated cultural meanings and embodied practices that may contribute to particular places becoming known or used as locations for suicide. This is despite a ready acknowledgement that such meanings are vital in understanding how some areas, rather than others, may acquire 'cultural significance' as places where suicides are imagined to occur (Chen, Wu, Wang, & Yip, 2016).

While some studies are beginning to engage with the qualitative meanings that particular places may hold (Ross, Koo, & Kõlves, 2020), overall engagement with cultural meaning and embodied space/place has been limited in suicide studies. This limitation extends to a consideration of suicides that occur in places *not* considered locations of concern. Indeed, the contribution of geography to suicide research, particularly cultural geography, has been limited (though see Balayannis & Cook, 2015; Stevenson, 2016 for important exceptions). In contrast, our multidisciplinary team (which incorporates anthropology, critical psychology, sociology and geography) has sought to pay closer attention to the role of place and space in shaping practices relating to suicide and suicide prevention, the meanings that these practices hold, as well as affective aspects of suicide, and its aftermath.

To help focus our analytic gaze, we developed the concept of the *suicidescape*. This novel concept is derived from that of the *deathscape*, which was designed to draw attention to the role of space and place as integral sites through which mourning, remembrance, and indeed death are shaped (Maddrell & Sidaway, 2010; Stevenson, 2016). Informed by Appadurai (1996), the suffix 'scape' points to the constructed and subjective nature of death, and of suicide, and of the places where these occur (Maddrell & Sidaway, 2010). While suicide research often seeks to create objective and universal objects of study, the concept of suicidescapes invites a more complex, contextual and culturally sensitive engagement. Our use of suicidescapes addresses three facets: a) the situated and emplaced nature of suicides, and of knowledge about suicides; b) the affective or emotional aspects of emplaced knowledge about suicide; c) the role of politics in shaping meaning making around suicide. We see this concept as deliberately open to change /development in response to our own and other research in this area.

In the following sections, we draw on data from our ongoing ethnography of suicide and suicide prevention across diverse regions of Scotland, in order to illustrate how the concept of suicidescapes can be employed to inquire into the embodied and emplaced practices and effects of suicide and suicide prevention. We focus on the way in which 'locations of concern' and 'places of safety' are made sense of by our participants and through our analysis of these accounts.

Troubling locations of concern: into the woods

At a meeting of the Feldry Suicide Prevention Group, which is located within the broader Burnsvale area, a discussion emerges about a possible 'location of concern'. Anecdotally a number of incidences had been reported there, but there was no 'firm data'. The group noted that a location of concern could be defined as a site in which two or more deaths had occurred in a 12 month period. In response to this potential location of concern, two members of the suicide prevention group had visited the area, to explore what kind of intervention would best suit. They reported that this was difficult given the nature of the location (a stretch of woodland, with various entrances). One suggestion had been to have Samaritans (a suicide prevention helpline) signs at the entrances, but given that there were various entrances and different ways to access the wood, this was not deemed feasible. Another group member wondered whether it might be helpful to start a walking group, to try to develop more positive associations with the area, as well as increasing the amount of people walking through.

These fieldnotes from RH note some of the practical challenges faced by suicide prevention practitioners as they attempt to interpret guidance on locations of concern in their local areas. While woods are often noted as a potential 'location of concern,' the types of interventions most often advocated are shown to be nonsensical in this particular setting – a 'wild' area of woodland, with multiple entrances. The challenges that the suicide prevention group faced in intervening into this particular location underline the potential attraction of such places as sites of suicide. The secluded, wild nature of woods offers a greater chance of 'not being found', which as Stevenson's (2016) analysis of the stories of people who attempted suicide suggests, can be vital in understanding why places are chosen as sites of death. Further, in Burnsvale, ethnographic research with community members has identified a recurring motif associated with shared stories of suicides in the community: 'going up to the woods' was a well-known and recognisable emplaced metaphor for suicide.

In another of our three fieldsites, pseudonymised as Tir Ard, JA spent time with Lucy, a youth worker for a local charity who had grown up in the rural Lakemouth area, and who now worked in a role which involved supporting those at risk of or affected by suicide. Lucy shared that in recent years a young person had died by suicide in the local forest, and told of how she and the person's sister had found the body during a large-scale, locally run search effort. Lucy said emphatically, "You don't forget a thing like that, you know." She and the young person's sister returned sometimes to the forest, and described how both found themselves frightened by shadows moving in trees, imagining them to represent the slow creak of a hanging body.

This ethnographic encounter reflected a very different engagement with the woods or forest as a potential suicidescape. While suicide prevention practitioners in Burnsvale were engaged with the practicalities of enacting a policy about a 'location of concern', Lucy describes a more affecting engagement with a concerning location, underlining the way in which suicides can haunt or linger in a particular place, and the impact on first responders of finding the bodies of those who have died. Later, Lucy went on to describe the local efforts in Lakemouth to respond to this 'concerning location'; telling JA that one local council member suggested cutting down all of the trees near a notorious social housing development. Lucy related the serious debate that ensued about how this could work with disdain, angry that they were avoiding dealing with what she suspected was the root cause of these deaths.

From Lucy's perspective, the high numbers of young people dying by suicide in Lakemouth had more to do with deprivation and a lack of opportunities for meaningful and positive futures in a local economy dominated by tourism. The jobs on offer for residents are largely seasonal and low paid, meaning the winter months can be hard for Lakemouth locals, who express contradictory feelings towards the tourists who bolster the local economy, while changing the face of their towns and natural landscapes with infrastructure designed for visitors, not residents. For Lucy, focusing on 'locations of concern' and removing trees from the most deprived communities where suicide is more common ignored the deficit in resources, dignity, and opportunities afforded to local people living at the margins of an industry that is designed to siphon money away from the community and towards those who own the tourist infrastructure.

Each of these examples demonstrate, in different ways, the problematic nature of solutions to the 'problem' of suicide that can result from focusing narrowly on locations of concern. In this case, the focus on forests and trees obscures the damaging socio-economic structural contexts in which people live. The suggestion of cutting down trees to prevent suicides focuses narrowly on acute prevention, whilst neglecting the potential value of natural environments for supporting or enhancing wellbeing. In both cases, though, we recognise a desire to 'do something' in the face of suicide deaths. The public location of these deaths, as well as being clearly affecting and haunting, also perhaps invites a sense that something 'must be done'. In these examples, it is clear that suicides are located within the geographical, social, and economic landscapes in which they take place. Forests and other natural features become associated with suicide when they occur there, but this link becomes further embedded when suicide prevention efforts are directed towards them. Efforts to address 'locations of concern' may obfuscate or even ignore how an area's broader affective, social, and economic make-up may explain why suicides take place there.

A site of sensation or a mundane, slow death: private dwellings

A focus on 'locations of concern' may reflect an interest in intervening and addressing deaths which are or may become 'spectacles'. Indeed, existing literature addressing locations of concern often notes that such locations only become so because of media reporting and 'sensationalism' in relation to suicides at these places (Pirkis et al. 2015). In contrast, and as Lucy highlighted when reflecting on the discussion of suicide prevention in Lakemouth, such discussions can be distracting – diverting attention from deeper causes of suicide, and the challenging social and political contexts in which they can take place. An additional distraction can be seen in the focus on 'public' suicides, when the majority of deaths by suicide actually occur in houses. Each of these considerations were drawn on by Donna, who worked in Burnsvale in mental health advocacy, as well as having her own experiences with suicidal thoughts from a young age. Here, she reflected with RH on the complexities of broader socio-political contexts of distress, as well as place itself. Donna highlighted a contrast between the 'spectacle' of public deaths via jumping from buildings, and the 'silent' deaths of those who took medication in their own homes, ground down by deprivation and in the context of ongoing threats to life and livelihood which result from over a decade of austerity policies from the UK government:

> I would go as far as saying, this is eugenics by deprivation. … I see vulnerable pensioners going 'I don't know how I'm going to survive'. And I think there will be an increase in silent suicides, and by silent, I mean older people in particular, who save their medication, and then just take a whole load. There will be very few people climbing to the top of buildings and throwing themselves off to make statements. This is going to be silent and deadly.

Donna's account can be read in multiple ways. Like Lucy, she points to the broader social drivers of misery, distress, and self-inflicted death. However, her account also underlines the contingent ways in which different embodied practices of suicides (overdoses, compared to jumping) enacted in different places (homes, or outside) are given meaning. In her account, Donna frames people jumping from tall buildings as potentially making 'statements', compared with vulnerable older people taking medication not because of a 'statement' but because of despair – "I don't know how I'm going to survive". Subtly, the location of death – and its public, or private, character – is drawn on by Donna to give meaning to suicide. This is a curious contrast, one that invites further reflection on the way in which sites of death, and the social identity of the person who died, may inform interpretation of different deaths – as political or not, statement or not. Considering Donna's account as an articulation of different suicidescapes facilitates engagement with the multiple interpretive resources through which suicides are understood.

Sites of connection and severance: bridges

Bridges have been identified as important geographical markers associated with suicide across each of our three fieldsites. Correspondingly, bridges have generated debates among an aware public about how to respond to suicide in particular areas. Not only are bridges known as 'locations of concern' within particular areas, they also act as discursive objects that draw in various stakeholders to debate what it might mean to safeguard a bridge from suicide attempts.

During our fieldwork, over a period of several weeks, one bridge in Tir Ard became the subject of local controversy when it was shut eight times in two weeks due to a series of incidents that were framed as attempted suicides. Author JA spoke with Rugbyman, the head of a local peer support group, who shared that while no-one died during these incidents, they had sparked intense debate among the police, third sector organisations, transport companies, medical doctors, as well as the local population, about how best to respond to the 'problem'. Some suggested installing phones with direct links to the Samaritans helpline, while others called for nets to be put up beneath the bridge.

Rugbyman raised concerns that people who had jumped from the bridge within this two-week period had been taken to police cells or a hospital bed only to be released a few hours later with – apparently – no offer of help or on-going support. Stories circulated about this, with local outrage played out in social media and in meetings among third sector organisations, who took it as an indicator of long-standing deficiencies and failures in how local services responded to suicide. Participants across Tir Ard consistently reported that the police and local hospital should do better to respond to these incidents; the removal of people recovered from the bridge to either police stations or hospitals, and the lack of follow-up care were framed as wholly insufficient, and lacking in compassion and care.

This example shows how the built physical landscape can evoke and provide a focus for social and cultural debates about suicide. Bridges are not just important geographic locations within a suicidescape, they also become a discursive centre for debates about how to respond to high rates of suicide. Thus, a physical landmark can become a discursive object in the affective, ethical, and political conversations/responses that follow its association with suicide.

We identify similar connections in Abhainnmouth, where residents of Witchhazel, a small town in a rural area, told researcher SH a complex story of their local 'suicide epidemic'. The stories of suicide in this town centred around social deprivation and the clear divide between the wealthy and deprived neighbourhoods, but also spoke of a particular bridge in the middle of the town. While talking about the role of deprivation in suicide, community members often noted the lack of 'things to do' for young people – growing up hanging out by the river, and the bridge, and in particular, drinking alcohol there. These places were envisioned as places of leisure for disaffected youth, and as sites of their suicides – even though many of the actual suicides discussed took place in individuals' homes.

The river and bridge loom large in the centre of this picturesque town, literally dividing people (as the deprived neighbourhoods and wealthy ones are on opposite sides of the river), and its notoriousness inflects what would be an attraction of the town with a sense of danger. The bridges and physical landmarks in both Witchhazel and Tir Ard are associated with suicide because of attempts or deaths that have occurred there. However, shared local stories, media coverage of deaths and attempts to intervene in and reduce suicides in these locations can be seen to further embed their association with suicide. As such, these bridges become a part of the 'suicidescape' in the region, which importantly incorporates stories of death and despair, as well as of inequalities and social injustice.

Places of safety, or sites of suicide: returning to homes

Within our interviews with people who have attempted suicide, private or family homes frequently feature as sites of attempted or imagined suicides. This troubles the focus on locations of concern, or hotspots: which in addressing locations outside the home, implicitly construct home as a 'place of safety'. In this section, we reflect further on the role of the 'private' home as a space where suicides happen, and inquire into the implications of considering such spaces as *also* locations of concern. We wonder what the implications for suicide prevention might be if homes and private spaces were taken more seriously as sites of death.

Goblin, who lives in Abbey City in Abhainnmouth, provided a complex and detailed account of many years of distress, including frequent suicide attempts and numerous interactions with services, including inpatient psychiatric care. For Goblin, home was both a place of safety and care, *and* a site where they often tried to take their own life. Goblin's account indicates some of the relational work that went into keeping them safe – describing family members checking on them, medication being locked away, and their mother watching and physically being nearby.

> Then there was an electric safe, [which] was the bane of my existence because I took power tools to that bad boy, it was not budging. I know there were points where my mum would, like, fall asleep right next to my bedroom door and I would be pissed at her, like, why the fuck are you doing that? Looking back it was very clear why she was doing that.

Goblin contrasted the relative safety and care they experienced at home, with the more challenging circumstances that others they met in inpatient psychiatric care experienced. "I was really lucky that I've always been protected". Goblin's relative safety at home did not prevent them from attempting suicide, and they emphasised that despite all of this it was 'luck' that led to them surviving these difficult years. Goblin's account draws attention to the complex way in which places of safety are experienced, reliant upon the relationships that occur within these places, as well as the limitations of safety, even in such a 'safe place'.

Goblin's awareness of the difficulties faced by others in relation to having a secure home is illustrated starkly in Gillian's account. Gillian's former partner had killed himself during an eviction process, and Gillian expressed anger and frustration that those evicting him had not called her, as next of kin.

> And I think the day it happened, that was the day of the eviction. And I know, housing arrived – this is what I've heard from people – so they arrived about 11 to evict him,

with a locksmith. He was arguing with them through the door. What I can't get my head around is why housing didn't phone me. I was next of kin, on his forms... why they didn't phone me to say, look we're here to do this, we can't get him out, would you kindly come up, you know. I work three minutes away.

(Gillian 48, works as office manager, lives in Burnsvale)

For Gillian's former partner, home was a site not just of his suicide, but also of a traumatic attempted-eviction. The situation leading up to this eviction underlines the precarious nature of 'home' for those living with financial difficulties, and with unstable housing. Gillian's account – like Goblin's – highlights the vital importance of relationships in generating safety – in making places 'safe'. The role of relationships in producing 'safety' is frequently absent in procedural approaches to removing people who pose a risk to themselves to a 'place of safety' such as those described in Tir Ard (often police cells or hospitals). Such removals focus on constructions of physical, rather than emotional, safety, and can often invite coercive practices, including restraints, or removal of personal items and clothing (Bendelow & Menkes, 2014). Gillian's story also provides a stark illustration of the material role the state can play in producing suicide (Mills, 2018). As such, the suicidescape in which Gillian's ex-partner died is made up of the precarious 'home' in which he lived, the relational tensions and absences – Gillian not being present, not being called – and the confrontational forced eviction, as well as the political contexts which produced or made possible these situations. Understanding suicides via the lens of suicidescapes requires attending to the multi-layered, meaning-laden spaces in which deaths occur, attending not just to the act of suicide and its psychological antecedents, but also to the cultural, political and economic contexts in which these play out and are given meaning.

Discussion

This chapter has explored different ways through which suicide can be approached as an embodied, and emplaced practice, attending to particular locations: forests, bridges, and homes. We have proposed the concept of suicidescape as a way of focusing this emerging analysis. Suicidescapes, we suggest, involve three inter-related aspects.

Firstly, suicidescapes are situated in space and time. This shapes the possibilities of suicide: the material possibilities, as well as the interpretive resources available to make sense of suicide. Forests, bridges, or homes become potential sites of suicide both through material possibilities – of bodies moving to or from places, engaging in particular practices that facilitate death – and through interpretive possibilities. These possibilities are enacted, or avoided, in diverse ways in space-time, so are not static and require constant re-interpretation. Importantly, the material and interpretive features which make up suicidescapes are socially mediated, and – potentially – subject to change (Abrutyn, Mueller, & Osborne, 2019).

Secondly, the concept of suicidescapes seeks to draw attention to the affective or emotional aspects of emplaced knowledge (and practices) of suicide. The accounts we drew on in this chapter are not neutral – they are infused with emotion; they speak to affect. Horror, anger, despair, frustration. Making sense of suicide cannot occur without attending to these emotional aspects. Crucially, via suicidescapes we attend to the way that such emotions are embodied and affective – places of death, including by suicide, are affecting, and can haunt (Gordon, 2008).

Finally, suicidescapes are always also political – the sites, meanings and affects associated with different deaths by suicide must be understood as part of a broader political context. These aspects have been starkly rendered in our illustrations, and in our ongoing ethnographic work in Scotland. In contrast to approaches to suicide which focus on 'cognitive distortions' or individual mental illness, our fieldwork invites a more complex and socially situated understanding of suicide, one taken up readily by participants in our ethnography and interviews. Part of this complexity comes from the "global power imbalances and socio-economic inequalities [that] are played out between people, within homes and on bodies" (Mills, 2014, p. 37), as evidenced by the discussions around social deprivation and inequity in our fieldwork. As Mills (2020) has noted, particular cultural and social contexts create "hostile environment[s]… that make life, for some, unliveable and that incite, elicit, and invite suicidality" (p.71).

Instead of suicide research that seeks to "chop, or decontextualise, mind and body from social, cultural, relational, and historical contexts" (Polanco, Mancías, & LeFeber, 2017, p. 526), our approach is intended to embrace all of the factors discussed above, to complicate our approach to thinking about suicide, incorporating 'messiness', constructedness, and subjectivity.

References

Abrutyn, S., & Mueller, A. S. (2019). Toward a robust science of suicide: Epistemological, theoretical, and methodological considerations in advancing suicidology. *Death Studies, 45*(7), 522–527.

Abrutyn, S., Mueller, A. S., & Osborne, M. (2019). Rekeying cultural scripts for youth suicide: How social networks facilitate suicide diffusion and suicide clusters following exposure to suicide. *Society and Mental Health, 10*(2), 112–135.

Appadurai, A 1996, *Modernity at large: cultural dimensions of globalization*, University of Minnesota Press, Minneapolis.

Balayannis, A., & Cook, B. R. (2015). Suicide at a distance: The paradox of knowing self-destruction. *Progress in Human Geography, 40*(4), 530–545.

Beautrais, A. (2007). Suicide by jumping. *Crisis, 28*(Suppl 1), 58–63.

Bendelow, G., & Menkes, D. (2014). Diagnosing vulnerability and "dangerousness": Police use of Section 136 in England and Wales. *Journal of Public Mental Health, 13*(2), 70–82.

Bendelow, G., Warrington, C. A., Jones, A. M., & Markham, S. (2019). Police detentions of 'mentally disordered persons': A multi-method investigation of section 136 use in Sussex. *Medicine Science Law, 59*(2), 95–103.

Chandler, A. (2016). *Self-Injury, Medicine and Society: Authentic Bodies*. Basingstoke: Palgrave Macmillan.

Chandler, A. (2019). Boys don't cry? Critical phenomenology, self-harm and suicide. *The Sociological Review, 67*(6), 1350–1366.

Chen, Y.-Y., Wu, K. C.-C., Wang, Y., & Yip, P. S. F. (2016). Suicide Prevention Through Restricting Access ot Suicide Means and Hotspots. In R. O'Connor & J. Pirkis (Eds.), *The International Handbook of Suicide Prevention* (2nd ed., pp. 609–636). Oxford: John Wiley & Sons.

Cox, G. R., Owens, C., Robinson, J., Nicholas, A., Lockley, A., Williamson, M., … Pirkis, J. (2013). Interventions to reduce suicides at suicide hotspots: A systematic review. *BMC Public Health, 13*(1). https://bmcpublichealth.biomedcentral.com/articles/10.1186/1471-2458-13-214

Gordon, A. F. (2008). *Ghostly Matters: Haunting and the Sociological Imagination*. Minneapolis: University of Minnesota Press.

Jaworski, K. (2014). *The Gender of Suicide*. Aldershot: Ashgate.

Linskens, E. J., Venables, N. C., Gustavson, A. M., Sayer, N. A., Murdoch, M., MacDonald, R., … Sultan, S. (2022). Population- and community-based interventions to prevent suicide. *Crisis*, 44(4), 330–340. doi:10.1027/0227-5910/a000873

Maddrell, A., & Sidaway, J. D. (2010). Introduction: Bringing a Spatial Lens to Death, Dying, Mourning and Remembrance. In A. Maddrell & J. D. Sidaway (Eds.), *Deathscapes: Spaces for Death, Dying, Mourning and Remembrance* (pp. 1–16). London: Routledge.

Marsh, I. (2020). The social production of psychocentric knowledge in suicidology. *Social Epistemology*, 34(6), 544–554.

Mills, C. (2014). *Decolonizing Global Mental Health: The Psychiatrization of the Majority World*. London: Routledge.

Mills, C. (2018). 'Dead people don't claim': A psychopolitical autopsy of UK austerity suicides. *Critical Social Policy*, 38(2), 302–322.

Mills, C. (2020). Strengthening Borders and Toughening Up on Welfare: Deaths by Suicide in the UK's Hostile Environment. In M. Button & I. Marsh (Eds.), *Suicide and Social Justice* (pp. 71–86). London: Routledge.

Oaten, A., Jordan, A., Chandler, A., & Marzetti, H. (2022). Suicide prevention as biopolitical surveillance: A critical analysis of UK suicide prevention policies. *Critical Social Policy*, 02610183221142544. doi:10.1177/02610183221142544

Owens, C. (2016). Hotspots and copycats: A plea for more thoughtful language about suicide. *The Lancet Psychiatry*, 3(1), 19–20.

Owens, C., Lloyd-Tomlins, S., Emmens, T., & Aitken, P. (2009). Suicides in public places: Findings from one English county. *European Journal of Public Health*, 19(6), 580–582.

Pirkis, J., Too, L. S., Spittal, M. J., Krysinska, K., Robinson, J., & Cheung, Y. T. (2015). Interventions to reduce suicides at suicide hotspots: A systematic review and meta-analysis. *Lancet Psychiatry*, 2(11), 994–1001.

Platt, S., & Niederkrotenthaler, T. (2020). Suicide prevention programs. *Crisis*, 41(Supplement 1), S99–S124.

Polanco, M., Mancías, S., & LeFeber, T. (2017). Reflections on moral care when conducting qualitative research about suicide in the United States military. *Death Studies*, 41(8), 521–531.

Ross, V., Koo, Y. W., & Kõlves, K. (2020). A suicide prevention initiative at a jumping site: A mixed-methods evaluation. *EClinicalMedicine*, 19, 100265.

Stevenson, O. (2016). Suicidal journeys: Attempted suicide as geographies of intended death. *Social & Cultural Geography*, 17(2), 189–206.

Sueki, H. (2021). Characteristics of train stations where railway suicides have occurred and locations within the stations. *Crisis*, 43(1), 53–58.

White, J., Marsh, I., Kral, M. J., & Morris, J. (Eds.). (2016). *Critical Suicidology: Transforming Suicide Research and Prevention for the 21st Century*. Vancouver: UBC Press.

21 The university as a lived space
The experience of students in distress

Emma Farrell and Sheena Hyland

Introduction

The university is a space aligned, for the majority, with that critical juncture of late adolescence/early adulthood. Marked by developmental, emotional and geographical transitions, this period in life is, as Forstenzer (2022) puts it, "fraught with fragility and peril, as well as promise and excitement" (p.87). It is a time of movement and discovery, a "time out of time" (Forstenzer, 2022, p.87), in which ideas of self and certainty are suspended and explored. The university is not a passive backdrop against which these moments of promise and peril unfold but rather, as Nørgård and Bengtsen (2016) suggest, is "itself a force of being":

> When we speak of the university as a place and not merely a space, we speak of it as a place where people, with Heidegger's term, 'dwell' … [i]t is not an empty container to be filled with the conceptual spirit or concrete flesh of the people occupying these spaces (Aaen & Nørgård, 2015). The university itself is a force of being, and by dwelling there we become 'absorbed' (Heidegger, 2000) into this being. Accordingly, the university is not just a space we occupy in a specific time span during the day, while we teach or attend classes, continue our research projects, and maintain and develop the infrastructure of our department or faculty. Rather, the university becomes part of our broader lifeworld.
>
> (Nørgård and Bengtsen, 2016, p. 9)

While the majority 'dwell' in this space with relative ease, we know that, at any one time approximately one quarter of the student population struggles with their mental health (Dooley and Fitzgerald, 2012; Dooley et al., 2019). Indeed, as inundated student counselling services report (Bermingham, 2022), early indications suggest that the return to a post-pandemic university environment has been one of increased dis-comfort and distress. Institutional responses to this increased need range from positive mental health and well-being campaigns to the provision of specialist psychological and psychiatric services on campus. Inherent within these responses, however, is an understanding of human distress as something separate, individual, isolable and identifiable.

In this chapter we explore the experience we describe as distress, but which others may refer to as mental health difficulties or mental illness, and the university. In particular, we aim to examine how the university, as 'a force of being', shapes student understanding and experiences of distress. We begin by exploring the positivistic heritage

DOI: 10.4324/9781003345725-23

of the university and highlight how this heritage continues to influence the provision, not just of education, but of support and accommodations to third level students. We seek, by drawing on the work of Husserl, Heidegger, Merleau-Ponty and others, to evoke the distinction between distress as objective and reducible, and distress as embodied and immersed in the 'worldly' and social aspects of the lifeworld. We then turn to first-person insights from students with mental health difficulties (Farrell, 2017, Farrell, 2022) to further illuminate this juxtaposition with a view to articulating the experience of distress as it is "absorbed into the being", as Nørgård and Bengtsen put it, of the university. We do so, not to settle or prove but, as phenomenology invites us, to simply return to the experience itself.

The university, positivism and the dogma of scientism

The modern western university, as we know it today, emerged at a time when church and state were intimately intertwined. The central role of the papacy in granting university charters and funding these educational institutions meant that, up until the seventeenth century, the university was dominated by Christian teaching and ideology. This changed dramatically during the seventeenth and eighteenth centuries when the scientific revolution began to undermine the church's influence. Underpinned by positivism, a philosophical perspective that suggests that unless something can be objectively verified (i.e. observed and measured in an unbiased, impersonal and rigorous manner) that it doesn't exist or is not logical, the scientific revolution led to advances in areas such as physics, chemistry and astronomy that radically and positively changed our understanding of the world. While undoubted in the natural sciences, the early success of the scientific method served to reinforce positivism's authority and led to the belief that the scientific method was the only legitimate path to knowledge. This 'dogma of scientism' (Klein and Lyytinen, 1985) extended to our understanding of mental health with Oxford's Sedlian Professor of Natural Philosophy, Professor Thomas Willis, in 1681 suggesting that the source of human distress could be located in the body and, more specifically, the nerves.

That the Anatomy of the Nerves yields more pleasant and profitable Speculations, than the Theory of any parts besides in the animated Body: for from hence the true and genuine Reasons are drawn of very many Actions and Passions that are wont to happen in our Body, which otherwise seem most difficult and unexplicable; and no less from this Fountain the hidden Causes of Diseases and their Symptoms, which commonly are ascribed to the Incantations of Witches, may be found out and clearly laid open.

(Willis, 1681 p. 102)

The influence of the scientific revolution and its ideas about the nature of distress can still be observed today. For example, in order to access additional support, a student who experiences distress in the Irish tertiary education system requires the validation of an expert in the form of a clinical diagnosis. This diagnosis is selected from a classification system – either the Diagnostic and Statistical Manual (DSM, now in its fifth edition) or the International Classification of Diseases (ICD, now in its tenth edition). This diagnosis is appointed following a clinical encounter with a qualified expert, who has received training in a science-based discipline such as psychiatry (medicine) or psychology. In this encounter, the expert assesses the patient's symptoms, or expressions of distress;

identifies disorder (diagnosis); ascertains a cause (aetiology); suggests treatment and; perhaps offers a prediction of the future course of the diagnosed disorder (prognosis). The validation offered by this process is deemed, by the university, to confirm the student's eligibility for access to supports and resources from additional learning assistance to flexible assessment options and exam accommodations. The structures and requirements of the university, as a world in which students 'dwell' in the Heideggerian sense, serve to shape student experiences of distress along positivistic lines.

Phenomenology, *Lebenswelt* and the meaning of distress

By the early twentieth century a new philosophical method and movement known as phenomenology began to emerge. Developed by Edmund Husserl, it is later shaped by philosophers such as Martin Heidegger, Maurice Merleau-Ponty, Jean-Paul Sartre and many others. Its influence extends far beyond the strict parameters of philosophical inquiry; its application can be seen across various disciplines and fields from cognitive science and psychology to nursing and the medical humanities. In short, phenomenology seeks to describe what it is like to experience the world from the first-person perspective.

Phenomenology refers to the study of *phenomena* as they are experienced in human consciousness. It does not focus on how things might objectively exist in the world, but rather aims to elucidate how things appear to us in lived experience. Husserl writes that phenomenology is a 'return to the things themselves' as they are originally encountered from the first-person perspective. This is in contrast to the impersonal 'objective' point of view of scientific inquiry. Phenomenology thus seeks to describe the structure of consciousness rather than to categorise, analyse and explain phenomena from the third-person perspective. In this way, phenomenology represents a 'return' to what is most intimately known to us: our lived experience.

Husserlian phenomenology arises in part as a critical response to the dominance of scientism across disciplines including psychology. Science, Husserl claims, proceeds from observation and produces causal explanations for phenomena including mental states, but fails to account for how its insights ultimately depend upon and are derived from human experience in the first place. Scientific investigation tends to overlook how human conscious experience structures the way the world appears to us, and fails to recognise its own origins in pre-objective lived experience in the world. This is a point later taken up by Merleau-Ponty who writes in the Preface to his magnum opus, *Phenomenology of Perception* (1945): "All my knowledge of the world, even my scientific knowledge, is gained from my own particular point of view, or from some experience of the world without which the symbols of science would be meaningless" (Merleau-Ponty, 2002, p.ix).

Merleau-Ponty argues that scientific knowledge is meaningful to us because it ultimately depends upon the first-person perspective. Science is the "second-order expression" (Merleau-Ponty, 2002, p.ix) of our originary lived encounter with the world. The phenomenological call to 'return to the things themselves' means:

> to return to that world which precedes knowledge, of which knowledge always *speaks*, and in relation to which every scientific schematization is an abstract and derivative sign-language, as is geography in relation to the country-side in which we have learnt beforehand what a forest, a prairie or a river is.
>
> (Merleau-Ponty 2002, p.x)

The task of phenomenology is to descriptively 're-awaken' or retrieve what it is like to exist in the world. This approach opens up the possibility of accessing the richness of human experience as it is lived before it is reduced to the limited terms of scientific inquiry. Rather than limit our understanding of ourselves and the world to measurable facts and events, Merleau-Ponty and others follow the descriptive methodology of phenomenology to elucidate the world in the manner in which it has lived significance for us as human beings.

The Husserlian concept of *Lebenswelt* or lifeworld refers to the perceptual setting that conditions and structures the way we experience the world. It is this dynamic lived scene where our engagement with the world (and others) plays out, and where we can forge our sense of self through the enactment of our human projects. The lifeworld is never fully one's own; it is always already intersubjectively constituted and shared with others. We belong to the lifeworld and collectively share its common 'worldly' features of temporality, spatiality and embodiment. The *Lebenswelt* also includes the social, cultural and historical dimensions of our lived experience in the world. We are continually immersed in the 'worldly' and social aspects of the lifeworld, including the phenomena of cultural norms and values. This may be experienced as familiar, accessible and immediately understood by us (homeworld), or as unknown, strange, foreign or different (alienworld).

To be human is to be able to purposefully act and engage in these 'worldly' projects. However, as the philosopher of illness Havi Carel (2008, 2016) points out, the experience of illness may shut off regions of possible action in the (life)world. While healthy experience is often characterised in terms of our capacity to act in the world and engage in various projects, Carel points out that illness may be experienced as dis-ability, as a state of being (more or less) unable to be, do and act freely. She argues (2008) that while the biomedical model of illness understood in terms of biological dysfunction has come to dominate our ways of understanding and making sense of what it means to be ill, the experience of illness cannot be adequately understood in these exclusively biological terms.

Being diagnosed with a chronic or terminal illness is, for Carel, a 'life-transforming process'. Along with other philosophers of illness such as Fredrik Sveneaus (2000) and S. Kay Toombs (1992) who draw on the phenomenological tradition, Carel 'returns' to the experience of illness in order to descriptively elucidate how it transforms our sense of self and the way we encounter the world. As such, the meaning of illness or pain is not fully reducible to biomedical explanation; as Elaine Scarry (1985) describes, in its extreme forms bodily pain shatters one's sense of self and capacity for language, violently rupturing any prior ease with which we might have encountered the world. As a methodology, phenomenology affords a descriptive 'return' to what it is like to experience illness before the 'second-order expression' of biological explanation.

In recent years, philosophers such as Matthew Ratcliffe have directed their attention to the phenomenological description of mental illness (see for instance Ratcliffe and Stephan, 2014; Ratcliffe, 2015). Similar to the experience of somatic illness, they describe distress as "akin to inhabiting a different world, a suffocating, alien realm that is isolated from the rest of social reality" (Ratcliffe et al., 2014, p.iii). This rupturing of the structure of ordinary experience in mental illness or distress has the capacity to profoundly impact one's sense of self and to diminish one's ability to enact projects in the world. It may disrupt our relationship to time, to others, and even our sense of being present. Ratcliffe et al. note that distress and suffering is often compounded by the challenge of describing the experience itself. Language falters as it comes up against the ineffability of pain. Indeed, even as "we turn to diagnostic manuals" in an attempt to find a less impoverished language to describe mental distress, we find mere "skeletal descriptions of the various symptoms that are together sufficient for one or another diagnosis" (2014, p. iii).

Medicine, meaning and the university as "a force of being" in shaping student experiences of distress

The university as a lived environment in which students dwell serves to expect a certain experience of, and enact a certain response to, distress. If, in practical terms, a student goes through a period of distress, the university requires a diagnosis in order to validate access to support and accommodations which, in turn, involves subscribing to an understanding of distress as reifiable, reducible, diagnosable and treatable. It is important to note that not all mental health supports at university are predicated on diagnosis. Counselling, tutoring and peer support services, for example, tend to be available free-of-charge to all students. However, in order to access additional supports, a student requires a diagnosis. This requirement is largely an administrative one. In order to justify the allocation of limited resources (i.e. funding for moderators for separate exam centres or access to a disability support officer), a student's need must be validated by an expert according to pre-defined criteria (DSM or ICD). Regardless of whether or not a student wants a diagnosis, they are required to receive one in order to access the additional supports that they might need, if only temporarily, in order to engage fully in their education. Many students come to university with a pre-existing mental health diagnosis while others, such as Claire, receive a diagnosis while at university. A diagnosis was source of relief and clarity for Claire:

> When I was diagnosed with depression, straight away a big weight felt lifted because it was just, it's not just how I feel, it's like, it's something wrong with me and I can be fixed. (Claire)

For Claire, the positioning of her distress as a "medical problem", one with an associated course of treatment, was far more meaningful than a "let's talk about it" approach:

> I felt it was more clinical, like you go in say, "Oh, you have this medical problem and these are the ways that you can deal with it". [The psychiatrist] could prescribe stuff and talk about it with you and say, "Oh this will get better this way and take this long for things to start working". And this is how you can speed it up as opposed to just; you have a problem, let's talk about it. Kind of, I felt like it was like a medical thing, like a clinical thing that I need to sort out. (Claire)

Marie too described how medication was a helpful approach for her:

> I wasn't completely averse to the idea [of taking medication], because, I suppose, studying science I wouldn't be, 'Oh, no, I'm not going to touch medication.' Like, you know, depression has a biological side to it. (Marie).

Kingsley, in contrast, struggled with this reductive explanation of his distress. He described how, upon leaving hospital after a psychotic episode during the summer between his first and second years in university, he was left with "this sense that like my leg was broken and now it was fixed again. It was just making sure I didn't break it again".

> Anyway I walk out of [hospital name] on that Friday and I immediately think 'OK I'm totally cured. That was a crap seven weeks!' I was absolutely like 'that's it, that's it, I'm done, I'm out' but as I'm sure you know the episodes of mental health aren't sorted out that easily. (Kinsley).

For Kingsley, it was when he started working with a therapist who helped him process the enormity of his experience that he reached "a turning point":

> When I started seeing this psychologist he was like, " 'No, you are very much on the path of recovery" and he essentially helped me through it. ...the way he made me look at it which was a way I hadn't looked at it all before was that it was trauma, it really was, you know, just because, that was so different to anything I had experienced before...I mean that is all quite traumatic. ...That was a bit of a turning point. (Kinsley)

Sophie too described how the medical response she was presented with wasn't helpful for her in understanding or managing her distress:

> I got to see a psychiatrist, I was medicated, came back every – the time was adjusted in accordance to how well I was doing I suppose, but it was very much, I found it to be very much on the medical side of things and my actual stuff wasn't being dealt with. (Sophie).

Like Kinsley, it was meeting with somebody who "worked with" her to understand the underlying meaning of her distress that Sophie found "very, very helpful":

> I really knew I wasn't getting to the root of things. ...Until I found someone that worked with me and had the right kind of style for me I really found it unhelpful, because I wanted to know, it was very important to me to see the causes. Not all people need that, I think in cognitive behavioural therapy I'm pretty sure they just tell you how to fix it and they don't really go into the causes, but for me it was important, because I really needed to see what had, you know, caused this fall from grace for me. ...I wanted to see what had caused that. ...it was important to me to get to the bottom of it. So once I found someone who work with me to do that I found it very, very helpful (Sophie).

Kate described the help she was offered while struggling with an eating disorder while studying at university:

> I went to the [college] Health Centre and the doctor sent me to [psychiatric hospital] so I went to [psychiatric hospital] and they wanted to admit me and I was like "No fucking way". I went to keep him [college doctor] happy and I couldn't believe that they were going to admit me. I have never been in hospital and I don't want to be because the woman said, which I thought was hilarious, she said "we'll bring you in and you will eat and we'll get you at a proper weight to be physically healthy and then

after that we will assess you and see if you need to go on medication", which I thought was hilarious [...] I was like, if that is the way you are going to approach this, it's ridiculous because it's not about food ... it's not a solution. (Kate).

She went on to describe why food and feeding was not only not a solution but, for Kate, something quite harmful.

[Feeding someone] is not getting to the problem at all. To stuff somebody with food is almost like gagging them, as in, shutting up the mouth, and that is what you are doing, you are cutting off a very essential, perhaps the only way they have of communicating, so it's not going to result in their recovery. (Kate).

What these brief examples serve to highlight is that the university can validate or alienate students with mental health difficulties simply through its structures, practices and conceptual origins. For those students whose experiences and expectations align with the positivistic structure of service provision, the university as "a force of being" (Nørgård and Bengtsen, 2016) offers comfort and reassurance. For those whose experiences and expectations are not only misaligned but, as in the example of Kate in particular, undermined by these same structures, the university can be a space of isolation, disempowerment and alienation.

Conclusion

In this chapter we have sought to turn to the experience of third level students with mental health difficulties and illuminate itself can shape their experience of this "time out of time" (Forstenzer, 2022, p.87). More specifically, we described the positivistic origins of the university and how these structures, practices and conceptual origins continue to determine the provision of support and resources to students in distress. We turn to phenomenology, with its emphasis on experience as it is lived, to open up an understanding of encountering a lifeworld, or *Lebenswelt*, that is familiar, accessible and immediately understood by us (homeworld), as well as encountering a world that unknown, strange, foreign or different (alienworld). For students such as Claire or Marie, whose understanding aligns with its dominant, positivistic, structures, the university is an environment of support and endorsement. For those students for whom this reductionist approach, the 'broken leg' analogy as Kinsley describes it, does not fit, the university as "a force of being" (Nørgård and Bengtsen, 2016, p.9) can serve to inadvertently undermine, disempower and alienate. We conclude this chapter with a cautionary note. The university as 'a force of being' in shaping students experiences of distress has practical consequences as well as the consequence of shaping students' understanding of their experiences. University is a well-known time of transition and vulnerability for many young people. While a diagnosis may enable a student to access additional support in the immediate term, the longer term consequences of a psychiatric diagnosis are not inconsequential. Psychiatric diagnoses are notoriously tricky to shed. Even if a student has moved through a period of distress, their medical and other administrative records will continue to be marked with disorders that may limit their ability to obtain a mortgage, access life insurance, secure a visa to certain countries, and/or pursue certain careers

(Australian Government Department of Home Affairs, 2022). These careers include professional careers such as medicine or the military where a diagnosis may undermine a person's application for selection or fitness to practise (Government of Ireland, 2007; Ministry of Defence, 2018). We offer this chapter, not with a view to solve or prove but rather illuminate an aspect of the experiences of students' in distress that is often overlooked or lost in our efforts to provide support within the institutional lifeworld of the university.

References

Australian Government Department of Home Affairs (2022). Annual report 2021-2022. Available at URL: www.homeaffairs.gov.au/reports-and-pubs/Annualreports/home-affairs-annual-report-2021-22.pdf

Bermingham, D. 2022. Thousands of third-level students seeking support for anxiety, depression, and isolation. *Irish Examiner*, 09.10.2022.

Carel, H. 2008. *Illness: The Cry of the Flesh*, Stocksfield, Acumen.

Carel, H. 2016. *Phenomenology of Illness*, Oxford, Oxford University Press.

Dooley, B. & Fitzgerald, A. 2012. *The My World Survey: National Study of Youth Mental Health in Ireland*, Dublin, Headstrong The National Centre for Youth Mental Health.

Dooley, B., O'Connor, C., Fitzgerald, A. & O'Reilly, A. 2019. *My World Survey 2: The National Study of Youth Mental Health in Ireland*, Dublin, Ireland, UCD and Jigsaw.

Farrell, E. 2017. *Losing the plot: A hermeneutic phenomenological study of the natue and meaning of psychological distress amongst third level students in Ireland*. Ph.D., University of Dublin.

Farrell, E. 2022. *Making Sense of Mental Health: A Practical Approach Through Lived Experience*, Dublin, The Liffey Press.

Forstenzer, J. 2022. Re-Enchanting Undergraduate Education: On the Project of Metamorphosis in English Higher Education. *In*: Mahon, Á. (ed.) *The Promise of the University, Debating Higher Education: Reclaiming Hummanity, Humility, and Hope*. London: Routledge.

Government of Ireland (2007) Medical Practitioners Act 2007. www.irishstatutebook.ie/eli/2007/act/25/enacted/en/html

Klein, H. & Lyytinen, K. 1985. The Poverty of Scientism in Information Systems. *In*: Mumford, E., Hirschheim, R., Fitzgerald, G. & Wood-Harper, A. (eds.) *Research Methods in Information Systems*. Amsterdam: North-Holland.

Merleau-Ponty, M. 2002. *Phenomenology of Perception*, London, Routledge.

Ministry of Defence, (2018) *JSP 950 Medical policy: Joint Service Manual of Medical Fitness*. London: Ministry of Defence.

Nørgård, R. & Bengtsen, S. 2016. Academic citizenship beyond the campus: A call for the placeful university. *Higher Education Research & Development*, 35, 4–16.

Ratcliffe, M. 2015. *Experiences of Depression: A Study in Phenomenology*, Oxford, Oxford University Press.

Ratcliffe, M. & Stephan, A. (eds.) 2014. *Depression, Emotion and the Self: Philosophical and Interdisciplinary Perspectives*, Luton, Andrews UK.

Ratcliffe, M., Stephan, A. & Varga, S. 2014. Introduction. *In*: Ratcliffe, M. & Stephan, A. (eds.) *Depression, Emotion and the Self: Philosophical and Interdisciplinary Perspectives*, Luton, Andrews UK.

Scarry, E. 1985. *The Body in Pain: The Making and Unmaking of the World*, New York, Oxford University Press.

Svenaeus, F. 2000. *The Hermeneutics of Medicine and the Phenomenology of Health*, Dordrecht, Kluwer.

Toombs, S. K. 1992. *The Meaning of Illness: A Phenomenological Account of the Different Perspectives of Physician and Patient*, Dordrecht, Springer.
Willis, T. 1681. *Five treatises viz. [brace] 1. Of Urines, 2. Of the Accension of the Blood, 3. Of Musculary Motion, 4. The Anatomy of the Brain, 5. The Description and Use of the Nerves / by Thomas Willis*, London, Printed for T. Dring, C. Harper, J. Leigh, and S. Martin.

Section III

Creative spaces

22 Introduction to creative spaces

Candice P. Boyd

This section is concerned with the ways in which creative practices open up spaces which support (or diminish) mental health and wellbeing. More than just a form of self-expression, creative practices – like drawing, painting, dancing, and crafting – can be cathartic, meditative, and transformative, particularly for people with histories of trauma (Munt, 2012). While there is an established association between art making and mental health in the literature, very little attention has been given to the spatial dimensions of this relationship (Perkins, et al., 2021). Experienced as calm and safe spaces, creative spaces allow people with mental illness to share negative thoughts as well as 'contain' them in works of art (Abramson & Abramson, 2020). Such spaces also have the potential to be inclusive for people who feel marginalised by society (Parr, 2008), but they are perhaps better conceptualised as liminal spaces that require careful management to harness their transformative potential (Atkinson & Robson, 2012; Sunderland, Stevens, Knudsen, Cooper, & Wobcke, 2022).

Recent research also suggests that vernacular creativity and everyday creative habits maintain mental health and well-being more generally, as well as providing important sources of community connection (see Edensor, Leslie, Millington, & Rantisi, 2010). Beyond representation, cultural geographers and contemporary philosophers suggest that therapeutic art making can be generative of new modes of existence by reclaiming therapeutics as spatial, material, and ecological (Boyd, 2017; Manning, 2012). In this sense, the generative character of creative space is contingent and emergent rather than structured or pre-determined (McCormack, 2003; McCormack, 2013).

Contributors to this section reflect on a range of creative spaces from festivals spaces, the artist's studio, spaces of improvised performance, community spaces, cultural spaces, and other spaces of vernacular creativity that are sustaining or transformative for those who participate in them. Overwhelming affirmative, a notable exception is McPhie and Clarke's thought-provoking piece on the complex creative spaces of social media and the digital, which reminds us of the ever-increasing challenges of negotiating our public subjectivities as well as some of the negative forces at work in online environments. A similar caution is contained within recent scholarship on negative geographies (see Bissell, Rose & Harrison, 2021; Harrison, 2015; Philo, 2017) which contends that scholarship valorising the affirmative need not be at the expense of critically attending to 'bad feelings' (DeKeyser, Zhang, Bissell, 2023). Nonetheless, the central theme of this section of the *Routledge Handbook on Spaces of Mental Health and Wellbeing* is the affirmative potential of creativity.

DOI: 10.4324/9781003345725-25

The section begins with a contribution from Worimi man, Paul Callaghan, and Jesse Hodgetts, descendant of the Wangaaupuwan and Wiradjuri First Nations People of Australia. These scholars and cultural practitioners discuss how song and dance as essential to the mental health and wellbeing of Aboriginal Australians, and how cultural reclamation through dance promotes resilience to the harmful and on-going impacts of colonisation. Diti Bhattachayra's chapter follows, and resonates with the first, wherein she examines the collective practices of wellbeing that are intimately entangled with the *boipara* – the second-hand book market of College Start in Calcutta, India. Bhattachayra demonstrates how the *boipara* acts as a space of emotional refuge, kinship and care. Keller then introduces us to BAJO EL OLIVO – an immersive arts residency located on the outskirts of Alhaurín el Grande, Spain – where artists in residence are prompted to explore their coexistence with other species and experiment with creative methodologies that attune to the infrastructure of the residency's environment. Inspired by eco-feminism and nomadic theory, Keller's chapter is also an excellent overview to some of the key concepts involved in posthuman understandings of mental health and wellbeing. Extending on the posthumanist theme, Jamie McPhie and David Clarke consider the distributed assemblages of cognition and health in relation to social media. The chapter itself is a creative act which grapples with the agency of *person-computer-environment* and the ethical consequences of this when it comes to the proliferation of malignant forms of social interactions, such as misogyny and fascism, through these cognitive assemblages.

The remaining three chapters in this section are decidedly more place-based. Christian Edwardes takes us through a history of the artist's studio in Europe from a time when it was a privileged, solitary and often rural space to the contemporary experience of the studio as spatially distributed, mobile, social and urban. Kate Douglas provides a 'case in point' for these developments, describing how participatory, creative spaces operate as key sites of recovery in the post-disaster city, focusing in particular on Ōtautahi Christchurch, Aotearoa New Zealand. The section ends with a co-authored contribution from Michelle Duffy, Judith Mair, and Elaine Stratford whose work on regional festivals in Australia demonstrate their capacity for transformation, conceptualising them as complex infrastructures of care.

In summary, this section of the *Routledge Handbook of Mental Health and Wellbeing* on creative spaces illustrates the importance of space and relationality to mental health and wellbeing. Resolutely geographical, these perspectives describe the sorts of assemblages, entanglements, and atmospheres that are generated by creative activity and the ways in which these strengthen community connections and contribute towards collective 'hope'. Although the examples are diverse in this section, what they emphasise together is the opportunities for experience and experiment granted by the fluidity of creative space. Not necessarily ethical or affirmative, vernacular and amateur creativities (see Hawkins, 2018) may be public or very private endeavours but they nonetheless create moments for pause and reflection on the human condition, our modern lives, and our posthuman futures.

References

Abramson, P.R., & Abramson, T.L. (2020). Visual and narrative comprehension of trauma. *AMA Journal of Ethics, 22*(6), E535–E543. doi: 10.1001/amajethics.2020.535.

Atkinson, S., & Robson, M. (2012). Arts and health as a practice of liminality: Managing the spaces of transformation for social and emotional wellbeing with primary school children. *Health & Place, 18*(6), 1348–1355. DOI: https://doi.org/10.1016/j.healthplace.2012.06.017

Bissell, D., Rose, M., & Harrison, P. (2021). *Negative geographies: Exploring the politics of limits.* Lincoln: University of Nebraska Press.

Boyd, C.P. (2017). *Non-representational geographies of therapeutic art making: Thinking through practice.* London: Palgrave.

Dekeyser, T., Zhang, V., & Bissell, D. (2023). What should we do with bad feelings? Negative affects, impotential responses. *Progress in Human Geography,* Online First. DOI: https://doi.org/10.1177/03091325231213513

Edensor, T., Leslie, D., Millington, S., & Rantisi, N. (2010). *Spaces of vernacular creativity: Rethinking the cultural economy.* New York: Routledge.

Harrison, P. (2015). After affirmation, or, being a Loser: On vitalism, sacrifice, and cinders. *GeoHumanities, 1*(2), 285–306. DOI: 10.1080/2373566X.2015.1109469

Hawkins, H. (2018). Geography's creative (re)turn: Toward a critical framework. *Progress in Human Geography, 43*(6), 963–984. https://doi.org/10.1177/0309132518804341

Manning, E. (2012). *Relationscapes: Movement, art, philosophy.* Minneapolis: MIT Press.

McCormack, D. P. (2003). An event of geographical ethics in spaces of affect. *Transactions of the Institute of British Geographers, 28*(4), 488–507. DOI: https://doi.org/10.1111/j.0020-2754.2003.00106.x

McCormack, D.P. (2013). *Refrains for moving bodies: Experience and experiment in affective spaces.* Durham: Duke University Press.

Munt, S.R. (2012) Journeys of resilience: The emotional geographies of refugee women. *Gender, Place & Culture, 19*(5), 555–577, DOI: 10.1080/0966369X.2011.610098

Parr, II. (2008). *Mental health and social space: Towards inclusionary geographies?* Oxford: Blackwell. DOI: 10.1002/9780470712924

Perkins, R., Mason-Bertrand, A., Tymoszuk, U. *et al.* (2021). Arts engagement supports social connectedness in adulthood: Findings from the HEartS Survey. *BMC Public Health, 21,* 1208. DOI: https://doi.org/10.1186/s12889-021-11233-6

Philo, C. (2017). Less-than-human geographies. *Political Geography, 60,* 256–258.

Sunderland, N., Stevens, F., Knudsen, K., Cooper, R., & Wobcke, M. (2022). Trauma aware and anti-oppressive arts-health and community arts practice: Guiding principles for facilitating healing, health and wellbeing. *Trauma, Violence, & Abuse, 24*(4), 2429–2447. DOI: https://doi.org/10.1177/15248380221097442

23 Spaces of Australian Indigenous song and dance

Paul Callaghan (Worimi), Jesse Hodgetts (Wangaaypuwan and Wiradjuri)

<u>Cultural Terminology</u>

Corroboree: an Aboriginal English term for song, dance and gathering.
Country: Land, water, sky and everything that exists within it
Gathang: An Aboriginal language on the mid-north coast of NSW.
Gurri: Aboriginal person in Gathang
Kuthi/Guthi: Song, dance and ceremony in Ngiyampaa and Gathang
Mayi: Aboriginal person in Ngiyampaa
Mob: A colloquial term used by Aboriginal people to identify a group of Aboriginal people associated with a particular place or Country
Ngiyampaa: An Aboriginal language in the central west of New South Wales.
Ngurrampaa/Ngurrabaa: Homeland, tribal territory, my place and my connections to my place
Tyirr: Ancestor spirits who have passed on. Someone's spirit when they are dead

Dance from a mainstream perspective

According to Laird et al. (2021) meta-analyses suggest that dance has the potential to decrease psychological distress, increase trait mindfulness, and enhance quality of life. This chapter suggests conscious dance can be defined as unchoreographed, intentionally nonevaluative mindful movement commonly practiced in a group setting for purposes of authentic self-expression, self-discovery, interpersonal connectedness, and personal healing or growth.

Dance is one of several performing arts that include music, opera, drama and spoken words. In his book, *Arts with the Brain in Mind*, Eric Jensen states that the kinesthetic arts (including dance, drama, mime, theatre and musicals) contribute to the development and enhancement of critical neurobiological systems including cognition, emotions, immune, circulatory and perceptual-motor (Jensen 2001, p. 71). Other benefits identified by Jensen relate to creativity, self-concept, improved learning, vestibular activation, following direction, timing, personal mastery, playful expression, social skills, cognition and emotional attunement (pp. 76–82). Dancing in particular is recognised to improve the condition of your heart and lungs; increase muscular strength, endurance and motor fitness; increase aerobic fitness; improve muscular tone and strength; manage weight; create stronger bones and reduce the risk of osteoperosis; support better coordination,

DOI: 10.4324/9781003345725-26

agility and flexibility; improve balance and spatial awareness; increase physical confidence; improve mental functioning; improve general and psychological wellbeing; increase self-confidence and self-esteem and improve social skills (Victoria Department of Health 2022).

Dance from an Aboriginal perspective

For Aboriginal and Torres Strait Islander peoples, dance can also have physical, social, and mental health benefits, but what escalates the importance of dance to Aboriginal and Torres Strait Islander people is that dance is embedded in a framework that underpins cultural identity, meaning and purpose. This framing of dance from our Old People which has been transmitted across generations, comes from our *Ngurrampaa* or *Ngurrabaa*. Non-Indigenous people often call this *The Dreaming* but we translate Ngurrampaa as camp-world, homeland or my place. The Ngurrampaa tells of the journey and the actions of Tyiirr (Ancestral Beings) who created the natural world and laid down laws of social and religious behaviour. The connection to our Ngurrampaa continues today through various ceremonies. Warlpiri man Wanta Jampijinpa Pawu calls this Manyuwana (Corn & Curkpatrick 2014, p.11):

> Manyuwana (Ceremony), is the constitutive mechanism for observing Warlpiri law through the ritual execution of esoteric repertoires of song, dance and design that express Warlpiri polity, record jukurrpa connections between ancestors and land, maintain social order in balance with nature and prepare the young for adult responsibilities.

For us, dancing is far more than a way to stay fit and feel good. One of the major purposes of song and dance is to pass on story. Unlike Western society where dance is primarily an activity that is separated from other aspects of everyday lives, dance is a critical element of cultural practice that does not stand alone. Dance is interwoven with other forms of expression to support a traditional pedagogy and epistemology that has been actively maintained for tens of thousands of years and is essential in growing our children to be well. Ngarinyin senior songmen Mathew Dembal Martin (Treloyn & Martin 2012) explains:

> When they [the dancers] listen to this [the clapsticks], it's just like they hitting their bone. The spirit hitting their bone, they [the young dancers] get strong. Strong bone. That's why you see them kids real happy and thing. They're not looking sad, they're looking forward for dancing or anything, they'll do anything. Now the bone, that ornorr, is strong to do anything, dance. They can run all day too if they want to… They have the Country and for themselves they feel strong, they not weak. The spirit, the singing, the dancing, that makes them healthy. It's always been there.

Like our emu dance and our pelican dance, they exist to inform the dancers of the story, how to be on Country and includes morals in maintaining health and wellbeing. This transfer of knowledge and tradition is also called *Ngurrampaa*, but in English, has often been termed the *Lore*. *Ngurrampaa* is comparable with the ten commandments. It has rules regarding homicide, sacrilege, sorcery, incest, abduction of women, adultery, physical assault, theft, insult and the usurpation of ritual privileges and duties (Working with

Indigenous Australian First Nations People 2020). *Ngurrampaa* is also very much about an individual's connection to their place and their Country (Callaghan & Gordon 2022, p. 22). Like Manyuwana's function to maintain social order and balance with nature and prepare the young for adult responsibilities (Corn & Curkpatrick 2014), our songs and ceremonies hold knowledge of Kinship, which supports wellness.

Song and dance is essential to the creation, growth and maintenance of cultural identity, and therefore overall identity, for both the individual and their community. On the North Coast of NSW, the Bundjalung used Yawahr songs (Gummow 2002, p. 55) to support collective community participation and establishing cultural identity:

> Each specific group of people throughout the Bundjalung area had their own Yawahr songs and dances that were unique to their own particular community. These Yawahr songs and dances helped communities to establish their own separate identities and were performed to people from different areas at larger gatherings.

Song and dance maintain connection to our ancestors and therefore our way of living that protects us. Corn and Gumbula (2007, p. 117) describe how Yolngu, Gupapuyngu singers in north-East Arnhem land could feel the presence of their Waŋarr (ancestors) while they recorded their Manikay (songs):

> The musicians would later describe how they could feel the napes on their necks tingle as the waŋarr, who remain eternally present and sentient in Djiliwirri, observed from the stream behind. This is one way that waŋarr can recognise their human descendants before extending their protection to them. The lyrics of each manikay series record the original observations of waŋarr as they named, shaped and populated each Yolŋu homeland. Their faithful re-performance, generation after generation, is the cornerstone of upholding Yolŋu rom (law, culture, correct practice, the way) both through formal ceremonial actions and the esoteric knowledge that they convey.

Mathew Dembal Martin (Treloyn & Martin 2012) gives his perspective of how singing and dancing connects his people to his ancestral spirits and in turn supporting health and wellbeing.

> As you're dancing, you're stamping on the ground, you're waking up the spirit. [As] you're singing, and you're hitting this then [striking clapsticks], that echo goes everywhere... when the spirit comes up you'll see everything, like fruit, bush fruit and everything is healthy.

The singing of ancestral songs can assert rights and responsibilities associated with our Country, which has been used to assert ownership in native title land claims (Koch 2013). This is an important demonstration of the centrality of song (and dance) in Aboriginal and Torres Strait Islander people's continuous connection to country through cultural practice.

The impacts of colonisation including on dance

Although there is little research available to provide a snapshot of the health status of Aboriginal people prior to the British invasion in 1788, Aboriginal Elder Uncle Paul Gordon (Callaghan & Gordon 2022, p. 22) describes the wellbeing of traditional Aboriginal people as follows:

> Imagine a world where people have all they need to be contented. Where they live to be old and are happy in mind, body, and spirit. That is the way our people lived for a very, very long time. Life could sometimes be hard, but our knowledge of the land meant that we always had what we needed.

Aboriginal traditional ways of knowing, being and doing (including knowledge systems, *Lore*, value systems, connection with Country and cultural practices) have been passed down from generation to generation from time immemorial. As current recipients of this knowledge and the histories that underpin it, we have a lived understanding of how the creative arts of story, dance, song, and art are critical to the maintenance and evolution of this ontology. However, the first century and a half of European-Aboriginal relations in Australia was a time of major disruption to this way of life, described by Gardiner (1999) as a period of dispossession, physical ill-treatment, social disruption, population decline, economic exploitation, codified discrimination, and cultural devastation. Aboriginal loss of life over the period 1788–1920 is estimated to be somewhere between 80% and 96% (Harris 2003, p. 81). Figure 23.1 provides a chronology of Aboriginal people's collective experience since 1788 including the impacts of government acculturation policies, racism and transgenerational trauma leading to socio-economic disadvantage, reliance on government programs and services and targeted programs that target symptomatology rather than cause.

Since the colonisation of Australia by European settlers, Aboriginal and Torres Strait Islander Australians have experienced extreme hardships, ranging from the loss of traditional culture and homelands to the forced removal of children and denial of citizenship rights (Australian Human Rights Commission n.d.). Zubrick (2014, p. 99) suggests that colonisation has impacted on all dimensions of the holistic notion of Aboriginal wellbeing including psychological, social, spiritual and cultural aspects of life and connection to land. The term 'cultural genocide' is sometimes used to describe what has occurred. Dondors (2012) describes 'cultural genocide' as follows:

> The destruction by the State of State organs of the culture of a community in its broad sense of the term, including the distinctive spiritual, material, intellectual and emotional features of a society or social group, encompassing 'in addition to art and literarture', lifestyles, ways of living together, value systems, traditions and beliefs.

Aboriginal dance was a victim of cultural genocide in many communities for a prolonged period along with other interconnected elements of culture relating to land, family, *Lore,* ceremony and language which in turn had a profound impact on a person's sense of identity, belonging and purpose (Australians Together 2019). Atkinson (2002, p. 71) reinforces the impact of cultural genocide on the wellbeing of Aboriginal people today:

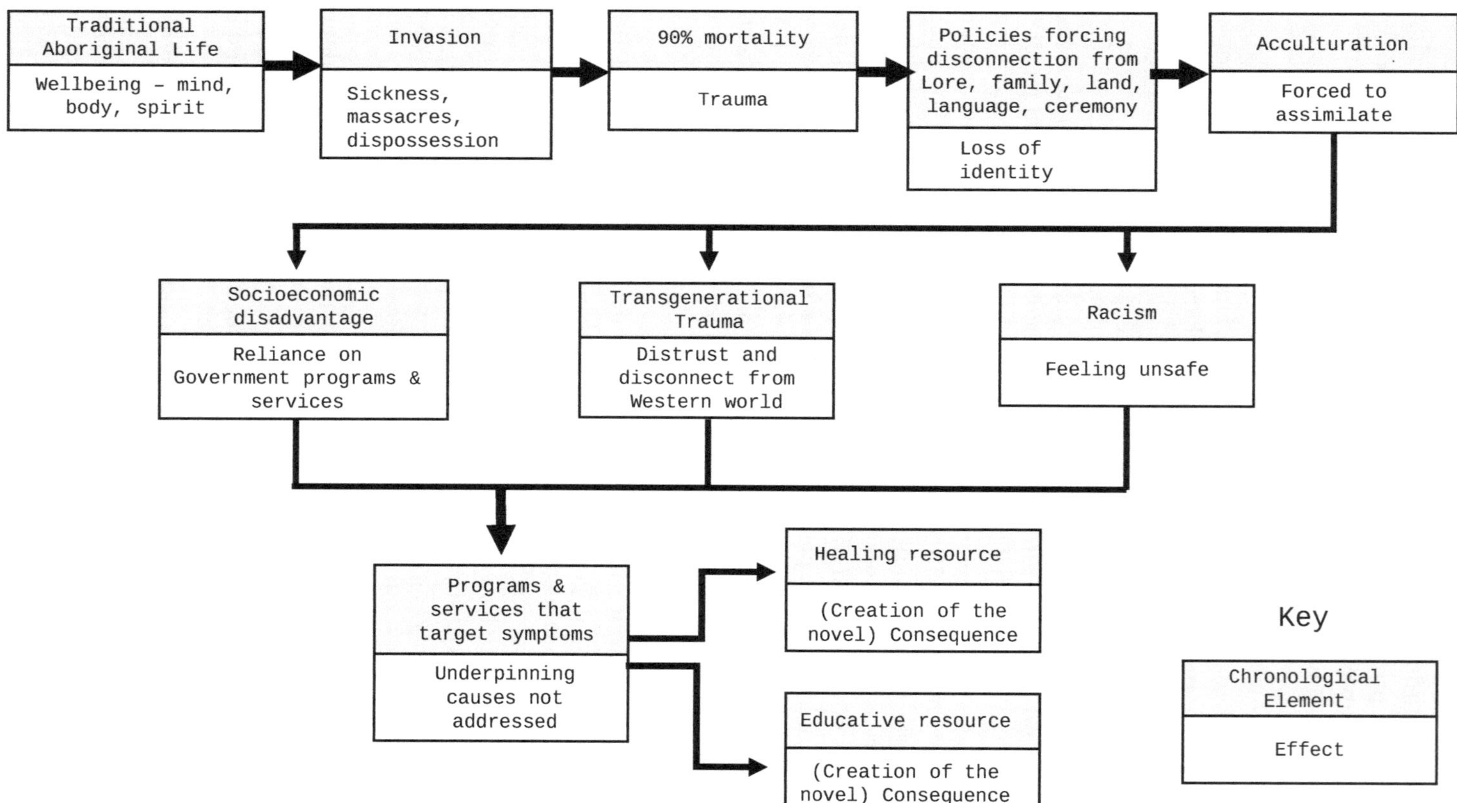

Figure 23.1 Chronology of Aboriginal people's collective experience (Callaghan, 2022).

Cultural genocide not only works to destroy the cultures of oppressed peoples, it also eradicates the sense of self, of self-worth and of wellbeing in individuals and groups so that they are unable to function from either their own cultural relatedness, or from the culture of the oppressors. They feel in a world between, devalued, and devaluing who they are.

The cumulative effect of colonialism, cultural genocide, transgenerational trauma, and racism over the past 230 years is that Indigenous Australians remain the most disadvantaged and marginalised group in Australia. Indigenous Australians experience widespread socioeconomic disadvantage and health inequality (Australian Institute of Health and Welfare 2017). A report by the Australian Institute of Health and Welfare (2022) also acknowledges the devastating impact of colonisation on Aboriginal and Torres Strait Islander communities and culture and then identifies the importance of participation in cultural activities as a protective factor that can positively influence the overall health and wellbeing of Aboriginal and Torres Strait Islander peoples (Corn & Curkpatrick (2014, p. 159) share an example from Lajamanu of the pressing need for reconnection to culture and kinship:

> By the twenty-first century, an entire generation of young adult Warlpiri had been raised at Lajamanu with no clear understanding of classical kinship and limited exposure to traditional ceremonies. These radical social changes had severely threatened the continuation of Ngurra-kurlu as a way of life for future generations, and they had also begun to endanger young lives.

Reconnection with culture including dance, is therefore critical in addressing the cultural determinants of wellbeing that have been taken from us.

Song and dance as resilience to the impact of colonisation and intergenerational trauma

Historically, it has been a common practice for Aboriginal people to sing and dance in response to the impact of colonisation. In 1967, Ngiyampaa man Peter Burke was recorded by musicologist John Gordon singing a song in response to his mob not living like black fullas and getting "randy on their food" (Burke 1967). He sings "yatamagila yuwan tharrinyi wirruumburay yaraybiyan", which translates to "I reckon the good food is disappearing" and then names the bush foods like mushrooms and wild apples.

Another song by Ngiyampaa man Jack King, tells the story of a woman who took a fancy to a man from Ivanhoe. The song was recorded in 1972 and 1975, sung by Ngiyampaa woman Sarah Johnson and recorded by linguist Tamsin Donaldson (Johnson 1972; 1975). The significant part of this song was that the man was "right meat" for her, meaning that he was the correct kin for her to marry under Aboriginal law. This was highlighted because kinship and marriage laws were breaking down and people were rarely marrying correctly.

In both Ngiyampaa song examples, the composer was recording the tragic events during cultural genocide that led to the decline of traditional Aboriginal ways. This provides history for us to understand why and how we have lost so much of our cultural knowledge due to colonial violence and cultural genocide. This also means we have an insight into how to learn from the past and revitalise our culture.

A more recent example of song and dance being used as a means to coping with the hardship created by colonisation relates to the problems mentioned earlier in the Lajamanu community. In 2005, in response to the challenges their young people faced due to lack of connection to culture, identity and kinship, song and dance was introduced as a solution through the establishment of the "Milpirri Festival", a festival of contemporary song and dance that embeds key principles of Warlpiri law for Warlpiri youth to learn. As explained by Corn and Patrick (2014, p. 160), "The 2005 and 2007 festivals respectively focused on the Jardiwarnpa and Kurdiji ceremonies. The 2009 festival focused on the Jurntu purlapa (public ceremony), which teaches responsibility, respect, justice and discipline to be key principles of Warlpiri law."

The importance of cultural reclamation including dance

As suggested by Murray (2021), to restore our nations and Country we need more of our lands and waters back. As the old man sang in the Ngiyampaa song (Burke 1967), "Yatamagila yuwan tharrinyi" – I reckon the good food (traditional bush food) is disappearing, which reinforces the value of land and our connection to it. We need healing – our nations, our people, our families, our children. Healing is a holistic process, which addresses mental, physical, emotional, and spiritual needs and involves connections to culture, family and land (The Healing Foundation 2023). Feeney (2009) asserts that projects need to be funded that integrate Indigenous values and world views that support three pillars of healing – reclaiming history, cultural interventions, and therapeutic healing. It is hard to feel optimistic about healing programs that reclaim history and culture being given government funding priority when the Australian Government Department of Education (2022), states as follows:

> The gap between the knowledge generated in the education system and the skills demanded by employers and individuals is widening. Overcoming these limitations requires a priority focus on science, technology, engineering and mathematics (STEM).

Aboriginal people require healing as a pre-requisite to engagement in the employment/ STEM paradigm being driven by government. Dance is a critical component of the healing process.

Fortunately, many Aboriginal groups across Australia are revitalising their cultural songs and dances through both reclamation as well as continuation of unbroken stories and knowledge. In New South Wales one example is the holding of regular Corroborees, to share song, dance and story from many different Aboriginal mobs across NSW (Hodgetts 2020). Some of these mobs include the Ngiyampaa, Wiradjuri, Gamilaraay, Barkandji, Gathang, Dharug and Gumbayngirr, who perform their songs and dances in Kinship with one another.

In Western Australia, the Nyungar have reclaimed their historical songs through the 'Mobilising Song Archives to Nourish and Endangered Aboriginal Language' project (Bracknell 2019). Reclaiming ancestral songs and dances can assist Aboriginal people in reconnecting with their heritage and identity, as Bracknell (2020, p. 150) explains:

> Community workshops undertaken from 2017 to 2019 to recirculate archival audio recordings of Noongar songs from the south coast of WA as part of the Australian Research Council funded project 'Mobilising Song Archives to Nourish an Endangered

Aboriginal Language' have involved both the interpretation of lyrics and intensely emotional reconnection between people and the songs of their deceased fathers, grandfathers and uncles.

This reclamation process and reconnection with Country and Ancestors, fulfils our identity and pride, and song and dance is a key component to express this. It is also essential to acknowledge that song and dance can not only heal people but heal Country, as demonstrated in the 2019 drought. Many Aboriginal communities through their Kinship with Country, responded to the drought through song and dance to break the drought and heal Country (Hodgetts 2020).

Testimonials

To reinforce the theoretical argument of the importance of dance to the mental health and well being of Aboriginal people, several Aboriginal community members throughout New South Wales, whom we have Kinship and relationship with, wished to contribute to this article by giving a perspective as to what dance means to them in the context of mental health and wellbeing. All of these dancers have participated in large scale Corroborees across NSW with a view to sharing traditional culture as a means of generating community connection and healing. The following quotes demonstrates how this form of cultural immersion can be both a protective factor and a healing factor in an individual's life. The intervention of dance and song can be transformative at an individual, family, community and generational level:

Dance and song has helped me become more confident, whether it be with body image or being able to stand up in front of 2,000 people and first tell the story of the dance, then sing that story, then dance that story. When you paint up in our ochre and put on that head dress, all the fear, all the stress, all the worries of our lives is taken away. All you focus on is the old ancestors and the story they left for us to share. Dance has helped me become more spiritually connected to the world around us. When we dance kangaroo, we become the kangaroo. When we dance emu, we become the emu. A spiritual connection is what many of us are searching for in our lives whether we go to church or start meditation, but as you learn more dance, this helps you become more connected as it has done with me.

(Marty Gordon – Ngemba, Wongibon, Gurrulgeerlu)

Dancing helps me connect with and build relationship with Country. Especially when we dance strong with all women for mother. It allows for strong feminine energy to grow. When we dance, it is essential we dance as one mob men, women, family. This gives strength, balance and helps strengthen our identity. Song and dance connects us to language, Mother and the old people. Dancing together as one mob makes me feel whole and nurtured.

(Leanne King, Dharug)

Dancing has connected me on so many levels to the Country, to my people, and to my ancestors.

(Steve Taylor, Wailwan)

Being able to learn traditional dance keeps me not only connected to my own Country but to mobs all over. When people feel connected, they have lower levels of social isolation, anxiety and depression.

(Tina Taylor, Ngiyampaa, Wailwan)

Dance has been a teacher for me. It's helped me overcome a lot of internal battles and overcome shame and that fear of failure. Dancing frees up all of the worry and stress because you are always dancing with brothers and sisters who are celebrating the stories with you.

(Adam Ridgeway, Worimi)

As soon as you start to dance you feel all your stress and worries from the modern world instantly go away and then you feel connected to the songs and dances and everyone else there. At that time, nothing else matters.

(Gavin Kelly, Worimi)

Dance is the connection to my being, my spirit, she needs me to move to feel energy, to release energy, to stay connected to Mother and to stay connected to myself. Dance is an expression. It tells a story, the telling of my story, the telling of my ancestors. If I can't dance, I can't breathe and I become sick.

(Talara Freeman, Wiradjuri)

For me, doing cultural dance strengthens my connection to my ancestors; to Country; to culture; to lore and to my community. When I feel connected, I feel emotionally, mentally, physically, and spiritually strong. What fills my cup up even more is seeing the thrill on my son's face when we paint up in ochre and have a stomp, knowing that he is connected to his culture from birth and being able to express his connection, through dance.

(Nathan Bramston, Wonnarua)

The things that have given me the most in my life have all been those where you are in the moment, and nothing is interrupting that time and place. This is a place of purity. Dancing gives me the same feeling and it has enabled me to face fears and shed them at the same time.

(Marcus Rowsell, Biripi, Dunghutti)

My power to walk this life rests in the harmony of Country, Law, Ancestors & Kin. When we dance, we become those things woven together, balanced & interconnected. Earth on our feet, ochre on our bodies, wind and rain on our skin. The song moves through us and we embody the story as one in Corroborree – my sisters and brothers next to me, our old people past, the stars, the animals, the trees, the earth – we become one body, held in the song & dancing our story, woven together as one dilly bag, connected by unbreakable strings to our mother and carrying our children for generations past and generations to come.

(Jazlie Davis, Birrbay, Dhanggati)

Dance for me is like a movie of the Country. It's the perfect way to articulate Lore. It's born directly from and belongs to Country like a fingerprint. Dance incorporates story, language, responsibility, obligation and how we need to interact with the world. It gives me purpose and lets me know exactly where I sit within time and place. When I know my dance, I know my Country. Knowing my Country is what makes me whole.

(Tom Flanders, Gomeroi, Gumbayngirr, Bunjalung)

Cultural dance practice has given me sense of identity, belonging and connection. I have witnessed young Aboriginal people literally transform from shy and withdrawn individuals to confident and proud people through cultural dance.

(Den Barber, Wiradjuri)

Being able to dance and live my culture gives me purpose, to learn, share and pass on to my babies, the next generation. When I dance ,I feel connected to my ancestors, which grounds me and gives me strength to draw on when I need it in difficult times.

(Sara Hooper, Biripi)

For me, traditional dance plays a central role in the maintenance of my mental health and wellbeing. It is not just the dancing alone, but the whole experience of cultural practice that surrounds the dancing. The preparation, mindset and learning is all part of the lead up to activating dances we have been taught that were handed down to us by our teachers along with millennia old creation stories. The cultural practice of going bush and learning these stories, the symbology associated with our ochre paint up and action of dancing in unison with our cultural brothers, in front of our Elders, is such a special feeling it really is hard to put into words. The whole experience is grounding. Physically, mentally, and spiritually. When we dance, we are not 'performing' but 'enacting' our cultural practice. We are not performing for an audience; we are dancing for our mother and for each other. This cultural practice is part of switching off the head noise of town and work life and connecting with our ancestors. When we dance, we connect to a practice as old as time itself. We go bush, and we disconnect to connect. This is the most valuable reset for mind, body, and soul.

(Robert Kelly, Yirandali, Ngati Maru)

Conclusion

Connection to land, spirituality and ancestry, kinship networks, and cultural continuity are commonly identified by Aboriginal people as important health protecting factors. These are said to serve as sources of resilience and as a unique reservoir of strength and recovery when faced with adversity, and can compensate for, and mitigate against, the impact of stressful circumstances on the social and emotional wellbeing of individuals, families, and communities (Zubrick et al. 2014, p.104).

Kuthi – song and dance, may support wellbeing for Aboriginal people, however, it is essential that the dancers feel connected to the song through their own Kinship and in relationship with their Country. This is strengthened when the songs hold stories of Ancestors, morals, laws and ways of being and when we have access to land and waters and can perform our songs and dances on Country. For our wellbeing, Country and Kinship are the core components, and through song and dance, we are able to express this.

References

Atkinson, J. (2002) *Trauma Trails: Recreating Songlines, the Transgenerational Effects of Trauma in Indigenous Australia*, Spinifex Press, North Melbourne, VIC.

Australian Human Rights Commission (n.d.) *Aboriginal and Torres Strait Islanders: Australia's First Peoples*, Australian Human Rights Commission, Accessed: 12 May 2023, https://humanrights.gov.au/our-work/education/aboriginal-and-torres-strait-islanders-australias-first-peoples#:~:text=Since%20the%20colonisation%20of%20Australia,and%20denial%20of%20citizenship%20rights

Australian Institute of Health and Welfare (2017) *Australia's Welfare 2017: In Brief*, Australian Institute of Health and Welfare, Accessed: 4 January 2023, www.aihw.gov.au/reports/australias-welfare/australias-welfare-2017-in-brief/contents/indigenous-australians

Australian Institute of Health and Welfare (2022) *Determinants of Health for Indigenous Australians*, Australian Institute of Health and Welfare, Accessed: 4 January 2023, www.aihw.gov.au/reports/australias-health/social-determinants-and-indigenous-health

Australian Government Department of Education (2022) *Why is STEM Important?*, Australian Government Department of Education, Accessed: 21 December 2022, www.education.gov.au/australian-curriculum/national-stem-education-resources-toolkit/introductory-material-what-stem/why-stem-important.

Australians Together (2019) *Why are Culture and Identity Important?* Australians Together, Accessed: 10 March 2020, https://australianstogether.org.au/discover/indigenous-culture/culture-identity/.

Bracknell, C. (2019) 'Connecting Indigenous song archives to kin, country and language', *Journal of Colonialism and Colonial History*, vol. 20(2), https://doi.org/10.1353/cch.2019.0016.

Bracknell, C. (2020) 'Maya waabiny: Mobilising song archives to nourish an endangered language', *Humanities Australia*, no. 11, pp. 19–27.

Burke, P. (1967) Australian Institute of Aboriginal and Torres Strait Islander Studies, archive recording, call number GORDON_J02.

Callaghan, P. (2022) Marruma ginyaang ngurra ngarra' (creating a better place through knowing), PhD thesis, University of New England, Armidale.

Callaghan, P. and Gordon, P. (2022) *The Dreaming Path*, Pantera Press, Neutral Bay, NSW.

Corn, A. and Gumbula, J. (2007) 'Budutthun ratja wiyinymirri: Formal flexibility in the Yolngu Manikay tradition and the challenge of recording a complete repertoire', *Australian Aboriginal Studies*, no. 2, pp. 116–127.

Corn, A. and Curkpatrick, S. (2014) 'Singing the winds of change: Ethnomusicology and the generation of new collaborative contexts for the teaching of Warlpiri knowledge across generations and vultures', In Barney, K. (ed). *Collaborative Ethnomusicology: New Approaches to Music Research between Indigenous and Non-Indigenous Australians*, Lyrebird Press, Melbourne.

Dondors, Y. (2012) 'Old cultures never die: Cultural genocide in International Law', In Ineke Boerefyn et al. (eds). *Human Rights and Conflict, Essays in Honour of Bas de Gaay Fortman*, Cambridge, Intersentia Publishing, pp. 290–291.

Feeney, M. (2009) Reclaiming the spirit of well being: promising healing practices for Aboriginal and Torres Strait Islander people. The Stolen Generations Alliance, Canberra. https://earlytraumagrief.anu.edu.au/files/Feeney_HealingDiscussionPaper_2009-1.pdf

Gardiner, J. (1999) *From Dispossession to Reconciliation*, Parliament of Australia, Accessed: 28 January 2022, www.aph.gov.au/About_Parliament/Parliamentary_Departments/Parliamentary_Library/pubs/rp/rp9899/99Rp27

Gummow, M. (2002) 'Yawahr: A corroboree for everybody', *Musicology Australia*, vol. 25(1), pp. 48–75, DOI: 10.1080/08145857.2002.10415994

Harris, J. (2003) 'Hiding the bodies: The myth of the humane colonisation of Australia', *Aboriginal History Journal*, vol. 27, pp. 79–104.

Hodgetts, J. (2020) 'Yama Karra Paay? When is it going to rain? The regrowth and renewal of old Ngiyampaa and Wiradjuri songs to empower the cultural identity of Ngiyampaa and Wiradjuri people of New South Wales Today', *Musicology Australia*, 42(2), pp. 108–122.

Jensen, A. (2001) *Arts with the Brain in Mind*, Association for Supervision and Curriculum Development, Alexandria, Virginia.

Johnson, S. (1971–1972) Australian Institute of Aboriginal and Torres Strait Islander Studies [archive recording], Items 002815C and 002816D, Call number DONALDSON_T01.

Johnson, S. (1973–1975) Australian Institute of Aboriginal and Torres Strait Islander Studies [archive recording], Items 003898B and 003899A, Call number DONALDSON_T02.

Koch, G. (2013) 'We have the song, so we have the land: song and ceremony as proof of ownership in Aboriginal and Torres Strait Islander land claims', AIATSIS Research Discussion Paper no. 33, AIATSIS Research Publications, Canberra.

Laird, K., Vergeer, I., Hennelly, S. and Siddarth, P. (2021, August) 'Conscious dance: Perceived benefits and psychological well-being of participants', *Complementary Therapies in Clinical Practice*, vol. 44, 101440. Accessed: 24 December 2022, https://radar.brookes.ac.uk/radar/file/9e94163d-40c8-4705-9d9a-439fe6d254ac/1/Conscious%20dance%20-%202021%20-%20Laird%20Vergeer%20Hennelly%20Siddarth.pdf

Murray, N. (2021) 'Australia's First Nations people need healing – of our families, our lands and our waters', *The Guardian*, Accessed: 4 January 2023, www.theguardian.com/commentisfree/2021/jul/08/australias-first-nations-people-need-healing-of-our-families-our-lands-and-waters

The Healing Foundation (2023) *Community Healing*, Accessed: 4 January 2023, https://healingfoundation.org.au/community-healing/#:~:text=For%20Aboriginal%20and%20Torres%20Strait,to%20culture%2C%20family%20and%20land

Treloyn, S. & Martin, M. (2012) 'Australia's endangered song traditions', Paper presented at the Music, Mind and Wellbeing Public Seminar Series, Accessed: 19 March 2013, www.melbournerecital.com.au/podcasts

Victoria Department of Health (2022) *Dance – Health Benefits*, Better Health Channel, Accessed: 11 May 2023, www.betterhealth.vic.gov.au/health/healthyliving/dance-health-benefits

Working with Indigenous Australian First Nations People (2020) *The Law and the Lore*, Working with Indigenous Australians First Nations People, Accessed: 20 December 2022, www.workingwithindigenousaustralians.info/content/Culture_4_The_Law_and_the_Lore.html

Zubrick, S., Shepherd, C., Dudgeon, P., Gee, G., Paradies, Y., Scrine, C., and Walker, R. (2014) *Working Together: Aboriginal Torres Strait Islander Mental Health and Wellbeing Principles and Practice*, 2nd edn, Department of Prime Minister and Cabinet, Canberra.

24 Caring through circulation

Reflections on affect and materiality at the second-hand book market of College Street, Calcutta

Diti Bhattacharya

Introduction

I have been a regular of the boipara for about thirteen years since my university days. At that time, it was more about my keen interest in scouting for rare second-hand books. Now I just like coming into the market every now and then, once in a few weeks' time. I do not buy as many books as before, I just like coming back here – chatting with some of my book seller friends, walk around the lanes and by-lanes. The books here are different to new books that you can buy at a regular bookshop – they carry memories, stories, hope and care – its unique to this place – where we see ourselves surrounded by second-hand books. It is the multiple circulation of the books, with scribbles, notes on the margins, folded pages from its many owners that creates a sort of unspoken friendship between us – strangers in real world but friends through our shared ownership of the book across temporalities. (can you cite your study here, either thesis or publication?) (Interview from doctoral thesis, September, 2016)

Vineeta, the respondent of the above excerpt, is a regular of the *boipara* for the last thirteen years. A mechanical engineer by profession, she shares in her extended interview how the second-hand books taught her how to read for pleasure and not for academic advancements. She notes how imagining the reading experiences of previous owners through the notes and scribbles made the process enjoyable, through a sense of curiosity. Her observations point towards a continual process that has enabled the *boipara* to become a space of sustainability but also emotional refuge; of kinship and care; of curiosity and scholarship.

Philips, Evans and Muirhead (2015, p. 2340) note that even though geographies of health have established important relationship between place, placemaking and well-being, there is further scope of research that examines the processes and practices that enables achieving a sense of being well within space. Atkinson suggests that 'a movement away from a focus on wellbeing as an outcome to think instead of wellbeing as process; and a concurrent shift in understanding of place as more than simply physical location or material setting but as "profoundly relational"' (Atkinson et al., 2012, p. 7). Situating this research within these lines of thinking, this chapter focuses on the materialities and immaterialities of second-hand books in the *boipara*.

The *boipara* is a kilometre and a half long stretch of College Street in the northern part of the city of Calcutta (now known as *Kolkata*). This precinct is comprised of an extensive series of makeshift book stalls and book shops stretching in different directions.

DOI: 10.4324/9781003345725-27

In addition, the area has a cluster of Calcutta's major and small-scale publishing houses; new and established bookstores; a coffee house which has retained the name 'the Albert Hall' since the British era; the prestigious Presidency College (now a university); Calcutta University; Sanskrit College; Hare School; and Hindu School. College Street is justifiably regarded as the educational and literary quarter of the city. For an extensive period in the past a breeding ground for leftist, progressive intellectual life, and consciously ideological, aggressive cultural, social and political practices, College Street today is still known as *the* space where art, culture, theatre, cinema, literature and other forms of creative expression thrive in Calcutta (Chakarborty, 1999; Bandyopadhay, 2011; Bose, 2013; Chatterjee, 2013).

Disrupting the attempt at spatial regulation that is colonial College Street is an aggregation of formal book shops, informal book stalls, formal printing and publishing houses, prominent educational institutions, the historically and politically significant Albert Hall coffee house as well as numerous shanty tea-stalls and other informal eateries. In material terms, an everyday regular thinks of the College Street *boipara* as a space where one establishes, experiences and practices certain relationships with certain things and their associated practices (Anderson and Wylie, 2009). Yet, this is a site in which the intersections between temporariness and permanence oscillate daily (Bhattacharya, 2023). For example, the physical positions of the books, the kettles, the bench, the motor scooter, in and around the makeshift stalls, although rearranging themselves daily, nevertheless make a regular appearance, in the same position on the footpath every day. In the everyday habits of sitting on the benches, tea-drinking and browsing among the books, the regulars of the space align themselves to the thingness hidden behind the garb of objects instead of simply using them. This is the kind of process through which the secret lives of objects make a final and irreversible transformation into things. The space invites certain habitual, romantic, and at times fleeting relationships with its materialities. For most regulars, such relationships are often with coffee tables, cigarettes, second handbooks, old diaries, yellow musty pages of someone's university notes, and the ever-the-same and ever-mobile character of the bookstalls (Chattopadhay, 2005; Das, 2013). Even though the regulars change over time, the affective, sensorial movements that people experience when they become a part of the space remains an apparent constant. In this sense there an affective atmosphere created by mobile negotiations between objects, things and subjects (Anderson and Wylie, 2009).

On caring and materialities

The reflections on this chapter are drawn from my doctoral research project that examined spatial movements of the second-hand book market in Kolkata, India. The research examined the spaceusing personal experience and extensive interviews of fifty book stall owners over three years, attending to movements between the material, the sensory and the human, and between experience, memory and imagination. In undertaking this project, this research reconsidered the ways in which affective attachments can be reimagined through reuse and sustainability through material entanglements with second-hand materials. This is intended to initiate a conversation about the value of thinking of intangible experiences of spaces of heritage through these sensorial registers. This work is centrally focused on experiencing the *boipara* as a cultural practice, rather than revisiting a cultural idea.

This particular chapter takes inspiration from Middleton and Sammanani in noting that 'care' as a framework or a 'normative ideal, rather thtan an ethos for doing geographical research more generally' (2021: 30). However, the political potential of care lies in catalyse to impart a sense of wellbeing and kinship within spaces of collective participation and community building as a process. In the excerpt used in this chapter, for example, the respondent notes that ways in which she gravitated to the second-hand book market – even when she was not buying books as regularly as she did before. She reflects on her desire to '*chat*' to relive the connections that she had made over the years with '*book seller friends, walk around the lanes and by-lane*'. For her, the boipra is a 'landscape of care' and in the process 'landscape of wellbeing' (Williams, 2007; Duff, 2011). The nature of marketplaces like that of the *boipara* is continually mobilised through their perpetual circulation of books but more important of affective energies of care – through memories of tactile and sonic interactions with the materialities of the books, the conversations in tea-stalls and the bypassing traffic (Bhattacharya, 2023).

Developing their ideas from health geography, Milligan and Wiles (2020) invite us to think of care as a networked landscape. In distinguishing between the practical idea of 'care for' and the emotional aspect of 'caring about' they centre how 'geographers ought to pay greater attention to how these two forms of care are distributed, supported, and governed' (Lawson, 2007; Milligan and Wiles, 2010). Landscapes of care are created by weaving in not only material space but also emotional registers of the space 'with each form of spatiality producing new relationships between the up-close, interpersonal experience of care and the broader ideological frameworks and public policies that shape this experience' (Middleton and Samanani, 2021, p. 31). They emerge because of spatial engagement with realities that come to verge on the mythic through nostalgia, memory and desire as a productive connection with anticipated futures.

Observational research formed a central aspect of my research methodology, which was conducted in various phases over three years. The *boipara* is marked by circulation, change, to-ing and fro-ing of bodies and books. People daily come to the *boipara* to buy second-hand books and bring other books for reselling. Those who buy books take them back to their home, make them part of their own lives. They use the books in diverse ways in their personal contexts. They read them, scribble on them, make notes in the margins, put in chits of paper as bookmarks and as notes to self for study or remembrance, and sometimes, much to the dismay of the booksellers, they tear pages from them. After various periods, they will probably return books to the *boipara* for further use and circulation. Similarly, the contents of the book stalls change regularly. As the existing second-hand supply goes out, batches of other second-hand books with their notes and other supplements come in. They are rarely placed in the same order in the stalls: they are put in different piles, on different racks and are produced for customers in new contexts and for new and different needs. In their unpacking each morning and packing away each night, the books daily experience 'mobile-spatial encounters' (Barry 2016). Similarly, the stalls themselves change. The yellow and blue paint with which many of their tin walls are painted needs to be renewed now and then. Some stalls are whitewashed. Some book sellers like to have wooden stools and chairs in their stalls, some simply sit on a pile of books. The booksellers often have other random materials and objects, or as they call them, tools that help to change the boundaries of their stalls. For example, sometimes they will use bamboo sticks and plastic sheets to extend a stall's perimeter. This usually happens at those times of the year when the buying and selling frequency is higher than usual – at the beginning and end of the academic year, or a new term, for instance. Sometimes they make these changes because of the weather, as described earlier.

The stalls are not used only to store and display the books, they are also for regulars to spend time in, an arrangement that meets a sentiment and understanding shared by booksellers and buyers. Thus, the booksellers are continually organising and rearranging the interiors of their stalls to make them more usable. Similarly, the customers do not merely come, collect their books and leave. They spend time, browsing, chatting with the stall owner and other customers, drinking tea, and clearly creating an experience for themselves. For the booksellers, how they experience the customers experiencing their stalls changes with each of the changes they make in the structural layout, the positioning of a stool or bench and the arrangements of books. Taken together, the book stalls, the neighbouring eateries, the shanty tea-stalls, the outer edges of the walls of the universities and other buildings, the railings along the footpaths seem to express a shared spatial understanding. It is as if no-one ever has to stop and think about whether they are encroaching on someone else's space. For example, the tea-stall owner never complains about a customer who always sits and reads the daily newspaper or books from a neighbouring stall in his meagrely sized space. Similarly, it is completely against the culture of the coffee house to ask someone to leave on account of their having spent too much time occupying a table. There are no formal rules to how the space should be used; but there are deep-rooted tacit agreements, affective understandings, emotional investments and conscious actions always in play about how the spatiality of the *boipara* is created and recreated. It is a vernacular understanding and production of spatiality grounded in practice, repetition and difference that creates a unique 'atmospheric' environment (Ray, 2015; Mazumdar, 2015).

My visits to the *boipara* as a student, as a graduate and as part of this fieldwork, often involved remembering the space: recollection of stories, anecdotes, events, moments – some of it had happened and some of it was imagination. The act of remembering is not just bringing the memory of the past into the present. It involves a close knitting of the imagined and the actual, both experienced in the past. Donald observes, 'notoriously, the vivid events recalled from childhood may or may not have taken place, and yet the reworking of the past plays a crucial role in our sense of who we are' (1999, p. 184). The affective resonances experienced during my first few visits as a college student were a combination of what was anticipated the *boipara* to be like before and re-imaginings of the multiple stories, anecdotes about it. This contributed a sort of creation of impressions and events to my imagination, bringing into my imaginary life recollections of moments that I may not have actually lived in that past time but had regularly shared through *their* storytelling and *their* lived experiences. There is also a very strong material connection – I have often reflected on why it was important for me to explore the book stall to which my *Dadu* (grandfather in Bengali) sold my second-hand books when I was at school. It was almost as if a part of my then self-had made the visits to those book stalls and to the *boipara* in general. My later actual visits were thus mediated through a series of affective, mobile flows of memories, material associations and cultural, political and social associations I had developed with it through the stories I had been told and the histories I came across. That is, each time the space is engaged in a process of reworking that add multiple layers to the fabric of the space through the actual presence of, my affective imaginings, family history, collective memories, written histories and numerous other trajectories of sensorial, intellectual, creative and material experiences.

The *boipara* involves ongoing emergences from the *milieu* (here, the middle, the in-between) of material, sensory and narrative elements. This, in turn, can impel a sense of the coming together of segments of space-time (as collisions, occasional contacts or flows) which can produce vectors that take off in all kinds of directions; have the potential to produce different speeds and intensities; and are likely to become implicated in the rhizomics of the *boipara*, which will probably be part of the assemblages that constitute it.

Conclusion

This chapter draws attention to the value of transdisciplinary, flexible and open ways of creating and occupying spaces that have a positive value in collective wellbeing. In exploring the characteristics and stories of the spatiality of the *boipara*, the chapter explores how complex temporal, material and socio-cultural relations between the books and the bookstalls can provide healing, kinship and joy through a shared collective experience. Books that find their way to the *boipara*, and spend years coming and going, to and from it, become, in a sense, hyper-capable of fulfilling these functions of '*the* book'. The capacity of books to form emotional attachments 'with the world' is intensified and re-intensified again and again by the *boipara* itself, the stall owners, their customers, the *adda*, the additions to the books that accumulate over time as a result of the books' movements through many spaces and many hands, and so on. The sense of intensity is surely part of the appeal of the *boipara*, its 'special' atmosphere, its role in cultural and political transformations.

I suggest that these can help us to consider the ongoing production and reproduction, occupation and narrativisation, valuing and revaluing of spaces without over-reliance on particular theories of spatial representation and conceptualisation developed in particular disciplinary contexts. I wanted to attend to the relational nature of all space – a perspective on 'space as a product of interrelations' (Massey, 2005, p. 9). Through my focus on the spatiality of the *boipara* the chapter focuses on how spatial relations can be revealed, reimagined, unfolded, and appreciated for their complexities. Relationality therefore is central to paying attention to the unique and differential experiences of the regulars of the space. In particular, it is an argument for how the kinds of approaches and processes can provide particularly nuanced and insightful engagements with spaces and spatiality. It points towards a mode of dealing with the multiplicities of spaces as complex and dynamic as the *boipara* in ways that avoid reductive or over-simplifying 'readings' and instead enable the spatiality of the area to reveal itself, with a greater degree of resistance to disciplinary, political, social or cultural preconceptions than might be made available by other approaches.

The wider research focuses on exploring, through the writing of it, different ways of opening out our thinking about spaces, between the human and the material through affordances of care. One of several ways of approaching this is to think of spatial relations in terms of conversations open between concepts and practice; between the stories that emerge from landscapes of care and wellbeing. Centring care and wellbeing with the material and the human then becomes an enabler or catalyst for further imaginary engagements (and not simply a representational practice). The second-hand book market provide a sense of calm, comfort through collective and individual and intimate revisiting of past memories – it is these moments that provide a sense of wellbeing and emotional safety. One of the foundational tenents of geographical research is the idea that places affect people – markets with complex materialities like that of second-hand books intensifies these affects in bringing back the regulars of space. The messy temporalities, multiple trajectories, heterogeneous components and crisscrossing flows and strata of histories, affects and memories create a place of warmth – the spatial energy that generates in and emanates from the *boipara* when the stories-so-far (Massey 2005) of this space meet the stories that the space is producing and can potentially produce.

References

Anderson, B. and Wylie, J., 2009. On geography and materiality. *Environment and Planning A*, *41*(2), pp. 318–335. doi:10.1068/a3940

Atkinson, S., 2013. Beyond components of wellbeing: The effects of relational and situated assemblage. *Topoi*, *32*, pp. 137–144.

Atkinson, S., Fuller, S., and Painter, J., 2012. Wellbeing and place, in S. Atkinson, S. Fuller and J. Painter (Eds.), *Wellbeing and Place* (pp. 1–14), Ashgate, Farnham.

Bandhyopadhay, R., 2011. Politics of archiving: hawkers and pavement dwellers in Calcutta. *Dialectical Anthropology*, *35*(3), pp. 295–316.

Barry, K., 2016. Packing as practice: Creative knowledges through material interactions. *Tourism Analysis*, *21*(4), pp. 403–415.

Bhattacharya, D., 2023. *Unfolding Spatial Movements in the Second-Hand Book Market in Kolkata: Notes on the Margins in the Boipara*, Taylor & Francis.

Bose, D., 2013. College street, in S. Chaudhuri (ed.), *Calcutta: The Living City: Volume II: The Present and Future*, Oxford University Press, New Delhi.

Chakraborty, D., 1999. Adda, Calcutta: Dwelling in modernity. *Public Culture*, *11*(1), pp. 109–145.

Chatterjee, P., 2013. The political culture of Calcutta, in S. Chaudhuri (ed.), *Calcutta: The Living City: Volume II: The Present and Future*, Oxford University Press, New Delhi.

Chattopadhyay, S., 2005. *Representing Calcutta: Modernitiy, Nationalism and the Colonial Uncanny*, Routledge, London and New York.

Das, S., 2013. The politics of agitation: Calcutta 1912–1947, in S. Chaudhuri (ed.), *Calcutta: The Living City: Volume II: The Present and Future*, Oxford University Press, New Delhi.

Donald, J., 1997. This, here, now: Imagining the modern city, in S. Westwood and J. Williams (eds.), *Imagining Cities: Scripts, Signs, Memory*, Routledge, London and New York.

Duff, C., 2011. Networks, resources and agencies: On the character and production of enabling places. *Health & Place*, *17*(1), pp. 149–156 doi: 10.1016/j.healthplace.2010.09.012

Lawson, V., 2007. Geographies of care and responsibility. *Annals of the Association of American Geographers*, *97*, pp.1–11.

Massey, D., 2005. *for space*, SAGE, London.

Mazumdar, A., 2013. Barnaparichoy: A mall in progress, a street in transition. *Subversions*, *1*(1), pp. 122–145.

Middleton, J. and Samanani, F., 2021. Accounting for care within human geography. *Transactions of the Institute of British Geographers*, *46*(1), pp. 29–43. doi:10.1111/tran.12403

Milligan, C. and Wiles, J., 2010. Landscapes of care. *Progress in Human Geography*, *34*(6), pp. 736–754.

Phillips, R., Evans, B. and Muirhead, S., 2015. Curiosity, place and wellbeing: Encouraging place-specific curiosity as a 'way to wellbeing'. *Environment and Planning A*, *47*(11), pp. 2339–2354. doi: 10.1177/0308518X15599294

Ray, P., 2013. The Calcutta adda, in S. Chaudhuri (ed.), *Calcutta: The Living City: Volume II: The Present and Future*, Oxford University Press, New Delhi.

Roy, A., 2014. Reading spaces: Calcutta's daftaripara, in N. Gupta (ed.), *Strangely Beloved: Writings on Calcutta*, Rupa Publications, New Delhi.

Williams, A., ed., 2017. *Therapeutic Landscapes*. Routledge, London.

25 Bajo el Olivo (Under the Olive Tree)

Experimenting with a posthuman life and landscape with radical affection in an artist residency

Juliana España Keller

Inception

This chapter is designed to foster the theoretical and creative ways that an artist residency is intra-connected with a situated perspective: one that flourishes as a transversal site for artistic events; building resilience in ecological continuity, local community building and social engagement. Most importantly, bringing other forms of life into a creative proposition suggesting that we have become 'post human', since our mode of being is dependent on complex entanglements with multi-species, ecosystems, and technology.

Visiting guest residents are creative protagonists contributing to the artistic, philosophical, methodological, and sociocultural matter that takes place in a transformative site for creative practice. This method of thinking suggests that (re)working the relational thought of working with other(s) in performative fieldwork can produce unexpected ruptures in dominant thinking about nature and culture. In our post-pandemic future, to walk mindfully is to converse with 'vital matter' as American theorist and Author, Jane Bennett proposes (Bennett, 2010). In its emergent growth, the vitality of the artist residency is rooted in a circular relationship for the practice of research-creation artworks where artists are using the residency as a speculative thinking space for practice-led research merging with a 'slow' infrastructure – in the doing and making of artwork; inclusive of how humans can slow-ly listen and relate with the articulations of nonhuman beings and living systems in a complex, interdependent world.

Thus, the projects and processes amplify both the tangible and the intangible qualities of a post-pandemic spatial experience by listening to the mind-body relation reaching for and extending out across the geographical and epistemological conditions of our current terrain. What is meaningful here are the radical diverse approaches for tender acts of individual and collective imagination through which new forms of caring and resilience might emerge. The residency engages in a slow-ness that integrates a range of scales, tempos, and durations to open pathways toward deep listening, learning or even unlearning.

The (post)colonial logics of speed and convenience are also manifest in much of the art world creating ease for some and harm for others in a hierarchal, elitist infrastructure. Many of the environmental crises that we are now entangled with require a 'slowing down' to grasp the notion of labour. For example, from a creative perspective, the performative act of practicing the context of "working from the gut", the process of 'slow' metabolism opens possibilities that consider an attunement to the earth as rather

DOI: 10.4324/9781003345725-28

a relation of 'co-composing' with the more-than human. This could reflect on how our relationship with other forms of life can be (re)configured and accountable as a site of transformative potential for creative practitioners through direct engagement with the earth, community – the contact with local artists, artisans, gardeners, beekeepers, farmers where storytelling in time, space mattering and the future architecture of "home" as a refuge is a becoming that enforces a (re)imagining that is rooted in participatory art practices (Springgay, 2022).

Artists that become a part of this residency can intra-sect and converge with deep ecologies that are relational to the concerns of a rapidly changing environment, shrinking natural resources and the realities of climate action. Far from perfect, this refuge is not immune to the rest of the world. This small parcel of land is being used to experiment, create, explore and share stories for a future world; to imagine posthuman futures and critically challenge pre-existing structures of thought where complex assemblages of matter exist and intra-act to challenge the discordant systems of city life and the dynamics in which we are currently entangled in.

From an ecofeminist position, art and the natural environment can create a participatory collective model or working with, rather than, working for. This method of collaboration forms a transdisciplinary perspective inhabited by varied and vibrant forms of matter and like-minded intersectional practitioners and thinkers in a dialogical exchange. In turn, environmental activism, which advocates for a world with biodiversity, avoiding toxic impacts, can be adopted as an underlying ethos to transdisciplinary and intersectional approaches within the fields of visual arts, the critical humanities and other hybrid media practices. For example, weaving queer studies and disability studies into self-guided explorations can render bodies in flow in nature, by model in relation to disability culture or queering space as a sensitivity to living in a shared world, oriented toward more socially just futures (Kuppers, 2022).

Key concepts

In this section of the chapter, key words are defined for the reader that are frequently mentioned in this critical text. In addition, there are key concepts that shape and sustain the theoretical nature of this chapter to expand on the essential qualities of each section as follows: (1) an artistic residency is an opportunity for change as it opens up possibilities for processes of ecological reparation and mental health and well-being. (2) a posthumanist approach is necessary for exploring the interplay between ontologically diverse entities in these reparatory processes – that which relates to the branch of metaphysics dealing with the nature of being in the world; and (3) there are theoretical and methodological challenges to practicing a post-human approach to repairing ecologies and "Affect" theory plays an important role to culture, history, and politics that addresses nonlinguistic forces, or affects.

"Affect" as a conscious subjective aspect of feeling or emotion that makes us what we are, but affects are neither under our "conscious" control nor even necessarily within our awareness – and they can only sometimes be captured in language (Seigworth, 2011). According to French philosopher, Gilles Deleuze and his reading of the critical texts of Dutch philosopher, Baruch Spinoza (Benedict de Spinoza), the mode (or affection, or intensity), is a state, and the affect is a passage or transition from one state to another. This is why Deleuze and French philosopher, Felix Guattari attribute *affects* as *becomings* (Deleuze and Guattari, 1988).

These key concepts come into view through a 'post-humanist' perspective, taking full consideration of the all non-human agencies that are a result of the on-going industrial extraction shaping the world. "Agency" identifies with a common sense of something that refers to the relationality of a political, cultural position that and by which matter and things are defined, distributed, and organised. For feminist practitioners, agency points towards how matter and things can be imagined; in new forms, or in ways that are different to the patriarchal structures of the world with a focus on the agency that *engenders* other ways of being. Consequently, this concept of agency spills over into human relations with mental health and well-being.

Simultaneously, the dire ecological outlook is also of essence to the mental health and wellbeing of the planet as a whole. Humans have set in motion a "sixth mass extinction" that may one day be our undoing. This is defined as a consequence of human-created global warming and ocean acidification, the destruction and fragmentation of forests, and our spread of invasive species around the world according to American journalist, Elisabeth Kolbert (Kolbert, 2014). What's more, these actions will determine the course of life on the planet long after our species is gone.

Agency is also conjured here through geographical space and place as the becoming of the human–non-human relationship. By resonating with agency, the residency at *Bajo el Olivo* is experiential and is intensely experienced as *creating together*, foregrounding a way to move forward in our creative processes and into our posthuman future. As Bennett writes: "Ecology can be defined as the study or story of the place where live, or better, the place that we live…that place is a dynamic flow of matter-energy that tends to settle into various bodies that often join forces, make connections, form alliances" (Bennett, 2010, p. 365). Therfore, an "Ecophilosophy" moves us to understand that humans must radically change their relationship to nature from one that values nature solely for its usefulness to human beings to one that recognises that nature has an inherent value and its value can be inclusive as part of the artmaking process.

When discussing "more-than-human" natures are refered to as all entities that compose the understanding that humans *are also nature* and relationally constituted into an eco-philosophy. If holistic health is an approach to wellness that concurrently addresses the physical, mental, emotional, social, and spiritual components of health and well-being; it is also dependent on the relation to reparative situations that include other-than-human natures. This also points to exploring and understanding both radical ontological differences and the immanent as permanently pervading and sustaining the universe (Deleuze and Guattari, 1988). The expressions of these differences are embedded in the concept of "radical affection" in this critical text and proposes the given indeterminate character of many of the relations that produce them as French Philosopher, Édouard Glissant proposes (Glissant, 1997).

Multispecies investigations of social and cultural phenomena are attentive to the agency of other-than-human species, whether they are plants, animals, fungi, bacteria, or even viruses, which confound the species concept (Kirksey, 2014). The platform of this artistic residency not only acknowledges that humans dwell in a world comprising of other life forms but also opens up the potential of how they are entangled with human lives, landscapes, and technologies and must be theoretically integrated into any account of existence. Thereby, the experimental artwork produced in the residency is mutual and reciprocal. This deeply textual analysis is not centered on explaining how crises are produced, but on understanding what they produce, mainly in their dimension of ecological and creative reparation guided towards mental health and wellbeing.

The notion of "assemblages" flourishes in situated forms and creative practices of reparation so as to manifest a (re)composition of life. The concept of assemblage is key to the ecologies of repair to provide theoretical reflections on recent processes of intense damage or affectation that seek to rebuild our mental spirit and wellbeing. Here, "reparation" is understood broadly as open-ended actions, practices, and modes of amendment of what is seen or felt as broken. It is within this process of "care" where life emerges with creative intensity despite destruction and ecological damage; to conceptually explore the ways in which we, as artists, in contexts of socio-environmental conflict or crisis, relate to nature, seeking to repair the damage provoked by the effects of a dying planet.

In writing this chapter, post-humanist and new materialist thinking are explored so that they can be put to work in order to (re)imagine a more open perspective in approaching and pursuing artist residency practices with fluidity, flux, expansion and understanding of difference. This may be regarded as performative cross-platform phenomenon where humanity is something that needs more humanising as we move forward to challenging times ahead, where participation is risky and where research-creation can be contextualised performatively as co-constructed. In this way, human–non-humans, actions, or events are defined by their relations and function as part of an assemblage that is concerned with processual work and self-transformation.

Thereby, human–non-human "intra-actions" are made apparent due to the doing of the action by the subject, paraphrasing American philosopher, Karen Barad, being the context of the work; this makes the effects of the action relational in the real world (Barad, 2003). Intra-action should not be confused with 'interaction', where elements exist first and then interact. Instead, an intra-action conceptualises that it is the action between (and not in-between) that which matters; it is in the action that the elements themselves are produced interdependently.

"Nomadic thought" is a concept used to describe ideas and identities that exist outside established frameworks or hierarchical categorisations, and are in a state of perpetual fluctuation as defined by Australian scholar and philosopher, Rosi Braidotti. (Braidotti, 2011). It is in (re)configuring our mental health and well being in relationship with the world that is often not a direct, elementary trajectory; it can entail messy and disquieting encounters, which embrace the indeterminate and manifest through negotiation and contradicting emotions as we seek a way forward.

Relationally, feminist power relations are also rooted in eco-feminism and are located within the live enactment or research-creative processes. Therefore, affirmative ethics are part of this notion that are defined as a relational matter of human and non-human powers of acting in pursuit of affirmative values. Affirmative ethics focuses on relations, forces and affects as described by Braidotti (Braidotti, 2019). In contributing to social change, activating a feminist ethico-politic must fundamentally emerge from work done at the transformative, energetic layer of the body, activated by doing-making processes in nurturing moments of connection and movement. Cooking. Playing. Making art. Resting. Working. Sharing touch. Sharing food. Gathering to remember. Growing up. Growing old. Grieving loss and oppression. Resisting. Empowering humans. Performing ritual after ritual as an affirmative politic in action. All of these processes (and more) could be seen to fall into the 'doing-making' constellation of performativity within a creative arts residency such as *Bajo el Olivo*.

To be clear, I also maintain and reiterate that as a feminist materialist, cultural space is not defined as around and between objects. It is considered already embedded in these objects (the human–non-human), spaces and things, as well as in "spacetimemattering" which is to define things and humans as consequently entangled with one another in complex and unexpected ways. We co-produce the world through *intra-actions* as Barad describes that are simultaneously material and discursive (Juelskjær and Schwennesen, 2012). Furthermore, what we take to be bounded entities are in fact complex phenomena that extend across time and space, in what Barad calls entanglements of 'spacetimemattering'— and this is where 'home' is a mutual relation of things and bodies.

(Re)newed speculation on 'home'

May the spring of a foreign river be your navel. May your soul be at home where there are no houses.

(Le Guin, 2016 p. 404)

'Home', has become a 'refuge' in our post-pandemic time and speaks to the future of human life, mental health, and wellbeing. The residency, *Bajo el Olivo* is situated on private land (2136 sqm) in the quiet annex of a mediterranean villa that houses three furnished guest rooms. *Casa Mia* is easily accessible by car and nestled in a small community on the outskirts of the pueblo (small village) of Alhaurín el Grande, inland from the city of Malaga.

This small parcel of land is a model of sustainability, and an exploration of non-exploitative methods of production to connect, to exchange, to consider traditional knowhow, sense, and insights as ways of understanding ecologically embedded perspectives on embodiment and create connections between embodiment, rural labour, and ecological sensibility.

The residency at *Bajo El Olivo* promotes deep listening to the earth and is situated as a 'becoming' by thinking with the ecologies of making kin (Haraway, 2016). What this mind body connection puts into motion is a speculative process that seeks the all-too-human desire to see concordance between two propositions – the desire, that we happen to occupy a privileged place within this spatial relation and two: the residency becomes an expanding network of users, collaborators and partners who come together to work on the land, share resources and local knowledge around a community economy. To keep it 'local' as an ecophilosophy is indicative to connecting the invisible majority where 'labour', whether artistic production in the studio or outside in nature, is a profound connection to the land (Guattari, 2005). How can we generate a (re)newed approach to creation, sustainability, and creative methods of artistic practice as a site of ecofeminist imaginative space-making and radical change? To (re) generate creative possibilities for emergent relational forces that are situated in rural places and where 'play' and 'thinking', 'doing' are working and possible (Thompson and Harney, 2018).

Where the meaning of entanglement meets the more-than-human

An affirmative ethic upholds that there is a way to bring farmers, scientists, creative artist/researchers, and even artisanal bakers together to connect to exchange processes as a transdisciplinary approach in a 'nomadic encounter', not a solution (Braidotti, 2011). Our sense of being in the world, and our sense of the natural world is motivated and made meaningful not merely by unconscious reaction and instinct, but by individually imagined and collectively produced symbolic structures, which is to say beliefs and

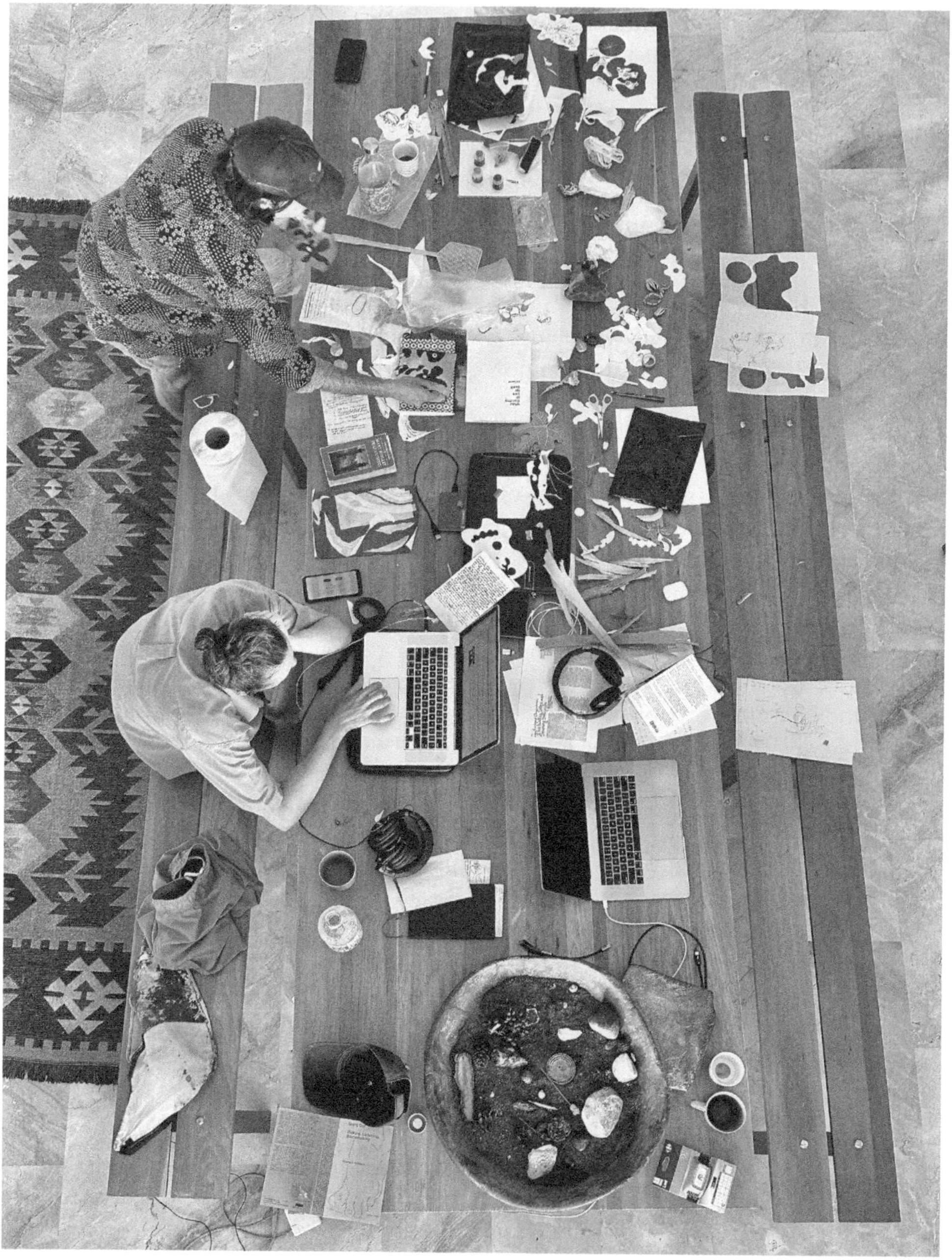

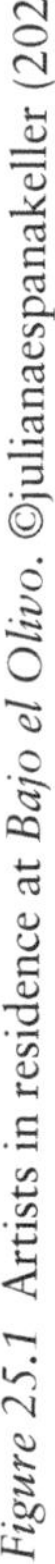

Figure 25.1 Artists in residence at *Bajo el Olivo*. ©julianaespanakeller (2022).

'more-than-human' stories between the earth and our bodies, indigenous knowledges, historicides weaving sensory data, feelings, and a desire to merge into a composite spatial, temporal, and social world that is entangled with micro-communities and the natural world.

By experimenting with different modes of storytelling, the human species is now exploring ways to being other species and ways of thinking into an interspecies relationship (Haraway, 2016). As Australian cultural anthropologist, Eben Kirksey asserts: "which beings flourish, and which fail, when natural cultural worlds intermingle and collide?" (Kirksey, 2014, p. 4). In this regard, the residency at *Bajo el Olivo* takes on a more cosmic point of view where our mutually constituted sense of the collective now – is changing into something else, perhaps no more or less than a new world, a new now, a different collective sense of human life (Bridle, 2022).

Our human dependence on environmental health and ecological diversity as a communitarian vision of small-scale non-hierarchical social organism such as an artist retreat offers, at such, a robust fiction as a strain of radical ecological thought in an environmentally attuned philosophy or deep ecology. Canadian scientist, Suzanne Simard proposes that the kind of stories we need to be telling propose a new way of communicating that the world desperately needs to hear. This becomes a reminder through an attuned philosopy to listen to our wilder selves, and to remember, with humility, how little we know of the complexities of the natural world (Simard, 2021).

In the book: "Ways of Being", writer and artist, James Bridle considers the fascinating, uncanny and multiple ways of existing on earth as a deep ecology (Bridle, 2022). What can we learn from other forms of intelligence and personhood, and how can we change our societies to live more equitably with one another and the non-human world? Bridle emphasises a radical new story about ecology, technology and intelligence. We must, he argues, expand our definition of these terms to build a meaningful and free relationship with the non-human, one based on solidarity and cognitive diversity since we have so much to learn, and many worlds to gain. To be become entangled in this proposition, American Theorist, Donna Haraway roots her co-existence with the human-non-human world as a "radical hope" (Haraway, 2016). In this critical context, *Bajo El Olivo* offers a timely approach of "radical affection" that is a commitment to a future existence and should be explored explicity, inclusive of mental health and wellbeing.

Embodying radical affection for mental health and wellbeing

At *Bajo el Olivo*, 'radical affection' can be expanded on as not necessarily beginning anywhere, in time, space, mattering, it can be thought of as present, mindful, and emergent and proposes a 'becoming', paraphrasing the American Quantum theorist and American philosopher, Karen Barad (Barad, 2007, p. 393). In addition, when Dutch Philosopher and Mystic, Baruch Spinoza speaks of "affections" in his "Book of Ethics", he is referring to modalities, or "that which exists in and through another; or that which is an affection (modification)" (Curley and Spinoza, 2020, pp. 85–87).

Thus, "radical affection" in this critical text is not urging one to press, to insist on hoping for (as a constant craving) or holding onto the perpetual axis of human exceptionalism, it is rather the proposition of a radical shift of focus that emerges from a key perspective of Indigenous praxis. One that springs forth from the key position that humans take care of the land and the spiritual world, and it will take care of us (Kimmerer, 2013).

In the midst of the nature/culture divide within the discourse of posthuman knowledge, humans are dependent on one another not just for mutual survival but also in experiencing joy, happiness, and wellbeing with an affirmative ethic (Braidotti, 2019). Moreover, this artist residency becomes a releasing of thoughts, in and through bodies in ways that support all of us in meeting the urgencies of our posthuman life – to decentre from binary belief systems, to release preconceptions, to start in the middle. When do our feet *feel* the ground beneath us to become rooted from the navel (In Chinese Eastern philosophy, the 'dantian' is a central core meridian to health and vitality) as Ursula K. Le Guin states in her book: "Always Coming Home" (Guin, 2016). The aim is to have the heart open, vision clear and actions that are grounded in the essence of our lower dantian – where we can strengthen our lower dantian to build and hold our Qi. Lower dantian breathing benefits us by helping us feel healthier, less stressed and happier according to Chinese medicine tradition and the practices of Tai Chi and Qi Gong. American musician and experimental composer, Pauline Oliveros was a Tai Chi and Qi Gong practitioner and has described in her *deep listening* workshops that by attuning to the mind body relationship; that by having a stronger core, proposes that you are less vulnerable to falling off balance (Oliveros, 2002). This means we can be physically, emotionally and mentally more stable if we allow for a healthier, more purposeful existence in that which radiates adventitiously and emerges elsewhere, unexpectedly in time (Oliveros, 2005).

Poetic resonance through quantum energies of co-composing with living matter

In that our conceptual bodies are porous as sentient beings, we are weaving stories by intra-acting with the flows and pulses of quantum energies (asserting that quantum phenomena govern health and wellbeing) and co-composing with matter of living and non-living forms, relations, human and the "more-than-human" as defined in the section on key concepts. It is in these entanglements (to create a place of connection) by thinking, knowing, feeling in space, time, matter. Proceeding slow-ly, in French philosopher, Édouard Glissant's book *Poetics of Relation* (Glissant, 1997) speaks to a dynamic form of gifting that operates beyond the confines of neo-capitalist logic – one that tries to support a balance between the economic growth, lower inflation, low levels of unemployment, good conditions of work, social assistance and good public services, across the intervention of the state in the economy.

Glissant asks us to bring forth an expanded unfolding, multitemporal, post-filial and posthuman approach to worlding. Glissant proposes that which finds expression in gestures of abundance, reciprocity and radiance through the opaque (opacité) is to enter into subtler and also more profound resonances within a vast field of planetary entanglements and multivalent expression (Glissant, 1997, p. 151).

In an affective framework (using Affect theory that seeks to organise affects, sometimes interchangeably with emotions or subjectively experienced feelings to typify their physiological, social, interpersonal, and internalised manifestations), bodies and spaces will be de-corporealised and (re)defined as molecular forces, intensities, capacities, and relationalities. What is fascinating is within the mind/body relation (paraphrasing French philosopher, Giles Deleuze and Dutch philosopher and mystic, Baruch Spinoza), to describe "affective cracks" of the conceptual human body, it can be argued, when stranded, withdrawn, disjunct, marginalised, are the substances of our sentient consciousness that lets attributes of the conceptual body fall away to become modes of the unfelt, the unprotected, and untended (Seigworth, 2011).

In simpler terms, it is as if a bird leaves the forest to never return. As humans, we do not notice the bird but only remember the bird song is not there anymore and has been disassociated from our field of perception. The conceptual body, is then rather entangled with sentient matter that is dimmed, drained, and exhausted, depleted and so in this instance, the relation to Glissant's concept of a 'poetic relation' is propositionally conducive to widen our liveable relations, to open up spaces to connect us to (re)enchantment, perhaps as offerings that shed light on how bodies and spaces can be (re)imagined and held together respectfully (Glissant, 1997). This emergence of a collective consciousness through relations of reciprocity, respect, and faith in each other and of our relations with everything human to non-human that surrounds us and gives us life as it proposes a (re) emergence of radical affection.

This radical contrast can carry multiple *felt* meanings which could translate as: love, compassion, mercy, sympathy, grace, charity, compassion, kindness, mercy, pity, charity (cite). An example that can illuminate our interconnection to the natural world is that different plant species find it possible to thrive together in nature in a wild celebration of life, relational to ways and practices in caretaking and kinship, as considerations of 'agency' are manifested within the landscape, despite the Anthropocene and on-going 'Sixth Extinction' (Kolbert, 2014). Through our entangled life, Glissant calls the post-postcolonial condition a life that we must all continue to strive for. For artists, it becomes a way of understanding connections that allows us to use the creative imagination to peer below the surface of human life, to imagine what is going on in our cells and below the soil, where tree roots and mycelium networks communicate. To think deeply, to suggest the intra-relation of a humans to galaxies, life and atoms and everything in between as if on a sound walk as we deep listen to the earth and sky and all its critters and creatures around us.

Creating a sensory, more-than-human world in an artist residency

Canadian Affect theorist, Brian Massumi puts forward the idea of "touching" as affecting and being affected by what a body can be or do and illustrates intra-textually the capacity to act and be acted upon. For Massumi, affect involves the transitions a body takes when it steps over a threshold and is a dimension of life enacted in such processes. Reading, writing, and creating in the world as sensory, intimate, and of the body is propositionally about intensities, moving toward the other, and being open to the "more-than" (Manning, 2013). In the *Bajo el Olivo* creative residency, guest residents are asked to propose how these concepts excite the senses which expand the body and its abilities, to exercise how we perform with each other and co-create on the earth.

Furthermore, Barad proposes that matter matters – it is both of substance and significance and views/sees matter and discourse as inextricably entangled (Barad, 2003). For Barad, matter is not passive and inert, but a lively participant in the world's becoming. In this way, radical entanglement for artists working out in the field, closer to nature; can explore how the experience of embodiment is embedded within the larger body of the earth through art works that sow seeds between somatic, performative, audio-visual, and intra-textual material ways of knowing in attuning to the human senses and the non-human world. This movement towards a deep ecology of thinking can include the sentient presence of food production and food security – the creative baking and breaking of bread collectively, to gut metabolism (working from the gut), and other nonhuman ecologies of nature such as collaborative beekeeping and co-producing honey as food.

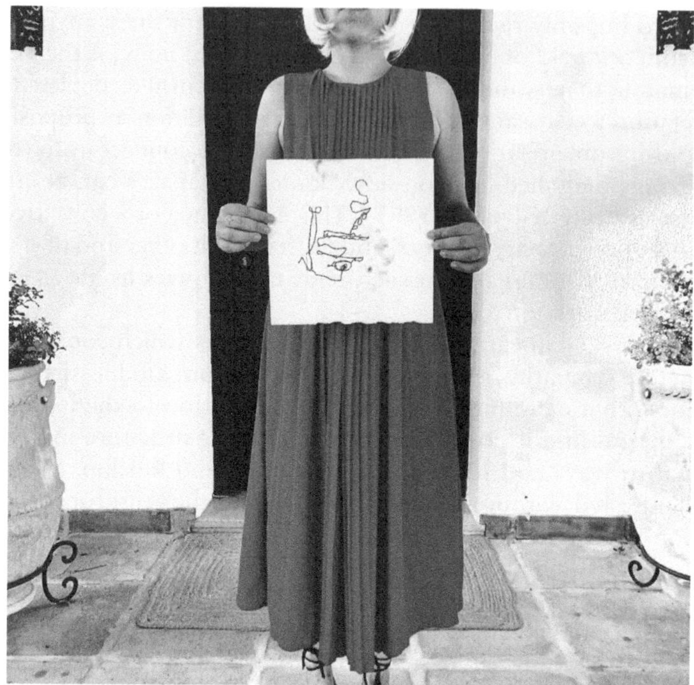

Figure 25.2 Working from the gut. A "gut metabolism" drawing exercise with a local Spanish artist. ©julianaespanakeller (2022).

Thus the interconnected ecosystems of the biosphere to networked biological processes at the microscopic level links ideas and energies with infinite signals rippling and resonating to come together in new ways. The residency seeks artist propositions that document and articulate the shifts of perception unfolding in space and place to attune our human senses to the sentient presence of the topography of the land, colonial histories, traditions, rituals, weather patterns, soil, food practices, food production, food security, manual labour, women's labour, and the many other nonhuman living systems within this assemblage of performative activisms and choreographies. In a performative and somatic sense, mental health and wellbeing, comes from a place in the body that is so deep, that making art as a form of healing does not create a kind of abstraction as an escape from reality. It is more about movement and bringing things to their essence and creating art projects that have a multitude of dimensions (Kuppers, 2022). The aim here is to respond to the times we are living in and helps artists define, organise and make sustainable goals and priorities visible.

Conclusion

This chapter reveals many related theoretical concepts that are integrated in order to give account to a slow-ness of critical performative engagement within creative practices as a method for supporting artist practitioners in spaces of wellbeing and most importantly, wellness as a methodology of caring and felt relations – that which opens into an ecophilosophy. A deep ecology that is rooted in a commitment to caring for the very conditions that enable nurturing posthuman life into the future and two, the desire that continues to occupy us, gnaw at us, to being open to the more-than and occupying a privileged place on this planet. Our sense of self is then, propositional to a becoming where flourishing and attuning to the human-non-human world is a form of radical hope manifested as an affirmative ethic.

The artist residency empowers guest residents to use the *sensing* body to explore the potential thousands of distinct material ecologies embodying a symbiotic relationship with the natural world and its creatures and multi-species. This creative convergence sets up an alternative ecology of matter and meaning in a site-specific latitude on a small parcel of land in Spain, which finds creative expression in gestures of abundance, reciprocity, and radiance as forms of multivalent expression where considerations of agency are manifested within our entangled lives that we must all continue to strive for as active hope.

Healing by which through the natural processes of which the mind/body repairs itself, can be generative and at times unpredictable. As one walks, crosses, stumbles, over this rugged terrain through rhizomatic pathways that curve through mountains and cut down to the sea – a sense of occupation rises. These affective intensities ascend when the land and its multi-species relations are threatened more-often than not by wildfires, drought, and extreme weather patterns. A place where ancient olive trees speak of unbearable thirstiness and tomato fruit plants are drying up because they are living, feeling, sweltering with us in these current climate conditions; we must all live vicariously together.

Therefore, a sense of place and belonging is of vital significance towards mental health and wellbeing. Following Glissant's lead, by taking stock of others, things, creatures, critters who inhabit this earth and asking what conditions are needed to nurture others; may sustain those relations that make 'caring' and 'creating' a sensory, more-than-human world possible. In doing so, this may include not losing sight of the complexities and complicities inherent in our own wellbeing.

As artists, *staying with the trouble,* is propositionally not only casting our lot with other animals and plants and ecological communities, but moving us to reflect on the stakes of what we are doing, what is being created as artist-practitioners as to when to stop and observe – even with the best intentions – to influence the conditions of earthly coexistence, wellbeing for others and vital self-care – a provisional condition for the future of this planet. Why not strive to live with gestures of radical entanglements, multivalent creative expressions, and everything *felt* in between, because we are all in this together?

References

Barad, K. (2003) 'Posthumanist Performativity: Toward an Understanding of How Matter Comes to Matter', *Signs: Journal of Women in Culture and Society*, 28(3), pp. 801–831. Available at: https://doi.org/10.1086/345321.

Barad, K. (2007) *Meeting the Universe Halfway: Quantum Physics and the Entanglement of Matter and Meaning.* Duke University Press.

Bennett, J. (2010) *Vibrant Matter: A Political Ecology of Things.* Duke University Press.

Braidotti, R. (2011) *Nomadic Theory: The Portable Rosi Braidotti.* Columbia University Press.

Braidotti, R. (2019) 'Affirmative Ethics and Generative Life', *Deleuze and Guattari Studies*, 13(4), pp. 463–481. Available at: https://doi.org/10.3366/dlgs.2019.0373.

Bridle, J. (2022) *Ways of Being: Beyond Human Intelligence*. Penguin UK.

Curley, E. and Spinoza, B. de (2020) *A Spinoza Reader: The Ethics and Other Works*. Princeton University Press. Available at: https://muse.jhu.edu/book/73619 (Accessed: 13 October 2022).

Deleuze, G. and Guattari, F. (1988) *A Thousand Plateaus: Capitalism and Schizophrenia*. Bloomsbury Publishing.

Glissant, É. (1997) *Poetics of Relation*. University of Michigan Press.

Guattari, F. (2005) *The Three Ecologies*. London: Bloomsbury.

Guin, U.K.L. (2016) *Always Coming Home*. Hachette UK.

Haraway, D.J. (2016) *Staying with the Trouble: Making Kin in the Chthulucene*. Duke University Press.

Juelskjær, M. and Schwennesen, N. (2012) 'Intra-Active Entanglements – An Interview with Karen Barad', *Kvinder, Køn & Forskning* [Preprint], (1–2). Available at: https://doi.org/10.7146/kkf.v0i1-2.28068.

Kimmerer, R. (2013) *Braiding Sweetgrass: Indigenous Wisdom, Scientific Knowledge and the Teachings of Plants*. Milkweed editions.

Kirksey, E. (2014) *The Multispecies Salon*. Duke University Press.

Kolbert, E. (2014) *The Sixth Extinction: An Unnatural History*. A&C Black.

Kuppers, P. (2022) *Eco Soma: Pain and Joy in Speculative Performance Encounters*. University of Minnesota Press.

Manning, E. (2013) *Always More Than One: Individuation's Dance*. Duke University Press.

Oliveros, P. (2002) 'Quantum Listening: From Practice to Theory (To Practice Practice)', *Culture and Humanity in the New Millennium: The Future of Human Values*, pp. 27–41.

Oliveros, P. (2005) *Deep Listening: A Composer's Sound Practice*. IUniverse.

Seigworth, G.J. (2011) 'Pt. III. Folds. From Affection to Soul', in C.J. Stivale (ed.) *Gilles Deleuze: Key Concepts*. McGill-Queen's University Press.

Simard, S. (2021) *Finding the Mother Tree: Uncovering the Wisdom and Intelligence of the Forest*. Penguin UK.

Springgay, S. (2022) *Feltness: Research-Creation, Socially Engaged Art, and Affective Pedagogies*. Duke University Press.

Thompson, T.S. and Harney, S. (2018) 'Ground Provisions', *Afterall: A Journal of Art, Context and Enquiry*, 45, pp. 120–125. Available at: https://doi.org/10.1086/698401.

26 Distributed assemblages of cognition and health (or) how TikTok ate my mind

Jamie Mcphie and David A. G. Clarke

Introduction

Relax. Drop your shoulders. Breathe deeply. How do you feel? Imagine for a moment that health is not a thing confined within your dermatological boundary – beneath your skin. And that mental health[1] is not confined to wherever you believe your mind to exist – in your head?

Take stock of the event. Your fingers, resting on the laptop keys. Clasping your phone. Holding the page. Or are you listening to this? Is someone reading it aloud? Or is there an automated voice, produced by a computer? The words you read or hear, they're not poured out of an author, but are wrestled onto/out of/through the making of this chapter. Thoughts grapple, tripping breaths, slippery conversations, scuffled rewritings and clashing tracked changes, struggled readings, layering the forces that move, and move through. Words bruised by and locked in with many things. Laid here, waiting for all you come with, all that becomes, to read and wrestle. And if on your phone, are you pulled to another app? An app that knows you? That is you? Tick tock, tick tock, tick tock, tick…

Now imagine this becoming exists on a plane of immanence – you are (all of you) 'of' the environment. Lose yourself to it now. You are entirely ecological, including the laptop, phone, page, human or computer voice, and the concepts you think you think. Now, ~~your~~ cognition becomes a 'transcranial' (Clarke and Chalmers, 1998) and 'transcorporeal' (Alaimo, 2010) process, with fluid boundaries – ~~your~~ agency is distributed and fully embodied around the environment you are currently 'plugged into' (Deleuze and Guattari, 2004). You are environ(mental). This is not (merely) a meditative exercise. This is not (only) a class-based mindfulness retreat into, or out of oneself. That self was never *one* to begin with. This is an ontological shift from transcendent thinking to that of immanence. You are not *in* the world, or *on* it, you are (all) *of* it. You might think you're thinking your own thoughts, well, you are, but those thoughts just so happen to be your environment's thoughts, because you *are* your/an environment.

Don't forget to breathe.

What is a breath? I suppose there is the 'what is in a breath?' question, and then there is the 'what is it to breathe question?'. I feel like this is how I want to divide the question, 'what is a breath'. But then, can we think this differently? Can a breath be assembled differently; a breath is a chance at (inorganic) life. It is relief. It is plastic particles and second-hand smoke, dodged in the wet greyness of the street. The new

DOI: 10.4324/9781003345725-29

November air, crisp in your lungs, as the weather finally turns a little colder. So late in the year. And the streetlights glow orange through the windows of the passing bus, and through this there is a burnt blush to your breath's vapour. And you worry about what is to come; the day's tasks, and burdens, about that ever-climbing line, plotted exponentially, rising as another COP[2] seems to do nothing, and your phone in your hand speaks with you to say something like 'let's escape together', and you do. And the screen is bright, and you turn it down. And you breathe, with it. Environ(mental).

We think with our immediate environment and ecology, and sometimes with distant environments and ecologies, with the aid of extended sensory limbs; satellites, radio waves, X-ray's, your 3G signal – we hunt for reception – one bar, two bars, three…now we can *be*.

And telegraph wires with bird song.

If the community of life that we are *of* is not healthy, how can we be?

Rather a lot of our memory is stored not in our heads, but in our phones and on our laptops. If we need to recall a phone number, we will need to cognise with our phones. We think *with* it, not over-and-against it. Our calendars are on our laptops. We find it hard to remember what we're doing without thinking *with* our laptop (which used to be our Filofax – *File of Facts*; which used to be our Lefax; which used to be an agenda – from the Latin *things to do;* which used to be pictographs, logograms, proto-writing, etc.). We infect it as it infects us.

We are not suggesting that the computer 'thinks' by itself. Rather:

What "thinks" and engages in "trial and error" is the man [sic] plus the computer plus the environment. And the lines between man, computer, and environment are purely artificial, fictitious lines. They are lines across the pathways along which information or difference is transmitted. They are not boundaries of the thinking system. What thinks is the total system which engages in trial and error, which is man plus environment.

(Bateson, 2000, pp. 490–491)

(Or woman, person?). *Person-computer-environment.* A cognising assemblage. Annalee Newitz (2011, p. 90) suggested that her laptop was, 'practically a brain prosthesis' as she recalls her relationship with her computer was determined by the affection she felt for someone she fell in love with online, so that 'every time [she] boot[s] up [her] machine, [she could] see a shadow of him flicker past' (cited in Mcphie, 2019, p. 149). But this prosthesis doesn't stop at a cold, hard screen of a laptop (or phone). The screen is not really a screen at all, but is a stage, conducting performances choreographed by different posthuman authors: here we think with algorithms.

Again, we don't simply *associate* memories with 'objects' such as laptops and algorithms. Again, we think *with* them as events:

We have to understand ourselves—our "self"—as such a "digital distribution," as a realization of possibilities thanks to dense distribution […] Computers are apparatuses for the realization of inner-human, interhuman, and trans-human possibilities […] We are no longer the objects of a given objective world, but projects of alternative worlds. […] The existential transformation from subject into project is clearly not the result of a "free decision." We are forced into it, just as our distant ancestors found themselves forced to stand up on two legs because the ecological catastrophe of the period compelled them somehow to cross the spaces between the more widely scattered trees [...] We can no longer be subjects, because there are no more objects whose subjects we might be, and no hard kernel which might be the subject of some object.

(Flusser, 1996, pp. 244–245)

But if we are 'forced into it', what might this mean – or rather 'do' – when considering the ethical consequences of such things as algorithmically driven social media on cultural constructions, behaviour, or what we might think of as individual actions? One of the issues here is that we tend to think linearly about cause-and-effect. One →direction. As if the decision has begun from one point and ends at another. Karen Barad (2007) contends that, 'we tend to think about causality and questions of agency in terms of either determinism on the one hand, or free will on the other' but insists 'agency is not something possessed by humans, or non-humans for that matter. It is an enactment. And it enlists, if you will, "non-humans" as well as "humans"' (pp. 54–55).

Perhaps we could imagine agency to be more like Tim Ingold's description of 'life' (see Ingold, 2011), in which case laptops don't 'possess' agency, but co-produce it, even without the 'human', as all things can be articulated in life – at least *inorganic life*. Human agency and behaviour 'can no longer be localized in individuals [...] but has to be treated [...] as a function of complex material systems which cut across individuals (assemblages) and which transverse [...] organismic boundaries (rhizomes)' (Ansell-Pearson, cited in Tiessen, 2011, p. 137). This requires what Karen Barad (2007) calls a distributed conception of agency.

Health is no different to agency in this respect. It is spread in lively environmental clusters. Assemblages of health (see Duff 2014; Fox 2011; McLeod 2017; Mcphie, 2019) can be plugged into and out of, depending on spatial and temporal context.

Don't forget to breathe. Environ(mental).

TikToky assemblages of health

If we imagine our body as political, and as a political battleground, then particular organs might influence us to think a certain way, depending on a host of other multi-directional influencers, such as cultural constructions, what you had for breakfast, how tall you are, whether you are impoverished or not, the weather, etc. For example, your uterus might play a central role in determining the next presidential election in the US. Who controls that organ, or who has the right to control that organ, can determine many health outcomes, some of which verge on gendered enslavement. 'Bodies are not the locus at which forces act, they are the production of the interactions of forces' (Fox, 2011, p. 368).

As Masny (2013, p. 341) states

[a]n assemblage can be constituted by teachers, classmates, researcher, computers, classrooms, and more [sic]. The subject is in the assemblage no more, no less important than the other elements in the assemblage. The elements in the assemblage construct relationships to each other once they come together in the actual. There is no a priori or pre-given relationship among elements in the assemblage.

Assemblages of health are constantly (co)created, near and far, in a topology. This moves conceptions of health away from boundaried views. Rather, '[w]ellbeing and illbeing are generally seen as interior states of the individual, which can readily be linked to individuals being blamed for the status of their wellbeing' (McLeod, 2017, p. xv). Instead of thinking of health as trapped beneath the skin, we could think with Deleuze and Guattari's ontology 'in which the body is no longer individual and organic; in which health and ill-health are marked not by aspects of an individual body but by connectivities and relations between bodies, objects and ideas' (Fox, 2011, p. 372).

Assemblages of Health 'ventures to explain how health may be reframed in the absence of conventional ontological distinctions such as human/nonhuman, nature/culture and body/society' (pp. ix–x) and refashions health, 'in the context of a posthuman, more-than-human, assemblage of spaces, forces and bodies' (Duff, 2014, p. x).[3] Duff (2014) asks us 'to be more alert to the multiple, overlapping and endemic imbrications of biology and technology, the human and the nonhuman in contemporary life' (p. 2).

So, what does a social media assemblage such as TikTok 'do' when humans think *with* it – plug into it? What hidden materials and creative ecologies does this digital distribution co-produce? Are monsters being made?

My phone and I often escape together. To new apps, and to games – Grand Mountain Adventure, and various 'Ordles' (Wordle, Worldle, Heardle, Quordle, etc). To photos of my boys, to property I can't afford. To 'the Socials'; to Facebook, and, mainly, Twitter. And for a time, TikTok. I had no reason to download TikTok, other than curiosity. I had seen a PhD stipend advertised, the intention of which was to research the potential of TikTok for climate change education. I was intrigued to see TikTok mentioned within my sphere of interest, as I didn't really know what it was. Before then I was vaguely aware of the name, but as a middle-aged man I had lumped it in with all the others I had heard of but had no interest in engaging with, such as Snapchat and Tumblr. So, one afternoon I downloaded it.

For the next few days TikTok consumed my life. In spare (and not so spare) moments I was on the app, watching inane but captivating videos. For tens of minutes at a time I would disappear with TikTok. And as we learned more about each other, the TikTok algorithm and I created a new world, reinforcing prejudices and delectations across our burgeoning assemblage.

Within the week I was feeling an uncanny sentience in this app, but it was the compulsion to be with it that led me to delete it.

Created in China in September 2016, *DouYin* (in China) or *TikTok* (it's twin app on the global market), previously known as musical.ly, now has over 750 million active users. Montag, Yang and Elhai (2021) listed a range of psychological theories to explain TikTok's highly addictive usage, such as Gratification Theory (GT), Social Impact Theory (SIT) and Self-Determination Theory (SDT), highlighting the motivations of young people to keep using it – expanding their social network, seeking fame, expressing themselves creatively, escapism, self-expression, fear of missing out, feelings of competence and autonomy, and being connected with others. But the field of psychology can only take us so far. Beneath the skin. Psychology often performs within the head, rather than dancing between dermatological boundaries (see Boyd, 2017; Mcphie, 2019).

There is a 'cognitive ecology of the internet' which 'enables new kinds of embodied interaction', extends embodiment and distributes cognitive processes, as well as facilitating collective cognition (Smart, Heersmink and Clowes, 2017, p. 251). In light of this, aside from people's motivations to engage with TikTok, it's perhaps more urgent to explore where the runaway platform may take you. What does it do to think *with* it? There is an obvious creativity that co-emerges via a TikTok-phone-human assemblage. Healthy artful expressions may be co-produced and felt, emerging from numerous creative and joyful explorations that heighten feelings of self-efficacy or self-worth, for example. But there are other, more insidiously creative paths that seem to be (co)emerging that might have more serious health consequences. For example, Weimann and Masri's (2020) 'findings reveal the disturbing presence of Far-right extremism in videos, commentary, symbols and pictures included in TikTok's postings' (n.p.). This is worrying, especially with the rise of misogynistic, fascist ideologies and their negative impacts on health for many people/assemblages who don't 'fit' the ideological criteria. However, whether TikTok 'itself' is healthy or not, is a matter of context. It depends what, where and when we are referring to when we think *health*. Health of an individual person? Health of an audience? Health of a nation? Health of an ecosystem? Health of an idea? It can be both healthy and unhealthy at the same time, depending on your situatedness. If we think with the concept of distributed assemblages of health, then we can plug in and out of a variety of possibilities, rather than dissecting adverse health consequences of TikTok, as if we could essentialise 'the problem' to a psychological state. If we think of it as an extended limb, organ or cognitive apparatus (whether conceived as inorganic or alive, for example), we would be more careful with its manipulative potential.

'Massively popular social media platforms have become a critical site for the joining of power and desire over the last decade, and it is here that contemporary fascist impulses are seeded' (Crano, 2022, p. 279). It is difficult to pinpoint where and when this seeding begins, as it is multidirectional. Yet, once it is established more coherently, as a *thing*, it performs as an assemblage of (at least) *internet-desire-body* that may become *internet-desire-body-fascism*. And rather than simply perceiving *hatred* as the impelling motivational affect/emotion, there seems to be an element of *exhilaration* driving the formation of hateful rhetoric on such sites. 'As fascistic power relations spread anew through digital cultures' newly evolving modes of visuality, hapticity, vibration and expression, one can observe something of what Deleuze calls 'sad joy', a sort of joy rooted in conquest and domination' (Crano, 2022, p. 278). There seems to be an intense material potential of certain social media sites, such as TikTok, to attract and addict creative affective capacities, the capacities to affect and be affected (one move). This capacity 'reaches into the very grain of individuals, touches their bodies and inserts itself into their actions and attitudes, their discourses, learning processes and everyday lives' (Foucault, 1980, p. 39).

> [T]he conditions for comparing our current political climate and socio-economic prerogatives to those of historical fascisms are to be found in the myriad ways in which such a network can possess a potent affective and imagistic pull comparable to that accompanying the first waves of European fascism.
>
> (Crano, 2022, p. 301)

Yet, it is not simply an imagistic pull, it is pull-and-push, at the same time, a plug-in and out of conceptual virtual material (literally). It (e)merges with our extended corporeal self as we cognise and embody the affective qualities of the conjoining engagement.

Bhandari and Bimo (2020) found that, unlike other social networking sites, 'the experience of using Tik Tok is one of repeatedly engaging with one's own self: intra rather than interpersonal connection', an experience directed towards the individual rather than an audience, something they call an 'algorithmized version of self' (n.p.). But where is this algorithmized version of self located?

Take Sandy Stone's description of encountering the physicist Stephen Hawking, whose voice was partly co-generated by a speech synthesiser and a single muscle in his cheek due to contracting amyotrophic lateral sclerosis (ALS):

> Exactly where, I say to myself, is Hawking? [...] Who is doing the talking up there on the stage? In an important sense, Hawking doesn't stop being Hawking at the edge of his body. There is the obvious physical Hawking, vividly outlined by the way our social conditioning teaches us to see a person as a person. But a serious part of Hawking extends into the box in his lap. No box, no discourse; Hawking's intellect becomes a tree falling in the forest with nobody around to hear it. Where does he stop? Where are his edges?
>
> (Stone, cited in Barad, 2007, p. 159)

If, as Manzotti (2008) says, 'the mind is larger, both in time and in space, than the body of the subject' (n.p.), surely the environment where we find ourselves located influences our cognition in the same way that it would 'inside our heads'. In fact, we could say that our wider environment is our inorganic head, in that we think *with* it, not over-and-against it. That includes our virtual environment too, as it is no less physical/material/ecological. It just means that our cognition is distributed over a larger area, even bouncing back from satellites in the outer atmosphere. In other words, we also think with other stuff – stuff like phones, computers, social media, crisp packets. 'In Hawking's case, the speech synthesiser pushed back, influencing the thoughts themselves. In this way, we cognise with external components, from computers to walls. These cognising human-object intra-actions are also interlaced with embodied memories' (Mcphie, 2019, pp. 175–176).

Two weeks ago I found the TikTok app back on my phone (I had deleted it several months earlier). I was just scrolling sideways, past my apps, looking for my weather app, and there it was. It was squatting, proudly, alone, – the last of the apps. I don't remember downloading it again. Maybe I did? But, why would I? It had been so scary the first time.

Is this a real memory? Did I dream this? Can apps just appear? No doubt someone more tech informed that me can reassure me that this is fine. This is normal. I hadn't deleted it properly, or something. It was only apparently gone, but it was residually there, and then it came back. Because that's what it's supposed to do, and that's fine. Nothing to see here.

But, I don't know if any of these things are the case, and its sudden appearance feels creepy, and revives the feeling of insidiousness I felt when, several months earlier, I had experienced TikTok for the first time.

Our cognitive functions, our algorithmic selves, can be manipulated by those who own the rights to our extra-sensory inorganic organs – TikTok, Twitter, Facebook, Instagram. If our extended memories are partially stored in these ever-shifting online podiums/organs, Elon Musk can engineer the pathways that are co-created (with the agency or will of the algorithms) in a way which mirrors and physically extends our chemical and electrical neural pathways. Thus, the online platforms are imbricated as part of our embodied cognitive processing. Elon Musk's, Andrew Tate's, Jordan Peterson's, Alex Jones' political affiliations, temperaments, whims and ideologies can enter and alter our very selves[4]. Of course, our pre-existing affiliations and ideologies are ready to meet those pathways to redirect or consume them, but we will nevertheless be transformed if we engage (actively or passively). The virtual hands that manipulate us may be invisible but they are still physical and perform ecologically, as trophic cascades (Mcphie and Clarke, 2020). After all,

> one's success on TikTok hinges on how cleverly and convincingly one exhibits what we might call the will of the platform [...] In network fascism, one's life rather becomes an expression of the will of the network [...] the self as brand [...] to be marketed, built up and invested in.
>
> (Crano, 2022, pp. 287–288)

Ever-increasing algorithmic selves enable misogyny and embodied fascism to become marketable products. Within and beyond the assemblages discussed in this chapter, public subjectivities are products of iterative intensifications within echo-chambered markets. We see the 'unhealthy' unidirectional effects of these public subjectivities in the news daily. And they're increasing.

Don't forget to breathe.

Notes

1 Throughout this chapter, when we say 'health', we mean mental health and wellbeing. We choose not to describe it as 'mental health' due to the invented and problematic mind-body dualism it induces. Following Spinoza, we see the mind as an idea of the body (see Mcphie, 2019, p.295). 'If the concept of "mind" does not stand in opposition to the concept of "body", then there is little justification for distinguishing between "mental" and "physical" health' (McGann & Cummins, 2013, p.2). Therefore, we will call it *health*.
2 'Conference of the Parties' (United Nations Climate Change Conference).
3 Also see, Andrews and Rishworth (Eds.) (2023), for a recent special issue on the subject.
4 We choose these particular Tweeters and TikTokers for their popular versions of what we deem to be unhealthy misogynistic rhetoric.

References

Alaimo, S. (2010). *Bodily Natures: Science, Environment, and the Material Self*. Bloomington & Indianapolis: Indiana University Press.

Andrews, G. & Rishworth, A. (Eds.) (2023). New Theoretical Terrains in Geographies of Wellbeing: More-Than-Human and More-Than-Representational Elements, Processes and Registers of Wellbeing. *Wellbeing, Space and Society*. 4, 100130 Available online at: www.sciencedirect.com/journal/wellbeing-space-and-society/special-issue/10CQFTS8J8V

Barad, K. (2007). *Meeting the Universe Halfway: Quantum Physics and the Entanglement of Matter and Meaning*. Durham & London: Duke University Press.

Bateson, G. (2000). *Steps to an Ecology of Mind*. Chicago: The University of Chicago Press.

Bhandari, A., & Bimo, S. (2020) *Tiktok And The "Algorithmized Self": A New Model Of Online Interaction*. AoIR Selected Papers of Internet Research. Available online at: https://journals.uic.edu/ojs/index.php/spir/article/view/11172

Boyd, C. P. (2017). *Non-Representational Geographies of Therapeutic Art Making: Thinking Through Practice*. Singapore: Palgrave Macmillan.

Clark, A., & Chalmers, D. (1998). The Extended Mind. *Analysis*, 58(1), 7–19.

Crano, R. (2022). The Joy of Following: Network Fascism and the Micropolitics of the Social Media Image. *Deleuze and Guattari Studies*, 16(2), 277–307.

Deleuze, G., & Guattari, F. (2004). *A Thousand Plateaus: Capitalism and Schizophrenia* (B. Massumi, Trans.). London: Continuum.

Duff, C. (2014). *Assemblages of Health: Deleuze's Empiricism and the Ethology of Life*. Dordrecht, Heidelberg, New York & London: Springer.

Flusser, V. (1996). Digital Apparition. In T. Druckrey (Ed.), *Electronic Culture: Technology and Visual Representation* (pp. 242–245). New York: Aperture.

Foucault, M. (1980). Prison Tal. In C. Gordon (editor), *Power/Knowledge: Selected Interviews and Other Writings*. 1972-1977. New York: Pantheon, pp. 37–54.

Fox, N. J. (2011). The Ill-Health Assemblage: Beyond the Body-with-Organs. *Health Sociology Review*, 20(4), 359–371.

Ingold, T. (2011). *Being Alive: Essays on Movement, Knowledge and Description*. Oxford, UK: Routledge.

Manzotti, R. (2008). A Process Oriented Externalist Solution to the Hard Problem. *The Reasoner*, 2(6), 13–20.

Masny, D. (2013). Rhizoanalytic Pathways in Qualitative Research. *Qualitative Inquiry*, 19(5), 339–348.

McGann, M., & Cummins, F. (2013). *No Mental; Health*. Conference Publication. Available online at: http://cspeech.ucd.ie/Fred/docs/NoMentalHealth.pdf

McLeod, K. (2017). *Wellbeing Machine: How Health Emerges from the Assemblages of Everyday Life*. Durham, NC: Carolina Academic Press.

Mcphie, J. (2019). *Mental Health and Wellbeing in the Anthropocene: A Posthuman Inquiry*. Basingstoke, UK: Palgrave Macmillan.

Mcphie, J. & Clarke, D. A. G. (2020) Nature Matters: Diffracting a Keystone Concept of Environmental Education Research – Just for Kicks. *Environmental Education Research*, 26(9–10), 1509–1526.

Montag, C., Yang, H. and Elhai, J. D. (2021) On the Psychology of TikTok Use: A First Glimpse From Empirical Findings. *Frontiers in Public Health*, 9, Sec. Digital Public Health https://doi.org/10.3389/fpubh.2021.641673

Newitz, A. (2011). My Laptop. In S. Turkle (Ed.), *Evocative Objects: Things We Think with* (pp. 86–91). Cambridge, MA & London: MIT Press.

Smart, P., Heersmink, R., Clowes, R.W. (2017). The Cognitive Ecology of the Internet. In: Cowley, S., Vallée-Tourangeau, F. (eds) Cognition Beyond the Brain. Springer, Cham. https://doi.org/10.1007/978-3-319-49115-8_13.

Tiessen, M. (2011). (In)Human Desiring and Extended Agency. In T. K. Davidson, O. Park, & R. Shields (Eds.), *Ecologies of Affect: Placing Nostalgia, Desire, and Hope* (pp. 127–142). Waterloo, ON: Wilfrid Laurier University Press.

Weimann, G. & Masri, N. (2020) Research Note: Spreading Hate on TikTok. *Studies in Conflict & Terrorism*, 46(5), 752–765. https://doi.org/10.1080/1057610X.2020.1780027

27 Distance and belonging in the studio

Christian Edwardes

Introduction

One major group exhibition at the ICA Miami recently declared, 'the studio is "everywhere"' (Gartenfield, 2017, p. 20), not just in the variety of physical spaces: the shed, the street, the repurposed factory or light industrial complex, but also in the technologies – the computers, tablets or mobile devices, and creative software through which artists both produce creative work, and the idea of what it is to *be* a contemporary artist. This re-ignition of interest in the studio comes at a time when discourse around how and where artists work has largely followed a narrative of dispersal (Davidts & Paice, 2009; Relyea, 2013). But, whilst few artists today make work in one place, the studio as site and metaphor continues to hold fascination both as a subject of study and a marker of artistic legitimacy for artists and scholars (Davidts & Paice, 2009; Jacob & Grabner, 2010).

In the last decade, the emergence of an interdisciplinary field of 'studio studies' has reaffirmed a need to bring renewed critical attention to both the situated and distributed modalities of art working. Following a broader material turn in the humanities, the scholarship in this field often takes inspiration from the pioneering work of Latour and Woolgar in the field of science and technology studies (Farías & Wilkie, 2016; Sjöholm, 2018), and parallel explorations of production in within media studies (Lehmann, 2013, p.251). As an approach to research, studio studies incorporates the knowledge and methods of historians, anthropologists, sociologists, cultural geographers, and cultural theorists to develop ways of accounting for the complexities of human and non-human actors, alongside the cultural, social, and economic constituents that are integrated in, and affect, the creation of art.

The routines, organisation, and distribution of these spaces have been central to the work of geographers too, where studio visits, interviews, and participatory research has provided insights into the complex relations between human and non-human actors (Engelmann, 2017; 2019; Sjöholm, 2014), atmospheres (Ash, 2016), and creative and professional identities (Bain, 2004, 2005). Geographers have also concerned themselves with the broader political and economic agency of the studio and its interrelations with creative economies and urban planning (Harris, 2012; Ley, 2003; Mathews, 2010; Moreton, 2013, Bain and Landau, 2019). Yet, given the diversity places in which creative work is made, the term 'studio' may aptly describe the multi-floor headquarters of an international artist such as Olafur Eliasson (Coles, 2012; Jellis, 2015), the teaching spaces in a creative university department (McHugh, 2014), a rented desk and laptop screen (Busta, 2017), or the corner of a room in an apartment.

DOI: 10.4324/9781003345725-30

Here, the focus is predominantly on the art studio and the ways in which the studio has been enrolled in emotional, professional, moral, and economic notions of health. Nevertheless, it is important to acknowledge that the art studio is only one method in which creative work is practiced. Artistic and creative making is not exclusively practiced in the studio (Adamson, 2007; Luckman, 2015; Price and Hawkins, 2018), nor is the studio the exclusive domain of the trained artist or designer (Leone, 2021; Miller, 2020). In drawing attention to histories of professional arts practices, I also acknowledge the large gap in accounting for the histories of 'open studio' approaches in art therapy (Moon, 2015), and some of the breadth of community based models of group studio practice.

The following sections outline a number of approaches to studio research around two loose but established themes: the studio as both a social space and a space of retreat or isolation. Each section takes these tropes and considers the ways in which they have been connected to notions of health, wellbeing, care, morality, and other value-laden geographies that map the condition of the individuals, environments, or communities involved in artistic labour.

Beginning with the psychic chambers of the Romantic studio-garret that has captured the European imagination of both writers and artists from the early nineteenth century, and through which the studio becomes the backdrop to the psychological travails of the figure at its centre. From the early professionalisation of art and the role of the studio in identity-construction, the examples progress from the realm of the authorial to those of social and collective studios. Here, I also touch on studio research that examines human/non-human relations between occupants, objects, and materials, that offer modes for caring, mnemonic reflection, and recuperation. Studios and studio communities, in turn, become objects in urban regeneration strategies – tools for improving social and economic health.

The chapter is presented in the form of vignettes, each briefly offering an illustration of the intersections between creative making spaces and morality and degeneracy, purity and "gross" materiality, mania, anxiety, recuperation and belonging.

A room of one's own

Arguably, one of the most enduring tropes of the studio is that it is the space in which the solitary artist, lost in uneasy contemplation or obsessive production, cements their individual vision (Jones, 1996; Grabner, 2010). As Michelle Grabner describes, these depictions often demonstrate 'the mind at work, not the hands' (p.2), a reminder that the studio is as much a space that is associated with the mental travails of the artist as it is for a specialised kind of practising (Cole & Pardo, 2005; Waterfield, 2009).

This notion of the studio as a retreat is often prefaced on the individuality of its occupant. It is 'the domain of X's authorship, the space in which a given X constructs himself as the independent creator/author of a unique product identified with his name' (Jones, 1996, p.3). In this respect, the studio takes on a double-inflection in which the space is seen as both imbued with an interiority that is uniquely connected to the occupant's 'psyche', and the originary location for professional validation – the first space that 'critics and other specialists' (Buren, 1979, p.53) may be invited into.

In Europe, representations of the studio as a space of specialised practice and unique artistic persona are rooted in the seventeenth century. The weakening of the guild system and changes in patronage created a market for art that could no longer rely on commissions (Bellony-Rewald & Peppiatt, 1983, p.20). Dutch artists like Rembrandt began to put themselves and their studios on display in ways that attended to both their artistic needs and those of self promotion (Chapman, 1990; 2005). Scenes of the artist at work in their studio grew rapidly, marketing the artist's intellectual and professional skills in an increasingly competitive market. The studio also became entangled with the persona of *being* an artist, defining 'a ground that [was] the painter's own, a license to be a self or a way to take on the identity of being a painter' (Alpers, 2005, p.34).

With the establishment of arts Academies in the eighteenth century, artists were further elevated to the status of professionals: 'equal to the philosophers and men (sic) of letters of other sections of the Institute' (White & White, 1965, p.18). Changes in the status of artists brought with it additional pressures, an emphasis as much on the artists 'social image' as their academic standing.

In 1835, the relationship between the private and professional persona of the artist found a particularly grim manifestation in the suicides of painters Léopold Robert and Antoine-Jean Gros. Whilst achieving significant recognition as painters, both also received scathing public criticism in the last years of their lives. Painted the following year, Alexandre-Gabriel Decamps' *The Suicide* (1836) was rumoured to be inspired by these untimely deaths (Gotlieb, 2005). It depicts the lifeless body of an artist shrouded in the semi-darkness of his empty studio, his palette hanging from the wall and a pistol on the floor at his side. Presented as a deliberate challenge to the businesslike orthodoxies of market-driven practices, the image was intended to conjure up 'the failed, melancholy, reclusive, impoverished, secretive, mad, and suicidal artist' (Gotlieb, p.164). The romanticism of this studio *topos,* in which the artist sacrifices everything for their art, reanimates antiquarian associations between creativity, melancholy and 'madness' (Ross, 2006; Witkower & Witkower, 2007). But it also forms as a continuing tension between ideas of professionalism and failure. In its wake, associations with the occupant's health and mental wellbeing are caught up in the mythology of the studio interior.

Moral hygiene and bohemian squalor

From the mid-nineteenth century, evocations of the artist's studio began to flourish in illustrated press, literature, and the theatre (Esner, 2018; Lamb, 1993), and the studio provided a stage set for the public appetite for contemporary art and their fascination with the private lives of artists. Cultivating a studio persona was as much a part of the artists professional life as the works being produced, and carefully choreographed photographs and studio visits demonstrated social standing and artistic success (Codell, 2003; Esner, 2018).

In Victorian London, the most respected artists commissioned studio-houses (Dakers, 1999) the floor plans of which would appear in professional architectural magazines. The representation of the artist in grand home-studio settings was intended to remove any suspicion of amateurism, and eradicate the moral ambiguities associated with bohemianism – an environment in which '[s]tudios were professional *and* morally hygienic sites of work *and* of "heavenly" domesticity' (Codell, 2003, p.48). The professional 'show studios' of artists such as Lord Leighton (Bellony-Rewald & Peppiatt, 1983; Dakers, 1999; Esner, 2013), were as much an expression of personal taste as working or commercial spaces, and magazines such as the *L'Illustration*, the *Magazine of Art* and *The Studio* would offer exclusive access to their readership in the form of illustrated editorials.

Despite their decidedly social operation, photographs and engravings of nineteenth century studios routinely featured images of the artist alone at their easels surrounded by exotic objects, carefully arranged furniture, and the paintings that were the results of their labour. These carefully constructed representations were intended to reassure the readers of the sober, hard-working, characters of successful artists (Esner, 2018, p.29), or to emphasise the ostentatious luxury and mild eccentricity that positioned them as celebrities and "taste makers" (Dakers, 1999; Esner, 2018; see also Burns, 1996). Whilst female artists such as Louise Joplin and Kate Greenaway were among the clients for studio houses (Codell, 2003, p.49) the studio was largely cast as a masculinised space – one that, whilst located in the domestic realm of the family home, was able to exude a paterfamilial authority (Codell, 2003, p.70). These palaces of artistic professionalism were positioned as robust defences against the licentious and degenerate reputation of the mad and failed bohemian artists of nineteenth century fiction.

Only a small few Victorian artists sustained such luxury, and their ideals of a morally hygienic gentleman artist were not universally shared. A short distance from the Holland Park studio-homes of George Frederick Watts and Lord Leighton, the cheap flats and seedy bedsits of Camden provided the working lodgings and subject matter for painters such as Walter Sickert, and Gwen and Augustus John (Postle, 2009). The sparse interiors of rented rooms that provided the atmospheric backdrop for portraits of friends, lovers, and acquaintances, were not just the result of poverty. These were an expression of artistic integrity and a devotion to a form of realism that positioned itself at some distance from the formal orthodoxies of society painters. In Sickert's words: 'the more our part is serious, the more it will tend to avoid the drawing room and stick to the kitchen. The plastic arts are gross arts, dealing joyously with gross material facts' (Sickert quoted in Wedd, 2001, p.116).

'Gross material facts' might describe Francis Bacon's studio at Reece Mews in Kensington, a space in which squalor was not just tolerated but encouraged (Turner, 2009). Bacon's self-presentations in this chaos of paint-encrusted magazines and rags was part of an expression of creative turmoil that the artist cultivated (Postle, 2009), and a display of the evidence of physical labour. Nicholas Chare (2006) remarks on the swell of 'cluttered incoherence' (p.85) and material 'noise' that filled Bacon's studio, in contrast to the quiet tidiness of the rest of the flat. But it is perhaps equally remarkable the meticulous (Herculean, even) effort that went into painstakingly reconstructing the studio at the Hugh Lane Gallery in Dublin. The studio, and the material it contained, are often seen as 'an extension of his inner being' (Postle, p.59); 'a mirror of his inner mind' (Peppiatt, 1984, p.86) in which the substance of his studio practices, '[l]ike Bacon… grew old and fragile, was trampled on, torn and decayed' (Dawson, 2009, p.67). It is perhaps not surprising that texts are dedicated to psychologically analysing and interpreting not only the works he created (Harrison, 2019) but also the fragments of studio detritus that he worked with (Dawson & Harrison, 2009)

Psychic chambers

Picturing the studio has played a significant role in maintaining its mythos, whether as an autobiographical account or at the hands of the visiting photographer. Caroline Jones's (1996) notes the particular "pull" that European Romanticism had on post-War American artists like Barnett Newman and Mark Rothko, who recognised 'a shared search for transcendence, and an overwhelming sense of isolation in an increasingly crowded, explosive, aggressive world' (8). Photographer and filmmaker Hans Namuth produced images of Newman and Rothko in silent contemplation, smoking and staring into the middle-distance. In composing the sparseness of the studio with the apparent silence and solitude of the sitter, Namuth constructs an analogue between the working space and state-of-mind of the artist. Poised in moments of introspective self-absorption, the artists present expressions of distance and indifference. These disaffected poses are themselves reflective of longstanding associations between melancholy and creativity (see Ross, 2006; Dixon, 2013; Bubenik, 2019).

The photographs of Newman and Rothko are a marked difference to Namuth's earlier documentation of Jackson Pollock at work. Filmed and photographed at the artists studio barn in Long Island, Namuth records Pollock's furious actions around canvases laid out on the floor. Rather than distanced contemplation, Namuth captures Pollock as a rapt and manic artist, consumed in the iterative and ritualistic performances of his painting. Witnessing his compulsive attention to the acts of curling and whipping threads of paint, however, we are expected to be left in no doubt of his 'supreme indifference' to the people and the world that surrounds him (Jones, 1996, p.75).

Both these depictions of the artist, lost in work or in thought, generate visions of creative mastery and autonomy that separate and elevate the artist from the social and material worlds that produce them. In the photographs of Hans Namuth, the sparse or paint splattered studios of Barnett Newman and Jackson Pollock are intended to represent more than just the spaces in which they work. They are presented as the material expressions of a singular, and often hyper-masculinised, energy (Bergstein, 1995) – a form of psychic mirror.

Privilege, professionalism, and pragmatism

These "framings" of the studio, which artist, work, and studio are expressive of a distancing from the world, play down both the materiality and bodily engagement with the acts of painting, and some of the pragmatic arrangements that make the studio a functioning experimental space. Morgan Thomas's (2009) analysis of Rothko's studio practice extends beyond romantic determinations, focusing on the social and material networks of assistants, devices, and systems, that came together in the production of works, and on the various changes in studio real estate. For Thomas, it was the effects of the paintings that were most important to Rothko, and as such the studio 'became a vehicle for producing effects, an instrument' (2009, p.33). Whilst this does not entirely escape the biography that privileges a version of the studio as the domain of singular male mastery, it opens out some of the overlooked dynamics of studio work.

The double-inflection between the private and the professional is evident in several geographic studies of artists in their studios at the turn of the millennium. Despite radical critiques of the studio and studio practicing that emerged in the latter decades of the twentieth century, the connection between dedicated spaces for practicing and claims to professionalism remain very much alive (Davidts & Paice, 2009). In Alison Bain's examinations of the role of artistic, professional and community identities in Toronto (Bain, 2004) the studio is as much as a nexus of *feelings* about self-worth, personal independence, and professional validation as it is a space to work. For the occupants it can be a place of safety and 'deep personal significance' (2004, p.179), separated from the obligations of other social, domestic, or work routines.

For women artists, the studio continues to be 'a hard-won resource' (2004, p.171) and one that has been essential in reinforcing artistic identities, and in a reputational and political claim to professionalism. Access to a fixed studio address is often still the way for artists to 'carve out a space in which they can seek and maintain continuity and stability' (Sjöholm, 2018, p.43), and to establish a sense of professional autonomy. In Bain's research the studio is a promise and a commitment to the production of art, but a dedicated personal space is often temporary, precarious, or squeezed from a corner of domestic space. Bain's work still carries echoes of the experiences of women artists working three decades earlier, whose visibility was conditional on erasing any suggestion of a lack of seriousness by allowing home and professional life to collide (Chicago, 1982; Gouma-Peterson, 1997; Stobbs, 2022).

Recently, however, the line between the two has seems increasingly hard to define, as an always-on, networked world demands flexibility alongside the need to construct and present a cohesive identity: 'a constant source of anxiety… [summed] up [in] the ideal of a successful life as *becoming oneself*' (Boltanski & Chiapello, 2018, p.461). Katy Seigel has argued that the conditions of contemporary creative autonomy are more likely to be staged in 'small room[s] with plywood or sheet rocked walls … a row of doors, one after another, with names on each one, along a wall of un-sheetrocked studs' (2010, p.314), than in the cavernous lofts of mid-century artists; and, as working lives have shifted from permanent 9-to-5 jobs to shift-work and gig economies, artists are no longer afforded same separation they once sought from domestic life and waged labour.

Within geography, the 'dark side of creativity' is marked out through the not-so-gradual turns towards a neoliberal framings of entrepreneurial "creativity" and creative economies (Bain, 2017; Hawkins, 2018; Moreton, 2013; Mould, 2018). Following Luc Boltanski and Eve Chiapello's (2018) work on the development of contemporary management language, many of the values once aligned to claims for the autonomy and authenticity of artistic labour: creativity, flexibility, and self-fulfilment, have become central motifs of entrepreneurial capitalism and the central theme in the marketing of urban regeneration strategies (Mathews, 2010; Mould, 2015).

Where artistic 'success' becomes a measure of one's capacity for self-realisation in an increasingly decentralised, temporary, and precarious working world, notions of 'professionalism' realign around 'the individual who is constantly engaged, interfacing, interacting, communicating, responding, or processing within some telematic milieu' (Crary, 2014:15). So, whilst it might be tempting to see the studio as entirely dematerialised within these transitory spaces of contemporary art-working, Caroline Busta sees this increased connectivity as an infinite reproduction of the studio 'literally everywhere … psychologically and operationally intermeshed and omnipresent… [the] everywhere studio exists on the screens in our hands and the sites they access' (Busta, 2017, p.254).

Social studios

Whilst studios carry the promise of affording a separation from the worlds of work and life, or a dubious autonomy from routines of waged labour, they can also be places of belonging, providing retreat and respite of a less individualistic kind. Up to now, the focus has been on the role of the studio as an apparatus for constructing and presenting artistic subjectivities and mythologies. Stories of isolated practice prioritise the individual at the expense of the social and material interrelations from which works, and creative identities emerge.

Even the studios associated with an individual artist are home to a plethora of assistants, administrators, visiting clients, and gallerists. Studio Olafur Eliasson, for example, offer examples of a networked model of transdisciplinary research that involves a studio staff 'made up of fabricators, architects, archivists, and art historians, with scientists, theorists, and curators invited to collaborate on selected projects' (Coles, 2012, p.9; see also Jellis, 2015). Geographer Sasha Engelmann's situated observations of artist Tomás Sareceno's at his studio in Berlin accounts not only for the *social* presence of the artist and those who assist him, but also for the spiders that are at the centre of his practice (Engelmann, 2017; 2019). In parallel research in the fields of design (Leclair, 2023) and media production (Ash, 2016), the objects that mediate studio interactions are seen to affect the organisation of the studio: generating localised anxieties and 'emotionally charged atmospheres' (p.98).

With a similar interest in the care and connection between human and non-human studio objects, Jenny Sjöholm (2014; 2018) directs focus to the embodied and material constitution of the studio as archive, approaching it as a series of relations between bodies, technologies, and materials. The studio becomes a register of re-encounterings between artist, the space, and the archive of 'collected materials, sketches, memories, and references' (2018, p.31.) through which relationships between artist and studio are continually placed under negotiation. For Sjöholm's interviewees, archives become mnemonic devices that are both recuperative and productive mnemonic devices. These investigations by Engelmann and Sjöholm move beyond the social towards other forms of material 'care', opening out the affective potential of artefacts and atmospheres as co-producers.

Studio communities

Historically, it has not been unusual for artists to cluster together: shared values, ideas, and expectations often provide the social glue for organising arts communities and studio complexes. Strategically, the sharing of technical resources, professional expertise, and critical judgement, are significant components in binding these communities together (Bain, 2005). They are also spaces in which artists, critics, gallerists, and their admirers cultivate their milieu (Dakers, 1999); develop 'radical aesthetics' (Peppiatt & Bellony-Rewald, 1982); make visible collective identities (Kellie, 2017; Blazwick, 2022); and forge acts of resistance (Raven, 1994, Costa, 2022).

Group studios and complexes can also be the catalyst for the construction and expression of underrepresented identities, where the sharing of practices and knowledges is not only a means of professional accreditation, but also a means of challenging professional orthodoxies and shaping international art scenes. Centres such as the *Studio Watts Workshop*, Studio Z's *The Studio*, and *Womanhouse*, for example, were instrumental not only in shaping the Los Angeles art scene in the 1970s and 1980s, but also acted as conduits for establishing art histories and identities that were not reflected in the mainstream arts programmes (Raven, 1994; Kellie, 2017). Collectivism and shared studio resources are vital in creating not just individual subjectivities, but forms of resistance (Costa, 2022).

The nurturing of artistic communities has been seen as a means of developing the economic health of neglected urban centres (Harris, 2012; Ley, 2003; Lloyd, 2002; Mathews, 2010). In America and Europe, the movement of artists into former industrial areas (or areas seen need revitalisation), and the conversion of manufacturing buildings into mixed use properties during the 1970s, started to shape real estate markets (Zukin, 1989). By the 1980s, these communities were already part of urban planning and redevelopment proposals (Cole, 1987). Often, the provision of affordable artists' studios formed part of a regeneration bid, in the hope that the creation of cultural quarters brings with it further stages of reinvestment (Moreton, 2013). Changes in the symbolic meaning of 'upcoming' neighbourhoods carry with them social costs, too. The displacement of (Catungal et al., 2009; Deutsche & Ryan, 1984) and disaffiliation with (Bain, 2017) existing communities can foster local resentment, and act as a polarising force in the relationships between influxes of cultural workers and existing residents.

At the more precarious end of work/live studio complexes, this make-shift arrangement can also lead to the devastation of communities. In 2016, a fire at the Ghost Ship warehouse in Oakland, California, claimed the lives of thirty-six people. Rising rent and real estate values had pushed artists into illegally adapted live-work spaces in a building that, following the fire, was described as a '10,000 square foot tinderbox' (Campbell, 2022, p.1). Small-scale DIY live-work artists' spaces are not uncommon, and in many cases, they form part of the neo-bohemian attraction that draws artists to a location (Lloyd, 2002). They can be 'safe spaces for the inclusive cultures they can foster' (Campbell, 2022, p.3): the Ghost Ship was not just a studio complex and venue, but a central hub for communities of LGBTQ+ and underrepresented artists.

The creation of affordable studio complexes and creative spaces in former industrial zones, or on existing (but often neglected neighbourhoods), has generated tensions around the co-existence and displacement of communities. Writings on the gentrification of urban areas regularly raise questions about the roles and agency of creatives (Deutsche & Ryan, 1984; Ley, 2003; Bain, 2004; 2017) and the implied benefits of artistic economies on the health of neighbourhoods. Creativity has been closely bound to the lexicon of urban planning, bringing with it a sense of entrepreneurial opportunity, and a belief in the affective power of the artists' presence to reinvigorate, rejuvenate, and (re)invent communities.

The urban-pastoral

Just as studio *topoi* mythologise the interiority of creative spaces, the notion of creative communities can mythologise connections between artistic groups and the neighbourhoods they inhabit. Studios, like parks and open spaces, are often value-laden and, subject to processes of evaluation and calculation through which social benefit is measured (Moreton, 2013, see also Bain & Landau, 2019). In Harris's (2012) analyses of the the arts scene in Hoxton, London, and Catungul et al.'s (2009) examination of the Liberty Village development in Toronto, both emerging artists and developers made use of a pastoral imaginary to generate and promote alternative notions of community. In different ways, the creation of pseudo-bucolic associations between the artists and neighbourhood fed a romanticised, nostalgic, and good-feeling sentiment around the repurposing of former industrial buildings as live-work studios. A notional rebranding that focused on an idyllic 'urban village' feel separated the emerging creative centres from business districts or longstanding residents nearby.

The aestheticisation of often ethnically diverse, economically neglected, or socially excluded neighbourhoods, involves selective control over what is representable: what offers a 'spectacle of slumming delectation' (Deutsche & Ryan, 1984), and what is considered "hazardous". Bain's examination of artistic regeneration in Ontario points to the use of 'selective practices of sanitisation and ordering' (2017, p.12), in the form of "clean-ups" and clearances, that reproduce class relations and displace street-based cultures. Recently, critical reevaluations of the discriminatory aesthetics of gentrification have pushed for the building of creative visibilities from within the communities. In comparing two examples of cultural gentrification in Los Angeles, Jonathan Jae-an Crisman (2021) argues for an 'aesthetics of engagement' that aligns with participatory arts practices, and counter to the privileging of autonomous modes of creative production. Just as Sjöholm (2014) reflects the value of the individual studio as an archive-space for recollection and recuperation, Crisman's study of event-spaces in Little Tokyo offers both a collective archive and an example of grass-roots activism aimed at preserving and caring for the cultural visibility of existing communities.

Summary

I have connected together a diverse range of historical and contemporary versions of the art studio in order to outline a series of links between ideas of physical, moral, psychological, and economic health and the spaces in which artists and artists' communities work in this chapter. The examples provided progress an idea of the studio from the isolated "psychic chamber" of Romantic-era bohemianism to the community studios and complexes are both spaces for sharing common values and strategic implements in an urban planner's toolbox.

The construct of studio is also nebulous. They arc both physical environments and metaphorical ideas about space and bodily performances; a "state of mind" as much as a room set aside for making and thinking (see Daniels, 2011; Hawkins, 2014; Sjöholm, 2018). Historically, the studio as a space to work, or to reclaim creative autonomy, has played a key role in notions of artistic "professionalism". These claims have not just been vital in validating artistic identities but also in achieving levels of visibility. In some cases the studio has not only become a backdrop to the projected identities of the artists who work there, but also a cipher for decoding a particular "state of mind". However, as a number of the illustrations here show, studios are more than isolated, amniotic, and self-absorbed enclaves of work, they are places of recuperation, gathering, remembering, and collaborating. Artists often cluster and studio communities offer a degree of cohesion, a sharing of professional knowledge and 'a sense of self that comes with knowing others' (Price & Hawkins, 2018).

To extend these relations beyond this text, I return to the statement made at the beginning of this chapter – to the diffuse nature of a contemporary studio emphasised in the idea of the 'everywhere studio' (Gartenfield, 2017). It refers to a transient, mobile, networked version of artistic labour that reflects a normalisation of precarity and instability that is already common to a good deal of creative work. Yet it also illustrates the degree to which artistic identity and community are forged in other ways and on other platforms, than the physical spaces that have formed the majority of current research in the fields of geography and studio studies. Alongside the studio *topoi* that have defined the living conditions of artists and art communities, these spaces of production and presentation offer equally complex topologies of anxiety, precarity, collaboration, and care.

References

Adamson, G. (2007) Craft and the Romance of the Studio. *American Art*, 21(1), 14–18.

Alpers, S. (2005) *The Vexations of Art*. Yale University Press, New Haven.

Ash, J. (2016) Theorizing Studio Space. In *Studio studies: Operations, topologies and displacements*, (Eds, Farias, I. & Wilkie, A.) Routledge, Abingdon, Oxon; New York, pp. 91–104.

Bain, A.L. (2004) In/visible geographies: Absence, emergence, presence, and the fine art of identity construction. *Tijdschrift voor economische en sociale geografie*, 95(4), 419–426.

Bain, A.L. (2005) Constructing an artistic identity. *Work, Employment and Society*, 19(1), 25–46.

Bain, A.L. (2017) Neighbourhood artistic disaffiliation in Hamilton, Ontario, Canada. *Urban Studies*, 54(13), 2935–2954.

Bain, A.L. & Landau, F. (2019) Artists, temporality, and the governance of collaborative place-making. *Urban Affairs Review*, 55(2), 405–427.

Bain, A.L. (2004) Female artistic identity in place: The studio. *Social & Cultural Geography*, 5(2), 171–193.

Bellony-Rewald, A. & Peppiatt, M. (1983) *Imagination's Chamber: Artists and Their Studios*. Gordon Fraser, London.

Bergstein, M. (1995) "The artist in his studio": Photography, art, and the masculine mystique. *Oxford Art Journal*, 18(2), 45–58.

Blazwick, I. (2022) Making the Studio Public. In *A century of the artist's studio 1920–2020*, (Eds, Blazwick, I., Costa, I. & Stobbs, C.) Whitechapel Gallery, London, pp. 16–21.

Boltanski, L. & Chiapello, E. (2018) *The New Spirit of Capitalism*. Verso, London; New York.

Bubenik, A. (2019) *The Persistence of Melancholia in Arts and Culture*. Routledge, Abingdon, Oxon; New York.

Buren, D. (1979) The Function of the Studio. *October*, 10, 51–58.

Burns, S. (1996) *Inventing the Modern Artist: Art and Culture in Gilded Age America*. Yale University Press, New Haven.

Busta, C. (2017) Studio Domains. In *The everywhere studio*, (Eds, Gartenfield, A., Moreno, G. & Seidel, S.) Institute of Contemporary Art, Miami and DelMonico Books/Prestel, Miami, FL, pp. 253–260.

Campbell, M. (2022) *Reimagining the Creative Industries: Youth Creative Work, Communities of Care*. Routledge, Abingdon, Oxon; New York.

Catungal, J.P., Leslie, D. & Hii, Y. (2009) Geographies of displacement in the creative city: The case of Liberty Village, Toronto. *Urban Studies*, 46(5–6), 1095–1114.

Chapman, H.P. (1990) *Rembrandt's Self-Portraits: A Study in Seventeenth-century Identity*. Princeton University Press, Princeton, NJ.

Chapman, H.P. (2005) The Imagined Studios of Rembrandt and Vermeer. In *Inventions of the studio, renaissance to romanticism*, (Eds, Cole, M.W. & Pardo, M.) University of North Carolina Press, Chapel Hill.

Chare, N. (2006) Passages to paint: Francis Bacon's studio practice. *Parallax*, 12(4), 83–98.

Chicago, J. (1982) *Through the Flower: My Struggle as a Woman Artist*. Anchor Books, Garden City, NY.

Codell, J.F. (2003) *The Victorian Artist: Artists' Lifewritings in Britain, ca. 1870–1910*. Cambridge University Press, Cambridge, UK; New York, NY, USA.

Cole, D.B. (1987) Artists and urban redevelopment. *Geographical Review*, 77(4), 391–407.

Cole, M.W. & Pardo, M. (Eds.) (2005) *Inventions of the Studio, Renaissance to Romanticism*. University of North Carolina Press, Chapel Hill.

Coles, A. (2012) *The Transdisciplinary Studio*. Sternberg Press, Berlin.

Costa, I. (2022) The collaborative studio: Art, resistance, exchange arpilleras workshops and Laboratoire Agit'art. In *A century of the artist's studio 1920–2020*, (Eds, Blazwick, I., Costa, I. & Stobbs, C.) Whitechapel Gallery, London, pp. 22–26.

Crary, J. (2014) *24/7*. Verso, London; New York.

Crisman, J.J. (2021) Art and the Aesthetics of Cultural Gentrification: The Cases of Boyle Heights and Little Tokyo in Los Angeles. In *Aesthetics of gentrification: Seductive spaces and exclusive communities in the Neoliberal City*, (Eds, Sandoval, G.F. & Lindner, C.) Amsterdam University Press, Amsterdam, pp. 137–154.

Dakers, C. (1999) *The Holland Park Circle: Artists and Victorian Society*. Yale University Press, New Haven, CT.

Daniels, S. (2011) *Art Studio*. SAGE Publications Ltd, London, pp. 137–148.

Davidts, W. & Paice, K. (Eds.) (2009) *The Fall of the Studio: Artists at Work*. Antennae; Valiz, Amsterdam.

Dawson, B. (2009) Francis Bacon: A Terrible Beauty. In *Francis Bacon: A Terrible Beauty*, (Eds, Dawson, B., Harrison, M. & Sisley, L.) Steidl, Göttingen, Germany, pp. 50–69.

Dawson, B. & Harrison, M. (2009) *Francis Bacon: A Terrible Beauty*. Steidl, Göttingen, Germany.

Deutsche, R. & Ryan, C.G. (1984) The Fine Art of Gentrification. *October*, 31, 91–111.

Dixon, L.S. (2013) *The Dark Side of Genius: The Melancholic Persona in Art*. Pennsylvania State University Press, University Park, PA.

Engelmann, S. (2017) Social spiders and hybrid webs at Studio Tomás Saraceno. *Cultural Geographies*, 24(1), 161–169.

Engelmann, S. (2019) Of spiders and simulations: Artmachines at Studio Tomás Saraceno. *Cultural Geographies*, 26(3), 305–322.

Esner, R. (2018) 'Ateliers d'artistes'(1898): An advertorial for the 'lady readers' of the Figaro illustré. *Early Popular Visual Culture*, 16(4), 368–384.

Esner, R., Kisters, S. & Lehmann, A.-S. (Eds.) (2013) *Hiding Making, Showing Creation: The Studio from Turner to Tacita Dean*. Amsterdam University Press, Amsterdam.

Farias, I. & Wilkie, A. (Eds.) (2016) *Studio Studies: Operations, Topologies, Displacements*. Routledge, Abingdon, Oxon; New York.

Gartenfield, A. (2017) Introduction. In *The everywhere studio*, (Eds, Gartenfield, A., Moreno, G. & Seidel, S.) Institute of Contemporary Art, Miami and DelMonico Books / Prestel, Miami, FL.

Gotleib, M. (2005) Creation and Death in the Romantic Studio. In *Inventions of the studio, Renaissance to Romanticism*, (Eds, Cole, M.W. & Pardo, M.) University of North Carolina Press, Chapel Hill, pp. 147–184.

Gouma-Peterson, T. (1997) Miriam Schapiro: An Art of Becoming. *American Art*, 11(1), 10–45.

Grabner, M. (2010) Introduction. (Eds, Jacob, M.J. & Grabner, M.) The studio reader: On the SPACE OF ARTISTS University of Chicago Press, Chicago, IL, London, pp. 1–16.

Harris, A. (2012) Art and gentrification: Pursuing the urban pastoral in Hoxton, London. *Transactions of the Institute of British Geographers*, 37(2), 226–241.

Harrison, M. (Ed.) (2019) *Bacon and the Mind: Art, Neuroscience and Psychology*. Thames and Hudson, London; New York.

Hawkins, H. (2014) *For Creative Geographies: Geography, Visual Arts and the Making of Worlds*. Routledge, Abingdon, Oxon; New York.

Hawkins, H. (2018) Geography's creative (re)turn: Toward a critical framework. *Progress in Human Geography*, 43(6), 963–984.

Jacob, M.J. & Grabner, M. (Eds.) (2010) *The Studio Reader: On the Space of Artists* University of Chicago Press, Chicago.

Jellis, T. (2015) Spatial experiments: Art, geography, pedagogy. *Cultural Geographies*, 22(2), 369–374.

Jones, C.A. (1996) *Machine in the Studio: Constructing the Postwar American Artist*. University of Chicago Press, Chicago.

Lamb, J. (1993) 'The way we live now': Late Victorian studios and the popular press. *Visual Resources*, 9(2), 107–125.

Leclair, M. (2023) The atmospherics of creativity: Affective and spatial materiality in a designer's studio. *Organization Studies*, 44(5), 807–829.

Lehmann, A.-S. (2013) "Good Art Theory Must Smell of the Studio". In *Hiding making, showing creation: The studio from Turner to Tacita Dean*, (Eds, Esner, R., Kisters, S. & Lehmann, A.-S.) Amsterdam University Press, Amsterdam, pp. 245–255.

Leone, L. (2021) *Craft in Art Therapy: Diverse Approaches to the Transformative Power of Craft Materials and Methods*. Routledge, Abingdon, Oxon; New York.

Ley, D. (2003) Artists, aestheticisation and the field of gentrification. *Urban Studies*, 40(12), 2527–2544.

Lloyd, R. (2002) Neo-bohemia: Art and neighborhood redevelopment in Chicago. *Journal of Urban Affairs*, 24(5), 517–532.

Luckman, S. (2015) *Craft and the Creative Economy*. Palgrave Macmillan, Houndmills, Basingstoke, Hampshire; New York, NY.

Mathews, V. (2010) Aestheticizing space: Art, gentrification and the city. *Geography Compass*, 4(6), 660–675.

McHugh, C. (2014) 'I've not finished': Why studios are still a fundamental requirement in the study of fine art. *Journal of Visual Art Practice*, 13(1), 30–40.

Miller, S.M. (2020) Disability art: Potential intersections in studio practice with artists labeled/with intellectual and developmental disabilities. *Art Therapy*, 37(2), 93–96.

Moon, C.H. (2015) Open Studio Approach to Art Therapy. In *The Wiley handbook of art therapy*, (Eds, Gussak, D.E. & Rosal, M.L.) print reference, pp. 112–121. www.wiley.com/en-us/The+Wiley+Handbook+of+Art+Therapy-p-9781118306598

Moreton, S. (2013) The promise of the affordable artist's studio: Governing creative spaces in London. *Environment and Planning A: Economy and Space Environ Plan A*, 45(2), 421–437.

Mould, O. (2018) *Against Creativity*. Verso, London; New York.

Mould, O. (2015) *Urban Subversion and the Creative City*. Routledge, Abingdon, Oxon; New York.

Peppiatt, M. (1984) Francis Bacon: The Studio as Symbol. *Connoisseur*, 214, 84–93.

Peppiatt, M., & Bellini-Rewald, A. (1982). Imagination's chamber: Artists and Their Studios. New York: New York Graphic Society.

Postle, M. (2009) The Artist's Studio, Everything, including the kitchen sink: Studio squalor from Barry to Bacon. (Ed, Waterfield, G.) Hogarth Arts, Compton Verney, pp. 42–63.

Price, L. & Hawkins, H. (2018) *Geographies of Making, Craft and Creativity*. Routledge, Abingdon, Oxon; New York.

Raven, A. (1994) Womanhouse. In *The power of feminist art: The American movement of the 1970s, history and impact*, (Eds, Broude, N. & Garrard, M.D.) H.N. Abrams, New York, p. 318.

Relyea, L. (2013) *Your Everyday Art World*. The MIT Press, Cambridge, Mass.

Ross, C. (2006) *The Aesthetics of Disengagement: Contemporary Art and Depression*. University of Minnesota Press, Minneapolis.

Seigel, K. (2010) Live/Work. In *The studio reader: On the space of artists*, (Eds, Jacob, M.J. & Grabner, M.) University of Chicago Press, Chicago; London, pp. 311–316.

Sjöholm, J. (2014) The art studio as archive: Tracing the geography of artistic potentiality, progress and production. *Cultural Geographies*, 21(3), 505–514.

Sjöholm, J. (2018) Making bodies, making space and making memory in artistic practice. In *Geographies of making, craft and creativity*, (Eds, Price, L. & Hawkins, H.) Routledge, Abingdon, Oxon; New York, pp. 40–51.

Stobbs, C. (2022) This is Where I Live: The Studio as Subject for Women Artists. In *A century of the artist's studio 1920–2020*, (Eds. Blazwick, I., Costa, I. & Stobbs, C.) Whitechapel Gallery, London, pp. 32–36.

Thomas, M. (2009) Studio Vertigo: Mark Rothko. (Eds, Davidts, W. & Paice, K.) Antennae; Distribution, D.A.P., Valiz, Amsterdam; New York, NY, pp. 23–42.

Turner, C. (2009) Bacon Dust. *Cabinet*, Fall 2009 (35) n.p.

Waterfield, G. (Ed.) (2009) *The Artist's Studio*. Hogarth Arts, Compton Verney.

Wedd, K. (2001) *Artists' London: Holbein to Hirst*. Merrell, London.

White, H.C. & White, C.A. (1965) *Canvases and Careers; Institutional Change in the French Painting World*. Wiley, New York.

Wittkower, R. & Wittkower, M. (2007) *Born Under Saturn: The Character and Conduct of Artists*. New York Review Books, New York.

Zukin, S. (1989) *Loft Living: Culture and Capital in Urban Change*. Rutgers University Press, New Brunswick, NJ.

28 Creative spaces of disaster recovery

Kate E. W. Douglas

(re)Creating the boundaries

As it stands, a unanimous definition for 'disaster recovery' is absent in geographic scholarship (Wisner, Gaillard & Kelman, 2012; McGee & Penning-Rowsell, 2022). This is symptomatic of the discipline's seemingly endless struggle to define the boundaries of disaster recovery; what it looks like, where and when it occurs, who can participate, and how long it takes to 'recover'. There are, however, points of agreement. Geographers of various specialisations have long advocated for disaster recovery programmes that support the specific needs, strengths, and goals of affected communities, particularly those led *by* community, *for* community (Cutter et al., 2008; Khasalamwa, 2009; Silva, 2009; Pelling & Dill, 2010; Howitt, Havnen & Veland, 2011; MacKinnon & Derickson, 2013; Cutter et al., 2014; Clissold, Westoby & McNamara, 2020). This perspective is in keeping with a broader multidisciplinary reconceptualisation of recovery as a "non-linear and relational" (Mika & Kelman, 2020, p. 646; see also Duff, 2016; Andrews & Duff, 2020), embodied and lived (de Vet et al., 2020) experience that "engages and empowers" (Glavovic, 2014, p. 208) disaster-affected individuals and communities. Ultimately, this push for *community-led recovery* points to a number of troubling gaps in the boundaries imposed by state-sponsored recovery models. While the specificities of these gaps will manifest in different ways for different individuals, most can be traced to a broader need for communities to establish and maintain autonomous spaces of *hope* (see Anderson, 2006; 2017; Head, 2016) during their recovery journeys.

Following disaster, the mental health and wellbeing of affected individuals is compromised by personal experiences of grief, loss, distress, and hurt (Whittle et al., 2012; McKinnon, Gorman-Murray & Dominey-Howes, 2016; Cloke et al., 2023). As evidenced in Eriksen and de Vet's (2021) study of insurance claims following the October 2013 bushfires in New South Wales, Australia, governments are responsible for some of the most critical recovery services – some of which are specifically designed to alleviate the impacts of these experiences. In many cases, these services are, however, inescapably bureaucratic; they are pre-determined within a web of neoliberal and capitalist agenda (MacKinnon & Derickson, 2012). This underlying mode of operation largely manifests as rigid spatiotemporal parameters, within which recovering individuals and communities must fit to receive the support on offer. Consequently, fraught with demanding eligibility measures, deadlines, and paperwork, the time between applying for and receiving government support requires a significant amount of emotional and intellectual labour from recovering individuals (de Vet, Eriksen & McKinnon, 2020). For some individuals,

DOI: 10.4324/9781003345725-31

the pressure of these processes can exacerbate underlying "post-disaster exhaustion" (Eriksen & de Vet, 2021, p. 232) and traumas. For others, being relegated to these "passive" roles (Clissold et al., 2020, p. 101) ignites a desire for self-autonomy and control over the trajectory of their recovery journeys. In each of these scenarios, there is a need to *feel* or *do more* in order to imagine and enact *hopeful* futures.

Community-led recovery is predicated on community participation and leadership. As such, community-led recovery *projects* emerge with and through the desires of a recovering community (Dionisio & Pawson, 2016). The implications of this emergent quality are twofold. Firstly, it enables projects to identify and facilitate immediate enactments of "hopeful imaginaries" (Dickinson, 2018, p. 637) that arise post-disaster. Secondly, as hopeful subjectivities evolve through time and space (Popke, 2003; Cloke & Conradson, 2018), this symbiotic relationship ensures projects can depart from or advance these initial enactments in accordance with the progress of a community's recovery journey. For this reason, it is common to see a multiplicity of "ephemeral, short-term, transitory and temporary" (Dionisio & Pawson, 2016, p. 111) community-led recovery projects at work across a post-disaster landscape.

Whether they be short- or long-term, improvised or pre-existing, geographic scholarship has routinely regarded community-led recovery projects as legitimate and *political* spaces of participation in the aftermath of disaster (Cretney & Bond, 2014; Cretney, 2017; 2018; Dickinson, 2018; 2021; Cloke & Dickinson, 2019). According to Cretney (2018), disaster events disrupt and, subsequently, suspend the status quo, leaving behind a "blank canvas" (p. 504) upon which various political contestations can ensue (see also Pelling & Dill, 2010). At first glance, the activities occurring within community-led projects may appear inconsequential against the backdrop of top-down recovery politics. However, as governments use this period of suspension to entrench centralised, neoliberal modes of governance, community-led projects offer persistent and experimental spaces of democratic participation in the face of de-politicising strategies (Cretney, 2016; 2018; Dickinson, 2018). As such, these projects "rupture" (Cretney, 2018, p. 497; see also Deleuze, Guattari & Polan, 1986; Head & Gibson, 2012; Head, 2016) and expand the boundaries of recovery politics, to embed participatory spaces of "progressive possibility" (Dickinson, 2018, p. 623; see also Wilson, 2013).

(re)Creating along the boundaries

Underpinning much of the preceding analyses are case studies of *creative* community-led projects based in the city of Ōtautahi Christchurch, Aotearoa New Zealand (Dionisio & Pawson, 2016; Cretney, 2018; Dickinson, 2018). Following the 2010-11 earthquakes in Ōtautahi Christchurch, these projects were largely established by third-sector organisations, namely Gap Filler, Project Lyttelton, Life in Vacant Spaces, and Greening the Rubble. Dickinson (2018) lists "temporary art, large-scale murals, sport and entertainment installations, novel attractions (such as a cycle-powered cinema) and ever-changing participatory activities (such as book exchanges, public poetry and community gatherings)" (p. 626) as some of the key projects facilitated by these organisations. The same case studies are also found in Cloke and colleagues' (Cloke, Dickinson & Tupper, 2017; Cloke & Conradson, 2018; Cloke & Dickinson, 2019; Cloke et al., 2023) work on *transitional organisations* and *urbanism* (e.g., Yeh & Wu, 1999; Cloke, May & Johnsen, 2008; Cupples & Glynn, 2009). Throughout these works, creative recovery projects are deemed 'transitional' in that they depart from "neoliberalised" values and practices of urbanism and offer "a new imagination of how things can be, and a new set of practices and performances that enact that imagination within a wider environment characterised by both *hopefulness* and difficulty" (Cloke & Conradson, 2018, pp. 362–365; emphasis added; see also Aiken, 2017; Gill, Johnstone & Williams, 2012).

As stated by Cloke and Dickinson (2019), this departure is "simultaneously real, imagined, and affective" (p. 1931). Just like other formations of community-led recovery, creative recovery projects offer 'real' opportunities for participation; they provide a geophysical site in which like-minded individuals can gather and renegotiate the post-disaster landscape. There are, however, notable distinctions between gathering to rebuild what has been destroyed during a disaster (e.g., a wall or building) and gathering to transform a vacant lot into a performance space. While both instances represent a form of "being-in-common" (Cloke & Conradson, 2018, p. 363; see also Nancy, 1991) following a disaster, they are underpinned by different ethics (Popke, 2003; Bennett, 2001; McCormack, 2003). By repairing what once was, using the same practices, for the same purpose, the 'rebuild' project upholds an ethics of conservatism (Cloke et al., 2017; Cloke et al., 2023). For such a project, participants are more likely to be local to a specific suburb and skilled in a related area of trade. Conversely, by establishing an entirely new place in the city, the creative project releases an ethics of "experimental generosity, hospitality and compassionate interconnectedness" (Cloke & Conradson, 2018, p. 371). This ethical sensibility is entwined in the emergent nature of creative recovery projects; their 'newness' leaves them without preconceived (pre-disaster) ideas regarding precisely who, how, and what purpose they serve. Accordingly, participation untethers from all prerequisites, leaving the creative recovery projects of Ōtautahi Christchurch able to welcome and accommodate a diverse demographic of participants (Cloke et al., 2023). Across the literature, this is traced to a "fidelity to the earthquake event" (Cloke & Dickinson, 2019, p. 1931; see also Badiou, 2005), through which creative recovery projects become:

> [...] markers of the *continuing* event of the earthquakes. Their continuing fidelity to the event not only prompts memorial practices for remembered pasts, and prophetic gaze on the *future* (Willis, 2014), but also highlights the possibility of new subjectivity embodying an excess over what previously 'counted'– in other words a new form of *collective creativity*.
>
> (Cloke et al., 2017, p. 71; emphases added)

Once these creative recovery projects and associated situated ethics (see Massey, 2005) are at work in the city, their deviation from the norm becomes increasingly 'real'. Most immediately, the projects encourage disaster-affected citizens to experiment with "new and more improvised performances of social life" (Cloke & Conradson, 2018, p. 362). By entering these public and communal spaces, participants are offered unique opportunities to *encounter* (see Wilson, 2017) and interact with unfamiliar people. Encounters and interactions with these 'others' (see Popke, 2006) are shaped by shared experiences of disruption and, in turn, the realisation of shared mind-sets (values, morals, and sensibilities). When coupled with a creative project's "practices of meeting, listening, interacting, performing and caring together" (Cloke & Conradson, 2018, p. 371), this "in-commonness" (Cloke et al., 2017, p. 78) quickly inspires new interpersonal relationships between participants; as the community of the project grows, so too do the communities of the individuals therein.

Creative recovery projects also leave material and aesthetic imprints in the cityscape. In Ōtautahi Christchurch, these imprints are encountered by project participants and spectators alike. For example, Gap Filler's 'The Commons' oversaw the transformation of a vacant car lot into a sprung dancefloor with "a coin operated washing-machine-turned-jukebox" (Cloke & Dickinson, 2019, p. 1929) (the 'Dance-O-Mat'), as well as the installation of a large Monopoly boardgame square over the foundations of a demolition area (Cloke et al., 2017). In each of these cases, the materiality of the city is altered; rubble is replaced by art, vacant space is filled with objects, and the grey of the city is embellished with colour. These material and aesthetic alterations are more than "colourful band aids" (Cloke & Dickinson, 2019, p. 1930) overlaying the material ruptures of a disaster event. The products of creative recovery projects are, in and of themselves, material ruptures across the cityscape (Dickinson, 2018). Unlike those caused by the earthquakes, these ruptures are borne out of collaborative practices of place- and memory-making and mature as "material and emotional homages" (Dickinson, 2018, p. 284) designed by and for the citizens of Ōtautahi Christchurch (Cloke et al., 2017; Cloke & Conradson, 2018).

Cloke and colleagues (Cloke & Conradson, 2018; Cloke & Dickinson, 2019) illustrate the 'imagined' and 'affective' dimensions of creative recovery projects through the lens of *affective atmospheres*. Mainly referring to the non-representational (e.g., Thrift, 2000; 2008; Lorimer, 2008) framings of Anderson (2006; 2009; 2014; 2016), *affect* is presented as a "set of pre-personal intensities which may nonetheless shape and inform the experiences of individuals" (Cloke & Conradson, 2018, p. 362). When these intensities are generated, reiterated, and felt by a collective of bodies in-situ, they come to constitute an affective atmosphere (Cloke & Conradson, 2018; Bissell, 2010; Closs Stephens et al., 2017). Importantly, these 'bodies' are both human and non-human. As such, in the context of post-disaster Ōtautahi Christchurch, attention is paid to the ways in which affective atmospheres seem to "envelop" (Anderson, 2009, p. 78) not only the participants of creative recovery projects, but also the social and material interactions in which they engage. Here, the 'real' and the 'imagined' combine with co-constitutive consequences. The "vibe" (Cloke & Dickinson, 2019, p. 1932) of the affective atmosphere is sustained by the "tentacular" (Dickinson, 2018, p. 285) relationship between human and non-human – each embodying the vibe, and each informed by the other. Ultimately, Cloke et al., (2023) suggest these affective atmospheres cultivate and diffuse the sense *hopefulness* arising from the creative, social, and aesthetic experimentations of the creative recovery projects "in amongst the landscapes of urban disaster" (p. 141).

(re)Creating beyond the boundaries

> Hopefulness, therefore, exemplifies a disposition that provides a dynamic imperative *to action* in that it enables bodies to *go on*.
>
> (Anderson, 2006, p. 744)

Throughout much of the aforementioned literature are implicit references to the ways in which creative recovery projects provide spaces of mental health and wellbeing for disaster-affected communities and individuals. In Ōtautahi Christchurch, this capacity is largely a consequence of the real, imagined, and affective avenues of *hope* these spaces inspire. As illustrated by Cloke and colleagues (Cloke, Dickinson & Tupper, 2017; Cloke & Conradson, 2018; Cloke & Dickinson, 2019; Cloke et al., 2023), creative recovery projects support activities of collective creativity, social networks of in-commonness, sites of re-materialisation, and diffusions of affective atmospheres. Each of these avenues have clear implications at the community-level; they promote diversity, inclusion, pride, and unity. Amidst these collective experiences also lie individualised avenues for personal development and respite. For instance, while painting a mural, constructing a temporary performance space, or dancing at the Dance-O-Mat may draw upon pre-existing skillsets or interests for some participants, these same experiences provide novel opportunities to develop new skills, new forms of expression, and new sources of recreation for others (Wesener, 2015; Cloke & Dickinson, 2019). Underpinning all these experiences (and many others) is an opportunity to *do* and *feel more*. Creative recovery projects in Ōtautahi Christchurch offer new and exciting spaces in which both communities and individuals can engage activities, relations, and atmospheres geared towards an alternative, experimental, and *hopeful* future. In doing so, these creative spaces of disaster recovery can achieve both immediate and ongoing impacts that "endure beyond the time-scale of the temporary" (Cloke et al., 2023, p. 137).

References

Anderson, B. (2006). "Transcending without transcendence": Utopianism and an Ethos of hope. *Antipode*, *38*(4), 691–710. https://doi.org/10.1111/j.1467-8330.2006.00472.x

Anderson, B. (2009). Affective atmospheres. *Emotion, Space and Society*, *2*(2), 77–81. https://doi.org/10.1016/j.emospa.2009.08.005

Anderson, B. (2014). *Encountering affect: Capacities, apparatuses, conditions*. Farnham, UK: Ashgate.

Anderson, B. (2016). Neoliberal affects. *Progress in Human Geography*, *40*(6), 734–753. https://doi.org/10.1177/0309132515613167

Anderson, B. (2017). Hope and micropolitics. *Environment and Planning D: Society and Space*, *35*(4), 593–595. https://doi.org/10.1177/0263775817710088

Andrews, G. J., & Duff, C. (2020). 'Whole onflow', the productive event: An articulation through health. *Social Science & Medicine*, *265*, 113498. https://doi.org/10.1016/j.socscimed.2020.113498

Badiou, A. (2005). *Being and event*. Continuum.

Bennett, J. (2001). *The enchantment of modern life: Attachments, crossings, and ethics*. Princeton, N.J: Princeton University Press.

Bissell, D. (2010). Passenger mobilities: Affective atmospheres and the sociality of public transport. *Environment and Planning D: Society and Space*, *28*(2), 270–289. https://doi.org/10.1068/d3909

Clissold, R., Westoby, R., & McNamara, K. E. (2020). Women as recovery enablers in the face of disasters in Vanuatu. *Geoforum*, *113*, 101–110. https://doi.org/10.1016/j.geoforum.2020.05.003

Cloke, P., & Conradson, D. (2018). Transitional organisations, affective atmospheres and new forms of being-in-common: Post-disaster recovery in Christchurch, New Zealand. *Transactions of the Institute of British Geographers*, *43*(3), 360–376. https://doi.org/10.1111/tran.12240

Cloke, P. J., Conradson, D., Pawson, E., & Perkins, H. C. (2023). *The post-earthquake city: Disaster and recovery in Christchurch, New Zealand* (1st ed.). Routledge.

Cloke, P., & Dickinson, S. (2019). Transitional ethics and aesthetics: Reimagining the postdisaster city in Christchurch, New Zealand. *Annals of the American Association of Geographers*, *109*(6), 1922–1940. https://doi.org/10.1080/24694452.2019.1570838

Cloke, P., Dickinson, S., & Tupper, S. (2017). The Christchurch earthquakes 2010, 2011: Geographies of an event: Christchurch earthquakes: Geographies of an event. *New Zealand Geographer*, *73*(2), 69–80. https://doi.org/10.1111/nzg.12152

Cloke, P., May, J., & Johnsen, S. (2008). Performativity and affect in the homeless city. *Environment and Planning D: Society and Space*, *26*, 241–263. doi:10.1068/d84j

Closs Stephens, A., Hughes, S. M., Schofield, V., & Sumartojo, S. (2017). Atmospheric memories: Affect and minor politics at the ten-year anniversary of the London bombings. *Emotion, Space and Society*, *23*, 44–51. https://doi.org/10.1016/j.emospa.2017.03.001

Cretney, R. (2018). "An opportunity to hope and dream": Disaster politics and the emergence of possibility through community-led recovery. *Antipode*, *51*(2), 497–516. https://doi.org/10.1111/anti.12431

Cretney, R., & Bond, S. (2014). 'Bouncing back' to capitalism? Grass-roots autonomous activism in shaping discourses of resilience and transformation following disaster. *Resilience*, *2*(1), 18–31. https://doi.org/10.1080/21693293.2013.872449

Cretney, R. M. (2016). Local responses to disaster: The value of community led post disaster response action in a resilience framework. *Disaster Prevention and Management*, *25*(1), 27–40. https://doi.org/10.1108/DPM-02-2015-0043

Cretney, R. M. (2017). Towards a critical geography of disaster recovery politics: Perspectives on crisis and hope: Towards a critical geography of disaster recovery politics. *Geography Compass*, *11*(1). https://doi.org/10.1111/gec3.12302

Cretney, R. M. (2018). Beyond public meetings: Diverse forms of community led recovery following disaster. *International Journal of Disaster Risk Reduction*, *28*, 122–130. https://doi.org/10.1016/j.ijdrr.2018.02.035

Cupples, J. and Glynn, K. (2009). Countercartographies: New (Zealand) cultural studies/geographies and the city. *New Zealand Geographer*, *65*(1), 1–5. https://doi.org/10.1111/j.1745-7939.2009.01143. x

Cutter, S. L., Ash, K. D., & Emrich, C. T. (2014). The geographies of community disaster resilience. *Global Environmental Change*, *29*, 65–77. https://doi.org/10.1016/j.gloenvcha.2014.08.005

Cutter, S. L., Barnes, L., Berry, M., Burton, C., Evans, E., Tate, E., & Webb, J. (2008). A place-based model for understanding community resilience to natural disasters. *Global Environmental Change*, *18*(4), 598–606. https://doi.org/10.1016/j.gloenvcha.2008.07.013

De Vet, E., Eriksen, C., & McKinnon, lS. (2020). *Dilemmas, decision-making, and disasters: Emotions of parenting, safety, and rebuilding in bushfire recovery.* https://doi.org/10.1111/area.12696

Deleuze, G., Guattari, F, & Polan, D. (1986). *Kafka: Towards a Minor Literature.* University of Minnesota Press.

Dickinson, S. (2018). Spaces of post-disaster experimentation: Agile entrepreneurship and geological agency in emerging disaster countercartographies. *Environment and Planning E: Nature and Space*, *1*(4), 621–640. https://doi.org/10.1177/2514848618812023

Dickinson, S. (2021). Alternative narrations and imaginations of disaster recovery: A case study of relocatees after the Christchurch, New Zealand, earthquakes. *Social & Cultural Geography*, *22*(2), 273–293. https://doi.org/10.1080/14649365.2019.1574883

Dionisio, M. R., & Pawson, E. (2016). Building resilience through post-disaster community projects: Responses to the 2010 and 2011 Christchurch Earthquakes and 2011 Tōhoku Tsunami. *Australasian Journal of Disaster and Trauma Studies*, *20*, 107.

Duff, C. (2016). Atmospheres of recovery: Assemblages of health. *Environment and Planning A*, *48*(1), 58–74. https://doi.org/10.1177/0308518X15603222

Eriksen, C., & de Vet, E. (2021). Untangling insurance, rebuilding, and wellbeing in bushfire recovery. *Geographical Research*, *59*(2), 228–241. https://doi.org/10.1111/1745-5871.12451

Gill, N., Johnstone, P., & Williams, A. (2012). Towards a geography of tolerance: Post-politics and political forms of toleration. *Political Geography*, *31*, 509–518. https://doi.org/10.1016/j.polgeo.2012.10.008

Glavovic, B. (2014). Disaster recovery: The particular governance challenges generated by large-scale natural disasters. In J. Boston, J. Wanna, V. Lipski, & J. Pritchard (Eds.), *Future-Proofing the State: Managing Risks, Responding to Crises and Building Resilience* (1st ed.). ANU Press. https://doi.org/10.22459/FPS.05.2014.17

Head, L. (2016). *Hope and grief in the anthropocene: Re-conceptualising human-nature relations.* Routledge.

Head, L., & Gibson, C. (2012). Becoming differently modern: Geographic contributions to a generative climate politics. *Progress in Human Geography, 36*(6), 699–714. https://doi.org/10.1177/0309132512438162

Howitt, R., Havnen, O., & Veland, S. (2011). Natural and unnatural disasters: Responding with respect for indigenous rights and knowledges. *Geographical Research, 50*(1), 47–59. https://doi.org/10.1111/j.1745-5871.2011.00709.x

Khasalamwa, S. (2009). Is 'build back better' a response to vulnerability? Analysis of the post-tsunami humanitarian interventions in Sri Lanka. *Norsk Geografisk Tidsskrift – Norwegian Journal of Geography, 63*(1), 73–88. https://doi.org/10.1080/00291950802712152

Lorimer, H. (2008). Cultural geography: Non-representational conditions and concerns. *Progress in Human Geography, 32*(4), 551–559. https://doi.org/10.1177/0309132507086882

MacKinnon, D., & Derickson, K. D. (2013). From resilience to resourcefulness: A critique of resilience policy and activism. *Progress in Human Geography, 37*(2), 253–270. https://doi.org/10.1177/0309132512454775

Massey, D. B. (2005). *for space.* SAGE.

McCormack, D. P. (2003). An event of geographical ethics in spaces of affect. *Transactions of the Institute of British Geographers, 28*(4), 488–507.

McGee, T. K., & Penning-Rowsell, E. C. (2022). *Routledge handbook of environmental hazards and society* (1st ed.). Routledge. https://doi.org/10.4324/9780367854584

McKinnon, S., Gorman-Murray, A., & Dominey-Howes, D. (2016). 'The greatest loss was a loss of our history': Natural disasters, marginalised identities and sites of memory. *Social & Cultural Geography, 17*(8), 1120–1139. https://doi.org/10.1080/14649365.2016.1153137

Mika, K., & Kelman, I. (2020). Shealing: Post-disaster slow healing and later recovery. *Area, 52*(3), 646–653. https://doi.org/10.1111/area.12605

Nancy, J.-L. (1991). *The inoperative community.* Minneapolis MN: University of Minnesota Press.

Popke, E. J. (2003). Poststructuralist ethics: Subjectivity, responsibility and the space of community. *Progress in Human Geography, 27*(3), 298–316. https://doi.org/10.1191/0309132503ph429oa

Silva, K. T. (2009). 'Tsunami third wave' and the politics of disaster management in Sri Lanka. *Norsk Geografisk Tidsskrift – Norwegian Journal of Geography, 63*(1), 61–72. https://doi.org/10.1080/00291950802712145

Thrift, N. (2000). Still Life in Nearly Present Time: The Object of Nature. *Body & Society, 6*(3–4), 34–57.

Thrift, N. J. (2008). *Non-representational theory: Space, politics, affect.* Routledge.

Wesener, A. (2015). Temporary urbanism and urban sustainability after a natural disaster: Transitional community-initiated open spaces in Christchurch, New Zealand. *Journal of Urbanism: International Research on Placemaking and Urban Sustainability, 8*(4), 406–422. https://doi.org/10.1080/17549175.2015.1061040

Whittle, R., Walker, M., Medd, W., & Mort, M. (2012). Flood of emotions: Emotional work and long-term disaster recovery. *Emotion, Space and Society, 5*(1), 60–69. https://doi.org/10.1016/j.emospa.2011.08.002

Wilson, G. A. (2013). Community resilience, social memory and the post-2010 Christchurch (New Zealand) earthquakes: Community resilience, social memory. *Area, 45*(2), 207–215. https://doi.org/10.1111/area.12012

Wilson, H. F. (2017). On geography and encounter: Bodies, borders, and difference. *Progress in Human Geography*, 41(4), 451–471. https://doi.org/10.1177/0309132516645958

Wisner, B., Gaillard, J. C., & Kelman, I. (Eds.). (2012). *Handbook of hazards and disaster risk reduction* (0 ed.). Routledge. https://doi.org/10.4324/9780203844236

Yeh, A., & Wu, F. (1999). The transformation of the urban planning system in China from a centrally-planned to transitional economy. *Progress in Planning*, 51(3), 167–252. https://doi.org/10.1016/S0305-9006(98)00029-4

29 Regional arts festivals as infrastructures of care

Michelle Duffy, Judith Mair, and Elaine Stratford

Introduction

Research in human geography has found that participation in arts and cultural activities is important for enhancing individual and community wellbeing (Fancourt & Finn, 2019; Hancox *et al.*, 2022). Arts engagement and creative participation facilitate flourishing across the life span in a variety of ways. Several studies have shown that arts and cultural activities improve mental wellbeing by decreasing anxiety and depression and increasing feelings of wellbeing and social inclusion by building and deepening relationships, facilitating social inclusion, and overcoming stigma by empowering participants (Bennett *et al.*, 2022; Davies *et al.*, 2016; Shakespeare & Whieldon, 2018). The importance of the arts sector to individuals and communities was made evident during the global lockdowns of 2020 and 2021 in terms of how they regulated negative emotions and found new and creative ways to reconnect and create feelings of belonging (Katczynski *et al.*, 2022a; Kiernan *et al.*, 2021).

In Australia, as elsewhere, to address existing, primarily economic, policy imperatives for economic development, to boost local business, and to attract tourist festivals are promoted and used by local and especially non-metroplitan governments (the equivalent to municipalities, county or district councils). In this context, arts festivals are used to frame the communities they celebrate. In terms of creating a sense of belonging to a community, festivals can facilitate how people to meet and interact and, if generated and shared successfully, such interactions contribute to individuals' and communities' broad social, civic, and economic wellbeing (Duffy & Mair, 2023). The promise of these positive outcomes prompts local governments to use festivals to increase meaningful social interactions and enhance cohesion, resilience, inclusion, and connectedness and foster creativity and diversity (Gibson & Connell, 2011; Gibson & Stewart, 2009).

Richard Florida's (2002) creative classes hypothesis, especially in urban locations, has informed conceptualisations of the role of festivals in local economic development (Cudny, 2014). Researchers have used this framework to explore the significance of rural creativity in regional redevelopment strategies and have uncovered diverse networks within rural areas that interconnect with urban areas and also operate in different and independent contexts (Anwar McHenry, 2011; Harvey *et al.*, 2012; Gibson, 2012; Waitt & Gibson, 2013). Despite the crucial importance arts festivals have for enhancing wellbeing, little research has considered how regional arts festivals can be leveraged to optimise their contributions to rural and regional wellbeing.

DOI: 10.4324/9781003345725-32

This chapter offers a conceptual framework different from that provided by the creative cities hypothesis, with its agenda for economic regeneration. Instead, we argue that festivals 'make visible, re-vision and re-value the caring possibilities of community (Power & Mee, 2020: 486). This perspective has yet to be taken up in festival studies, which we argue has been a significant barrier to understanding the full importance of arts festivals for wellbeing in regional communities.

The role of festivals in place-making, community identity, and wellbeing

Festivals exemplify complex, diverse processes of place-making and identity-formation in local and global contexts. These events have grown in number and variety in response to social and planning policies that encourage participation and encounters with others to minimise social isolation and facilitate greater understanding of difference (Duffy & Mair, 2018; Fincher & Iveson, 2008; Mair & Duffy, 2018, 2014). This broad objective is built on an underlying assumption that festivals build community, whether among groups with long-established connections to particular places, among those of more recent migration and settlement experiences, or arising from shared interests or values – including by differing from a dominant group. Festivals offer a means for communities to express and celebrate core values, and representations of community identity are mediated by distinctive artistic and cultural artifacts and activities such as music, food, and dance. Event organisers and funders position such celebrations of identity and community as important for health and wellbeing. Festivals are, therefore, complex sites for localness and belonging, that nonetheless also celebrate diversity and connections beyond locally defined communities.

While hosting a festival is a common strategy to create or re/affirm sense of community, questions arise about how tolerance, recognition, and accommodation of minority rights are generated, not least because such ideas assume a dominant social group whose members allow difference (Hage, 1998). Festivals celebrating cultural diversity encourage those recently arrived in communities to maintain their heritages and cultural traditions and help reframe social relations and connections in new places. Yet there are concerns about and even instances of gatekeeping by members of communities themselves as well as by local authorities – especially with respect to notions of "authentic" practices that tap into assumptions about some essential identity expressed and maintained through cultural and ethnic characteristics. These assumptions can be damaging (Duffy, 2005; Waitt, 2008). As the Australia Council for the Arts (2020: 88) has noted, social cohesion remains a pressing public policy concern, yet participation in creativity and the arts has 'a unique capacity to connect us all, irrespective of our life circumstances and experiences'.

The arts and culture components of festivals generate benefits for the economy but often are promoted as ways to express, challenge, and create notions of belonging, identity, and community (Fincher & Iveson, 2008). The arts are understood as significant to mental health and wellbeing (Crossick & Kaszynska, 2016), but less well known is what these benefits may mean within festival structures. Studies have explored the role of the arts within festival structures in creating and enhancing social connectedness, community building, identity, and belonging (Duffy & Mair, 2018). And while festivals are now perceived as part of everyday social infrastructure, we argue that these studies and perceptions inadequately capture the significance of arts festivals specifically as infrastructures of care.

The role of infrastructure in shaping and supporting community wellbeing

Infrastructure refers mostly to physical structures and systems that underpin and support diverse processes and production of goods and services. Examples are factories, roads, schools, Wi-Fi, and the electricity grid. Such infrastructure is essential to maintain contemporary ways of life. However, Klinenberg (2018) has extended views of infrastructure to include those institutions, facilities, spaces, and groups enabling social connection. Such "spaces of sociality" consist of:

> Places that allow people to gather. Places that support community life. Places that allow friends to spend time together, and care for each other. Places that allow people to crowd together, experience culture together. Places that encourage people to exercise, play sport, dance.
>
> (Layton & Latham, 2022: 659)

Layton and Latham (2022) name four ways in which social infrastructure can be conceptualised. First, people as social infrastructure refers to the idea that where physical infrastructure is unreliable or insufficient, people band together to overcome these shortcomings or limitations (Simone, 2004). Nevertheless, and second, even where physical infrastructure is sound, people need to ensure that it functions; therefore, the sociality of working with physical infrastructure is another way of understanding infrastructure in terms of socio-technical systems (Graham & McFarlane, 2015; Alam & Houston, 2020). Third, the term "social infrastructure" is sometimes used to denote the infrastructures of social care; those spaces that provide care for a range of people, such as hospitals, care homes, mental health services and others (Layton & Latham, 2022). Fourth, and most relevant here, is the idea that social infrastructure refers to public, quasi-public, and community spaces and places that support social connection, among them libraries, parks, gyms, community halls, and town squares (Klinenberg, 2018).

Inherent to festivals are all the hallmarks of social infrastructure—co-presence, sociability and friendship, care and kinship, kinesthetic practices, the carnivalesque, collective experiences, and civic engagement. Research has examined the important roles festivals play in communities by establishing how these events may facilitate sociability and friendship through encounters and co-presence with others (Duffy & Mair, 2018; Layton & Latham, 2022); questioning and disrupting social norms (Bakhtin, 1984; Falassi, 1987); and showing the significance of collective experience to enhance sense of belonging or communitas.

Feminist urban scholars argue that greater consideration be given to the role care plays in the provision of infrastructure (Power & Mee 2020; Alam & Houston, 2020; Williams & Tait, 2023). Unlike a social infrastructure approach, which seeks to understand how particular spatial arrangements in public space 'affords and supports all kinds of social life' (Layton & Latham, 2022: 756), the introduction of care, and more specifically a feminist care ethics, shifts attention to the ways 'existing care practices … both exceed and mobilise publics to potentially generate more inclusive and ethical infrastructural spaces' (Alam & Houston, 2020: 1–2). Caution is nevertheless needed because the quality of these socio-technical relations can enable, facilitate, and re/produce justice and injustice and care and neglect (Williams & Tait, 2023), such as when privileged institutions circulate care as 'forms of social control and (sometimes) oppression' (Rodgers & O'Neill, 2012: 402). An infrastructure of care framework has yet to be taken up in festival studies research, and we argue it could support critical consideration of the claims made about community arts festivals as sites of community building and belonging.

Regional arts festivals as practices of care

Our work on regional Australian festivals has demonstrated the complex and competing roles attributed to regional festivals. Drawing on an infrastructures of care framework, we argue that the significance of regional festivals involves determining impacts beyond the time and location of the festival because of the role they may offer for regional places and communities. Such communities are facing challenges such as a just transition to low or zero carbon emissions; out-migration of youth and population decline; lack of essential services; and the impacts of climate change. Underpinning this argument is the premise that the value and impact of festivals are better understood if we consider how they may strengthen and/or re-arrange economic, environmental, social, health and cultural relations in communities within and beyond the festival's events (Duffy & Mair 2023).

Berlant's definition of infrastructure as comprising assemblage, inventiveness, and dynamic reciprocity mirrors how arts and creative practices sustain participation in arts and cultural activities and can both tackle public issues such as health and enhance individual and community wellbeing (Hancox *et al.*, 2022). Indeed, arts engagements and interventions address the social determinants of health because they afford opportunities to engage motor, cognitive, social, and emotional functions, skills, and experiences that are 'all known to be health promoting' (Fancourt & Finn, 2019: 2). Festivals garner social, cultural, and material relations and create a sense of collective identity and connections with and sense of belonging in festival and other, associated places (Katczynski *et al.*, 2022b). Such creative participation facilitates flourishing across the life span by enabling "purposeful togetherness" (Wood & Dashper, 2020; see also Duffy & Mair, 2018; Jepson & Stadler, 2017; Quinn, 2019). In addition, the festival's powerful and intoxicating effect sustains but also has the potential to transform social life (Mackley-Crump, 2015). Such transformational potential, and how this may be better understood in terms of an infrastructures of care, can be observed in the example of Clunes, a small regional town located in around 20 kilometres outside the city of Ballarat, and just over one hour's drive north of Victoria's capital, Melbourne.

Clunes was one of the first places where gold was discovered in Victoria and at the centre of the gold rush of the late nineteenth-century. Nonetheless, by the early 2000s, Clunes was faced with population decline, a longstanding drought, weakened local agriculture, high unemployment, an ageing population and a resultant struggling local economy (Duffy & Mair, 2018). This was changed in 2007 when recently arrived "tree-changers" (the Australian term for amenity-led migrants) decided on an arts-focused renewal strategy to address what they defined as issues of social justice (personal communication with the original festival director, 2015). As the original Clunes Book Town director explained, the severe drought effecting the region at the time had 'reinforce[d] helplessness, a knowledge that the *individual* cannot act or make a difference' and that 'a willingness to dream, to imagine, and to act' in the face of this drought was what drove the group to seek to bring about social change (Brady 2012: 2, quoted in Johnston 2016: 139; emphasis added). The plan was to use books and literature to transform the economy rather than permitting fast-food chains into the town as a means to renew economic and social development (personal communication with first festival director,

2015). This plan also aligned with acknowledging Clunes as having one of the best preserved nineteenth-century towns in Victoria's Central Goldfields area (Clunes Tourism and Development Association 2017), which has made it a popular location for film and television, particularly its main street, Fraser Street, which became 'Wee Jerusalem' in *Mad Max* (1979) and transformed into 1880s versions of Euroa and Jerilderie in *Ned Kelly* (2003).

The first Book Town event was held in order to test the idea that books would generate tourism, and as part of a branding exercise for broader cultural renewal proposed by the parent organisation behind the festival, Creative Clunes (Kennedy 2011). Annual reports from Creative Clunes estimate that the event generates an extra AUD\$2–4 million of additional funds in the region (noting that COVID-19 lockdown effected revenue; Creative Clunes Inc., 2013: 1–2, cited in Driscoll 2018: 406). For some local businesses, the festival represents over a third of their annual income, allowing them to get through the winter, traditionally a quiet time, and thus remain financially sustainable (personal communication with a Clunes bookshop owner, 2015; Mair & Duffy 2018). What is now known as the Clunes Booktown Festival is primarily an annual weekend event, with numerous second-hand bookstalls located along the main street and in public buildings throughout the town, as well as a program of writing workshops and author talks and attractions for children. This model has been so successful that this weekend event is now part of a series of other, book-related events throughout the year, such as writing retreats, and in 2014, a separate weekend festival, Clunes Booktown for Kids, was held.

As Brady's insight (quoted above) suggests, an event like Book Town is significant to facilitating meaningful economic *and* social relations with others in order to address broader community challenges, and that those involved in initiating this festival did so through a commitment to care. An infrastructures of care can bring into consideration 'the patterns, habits, norms, and scenes of assemblage and use. Collective affect gets attached to it too, to the sense of its inventiveness and promise of dynamic reciprocity' (Berlant, 2016: 403). Thus, this regional arts festival exemplifies the invitation to connect with particular places and communities – not by setting up boundaries between who belongs and who does not, but rather in terms of 'the specificity of the mix of links and interconnections to that "beyond". Places viewed this way are open and porous' (Massey, 1994: 5). As a performer from other research we have conducted explains, participating in a festival event:

> *changes the nature* of the place where I conduct my daily life. Where I walk to pay bills or do the shopping becomes a place infused with memories of people dancing, playing music, sitting in the sunshine chatting, meeting friends. It adds to the quality of life by adding a new and pleasant dimension to what Sydney Road means to me (interview with performer, 1998; emphasis added).

The publicness of festivals is important in this respect because these events are sites for social relations, and it is in public spaces that different types and forms of relational networks overlap and meet. Even so, being present together in one space does not necessarily translate into care for others. As Amin (2002) has noted, social cohesion and cultural interchange can be prevented by all sorts of prejudice.

More specifically, the arts may attune participants to practices of care and help them express and share such lived experiences (Bennett *et al.*, 2022) because they are 'fundamental practices of meaning-making … uniquely powerful for exposing root issues, centring under-represented voices and shifting sociocultural norms' (Hancox *et al.*, 2022: 64). Even so, while studies have explored how arts and creative practices may bring about feelings of connection and belonging during festivals, they have yet to critically consider how such emotional responses – and others such as disconnection and alienation – engender practices that inform the development of infrastructures of care.

Conclusion

As Blichfeldt and Halkier (2014: 1587) point out, there is a flaw in development strategies due to poorly understood spatial relations:

> Rural areas are facing the prospect of marginalization and peripherality in an age of globalization where the attention of governments and media focuses increasingly on the (lack of) competitiveness of urban and metropolitan regions.

We argue the festival has an inherent capacity for transformation, which is particularly important in places undergoing crisis and transition. It is not enough simply to bring people together for any positive outcomes to ensue. A festival can contribute to changing people's capacities to act, and this is where its significance in generating sustainable and resilient communities lies. In this framing, the festival is no longer the focus, rather, its purpose is to catalyse encounters (O'Grady & Kill 2013).

Scholars propose that festival times and spaces provide encounters: 'common ground where civility and our collective sense of what may be called "publicness" are developed and expressed' (Francis 1989: 149). Festivals may be spaces of social interaction, conviviality, and co-presence, yet such framing ignores how 'competing narratives, ideologies and ideas inform who (and what) constitutes a place and community' (Duffy & Mair, 2018: 51–52; Fincher & Iveson, 2008). In the final analysis, we argue that festivals provide spaces for chance encounters in the specific timeframes and, crucially, are also about ongoing exchanges in economic terms and in ways that enable participants to acknowledge, experience, feel, debate, and engage (Amin, 2008; Duffy & Mair, 2018). In that framing, festivals are no longer the sole focus; instead, their purpose is to catalyse exchanges that may go on to shape ideas of and practices related to community and place and to spill out beyond their original temporal and spatial boundaries (Duffy, 2014). This proposition merits a new way to explore the ongoing impacts of regional arts festivals, and we argue that best provided by thinking of festivals as social infrastructures and, more specifically, as infrastructures of care.

References

Alam, A., Houston, D. (2020). Rethinking care as alternative infrastructure. *Cities*. 100: 102662.

Amin, A. (2008). Collective culture and urban public space. *City*. 12(1): 5–24.

Amin, A. (2002). Ethnicity and the multicultural city: Living with diversity. *Environment and Planning A*. 34(6): 959–980.

Anwar McHenry, J. (2011). Rural empowerment through the arts: The role of the arts in civic and social participation in the Mid West region of Western Australia. *Journal of Rural Studies*. 27(3): 245–253.

Australia Council for the Arts. (2020). *Creating Our Future Results of the National Arts Participation Survey*. Retrieved on October 25, 2022 from https://australiacouncil.gov.au/advocacy-and-research/creating-our-future/.

Bakhtin, M. (1984). *Rabelais and his world*. Trans. Hélène Iswolsky. Bloomington: Indiana University Press.

Bennett, J., Boydell, K., Davidson, J., Hooker, C. (2022). Discussion paper: *Arts, creativity and mental wellbeing policy development program*. Sydney: Australia Council for the Arts.

Berlant, L. (2016). The commons: Infrastructures for troubling times. *Environment and Planning D: Society and Space*. 34(3): 393–419.

Blichfeldt, B.S., Halkier, H. (2014). Mussels, tourism and community development: A case study of place branding through food festivals in rural North Jutland, Denmark. *European Planning Studies*. 22(8): 1587–1603.

Brady, T. (2012). Clunes Address. *World Booktown Symposium*, Paju Booksori.

Clunes Tourism and Development Association. (2017). Welcome to Clunes [online]. www.clunes.org/index.php [Accessed 31 March 2017].

Crossick, G., Kasznska, P. (2016). *Understanding the value of arts and culture: The AHRC Cultural Value Project* [Online]. https://apo.org.au/node/199546.

Cudny, W. (2014), Festivals as a subject for geographical research. *Geografisk Tidsskrift-Danish Journal of Geography*. 114(2): 132–142

Davies, C., Knuiman, M., Rosenberg, M. (2016). The art of being mentally healthy: A study to quantify the relationship between recreational arts engagement and mental well-being in the general population. *BMC Public Health*. 16(1): 1–10.

Driscoll, B. (2018). Local places and cultural distinction: The booktown model. *European Journal of Cultural Studies*. 21(4): 401–417.

Duffy, M. (2014). The emotional ecologies of festivals. In A. Bennett, I. Woodward, J. Taylor (eds). *Festivalisation of Culture: Identity, Culture and Politics*. Farnham: Ashgate; pp. 229–250.

Duffy, M. (2005). Performing identity within a multicultural framework. *Social and Cultural Geography*. 6(5): 677–692.

Duffy, M., Mair, J. (2023). Regions in recovery? The significance of festivals for regenerating and reimagining regional community life. In I. Woodward, J. Haynes, P. Berkers, A. Dillane, K. Golemo (eds). *Remaking Culture and Music Spaces: Affects, Infrastructures, Futures*. London & New York: Routledge; pp. 235–247.

Duffy, M., Mair, J. (2018). *Festival encounters: Theoretical perspectives on festival events*. Oxon & New York: Routledge.

Falassi, A. (1987). *Time out of Time: Essays on the Festival*. Albuquerque: University of New Mexico.

Fancourt, D., Finn, S. (2019). *What is the Evidence on the Role of the Arts in Improving Health and Well-Being? A Scoping Review*, Health Evidence Network synthesis report 67, Copenhagen: World Health Organisation. https://apps.who.int/iris/handle/10665/329834 [Accessed 14 November 2022].

Fincher, R. and Iveson, K. (2008). *Planning and diversity in the city: Redistribution, recognition and encounter*. Hampshire, UK: Palgrave Macmillan

Florida, R. (2002). *The rise of the creative class: And how it's transforming work, leisure, community and everyday life*. New York: Basic.

Francis, M. (1989). Control as a dimension of public space quality. In: M Sorkin (ed). *Variations on a Theme Park*. New York: Hill and Wang, pp. 147–172.

Gibson, C. (ed.). (2012). *Creativity in peripheral places: Redefining the creative industries*. Routledge, London and New York.

Gibson, C., Connell, J. (2011). *Festival Places: Revitalising rural Australia*. Bristol, Buffalo, Toronto: Channel View Publications.

Gibson, C., Stewart, A. (2009). *Reinventing rural places. The extent and impact of festivals in rural and regional Australia*. Research Report. University of Wollongong

Graham, S., McFarlane, C. (2015). *Infrastructural lives: Urban infrastructure in context*. Oxon & New York: Routledge.

Hage, G. (1998). *White nation: Fantasies of white supremacy in a multicultural society*. Annandale, NSW: Pluto Press.

Hancox, D., Gattenhof, S., Mackay, S., Klaebe, H. (2022). Pivots, arts practice and potentialities: Creative engagement, community well-being and arts-led research during COVID-19 in Australia. *Journal of Applied Arts & Health*, 13(1): 61–75.

Harvey, D.C., Hawkins, H., Thomas, N.J. (2012). Thinking creative clusters beyond the city: People, places and networks. *Geoforum*. 43: 529–539.

Jepson, A., Stadler, R. (2017). Conceptualizing the impact of festival and event attendance upon family quality of life (QOL). *Event Management*. 21(1): 47–60.

Jepson, A., Stadler, R. (2017). Conceptualizing the impact of festival and event attendance upon family quality of life (QOL). *Event Management*. 21(1): 47–60

Johnston, J. (2016). *Public relations and the public interest. New York & Oxon:* Routledge.

Katczynski, A., Stratford, E., & Marsh, P. (2022a). Absence and distance: Reflections on festival landscapes in a pandemic. *Social & Cultural Geography*. 24 (10): 1808–1826. https://doi.org/10.1080/14649365.2022.2107230

Katczynski, A., and Stratford, E., & Marsh, P. (2022b). Tracing memories and meanings of festival landscapes during the COVID-19 pandemic, *Emotion. Space and Society*, 44. https://doi.org/10.1016/j.emospa.2022.100903

Kennedy, M. (2011). Binding a sustainable future: Book towns, themed placebranding and rural renewal; A case study of Clunes' back to Booktown. In J. Martin & T. Budge (eds). *The Sustainability of Australia's Country Towns: Renewal, Renaissance, Resilience*. Victorian Universities Regional Research Network (VURRN) Press. pp. 207–226.

Kiernan, F., Chmiel, A., Garrido, S., Hickey, M., Davidson, J. (2021). The role of artistic creative activities in navigating the Covid-19 pandemic in Australia. *Frontiers in Psychology*. 12: 696202. https://doi.org/10.3389/fpsyg.2021.696202.

Klinenberg, E. (2018). *Palaces for the people: How to build a more equal and united society*. New York: Penguin Random House.

Layton, J., Latham, A. (2022) Social infrastructure and public life – notes on Finsbury Park, London, *Urban Geography*. 43(5): 755–776

Mackley-Crump, J. (2015). *The Pacific festivals of Aotearoa New Zealand: Negotiating place and identity in a new homeland*. University of Hawaii Press.

Mair, J., Duffy, M. (2018). The role of festivals in strengthening social capital in rural communities. *Event Management*. 22(6): 875–889.

Mair, J, Duffy, M (2014) Social cohesion and local festivals. *Journal of Policy Research in Tourism, Leisure & Events*. 7(3): 282–298

Massey, D. (1994). Double articulation. In A. Bammer (ed.) *Displacements*. Bloomington: Indiana University Press; pp. 110–121.

O'Grady, A., Kill, R. (2013). Exploring festival performance as a state of encounter. *Arts & Humanities in Higher Education*. 12(2-3): 268–283.

Power, E., Mee, K. (2020) Housing: An infrastructure of care. *Housing Studies*. 35(3): 484–505

Quinn, B. (2019). Festivals and social sustainability. In: Mair, J. (ed.) *The Routledge Handbook of Festivals. Routledge*, Abingdon. pp. 53–61

Rodgers, D., O'Neill, B. (2012). Infrastructural violence: Introduction to the special issue. *Ethnography*. 13(4): 401–412.

Shakespeare, T., Whieldon, A. (2018). Sing your heart out: Community singing as part of mental health recovery. *Medical Humanities*. 44(3): 153–157.

Simone, A. (2004). People as infrastructure: Intersecting fragments in Johannesburg. *Public Culture. 16*(3): 407–429. https://doi.org/10.1215/08992363-16-3-407

Waitt, G. (2008). Urban festivals: Geographies of hype, helplessness and hope. *Geography Compass*. 2(2): 513–537.

Waitt, G., Gibson, C. (2013). The spiral gallery: Non-market creativity and belonging in an Australian country town. *Journal of Rural Studies*. 30: 75–85

Williams, M., Tait, L. (2022). Diverse infrastructures of care: Community food provisioning in Sydney. *Social & Cultural Geography*. 24 (8): 1362–1382. https://doi.org/10.1080/14649365.2022.2056630.

Wood, E., Dashper, K. (2020). "Purposeful togetherness": Theorising gender and ageing through creative events. *Journal of Sustainable Tourism*. 29(11–12): 2008–2024.

Section IV
Spaces of work and home

30 Introduction to spaces of work and home

Joshua Evans and Alak Paul

Spaces of home and work are powerful determinants of mental health and wellbeing and critical dimensions of community-based recovery. How people recover from trauma, illness, or hardship and live meaningful, flourishing lives depends upon the spaces of home and work afforded to them. Safe, adequate and affordable housing promotes wellbeing (Gregory 2022) and is inextricably linked to recovery-affirming psychosocial processes such as the development of social connection, optimism about the future, positive sense of identity, meaning in life, and self-control (Leamey et al. 2011). Feeling at home in a community is equally important for wellbeing. Both community integration, at the neighborhood level, and participation in meaningful activities, are central to reestablishing social roles and rebuilding a positive identity (Price-Robertson et al. 2017). Alongside stable housing and inclusive neighborhoods, the workplace is another site of significance for mental wellbeing. Generally speaking, employment can provide the economic means to purchase basic necessities, such as housing, which are themselves essential to health and wellbeing. Employment also structures day-to-day life and serves as a core component of identity. In the field of mental health treatment, employment is commonly viewed as a key marker of personal recovery in this regard (Drake and Wallach 2020).

These are just some of the ways in which housing and the workplace have been associated with health and wellbeing. Such understandings have profoundly influenced the normative orientation of mental health treatment, as well as more recent recovery-orientated discourses, which have placed an emphasis on stable housing and participation in paid employment as an indicator of recovery. Yet, both housing and workplaces are inherently contradictory: the home can be both a site of refuge and trauma while the workplace can be both a site of empowerment and exploitation. Negative experiences of the home or workplace, be it in terms of the loss of housing or the growing precariatisation of employment, have been associated with enduring mental ill-health (Strauss 2018; Nowicki et al. 2019). Historically speaking, spaces of home and work have long served as powerful 'geographies of mental difference' (Evans and Wilton 2019). Looking to the past, differences between the supposedly 'sane' and the allegedly 'insane' emerged out of specific ways of spatially separating the domestic and working lives of the ill and the well, most notoriously through institutional approaches such as the 'asylum' (see *Institutional and Post-Institutional Spaces* in this edited collection). Today, these spatial processes of differencing are still a prominent feature of everyday life where spaces of work and home play an important role.

This section on the *Spaces of Home and Work* critically analyses and evaluates the relationship between home, work, mental health and wellbeing while remaining sensitive

DOI: 10.4324/9781003345725-34

to the broader experience of social and cultural difference as it has impacted people experiencing mental ill-health. In keeping with the central theme of *Spaces of Mental Health and Wellbeing*, each chapter in this section explores how spaces of home and work, which are themselves products of wider social, economic and political forces, are experienced, negotiated and in some cases resisted as part of people's efforts to live well in the world. A common thread running through all the chapters is that homeplaces and workplaces can serve as an important milieu for personal recovery, interpreted by many to mean 'living a fulfilling life in the community in the presence of mental ill health.' Instead of the alleviation of symptoms and return to a 'normal' state, personal recovery is viewed as an individualised journey during which individuals build a meaningful life despite the disruption and restrictions of illness.

The relational connections between home, broadly understood, and the lived-experience of recovery are theoretically foregrounded by Doroud and Fossey (Chapter 31) who draw attention to the importance of doing, being-in, becoming and belonging-in 'everyday places.' In distinguishing these processes, Doroud and Fossey draw attention to the multidimensionality of everyday places in the community. Using examples drawn from the lives of individuals living with mental illness, Doroud and Fossey show how places in the community and the on-going process of recovery are connected through participation in everyday activities, such as doing chores, going for a walk or meeting a friend for coffee, all of which help position individuals in the world in enabling ways.

Participation in everyday activities in the community, including employment, was very much the goal of community integration strategies implemented in the era of deinstitutionalisation (see *Institutional and Post-Institutional Spaces*); however, this integration has been difficult to achieve in practice, particularly in the realm of housing. For decades, people with serious mental ill-health have been disproportionately represented in unhoused populations, a trend that is indicative of the failure of deinstitutionalisation policies and the implications of homelessness for mental wellbeing. Efforts to address this homelessness pathway through housing interventions are reviewed by Padgett (Chapter 32) who provides a history of Permanent Supportive Housing, a model that originated in New York City in the 1980s, came to be reformulated through the discourse of 'Housing First' in the 1990s, and has since spread to cities around the world. As Padgett shows, by offering greater stability and support services attuned to individual needs, the Permanent Supportive Housing model increases individual 'ontological security,' thus offering a "foothold on recovery from the multiple traumas of homelessness and disability."

Drawing on this same notion of 'ontological security,' Woodhall-Melnick, Monette, and MacKenney (Chapter 33) explore ways in which the built environment can be reimagined through Trauma-Informed Design to promote place-based healing from a wide range of adverse experiences that can cause toxic stress and instability across the life course. Foregrounding efforts to promote such healing, the authors begin by acknowledging the contradictory nature of the home itself, noting that home can be "hell" for some, whereas for others it can be "a haven where people can go to escape the outside world, relax, restore calm, heal and grow." In their survey of Trauma-Informed Design they detail how connections between the built environment and wellbeing can be intentionally fostered to encourage recovery from trauma. In the following chapter, Herron (Chapter 34) also problematises the home, drawing attention again to its contradictory nature, but this time in the context of aging in place. Here the home is a complex and multifaceted site that is continually negotiated by older people, some of whom live with mental health problems or care for individuals living with mental health problems. Drawing on the lived experiences of older people, Herron explores how the home can simultaneously be a site of refuge, care, and confinement. Moreover, the experience of home is always connected to other places beyond the home, a relationality demonstrated most clearly during the COVID-19 pandemic.

One place that is beyond the home, so to speak, and which has equal significance for mental wellbeing is the workplace. As noted above, paid employment and the workplace is one sphere that has functioned to facilitate processes of differencing, separating the able-bodied from disabled, and the mentally well from the unwell. Employment outside the home and productivity in the workplace has long been a marker of 'normalcy' in this regard. Additionally, participation in paid employment and visibility in the workplace has been highly gendered. In their chapter, Wilton and Fudge Shormans (Chapter 35) explore the complex interplay between employment outside the home and culturally valued understandings of masculinity in the lives of men living with mental ill-health. Using arts-based methodologies, Wilton and Fudge Shormans explore how men negotiate gender-based expectations related to work undertaken outside and within the home and the implications of these expectations for processes of recovery. This brings to mind the very nature of work itself as a process with far reaching consequences for mental wellbeing. For example, care work in mental health contexts, such as psychological counseling, benefits millions of people around the world. This 'doing' of mental health care is the focus of the chapter by Boyd (Chapter 36) who explores the shift of mental health care online, a practice that is becoming increasingly common in the post-COVID-19 world. Rather than focus on the online platform as a space of care work, Boyd draws upon personal experiences as a clinician to highlight what therapists do in online environments to create therapeutic spaces and how such practices impact the therapeutic relationship. Our final chapter by Proudfoot (Chapter 37) returns to the discourse of trauma. The discourse of trauma is often employed in descriptions of the contradictory nature of the home and workplace, both of which can operate as sites of on-going, everyday harm. Proudfoot challenges us to resist the tendency to view trauma as an individual concern and/or an exceptional event; instead, we must grapple with the everyday nature of trauma and locate its origins in large-scale structural forces.

References

Drake, R. and Wallach, M. 2020. Employment is a critical mental health intervention. *Epidemiology and Psychiatric Sciences*, 29, pp. 1–3.

Evans, J. and Wilton, R. 2019. Well Enough to Work? Social Enterprise Employment and the Geographies of Mental Health Recovery. Annals of the American Association of Geographers, 109(1), pp. 87–103

Gregory, J. 2022. *Social Housing, Wellbeing, and Welfare*. Bristol, UK: Bristol University Press.

Leamy, M., Bird, V.C., Boutillier, L., Williams, J. and Slade, M. 2011. A conceptual framework for personal recovery in mental health: *Systematic review*. British Journal of Psychiatry 199(6), pp. 445–452.

Nowocki, M., Brickell, K., and Harris, E. 2019. The hotelisation of the housing crisis: Experiences of family homelessness in Dublin hotels. *Geographical Journal*, 185(3), pp. 313–324.

Price-Robertson, R., Obradovic, A., and Morgan, B. 2017. Relational recovery: Beyond individualism in the recovery approach. *Advances in Mental Health*, 15(2), pp. 108–120.

Strauss, K. 2018. Labour geography I: Towards a geography of precarity. *Progress in Human Geography*, 42(4), pp. 622–630.

31 Recovering place and wellbeing for individuals with mental illness

Nastaran Doroud and Ellie Fossey

Introduction

Recovering is a lived experience for people experiencing mental illness; one that occurs in the context of everyday living (Borg and Davidson, 2008) and that is often described as a journey or a process of healing and restoring or developing a meaningful and satisfying life (Slade and Wallace, 2017, Anthony, 1993). It may also involve unique experiences of growing beyond persistent and recurring psychiatric symptoms, overcoming adversity and finding one's place in the world (Bradshaw et al., 2007; Van Weeghel et al., 2019). As contexts for recovery, places are not only the geographical locations or environments where people live but also important as resources and arenas for social interactions, collective meaning-making and connectedness fundamental to wellbeing. Before exploring how places can offer possibilities for recovery and wellbeing, it is useful to consider how recovery is understood in the context of mental illness.

Recovery for people experiencing mental illness

The term 'recovery' has been widely embraced in the mental health field (Slade et al., 2014). Historically, it was assumed that only a small proportion of individuals experiencing persistent mental illness could recover *from* their illness in the sense of full symptom remission and restoration of previous functioning (e.g. independent living, work and so on), or what is referred to as *clinical recovery* (Davidson and Roe, 2007, Slade and Wallace, 2017). Overemphasis on clinical recovery is increasingly recognised as problematic because it fails to explain the heterogeneity of outcomes observed in longitudinal studies (Carpenter and Strauss, 1991, Slade and Wallace, 2017) and because it disregards the subjective experiences of the everyday worlds in which people live (Slade and Wallace, 2017, Davidson and Roe, 2007). A different perspective of recovery originates in the psychiatric survivor/consumer movement (Byrne et al., 2015), and is reflected in the influential work of Patricia Deegan (1996, 1997) and many other individuals' own lived experiences, which highlight that recovering does not necessarily require alleviation of psychiatric symptoms. This rich experiential evidence has led to current understandings of personal and social recovery (Llewellyn-Beardsley et al., 2019).

Personal recovery involves an individualised, ongoing journey of establishing a meaningful life, a sense of hope and purpose, pursuing goals and growing beyond the limitations of mental illness (Slade and Wallace, 2017, Anthony, 1993). Based on a narrative review (Leamy et al., 2011, Van Weeghel et al., 2019), the CHIME framework provides a useful way to describe five key elements of personal recovery: Connectedness, Hope, Identity,

DOI: 10.4324/9781003345725-35

Meaning and Empowerment. While these elements may vary in meaning and importance for people, they include:

a) **Connectedness**: connecting with family, friends and supports, such as peer support; working in partnership with mental health and other practitioners; establishing social roles and a sense of belonging (Bradshaw et al., 2007, Topor et al., 2011, Leamy et al., 2011)

b) **Hope**: having a sense of purpose and optimism, holding hopes or dreams for the future, pursuing aspirations, feeling motivated and believing in one's own capabilities in moving forward (Van Weeghel et al., 2019, Leamy et al., 2011)

c) **Identity**: building a positive sense of self connected to a valued identity, beyond pessimistic labels and the stigma of an illness-identity (Van Weeghel et al., 2019, Leamy et al., 2011)

d) **Meaning**: making meaning of one's experiences, engaging in meaningful roles and activities that support discovering new skills, interests and purpose in life (Van Weeghel et al., 2019, Leamy et al., 2011, Doroud et al., 2022)

e) **Empowerment**: Taking an active role, leading one's recovery journey, focusing on strengths and rebuilding one's sense of determination, responsibility and power (Van Weeghel et al., 2019, Leamy et al., 2011, Treichler et al., 2019)

As summarised in Table 31.1 below, the process of personal recovery may also include managing ongoing symptoms, difficulties and challenges (Treichler et al., 2019, Van Weeghel et al., 2019, Slade and Wallace, 2017). In comparison, the term *social recovery* acknowledges the social and cultural dimensions of recovery, placing greater emphasis on involvement in one's community, inclusion and citizenship (Slade and Wallace, 2017, Mezzina et al., 2006, Topor et al., 2011, Whitley and Drake, 2010, Reis et al., 2022).

Recovery can also be considered a 'journey of living' that is intertwined with and unfolds through everyday experiences. Naming this an "occupational recovery" (Doroud

Table 31.1 Summary of the dimensions and key elements of recovery

Dimensions of recovery	Key elements
Clinical Recovery	Remission of psychiatric symptoms Functional improvements Independent living
Personal Recovery	Deeply personal Ongoing and non-linear Connectedness Hope Identity Meaning Empowerment Managing symptoms and facing challenges
Social Recovery	Cultural and social dimensions Participating in and contributing to the community Engaging in valued social roles Citizenship
Occupational Recovery	Engaging in meaningful activities Balancing between taking an active role, being easy on oneself, learning about oneself, making use of the resources and developing strategies to navigate barriers to participation

et al., 2015, Doroud et al., 2022), we argued that establishing a meaningful life is inherently a process of engaging in activities and relationships that enable the CHIME elements of recovery. Similarly, Hammell and Iwama (2012) and Hammell (2014, 2015, 2017) have discussed opportunities for 'doing' as imperative to wellbeing and a basic human right. 'Doing' is a vehicle to pursue aspirations, flourish and shape one's own life. Individuals need to engage in activities to meet their basic wellbeing needs (e.g. food, shelter, security); to exercise control; to develop a sense of worth, identify, purpose and meaning; to connect with others and to belong (Hammell, 2017). Engagement in meaningful activities and "ordinary" life experiences have been identified as a key priority by people experiencing mental illness (Piat et al., 2017; Waks et al., 2017), precisely because these everyday experiences offer opportunities to connect with other people, develop a sense of hope and growth, regain a sense of autonomy and self-determination, and establish socially valued roles and to grow beyond the illness (Doroud et al., 2015, Doroud et al., 2022, Borg and Davidson, 2008, Slade, 2012, Sutton et al., 2012, Sells et al., 2006).

To illustrate, in a qualitative photo-elicitation study involving adults experiencing mental illness in Australia (Doroud et al., 2022), we identified a highly individualised and non-linear process constructed by individuals as they experience the ebbs and flows of everyday life. Almost all participants spoke about recovery as embedded in their everyday experiences such as doing things that they enjoyed, keeping up with the chores, going for a walk or for coffee. One participant, for instance, shared a photograph of a tennis match and passionately talked about engaging with her love of tennis (Figure 31.1). Another

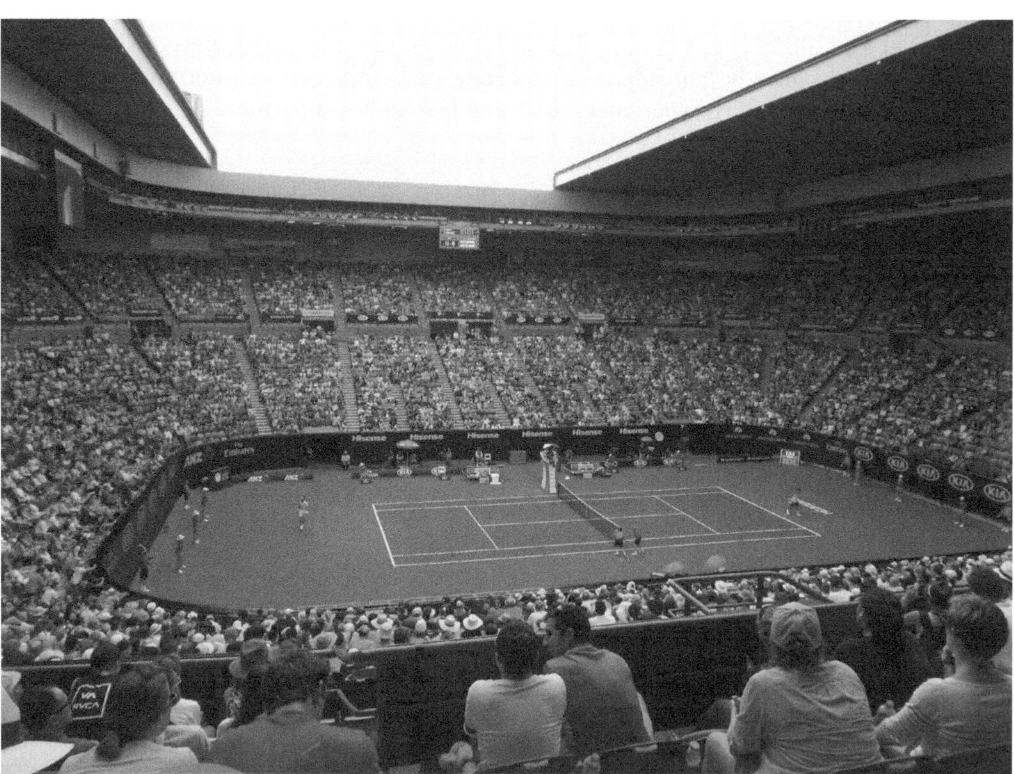

Figure 31.1 Participant photo: A tennis match.

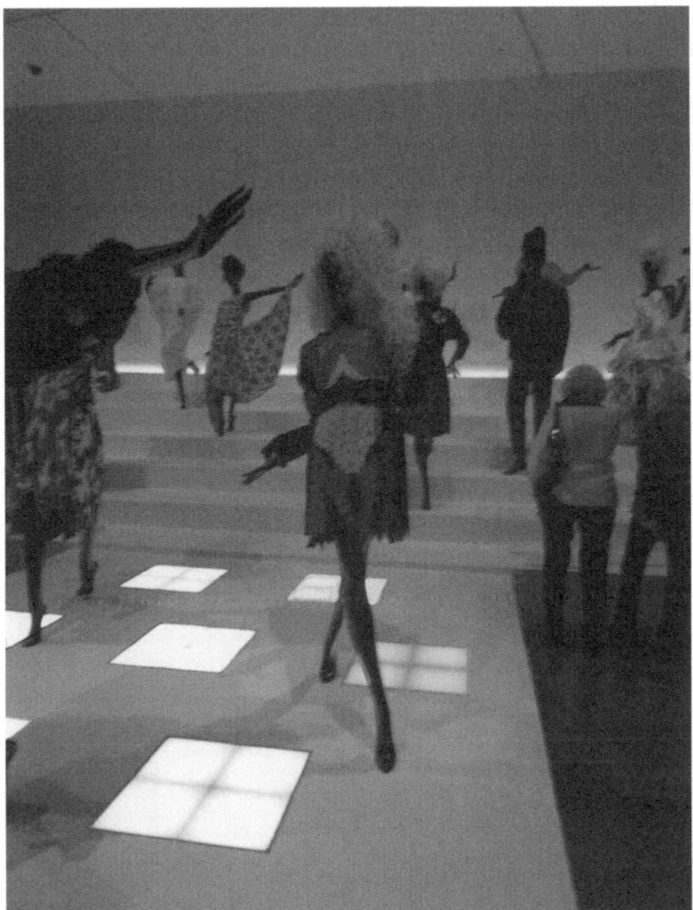

Figure 31.2 Participant photo: A fashion show.

participant took a photograph while visiting a fashion show and spoke about connecting with her interest in fashion and clothing (Figure 31.2) (Doroud, et al., 2022). Occupational recovery then is situational, unfolding in the places where individuals live and engage in taking on active roles, being easy on oneself, learning about oneself, making use of the resources and developing strategies to navigate barriers (Doroud et al., 2022).

The role of everyday places in recovery

Place offers an array of opportunities, resources and challenges that pave the way towards a meaningful, satisfying and contributing life (Doroud et al., 2022, Doroud et al., 2018). Yet, this is not a unidirectional or a causal relationship; as individuals with mental illness create places in the course of their recovery, they explore opportunities and resources, and navigate ways to face constraints. Recovery is situated within place as individuals interact with and position themselves within the contexts of their living (Milasan et al., 2022, Bierski, 2016). In turn, recovery can be cultivated within ordinary places, given that places offer 'arenas' for connection and participation with potential over time for personal development and growth (Borg and Davidson, 2008, Duff, 2015, Sells et al., 2006). The question here, however, is how does the objective environment become an 'enabling place' (Duff, 2012, Duff, 2015)?

In a review of qualitative studies exploring the role of place in recovery (Doroud et al., 2018), we discussed how this occurs through processes of being, doing, becoming and belonging, and through interacting with characteristics of place, particularly secure housing, material resources, local facilities, natural environment and social dimensions of environment (Doroud et al., 2018). Below we further elaborate on these processes with attention to place as an experiential and relational construct. Figure 31.6 illustrates these processes. It is noteworthy that the 'types' of places that we discuss below are not static or universal; rather, they are dependent on how individuals and communities interpret and make meaning of places available to them. A local café, for example can be a quiet place to relax, an enabling environment, or a meeting place to socialise. Equally, cafés may be experienced as noisy, making conversation difficult, or as intimidating if a person feels 'different' to others present in some way. To illustrate, several participants in our aforementioned qualitative photo-elicitation study (Doroud, et al., 2022) shared their experiences of meaningful places in their recovery. One participant spoke of going for walks along the beach, describing it as a "magical place" where she could find peace and unwind (Figure 31.3). Other participants, similarly, talked about

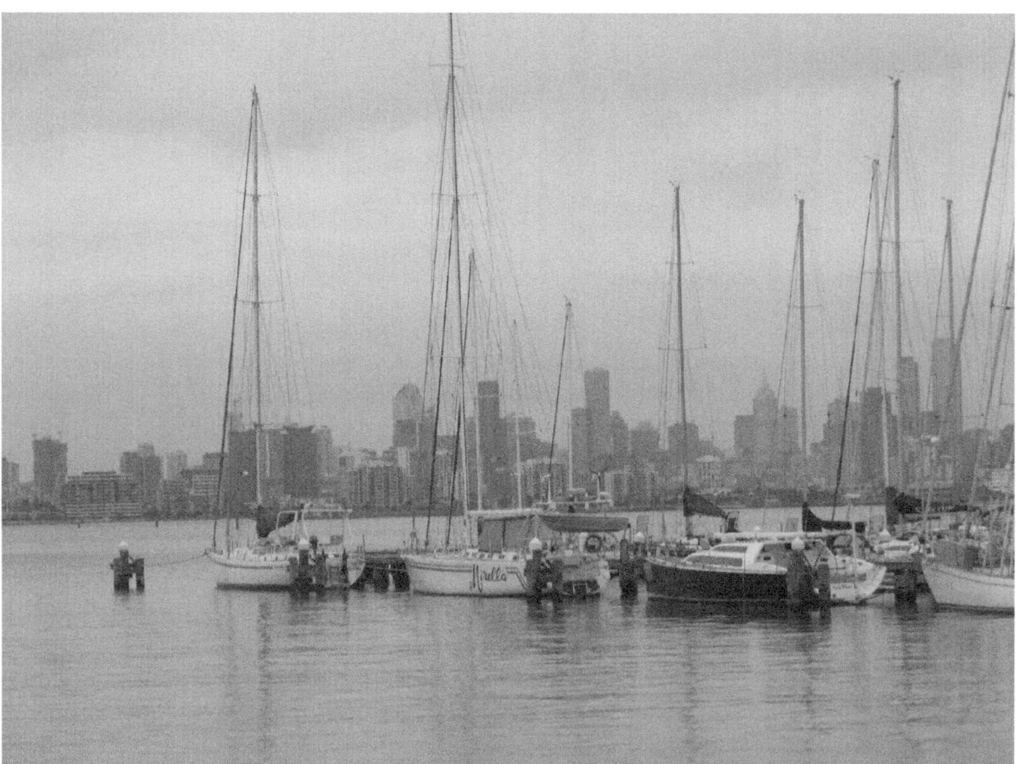

Figure 31.3 Participant photo: Sailboats in a harbor.

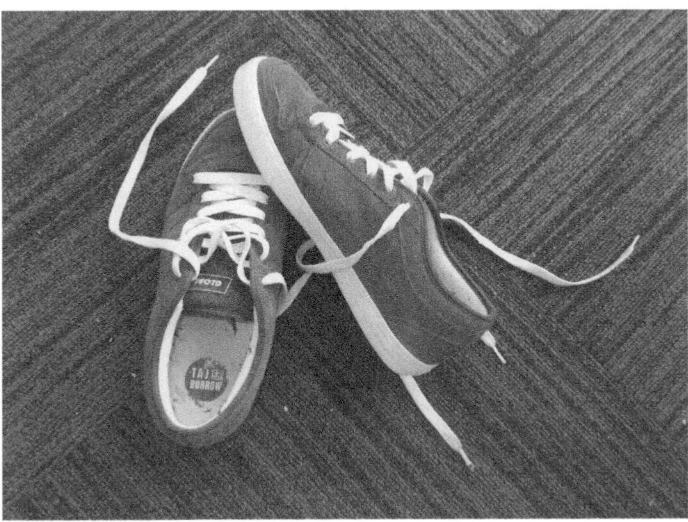

Figure 31.4 Participant photo: Sneakers.

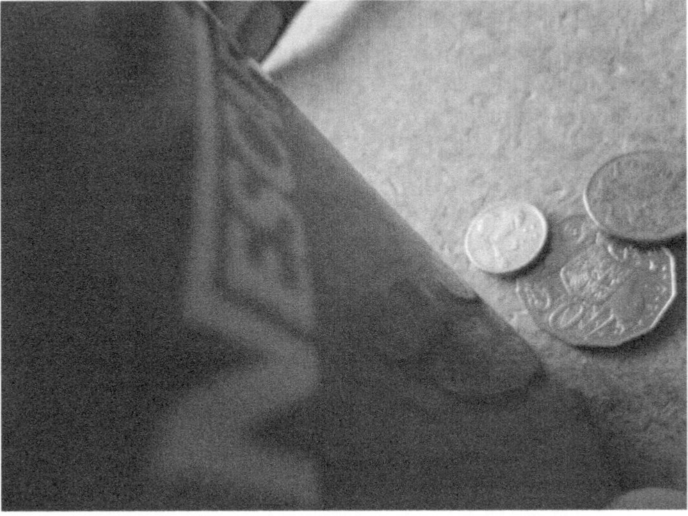

Figure 31.5 Participant photo: Coins next to a mug.

creating places to reflect, to engage in activities, to connect with others in their community. For instance, photographs of his sneakers (Figure 31.4) and a coffee mug were taken by another participant to describe his recovery in terms of living a "normal" life; creating his own niche to connect and participate in the community. This participant also put the coins next to the mug to emphasise the importance of financial resources in recovery (Figure 31.5).

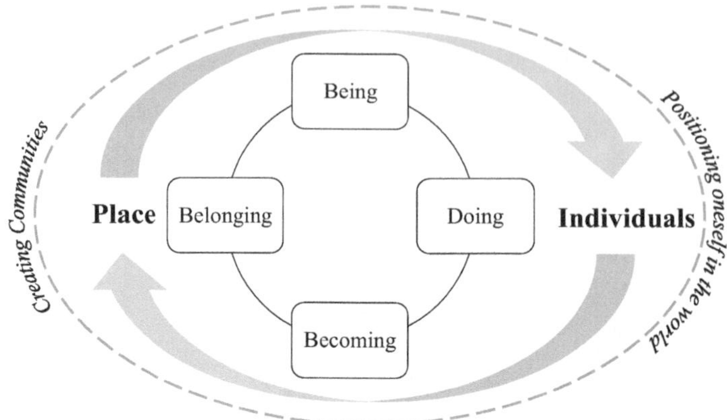

Figure 31.6 Recovery and place are interconnected through opportunities for being, doing, becoming and belonging.

Being-in a safe place

'Being-in' place, according to Heidegger (2010), can represent the individual's presence in relation to the characteristics of place. It comprises mutually interconnected processes of creating a lived-environment by being present in time and space. Safe and private places encourage an opportunity to reflect and to integrate with sense of self (Doroud et al., 2018). Access to secure and a private housing, a place to call home, has been the emphasis of most place-related research (Vansteenkiste et al., 2021, Duff, 2012, Piat et al., 2020, Smith et al., 2015, Kirst et al., 2014, Watson et al., 2019). A nearby park to connect with self and nature, financial and material resources to feel empowered, a safe neighbourhood that brings a sense of normality, and a personalised place that has emotional significance are some other examples (Doroud et al., 2018, Duff, 2015). Referring to "atmospheres of safety and belonging" (p.11), Duff (2015) explains that the physical boundaries of a house may help to draw a line between social and private selves by giving freedom to be "totally oneself". Through 'being-in' place, individuals develop emotional bonds and create an affective structure to feel safe (Duff, 2015). Given recovery includes dealing with ups and downs, vulnerabilities and challenges (Vansteenkiste et al., 2021, Van Weeghel et al., 2019), 'being-in' a safe place can act as an escape from demands and difficulties, to reflect and to be easy on oneself (Doroud et al., 2018, Sutton et al., 2012).

In contrast, places that are "too sterile" (Chesters et al., 2005) (p. 5), restrictive and institutionalised offer limited or no opportunities for emotional connection, self-expression, control and power; and can be counterproductive to recovery (Smith et al., 2015, Leviten-Reid et al., 2014, Yates et al., 2012). Temporary and unstable housing, or those in unsafe neighbourhoods, too, can cause distress and are unhelpful in recovery (Smith et al., 2015). This highlights the primacy of understanding the lived experience of place and has implications for partnering with individuals experiencing mental illness in co-design of supported housing, therapeutic spaces and local facilities.

Doing in an enabling place

Place offers enabling characteristics that may support individuals to undertake day-to-day activities, establish structure and daily routines, engage in activities of their choosing and lead their recovery journeys (Doroud et al., 2018, Duff, 2015). As a vehicle to engage in a meaningful and fulfilling life, 'doing' is essential to wellbeing, that is, not only to meeting basic needs (e.g. eating, showering) but also to develop autonomy, positive sense of self and esteem, meaning and purpose, and new ways to connect with the very features of place (Doroud et al., 2022, Hammell, 2017). Living in stable housing, for example, creates opportunities to form routines and engage in activities in the neighbourhood (Beal et al., 2005, Söderström et al., 2016, Doroud et al., 2018). Access to local facilities and transport, proximity to nature, adequate financial resources and availability of services also play important roles in recovery (Doroud et al., 2018, Borg et al., 2005, Duff, 2015, Beal et al., 2005). We discussed earlier that taking an active role and engaging in meaningful activities are essential in recovery. Individuals with mental illness often talk about trying something new, stepping out of comfort zone and exploring possibilities as important in their recovering (Doroud et al., 2022). How will these be possible if one lives in an area with no parks, cafés or shops or with limited public transport options, especially for those who do not have a car? Or if there are no neighbourhood facilities or nothing of relevance on offer in the places where people might gather in a community?

Caution should nonetheless be taken not to be 'prescriptive' about the enabling features of place as these are sculpted by the individuals (Söderström et al., 2016, Bierski, 2016, Bromley et al., 2013). As an example, one person may enjoy the discounted public transport on the weekends and find it 'enabling' to go around and do things, whereas another person may identify busy and unreliable weekend trains as too stressful and discouraging. Thus, to better understand the experiences of enabling places, it is important to work in partnership with individuals with lived experience of mental illness to engage in 'doing-in' place and exploring their features collaboratively, for which empowering and emergent modalities such as filmmaking or photo-elicitation may be useful (Kemp, 2011, Milasan et al., 2022).

Becoming; a catalyst place

Hope, optimism and growth are pivotal to recovery (Leamy et al., 2011). Place offers new possibility when it supports a sustained engagement to pursue goals. Secure housing and material resources, in particular, can pave the way towards achieving aspirations (Doroud et al., 2018, Kirst et al., 2014, Macnaughton et al., 2016). A permanent address and phone number, work clothes and transport, for example, are the rudiments for seeking and maintaining employment and can go a long way for individuals with long histories of homelessness (Patterson et al., 2015, Poremski et al., 2016, Sample and Ferguson, 2020). Individuals with mental illness often talk about stable housing as a turning point in their recovery that made them feel prepared to seek new challenges (Watson et al., 2019, Kirst et al., 2014, Patterson et al., 2015). The role of place in growth and recovery is dynamic and emergent too. Places can become indicators of success or recovery milestones. Leaving an inpatient unit, being sheltered after years of sleeping rough or moving from supported housing to one's own rental accommodation (e.g. Kirst et al., 2014, Macnaughton et al., 2016) provide a few examples of what Duff (2015) refers to as establishing "atmospheres of hope and belief" (p. 11). As Duff (2015) explains, hope is established and sustained when the physical, social and material aspects of place create a springboard for new possibilities, healing and transformative potential. While this can apply to housing, it also applies to natural environments. For example, a walk in the park, fresh air and green spaces are examples that can encourage individuals to create their unique healing places (Bierski, 2016). On the other hand, certain characteristics of place can result in moving backward and limit opportunities for growth and recovery. Reported examples include unsafe neighbourhoods, mixing with individuals who use illicit substances (Smith et al., 2015, Pahwa et al., 2019), and temporary or insecure accommodation (Poremski et al., 2016).

Belonging to an affirming place

Place is where people connect, participate in the community, and grow a sense of belonging. Belonging is central to recovery, in that it brings together and strengthens being, doing and becoming (Doroud et al., 2018). Access to private and stable housing, for example, is where an individual can draw a line between their "domestic" (Borg et al., 2005, p.247) and social identities, invite friends and family, and develop relationships with neighbours (Duff, 2012, Smith et al., 2015, Macnaughton, 2008). Spending time with other people (e.g. in a café or a barbershop) or taking a stroll at a park without the pressure to connect ("Undemanding Sociality" (Bierski, 2016) p. 142) are other examples.

Developing relationships, engaging in meaningful activities, interacting with the characteristics of place and developing emotional ties encourage a sense of belonging and affirmation (Bromley et al., 2013, Rebeiro, 2001, Yanos, 2007). A body of evidence has identified the role of affirming and inclusive places in promoting recovery and community participation (Sells et al., 2006, Topor et al., 2011, Reis et al., 2022), with an emphasis on dynamic interconnections between place, individuals, community and recovery. Most importantly, communities are co-created and shaped through the possibilities for people to interact within their everyday worlds. For example, in Duff's (2015) words, cafes, libraries, bookshops and parks can represent gathering places that endorse social connection and foster recovery through enabling individuals to contribute to:

> "...co-constitution of a receptive atmosphere that promotes sociality by assembling a mix of affective forces (security, wonder, reflection), dispositions (comfort, relaxation) and social skills (allocentrism, conversational nous)" (p.68).

On the negative side, when a place lacks opportunities for reciprocity, connection and inclusion it may lead to isolation, stigma and potential conflict. Therefore, careful attention should be paid to characteristics of places that can transform them into communities (e.g. environmental and social infrastructures, opportunities for meaningful activities, membership and affiliation). Interactive and transformative methods such as photo-elicitation can help co-creation of recovery-promoting communities (Milasan et al., 2022, Vansteenkiste et al., 2021, Doroud et al., 2022).

Conclusion

Place plays an essential role in promoting recovery. Place comprises experiential, dynamic and relational dimensions that are created as individuals pave their way through recovery. This chapter discussed that being in a safe place, doing in an enabling place, becoming through a catalyst place and belonging to an affirming place are essential mechanisms through which individuals interact with and position themselves in the world. Acknowledging the lived-experience and social meanings of place, the chapter urges collaborative and interactive methods for working alongside people with lived and living experiences of mental ill-health to co-create recovery-promoting places.

References

Anthony, W. A. 1993. Recovery from mental illness: The guiding vision of the mental health service system in the 1990s. *Psychosocial Rehabilitation Journal*, 16, 11.

Beal, G., Veldhorst, G., Mcgrath, J.-L., Guruge, S., Grewal, P., Dinunzio, R. & Trimnell, J. 2005. Constituting community: Creating a place for oneself. *Psychiatry: Interpersonal and Biological Processes*, 68, 199–211.

Bierski, K. 2016. Recovering mental health across outdoor places in Richmond, London: Tuning, skill and narrative. *Health & Place*, 40, 137–144.

Borg, M. & Davidson, L. 2008. The nature of recovery as lived in everyday experience. *Journal of Mental Health*, 17, 129–140.

Borg, M., Sells, D., Topor, A., Mezzina, R., Marin, I. & Davidson, L. 2005. What makes a house a home: The role of material resources in recovery from severe mental illness. *American Journal of Psychiatric Rehabilitation*, 8, 243–256.

Bradshaw, W., Armour, M. P. & Roseborough, D. 2007. Finding a place in the world: The experience of recovery from severe mental illness. *Qualitative Social Work*, 6, 27–47.

Bromley, E., Gabrielian, S., Brekke, B., Pahwa, R., Daly, K. A., Brekke, J. S. & Braslow, J. T. 2013. Experiencing community: Perspectives of individuals diagnosed as having serious mental illness. *Psychiatric Services*, 64, 672–679.

Byrne, L., Happell B. & Reid-Searl, K. 2015. Recovery as a lived experience discipline: A grounded theory study. *Issues in Mental Health Nursing*, 36:12, 935–943.

Carpenter, T. W. & Strauss, S. J. 1991. The prediction of outcome in Schizophrenia IV: Eleven-year follow-up of the Washington IPSS cohort. *The Journal of Nervous and Mental Disease*, 179, 517–525.

Chesters, J., Fletcher, M. & Jones, R. 2005. Mental illness recovery and place. *Advances in Mental Health*, 4, 89–97.

Davidson, L. & Roe, D. 2007. Recovery from versus recovery in serious mental illness: One strategy for lessening confusion plaguing recovery. *Journal of Mental Health*, 16, 459–470.

Deegan, P. 1996. Recovery as a journey of the heart. *Psychiatric Rehabilitation Journal*, 19(3), 91–97. https://doi.org/10.1037/h0101301

Deegan, P. E. 1997. Recovery and empowerment for people with psychiatric disabilities. *Social Work in Health Care*, 25, 11–24.

Doroud, N., Fossey, E. & Fortune, T. 2015. Recovery as an occupational journey: A scoping review exploring the links between occupational engagement and recovery for people with enduring mental health issues. *Australian Occupational Therapy Journal*, 62, 378–392.

Doroud, N., Fossey, E. & Fortune, T. 2018. Place for being, doing, becoming and belonging: A meta-synthesis exploring the role of place in mental health recovery. *Health & Place*, 52, 110–120.

Doroud, N., Fossey, E., Fortune, T., Brophy, L., & Mountford, L. 2022. A journey of living well: A participatory photovoice study exploring recovery and everyday activities with people experiencing mental illness. *Journal of Mental Health*, 31(2), 246–254.

Duff, C. 2012. Exploring the role of 'enabling places' in promoting recovery from mental illness: A qualitative test of a relational model. *Health & Place*, 18, 1388–1395.

Duff, C. 2015. Atmospheres of recovery: Assemblages of health. *Environment and Planning A, Economy and Space*, 48(1), 58–74. https://doi.org/10.1177/0308518X15603222.

Hammell, K. W. 2014. Belonging, occupation, and human well-being: an exploration. *Canadian Journal of Occupational Therapy*, 81, 39–50.

Hammell, K. W. 2015. Participation and occupation: The need for a human rights perspective. *Canadian Journal of Occupational Therapy*, 82, 4–8.

Hammell, K. W. 2017. Opportunities for well-being: The right to occupational engagement. *Canadian Journal of Occupational Therapy*, 84, 209–222.

Hammell, K. W. & Iwama, M. K. 2012. Well-being and occupational rights: An imperative for critical occupational therapy. *Scandinavian Journal of Occupational Therapy*, 19, 385–394.

Heidegger, M. 2010. *Being and time*. Albany: State University of New York Press.

Kemp, S. P. 2011. Place, History, Memory: Thinking Time Within Place. *In:* Burton, L. M., Kemp, S. P., Leung, M., Matthews, S. A. & Takeuchi, D. T. (eds.) *Communities, neighborhoods, and health: expanding the boundaries of place*. New York: Springer Science & Business Media.

Kirst, M., Zerger, S., Harris, D. W., Plenert, E. & Stergiopoulos, V. 2014. The promise of recovery: Narratives of hope among homeless individuals with mental illness participating in a Housing First randomised controlled trial in Toronto, Canada. *BMJ Open*, 4(3), e004379.

Leamy, M., Bird, V., Le Boutillier, C., Williams, J. & Slade, M. 2011. Conceptual framework for personal recovery in mental health: Systematic review and narrative synthesis. *The British Journal of Psychiatry*, 199, 445–452.

Leviten-Reid, C., Johnson, P. & Miller, M. 2014. Supported housing in a small community: Effects on consumers, suggestions for change. *Canadian Journal of Community Mental Health*, 33, 57–69.

Llewellyn-Beardsley, J., Rennick-Egglestone, S., Callard, F., Crawford, P., Farkas, M., Hui, A., Manley, D., McGranahan, R., Pollock, K., Ramsay, A., Sælør, K. T., Wright, N. & Slade, M. 2019. Characteristics of mental health recovery narratives: Systematic review and narrative synthesis. *PloS One*, 14(3), e0214678.

Macnaughton, E. 2008. *Understanding insight development in early psychosis: A narrative approach*. University of British Columbia, Canada.

Macnaughton, E., Townley, G., Nelson, G., Caplan, R., Macleod, T., Polvere, L., Isaak, C., Kirst, M., Mcall, C. & Nolin, D. 2016. How does Housing First catalyze recovery?: Qualitative findings from a Canadian multi-site randomized controlled trial. *American Journal of Psychiatric Rehabilitation*, 19, 136–159.

Mezzina, R., Davidson, L., Borg, M., Marin, I., Topor, A. & Sells, D. 2006. The social nature of recovery: Discussion and implications for practice. *American Journal of Psychiatric Rehabilitation*, 9, 63–80.

Milasan, L. H., Bingley, A. F. & Fisher, N. R. 2022. The big picture of recovery: A systematic review on the evidence of photography-based methods in researching recovery from mental distress. *Arts & Health*, 14, 165–185.

Pahwa, R., Smith, M. E., Yuan, Y. & Padgett, D. 2019. The ties that bind and unbound ties: Experiences of formerly homeless individuals in recovery from serious mental illness and substance use. *Qualitative Health Research*, 29, 1313–1323.

Patterson, M. L., Currie, L., Rezansoff, S. & Somers, J. M. 2015. Exiting homelessness: Perceived changes, barriers, and facilitators among formerly homeless adults with mental disorders. *Psychiatric Rehabilitation Journal*, 38, 81–87.

Piat, M., Seida, K. & Padgett, D. 2020. Choice and personal recovery for people with serious mental illness living in supported housing. *Journal of Mental Health*, 29(3), 306–313.

Piat, M., Seida, K., & Sabetti, J. 2017. Understanding everyday life and mental health recovery through CHIME. *Mental Health and Social Inclusion*, 21(5), 271–279.

Poremski, D., Woodhall-Melnik, J., Lemieux, A. J. & Stergiopoulos, V. 2016. Persisting barriers to employment for recently housed adults with mental illness who were homeless. *Journal of Urban Health*, 93, 96–108.

Rebeiro, K. L. 2001. Enabling occupation: The importance of an affirming environment. *Canadian Journal of Occupational Therapy*, 68, 80–89.

Reis, G., Bromage, B., Rowe, M., Restrepo-Toro, M. E., Bellamy, C., Costa, M. & Davidson, L. 2022. Citizenship, social justice and collective empowerment: Living outside mental illness. *Psychiatric Quarterly*, 93, 537–546.

Sample, K. & Ferguson, K. M. 2020. It shouldn't be this hard: Systemic, situational, and intrapersonal barriers to exiting homelessness among homeless young adults. *Qualitative Social Work*, 19, 580–598.

Sells, D., Borg, M., Marin, I., Mezzina, R., Topor, A. & Davidson, L. 2006. Arenas of recovery for persons with severe mental illness. *American Journal of Psychiatric Rehabilitation*, 9, 3–16.

Slade, M. 2012. Everyday solutions for everyday problems: How mental health systems can support recovery. *Psychiatric Services*, 63, 702–704.

Slade, M., Amering, M., Farkas, M., Hamilton, B., O'Hagan, M., Panther, G., Perkins, R., Shepherd, G., Tse, S. & Whitley, R. 2014. Uses and abuses of recovery: Implementing recovery-oriented practices in mental health systems. *World Psychiatry*, 13(1), 12–20. https://doi.org/10.1002/wps.20084

Slade, M. & Wallace, G. 2017. Where are we now? Recovery and mental health. *In:* Slade, M., Oades, L. & Jarden, A. (eds.) *Wellbeing, recovery and mental health.* Cambridge: Cambridge University Press.

Smith, B. T., Padgett, D. K., Choy-Brown, M. & Henwood, B. F. 2015. Rebuilding lives and identities: The role of place in recovery among persons with complex needs. *Health & Place*, 33, 109–117.

Söderström, O., Empson, L. A., Codeluppi, Z., Söderström, D., Baumann, P. S. & Conus, P. 2016. Unpacking 'the City': An experience-based approach to the role of urban living in psychosis. *Health & Place*, 42, 104–110.

Sutton, D. J., Hocking, C. S. & Smyth, L. A. 2012. A phenomenological study of occupational engagement in recovery from mental illness. *Canadian Journal of Occupational Therapy / Revue Canadienne D'Ergothérapie*, 79, 142–150.

Topor, A., Borg, M., Di Girolamo, S. & Davidson, L. 2011. Not just an individual journey: Social aspects of recovery. *International Journal of Social Psychiatry*, 57, 90–99.

Treichler, E. B. H., Li, F., O'hare, M., Evans, E. A., Johnson, J. R. & Spaulding, W. D. 2019. Psychosocial and functional contributors to personal recovery in serious mental illness. *Journal of Mental Health*, 28, 427–435.

Vansteenkiste, T., Morrens, M. & Westerhof, G. J. 2021. Images of recovery: A photovoice study on visual narratives of personal recovery in persons with serious mental illness. *Community Mental Health Journal*, 57(6), 1151–1163.

Van Weeghel, J., Van Zelst, C., Boertien, D. & Hasson-Ohayon, I. 2019. Conceptualizations, assessments, and implications of personal recovery in mental illness: A scoping review of systematic reviews and meta-analyses. *Psychiatric Rehabilitation Journal*, 42, 169.

Waks, S., Scanlan, J. N., Berry, B., Schweizer, R., Hancock, N. & Honey, A. 2017. Outcomes identified and prioritised by consumers of partners in recovery: A consumer-led study. (Report). *BMC Psychiatry*, 17(1). https://doi.org/10.1186/s12888-017-1498-5

Watson, J., Fossey, E. & Harvey, C. 2019. A home but how to connect with others? A qualitative meta-synthesis of experiences of people with mental illness living in supported housing. *Health and Social Care in the Community*, 27, 546–564.

Whitley, R. & Drake, R. 2010. Recovery: A dimensional approach. *Psychiatric Services*, 61, 1248–1250.

Yanos, P. T. 2007. Beyond "Landscapes of Despair": The need for new research on the urban environment, sprawl, and the community integration of persons with severe mental illness. *Health & Place*, 13, 672–676.
Yates, I., Holmes, G. & Priest, H. 2012. Recovery, place and community mental health services. *Journal of Mental Health*, 21, 104–113.

32 Permanent supportive housing
A safe space for mental health recovery and healing

Deborah K. Padgett

Introduction

In the decades since deinstitutionalisation and the closing down of mental hospitals in many Western nations, the goal of community integration became paramount in the treatment of persons with serious mental illnesses (SMI) such as schizophrenia and bipolar disorder (Flynn, 1985). Unfortunately, inadequate outpatient treatment facilities combined with a looming housing affordability crisis in the 1970s set the stage for widespread homelessness among individuals with SMI. Stigmatised by a society with little understanding of mental illness and recovery, these men and women were highly visible reminders of a promise unkept and a troubled existence in full public view. In response, some cities and states had the funding and political will to adopt a new form of treatment-plus-housing known as permanent supportive housing (PSH).

This chapter is about PSH, including its origins and operations and its impact on the growing crisis of homelessness that engulfed the United States and many other Higher Income Countries (HICs) beginning in the 1980s. Since New York City and State are arguably responsible for the early iterations of PSH, the chapter's focus will be on the New York experience with concurrent awareness of PSH in other states and nations. Our concern is with the role of PSH in providing a safe space for mental health recovery and healing that makes community integration possible.

The rise of PSH

PSH occupies an important place in the array of services for persons experiencing homelessness and needing medical or mental health services. Indeed, the combination of having a stable place to live and access to needed services – most often intended for persons with a serious mental illness – is a defining characteristic of PSH. As a result, PSH is not suitable for homeless families or individuals without disabling conditions. For these groups, the end of homelessness might come in the form of a rental voucher or a moderate sum of money to avoid eviction (or to rapidly re-house if already evicted).

The significant increase in and dependence on PSH in recent decades is directly related to the rising numbers and associated costs incurred by the 'chronically homeless' who have physical or mental disabilities or both. The US government definition of 'chronic' homelessness is having been unsheltered continuously for a year or having four episodes of homelessness in the previous four years (US Department of Housing and Urban Development 2024).

DOI: 10.4324/9781003345725-36

The annual point-in-time count in 2017 in the United States revealed 550,000 individuals were homeless and 86,962 were classified as chronically homeless; 70 percent of the latter were unsheltered. It is this sub-group of 60+ thousand individuals (certainly an under-count) who challenge homeless services, police departments and medical personnel to contain 'anti-social' behaviour and de-escalate crises of psychosis in combination with potent illicit drugs. Deinstitutionalisation (the national trend of closing psychiatric hospitals in favour of mental health care in the community beginning in the 1960s) is believed to play a prominent role in contributing to the urgent need for PSH as ex-patients struggled with life on the outside. As community mental health care did not increase to meet the needs of these discharged patients, thousands of ex-patients (and newly diagnosed) found themselves without housing.

Defining permanent supportive housing

PSH units are typically studio or one-bedroom apartments. They may be 'single site' (all or most of the units in a building are PSH) or 'scatter site' (individual units are scattered throughout a city or other municipality). A sub-category of the single site model is when the building has mixed income tenants, mingling programme clients (formerly homeless) with low-income single adults. One of the earliest and largest examples of mixed income PSH was The Times Square Hotel in the heart of New York City operated by a non-profit organisation. With 652 rooms and an ornate lobby, the deteriorating building was converted in 1990, early in the homeless 'crisis.' Formerly homeless men and women – most with mental disabilities – shared the building with actors who could live near the theatre district and other artists (Breaking Ground, 2024). Converting aging hotels was costly but at least contributed supported housing apartments to the dwindling housing stock in New York City and elsewhere.

Regardless of housing arrangements, a defining feature of PSH is the availability of support services, whether on-site (locating offices for staff in the single-site building) or off-site where staff travel to client's apartments and help to schedule them to receive varied services and treatment. The 'permanent' in the title of PSH is not an absolute guarantee – a severely disabled resident may need institutional care, the PSH programme may evict a particularly troublesome tenant, or a tenant may go 'AWOL' and leave the programme. In the latter case, the reason is often the decrepit conditions of the apartment or the rules and restrictions imposed by the PSH provider.

PSH remains an aspirational goal for many homeless persons by fulfilling an essential need for a sense of 'place' and security (Padgett, 2007). This sets PSH apart from transitional housing (or night shelters) run by programmes that focus on temporary service provision with end dates (usually one or two years maximum). Persons eligible for PSH often languish in temporary accommodations for years – available PSH units meet only 1/3 of demand (United States Interagency Council on Homelessness 2024).

Background: Historic precedents and a growing need

Early versions of PSH arose in the 1960s when charity services were co-located with SRO (single room occupancy) hotels to help residents who were impoverished elders, substance-dependent users and disabled men and women (Hopper, 2003). As SROs were torn down and virtually disappeared due to gentrification, older and disabled inhabitants became homeless and community-based support services were scattershot.

When homelessness reached record levels in the late 1980s, service providers pivoted to screening homeless persons on the street or in shelters to identify those with disabilities (usually mental illness) requiring more attention and assistance. Though incurring costs to provide necessary support services, these programmes were eventually shown to be cost-effective when compared to the expensive 'institutional circuit' of hospitalisations, jail stays and emergency visits incurred by those deemed chronically homeless (Culhane & Kuhn, 1998; Gladwell, 2006; Hopper, 2003).

With the numbers of chronically homeless steadily rising in the 1990s, PSH programmes filled an important gap in service provision. In addition to SROs, this gap had previously been addressed by adult homes or nursing homes. Neither of these options was satisfactory, the former often poorly run with few services and the latter inappropriate for younger individuals suffering from mental illness (yet reimbursable by Medicaid as the nursing home setting is the only housing Medicaid covers).

One of the early initiatives to expand PSH for those with SMI was an unprecedented agreement between New York State and City (the NY/NY agreement) beginning in 1990 (Houghton, 2001). With state and city governments working in tandem, over 3,000 units of PSH were budgeted for using monies earmarked for mental health services. This conflation of mental health and housing was shown to save money but it also had salubrious non-monetised effects in stabilising and enriching the lives of inhabitants (Houghton, 2001). In short, PSH was viewed as a win-win approach, benefiting individuals and governments charged with their care and rescuing disabled people from life on the streets. The concept of 'housing improving health' was novel in the early 1990s but the connection between the two, i.e., the notion that one's health is improved by having stable housing, formed the basis for declaring housing a social determinant of health (Rolfe et al., 2020).

By the end of 2000, 7,774 clients had been placed in NY/NY housing (Houghton, 2001).As of this writing 23 years later, New York City has 35,000 supported housing apartments – of these 16,000 are scatter-site. All are run by a variety of non-profit programs who either own the building or rent apartments from private landlords (Supportive Housing Network of New York). The 'supportive' part of the arrangement usually consists of case managers who make apartment visits to link residents with needed services. Most PSH units are locating in low-income areas of New York City.

The idea of cooperating to fund housing by government authorities reversed a trend dating to President Reagan's administration whose policies worsened an already struggling housing market for working poor and unhoused alike. The demand for PSH units far exceeded the supply. The context of this dilemma made this dire situation inevitable as the Reagan era policies put a virtual stop to funding for new public housing and sharp decreases in housing rental vouchers. Instead, the housing market became privatised and for-profit developers were hardly motivated to build for low-income residents. Some 40 years later, the situation has worsened, with expensive condominium buildings attracting affluent buyers while the less fortunate are consigned to aging buildings where rents have risen disproportionately (Desmond, 2023). It is in this chasm of privilege juxtaposed against deprivation that PSH has a niche.

To assist in the spread of PSH, the Corporation for Supportive Housing (CSH) was founded in 1991 to operate as a technical assistance go-between joining varied stakeholders – non-profit homeless service providers, real estate boards, and private philanthropists – in breaking down barriers to building and maintaining PSH units locally. CSH staff were versed in zoning regulations, tax incentives, and urban planning priorities to enable cooperation (Corporation for Supportive Housing, 2011). Though barriers often appeared – especially in the form of NIMBY (not-in-my-backyard) attitudes by neighbours of PSH sites – CSH became a national entity dealing with the myriad of laws, ordinances, funding streams and other information needed by nonprofits seeking to expand their PSH capabilities (Houghton, 2001).

Housing first: Making PSH more empowering and effective

As PSH became an enduring feature in the landscape of homeless services in cities having densely developed apartment housing (most in the Eastern US), it was hardly flawless. Some apartments were sub-standard, rented from unscrupulous landlords whose properties were located in dangerous neighbourhoods. Support services supplied by low-paid poorly trained case managers, often consisted of little more than medication checks, drug tests and rules enforcement, i.e., prohibiting visitors, requiring day treatment for mental patients and 12-step programme attendance to achieve sobriety.

In 1992 in New York City, a new form of PSH was established that reversed the 'staircase' approach that characterised homeless services throughout the US Known as the "housing first" (HF) approach taken by Pathways to Housing, Inc., the programme provided immediate access to one's own apartment with few conditions beyond accepting case manager visits and contributing one-third of any income toward payment of rent. Pathways up-ended the continuum of care in which the homeless person traverses a staircase beginning with a shelter, then transitional housing then PSH – a staircase where people could languish for years in temporary residences. Moving up the staircase required a host of conditions – medication compliance, sobriety and drug-free living and other accoutrements of being 'housing worthy' i.e., able to access PSH (Padgett, Henwood & Tsemberis, 2016).

Homeless persons eligible for HF had to have a diagnosed serious mental illness such as schizophrenia, bipolar disorder or major depression. Many of these persons also had substance use problems, but this was not disqualifying as Pathways to Housing practiced harm reduction rather than require sobriety or remaining drug-free. Not surprisingly, Pathways accepted many individuals who had been evicted from a variety of programmes due to substance use, active psychosis, and criminal records (often a combination of these).

What was surprising was the ease with which these individuals became habituated to having a home of their own. Pathways provided furniture, linens and other necessities so moving in was an occasion for celebration mixed with a measure of disbelief at their good fortune. To be sure, a small proportion of Pathways tenants did not do well, either too sick or too actively addicted to adapt to independent living. Pathways responded to landlord complaints and, if necessary, moved the troubled tenant to another apartment urging them to seek rehabilitation or hospitalisation (with the promise of having their apartment upon release). A jail stay was not cause for eviction from the programme. For the majority of tenants, having a home was the first step in reaching for recovery – over 80 percent were still housed stably after one year (Tsemberis, Gulcur and Nakae, 2004).

Benefiting from NY/NY funds as well as Federal grants, Pathways pursued what was considered dangerous and doomed to failure. With research showing consistently favourable findings of 80-90 percent housing stability after one year at a cost-saving compared to 'usual care' (living on the streets, shelters and transitional housing), Pathways-PSH gradually gained momentum and has since become the recommended approach by the

Department of Housing and Urban Development, the Veteran's Administration and homeless advocates. Pathways' "housing first" model is the national policy of Canada. It is in wide use throughout Western Europe and is also being used in South America (Chile and Brasil).

HF tenants proudly cite the advantages of the approach – having a key and locked door for privacy, a refrigerator to aid in storing nutritious food, a bathroom for personal hygiene, and a bed where one can finally have uninterrupted sleep. Having voluntary access to services for health care, substance dependence, and mental health helped to restore trust. Leaving behind a life spent searching for safe spaces and finding a permanent haven enhances 'ontological security' (Padgett, 2007).

The term ontological security is derived from the writings of psychiatrist R.D. Laing (1965) and social scientist Anthony Giddens (1990) to connote a sense of meaning and constancy in one's life that is stabilising and helps to cope with life in an ever-changing modern era. Padgett (2007) examined this conception as applied to the transition from homelessness to having a home in a HF programme. Following the four-part operationalisation of Dupuis and Thorns (1998), ontological security resulting from having a home is marked by: 1) constancy in the daily environment; 2) a place to carry out day-to-day routines; 3) feeling control in one's life and free of the surveillance commonly found in public domains; and, 4) a secure base around which identities are constructed.

In-depth interviews with individuals in a HF apartment, when compared to their peers still living in shelters or transitional housing, were striking in their alignment of having vs. not having ontological security. Both interviews and ethnographic observation revealed the tremendous relief of having a home of their own including the sensory delights of having fresh food available at all hours and the joy of a bubble bath. A life without constant bed checks, drug tests and other interruptions was noted with gratitude (Padgett, 2007). The fourth marker of ontological security was both compelling and challenging, as 'identity' development is a cognitive process of negotiating external cues with an internal sense of the self (Goffman, 1963). Study participants revealed a desire to shed earlier stigmatising identities such as 'addict', 'mentally ill', 'homeless' and replace them with positive identities such as 'grandparent', 'trusted confidant', 'religious believer' and 'reliable worker'.

Moving on initiatives: 'Graduating' from PSH

With apartments becoming scarce and PSH programs struggling to find available units, the question arose – is permanence necessary if the tenant is doing well and would like to leave? Could these 'high-functioning' tenants combine disability income with a rental voucher and move on from programme housing to an apartment on their own? Some PSH residents have a job – typically low-paid and part-time – that generates modest income to help them achieve independence.

Moving On Initiatives (MOIs) emerged to address the dual goals of tenant independence and reducing the shortage of PSH apartments (Tiderington, Goodwin and Noonan, 2022). According to federal data, the number of PSH units doubled after 2007 with 373,000 units available nationally, but this represents about one-third of extant need being met (U.S. Government Department of Housing and Urban Development, 2024). In a scoping literature review of MOIs, Tiderington et al. (2022) found positive outcomes of MOI (less or no reliance on case management services) and post-PSH housing retention for 17 MOI studies that met scoping review criteria. Given the relatively few MOIs studied thus far, these findings are encouraging but not conclusive.

Outcomes from PSH Programmes

As mentioned earlier, the research on HF has yielded positive outcomes in terms of housing stability, fewer hospitalisations, and enhancing tenants' sense of ontological security. In 2018, the National Academy of Sciences, Engineering and Medicine (NASEM) released a report on the effectiveness of PSH for health outcomes (National Academies Press, 2018). Acknowledging the lack of research in this area, the NASEM report nonetheless concluded that there was no evidence of benefit and cost-effectiveness of PSH with the possible exception of PSH for persons with HIV/AIDS. This negative take on PSH addressed outcomes that PSH was not designed to improve (but presumably would show benefits given the overall positive outcomes of PSH in non-health conditions such as housing stability and engagement with service providers).

The evaluation of PSH for tangible improvements in health overlooks the chronicity of many health problems (diabetes, high blood pressure, arthritis) and the length of time needed to demonstrate substantive changes in health given months or years spent in survival mode. Nevertheless, this report carries the imprimatur of NASEM and as such has cast some doubt on at least one type of outcome (health) expected to improve under PSH residency.

Meanwhile, several PSH studies have produced positive findings. A randomised trial of PSH vs. non-PSH conducted by Raven et al. (2020) found PSH participants had fewer emergency psychiatric visits and higher rates of ambulatory mental health visits. A systematic review by Aubry et al. (2021) found significant positive effects of PSH in terms of six-year housing stability, improved quality of life and no adverse effects on health, mental health and substance use.

Studies of PSH longitudinally are very few in number. In one longitudinal follow-up study of 73 PSH residents by Roncarati et al. (2021), housing retention dropped from 82% to 36% at five years of follow-up. The study was located in Boston; the sample was predominantly white male (77%) and 63 (86%) had 'trimorbidity' (health, mental health and substance use disorders). Almost half (46%) died in the five-year period (average age was 52). Although the generalisability of these findings is limited given the sample characteristics (e.g., older age, absence of African-Americans, etc.) it nonetheless poses questions about the long-term stability of PSH residents.

In sum, PSH has consistently been found to be effective in ending homelessness and has no more negative health or mental health effects when compared to the 'staircase' approach. Meanwhile, some studies have shown reduced dependence on drugs or alcohol in PSH treatment compared to transitional/shelter approaches. A study by Padgett and colleagues (2011) used longitudinal (12 month) qualitative data that were quantified (yes/no on substance use in year after entry into the PSH or non-PSH programme) as dependent variables and subjected to logistic regression. The findings were not only quantitatively robust (participants in the PSH program were three times less likely to use drugs or alcohol compared to their peers) but offered insights from the qualitative interviews into how stable housing enabled recovery (Padgett et al. 2011) through harm reduction in combination with a sense of 'something to lose' if relapse occurs. The sturdiness of these positive findings, i.e., whether and how they last, requires further research – preferably with a comparison group.

The Olmstead decision, disability rights and PSH

The civil rights of persons with disabilities in the US were formally acknowledged with passage of the Americans with Disabilities Act (ADA) in 1990. The ADA had a profound effect in 'leveling the playing field' for persons with physical disabilities and reached its full potential with the Supreme Court's Olmstead decision in 1999. Olmstead extended ADA protections to (and required accommodations for) persons with psychiatric or mental disabilities. Put simply, institutional-like residential living was considered damaging to community integration and constituted unfair segregation.

The closure of hundreds of psychiatric hospitals in the US had already put in motion the principles of Olmstead. Moreover, the rise of Housing First with scatter-site housing in 1992 presaged the court decision. However, enforcement of the Olmstead decision was problematic since compliance would require fundamental systems change in homeless services where persons with serious mental illness or developmental disabilities were confined to adult homes, mental health shelters and long-term care facilities such as nursing homes. Since Olmstead was ordained by the highest court in the country, the door was opened for civil rights groups to file lawsuits against a city or state to demand compliance. One of the more egregious violations of Olmstead was revealed in a *New York Times* April 2002 report that generated outrage aimed at for-profit proprietors of adult homes, where residents were warehoused and received little/no care. Many died of suicide or untended health problems; bodies would lie unattended for days (Levy, 2002).

Adult home operators fought to protect their lucrative business interests (appropriation of residents' disability income plus funds from the State Office of Mental Health). A building with 350 beds at $1200 monthly disability per resident yields $420,000 and over 5 million dollars annually. The owners lost and an Olmstead-inspired legal settlement was overseen by a judge in which residents were to be transferred to private apartments and given support services as needed – many having spent decades languishing in filthy rooms without support services. Though progress has been slow – 800 rehomed when the target was 2500 – many adult home residents have found new lives in PSH (Sapien 2019).

Housing is health: A movement to end homelessness led by health providers

As homelessness continued some four decades after the crisis began in the 1980s, a new breed of health activists coalesced to demand greater attention be paid to the health benefits of housing. Emergency department physicians had for years seen a steady stream of patients with leg ulcers, high blood pressure, traumatic brain injuries and a host of other problems that were not always emergencies but still allowed admission for a homeless person pursuing health care and knowing the long wait brought benefits, i.e., a warm place to sleep while waiting. Two physicians – James O'Connell in Boston and Jim Withers in Pittsburgh – pioneered street medicine, going to encampments or individuals sleeping in doorways and providing medical care on site (Kidder, 2023).

Of all the options for homeless persons – shelters, safe havens, drop-in centers – PSH is by far the safest in guarding the health of inhabitants. This became abundantly clear during the COVID pandemic as shelters were prime sites for the virus due to crowding, poor sanitation and lack of air cleaners. Temporary re-housing to empty hotel rooms helped fend off major outbreaks but the return to 'normal' shelter life came a few months later in 2020. In this scenario, shelter residents with serious mental illness are manifestly not given their Olmstead rights.

The salience of PSH also rose as researchers pointed to the Baby Boom effects under-lying sharp increases in older homeless populations in recent years. Kushel (2024) notes that only 11% of homeless persons were older than 50 in 1990 but by 2020 over half were over age 50. The implications of this demographic shift are fairly easy to identify – changes in needs toward cognitive impairments and dementias, injurious falls, lack of mobility and/or inability to carry out activities of daily living (Brown et al., 2012). Given decreases in life expectancy, homeless persons of age 50 are considered to be 'old' due to the brutality of their existence. Accustomed to homeless clients of younger age, PSH staff are ill-prepared for such changes (Culhane et al., 2019).

Conclusion

This review of permanent supportive housing (PSH) began with its origins and growth as a means of combining housing with support services for homeless (or at-risk for homelessness) individuals. PSH has its roots in New York City in the 1980s as state and local governments cooperated in assisting the rising numbers of homeless adults with disabilities, primarily mental illness. Through philanthropic contributions, the Corporation for Supportive Housing (CSH) was established to assist in communities across the US as they struggled with growing numbers of homeless persons afflicted by disabilities. Whether relying on scatter-site apartments or entire buildings, PSH programs shared in common a commitment to helping clients achieve autonomy through providing support services as needed.

The emergence of the paradigm-shifting approach to PSH known as Housing First in New York City in 1992 positioned access to PSH as a 'right' where clients were not required to take all medications, maintain complete sobriety and follow a host of other rules common to PSH programs and shelters. HF set itself apart from the mainstream approach of adhering to these rules to become 'housing worthy' (Padgett et al., 2016). In the U.S. the success of HF propelled it to become a top priority in HUD funding of local homeless providers after 2009. This policy shift away from shelters and other forms of temporary accommodations was not altogether popular with non-profits unaccustomed to (and often uncomfortable with) HF precepts such as consumer choice, harm reduction (as opposed to 'clean and sober' requirements) and scatter-site independent living.

Overall, PSH – and HF in particular – offers greater stability, support and services attuned to individual needs and a foothold on recovery from the multiple traumas of homelessness and disability. Alternatives – night shelters, drop-in centres, outdoor camping – are linked to disconnects from needed services as well as physical and emotional harm. Though research on 'moving on' (leaving PSH to rent an apartment free of program enrollment) is still in its infancy, there is reason to believe that community integration is better served by having PSH as a way station than the alternatives – a return to the streets or long-term (costly) institutionalisation.

References

Aubry, T. et al. (2021). 'Effectiveness of permanent supportive housing and income assistance interventions for homeless individuals in high-income countries: a systematic review'. *Lancet Public Health*, 5, e342–e360.

Breaking Ground (2024). 'Breaking Ground: Who We Are.' Breaking Ground, New York. Available at: https://breakingground.org/who-we-are/ [Accessed March 14, 2024].

Brown, R. T., Kiely, D. K., Bharel, M., and Mitchell, S. (2012). 'Geriatric syndromes in older homeless adults'. *Journal of General Internal Medicine*, 27(1), 16–22.

Corporation for Supportive Housing (2011). *Ending homelessness among older adults and elders through permanent supportive housing*. New York: Author. www.csh.org/wpcontent/uploads/2012/01/Report_EndingHomelessnessAmongOlderAdultsandSeniorsThroughSupportiveHousing_112.pdf

Culhane, D., Treglia, D., Burne T., Metraux, S., Kuhn, J., Doran, K., and Johns, E. (2019). 'The emerging crisis of aged homelessness'. Retrieved from: https://works.bepress.com/dennis_culhane/223/

Culhane, D. P. and Khun, R. (1998). 'Patterns and determinants of public shelter utilization among homeless adults in New York City and Philadelphia'. *Journal of Policy Analysis and Management*, 17(1), 23–43.

Desmond, M. (2023). *Poverty, by America*. New York: Crown.

Dupuis, A. and Thorns, D. (1998). 'Home, home ownership, and the search for ontological security'. *The Sociological Review*, 46(1), 24–47.

Flynn, K. (1985). 'The toll of deinstitutionalization' pp. 189–190 in P. W. Brickner, L. K. Sharer, B. Conanan A. Elvy, and M. Savarese. *The health care of homeless people*. New York: Springer Publishing Company.

Giddens, A. (1990). *Consequences of modernity*. Oxford, UK: Polity Press.

Gladwell, M. (2006). 'Million dollar Murray'. *The New Yorker*.

Goffman, E. (1963. *Stigma: Notes on the management of spoiled identity*. New York: Simon & Schuster.

Hopper, K. (2003). *Reckoning with homelessness*. Ithaca, New York: Cornell University Press.

Houghton, T. (2001). *A history of the New York/New York Agreement to house homeless mentally ill individuals*. New York: Corporation for Supportive Housing.

Kidder, T. (2023). *Rough sleepers: Dr. Jim O'Connell's urgent mission to bring healing to homeless people*. New York: Random House.

Kushel, M. 'Aging and Homelessness: Margot Kushel'. *Geripal*, Available at: https://geripal.org/aging-and-homelessness-margot-kushel/ [Accessed 14 March 2024].

Laing, R. D. (1965). *The divided self: An existential study in sanity and madness*. London: Pelican Press.

Levy, C. (2002). 'Voiceless, defenseless and a source of cash'. Retrieved from www.nytimes.com/2002/04/30/nyregion/voiceless-defenseless-and-a-source-of-cash.html

National Academies Press (2018). *Permanent supportive housing: Evaluating the evidence for improving health outcomes among people experiencing homelessness*. Washington, DC:National Academies Press.

Padgett, D., Henwood, B. F., and Tsemberis, S. (2016). *Housing first: Endinghomelessness, transforming systems and changing lives*. New York: Oxford.

Padgett, D. K. (2007). 'There's no place like (a) home: Ontological security among persons with serious mental illness in the United States. *Social Science & Medicine*, 64(9), 1925–1936.

Padgett, D. K., Stanhope, V. Henwood, B., and Stefancic, A. (2011). 'Substance use outcomes among homeless clients with serious mental illness: Comparing Housing First with treatment first programs'. *Community Mental Health Journal*, 47(2), 227–232.

Raven, M., Niedzwiecki, M., and Kushel. M. (2020). 'A randomized trial of permanent supportive housing for chronically homeless persons with high use of publicly funded services.' *Health Services Research*, 55(suppl 2), 797–806.

Rolfe, S., Garnham, L., Anderson, I., Seaman, P., and Donaldson, C. (2020). 'Housing as a social determinant of health and well-being'. *BMC Public Health*, 20, 1138–1141.

Roncarati, J. et al. (2021). 'Housing Boston's chronically homeless population 14 years later'. *Medical Care*, 59, S170–S174.

Sapien, J. (2019). 'After failing mentally ill new yorkers, adult homes get second chance' *Propublic*, Available at: www.propublica.org/article/after-failing-mentally-ill-new-yorkers-adult-homes-get-second-chance [Accessed 14 March. 2024].

Tiderington, E., Goodman, J., and Noonan, E. (2024). 'Leaving permanent supportive housing: A scoping review of Moving On Initiative participant outcomes'. *Housing Studies*, 39, 203–226.

Tsemberis, S., Gulcur, L., and Nakae, N. (2004) 'Housing first, consumer choice, and harm reduction for homeless individuals with a dual diagnosis'. *American Journal of Public Health*, 94(4), 651–656.

United States Interagency Council on Homelessness (2024). Scale housing and supports that meet demand. United States Interagency Council on Homelessness, Washington, DC. Available at: www.usich.gov/federal-strategic-plan/scale-housing-and-supports-meet-demand [Accessed 14 March 2024].

US Government Department of Housing and Urban Development (2024). 'Definition of Chronic Homelessness.' US Government Department of Housing and Urban Development. Available at: www.hudexchange.info/homelessness-assistance/coc-esg-virtual-binders/coc-esg-homeless-eligibility/definition-of-chronic-homelessness/ [Accessed 14 March 2024].

33 Haven or hell?

An introduction to trauma informed design as a mechanism for place-based healing

Julia Woodhall-Melnik, Cassandra Monette, and Erin MacKenney

Introduction

Home as an emotive concept is different from the physical house. It is not windows and roofs, but rather an environment that can contribute to safety and permanence. It is often talked about as a place of refuge that offers privacy, protection, and a place to establish and build one's identity and life (Manzo, 2005; Padgett, 2007). Homes that offer this kind of safety and feelings of stability provide a myriad of psychosocial benefits that contribute to positive mental health and wellbeing (Kearns et al., 2000). They promote growth and healing and can provide a sense of cohesion and assurance of one's place in the world (Hiscock et al., 2001). However, not all experiences of home are positive (Mallet, 2004; Woodhall-Melnik et al., 2017a). Home can provide safety, comfort and refuge, but it can also be a site of instability, trauma, anger, stress, neglect and abuse. Research finds that negative experiences of home in early life can contribute to feelings of fear, trauma and instability within places of residence that persist throughout life (Woodhall-Melnik et al., 2018). Individuals who experience a variety of social structural and economic vulnerabilities are more likely to also experience trauma and dysfunction in the home (Crouch et al., 2020). This leads to the question: How do individuals who are housing insecure and associate home with trauma build positive associations of home within housing? Further, how can elements of physical space and the built environment contribute to the creation of positive associations with home that can promote healing from trauma?

Scholars and front-line workers are increasingly aware of the need to develop therapeutic environments that respond to trauma carried by persons with lived experience of housing instability. Newer housing models are beginning to recognise the need to consider experiences of trauma to increase housing stability and wellbeing in persons with lived experience of homelessness. Trauma informed design (TID) is an example of an emergent practice that utilises architectural design to create therapeutic spaces for individuals who have histories of trauma in previous home environments. Increasingly recognised as a promising practice for persons who have survived gender-based violence and homelessness, TID reorients built environments to provide spaces that focus on mental health promotion (Bollo & Donofrio, 2022; Shopworks et al., 2020). These spaces may align with positive understandings of home. In this chapter, we discuss TID as an emerging method to realise individualised spaces of home that contribute to mental health and wellbeing and promote healing, dignity, and empowerment through choice.

DOI: 10.4324/9781003345725-37

The importance of home

Researchers understand the importance of the built environment to human health and wellbeing (Kent & Thompson, 2012). Houses as physical structures are important to everyday wellness. They are relied on to provide shelter from natural elements and external threats; however, houses can also provide safe spaces that allow us to be ourselves and escape public surveillance or scrutiny (Mallet, 2004). The literature on home as an emotive concept focuses on the importance of the home to wellbeing and comfort and argues that home is fundamentally different from, although related to, the physical experience of housing (Woodhall-Melnik et al., 2017a; 2017b). The concept of home captures the emotional imprint of experiences that happen within the physical location of the house.

Although the home is often presented as a place of refuge, privacy and growth, experiences of home are not always positive. The concept of home as a place of domination, submission, violence and trauma stems from feminist literature on place. Herein, the concept of home is presented as a site of gendered violence, wherein women experience the emotional consequences of the expectation that they cater to the needs of others (Kay, 2020; Manzo, 2003). Further, home becomes more complex when it is viewed outside of the binary experiences of positive or negative. Manzo (2003) argues that these dichotomous views of home are often overly simplistic and do not represent the complexity and diversity of experiences that lead to one's understanding of place.

Home is a multifaceted concept and its meaning hinges on diverse human experiences, often influenced by structural factors of race, gender, class, and sexuality. These multifaceted, complex understandings are more recently discussed by scholars who examine experiences of housing instability and homelessness (Padgett, 2007; Rosenberg et al., 2021). For example, in their study of the meaning of home for men with histories of homelessness, Woodhall-Melnik et al. (2017b:369) quote a study participant who states that home can "be bingeing or bacon." This seemingly simple statement from a man who experienced long-term homelessness describes the stability and refuge that comes from the smell of bacon cooking in the morning; however, in the same breath, he describes experiences of home that are violent, traumatic, and tainted by his parents' substance use. This indicates that even when home is a site of trauma, individuals may still be able to derive comfort from positive home experiences.

Home as an emotive concept is often associated with ontological security (Gustafsson & Krickel-Choi, 2020). Proposed by R.D. Laing (1960) and popularised through Giddens' (1984) development of the term (Gustafsson & Krickel-Choi, 2020), ontological security describes the ability to feel whole and stable in the world and to experience a sense of continuity and consistency, established through routine, that ultimately leads to individual agency (Giddens, 1984). Individuals without ontological security are said to experience anxiety about their place in the world (Giddens, 1991). They are "preoccupied with preserving [themselves]" (Laing, 1969: 44), which leads to inaction on other less basic tenets of existence. Flockhart (2020) and Kinnvall et al., (2018) note that individuals who exist in a perpetual state of crisis or who often experience disruptive life events lack the cognitive consistency to ward off anxiety. This produces insecurity about the future (Flockhart, 2020; Kinnvall et al., 2018), and when adaptation to produce the conditions necessary for ontological security is not successful, it ultimately leads to diminished motivation and further limits the ability to take action to adapt to present circumstances (Flockhart, 2016; Flockhart, 2020). Individuals who lack strong connection to home and place often lack ontological security and may be unable to envision positive futures. This has negative implications for mental health and wellbeing and it perpetuates the cycle of housing instability experienced by individuals with lived experience of trauma.

Home is easily connected to the establishment of routine and the individual experience of safety and security (Woodhall-Melnik et al., 2017a). The home is supposed to be a place of refuge to rebuild and establish ontological security; however, when the home becomes a site of anxiety or produces significant trauma, a preoccupation with self-preservation can occur (Banham, 2020). Instability in home environments at a young age can have persisting impacts on one's ability to establish and maintain ontological security (Vaquera et al., 2017). Researchers find that the trauma produced by unstable home environments in early life can lead to housing instability in youth that persists into adulthood (Woodhall-Melnik et al., 2018; Hallett & Freas, 2018).

If home is associated with trauma and is also a necessity for the establishment of ontological security, individuals may lack a sense of permanence and self-identity which is necessary to develop future plans and meet normative goals and expectations within society (Kinnvall, 2004). This leads to the question: how can people with traumatic past experiences of home environments safely build a positive sense of home? In order to regain the benefits of being ontologically secure, the present authors argue that practices must be developed to house vulnerable populations in therapeutic spaces that respond to past views of home as traumatic.

Complex experiences of trauma

Trauma is complex and multifaceted. The American Psychiatric Association (2018) offers a simple definition of trauma as:

> Any disturbing experience that results in significant fear, helplessness, dissociation, confusion, or other disruptive feelings intense enough to have a long-lasting negative effect on a person's attitudes, behaviour, and other aspects of functioning. Traumatic events…often challenge an individual's view of the world as a just, safe, and predictable space.

Trauma can be the consequence of human interactions and victimisation, but it can also result from exposure to external environmental threats, such as natural disasters, and social structural conditions of disadvantage (APA, 2018). Comprehensive definitions of trauma recognise that it is often the result of interactions between social, economic, health, and environmental factors that produce toxic stress and instability across the life course (Shanks and Robinson, 2013). Exposure to toxic stress is linked to fundamental changes to genes and their expressions (Shonkoff et al., 2012) and often results in adverse outcomes that are persistent and capable of producing additional stressors and trauma over time (Franke, 2014; Shern et al., 2016).

Trauma may result from a singular event, a series of events, or a specific set of circumstances (SAMHSA, 2014) including systemic oppression and discrimination (Mihelicova et al., 2018). Many of the consequences of trauma are also causes. For example, housing insecurity, poverty, and experiences of violence or abuse may cause damage, but they are also consequences of living with unaddressed trauma (Beyerlein and Bloch, 2014). Hence, persons who experience trauma may become locked in a cycle wherein trauma begets more trauma and the cumulative impacts of these exposures leads to worsened outcomes that seem insurmountable. The effects of this accumulation are visible in the research on Adverse Child Experiences (ACEs), a specific set of harmful socioeconomic conditions, and/or exposures to abuse or neglect that occur under the age of 18. ACEs have a cumulative impact on a variety of health, social and economic outcomes. Further, certain combinations of ACEs (e.g. parental mental illness and poverty) place children at greater risk of poor health outcomes (Lanier et al., 2018).

Although home is often the primary site of early socialisation that plays an important role in shaping how people view themselves and others, it is also the primary site of early trauma for many individuals who later experience chronic homelessness (Hamilton et al., 2011; Woodhall-Melnik et al., 2018). Trauma that happens in the home has the potential to shape future experiences with housing (Mackelprang et al., 2014), which can make it hard for traumatised persons to form and maintain positive attachments to home and can impact their ability to frame home as a positive space for healing and growth.

Care for individuals and groups with place-based trauma

Trauma fundamentally changes the way that people understand and interact with the world. Although trauma may be difficult to recognise initially (Moses et al., 2003a), it plagues the minds and bodies of many individuals who experience homelessness (Davies & Allen, 2017; Mackelprang et al., 2014; Menzies, 2006; Zlotnick et al., 2007). Many frontline service providers recognise the importance of trauma as a contributor to homelessness and have adapted their programming and approaches to be trauma informed. The ultimate goal of this practice is to provide service that does not retraumatise individuals or contribute to additional experiences of distress.

Service providers who are trauma informed often integrate the practice of Trauma Informed Care (TIC) in their approaches to their work with persons who experience housing instability. TIC is a strengths-based approach that integrates awareness of the existence of trauma into all levels of policies, procedures, and elements of decision-making. Moses et al. (2003b) define TIC as "understanding, anticipating, and responding to the issues, expectations, and special needs that a person who has been victimised may have in a particular setting or service." The goal of TIC is to avoid retraumatisation, while recognising that trauma fundamentally alters the way that individuals and their brains respond to stimuli within their environments (SAMHSA, 2014). Trauma-informed service providers seek to recognise the strengths of clients as they put forth efforts to manage reactions to settings and experiences that arise from past experiences of trauma (Hooper et al., 2010). TIC does not strive to treat trauma (Mihelicova, 2018); rather, it aims to reduce the harm associated with navigating systems, services, relationships, and environments that have the potential to exacerbate distress related to past traumatic experiences. When distress is unavoidable, TIC providers respond with acceptance, compassion and referrals to appropriate supports while maintaining clients' rights to agency and choice.

The principles of TIC are highly effective when implemented with organisational commitment to cultural changes that promote sensitivity and awareness (CDC, 2023). The six guiding principles of TIC are to establish safety, promote trustworthiness and transparency, incorporate peer support, encourage collaboration and mutuality, promote empowerment through choice, and operate with awareness and understanding of cultural, historical and gender issues (SAMHSA, 2014). TIC uses a holistic approach to the provision of supports. It focuses on the strengths of traumatised persons while striving to limit distress in interactions with environments, systems, services, and people that may trigger adverse reactions.

Architects and social workers have adapted principles of TIC to inform physical aspects of built environments through the practice of Trauma Informed Design (TID). TID shows promise as a mechanism for building or reestablishing positive views of home as therapeutic and comfortable environments. Like TIC, TID acknowledges the harm that home environments have caused for many individuals and aims to prevent or minimise the potential for additional distress from exposure to triggers within housing environments (Bollo & Donofrio, 2022; Shopworks et al., 2020). However, unlike TIC, TID can be described as a therapeutic approach that integrates individuals' preferences and choices, and elements of nature into living spaces with the goal of promoting healing in place.

Trauma informed design as a mechanism for place-based healing

Physical housing for persons who experience socioeconomic and structural marginalisation largely reflects the crisis situations in which they live and does little to promote positive experiences of home. Those who struggle with housing precarity often end up in substandard living conditions marked by poor housing maintenance, overcrowding, pest infestations, environmental toxins and mould, a lack of physical security and safety, and little access to health promoting resources. Hernández (2014: pg. 13) describes the necessity of lower-income households to take up residence in substandard conditions as "affording housing at the expense of health." Consequently, poor conditions contribute to higher rates of injury, health complications, and mental health concerns (Krieger & Higgins, 2002; Novoa et al., 2015). Further, people who are provided with housing support are often offered little choice in the location, layout, and conditions of their own housing. The physical environment is itself in a state of crisis which can further aggravate any trauma residents face. These spaces perpetuate stigma and communicate to residents that their social and economic position makes them somehow unworthy, or undeserving of better living conditions. This kind of negative validation can exacerbate the trauma faced by these individuals and applies a seemingly punitive lens to the design of low-income housing.

Trauma-informed design (TID) places emphasis on the connections between the built environment and place-attachment, the emotive concept of home and identity formation. This approach to design incorporates TIC principles by limiting triggers that lead to distress within the environment. It goes further to create dignified, therapeutic spaces and invests in vulnerable communities as it moves beyond crisis responses to housing and offers choices for how residents interact with and engage in their home environments (Shopworks et al., 2020). TID integrates resident experiences of housing with biophilic design, which is described further below, to create housing options that embody the core principles of trauma-informed care. These spaces communicate to residents that they deserve quality housing, that they do in fact have agency over their lives, and that they are worthy of belonging and joy.

The process of design for TID buildings involves multiple forms of consultation. Architects and social service workers meet with individuals who meet the criteria for residence in the new building (e.g. women in need of housing following IPV, persons experiencing homelessness, etc.). These individuals are asked about safety, comfort, practicalities, daily routines, and triggering areas within housing. They are asked about elements that make them feel comfortable and about their past experiences with housing. This is often done in focus group settings to allow for the co-creation of communal and individual spaces that are not tailored to the needs of one individual, but rather meet the needs of the larger group (Shopworks et al., 2021a; b). Architect then work with the ideas collected during these focus groups to create preliminary housing designs. Preliminary plans are shared back to focus group participants and an iterative process ensues wherein the architect augments plans after each meeting until focus group participants are happy with the plans (Shopworks et al., 2021a; b).

Ideally, the focus group participants are the initial residents of the building; however, this is not always the case. Further, when the TID building offers transitional housing, it must be adaptable to meet the needs of future residents whose individual preferences and experiences are not captured in the pre-design focus groups. This creates a need for highly adaptable and dynamic spaces that allow for personalisation. Shopworks et al., (2020) recommends that TID buildings include a variety of features, such as movable walls to create protective nooks and areas, referred to as nested layers, sound barriers, and light dimmers that allow for individuals to make choices before and throughout their residencies. The managers of the building may also reserve money for furnishings, paint, and decor, among other things, that can be accessed by new residents as they set up their spaces.

Resident experiences

Resident experiences with the physical house and emotive home are central to, and guide, the process of TID. The integration of residents' experiences has multiple objectives. The first goal is to create places where residents feel empowered through their own decision making and respected in their abilities to make choices about their home environments. Bollo & Donofrio (2022) find that when residents exercise choice, such as using dimmer light switches, movable walls, and other flexible elements to construct the potential uses for different areas within their housing units, they feel greater place-attachment. In addition to input on the design of their own units, residents are asked to share their experiences on communal living spaces such as hallways, lobbies, laundry rooms, and elevators.

They discuss potential layouts, uses of common spaces, and identity anchors, such as culturally relevant art, which can be implemented in communal living spaces to further contribute to place-attachment and promote a sense of belonging and safety in physical environments (Bollo & Donofrio, 2022; Shopworks et al., 2020). Place-attachment, a concept used to describe the bonds people have with environments that hold meaning for them, is an important contributor to wellbeing (Lewicka, 2010; Scannell and Gifford, 2010). Strong attachments to place increase feelings of safety in dangerous environments, such as war zones (Billig, 2006) and may promote security for individuals with histories of trauma.

Buildings that are constructed to provide affordable, supported, and transitional housing for people who are housing insecure tend to be neutralising places, follow standardised templates, and can feel highly institutional. TID strives to create intentional spaces that follow the core values of trauma-informed care. The objective herein is to promote community, comfort, and prioritise resident choice (Shopworks et al., 2020). To accomplish this, architects work with residents to understand how they engage with physical spaces and the meanings that these spaces hold. In doing so, they recognise the need for environments to be personalised and reinforce the trauma-informed principle of choice (Bollo & Donofrio, 2022; SAMHSA, 2014; Hopper et al., 2010). Spaces are designed to be flexible to allow them to change and develop as residents' needs vary over time (Bollo & Donofrio, 2022; Shopworks et al., 2020). This further reinforces the objective of creating space for agency in how residents physically and emotionally engage with their homes.

TID aims to avoid retraumatisation and distress which is the primary aim of TIC. However, TID specifically focuses on the influences that physical spaces have on emotions and trauma. To avoid resident retraumatisation, TID architects work to remove or reimagine elements of physical housing that are associated with past trauma. If residents desire them, buildings can include intentionally placed supports to encourage feelings of safety and connection to self and others (Rai et al., 2020; Day, 2017; Shopworks et al., 2020). For example, The Elisabetta House, a TID building designed by Shopworks et al., (2020), has enhanced lighting and social spaces in the laundry room. This was done in response to residents' discussions of the stress produced when they are required to choose between leaving their belongings unattended or staying and feeling isolated in a poorly lit, unprotected space.

TID focuses on residents' descriptions of features of home environments that limit distress and enhance feelings of safety. These features often differ from what one would expect to find in a space that promotes positive feelings of home. For example, safety features, such as controlled entryways and common area cameras may be viewed as intrusive surveillance by untraumatised individuals; however, research finds that these features provide comfort and help establish a sense of home for women who have experienced intimate partner violence (Woodhall-Melnik et al., 2017a). If residents note that these features are important to their feelings of security and safety, architects work with them to incorporate these supports and features into the built environment. In doing so, they respect the communal choices of residents and provide autonomy while simultaneously enhancing feelings of safety and comfort which are factors that promote positive experiences of home.

Biophilic design

In addition to resident experiences, the TID process carefully considers the impacts of nature on human wellbeing. Biophilic design carefully and intentionally incorporates elements found in nature into the design of the built environment (Bollo, Donofrio, 2022). It has been shown to calm psychological and physiological responses associated with trauma and provides restorative benefits to individuals' physical and mental health (Bollo, Donofrio, 2022; Bakir-Demir et al., 2021; Jimenez et al., 2021; Ulrich, 1983). Evidence of diminished fight/flight/freeze responses, and reduced cortisol levels, blood pressure, mental fatigue, aggression, and perceived stress are all associated with exposure to nature (Bakir-Demir et al., 2021; Fry et al., 2020; Gifford, 2007). When designed to incorporate elements of nature, the physical environment can improve cognitive functioning, attention, mood, emotional regulation, social behaviours, creativity, working memory, learning, and psychological well-being (Alaqueel, 2019; Faber Taylor et al., 2002; Gifford, 2007; Wells, 2000). In simple terms, nature helps bodies and minds relax. By incorporating nature into the design of housing, improvements can be made to the capacity for healing and growth in individuals with histories of trauma.

The notion that environments contribute to wellbeing is not new. By using preferred spatial layouts and natural elements within the architectural design of a build, the housing structure itself can become a therapeutic tool and contribute to residents' comfort and positive attachment to home. A myriad of research findings demonstrate a human affinity for environments that offer the ability to prospect threats and resources, and produce opportunities to take refuge for moments of relaxation and safety (Appleton, 1975; Bollo & Donofrio, 2022; Joyce, 2007). Humans are drawn to specific types of spatial layouts, thought to resemble the natural landscapes that early humans evolved in (Kaplan & Kaplan, 1989; Ulrich 1983). These types of spatial layouts promote cognitive stimulation and captivate curiosity (Kaplan & Kaplan, 1989; Kaplan, 1995). When features of the built environment mirror these patterns and types of spatial layouts (e.g. repeated patterns and textures, easily accessible points of reference, curved pathways, open areas with clear visibility, semi-closed nested areas, etc.), individuals are better able to make sense of their physical spaces (Kallai et al., 2007; Kaplan, 1995; McLane & Pable, 2020; Ulrich, 1983).

In addition to patterns in spatial layouts, building designs that include elements found in nature such as plants, natural light, colours, textures, and sound, promote wellbeing and restorative impacts on physical, psychological, and emotional health (Bollo, Donofrio, 2022; Bakir-Demir et al., 2021; Jimenez et al., 2021; Ulrich, 1983). In the well-known study by Ulrich (1983), nature mitigated the impacts of physical pain and recovery time from a physical trauma. Hospitalised patients who see trees out of their windows have less need for pain relief medications and faster recovery times from medical procedures than those who cannot (Ulrich, 1983). In addition to pain relief and improved health outcomes, spaces with more greenery are linked to a stronger sense of safety and community membership and a reduction in aggressive and violent behaviours (Kuo et al., 1998; Kuo & Sullivan, 2001). It is clear that exposure to nature has a significant impact on physiological and psychological functioning of humans. When nature is found within the built environments, it enhances the environment's ability to be restorative and therapeutic. Once again, in simple terms, nature helps us heal.

To summarise, the main premise of TID is to build homes and social service agencies that consider residents' preferences and needs in order to avoid distress triggered by previous traumas in their built environments. It can be argued that nature should be incorporated into these designs when possible to promote healing, support wellbeing, and mitigate the effects of stress. TID represents a marked shift in the way that services and supportive housing respond to traumatised individuals. Rather than offering housing that is highly institutional or in poor repair, which is characteristic of punitive approaches to housing vulnerable populations, housing constructed through TID processes respects people's experiences of trauma with investments in buildings that meet their needs and promote restoration and calm. The combination of biophilic design and respect for people's experiences reduces their need to be on alert, restores attention, reinforces individual worth and promotes agency and dignity. TID transforms housing into an opportunity to move beyond crisis and build a new sense of home.

Creating Jerome's place: TID for youth with histories of trauma and homelessness

Youth is an extremely important period of development and transition that sets the stage for socioeconomic opportunities and outcomes that persist throughout adulthood. This life stage is a challenge to navigate for even the most well-supported youth who thrive within caring and comforting home environments. Persons who experience housing instability and homelessness often face the challenges of youth without access to supportive networks (Gaetz et al., 2018). Further, youth who are unhoused often enter homelessness as a direct result of trauma experienced in homes or custodial care arrangements (Schwan et al., 2018). Research finds that these youth live with the consequences of persistent exposure to Adverse Childhood Experiences (Barnes et al., 2021). They are often survivors of abuse and neglect, come from homes with adults with mental health and substance use concerns, and are more likely to have lived in poverty than their housed counterparts. For these youth, the experience of home is often a negative one, marred with trauma and violence.

In New Brunswick, Canada, there is an urgent need to address the trauma that youth experience prior to and after entry into homelessness. This is quite apparent in the city of Saint John, which has one of highest rates of childhood poverty in Canada (Human Development Council, 2021). Throughout the COVID-19 pandemic lockdowns, youth experienced significant upheaval and local social service providers grasped at straws to provide housing to youth whose significant past trauma made available options impossible to access. Saint John does not have a designated youth shelter and youth under the age of 19 are denied access to rapid rehousing initiatives through the homelessness registry as they are ineligible for provincial rent subsidies.

At the time of the lockdowns, the only programme that provided housing for youth in Saint John required enrollment in school and/or participation in employment which proved insurmountable for many unhoused youth who also grappled with poor mental health from years of unaddressed trauma and housing instability. Three local service providers received funding to pilot a Housing First for Youth program in early 2021. Throughout the two-year pilot, youth achieved housing stability in cohousing and scattered site units. These places provided stability, but the agencies recognised a greater need to explore mechanisms to address trauma from past home experiences that percolated into youth experiences of their established residences. In response, the local service providers began to explore TID.

With mentorship from Shopworks, a Colorado-based leader in TID, the agencies began the process to explore what a TID build would look like for youth in Saint John. They partnered with the Housing, Mobilisation & Engagement Research Lab (HOME-RL) at the University of New Brunswick to develop a research plan that captures the experiences and desires of youth who are housed through the Housing First programme. Through youth engagement in focus groups and youth-led tours of their current housing units, the team will assess the impacts of different elements of housing on youth trauma and wellbeing. Safety and comfort needs of staff who work with youth will also be captured in focus groups. Following the interviews and tours, the team will work with an architect to draft an initial building design. The youth and staff will then gather for a series of interactive and iterative meetings with the architect to refine these designs until consensus is achieved on the design features of the build. Once the building is erected and youth move in, the team will conduct research on their experiences of home, healing, and wellbeing in their new space. This building will be the first TID build in Atlantic Canada to attempt to actively promote healing and foster positive connections with home in youth with histories of homelessness. This research is ongoing, but initial reactions from the youth indicate that this process should provide immense benefit for youth with place-based trauma from past home experiences.

Conclusion

Home can be a site of hell, characterised by abuse, violence, trauma, instability and uncertainty. It can also be a haven where people can go to escape the outside world, relax, restore calm, heal and grow. Home can also be more complicated than presented in this common dichotomy. It can be traumatic in some situations and restorative in others (Mallet, 2004). For those who experience trauma through the home, the emotive concept of home may be suffused with uncertainty or promote feelings of distress linked to past experiences. In more recent years, many social and human service providers have operated as trauma informed; however, the majority of our physical spaces in the built environment are not intentionally designed to reduce triggers of distress and promote healing in persons who have experienced trauma.

TID offers an avenue to explore recovery from trauma through the physical environment of housing. However, this cannot be done in isolation from the emotive concept of home. Whether positive, negative, or hazy, experiences of home are shaped through relationships with physical spaces and their occupants. When the built environment is trauma informed, previous physical stressors and sites of trauma are reimagined in an attempt to limit distress and produce spaces that are restorative, comforting and stable. For individuals, such as the youth in Saint John, New Brunswick, who will live in a TID building, strengthening relationships to their physical environments can provide them with space to heal from trauma, develop and grow.

There is still a lot to learn about TID and its application. To date, TID has been largely employed by architects, social workers, and housing service providers who are focused on design features and wellness outcomes. However, from a theoretical standpoint, as social scientists begin to engage more with TID, discoveries on the emotive concept of home, alongside other related concepts like ontological security, attachment to place, and place-identity will emerge. Questions remain on who TID works best for and in what context. Perhaps more importantly, practitioners must never lose sight of the need to prevent trauma in the first place through stronger social programming and more just systems of wealth redistribution. Nevertheless, TID provides an avenue to empower individuals to think critically about the impact of place on their wellbeing. Further, it moves away from punitive models of housing and recommends the creation of housing as an intentional space for healing in individuals for whom home was not a haven.

References

Alaqueel, D. (2019). *Biophilic Design Contributions to Health and Wellness in Coworking Settings.* Washington DC: University of Oklahoma.

American Psychological Association (2018). *APA Dictionary of Psychology: Trauma.* https://dictionary.apa.org/trauma Accessed: January 14, 2023.

Appleton, J. (1975). *The Experience of Landscape.* New York: Wiley.

Bakir-Demir, T., Berument, S., and Akkaya, S. (2021). Nature connectedness boosts the bright side of emotion regulation, which in turn reduces stress. *Journal of Environmental Psychology,* 76, pp. 1–9.

Banham, R. (2020). Emotion, vulnerability, ontology: Operationalising 'ontological security' for qualitative environmental sociology. *Environmental Sociology,* 6(2), pp. 132–142.

Barnes, A. J., Gower, A. L., Sajady, M., and Lingras, K. A. (2021). Health and adverse childhood experiences among homeless youth. *BMC Pediatrics,* 21(1), pp. 1–10.

Beyerlein, B. A. and Bloch, E. (2014). Need for trauma-informed care within the foster care system. *Child Welfare*, 93(3), pp. 7–22.

Billig, M. (2006). Is my home my castle? Place attachment, risk perception, and religious faith. *Environment and Behavior*, 38(2), pp. 248–265.

Bollo, C. and Donofrio, A. (2022). Trauma-informed design for permanent supportive housing: Four case studies from Seattle and Denver. *Housing and Society*, 49(3), pp. 229–250. doi:10.1080/08882746.2021.1989570

Centre for Disease Control (2023). 6 Guiding Principles to a Trauma Informed Approach. www.cdc.gov/orr/infographics/6_principles_trauma_info.htm. Accessed March 4, 2023.

Crouch, E., Jones, J., Strompolis, M., and Merrick, M. (2020). Examining the association between ACEs, childhood poverty and neglect, and physical and mental health: Data from two state samples. *Children and Youth Services Review*, 116, 105155.

Davies, B. R. and Allen, N. B. (2017). Trauma and homelessness in youth: Psychopathology and intervention. *Clinical Psychology Review*, 54, pp. 17–28.

Day, C. (2017). *Places of the Soul: Architecture and Environmental Design as a Healing Art*. New York, NY: Routledge.

Faber Taylor, A. Kuo, F., and Sullivan, W. C. (2002). Views of nature and self-discipline: Evidence from inner city children. *Journal of Environmental Psychology*, 22(1–2), pp. 49–63. doi:10.1006/jevp.2001.0241

Flockhart, T. (2016). The problem of change in constructivist theory: Ontological security seeking and agent motivation. *Review of International Studies*, 42(5), pp. 799–820. doi:10.1017/S026021051600019X

Flockhart, T. (2020). Is this the end? Resilience, ontological security, and the crisis of the liberal international order. *Contemporary Security Policy*, 41(2), pp. 215–240. doi:10.1080/13523260.2020.1723966

Franke, H. A. (2014). Toxic stress: Effects, prevention and treatment. *Children*, 1(3), pp. 390–402.

Fry, C., Langley, K., and Shelton, K. (2020). Executive functions in homeless young people: Working memory impacts on short-term housing outcomes. *Child Neuropsychology*, 26(1), 27–53.

Gaetz, S., Schwan, K., Redman, M., French, D., and Dej, E. (2018). *Report 3: Early Intervention to Prevent Youth Homelessness*. A. Buchnea (Ed.). Toronto, ON: Canadian Observatory on Homelessness Press.

Giddens, A. (1984). *Elements of the Theory of Structuration*. Routledge.

Giddens, A. (1991). *Modernity and Self-identity: Self and Society in the Late Modern Age*. Stanford University Press.

Gifford, R. (2007). Environmental psychology and sustainable development: Expansion, maturation and challenges. *Journal of Social Issues*, 63(1), pp. 199–212.

Gustafsson, K. and Krickel-Choi, N. C. (2020). Returning to the roots of ontological security: Insights from the existentialist anxiety literature. *European Journal of International Relations*, 26(3), pp. 875–895. doi:10.1177/1354066120927073

Hallett, R. E. and Freas, A. (2018). Community college students' experiences with homelessness and housing insecurity. *Community College Journal of Research and Practice*, 42(10), pp. 724–739.

Hamilton, A. B., Poza, I., and Washington, D. L. (2011). "Homelessness and trauma go hand-in-hand": Pathways to homelessness among women veterans. *Women's Health Issues*, 21(4), pp. S203–S209.

Hernández, D. (2014). Affording housing at the expense of health exploring the housing and neighborhood strategies of poor families. *Journal of Family Issues*, 0192513X14530970.

Hiscock, R. *et al.* (2001). Ontological security and psycho-social benefits from the home: Qualitative evidence on issues of tenure. *Housing, Theory and Society*, 18(1/2), pp. 50–66.

Hopper, E. K., Bassuk, E. L., & Olivet, J. (2010). Shelter from the storm: Trauma-informed care in homelessness services settings. *The Open Health Services and Policy Journal*, 3(1), pp. 80–100.

Human Development Council (2021). New Brunswick's 2021 Child Poverty Report Card. https://campaign2000.ca/wp-content/uploads/2021/11/New-Brunswicks-2021-Child-Poverty-Report-Card.pdf Accessed: December 12, 2022.

Jimenez, M. P., DeVille, N. V., Elliott, E. G., Schiff, J. E., Wilt, G. E., Hart, J. E., and James, P. (2021). Associations between nature exposure and health: A review of the evidence. *International Journal of Environmental Research and Public Health*, 18(9), 4790.

Joyce, Y. (2007). Architectural lessons from environmental psychology: The case of biophilic architecture. *Review of General Psychology*, 11(4), pp. 305–328.

Kallai, J., Makany, T., Csatho, A., Karadi, K., Horvath, D., Kovacs-Labadi, B., Jarai, R., Nadel, L., and Jacobs, J. W. (2007). Cognitive and affective aspects of thigmotaxis strategy in humans. *Behavioral Neuroscience*, 121(1), p. 21.

Kaplan, R. and Kaplan, S. (1989). *The Experience of Nature: A Psychological Perspective.* Cambridge: Cambridge University Press.

Kaplan, S. (1995). The restorative benefits of nature: Toward an integrative framework. *Journal of Environmental Psychology*, 15(3), pp. 169–182. doi:10.1016/0272-4944(95)90001-2

Kay, J. B. (2020). 'Stay the Fuck at Home!': Feminism, Family and the Private Home in a Time of Coronavirus. *Feminist Media Studies*, 20(6), pp. 883–888. doi:10.1080/14680777.2020.1765293

Kearns, A., Hiscock, R., Ellaway, A., & Macintyre, S. (2000). 'Beyond four walls'. The psycho-social benefits of home: Evidence from West Central Scotland. *Housing Studies*, 15(3), pp. 387–410.

Kent, J. and Thompson, S. (2012). Health and the built environment: Exploring foundations for a new interdisciplinary prosfession. *Journal of Environmental and Public Health*, 2012, pp. 1–10.

Kinnvall, C. (2004). Globalization, identity, and the search for chosen traumas. *The Future of Identity: Centennial Reflections on the Legacy of Erik Erikson.* pp. 111–136, edited by Kenneth Hoover Lexington Books: Maryland, US.

Kinnvall, C. (2018). Ontological insecurities and postcolonial imaginaries: The emotional appeal of populism. *Humanity & Society*, 42(4), pp. 523–543.

Krieger, J. and Higgins, D. (2002). Housing and health: Time again for public health action. *National Library of Medicine*, 92(5), pp. 758–768. 10.2105/ajph.92.5.758

Kuo, F. E., Bacaicoa, M., and Sullivan, W. C. (1998). Transforming inner-city landscapes: Trees, sense of safety, and preference. *Environment and Behavior*, 30(1), pp. 28–59.

Kuo, F.E. and Sullivan, W.C. (2001). Environment and crime in the inner city: Does vegetation reduce crime? *Environment and Behavior*, 33(3), pp. 343–367.

Laing, R. (1960). The divided self: An existential study. *Sanity and Madness*. London: Tavistock.

Laing, R. D. (1969). Ontological Security. The Divided Self.

Lanier, P., Maguire-Jack, K., Lombardi, B., Frey, J., and Rose, R. A. (2018). Adverse childhood experiences and child health outcomes: Comparing cumulative risk and latent class approaches. *Maternal and Child Health Journal*, 22, pp. 288–297.

Lewicka, M. (2010). What makes neighborhood different from home and city? Effects of place scale on place attachment. *Journal of Environmental Psychology*, 30(1), pp. 35–51.

Mackelprang, J. L., Klest, B., Najmabadi, S. J., Valley-Gray, S., Gonzalez, E. A., and Cash, R. E. (2014). Betrayal trauma among homeless adults: Associations with revictimization, psychological well-being, and health. *Journal of Interpersonal Violence*, 29(6), pp. 1028–1049.

Mallett, S. (2004). Understanding home: A critical review of the literature. *The Sociological Review*, 52(1), pp. 62–89.

Manzo, L. C. (2003). Beyond house and haven: Toward a revisioning of emotional relationships with places. *Journal of Environmental Psychology*, 23(1), pp. 47–61.

Manzo, L. C. (2005). For better or worse: Exploring multiple dimensions of place meaning. *Journal of Environmental Psychology*, 25(1), pp. 67–86. doi:10.1016/j.jenvp.2005.01.002

McLane, Y. and Pable, J. (2020). Architectural design characteristics, uses, and perceptions of community spaces in permanent supportive housing. *Journal of Interior Design*, 45(1), 33–52. https://doi.org/10.1111/joid.12165

Menzies, P. (2006). Intergenerational trauma and homeless Aboriginal men. *Canadian Review of Social Policy*, 58(1), pp. 1–24.

Mihelicova, M., Brown, M., and Shuman, V. (2018). Trauma-informed care for individuals with serious mental illness: An avenue for community psychology's involvement in community mental health. *American Journal of Community Psychology*, 61(1–2), pp. 141–152.

Moses, D. J., Reed, B. G., Mazelis, R. and D'Ambrosio, B. (2003a). Creating trauma services for women with co-occurring disorders. Washington, DC: Substance Abuse and Mental Health Services Administration, 1(1), pp. 1–49.

Moses, D. J., Reed, B. G., Mazelis, R., and D'Ambrosio, B. (2003b). *Creating trauma services for women with co-occurring disorders: Experiences from the SAMHSA women with alcohol, drug abuse, and mental health disorders who have histories of violence study.* Delmar, NY: Policy Research Associates.

Novoa, A. M., Ward, J., Malmusi, D., Díaz, F., Darnell, M., Trilla, C., ... and Borrell, C. (2015). How substandard dwellings and housing affordability problems are associated with poor health in a vulnerable population during the economic recession of the late 2000s. *International Journal for Equity in Health*, 14(1), pp. 1–11.

Padgett, D. K. (2007). There's no place like (a) home: Ontological security among persons with serious mental illness in the United States. *Social Science & Medicine*, 64(9), pp. 1925–1936. doi:10.1016/j.socscimed.2007.02.011

Rai, S., Asim, F., & Shree, V. (2020). Biophilic Architecture for restoration and therapy within the built environment. *Visions for Sustainability*, 15(5104), 53–79.

Rosenberg, A., Keene, D. E., Schlesinger, P., Groves, A. K., & Blankenship, K. M. (2021). 'I don't know what home feels like anymore': Residential spaces and the absence of ontological security for people returning from incarceration. *Social Science & Medicine*, 272, (113734), pp. 1–8. doi:10.1016/j.socscimed.2021.113734

SAMHSA (2014). *SAMHSA's working concept of trauma and framework for a trauma-informed approach.* Rockville, MD: National Centre for Trauma-Informed Care (NCTIC), SAMHSA.

Scannell, L. and Gifford, R. (2010). Defining place attachment: A tripartite organizing framework. *Journal of Environmental Psychology*, 30(1), pp. 1–10.

Schwan, K., Gaetz, S., French, D., Redman, M., Thistle, J., and Dej, E. (2018). What would it take? Youth across Canada speak out on youth homelessness prevention. Toronto, ON: Canadian Observatory on Homelessness Press.

Shanks, T. R. W. and Robinson, C. (2013). Assets, economic opportunity and toxic stress: A framework for understanding child and educational outcomes. *Economics of Education Review*, 33, pp. 154–170.

Shern, D. L., Blanch, A. K., and Steverman, S. M. (2016). Toxic stress, behavioral health, and the next major era in public health. *American Journal of Orthopsychiatry*, 86(2), p. 109.

Shonkoff, Jack P., Andrew S. Garner, Committee on Psychosocial Aspects of Child and Family Health, Committee on Early Childhood, Adoption, and Dependent Care, and Section on Developmental and Behavioral Pediatrics, Benjamin S. Siegel, Mary I. Dobbins, Marian F. Earls, Andrew S. Garner, Laura McGuinn, John Pascoe, and David L. Wood. (2012) The lifelong effects of early childhood adversity and toxic stress. *Pediatrics*, 129(1), pp. e232–e246.

Shopworks Architecture, Group 14 Engineering, and the University of Denver Centre for Housing and Homelessness Research (2020). Designing for Healing Dignity and Joy. https://shopworks arc.com/wp-content/uploads/2020/06/Designing_Healing_Dignity.pdf

Shopworks Architecture, Group 14 Engineering, and the University of Denver Centre for Housing and Homelessness research (2021a). Implementing a Four Phased Trauma Informed Design Process. https://shopworksarc.com/wp-content/uploads/2021/10/TID-Four-Phase-Process-Man ual.pdf

Shopworks Architecture, Group 14 Engineering, and the University of Denver Centre for Housing and Homelessness research (2021b). Trauma Informed Design Manual: Promoting Physical

Health, Mental Health and Wellbeing through Trauma Informed Design. https://shopworksarc.com/wp-content/uploads/2021/10/TID_Process_10_12_2021.pdf

Ulrich, R. S. (1983) *Aesthetic and Affective Response to Natural Environment*, In: Altman, I., Wohlwill, J.F. (eds) Behavior and the Natural Environment. Human Behavior and Environment, vol 6. Springer, Boston, MA, pp. 85–125. https://doi.org/10.1007/978-1-4613-3539-9_4

Vaquera, E., Aranda, E., and Sousa-Rodriguez, I. (2017). Emotional challenges of undocumented young adults: Ontological security, emotional capital, and well-being. *Social Problems*, 64(2), pp. 298–314.

Wells, N. M. (2000). At home with nature: Effects of 'greenness' on children's cognitive functioning. *Environment & Behavior*, 32(6), pp. 775–795.

Woodhall-Melnik, J. *et al.* (2018). Men's experiences of early life trauma and pathways into long-term homelessness. *Child Abuse & Neglect*, 80, pp. 216–225. doi:10.1016/j.chiabu.2018.03.027

Woodhall-Melnik, J., Hamilton-Wright, S., Daoud, N., Matheson, F.I., Dunn, J.R. and O'Campo, P. (2017a). Establishing stability: Exploring the meaning of 'home' for women who have experienced intimate partner violence. *Journal of Housing and the Built environment*, 32, pp. 253–268.

Woodhall-Melnik, J. *et al.* (2017b). Finding a place to start: Exploring meanings of housing stability in Hamilton's male housing first participants. *Housing, Theory and Society*, 34(3), pp. 359–375.

Zlotnick, C., Tam, T., and Bradley, K. (2007). Impact of adulthood trauma on homeless mothers. *Community Mental Health Journal*, 43, pp. 13–32.

34 Exploring the complex negotiation of home, aging, and mental health

Haven or not?

Rachel Herron

Introduction

Home is a complex and significant place in the lives of older people. It is associated with powerful socio-cultural ideals and emotions. Traditionally, geographers viewed the home in largely positive terms associating the space with feelings of safety, comfort, belonging, calm, and control (Moore, 2000). Over the past 30 years a growing body of critical geography has shown that the home can also be a site of conflict, tension, contradiction, and violence (Blunt and Varley, 2004; Brickell, 2012; Herron et al., 2019). For many older adults, the complexity of the home is shaped by routines and relationships of care (Angus et al., 2005; Wiles, 2003) related to chronic illness – including physical, cognitive, and mental health problems.

Over the past half century, the home has become a more significant site in the treatment and recovery of chronic conditions throughout the life course. In Canada and other countries in the Global North, the process of deinstitutionalisation shifted much of the care offered to people living with mental health problems back into the community and domestic spaces and away from institutional settings because of concerns about the physical, spiritual and emotional harms associated with institutional care (Goffman, 1961; Herron et al., 2021). Parallel processes of healthcare restructuring aimed at reducing government responsibility and cutting costs associated with the provision of care as well as policies directed at aging in place have reinforced the idea that home is the ideal site of care for older people (Milligan, 2009; Wiles et al., 2012). More recently, the COVID-19 pandemic and related public health restrictions and discourses have further emphasised the idea that the home is the safest and best place for older people (Herron et al., 2021).

In this chapter, I explore the home as a complex, contradictory, and continually negotiated place for older people living with mental health problems. First, I briefly highlight the diversity of older adult experiences in relation to mental health problems and the particular mental health stressors that older people face. Drawing on research from health geography and environmental gerontology, I illustrate how the home can be a site of refuge, care, and confinement. Using two examples from a recent study of older people's experiences during COVID-19, I explore how older people living with mental health problems actively negotiate the contradictory nature of the home during a period of public health restrictions that strongly encouraged older people to stay home. In doing so, I show how the meanings, relationships, and resources in the home change and are influenced by what is happening outside the home globally and locally. I argue that the

DOI: 10.4324/9781003345725-38

home is only a haven to the extent that resources and relationships are adequate, accessible, and sustainable.

Mental health and mental health problems across the life course

Older people have diverse experiences of both mental health and aging. Some older people have lived with a diagnosis of a mental health problem for decades (Roger et al., 2021). Other older people may experience mental health problems as a more recent phenomenon. Increasingly, researchers recognise that mental health at any age is influenced by a broad array of stressors in our social and physical environments, including our homes, workplaces, neighbourhoods, regions and countries (WHO, 2022). Some older people have experienced accumulated stressors or disadvantages in relation to their gender, sexuality, race and immigration status, disabilities, and place of residence throughout their life course that undermine their mental health and overall wellbeing (Grenier et al., 2017). Older adults can face additional stressors as they age including caregiver burden, loneliness, isolation, ageism, and stigma that may increase the risk and persistence of mental health problems (Lyons et al., 2018; Penning and Wu, 2016). These stressors point to the need for structural and societal changes to promote the mental health of older people while also highlighting the need to pay attention to a broad range of social and physical environments that shape, and have shaped, older peoples' wellbeing over the life course.

Home as a refuge

The home is often understood as the social and physical environment closest to the person and central to their wellbeing. In the 1970s and 1980s humanistic geographers writing about place attachment identified the home as a haven, refuge or retreat (Moore, 2000). Gerontologists also studied attachment to home as a factor contributing to diverse experiences of aging (Rubinstein, 1989). Research in this area emphasised how older people experience their homes and the meanings they associate with this place (Rowles and Bernard, 2013). Having a home that acts as a haven or refuge may be particularly important for people living with mental health problems who face stigma in their everyday interactions outside the home (Herron and Rosenberg, 2017). Furthermore, older people living with mental health problems may face a double burden of mental and physical disability that makes the home a particularly important site of refuge. In this regard, the physical space of the home is critical as it can enable or hinder the independence, autonomy, and flourishment of older people.

The physical and material qualities of the home influence meanings and relationships within the home. For example, older people may draw on familiar objects in the home to connect with their past, reinforce their sense of who they are in the present, and renegotiate their ability to age in place. The material objects within the home may not always be experienced positively, such as in the case of bereavement, when objects reinforce a sense of loss and instability (Coleman and Wiles, 2020). Being aware of the material and symbolic dimensions of the home can facilitate interventions that are more supportive of the holistic wellbeing of older people.

In thinking about the physical, material, and symbolic features of the home, geographers have increasingly advocated for relational approaches to understanding aging, which recognise that places are connected to other influential sites (Skinner et al., 2015). For example, the meaning of the home is shaped by national aging in place policies that reinforce the idea that the home is a site of independence and autonomy as well as an ideal place to grow old. In addition, connection to the neighbourhood and surrounding resources may contribute to feelings of belonging and being at home, particularly for older people who live alone and lack meaningful social connections (Wiles et al., 2012). Thus, the meaning of home is never just a product of what happens within the isolated walls of the home.

Geographers and gerontologists have been increasingly interested in adjacent outdoor or green spaces and their value to older people. In a recent New Zealand study, Wiles and colleagues (2021) draw on the concept of enabling places (Duff, 2011) to explore the social, affective, symbolic, and material resources these spaces offer Maori and non-Maori older people. They explain that home gardens are enabling in that they can reinforce older peoples' sense of identity as resourceful, hardworking, skillful, contributors. Sharing knowledge and produce from their gardens can strengthen older peoples' social resources, while offering pleasure, an opportunity to reflect on the past, and a source of food. Older adults may also accept help from others to maintain their gardens, demonstrating adaptation and role negotiation while also maintaining attachment to this important part of their home and lifelong identity. This work highlights the many resources and relationships associated with spaces of the home and it challenges perceptions of older people as dependent care recipients.

Home as a site of care

Home is a site where older people enact various types of care, including care for self, care for others, and care for place. Care for self and care for place may be mutually supportive and essential to maintaining one's health. For example, older people may perform home maintenance tasks that contribute to the cleanliness and integrity of the home as well as their individual health and wellbeing. They may also provide informal and emotional support to family, friends, neighbours, and community members from their home or they may write letters to advocate for things that matter to them. Wiles and Jayasinha (2013) call this work 'care for place' and they challenge assumptions that older people are not actively involved in contributing to their communities. Care work for and from the home may reinforce older people's affirmative sense of place within their home and community.

Relationships and processes of care can also challenge affirmative feelings associated with the home. Mobility limitations, reduced capacity to perform self-care, and increasing medical needs may require older people to bring help into the home so that they can continue to age in place. Research has examined how home care practices, intended to support people to age in place, can undermine meanings and experiences of home (Angus et al., 2005, Wiles, 2003). For example, logics of cleanliness and order associated with home care may challenge long-established routines as well as meanings of the home. Mobility devices and technologies of care can also reorder the home and change how people feel within the space. Finally, relationships and power dynamics between members of the household may change as an older person becomes more reliant on a spouse or other family member for care. Whether home is a therapeutic place or site of loss and confinement depends on the nature of relationships and availability of resources inside and outside the home.

Home as confinement?

Rowles (1978) humanistic study of older people's relationships with place was a seminal exploration of the extent to which older people are confined or "imprisoned" in their homes as they age. His rich description of five older people's lifeworlds in New England revealed that these older people experienced some spatial constriction, but they also adapted their routines and practices to continue to remain engaged with the broader world, using the phone, writing letters, making new friends, watching TV, reading, and becoming more aware of features of the physical environment that may pose a risk to their wellbeing. Older people's adaptation and connection to a wider world is contingent on a wide variety of resources and strategies. Because of this contingency, geographers from different epistemological backgrounds, remain interested in the home as a space of confinement or, more aptly, lack of choice.

Indeed, feminist perspectives on the home have done much to enrich our understanding of the contradictory and often political nature of the home as a site where rights and responsibilities are continually negotiated (England, 2010). There is a large interdisciplinary body of research showing that women are often carers of choice but not carers by choice within the home; while low-paid, non-unionised, racialised workers provide the bulk of paid care in the home (Armstrong et al, 2008). Both paid and unpaid women providing care in the home are subject to violence in the provision of care in the home and may lack the ability to escape the role of carer because of societal expectations and lack of alternative resources in terms of work and care provision (Herron et al., 2019). In this respect, home remains a site of hidden injustices.

Disability scholars have also revealed the ways in which ablest home designs limit or challenge the choices and actions of impaired bodies (Imrie, 2004) as well as ableist conceptions of care. Often older people receiving care are repeatedly acted on rather than being respected as actors in their own care. Particularly in the context of the COVID-19 pandemic, researchers called attention to how ageism and ableism contributed to the confinement of older people, specifically those living with dementia, to care homes without rights to participate in basic activities that support human flourishing (Kontos et al., 2021). Importantly, feminist and disability scholarship remind researchers and the public that aging at home is political for both care providers and older people who receive care.

Home during COVID-19

Older people living with mental health problems navigate the complex politics, relationships, resources, and feelings associated with the home. The section below presents two examples of this complex negotiation in the midst of the COVID-19 pandemic in Manitoba, Canada. These examples were developed from a series of telephone interviews that took place with each of the older people in June 2020, July 2020, and April 2021. During this time, social gatherings outside individual households were restricted or discouraged and there was particular emphasis in the public discourse on the vulnerability of older people. Quotations from the interviews are used in the narratives below but the participants names have been replaced with pseudonyms.

Evelyn's story

Evelyn is a 71-year-old woman of mixed European heritage who lives in a small private dwelling in a rural community with her husband and her cat. She took some college courses, but she did not work outside the home for much of her life. She describes herself as a "domestic engineer… I'm the manager, I am the CEO of this house." As she jokes about her work life, she reveals a strong relationship between her home and her identity. She is now a caregiver to her 81-year-old husband who lives with dementia.

Home was not always a safe and comfortable place for Evelyn. She said, "I was born and raised in an alcoholic home, where there was a lot of violence and married young, and had children, and got divorced… and then I turned around and got married to another, to an alcoholic and that was highly abusive." Throughout Evelyn's life, relationships in the home had a profound impact on her wellbeing. However, she had only recently spoke to her family doctor about depression. Evelyn went to the doctor before our first interview for help. She explained,

> "…we [she and her husband] are together here, with no intimacy, there hasn't been for quite a while. And no anything. I just felt very much alone with him as his caregiver. I was actually feeling very resentful. Because I'm just here to cook and wash and be your caregiver? Like, [SCOFFS] Yeah. And I'm getting nothing in return to fill my cup, to fill my needs. So I ended up going to the doctor and, um, we did this little test that he gave me, and he says I am borderline anxiety and depression. Yeah, I believe you [she said to the doctor]. So he put me on medication…"

Evelyn explained that prior to public health restrictions, she had developed strategies and social resources outside the home to fulfill her needs and support good mental health such as going to community coffee groups, church, and other social clubs. These community resources influenced her wellbeing and compensated for a lack of social connection at home. She felt better at home because of resources outside the home in her community.

Although she lacked important social resources that influenced how she felt at home, Evelyn developed strategies to maintain social connection through sending out emails and cards to friends. She explained,

> "I do send out, I have a list of names and I send out a lot of emails to people with, uh, I find little inspirational things or, or jokes. I like jokes mostly. Or, uh, pictures, and things, you know. And that way, I keep in contact with my friends by sending them emails. And most of them respond, saying 'thank you' and you know, and send me something too."

In addition to Evelyn's strategies above, the research team also referred Evelyn to a telephone program run out of a social service organisation in a larger city in the province. This programme put her in touch with other older people to talk with from her home. When we spoke to her a second time, she explained that the telephone program helped her to gain some perspective. She said,

> "I began to realize how fortunate I was to live in a rural community… They [people in the city] seem to be more confined, where I have more freedom to walk if I want. I've got a yard to work in, and a lot of these people are literally confined to their apartment or very dependent on other people."

Evelyn made use of physical and material resources of the home to promote her wellbeing. She explained, "we are in a small home in a private dwelling. The same square footage as an apartment would be. But it's a home, and we have our privacy and we have our yard, and I have a little garden space and flowers, and there is a front deck to settle on." In warmer weather, Evelyn was able to wave and socialise with people walking by from her deck and she found purpose and meaning in outdoor work. She also found ways to spend time with her husband and recognise his abilities. She said,

> "Now that the weather is nice, I have been able to do some painting and things, you know, maintaining the steps. I was given a wooden lawn chair for Mothers' Day so I painted that yesterday. And I planted some flowers. And I put a few garden seeds in. I cleaned the yard. My husband, well he was able to help me there because I could clean it up and then we could go together to dump it at the compost."

When we talked to Evelyn a year later, she had some health problems that constrained her mobility, and she also did not feel as safe walking around her house in the winter. The value and meaning of different features of her home changed with the seasons.

Helen's story

Helen is a 73-year-old woman who was born in England and immigrated to Canada 35 years ago. She lives alone in a small apartment; she has one daughter who lives nearby but she has few visitors. She has poor eyesight and uses a walker to get around which limits her mobility. Helen receives home care to give her medications and to put her socks on in the morning and take them off at night. She says, "I appreciate them coming, that is the only contact I have with anybody right now." She described herself saying "Oh, I- I'm very bored… It's, uh, it's just very lonely and [PAUSE] um, and I get I get tired of watching TV."

For Helen, home is a site to be creative and attempt new things; however, in her state of loneliness and depression she is primed for negative reactions. She said, "I've been making suppers and I try and make a different meal every time. But … . I got the impression that she [daughter] didn't like what I cooked." Her daughter visits once a week, but she does not think she will keep visiting. She also has a mental health worker, but she worries she will not return her calls. She feels others in her building do not like her and do not want to talk with her. Overall, she lacks trusting relationships.

Like Evelyn, Helen longs to get out of the house to be with others. She hopes to take a trip on her scooter to a local coffee shop when the weather is nice. Helen's sense of hope and wellbeing is not simply associated with the building in which she lives; it is also tied to other meaningful places in the surrounding community.

Being unable or discouraged from visiting other places, Helen turned to caring for her home and precious objects to find purpose. She explained that she started a project naming her boxes of photographs. She said, that when she started thinking " 'Okay what am I going to do today? I got nothing to do.' Instead of getting down on myself, I go and pick up one of the albums and start looking through them." She has been cleaning and sorting through things in her storage area. In addition, she found a compact exercise machine she could sit and peddle on. She exclaimed, "I'm doing everything I can that I can think of" to promote her wellbeing at home.

When we spoke to her a year later, she had developed an additional strategy for meeting one of her affective needs during this period of isolation. She explained, "Actually bought myself, um, it's what they call a therapy doll. I bought a doll and I said she- I- I hug her lots of times 'cause that really brings me back up from being down." She said she came up with this idea herself and ordered the doll online. She was proud yet cautious about her resourcefulness. She said, "I'm afraid if I should tell somebody I bought a doll because they're gonna think I'm nuts." Helen is aware that people may judge her for her use of a doll, but she knows this object helps here to feel better and meet her affective needs.

One of Helen's greatest desires is to help others. She volunteers to do income tax returns for other older people in her community but she is still waiting for another community member to bring them to her home. She said, "I feel so useless [voice breaking a bit]… I don't know if I'll get any or not." Although Helen does not trust others and shares negative views of her situation, she continues to make concerted efforts to meet her social and emotional needs during a year of relative isolation at home demonstrating her ability to adapt and maximise resources that are available to exert agency over her situation.

Evelyn and Helen share the important relationships, resources, contingencies, and limitations of the home in supporting good mental health and wellbeing in times of isolation. Although they have different living situations, both women clearly rely on community spaces to address a lack of social connection at home. Their stories highlight a critical limitation of the home as a haven ideal – home can be a very lonely place without meaningful relationships. This can be further complicated by severe loneliness and depression which can make people less trusting and open to others when they experience social contact (Van Winkel et al., 2017). Being an older carer to a spouse at home can also challenge the idea of home as a haven and a site of care. Carers may feel they are no longer being cared for at home when their spouse is no longer able to participate in routines and rituals of reciprocity associated with a mutually supportive intimate relationship.

Despite these limitations, older people living with mental health problems during COVID restrictions sought out meaningful activities at home, they made use of a wide variety of material objects in their homes as well as communications technology to either keep busy on their own or connect with others. Evelyn's story illustrates the importance of outdoor home spaces for reinforcing sense of autonomy, connection with others, purpose and resourcefulness consistent with Wiles and colleagues (2021) recent work. Helen's story shows that material resources can be used to meet human and affective needs supporting more than human and non-representational approaches to aging, home, and mental health (Andrews et al., 2014). Both women also found there was a seasonality or temporality to the value and usefulness of different strategies. For example, Helen became less mobile and cleaning was no longer a purposeful and enjoyable activity and Evelyn found the outdoors spaces of her home were only safe in the warmer months. Despite the temporalities and contingencies of the home, both women demonstrated considerable agency and adaptation in navigating the relationships and resources they needed to improve their feelings and mental states at home.

That the older women living with mental health problems in the stories above were able to negotiate various resources and strategies to support their mental health and wellbeing at home, does not mean that they do not require further resources and strategies outside the home. Their depression and loneliness were worsened by a lack of care and social resources. The home was not always a haven; it was also a site of struggle for adequate, accessible, and sustainable resources to support wellbeing.

Conclusion

There are many new directions that could emerge in studying home, aging, and mental health, building on understandings of the home as a place rich with meaning, constantly being negotiated, and connected to other places beyond the home. Future research should explore the stories of older men, racialised and/or Indigenous older people, older people who identify as lesbian, gay, bisexual, transgender, intersex or queer (LGBTIQ), older people without a home, and older people with other mental health problems (e.g., schizophrenia and bi-polar). There is much diversity in aging, home, and mental health that has yet to be explored. Understanding this diversity will require additional conceptual and methodological approaches such as non-representational theory and visual methodologies that will enrich how researchers and the general public see older people, mental health problems, and the home. The home is not just how we talk about it; how we see and feel it also matters when understanding mental health. Finally, research must continue to critically examine the political discourses of the home as an ideal site of care for aging and mental health to identify gaps in resources and advocate for change.

References

Andrews, G. J., Chen, S., Myers, S. (2014). The 'taking place' of health and wellbeing: Towards non-representational theory. *Social Science & Medicine* (1982), 108, 210–222.https://doi.org/10.1016/j.socscimed.2014.02.037

Angus, J., Kontos, P., Dyck, I., McKeever, P., Poland, B. (2005). The personal significance of home: Habitus and the experience of receiving long-term home care. *Sociology of Health & Illness*, 27(2), 161–187. https://doi.org/10.1111/j.1467-9566.2005.00438.x

Armstrong, P., Armstrong, H., Scott-Dixon, K. (2008). *Critical to care: The invisible women in health services*. University of Toronto Press.

Blunt, A., Varley, A. (2004). Geographies of home. *Cultural Geographies*, 11(1), 3–6. https://doi.org/10.1191/1474474004eu289xx

Brickell, K. (2012). 'Mapping' and 'doing' critical geographies of home. *Progress in Human Geography*, 36(2), 225–244. https://doi.org/10.1177/0309132511418708

Coleman, T., Wiles, J. (2020). Being with objects of meaning: Cherished possessions and opportunities to maintain aging in place. *The Gerontologist*, 60(1), 41–49. https://doi.org/10.1093/geront/gny142

Duff, C. (2011). Networks, resources and agencies: On the character and production of enabling places. *Health & Place*, 17(1), 149–156. https://doi.org/10.1016/j.healthplace.2010.09.012

England, K. (2010). Home, work and the shifting geographies of care. *Ethics, Place and Environment*, 13(2), 131–150.

Goffman, E. (1961). *Asylums: Essays on the social situation of mental patients and other inmates*. AldineTransaction.

Grenier, A., Phillipson, C., Rudman, D. L., Hatzifilalithis, S., Kobayashi, K., Marier, P. (2017). Precarity in late life: Understanding new forms of risk and insecurity. *Journal of Aging Studies*, 43, 9–14.

Herron, R., Kelly, C., Aubrecht, K. (2021). A conversation about ageism: Time to deinstitutionalize long-term care? [Special issue] *University of Toronto Quarterly*, 9(2), 183–206. https://doi.org/10.3138/utq.90.2.09

Herron, R. V., Funk, L. M., Spencer, D. (2019). Responding the "wrong way": The emotion work of caring for a family member with dementia. *The Gerontologist*, 59(5), e470–e478. https://doi.org/10.1093/geront/gnz047

Herron, R., Kelly, C., Aubrecht, K., (2021). A conversation about ageism: Time to deinstitutionalize long-term care? [Special issue] *University of Toronto Quarterly*, 9 (2), 183–206. https://doi.org/10.3138/utq.90.2.09

Herron, R. V., Newall, N. E. G., Lawrence, B. C., Ramsey, D., Waddell, C. M., Dauphinais, J. (2021). Conversations in times of isolation: Exploring rural-dwelling older adults' experiences of isolation and loneliness during the COVID-19 pandemic in Manitoba, Canada. *International Journal of Environmental Research and Public Health*, 18(6), 3028. http://dx.doi.org/10.3390/ijerph18063028

Herron, R. V., Rosenberg, M. W. (2017). "Not there yet": Examining community support from the perspective of people with dementia and their partners in care. *Social Science & Medicine* (1982), 173, 81–87. https://doi.org/10.1016/j.socscimed.2016.11.041

Imrie, R. H. (2004). Disability, embodiment and the meaning of the home. *Housing Studies*, 19(5), 745–763. https://doi.org/10.1080/0267303042000249189

Kontos, P., Radnofsky, M. L., Fehr, P., Belleville, M. R., Bottenberg, F., Fridley, M., ... Whitehouse, P. (2021). Separate and unequal: A time to reimagine dementia. *Journal of Alzheimer's Disease*, 80(4), 1395–1399.

Lyons, A., Alba, B., Heywood, W., Fileborn, B., Minichiello, V., Barrett, C., Hinchliff, S., Malta, S., Dow, B. (2018). Experiences of ageism and the mental health of older adults. *Aging & Mental Health*, 22(11), 1456–1464. https://doi.org/10.1080/13607863.2017.1364347

Milligan, C. (2009). *There's no place like home: Place and care in an ageing society*. Ashgate Publishing.

Moore, J. (2000). Placing home in context. *Journal of Environmental Psychology*, 20(3), 207–218.

Penning, M. J., Wu, Z. (2016). Caregiver stress and mental health: Impact of caregiving relationship and gender. *The Gerontologist*, 56(6), 1102–1113.

Roger, K., Herron, R., Ahmadu, M., Allan, J., Waddell, C. (2021). Exploring ageing and time as resources in men's mental health experiences. *Ageing and Society*, 42(12), 1–15. http://doi:10.1017/S0144686X21000362

Rowles, G. (1978). *Prisoners of space? Exploring the geographical experiences of older people*. Westview Press.

Rowles, G. D., Bernard, M. (2013). The meaning and significance of place in old age. In G. D. Rowles & M. Bernard (Eds.), *Environmental gerontology: Making meaningful places in old age* (pp. 3–24). Springer Publishing Company.

Rubinstein, R. (1989). The home environments of older people: A description of psychosocial processes in linking person to place. *Journal of Gerontology*, 44, 45–53.

Skinner, M. W., Cloutier, D., Andrews, G. J. (2015). Geographies of ageing: Progress and possibilities after two decades of change. *Progress in Human Geography*, 39(6), 776–799.

van Winkel, M., Wichers, M., Collip, D., Jacobs, N., Derom, C., Thiery, E., Myin-Germeys, I., Peeters, F. (2017). Unraveling the role of loneliness in depression: The relationship between daily life experience and behavior. *Psychiatry*, 80(2), 104–117. https://doi.org/10.1080/00332747.2016.1256143

Wiles, J. (2003). Daily geographies of caregivers: Mobility, routine, scale. *Social Science & Medicine* (1982), 57(7), 1307–1325. https://doi.org/10.1016/S0277-9536(02)00508-7

Wiles, J., Leibing, A., Guberman, N., Reeve, J., Allen, R. E. (2012). The meaning of Aging in Place to older people. *The Gerontologist*, 52(3), 357–366. https://doi.org/10.1093/geront/gnr098

Wiles, J., Miskelly, P., Stewart, O., Rolleston, A., Gott, M., Kerse, N. (2021). Gardens as resources in advanced age in Aotearoa NZ: More than therapeutic. *Social Science & Medicine* (1982), 288, 113232. https://doi.org/10.1016/j.socscimed.2020.113232

Wiles, L. R., Jayasinha, R. (2013. Care for place: The contributions older people make to their communities. *Journal of Aging Studies*, 27(2), 93–101. https://doi.org/10.1016/j.jaging.2012.12.001

World Health Organization. (2022) *World mental health report: Transforming mental health for all*. World Health Organization.

35 Breadwinning, mental health and the geographies of masculinity

Robert Wilton and Ann Fudge Schormans

Introduction

As Laws (2011) notes, there is a long-standing fascination in the West with the therapeutic potential of work for people experiencing mental health difficulties. In recent decades, this fascination has been principally embodied in the professional field of vocational rehabilitation, where participation in employment is understood to be both a contributor to, and a key indicator of, mental health recovery (see Drake and Wallach 2020). In this sense, the meaning and experience of mental ill health is shaped in important ways by whether one is 'well enough to work' (Evans and Wilton 2019).

At the same time, socialist feminist scholarship has effectively demonstrated that the organisation and experience of paid work employment is profoundly gendered. Gender relations and identities are defined, in part, through the types of paid and unpaid work that people do and the sites in which this work is performed (i.e., within or beyond the home). The ideology of male breadwinning also remains key to the reproduction of a culturally valued or 'hegemonic' masculinity in many countries (Gonalons-Pons and Gangl 2021). By contrast, the absence of stable employment, and exclusion from workplaces, can force a rethinking of what it means to be a 'man' (Nayak 2006; Myers and Demantas 2016).

In this chapter, we are interested in how mental ill health and gender intersect in people's relationships to spaces of paid work. Our objectives are twofold. First, we want to critically examine the emphasis of psychiatric rehabilitation on job holding as a key marker of success for people living with, and recovering from, mental ill health. Second, we consider the gendered nature of these vocational priorities. Drawing on recent research, we consider how masculine norms of 'breadwinning' shapes men's experience of mental ill health and recovery in the absence of paid work.

Psychiatric rehabilitation and paid work

We begin with a statement from Corrigan and Mueser's (2016) *Principles and Practices of Psychiatric Rehabilitation* on the significance of paid work:

> As it does for most people, work serves many goals for those with psychiatric disabilities... It provides structure to the day, a place to be, and tasks to do, which can often help people manage psychiatric symptoms. Work may also augment a person's social support system; coworkers may evolve into friends or intimate

DOI: 10.4324/9781003345725-39

partners. Certainly, work is the foundation for a living wage and health benefits. And it is often an important part of one's identity: Social exchanges often begin with 'What do you do for a living?' (p.19).

This statement tells us a great deal about the importance accorded to employment and people's presence in workplaces for the field of psychiatric rehabilitation. For Corrigan and Mueser, and many other authors in the field, engagement in employment is a core pillar of successful rehabilitation (see also Evans and Wilton 2019; Drake and Wallach 2020; Krupa et al. 2020). Defining the field of psychiatric rehabilitation, Rutman (1993, p.1) states that it is about 'giving people with psychiatric disabilities *the opportunity to work*, live in the community, and enjoy a social life, at their own place, through planned experiences in a respectful, supportive and realistic atmosphere'. Rössler (2006), in an overview of the field, states that employment is understood to be health promoting, with links between work and health 'known for centuries' (also Modini et al. 2016; Krupa et al. 2020).

As Corrigan and Mueser note, employment is understood to provide structure, meaning, social connection, adequate income, and a core pillar of identity. Moreover, these and other authors cite evidence indicating that a majority of people living with mental ill health want to work (also Dunn et al. 2008; Vukadin et al. 2021). Given the benefits that supposedly accrue from paid work, it is not surprising that a majority of people might desire this outcome.

However, a more critical reading raises several concerns with the relationship between paid work and psychiatric rehabilitation. One issue is the extent to which people living with mental ill health can find and retain paid work in practice. The enthusiasm for vocational rehabilitation stems, in part, from the demonstrated success of supported employment programmes, in which people are provided with assistance to train and search for work, as well as follow-along supports to assist workers and employers over time. Yet the vast majority of those living with mental ill health do not have access to these intensive supports. Figures from the mid-1990s in the US suggested that only 2 percent of mental health consumers were receiving supported employment services (see Bond et al. 1999). Almost two decades later, Corrigan and Mueser note that vocational rehabilitation and supported employment remain grossly underfunded, and even when people do have access to supported employment programming, only around a third become 'steady workers' (Corrigan and Mueser 2016, p.201).

Beyond supported employment programmes, the reality is that people's efforts to find and engage in paid work often do *not* take place in the context of what Rutman (1993, p.1) specifies as 'supportive and realistic atmospheres'. Although disability rights legislation in countries like the US and Canada requires reasonable accommodations for workers with disabilities, including those with mental health disabilities, many employers remain resistant to greater flexibility with respect to 'where, when, and how work can be performed' (Molyneux 2023, p.2).

The resistance highlighted by Molyneux connects to a larger structural characteristic of the capitalist economy; namely, that the labour process and workplaces that make up the economy continue to be organised on the basis of able-bodied and able-minded norms. Looking back at Foucault's (2006) classic work on madness and society, it is the 'failure' to successfully embody these norms that informs the social meanings assigned to mental illness in the context of industrialisation. While contemporary service-dominated economies differ markedly from the industrial economies of the nineteenth century, studies highlight how able-bodied/minded norms continue to inform contemporary organisational understandings of the 'ideal worker' and the 'normal workplace' (Wilton 2004; Jammaers and Zanoni 2021). In this context, employment success – and the logic of vocational rehabilitation – hinges to a significant degree on the extent to which people living with and recovering from mental ill health can be trained and supported to approximate the able-bodied/minded norms desired by employers. For some people, this approximation may be possible but for many others this may be not only difficult, but also unhealthy. It is for this reason that Patricia Deegan, a key voice in the mental health recovery movement, cautioned that vocational programs based on:

> [T]raditional values of competition, individual achievement, independence, and self- sufficiency are oppressive. Programs that are tacitly built on these values are invitations to failure for many recovering persons (1988, p.17).

Other have argued against a disproportionate focus on employment, calling for greater focus on 'opportunities for activity and participation that have personal and social meaning' beyond paid work (see Krupa et al. 2020, p.956). Yet neo-liberalisation has in many ways amplified the extent to which ableist values of competition, individual achievement, independence, and self-sufficiency underlie and inform health and welfare services specifically, and the social field more broadly. For people living with mental ill health, negotiating a life in the absence of paid work remains difficult culturally given the importance accorded to work in relation to identity (Doroud et al. 2015). It is also more difficult materially, as the restructuring of income support programs has increasingly impoverished those without work (Lowe and Deverteuil 2020).

Breadwinning and masculinity

We now want to consider how the relationship between mental ill health and paid work is gendered, and what this means for experiences of recovery and rehabilitation. More specifically, we explore the intersection between employment outside the home as a marker of 'normalcy' with respect to psychiatric rehabilitation, and breadwinning as part of a culturally valued masculinity.

Socialist feminism has shown that the division of labour – the way in which different forms of paid and unpaid work are allocated to particular groups and places – is a key process underlying the gendering of social life and identities (McDowell 1999; Connell 2005). With industrialisation, the coding of production as a masculine sphere and men's disproportionate access to spaces of paid work outside the home was a critical source of male privilege and gender inequality. The division of labour facilitated what Connell (2005) called a gendered logic of accumulation, through which men accrued economic gains at the expense of women (also Crompton 2006). At the same time, access to paid work and the breadwinning role were critical to normative performances of masculinity and to men's identities (Zuo 2004; Crompton 2006).

In recent decades, a combination of economic restructuring and women's entry into the labour force have weakened the gender division between paid and unpaid labour. This has had a range of implications for men. In the labour force, post-industrial economies have produced a new gender order, in which 'increasing numbers of men are employed in the peripheral labour market… on terms and conditions that traditionally were regarded as female' (McDowell 1991, p.408). At the household level, far fewer men now earn a family wage (Bloome et al. 2019). An increasing reliance on multiple earners has, to some extent, eroded the material basis of male privilege, although some men resist the redistribution of unpaid work in the home despite the decline in their economic power (e.g., Gerson 2009).

While economic conditions have changed, breadwinning remains part of a valued masculine identity (Zuo 2004; Gerson 2009; Thébaud 2010; Damaske 2020), although the strength of the male-breadwinner norm varies culturally and geographically (Gonalons-Pons and Gangl 2021). This can create problems with respect to the 'doing' of gender for men who confront joblessness. For example, studies have looked at the experiences of young working-class men who do not have access to the industrial jobs and workplaces of their fathers and earlier generations (Connell 2005; McDowell 2011; Damaske 2020). As Connell (2005, pp.93–94) observes:

> Large numbers of youth are now growing up without any expectation of the stable employment around which familiar models of working class masculinity were organized... In such conditions, what happens to the making of masculinity?

While the specific labour market experiences of men living with mental ill health may be distinct from the young men described by Connell, the broader question about the *making of masculinity* in the absence of stable employment is directly relevant to a discussion of the role of paid work in psychiatric rehabilitation/recovery. Taking up this question allows us to consider how gendered expectations about paid work and the 'breadwinning' norm intersect with and mediate experiences of mental ill health and recovery.

To explore this intersection, we draw on data from a recent arts-informed, qualitative research project with men living with mental ill health. In this project eighteen men participated in one to two semi-structured interviews focused on experiences of mental ill health, contacts with treatment systems, recovery journeys, as well as their views on gender norms and the ways in which their everyday lives reflected particular notions of masculinity. Subsequently, participants were invited to attend one of three visual arts workshops organised in collaboration with a local artist/arts facilitator, who is herself a mental health service user. Fourteen men agreed and they were asked to create a picture 'that shows what it means to be a man based on your experience'. After the art was completed, we invited the men to talk about its meaning with the group, which produced valuable discussion about shared feelings and experiences. Interviews and groups sessions were recorded and transcribed for analysis.[1]

Making masculinity in the absence of paid work

While the topics covered in the project were diverse, employment and breadwinning figured centrally in many interviews and in some artwork. Many of the participants commented on the fact that more women were working in the contemporary economy, and this was seen, for the most part, as a positive development. As Alan[2] commented:

> Nowadays, they split it [work] both ways cause women want to be, like... you know, women want to have their rights and everything. I don't mind, you know. It's cool.

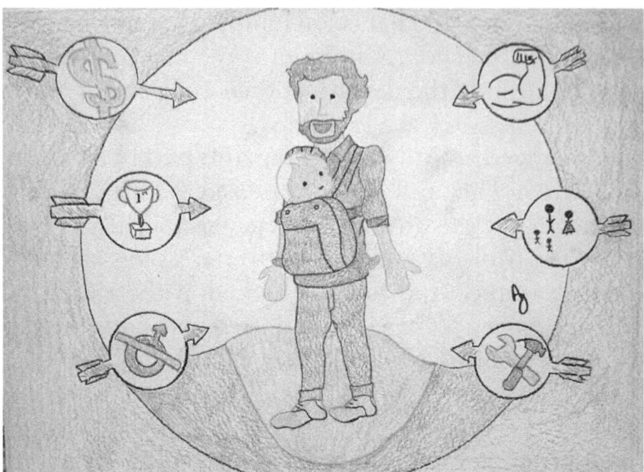

Figure 35.1 Stewart's artwork: 'Being me despite the distractions'.

At the same time, there was a strong sense that breadwinning and employment outside the home remained important to contemporary conceptions of successful masculinity. George, for example, commented: 'to be a man in society today, you'll have to have a job, a good job. You'll have to have a lot of money'. The yellow dollar sign in the top left corner of Stewart's artwork (Figure 35.1) signifies the way in which cultural expectations about wage earning press in on him in the context of family life.

Asked about the meaning of his artwork, Stewart explained that the pressure to be a breadwinner, as well as other normative gender expectations, impacted his sense of self-identity:

> I'm happiest when I'm at home with my kids, and just that kind of life. So that's my happy place, but then constantly there's these arrows that are flying at me to make sure that I'm the breadwinner, making sure I'm bringing in enough money to support my family because society has told us that guys are supposed to be the breadwinner, where it's not necessarily true anymore but it's just constantly, 'you need to bring in more money'.

It is significant that Stewart views the space of the home and relations with his children as constituting his 'happy place'. This speaks to the ways in which masculinity might be done differently in the context of mental health recovery, a point to which we return below.

While participants understood breadwinning and workplace participation as markers of normative masculinity, most had struggled to find and keep employment. Only one of the 18 participants was in full-time employment at the time of the interviews and one other was employed part-time. Fourteen participants reported disability support as their primary income, and two others were receiving general welfare assistance.

For many, their experience had been characterised by tenuous connections to the labour force, shaped by impacts of mental ill health and the difficulties of securing meaningful workplace accommodations. George, for example, talked about the difficulties he faced in handling the stresses of competitive employment:

> I've had jobs. I've had paid jobs, but none of them went well. They were all too stressful for me... I worked at [cable company] as a telephone technical support. That was a good job, it was almost full-time. At the beginning, I thought I knew what I was doing, but by the end, I had no clue... I had no personal experience with the equipment and the service, so I just fell behind. I began to dread going in there.

James, who was in his mid-twenties, had worked for a while collecting shopping carts at a grocery store. While he described it as an easy job, his anxiety made it difficult to sustain:

> I was just so anxious all the time and I couldn't (.) like when I get anxious, this is a big problem for me, when I get really anxious it makes me have the urge to use the washroom, so I'd be using the washroom like ten times a shift and that's not okay.

Often participants quit or were fired from employment rather than seeking accommodations at work. In part, this was linked to a reluctance to disclose mental illness to employers, as well as uncertainty about how to seek help. Mason had left a job at an auto-assembly plant when his anxiety worsened because 'I felt like no one, there was no on there to listen to me about it, you know, there was no outlet for help'.

Difficulties finding and keeping employment have immediate implications for the making of masculinity in the context of mental health recovery. On the one hand, participants recognised that problems in the labour market made it difficult to draw on the breadwinning norm as a basis for identity. On the other hand, participants were engaged in efforts to craft a valued sense of self in the absence of employment. One strategy used by some participants was an active rejection of paid work, something that they linked to better mental health. For example, George had left the labour market in his mid-fifties and believed that this decision had significantly reduced his anxiety levels.

> [Int: Did you make a conscious decision to stop looking for work?] Yeah, I decided that 'I'm retiring now' (chuckles) … When I left I was freed up to, you know, my time is my own. I decided I like that better and decided I was not going to look for work anymore.

After leaving the auto-assembly plant Mason had decided to stop looking for employment and was exploring opportunities for volunteer work as an alternative. Likewise, Gerald had decided to leave the labour market after several years of working as a teacher and in cosmetics. While he was upset at leaving employment, he acknowledged that 'I couldn't do it and it was all because of my anxiety and stress and just the terrible [work] environments that I was in.' Reflecting on his departure, Gerald said: 'having the luxury to do that helped my mental health tremendously.'

The active rejection of paid work was coupled with efforts to find forms of meaningful activity beyond the workplace. For some, this involved formal volunteer work outside the home. Others saw valuable opportunities in the provision of informal care at home

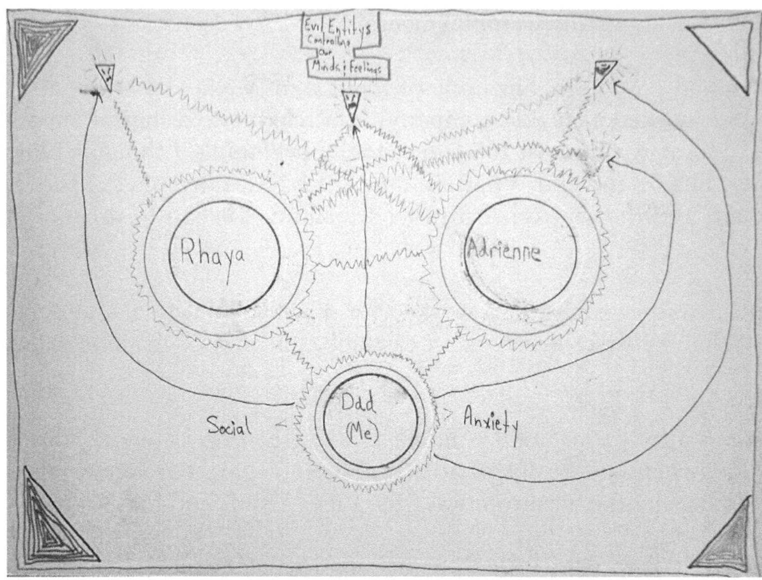

Figure 35.2 Charles' artwork: 'The Unholy Quintumvirate'.

and the practice of fathering. This was clear in Stewart's comments and artwork above. Likewise, Charles was in his early fifties and living with Schizoaffective disorder. He had been out of the labour market for a long time. In response, Charles had rejected the breadwinning norm as basis for his masculinity, focusing instead on his role as a father and his relationship with his daughters as a basis for enacting masculinity. This is visible in his artwork, which focuses on his role in safeguarding his children (Figure 35.2). Asked about the meaning of his artwork, Charles explained:

> I believe that anything masculine, except for one thing as far as I'm concerned, is due to social conditioning and stigma. The only thing that defines me as a man is the fact that I'm a father. So [in my art] I have my two daughters and me in this protective field with each other.

A final example comes from Mark, who was in his early thirties. Mark had worked a series of jobs, primarily in the service sector, but none had lasted more than a few months. He linked the challenge of keeping employment to his mental ill health, especially the high levels of anticipatory anxiety he experienced but he was also frustrated by employers' unwillingness to modify schedules and tasks so that he could fit in more easily at work. The departure from the labour force carried significant material penalties and Mark worried it would be hard for him to ever move out of his mother's house. At the same time, he thought that *not* working could provide new opportunities in other areas of his life. Talking about the future, he hoped to find a long-term partner and start a family. He explained he would be happy to take on the work of childcare while his partner worked outside the home:

Maybe she's better suited to be in the work force, and she has a better personality with other people. Maybe she's good with people and I'm not good with people. Maybe I'm better at being the parent, maybe I have more of the femininity, what people want to classify as femininity.

Mark's willingness to take on the position of stay-at-home father offers an important example of how some men may actively challenge masculine norms through unpaid care work at home (Latshaw 2015). This willingness aligns with his critique of the masculine norms and domestic division of labour he witnessed in his childhood home:

You know, masculine is 'I go get the bacon, I go, I work, I come home, I get to do whatever I want' ...That is a stereotypical man right there. That's how my Dad was. 'I went to work, I come home, shit better be done, house better be clean, if it isn't, I'm going to be a grouchy motherfucker for the rest of my day'.

Importantly, Mark links his motivation to rework gender relations within the space of the home to his experience of mental ill health. He argues that what makes him well suited to the supposedly 'feminine' task of caring for children is his capacity for empathy, something that has been strengthened through the challenges he himself has faced in relation to mental ill health. While dealing with the symptoms of mental ill health 'sucks', Mark recognises that: 'learning wise having mental health issues has helped me to um, to feel empathy.'

Conclusion

Psychiatric rehabilitation positions employment as a key marker of, and contributor to, successful recovery for people living with mental ill health. For those able to find and keep paid work, the benefits in terms of employment income, workplace relations, and self-esteem may be significant. For many, however, employment experiences can be stressful, characterised by ongoing struggle to 'fit in' at work in the absence of meaningful accommodations. Most of the participants in this project reported experiences of this nature; repeated cycles of hiring and firing gave many a sense that they were, at best, on the margins of the labour market. These experiences resonate with existing scholarship on the problems of positioning employment as a key marker of successful recovery. This reflects the *normative orientation* of psychiatric rehabilitation, endorsing dominant cultural values that may stand at odds with the lived experiences and capacities of some people living with mental ill health (see Corin and Lauzon, 1992).

At the same time, participants' experience also highlight how experiences of psychiatric rehabilitation and labour market participation take place in the context of an evolving gender division of labour mapped onto a gendered geography of home and work. By implication, the meaning and experiences of rehabilitation, and the identities people craft in the context of recovery, are gendered. In the sphere of paid work, enduring norms of breadwinning hold particular implications for the ways in which men living with mental ill health do gender. On the one hand, difficulties finding employment can signal a marginal or 'defective' masculinity. However, efforts to resist this breadwinning norm – for example, through deliberate withdrawal from the labour market – can create space for other ways of making masculinity.

Notes

1 More details about the project and colour versions of the artwork are available at www.negot iatingmasculinities.ca. Among the participants, seven reported living with Depression and Anxiety Disorders, while others reported Bipolar Disorder (5), Schizophrenia (4), Schizoaffective Disorder (1), and PTSD (1).
2 Pseudonyms are used throughout the chapter.

References

Bloome, D., Burk, D., and McCall, L. 2019. Economic self-reliance and gender inequality between U.S. men and women, 1970–2010. *American Journal of Sociology*, 124(5), pp.1413–1467.

Bond, G., Drake, R., and Becker, D. 1999. Effectiveness of psychiatric rehabilitation approaches for employment of people with severe mental illness. *Disability Policy Studies*, 101, pp.18–52.

Connell, R. 2005. *Masculinities* (Second Edition). Berkeley and Los Angeles: University of California Press.

Corin, E., and Lauzon, G. 1992. Positive withdrawal and the quest for meaning: The reconstruction of experience among schizophrenics. *Psychiatry*, 55(3), pp.266–278.

Corrigan, P., and Mueser, K. 2016. *Principles and practice of psychiatric rehabilitation: An empirical approach*. New York: Guilford Press.

Crompton, R. 2006. *Employment and the family: The reconfiguration of work and family life in contemporary societies*. Cambridge, UK: Cambridge University Press.

Damaske, S. 2020. Job loss and attempts to return to work: Complicating inequalities across gender and class. *Gender and Society*, 34(1), pp.7–30.

Deegan, P. 1988. Recovery: The lived experience of rehabilitation. *Psychosocial Rehabilitation Journal*, 11(4), pp.11–17.

Doroud, N., Fossey, E., and Fortune, T. 2015. Recovery as an occupational journey. *Australian Occupational Therapy Journal*, 62(6), pp.378–392.

Drake, R., and Wallach, M. 2020. Employment is a critical mental health intervention. *Epidemiology and Psychiatric Sciences*, 29, pp.1–3.

Dunn, E., Wewiorski, N., and Rogers, E. 2008. The meaning and importance of employment to people in recovery from serious mental illness. *Psychiatric Rehabilitation Journal*, 32(1), pp.59–62.

Evans, J., and Wilton, R. 2019. Social enterprise employment and the geographies of mental health recovery. *Annals, American Association of Geographers*, 109(1), pp.87–103.

Foucault, M. (2006) [1972]. *History of madness*. London and New York: Routledge.

Gerson, K. 2009. *The unfinished revolution: Coming of age in a new era of gender, work, and family*. Oxford: Oxford University Press.

Gonalons-Pons, P., and Gangl, M. 2021. Marriage and masculinity: Male-breadwinner culture, unemployment, and separation risk. *American Sociological Review*, 86(3), pp.465–502.

Jammaers, E., and Zanoni, P. 2021. Unveiling the varieties of ableism in employers' socio-ideological control. *Organization Studies*, 42(3), pp.429–452.

Krupa, T., Moll, S., and Fossey, E. 2020. Beyond employment: A broader vision linking activity and participation to well-being, and recovery. *Psychiatric Services*, 71(9), pp.956–958.

Latshaw, B. 2015. From mopping to mowing: Masculinity and housework in stay-at-home father households. *The Journal of Men's Studies*, 23(3), pp.252–270.

Laws, J. 2011. Crackpots and basket-cases: A history of therapeutic work and ocupation. *History of the Human Sciences*, 24(2), pp.65–81.

Lowe, J., and DeVerteuil, G. 2020. Austerity Britain, poverty management and the missing geographies of mental health. *Health & Place*, 64, pp.1–7. https://doi.org/10.1016/j.healthpl ace.2020.102358

McDowell, L. 1991. Life without father and Ford: The new gender order of post-Fordism. *Transactions, Institute of British Geographers*, 16(4), pp.400–419.

McDowell, L. 1999. *Gender, identity and place: Understanding feminist geographies.* Minneapolis: University of Minnesota Press.

McDowell, L. 2011. *Redundant masculinities? Employment change and white working class youth*. Hoboken: John Wiley and Sons.

Modini, M., Joyce, S., and Christensen, H. 2016. The mental health benefits of employment: A systematic meta-review. *Australasian Psychiatry*, 24(4), pp.331–336.

Molyneux, C. (2023). Why employer inflexibility matters for the recruitment, retention and progression of disabled workers. *Disability and Society*, 38(4), pp.1–6.

Myers, K., and Demantas, I. (2016). Breadwinning and bread-losing: Exploring opportunities to rework manhood. *Sociology Compass*, 10(12), pp.1119–1130.

Nayak, A. (2006). Displaced masculinities: chavs, youth and class in the post-industrial city. Sociology, 40(5), pp.813–831.

Rössler, W. 2006. Psychiatric rehabilitation today: An overview. *World Psychiatry*, 5(3), p.151.

Rutman, I. 1993. 'And now, the envelope please...' *Psychosocial Rehabilitation Journal*, 16(3), pp.1–3.

Thébaud, S. 2010. Masculinity, bargaining, and breadwinning: Understanding men's housework in the cultural context of paid work. *Gender and Society*, 24(3), pp.330–354.

Vukadin, M., Schaafsma, F., and Anema, J. 2021. Experiences with individual placement and support and employment: A qualitative study. *BMC Psychiatry*, *21*, pp.1–12.

Wilton, R. 2004. From flexibility to accommodation? Disabled people and the reinvention of paid work. *Transactions, Institute of British Geographers*, 29(4), pp.420–432.

Zuo, J. 2004. Shifting the breadwinning boundary. *Journal of Family Issues*, 25(6), pp.811–832.

36 Creating space for youth mental health online
A clinician's perspective

Candice P. Boyd

Introduction

Digital mental health care is often lauded for its accessibility – its ability to 'democratise' mental health and for the capacity to augment professional mental health services (Zimerman, Montezano, Dalla Vecchia, Kapczinksi, & Passos, 2023). Implicit in these claims is that accessing mental health care is prohibitive both in terms of limited access to a qualified mental health workforce and in the monetary cost of providing and receiving these services. Digital mental health addresses both concerns by substituting clinician-led care with clinician-supported care or wholly self-guided care in the form of an evidence-based programme delivered online or via a mobile phone application (apps) at low- or no-cost. The utility of artificial intelligence (AI or chatbots) as a way of helping clinicians monitor patients' symptoms is also being explored in the mental health care sector (see Lakhtakia & Torous, 2022). Zimerman et al. (2023) envisage a future where clinicians no longer rely on patients to remember or report clinical information in a session but, via continual patient self-monitoring, are provided with active and passive data which are 'curated' by scientists and engineers, leading to 'better clinical insights' (p.5).

For now, an experience of digital mental health care is mostly one that is mediated by technology rather than delivered by it. For example, telepsychiatry and telepsychology – the delivery of mental health services online via a dedicated 'telehealth' platform – has become mainstay in many countries as an alternative to face-to-face consultations (Baker & Bufta, 2011; Zimerman et al., 2023). In Australia, telehealth is covered by Medicare – a national insurance scheme that provides free or subsidised health care – and it is this practice which is the focus of this chapter. When it comes to the geographies of telehealth (also referred to as telemedicine in the literature), scholars have considered how the practice is regionalising healthcare but also how telehealth and its associated technologies are nested in 'the social' (Cutchin, 2002; Petersson, 2014). This work highlights the 'double-edged' nature of digital technologies in that by creating greater access, these technologies also produce 'virtual' regions of care that may not integrate well into existing, material systems as the ownership and control of digital systems often lies outside of local communities (Cutchins, 2002; Flore, 2023).

Digital geographies are an emerging sub-field of disciplinary practice within human geography which considers the digital as object and subject of inquiry (Ash, 2018). These interrogations go beyond the proliferation of the digital in our everyday lives by attending to '... the production of space, spatiality and mobilities; the processes, practices, and forms of mapping; the contours of spatial knowledge and imaginaries; and the formation

DOI: 10.4324/9781003345725-40

and enactment of spatial politics' in relation to the digital (Ash et al., 2016, p. 26). As Leszcynski (2018) points out, technology-society-space relations take place in 'hybrid spaces, digital spaces, and augmented realities' with their own space/time configurations. This mediation is a contemporary condition, Leszczynski (2018) argues, whereby we understand these spaces and interactions as *effects* of the digital and the human coming together. Rose (2018) further argues that digitally mediated spaces rely upon embedded notions of representation with their own cultural politics which put them at risk of caricature. In terms of telehealth, these cultural and spatial politics also raise ethical questions in regard to equality of care (Cutchins, 2002).

The COVID-19 pandemic accelerated the uptake of digital mental health as well as research into client's experiences of it (see Gruber et al., 2020). For example, a study by Razman et al. (2022) explored young people's experiences of online therapy for the emotional dysregulation common to people with a diagnosis of borderline personality disorder. While some of their experiences are likely attributable to their diagnosis, clients did raise issues of relevance to a more general experience of online therapy, e.g., a feeling of 'loss of connection', 'limited privacy', 'lack of a safe therapy space', and 'difficult endings' when comparing to therapy in person. On the positive side, they appreciated the 'convenience and accessibility' and 'home comforts' of the online format (see Razman et al., 2022 for details).

Therapists' experiences of and attitudes towards digital mental health care are also rapidly changing, post-pandemic lockdowns (Ojha & Syed, 2020). A qualitative survey of Australian psychologists found that their attitudes had shifted over the course of the pandemic to be less resistant and more positive about telehealth modalities (Scott et al., 2023). The psychologists who took part in this study indicated a preference for video conferencing and/or clinician-guided access to digital programmes rather than self-guided, standalone programmes. Concerns were cited about the potential for digital mental health care to create barriers to face-to-face support without '… appropriate steps to access other mental health support if online programs are not a good fit' (Scott et al., 2023 p. 348).

For the remainder of this chapter, I provide a first-hand account of the delivery of youth mental health services via telehealth from the unique vantage point of geographer and clinical psychologist. The objective is to present and examine some of the tensions that exist in the delivery of youth mental health online, particularly as they relate to the online environment as a space of work and a space of mental health and wellbeing. Where qualities of traditional face-to-face therapy are lost, others are gained, and this can impact the therapeutic relationship that is formed as well as the clinical information that needs to be gathered to properly assess clients' 'mental states'. This has implications for the client's overall experience but also the quality of their care. In the following sections, I attend to these concerns by first focusing on how online therapy is 'done' and then thinking through how online practice might impact mental health care more broadly.

'Doing' youth mental health care online

In reflecting on my practice as a clinical psychologist in a telehealth context, I am also cognisant of geographical notions of space and the manifold relations that unfold in any setting. In this respect, I find the following metaphor for space to be very useful to my online clinical practice:

> ... spaces are – at least in part – as moving bodies *do*. Think, for instance, of the difference between a football pitch with and without a game taking place on it. The presence of moving bodies is not only a physical transformation of the pitch: it also alters the imaginative, affective, sonic and social qualities of this space. (emphasis in the original; p. 1823)

How this metaphor helps is by shifting the focus in online work from the platform itself to what we *do* in online environments to create therapeutic spaces. In terms of therapeutic relationships, it is never just what we do as clinicians but what our clients do as well – what they bring to a session but also the extent to which they are willing to 'engage'. Our job as clinicians is to foster this engagement in ways that clients are empowered to make positive changes in their lives but also to create and maintain 'holding' spaces for clients to express and 'sit with' difficult emotions. These processes are less about the two-way exchange but how both people contribute to a third relation referred in the counselling tradition as the 'therapeutic alliance' and in the psychoanalytic tradition as the 'inter-subjective field' (Civitarese, 2021; Wolitzy et al., 2001). This is a 'felt' relation and so difficult to put into words but when therapy is 'working', this third relation is 'mobile' and when the therapy is not going well this third relation is weak (or weakened in the process) and relatively static.

A significant limitation of online therapy is the inability to make direct eye contact. Figure 36.1 illustrates how this works in my own practice context, i.e., if I look at the client's image then I am not looking at the camera, and if I look at the camera (which would simulate eye contact for the client) then I cannot look directly at the client. While looking at the camera might appear to the client as an attempt to make eye contact, they have the same dilemma if they want to 'return' the eye contact – they cannot do so and look at me at the same time. The problem is somewhat alleviated by minimising the image at each end and centring the image of the other party, but this tends to result instead in one or both parties directing their eyes downward rather than sideways.

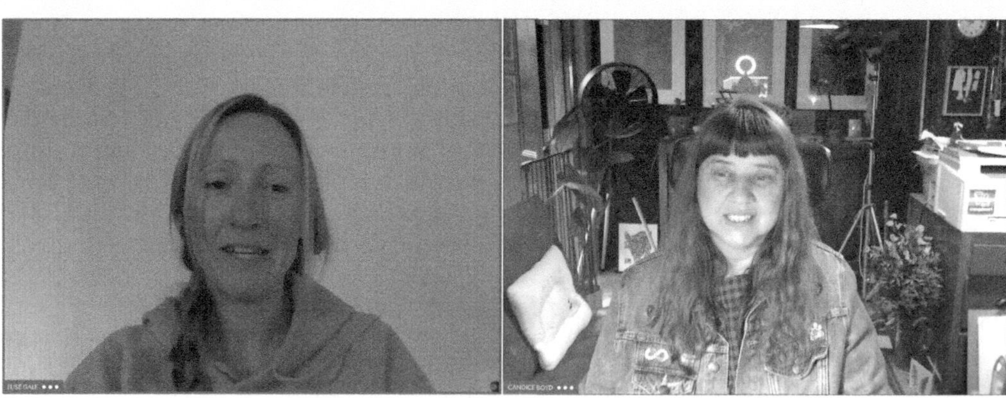

Figure 36.1 Inability to make eye contact during a telehealth session (Author photograph; with thanks to Elise Gale, Clinical Lead at headspace Bathurst, for assisting with the demonstration).

It could be argued that the use of mobile phones could reduce the amount of distance the eyes need to travel from camera to image in a video call, but there are other restraints in telehealth which limit the feasibility of this option. One is that it is preferred that clients come into the centre and have their telehealth appointments in a consultation room, so that there is technical help available if there are connection issues but more importantly that there is clinical 'back up' if they terminate a call while in clinical distress. From the clinician's end, the need to access multiple sources of digital information simultaneously with the video call, makes a mobile phone impractical. It has also been my experience that in attempting to share digital information with clients who 'dial in' from a mobile that it 'crashes' the call. As such, my clients and I have had to adapt to never making eye contact with one another.

While there are cultural differences in the social acceptability of making sustained eye contact, it is generally understood as a fundamental component of social interaction. As Jongerius, Hessels, Romijn, Smets and Hillen (2020) explain, direct eye contact between patient and physician is positively associated with patient's levels of trust, anxiety, and satisfaction with treatment. Furthermore, eye contact has been shown to trigger the release of oxytocin in the brain – a neurotransmitter responsible for interpersonal bonding. Auyeung et al. (2015) also demonstrate the reverse relationship whereby the administration of oxytocin will increase eye contact in 'real-time'. As such, the inability to make eye contact with clients at any point in a telehealth consultation is likely to negatively impact upon the client's experience of therapy and potentially therapeutic outcome. There is, however, an exception to this when direct eye contact is a source of anxiety for the young person and so the ability to avoid it in the telehealth environment may be productive in the short term.

Non-verbal behaviour is not only important in therapeutic relationships, but it can also provide essential 'data' for a mental status examination (MSE). While the notion of a mental state examination is fraught, especially from a philosophical perspective (see Descombes, 2001), it does provide useful 'diagnostic information'. For example, I saw a young person for 10 sessions via telehealth with his grandmother in attendance. His grandmother attended as a support person because he was nervous and uncertain about the process. While he was slowly able to engage with me over the 10 sessions, he usually kept to the side of the camera and wore a cap to cover his eyes. It was only during the last session, when his grandmother wasn't in attendance, that he allowed himself to appear fully on camera, although still covering his eyes with his cap. It was only in this last session that I could see that whenever he responded to me, he started muttering to himself in barely audible self-talk. The telehealth environment had prevented me from seeing or hearing what would have been readily observable in a face-to-face consultation. Although not cause for concern in this client's case, audible self-talk, and its content, is a clinically significant sign that would normally be recorded as part of an MSE and further explored in the session.

As Piper and Treyger (2010) argue, power and privilege are inherent in all social interactions and therapeutic relationships are no exception. Managing power imbalances, as well as acknowledging and attending to their unconscious effects, is usually the therapist's responsibility. Telehealth, however, tends to impart more opportunities for clients to exert power in sessions, particularly in how they present themselves. The example above relates to this tendency as clients can choose how to position the camera in the room and how much or how little they appear in the image. They can also turn the camera off without ending the call. Ultimately, it is in their power to 'hang up' and terminate the call whereby there is no way for the clinician to continue the session (if a client 'walks out' of a face-to-face consultation there is always the possibility for the clinician follow them out and to invite them back in). I recently had a session with a new client who turned off the camera and refused to speak for most of it but didn't hang up. She was there and listening, which was apparent from occasional vocalisations, but did not choose to end the session even though I invited her to do so whenever she wanted. This can happen in face-to-face consultations, too, where sitting in silence and 'holding' a space for clients without words can be meaningful, but in these instances a whole host of nonverbal behaviours like eye contact and an open posture come into play. In telehealth, even when both cameras are on, we are 'talking heads' and, as such, our ability to communicate nonverbally is severely restricted. In practice, this seems to force the therapy into a more didactic mode.

I have found that this slippage into a more didactic mode of working as a therapist has both positive and negative consequences for me as a practitioner. I have always struggled as a therapist with the phenomenon of projective identification – where emotions that are disowned by the client are projected onto the therapist – and the 'countertransference' that sometimes results from this (Báez-Powell, 2023). Since I've been practising online, however, I have not been consciously experiencing the phenomenon as much as I have in the past. Speculatively, I think that this is because the conscious experience of transference in therapy is largely somatic (Hobday, 2011), and that reducing the client to an 'image' or 'caricature' of a person (see Rose, 2018) avoids having to attend to the body in the same way. While the 'depersonalisation' of the client that inevitably takes place in online therapy might actually assist therapists in managing (or denying?) their vulnerabilities, I wonder what negative impacts this might be having on the therapeutic relationship and on my own professional development as a youth mental health practitioner.

To summarise, while telehealth platforms increase accessibility to youth mental health services this is not without impacts on the therapeutic process, most of which could be regarded as negative. Restricting the ability for both parties to communicate affectively through the full range of non-verbal body language normally available to them in a face-to-face consultation is the biggest drawback. While clients do have more control over how they present themselves and to what extent they engage in the process, this can also be detrimental by reducing the therapist's ability to make clinically relevant observations and/or to explore therapy's more dynamic processes. But perhaps ineffably, I have found that the ability to create, foster, and contribute to a therapeutic alliance/dynamic is diminished in online therapy, which, in my opinion, ultimately renders it suboptimal in terms of mental health care.

Conclusion

In this chapter, I have attended to the telehealth environment as a space of mental health care as a geographer and practising clinical psychologist. While there are great benefits to telehealth technologies for improving access to mental health services, especially in the regions, from a practitioner's perspective there are also downsides. While clients have greater flexibility and control, I can also see how this might not always be to their benefit. But most of all I see the greatest losses as those that relate to the embodied and dynamic experience of therapy which the online environment largely denies. Zimerman et al.'s (2023) vision of psychiatry's digital future might be one of 'improved mental health outcomes' but it might also be what Dekeyser (2023) describes as 'ontological murder'. In the rush to embrace the potential of digital mental health care, its subjective limitations should not be ignored.

References

Ardito, R. B. & Rabellino, D. (2011). Therapeutic alliance and outcome of psychotherapy: Historical excursus, measurements, and prospects for research. *Frontiers in Psychology, 2,* 1–11. DOI: 10.3389/fpsyg.2011.00270

Ash, J., Kitchin, R., & Leszczyinksi, A. (2018). Digital turn, digital geographies? *Progress in Human Geography, 42,* 25–43. DOI: 10.1177/0309132516664800

Ash, J., Kitchin, R., & Leszczyinksi, A. (2018). Introducing digital geographies. In J. Ash, R. Kitchin, and A. Leszczynski (Eds), *Digital Geographies.* London: Sage.

Auyeung, B., Lombardo, M. V., Heinrichs, M., Chakrabarti, B., Sule, A., Deakin, J. B., Bethlehem, R. A., Dickens, L., Mooney, N., Sipple, J. A., Thiemann, P., & Baron-Cohen, S. (2015). Oxytocin increases eye contact during a real-time, naturalistic social interaction in males with and without autism. *Translational Psychiatry, 5,* e507. DOI: 10.1038/tp.2014.146

Báez-Powell, N.N. (2023). Ramifications of client's use of projective identification, racism, and enactments of otherness: A nascent clinician's struggle inhabiting her identities in the therapy room. *Psychoanalalysis, Culture, and Society,* 28, 232–249. https://doi.org/10.1057/s41 282-023-00378-5

Baker, D. C., & Bufka, L. F. (2011). Preparing for the telehealth world: Navigating legal, regulatory, reimbursement, and ethical issues in an electronic age. *Professional Psychology: Research and Practice, 42,* 405–411. DOI: 10.1037/a0025037

Civitarese, G. (2021). Intersubjectivity and analytic field theory. *Journal of the American Psychoanalytic Association, 69,* 853–893. DOI: 10.1177/00030651211044788

Cutchin, M. P. (2002). Virtual medical geographies: Conceptualizing telemedicine and regionalization. *Progress in Human Geography, 26,* 19–39.

Dekeyser, T. (2023). Rethinking posthumanist subjectivity: Technology as ontological murder in European colonialism. *Theory, Culture & Society,* online early, DOI: 10.1177/ 02632764231178482

Descombes, V. (2001). *The mind's provisions: A critique of cognitivism.* [Translated by Stephen Adam Schwartz]. Princeton: Princeton University Press.

Flore, J. (2023). *The artefacts of digital mental health.* Singapore: Palgrave Macmillan.

Flückiger, C., Del Re, A. C., Wampold, B. E., & Horvath, A. O. (2018). The alliance in adult psychotherapy: A meta-analytic synthesis. *Psychotherapy, 55,* 314–340. DOI: 10.1037/ pst0000172

Gruber, J., Prinstein, M. J., Clark, L. A., Rottenberg, J., Abramowitz, J. S., Albano, A. M., Aldao, A., Borelli, J. L., Chung, T., Davila, J., Forbes, E. E., Gee, D. G., Hall, G. C. N., Hallion, L. S., Hinshaw, S. P., Hofmann, S. G., Hollon, S. D., Joormann, J., Kazdin, A. E… & Weinstock, L. M. (2020). Mental health and clinical psychological science in the time of COVID19: Challenges, opportunities, and a call to action. *The American Psychologist, 76,* 409–426. DOI: https://doi. org/10.1037/amp0000707

Hobday, G. S. (2011). Of two minds: Countertransference in contemporary psychotherapy. *Psychiatric Times, 28*(8), 29.

Jongerius, C., Hessels, R. S., Romijn, J. A., Smets, E. M. A., & Hillen, M. A. (2020). The measurement of eye contact in human interactions: A scoping review. *Journal of Nonverbal Behavior, 44,* 363–389. DOI: 10.1007/s10919-020-00333-3

Kinsley, S. (2018). Subject/ivities. In J. Ash, R. Kitchin, and A. Leszczynski (Eds), *Digital Geographies.* London: Sage.

Lakhtakia, T., & Torous, J. (2022). Current directions in digital interventions for mood and anxiety disorders. *Current Opinion in Psychiatry, 35,* 130–135. DOI: 10.1097/YCO.0000000000000772.

Leszczynski, A. (2018). Spatialities. In J. Ash, R. Kitchin, and A. Leszczynski (Eds), *Digital Geographies.* London: Sage.

McCormack, D. P. (2008). Geographies for moving bodies: Thinking, dancing, spaces. *Geography Compass, 2,* 1822–1836.

Ojha, R., & Syed, S. (2020). Challenges faced by mental health pro- viders and patients during the coronavirus 2019 pandemic due to technological barriers. *Internet Interventions, 21*, 100330. DOI: https:// doi.org/10.1016/j.invent.2020.100330

Petersson, J. (2014). *Geographies of eHealth: Studies of healthcare at a distance*. Doctoral dissertation: The University of Gothenberg.

Piper, J., & Treyger, S. (2010). Power, privilege, and ethics. In L. Hecker (Ed.), Ethics and professional issues in couple and family therapy (pp. 71–87). Routledge/Taylor & Francis Group.

Razman, N., Dixey, R., & Morris, A. (2022). A qualitative exploration of adoelscents' experiences of digital dialectical behaviour therapy during the COVID-19 pandemic. *The Cognitive Behaviour Therapist, 15*, e48. DOI: 10.1017/S1754470X22000460

Rose, G. (2018). Representation and mediation. In J. Ash, R. Kitchin, and A. Leszczynski (Eds), *Digital Geographies*. London: Sage.

Scott, S., Knott, V., Finlay-Jones, A. L., & Mancini, V. O. (2023). Australian psychologists experiences with digital mental health: A qualitative investigation. *Journal of Technology in Behavioural Science, 8*, 341–351. DOI: https://doi.org/10.1007/s41347-022-00271-5

Wolitzky, D. L., Eagle, M., & Luborsky, L. (2001). Dynamic psychotherapy in D. L. Wolitzky, M. Eagle, and L. Luborsky (Eds), *Advanced Abnormal Psychology*. New York: Springer.

Zimerman, A., Montezano, B. B., Dalla Vecchia, G. F., Kapczinksi, G., and Passos, I. C. (2023). The dawn of digital psychiatry. In I. C. Passos, F. D. Rabelo-da-Ponte, and F. Kapczinksi (Eds), *Digital mental health: A practitioner's guide*. Cham: Springer.

37 Landscapes of trauma and mental health

Jesse Proudfoot

In Cathy Caruth's genre-defining *Unclaimed Experience* (1996), she posits that trauma is an event that exists outside of history – an experience so overwhelming that the subject cannot assimilate it into their personal narrative. Janet Walker (2010), writing about hurricane Katrina's devastation of New Orleans, suggests that Caruth's temporal framing is suggestive of a geographical corollary – one in which trauma is an experience so disorienting that it cannot be located in a subject's cognitive map. Trauma's ahistoricism lies in its insistence and repetition, its unwillingness to be confined to the past. Likewise, trauma might be understood geographically as something that follows the subject wherever they go: an experience that refuses to be confined to the site of trauma, reappearing even though the subject has left the battlefield or the abuser's home. If the task of therapy for traumatised people has often been understood as integrating the exceptional event into a subjective history, rehistoricising an experience of time out of joint, we can similarly assert that this process is also spatial: that integrating trauma into a subjective 'history' is also one of remapping it, of *finding a place* for the experience that refuses to stay put. In this chapter, I review geography's engagement with trauma, focusing largely on the discipline's recent 'critical' engagement with trauma studies and situating this turn within earlier geographical work on trauma and memorialisation.

While 'geographies of trauma' now describes a coherent subfield, the term is also useful as a provocation to consider what other work might be captured by it. A capacious reading suggests that geographers have had much to say about the spatial production of 'trauma': from the urban geographical literature on slums and poverty (Dear and Wolch, 1987), to the literature on environmental racism (Pulido, 2000), and health geography's interest in unhealthy places (Wakefield and McMullan, 2005; Proudfoot, 2019). Understood in these terms, critical geography's interest in the spatiality of social problems can be read as long being invested in the intersection of trauma and place.

In a more narrow sense, the contemporary geography of trauma traces its lineage to the literature on landmarks and memorialisation of the 1990s. Drawing on Maurice Halbwachs's and Pierre Nora's work on collective memory and Hobsbawm's idea of the 'mass production of tradition', this literature explored the politics of memorialisation and the production of political narratives through landmarks. As Karen Till argues, "the study of landmarks offers us insights into the ways nationalist political discourses are articulated" (Till, 1999, p. 252), an insight which led scholars to examine a variety of nationalist monuments and contested landmarks (for a review see Till, 2003). Because of the traumatic nature of what was often memorialised, this work evolved to consider the

DOI: 10.4324/9781003345725-41

relationship between landscape, memorialisation and trauma. In Till's work on 'wounded cities' for example, she examined how cities can be "harmed ... by particular histories of physical destruction, displacement, and individual and social trauma resulting from state-perpetrated violence" (Till, 1999, p. 6). Cities are marked by their oppressive pasts, she argued, leaving scars in the landscape, such as the erasures of peoples' histories by displacement and gentrification.

Critical geographies of trauma

Critical geography's more recent interest in trauma has drawn largely on engagements with trauma studies beyond the discipline. The 1980s and 1990s saw an efflorescence of work related to trauma, most notably in the work of Cathy Caruth in literary studies (1995, 1996), and in psychiatry through work on traumatic memory by Bessel van der Kolk (2014). Caruth drew on psychoanalytic formulations of trauma as an experience that overwhelms the subject, such that it cannot properly be admitted to consciousness and is therefore split off, later returning in the form of nightmares, flashbacks, and other symptoms, to develop arguments about the impossibility of representing trauma and how this bears on theories of representation. In psychiatry, van der Kolk was instrumental in formulating new conceptualisations of traumatic experience and treatment, arguing that there was, in fact, a separate system in the brain for recording traumatic memories, and that treatment for trauma required accessing not just the mind via language but the body itself, via somatic therapies.

The turn towards trauma occurs in the aftermath of the recognition of Post-Traumatic Stress Disorder (PTSD) by mainstream psychiatry in the 3rd Diagnostic and Statistical Manual of Mental Disorders (DSM-III) in 1980. As many have argued (Young, 1995; Leys, 2000; Fassin and Rechtman, 2009), the recognition of PTSD as a disorder – like the removal of homosexuality before it – was the result of political activism. In the case of PTSD, the campaign for inclusion was waged initially by American veterans of the war in Vietnam and later by women's groups concerned with sexual violence, both of whom sought to have their experiences recognised by the medical establishment and to gain access to recognition and entitlements as a result. That such politics were at play in the field of trauma and mental health should alert us to the critical debates within trauma studies that have appeared since.

These critiques have been underpinned by important work historicising the concept of trauma and the diagnosis of PTSD. Allen Young (1995) provides a masterful histori-ography of the development of trauma as a diagnostic category and an ethnography of PTSD treatment. Rather than making claims about the authenticity of PTSD itself, Young devotes himself to "describing the mechanisms through which these phenomena penetrate people's life worlds, acquire facticity, and shape the self-knowledge of patients, clinicians, and researchers" (5-6). Such a claim does not mean that PTSD is not 'real' for Young; rather, he demonstrates how trauma has been understood differently at different points and how the diagnosis of PTSD makes visible certain aspects of experience while obscuring others.

Such critical reflection and historicisation lie at the heart of geographers' engagements with trauma in recent years. In the remainder of this chapter, I review this work, organising it around what I see as the two principal interventions made by this avowedly 'critical' scholarship. The first concerns the question of the medicalisation and individualisation of trauma and associated engagements with the diagnosis of PTSD. The second addresses debates over the question of exceptionality in trauma in comparison to more systemic, ongoing, or everyday forms of harm.

Individualisation and medicalisation

Nearly all of the recent work by geographers focusing on trauma makes the argument that our frameworks of trauma need to be expanded beyond a focus on the individual sufferer, and accordingly, that trauma has been unduly conflated with the psychiatric diagnosis of PTSD. As Rachel Pain puts it in a recent survey of the field, "...trauma is located not only within people's minds and bodies, but in the social, environmental and structural contexts around us" (2021, p. 974). This draws on two pillars of contemporary critical theory: the critique of the (neo-)liberal individual and the concept of medicalisation. The crux of both is that by focusing on trauma as an individual pathology, and especially by reifying it in a psychiatric diagnosis, we obscure the larger structural forces that have produced trauma to begin with. Similarly, the critique of medicalisation asserts that diagnoses such as PTSD render as *medical* and *individual* problems that are better understood as *political* and *social*. This argument holds that purely clinical attempts to resolve the problem will therefore falter if they fail to address root causes. As Pain argues: "...there is a political imperative for de-medicalizing our understanding" (2021, p. 973).

While these arguments emerge, it could be said, rhizomatically, from a number of different traditions, geography's recent use of them owes a particular debt to Ann Cvetkovich. Cvetkovich's project of reclaiming trauma for radical queer politics explicitly rejects "the authority given to medical discourses and especially the diagnosis of... PTSD" (2003, p. 4), in order to use trauma as a ground for constructing 'public cultures' rather than narrowly therapeutic ones. Trauma opens up space for discussing pain and oppression that is psychical rather than simply physical and makes possible new, collective forms of therapy, "...rather than a model in which privatized affective responses displace collective or political ones" (10).

Many aspects of this argument appear in geography's critical engagements with trauma, taking a variety of forms. Kate Coddington (2017) develops the idea of "contagious trauma" in her research with asylum seekers in Australia and the advocates working with them. Writing about the shifting affective exchanges between these groups, including the ways that trauma seeps into the lives and dreams of advocates, triggering their own traumas and leading to mental health crises and burnout, she argues that such relations should be understood as "contagious". The experience of hearing another's trauma produces "connections to other and unrelated traumas in other times and spaces" (68) in ways that complicate individualised conceptions of trauma (see too Adams-Hutcheson, 2017; Coddington and Micieli-Voutsinas, 2017).

Alison Mountz (2017) makes a similarly relational argument in her work on island detention centres. Mountz argues that the traumas encountered in contemporary struggles over asylum must be understood as "sedimented" in the sense that they are built upon and revive earlier traumas rooted in these places. Examining detention centres in places with long colonial histories, she argues that sedimented traumas 'affectively erupt' in the present, connecting bodies and histories in unpredictable ways. In an especially powerful illustration, Mountz interviews the manager of a detention centre in Guam, noting the deeply dehumanising language used to describe refugees – for example, referring to their meals as "feeding time". Yet, Mountz refuses to simplistically castigate her interviewee, instead reminding us that, "although in a position of power" over the detainees, the manager is himself a colonised person forced to implement the will of authorities, a worker who is largely unable to challenge the "long history of federal control" (80). In this way, the trauma of colonialism is repeated, cathected between different bodies, and across generations.

Perera (2010) examines the slippages and connections between traumas in her work on humanitarian aid following the Indian Ocean Tsunami of 2004 and its effects on Sri Lanka, already suffering from protracted civil war. When tragedies are layered on top of one another – natural disasters following human-made catastrophe in a context of engineered underdevelopment – they constitute what she calls a "tortuous dialogue" in which trauma functions as a "medium" (33), linking forms of suffering while also potentially reinscribing existing hierarchies. Such links are fraught, however, and Perera argues that forms of 'natural' suffering are acknowledged and mourned, while 'political' suffering is not. In this way, we see how trauma can function both as a bridge, building solidarities, and also as a barrier, shutting down connections between subjects (see too Linz, 2021).

In a series of articles focused on their work with Iraqi refugees in Turkey, Loyd, Ehrkamp and Secor draw together a number of these threads, developing what they call a 'geopolitics of trauma' (2018). The authors offer a "critical examination of the PTSD framework" (2018, 379) and the ways that the diagnosis has become integral to making legible claims for asylum. Refugees, they demonstrate, are often placed in an impossible double bind, in which UNHCR interviewers demand coherent narratives of suffering and latch onto inconsistencies as evidence of deception, even though confused narratives are a common element of trauma. At the same time, interviewers may be sceptical of overly clear narratives for these same reasons, even though such narrative coherence is a goal of the very PTSD treatment refugees are provided (2018). Following Cvetkovich, they argue that trauma must be depathologised and understood not as "a medical problem in search of a cure but as felt experiences that can be mobilised in a range of directions, including the construction of cultures and publics" (Cvetkovich 2003, quoted in Loyd, Ehrkamp, Secor 2018, 378). Ultimately, refugees' suffering cannot be solved by therapy alone; as one interviewee puts it simply: "war has to stop" (386).

Finally, Pratt et al. (2017) echo many of these themes in their ongoing work with Filipina migrant workers. Discussing the theatre production that they have developed with their interlocutors, they echo the idea that "trauma may serve as a medium of exchange ... linking different times and places" (2017, p. 84) while also wondering whether trauma can translate across national boundaries and positionalities: Will the traumas of Filipina live-in caregivers in Canada be legible as traumatic to those still living in the Philippines? Framing their intervention as part of broader efforts to decolonise trauma theory, they draw on earlier literatures (e.g. Fanon, 1967) to echo the critique of trauma theory as individualising and medicalising. As the source of trauma here is not accidental or exceptional but "systematic and planned", they argue, it is ultimately "unamenable to therapeutic resolution" and "it is only through collective struggle to alter the material conditions of colonial subjugation that trauma can be overcome" (85).

While these critiques of individualised trauma are essential, they also point towards thorny conceptual questions about the translation between the spheres of the individual and social. Despite the crucial importance of identifying the structural forces that lie behind individual traumas, it is another matter to insist, first, that such traumas should be understood using the same framework as for those that befall individuals, and second, that their remedy lies in collective action. In an essay discussing the differences between traumatic memory related to childhood sexual abuse and those of Holocaust survivors, the medical anthropologist Lawrence Kirmayer notes that when "whole communities" experience a trauma and are "able to talk about it openly or share tacit acknowledgement of its horrors" (1996, p. 189) it is more likely that it will be retained in memory and worked through. By comparison, traumas experienced by individuals that are not afforded a social space for working through are more likely to result in a "sequestration of memory in a virtual space shaped by the social demand [...] to remain silent... The difference is between a public space of solidarity and private space of shame" (1996, p. 189). In my own work with people who use drugs, I have encountered similar dynamics, in which people whose drug use is driven by intimate traumas such as sexual abuse often evince more complex and intractable addictions than those whose drug use appear to be a 'self-medicative' impulse related to large-scale social forces such as racism and poverty (Proudfoot, 2019). But, rather than simply opposing social traumas to individual ones, my work argues that the relationship between social oppression and individual traumas is itself fraught, and therapeutic work must be attentive to the ways that collective traumas are experienced through deeply personal, intimate forms of violence – a finding that both deepens and complicates calls for 'collective struggle' as the solution to a trauma (Proudfoot, 2023).

Exceptionality and the everyday

The second pillar of critical geography's engagement with trauma concerns the question of exceptionality. Classical trauma theory, from Freud and Janet through to Cathy Caruth, has emphasised the exceptional nature of experiences that produce trauma. Here, trauma is an experience that overwhelms the subject: an accident so shocking that we freeze in disbelief, an assault that disrupts our sense of safety, the chaos of the battlefield that lays bare the terrifying fragility of our bodies. From early in the critical turn, however, this aspect of trauma was singled out for reassessment. Why must trauma be reserved for exceptional events when there are so many forms of traumatic experience that are in fact extremely common? This question is, of course, eminently political, especially in reference to the sorts of gendered and racial traumas for which critical voices seek recognition.

In Caruth's first edited collection on trauma, the feminist psychotherapist Laura Brown argues that the DSM-III definition of trauma as an experience "outside the range of human experience" (quoted in Brown, 1995, p. 100) is responsible for the erasure of systemic trauma. Understood as exceptional, this framing ignores those traumas that disproportionately affect women and minorities such as sexual violence and oppression. Judith Herman, responsible for the expanded definition of 'complex PTSD' (1992) that better captures prolonged forms of trauma, deftly threads a needle through this discussion, arguing that "traumatic events are extraordinary, not because they occur rarely, but rather because they overwhelm the ordinary human adaptations to life" (2001, p. 33).

These evocations of more pervasive and systemic forms of trauma have been immensely productive for critics interested in the application of trauma beyond isolated events. Lauren Berlant (2011) develops the concept of "crisis ordinariness" as part of an attempt to critique an overreliance on trauma as an arch-metaphor of modernity. Situating trauma within this larger historical frame, they argue that trauma has been the dominant interpretive framework for conceptualising the 'cognitive overload' of modernity since the early twentieth century. Against trauma's focus on shock, Berlant argues instead for 'the ordinary' as the site of *systemic* crisis, within which people attempt to make lives under conditions more productive of "slow death" – shifting attention from the exceptional to the dispiritingly mundane.

Such arguments for the systemic nature of trauma are central to critical geography's engagements with the concept. Summarising much of this work, Rachel Pain's review of the field argues that while "most Western trauma theory" continues to conceptualise trauma as the product of a single (exceptional) event, interventions from Black, queer, postcolonial and indigenous scholars around concepts like cultural and structural trauma have highlighted how this model privileges "the suffering of white Europeans and the depoliticization and dehistoricization of trauma" (Pain, 2021, p. 976). In contexts where trauma is the product not of a single event but ongoing, pervasive oppression, the concept of a safe and secure period 'before' trauma is untenable. As Pain argues, "it is the commonness of experiences of gender-based, racist and homophobic violence that challenges assumptions of cohesion or security before or after trauma" (ibid).

Ehrkamp, Loyd, and Secor, in their work on refugees, reiterate the critique of this focus on "singular events rather than sustained, even multigenerational suffering" (2022, p. 715). Tying the problem of exceptionality to their critique of medicalisation, they assert that the diagnosis of PTSD is inappropriate not just for its Eurocentrism but because many of the most salient traumas in these refugees' lives are not *post*-traumatic in any meaningful sense of the term. Trauma, for these groups, is ongoing: it is not simply the product of the wars they are fleeing but also the arduous process of resettlement they are forced to undergo, including "structural racism… xenophobic hostility, language barriers, poverty, inability to continue working in one's profession… and government surveillance" (2019, p. 122).

Exceptionality also figures as a problem in more commonly recognised cases of PTSD where the sufferer's case history fails to conform to overly narrow diagnostic criteria. Moss and Prince (2017) recount the case of Corporal Stuart Langridge, a Canadian soldier whose 2008 suicide garnered widespread media coverage about traumatised veterans. Although clearly suffering mental distress following two tours of duty in Bosnia and Afghanistan, Langridge's attempts to access psychiatric help for PTSD were unsuccessful because military psychiatrists could identify "no *single event* … that caused a psychiatric breakdown" (2017, p. 63 emphasis added). Psychiatrists instead attributed his problems to his alcohol use disorder, seemingly mistaking a common symptom of PTSD for its cause.

This case provides another example of the very concrete politics at play in many struggles over trauma and diagnosis. Following the scholarship on medicalisation, we note that claims to PTSD are often also claims on entitlements from medical authorities and ultimately the state. Many struggles over who is entitled to claim trauma succeed or fail based on where claimants are situated in relations of power and whose interests are served by recognising experiences as traumatic. Fassin and Rechtman (2009) note the struggles of soldiers in World War One to have shell-shock recognised as a legitimate psychiatric condition against a medical establishment that largely accused them of cowardice and malingering to avoid being sent back to the front. They contrast this with the near-immediate acceptance that large numbers of New Yorkers who witnessed the attacks of September 11th, 2001 subsequently suffered from PTSD. More than the passing of time has elapsed between these two events: what distinguishes them is whose interests are served in recognising trauma. In the first, a belligerent state is loath to admit the horrors endured by its soldiers; in the second, the state is eager to tout the suffering of its citizens as it builds support for war. Thus, while recognition of trauma is generally seen as politically progressive – part of an openness to vulnerability and willingness to consider mental health that is still frequently attacked by a Right sceptical about the 'therapeutic' society – these examples remind us that acknowledging trauma is far from universally progressive (Sitman and Adler-Bell, 2023). This resonates with Judith Butler's argument about grief and mourning, in which "certain forms of grief become nationally recognized and amplified, whereas other losses become unthinkable and ungrievable" (2004, p. xiv). Trauma, clearly, is as much a question of power as pathology.

As these critics have demonstrated, forms of suffering that do not conform to the model of exceptional, singular, overwhelming events should be included in conversations about trauma. At the same time, it is worth considering whether our political efforts to expand trauma in this way raise additional problems. This political question is matched by the theoretical question of why it is, today, that there is such an imperative to recognise all forms of distress as trauma: why is it that concepts like *suffering* no longer suffice? While a thorough analysis of this question is beyond my scope here, I suggest that there is a case to be made for distinguishing trauma from something like suffering, without creating a hierarchy between them. Psychiatric and psychotherapeutic research suggests that events that are exceptional, shocking and overwhelming like assaults, accidents, and catastrophes tend to produce symptoms that are distinct from those that result from ongoing, everyday suffering and indicate that different mechanisms are involved in their psychical processing. This does not mean that the suffering that results from pervasive systemic oppression is any less serious (not least because exceptional traumas are themselves more common for those who are also oppressed), simply that different concepts may be required. To take just a few: Arline T. Geronimus's concept of 'weathering' (2023) describes the negative health effects of social exclusion from cumulative forms of intersectional oppression, leading to a wearing-down of populations through a variety of forms including disease, poor maternal and infant health, and physiological stress responses. Case and Deaton's 'deaths of despair' thesis seeks to explain increases in midlife mortality and morbidity among poor whites in the United States through increased rates of suicide, drug poisoning, and chronic liver disease, and ties these to the political economic shifts that have led to the "broad deterioration in the lives of Americans without a college degree" (2018, p. 2).

Alongside these, critical medical anthropologists have developed a host of frameworks for making sense of the subjective experience of socially and politically produced harms, from Kleinman, Lock and Das's (1997) 'social suffering' to Singer and Toledo's 'oppression illness' (1995; see also Bourgois, 1995; Garcia, 2010; Singer *et al.*, 1992). With such a robust array of concepts to choose from, why not reserve trauma for cases displaying its unique symptomatology? As critical scholars often remind us, trauma is, originally, a psychological account of suffering – with all the medicalisation and individualisation this implies. In these efforts to make trauma into something less psychological, it sometimes appears as if critics expend a great deal of energy making it conform to concepts like suffering that already exist, and in so doing, rob it of its analytic utility. At the same time, there is something essential in the political work done by the move towards systematic, everyday 'trauma'. As Cvetkovich (2003) persuasively argues, it is through the everyday that we grasp the structural production of trauma. Understood as something exceptional, trauma can only ever be an experience of individuals, and likely something over which medicine exercises authority. When we shift focus to the everyday, we can begin to conceptualise it as structural rather than individual. In doing so, we encounter the possibility of building more than therapeutic relationships around trauma: we raise the possibility of solidarity, what Cvetkovich calls a "public culture around trauma that does not involve medical diagnoses or victims" (2003, p. 1). This is the promise of trauma beyond the exception.

Conclusion

On the question of why there is so much effort to expand the concept of trauma, one answer, of course, is simply that trauma is having a moment. Writing in the *New York Times*, Danielle Carr observes that in recent years, between Trump, #Metoo, and reckonings with white supremacy, trauma has become 'the inflationary currency through which we transact our lives" (2023, n.p.). Much of trauma's appeal is undoubtedly to do with what Carr calls the "scientific sheen" that the diagnosis of PTSD provides. In its increasingly neurobiological framing, trauma now promises an objective, identifiable name for all manner of injury. In my own research with drug users, I remember vividly one man's bitter complaints about veterans from Iraq being afforded diagnoses of PTSD while his own suffering from childhood abuse and solitary confinement in prison was ignored or minimised. Here again we encounter the problem of whose suffering is recognised and whose is discounted.

There are also increasing signs of unease about the ubiquity of trauma, not just from the Right but also within progressive circles. Critical geographers often feel obliged to note, in otherwise approving engagements, that trauma is now an "overused" concept (Pain, 2021, p. 973), while cultural critics such as Parul Sehal (2021) argue that "the trauma plot" has become so omnipresent in fiction that human subjectivity is reduced to little more than the sum of our tragedies. Huw Green (2022), meanwhile, writes that "when mental health is given as a principal motivator for our choices… there is less room for moral or ethical considerations". To focus too much on mental health potentially obscures the political and ethical stakes of a situation and ignores how difficult experiences "can at times be part of what makes for a life worth living" (n.p.). Echoing many of the arguments of critical geographers, Danielle Carr argues that the broader turn towards mental health, of which trauma discourse is a part, risks reifying the political economic structures that actually produce harms. When economic insecurity, war, and pandemics upend every aspect of our emotional lives, we are forced to recognise that "a crisis that *affects* mental health is not the same thing as a crisis *of* mental health" (2022, n.p.). Indeed, if there are reasons to be concerned with the omnipresence of trauma, one might be that it shifts attention from the sources of suffering to how suffering *feels*, with all the potential losses of precision and culpability that this entails. Of course, there are progressive strategic reasons for shifting attention in this way, deploying mental health as a discourse for manoeuvring around ossified political debates – just as the health inequalities literature was able to draw renewed attention to economic inequality by focusing on the politically neutral good of 'health'. Beyond these questions of strategy, the question remains: What value is there in focussing on trauma – on how oppression feels – when critical geographers are most concerned with contesting that oppression? Trauma may well be an inherently individualising, psychologising framework, and its greatest value may lie in what that particular scalar lens can reveal. In our efforts to contest the structural sources of suffering, we might be best served by thinking of trauma as the affective medium through which structural forces are expressed: worth attending to, but only insofar as it illuminates rather than mystifies those forces.

References

Adams-Hutcheson, G. (2017) 'Spatialising skin: Pushing the boundaries of trauma geographies', *Emotion, Space and Society*, 24, pp. 105–112.

Berlant, L.G. (2011) *Cruel Optimism*. Durham: Duke University Press.

Bourgois, P. (1995) *In Search of Respect: Selling Crack in El Barrio*. Cambridge: Cambridge University Press.

Brown, L. (1995) 'Not Outside the Range: One Feminist Perspective on Psychic Trauma', in C. Caruth (ed.) *Trauma: Explorations in Memory*. Baltimore: Johns Hopkins University Press, pp. 100–112.

Butler, J. (2004) *Precarious Life: The Powers of Mourning and Violence*. London; New York: Verso.

Carr, D. (2022) 'Opinion | Mental Health Is Political', *The New York Times*, 20 September. Available at: www.nytimes.com/2022/09/20/opinion/us-mental-health-politics.html (Accessed: 3 August 2023).

Carr, D. (2023) *How Trauma Became America's Favorite Diagnosis, Intelligencer*. Available at: https://nymag.com/intelligencer/article/trauma-bessel-van-der-kolk-the-body-keeps-the-score-profile.html (Accessed: 2 August 2023).

Caruth, C. (ed.) (1995) *Trauma: Explorations in Memory*. Baltimore: Johns Hopkins University Press.

Caruth, C. (1996) *Unclaimed Experience: Trauma, Narrative and History*. 1st ed. Baltimore: Johns Hopkins University Press.

Case, A. and Deaton, A. (2018) 'Deaths of Despair Redux: A Response to Christopher Ruhm', 8 January. Available at: www.princeton.edu/~accase/downloads/Case_and_Deaton_Comment_on_CJRuhm_Jan_2018.pdf (Accessed: 24 September 2018).

Coddington, K. (2017) 'Contagious trauma: Reframing the spatial mobility of trauma within advocacy work', *Emotion, Space and Society*, 24, pp. 66–73.

Coddington, K. and Micieli-Voutsinas, J. (2017) 'On trauma, geography, and mobility: Towards geographies of trauma', *Emotion, Space and Society*, 24, pp. 52–56.

Cvetkovich, A. (2003) *An Archive of Feelings: Trauma, Sexuality, and Lesbian Public Cultures*. Durham, NC: Duke University Press (Series Q).

Dear, M.J. and Wolch, J.R. (1987) *Landscapes of Despair: From Deinstitutionalization to Homelessness*. Cambridge: Polity.

Ehrkamp, P., Loyd, J.M. and Secor, A. (2019) 'Embodiment and Memory in the Geopolitics of Trauma', in K. Mitchell, R. Jones, and J.L. Fluri (eds) *Handbook on Critical Geographies of Migration*. Cheltenham, UK: Edward Elgar Publishing.

Ehrkamp, P., Loyd, J.M. and Secor, A.J. (2022) 'Trauma as displacement: Observations from refugee resettlement', *Annals of the American Association of Geographers*, 112(3), pp. 715–722.

Fanon, F. (1967) *The Wretched of the Earth*. Translated by C. Farrington. London: Penguin.

Fassin, D. and Rechtman, R. (2009) *The Empire of Trauma: An Inquiry into the Condition of Victimhood*. Princeton: Princeton University Press.

Garcia, A. (2010) *The Pastoral Clinic: Addiction and Dispossession Along the Rio Grande*. Berkeley: University of California Press.

Geronimus, D.A. (2023) *Weathering: The Extraordinary Stress of Ordinary Life on the Body in an Unjust Society*. London: Virago.

Green, H. (2022) 'Opinion | We Have Reached Peak "Mental Health"', *The New York Times*, 20 September. Available at: www.nytimes.com/2022/09/20/opinion/us-mental-health-awareness.html (Accessed: 3 August 2023).

Herman, J.L. (1992) 'Complex PTSD: A syndrome in survivors of prolonged and repeated trauma', *Journal of Traumatic Stress*, 5(3), pp. 377–391.

Herman, J.L. (2001) *Trauma and Recovery*. London: Pandora.

Kirmayer, L.J. (1996) 'Landscapes of Memory: Trauma, Narrative, and Dissociation', in P. Antze and M. Lambek (eds) *Tense Past: Cultural Essays in Trauma and Memory*. New York: Routledge, pp. 173–198.

Kleinman, A., Das, V. and Lock, M.M. (eds) (1997) *Social Suffering*. Berkeley: University of California Press.

Leys, R. (2000) *Trauma: A Genealogy*. Chicago: University of Chicago Press.

Linz, J. (2021) 'Where crises converge: the affective register of displacement in Mexico City's post-earthquake gentrification', *Cultural Geographies*, 28(2), pp. 285–300.

Loyd, J.M., Ehrkamp, P. and Secor, A.J. (2018) 'A geopolitics of trauma: Refugee administration and protracted uncertainty in Turkey', *Transactions of the Institute of British Geographers*, 43(3), pp. 377–389.

Moss, P. and Prince, M.J. (2017) 'Helping traumatized warriors: Mobilizing emotions, unsettling orders', *Emotion, Space and Society*, 24, pp. 57–65.

Mountz, A. (2017) 'Island detention: Affective eruption as trauma's disruption', *Emotion, Space and Society*, 24, pp. 74–82.

Pain, R. (2021) 'Geotrauma: Violence, place and repossession', *Progress in Human Geography*, 45(5), pp. 972–989.

Perera, S. (2010) 'Torturous dialogues: Geographies of trauma and spaces of exception', *Continuum*, 24(1), pp. 31–45.

Pratt, G., Johnston, C. and Banta, V. (2017) 'Filipino migrant stories and trauma in the transnational field', *Emotion, Space and Society*, 24, pp. 83–92.

Proudfoot, J. (2019) 'Traumatic landscapes: Two geographies of addiction', *Social Science & Medicine*, 228, pp. 194–201.

Proudfoot, J. (2023) 'The dreamwork of the symptom: Reading structural racism and family history in a drug addiction', *Culture, Medicine, and Psychiatry*, 47(4), pp. 961–981.

Pulido, L. (2000) 'Rethinking environmental racism: White privilege and urban development in Southern California', *Annals of the Association of American Geographers*, 90(1), pp. 12–40.

Sehgal, P. (2021) 'The Case Against the Trauma Plot', *The New Yorker*, 27 December 2021. Available at: www.newyorker.com/magazine/2022/01/03/the-case-against-the-trauma-plot

Singer, M. *et al.* (1992) 'Why does Juan García have a drinking problem? The perspective of critical medical anthropology', *Medical Anthropology*, 14(1), pp. 77–108.

Singer, M. and Toledo, E. (1995) Oppression Illness: Critical Theory and Intervention with Women at Risk for AIDS'. *American Anthropological Association Meeting*, Washington, DC.

Sitman, M. and Adler-Bell, S. (2023) 'Know Your Enemy: Triumph of the Therapeutic, with Hannah Zeavin and Alex Colston', *Dissent Magazine*. Available at: www.dissentmagazine.org/blog/know-your-enemy-triumph-therapeutic/ (Accessed: 9 April 2024).

Till, K.E. (1999) 'Staging the past: Landscape designs, cultural identity and Erinnerungspolitik at Berlin's Neue Wache'.

Till, K.E. (2003) 'Places of Memory', in J. Agnew, K. Mitchell, and G. Toal (eds) *A Companion to Political Geography*. Malden, MA, USA: Blackwell Publishing, pp. 289–301.

Van der Kolk, B.A. (2014) *The Body Keeps the Score: Mind, Brain and Body in the Transformation of Trauma*. London: Penguin Books.

Wakefield, S. and McMullan, C. (2005) 'Healing in places of decline: (Re)imagining everyday landscapes in Hamilton, Ontario', *Health & Place*, 11(4), pp. 299–312.

Walker, J. (2010) 'Moving testimonies and the geography of suffering: Perils and fantasies of belonging after Katrina', *Continuum*, 24(1), pp. 47–64.

Young, A. (1995) *The Harmony of Illusions: Inventing Post-Traumatic Stress Disorder*. Princeton, NJ: Princeton University Press.

Institutional and post-institutional spaces

38 Introduction to institutional and post-institutional spaces

Ebba Högström

The provision of mental health care, support and service is tightly connected to *Institutional and post-institutional spaces*, the theme of this final section. Mental health care provisions belong to a history of treatment, care, support, ordering practices, and spatial arrangements – a history of how different modalities (Moon, Kearns, and Joseph, 2015) have succeeded each other, oscillating between notions of progress and 'not-fit-for-purpose'; e.g., care modalities (innovation in drugs vs. counselling therapies), location modalities (the rural vs. the urban), facilities modalities (huge institutions vs. small-scale facilities). It is a spatial story which has been largely labelled as a shift from 'asylum to post-asylum geographies' (Philo, 2000), and the word 'institution' itself embodies both 'space' – as buildings, rooms, premises, rooms, accommodations, grounds, landscapes, and 'organisation' – as ordering, habits, routines, norms. Space and organisation are thus intertwined, in reinforcing or hindering caring and supporting, or in coercive and controlling practices, as well as in affecting the lived experience, positively and negatively, of those inhabiting these.

Engagement in the overall theme of the handbook, in the spaces for mental health and wellbeing, is also an engagement in 'other spaces' – all those spaces designed and organised for situations when mental health and wellbeing is weakened and when more-or-less organised care, support and/or treatment is considered needed (voluntarily or not). How to best care, but also control and sometimes cure – or in the 'care in the community' vocabulary, to support and give service – has been on the mental health care agenda throughout its long history (Topp, 2016). This is a recurrent issue of both institutional and post-institutional mental health care with clear spatial connotations, especially for architecture (the way space is organised and designed) and localisation (relating to the urban fabric or rural context). All these spaces have varied dramatically by place and period in purpose, scale, and boundedness, from the isolated, sizeable, and often repressive 'lunatic asylum' of the eighteenth-century Global North, to the 'deinstitutionalisation' era (Kritsokaki, Long and Smith, 2016) which extended forward from the 1960s and was characterised by the opening of smaller-scale mental health facilities run by state, voluntary and private sectors as a new 'social infrastructure' in the local communities (Högström, Berglund-Snodgrass & Fjellfeldt, 2022). Even though severely critiqued, the institution has not entirely disappeared, as there is still a need (if disputed) for some people to get psychiatric inpatient treatment, for shorter and sometimes longer periods (what Curtis et al [2009] have called 'the rebirth of the clinic'). The institution thus

DOI: 10.4324/9781003345725-43

remains but in variant forms, as for example psychiatric inpatient clinics, mental health centres, user clubs, sheltered work and supported accommodations. The institutional characteristics are more (the clinic) or less (the supported accommodation) obvious and more (the clinic) or less (the accommodations) contested.

This section on *Institutional and post-institutional spaces* critically examines a variety of spatial arrangments of mental health care. As a point of departure from past and recent transformations – from ideas of a more humane care within the asylum system in the beginning of the twentieth century (Philo, 2004) to contemporary post-deinstitutionalised support and service in the community (Markström, Högström & Fjellfeldt, 2023), see also the section *Spaces of Home and Work* in this edited collection) to psychiatric survivor-led questioning of the entire global psychiatric system (Beresford, 2020) – different perspectives on institutional and post-institutional spaces are explored. At the centre stand nuanced empirical investigations, theoretical analyses and creative engagements of contemporary and historical spatial arrangements for people with mental ill-health, as well as a sensitivity to the lived experiences of people affected by these spatial arrangements. Furthermore, a sensitivity to the context of broader societal change, setting the frames for the development of institutional care and post-institutional support and service, permeates the chapters.

Contributors to this section reflect on institutional and post-institutional spaces, ranging from psychiatric clinics, asylums, islands, mental health care spaces in local communities to the mental health care system as a whole. These varied ways of looking at institutionalised and post-institutionalised spaces reflect the many starting points for approaching this topic as well as different research fields. In this section, scholars from organisation studies, geography, sociology, psychology, history, creative writing and architecture analyse and discuss a variety of cases in relation to the section's theme.

Visions of 'healing architecture' and the process of translating these to spatial organisation and design is discussed by **Simonsen** with the example of a newly opened psychiatric clinic in Denmark. He explores how this novel synthesis of ideas is developed in the design process and in what way the concept of 'healing architecture' makes a difference in practice. Simonsen aims to better understand how the spatial organisation of contemporary psychiatric clinics impacts the complex and contingent interactions between staff and patients, as well as processes of recovery and wellbeing. **Kearns and Connell** survey the links between islands, institutions and mental wellbeing, and point to islands' ambigious reputation, on the one hand sites for finding solitude and respite from the stressful mainland life (which relates this chapter to the section *Green/ Blue Spaces* of this edited collection) and on the other offering feelings of entrapment. There is a history of deploying islands as institutional spaces, as places of exile for recovery and restoration, whether chosen or imposed. As such, islands mirror asylums, they conclude, in their boundedness, separation and the idea that cure is more likely to be found in isolated and focused environments. The concept 'total landscapes', drawing from Goffman's (1961/1976) 'total institution', is coined by **Topor, Bøe, Hope, Ness & Friesinger** to characterise contemporary post-institutionalised spaces. Using as an example the social psychiatry services in a region of Norway, they describe the total institutional landscape as comprising a tight network of new social and cultural places, including elements of total institutions. This whole system of places for care in the community, they point out in the chapter, is building a rich network of potentially enabling places, yet also of tight control.

From the post-institutional space (or landscape) of today, we travel back to the early twentieth century and the first wave of modern psychiatric care where **Guillemain &** **Ferrari,** with the example of the village hospital, trace the transfer of ideas of the built and natural environment's role in 'curing madness'. Focusing on the circulation of the so-called Open Door model (the idea of 'healing architecture' of the time developed between Argentina and Europe, predominantly France) this global historical account of psychiatry shows what was generated and applied in both countries, and what didn't travel. **Repo** present an analysis based on her research on psychiatric clinics in Finland. In the chapter, she highlights the connection between care, risk and the carceral – as well as their spatial meaning in institutions – by introducing the concept of 'carceral riskscapes'. All these aspects are intertwined, influencing everyday life in care institutions. In the conclusion, Repo argues that acknowledging the mechanisms of inequality is a first step to supporting and consequently improving institutional care and advancing wellbeing in institutions.

In the chapter by **McDougall,** the creative project "Writing the Asylum" is presented. She invited 28 artist and writers to work creatively with the archive material from Gartnavel Royal Asylum in Glasgow, Scotland. The collaborative and public engagement project with the motto 'all voices are valued' is a celebration of asylum and post-asylum geographies taking as its starting point Gartnavel, a site of spatial change of specific historic cultural significance. Stories based on lived experience from the archive are mediated by poetry, fiction, and art leading to queries on what we would like to remember and hand down to subsequent generations. The final chapter of this section and the whole handbook take on a quite different perspective on institutional and post-institutional spaces – the problematic of whether the mental health system itself should exist, or conversely, be abolished. **Högström and Philo** explore this question in their chapter, recognising that answers necessarily acquire complexity and nuance due to the vulnerable and indeed often suffering character of people accessing mental healthcare provisions. Their conclusion is that mental health geography has tended to work – but also probably *should* work 'in the cracks' between abolition and reform, precisely because of what psychiatric 'user-survivors' often value about places where they have a sense of belonging *even* when those places have compromised origins, histories and functions.

To summarise, this section provides a thought-provoking overview of institutional and post-institutional spaces of different scales, geographies and situations and the different ways of organising and designing spaces for housing, treating, caring, controlling and recovering of people with mental ill-health. A theme that might be considered as the dark or at least more shaded side of mental health and wellbeing, as it concerns the spaces for (in one way or the other) people suffering from mental ill-health and illbeing – sometime through a recovery approach, sometimes directly intervening in curative and/ or controlling practices. All contributions in the section operate from a spatial perspective and examine the influence spatial organisation and design, in terms of architecture, localisation and landscapes, has had on institutions and the way care and support is/was supposed to be implemented. While the examples represent an array of different spatio-temporal engagements, when taken together in relation to the central theme of the handbook, Spaces of Mental Health and Wellbeing, they emphasise the impact institutional and post-institutional spaces have had, and still have, on how we look upon mental ill-health, recovery and liveable lives. A common thread running through the contributions in this section is that the spatial answers on the 'where', 'how' and 'why' in relation to the question of what good care, support and service comprise has changed over time and geography. This section shows that such questions are recurrently posed, and rightly so, yet the most important is that the answers should always be critically examined.

References

Beresford, P. (2020) 'Mad', Mad studies and advancing inclusive resistance. *Disability & Society*, 35(8), 1337–1342.

Curtis, S., Gesler, W., Priebe, S., & Francis, S. (2009) New spaces of inpatient care for people with mental illness: A complex 'rebirth' of the clinic? *Health Place* 15, 340–348.

Goffman, E. (1961/1990) *Asylums: Essays on the social situation of mental patients and other inmates*. New York: Doubleday.

Högström, E., Berglund-Snodgrass, L., & Fjellfeldt, M. (2022) Editorial: The challenges of social infrastructure for urban planning. *Urban Planning*, 7(4), 377–380. Editorial of special issue: Localizing Social Infrastructures: Welfare, Equity, and Community.

Kritsotaki, D., Long, V., & Smith, S. (Eds.). (2016) *Deinstitutionalisation and after: Post-war psychiatry in the western world*. London: Palgrave Macmillan.

Markström, U., Högström, E., & Fjellfeldt, M. (2023) Mental health supported accommodation services in a post-deinstitutionalised era, *Alter*, 17-3, 39–56.

Moon, G., Kearns, R. A., & Joseph, A. E. (2015) *The afterlives of the psychiatric asylum: Recycling concepts, sites and memories*. Farnham: Ashgate

Philo, C. (2004) *A geographical history of institutional provision for the insane from medieval times to the 1860s in England and Wales: 'The space reserved for insanity'*. Lewiston, Queenston and Lampeter: Edwin Mellen Press.

Philo, C. (2000) Post-asylum geographies: An introduction. *Health & Place*, 6, 135–136.

Topp, L. (2016) *Freedom and the cage: Modern architecture and psychiatry in Central Europe, 1890-1914*. University Park, Pennsylvania: The Pennsylvania State University Press.

39 'Healing architecture' and the spatial organisation of the psychiatric clinic

Thorben Peter Høj Simonsen

Introduction

From the early modern period to the present, designing alternative spaces and constructing purposive architecture, whether conceived of as custodial or curative, has been a predominant social response, epsecially in the West, for managing those deemed deviant or mentally troubled (Topp et al., 2007). In this way, psychiatric architecture is linked to changing patterns of psychiatric discourse and treatment and, thus, bound to the forms of medical theorising operant at the moment of construction (Prior, 1988), creating an inseparable "[…] relationship between social and cultural forms on the one hand, and built and spatial forms on the other" (King, 1980, p. 3). Michel Foucault's (1961) excavation of the relationships between epistemology and spatiality in psychiatry have been highly influential in this regard, and his work (e.g., 1973a, 1973b, 1961) demonstrates that the spatiality of any given situation is subject to various historical transformations within a public order of discourse and technology, making the architectural representations of a time contingent upon these.

Through a synthesis of functional demands and sensory impressions, the emergence of so-called 'healing architecture' is certainly transforming the institutional spaces of psychiatric care, producing what the German philosopher Peter Sloterdijk (2016) might recognise as the development of a novel 'alphabet of forms' (see also Simonsen and Højlund, 2018). While Sloterdijk does not refer to the development of 'healing architecture', he addresses how the broader architectural developments of modernity are all about the spatial production of an artificial milieu, a "spelling-out" or "explication" of particular living conditions (Sloterdijk, 2016), where natural environments are increasingly replaced by technical ones (Sloterdijk, 2017). Contemporary ideas of 'healing architecture' in psychiatric hospitals, rather than replace the natural with the technical, seek to create a sort of atmospheric composite in which the natural, or at least a version of the natural, is sustained by, and juxtaposed to, the technical.

Exploring such spatial transformations in considering the relations between hospital architecture and medical discourse entails navigating a "complex terrain" (McGrath and Reavey, 2018). While we might have witnessed a decline of the general hospital as a healing machine during the twentieth century due to the rise of especially neurobiological approaches that focused on biomedical rather than therapeutic means to support recovery (Theodore, 2017), contemporary developments are surely reanimating the idea of the hospital as a therapeutic operator, a "curing machine", as Foucault (1973b) would have it, built to work on both bodies and practices. Johannessen and Holm (2021),

DOI: 10.4324/9781003345725-44

however, have recently argued that the medicalisation of contemporary hospital architecture, rather than representing a return to, and a reinvigoration of, ideas from previous decades, marks an affective reformulation of the role of architecture as an instrument for healing (Johannessen and Holm, 2021). Contemporary hospital architecture is in other words designed to target not only the fleshy body but also its senses, marking what Johannesen and Holm (2021) conceptualise as a historical and biopolitical shift in architectural focus: from the somatic to the affective. This shifts the focus away from the body as immune system and towards the body as sensorium.

While no shared or operative definition of 'healing architecture' currently exists (Simonsen et al., 2022), its uptake in contemporary architectural practice nonetheless goes to show how hospitals are being designed to have an impact and to promote patient recovery by (re)imagining inpatient settings as therapeutic environments (see also Gesler et al., 2004). Although the notion of recovery expresses a variety of conceptual understandings and modes of practice (Hummelvol et al., 2015), and has been historically linked to processes of deinstitutionalisation (Spaulding, 2016), at the turn of the century, it became a widely accepted term in mental health care in Denmark, figuring in national standards, guidelines, and policies. In this chapter, rather than seek to define or specify the notions of healing and recovery, I consider how architects interpret them. In Denmark the interest in architecture with alleged recovery supporting and healing capacities became both apparent and possible with the 2007 Structural Reform. Here, the state massively invested in transforming and future-proofing the Danish hospital system, representing what Johannessen (2022, p. 311) identifies as a "historic opportunity to recalibrate the relationship between architecture, medicine and welfare on a large scale." Like the notion of the hospital as a healing machine, 'healing architecture' functions as a normative concept about the ideal hospital arrangement, and the hospital, as Theodore (2017, p. 187) describes it, should "be a place not just where a sick patient *might* get better, but the instrument or machine that would cause a cure."

Although the architecture of psychiatric hospitals has changed dramatically over the last 50 years (Nord and Högström, 2017a), due, especially, to a shift in psychiatric treatment from containment to recovery (Jovanović et al., 2019), changes in the way we think about medical spaces may be less profound than first assumed. As Nord and Högström (2017a) observe, far from simply replacing the old with the new, contemporary architectural designs may for instance draw simultaneously on medical and organisational ideas from the early twentieth century and current ideas about commercial environments. Importantly, as Adams (2008) has pointed out in relation to interwar hospital architecture, but which rings true of contemporary designs as well, hospital architecture does not simply reflect medical innovations. Rather, the relations between medicine and architecture are dynamic, with the ensuing building typologies an effect of intricate relations between heterogeneous stakeholders, such as architects, health-care professionals, and users (Adams, 2008). As opposed to the asylum era, contemporary developments do not reflect any one dominant building type (Bruun Petersen et al., 2013) and the confluence of modern architectural assumptions and current medical values create a "deceptively complex matrix of levels of engagement" (Astbury, 2016, p. 4) in which the architecture is thought to be a subtle facilitator and mediator.

In contrast to the disciplinary and closed institutions depicted by Foucault (1977, 1961) and Goffman (1961), new inpatient facilities are becoming ever more permeable (Quirk et al., 2006) and functioning as spaces of transition (Curtis et al., 2009; Wood et al., 2013). Quirk and colleagues (2006) suggest the notion of permeability as an ideal type to describe the increasingly open and flexible environments of contemporary inpatient settings, an idea which Wood (2013) and Curtis (2009) develop by proposing that such permable institutional settings encourage greater interaction with the surrounding community, indeed operatating as 'spaces of transition', where patients are prepared for the move from the institutional space to community living. These spatial reorganisations reflect interpretations of contemporary models of care (Bromley, 2012; Vaughan et al., 2018). As such, heavy opaque walls, and the sequestered spaces they enclose, have been progressively replaced by transparent glass structures and open flexible spaces, combined with an effort to bring 'Nature' into the built environment (Connellan et al., 2013; McGrath and Reavey, 2018; Reavey et al., 2017).

As this chapter will show, architects and other involved stakeholders have had the interpretative space to develop what 'healing architecture' in psychiatry might mean, "etching" (Gieryn, 2002) their interests into the hospital building itself. Put differently, and as Gieryn (2002) explains, the design (of 'healing architecture') is simultaneously a representation of a particular architectural form and the enrolment of allies necessary to make such form manifest. In the following, I consider the architectural visions and spatial forms of a new psychiatric hospital in Denmark, widely considered an inspiration, if not a standard, for healing architecture in the development of the future of psychiatric institutions in the Nordic countries. By exploring the architectural plans and documents and by drawing on interviews with the lead architect and key stakeholders involved in the process of design, I show how a novel synthesis of ideas is developed in the process of coming to terms with how 'healing architecture' is understood and how it is imagined to *work*. While I primarily focus on the conditions of production in this chapter – on how 'healing architecture' is a phenomenon rooted in the changing spatial formations of psychiatry – the implications of the conditions of possibility that follow are equally important to investigate. Indeed, coming to terms with how 'healing architecture' makes a difference *in practice* is key to better understanding how the spatial organisation of the psychiatric clinic of today shapes the complex and contingent interactions between staff and patients, as well as processes of recovery and well-being. I return to these questions in conclusion as I discuss how to study healing architecture in practice.

Designing 'healing architecture'

Ulrich's original work (1984, 2010, 2008b) on evidence-based-design has been a key reference guiding research on healthcare facilities and how these may be designed to support and promote wellbeing. This movement (Theodore, 2017), echoing the notion of evidence-based-medicine, seeks to measure and evaluate architectural, spatial, and material properties of the built environment based on evidence gathered from scientific studies. Ulrich's 1984 paper 'View through a window may influence recovery from surgery' is in this respect considered a turning point for healthcare design, shifting the focus towards the relations between the human and the environment, and especially towards how affective responses to both built and natural environments have an impact on recovery and healing. In later developments, a number of key design factors and spatial types have been identified and linked to improved mental health outcomes (Connellan et al., 2013; Reavey et al., 2017) as well as in relation to the development of therapeutic environments in hospital settings (Curtis et al., 2007; Gesler et al., 2004), including, but not limited to, single rooms, views to nature, wayfinding, personal control, privacy, and lighting (e.g., Frandsen et al., 2009; Lawson, 2010; Simonsen et al., 2022; Ulrich et al.,

2008b). Private rooms have become the norm (Folmer, 2014), just like facilitating social interactions has become a key component for the promotion of recovery in 'healing architecture' (Frandsen et al., 2009). While there is substantive evidence (Connellan et al., 2013; Curtis et al., 2007; Reavey et al., 2017; Ulrich et al., 2008a) that these different elements have a positive impact on health outcomes, their collective integration into specific architectural forms continue to be explored.

'The road to recovery': The psychiatric hospital in Slagelse

In the fall of 2015, approximately 650 employees from five psychiatric facilities in Region Zealand were relocated to the new psychiatric hospital at Slagelse. This new build reflects broader political interests in, and developments of, hospital buildings in Denmark, with 41,4 billion DKK currently invested in the construction of new healthcare facilities. The psychiatric hospital in Slagelse makes manifest the ambition to establish a world class psychiatric facility (Region Denmark, 2009) by making the 'road to recovery' manifest in built form (Astbury, 2016). Karlsson Architects and Vilhelm Lauritsen Architects spearheaded the project under the title A *lighthouse for the future of psychiatric building*, with the new building reflecting current trends in healthcare design, including access to and oversight of green spaces, proximity to the local community and the use of advanced lighting technology to reflect everyday rhythms. Since its inception, the design has won several awards, among others 'the Oscar of the real estate industry' – the MIPIM Award 2017 for Best Healthcare Development. As a reason for the award, the jury pointed to the innovative thinking and architecture's great role in healing patients. The building has thus been recognised as being at the frontline of redefining the way patients are treated in psychiatry today, with the architecture obviously being ascribed an important part of transforming what that means. The lead architect of the project explains in an interview I conducted how they were invited to consider and suggest new forms of treatment as part of the project proposal, which "in a way isn't a task for an architect", but, as he subsequently reflects, "you might make it one." (Interview 2017, Lead architect).

Karlsson Architects and Vilhelm Lauritzen Architects won the architectural competition for the Slagelse site with their project proposal *The house in the park, the park in the house* which, according to Project Director, had the "innovative approach they were looking for" (Interview 2017, Project director). During initial phases of development, the design office went looking for inspiration at other sites, nationally and internationally, but, as the lead architect explained, they returned disappointed:

> It was a disappointment. We expected to find the state of the art in Germany or in the US in terms of healing architecture, but we didn't and neither did the hospital management. We didn't find anything in Norway or Sweden, and what we encountered in Holland and in the UK was completely discouraging [...] We were forced to admit that we had to develop something ourselves. (Lead architect in Region Denmark n.d.)

Clearly this interpretation of the state of affairs of contemporary healthcare designs affords the architect a space of interpretation and, as a result, the design office developed its own approach to the question of what healing architecture might look like:

We started with the thesis that, what is good for all of us – is also good for those of us who are sick. It just needs to be scaled. And then suddenly it became quite simple to define healing architecture. (Lead architect in Region Denmark n.d.)

The lead architect clearly renders the notion of 'healing architecture' open to interpretation. Indeed, the architects are invited to imagine and develop the spatial circumstances for contemporary psychiatric treatment. However, it was important to the hospital management to create something that was different from the Victorian asylums, as the Vice-Director of Psychiatry in Region Zealand explains in an interview with the lead architect:

[…] something that can be a counterpart to the role psychiatry has had in society. Sct. Hans was built 150 years ago; it was placed outside the city, far away, and wasn't something people really knew about. Psychiatry was something that was hidden. Now we are placing it in the city, close by, and making it into something open, transparent. (Vice-Director of Psychiatry, Region Zealand in Karlsson Arkitekter/Vilhelm Lauritzen AS, 2015, p. 42)

The history of psychiatric architecture is evoked as something to avoid, with asylums of the past representing a crude spatial organisation that the new development should stand in contrast to. Symbolising openness towards the surrounding community was an explicit design goal from the outset of the building project, signaling a new direction for psychiatric practice in Denmark. In the words of the Director of Psychiatry in Region Zealand:

Here we get something [psychiatric hospital in Slagelse] open which is normally closed. It is transparent; it has glass that you can see through; you can see what's going on. That's openness, instead of the black box that characterizes psychiatry in many other places, and that we're struggling to combat and open up […] The physical environment treatment takes place in is given a completely different expression, showing openness, transparency, and that supports the changed attitude towards psychiatry we are trying to communicate to a society still living with a point of view dating back 30 years. (Director of Psychiatry, Region Zealand in Karlsson Arkitekter/Vilhelm Lauritzen AS, 2015, p. 43)

Placing the hospital near the surrounding community and directly across the general hospital was an important expression of the overall narrative of challenging existing ideas about psychiatric care as something dangerous or deviant. As the Director of Psychiatry in Region Zealand clearly indicates in the above quote, the notion of transparency follows both functional and symbolic lines, aiming to make psychiatry tangible and accessible to people outside the facility, as well as enabling intelligibility through visibility for people inside the facility.

A fundamental tenet of the overall design scheme was creating porous boundaries between the hospital and its surroundings, making visible what was once hidden. The building and its location thus aim to mark a shift in a particular discourse still shaping contemporary understandings of psychiatry, pushing a new narrative about an inclusive and transparent psychiatric practice enabled by an open and transparent architecture. More particularly though, Karlsson Architects and Vilhelm Lauritzen Architects developed four guiding principles during initial phases of development, which then

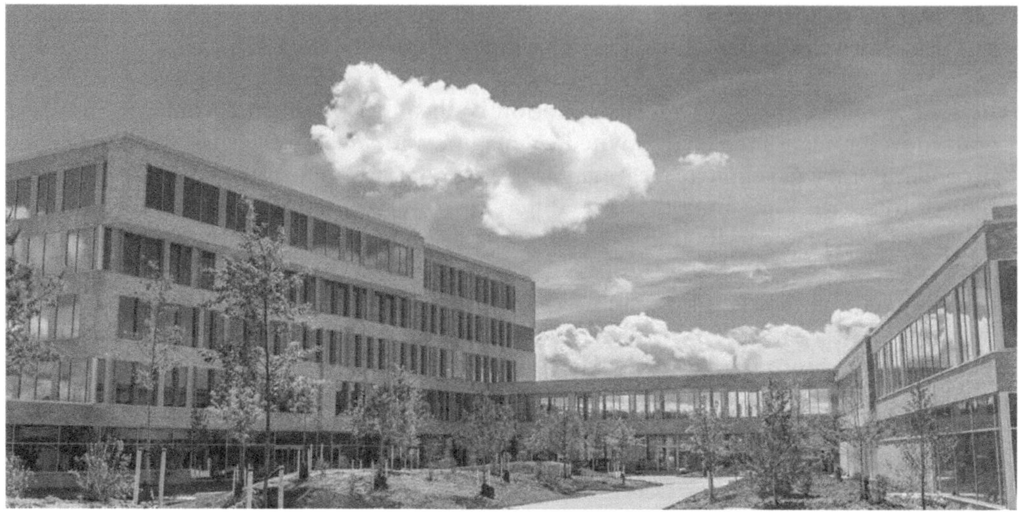

Figure 39.1 New Psychiatric Hospital Slagelse, Denmark. Photo by Karlsson Architects/Jens Linde.

informed all phases of construction. The design-principles guiding the development were: (i) Healing architecture and the principle of recovery; (ii) Transparency and proximity between people and functions; (iii) Generality and flexibility in rooms and sites; and (iv) Hierarchy of spaces and stimuli (Karlsson Arkitekter, n.d.). These principles are made manifest through a series of deliberate design interventions, including the widespread use of glass and open spaces.

The vision for the future of psychiatric treatment in Denmark (Region Denmark, 2009) is based on recent policy documents, explicating the importance of taking a recovery-oriented approach in inpatient and outpatient treatment (Region Zealand, 2008). Indeed, as Bruun Petersen and colleagues (2013, p. 45) contend, the recovery-oriented model poses new demands on the capabilities and capacities of contemporary psychiatric facilities, with the design of the psychiatric hospital in Slagelse seeking to to mirror the recovery-oriented model, now widely considered the prevalent psychiatric treatment paradigm (Hummelvol et al., 2015), also within inpatient care (Williams et al., 2012).

Transparency was considered crucial to the design, and enabling encounters between staff and patients ended up permeating the entire design based on the assumption that the architecture should facilitate meetings between people, with the hospital manifesting a meeting place in itself, "that is, a meeting place between people who need help and people who have the opportunity to help" (Interview, Lead architect, 2017). Helping people who need help is, one might argue, simply the organisational purpose, but the notion of meeting or encounter is extended well beyond this purpose, making it a key component in the hospital's spatial organisation.

Enabling encounters through architectural arrangements was closely tied to ideas of visibility; "that is, that you can find each other; see each other; that you are constantly present, but also that each individual can bring themselves best into play", as the lead architect explains (Interview, Lead architect, 2017). Designing meeting places entailed enabling visibility, as seeing each other, and ensuring that you are constantly present

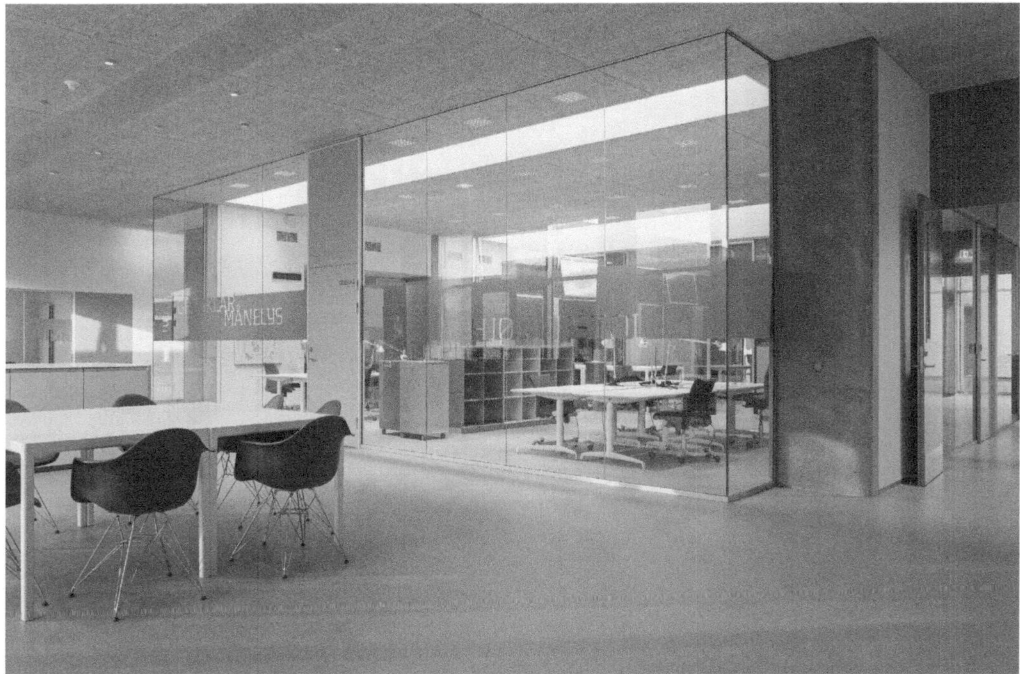

Figure 39.2 Nursing station within inpatient setting. Photo by Karlsson Architects/Jens Linde.

were considered important to psychiatric practice. This visibility was, furthermore, intended to facilitate predictability and intelligibility for patients during hospitalisation. Accordingly, the following definition of transparency was offered in a presentation of the project written by the architects' offices:

> [...] a precondition for understanding what is going on, overview and contact. Throughout the site, walls between common areas, living room spaces, conference rooms and work areas [are] made of glass from floor to ceiling. If necessary, a lightcurtain can change the transparency and character of the room. A sense of safety, for both patients and staff, is attained by being able to see and know that one isn't alone. (Karlsson Arkitekter/Vilhelm Lauritzen AS, 2015, p. 26)

According to the architects, being able to see what is going on and having an overview of spaces is deemed important for patients and staff. In an interview published by Region Denmark, the lead architect explained this sense of constant presence as being important for patients:

> Patients can see them [staff], sitting and working, having meetings, etc. They can see that when someone laughs, it's because someone said something funny [...] It's not because someone's laughing at me. That provides a sense of safety. And staff, on the other hand, can observe and see what's going on unhindered. They can quickly intervene if necessary. (Lead architect in Region Denmark, n.d., p. 5)

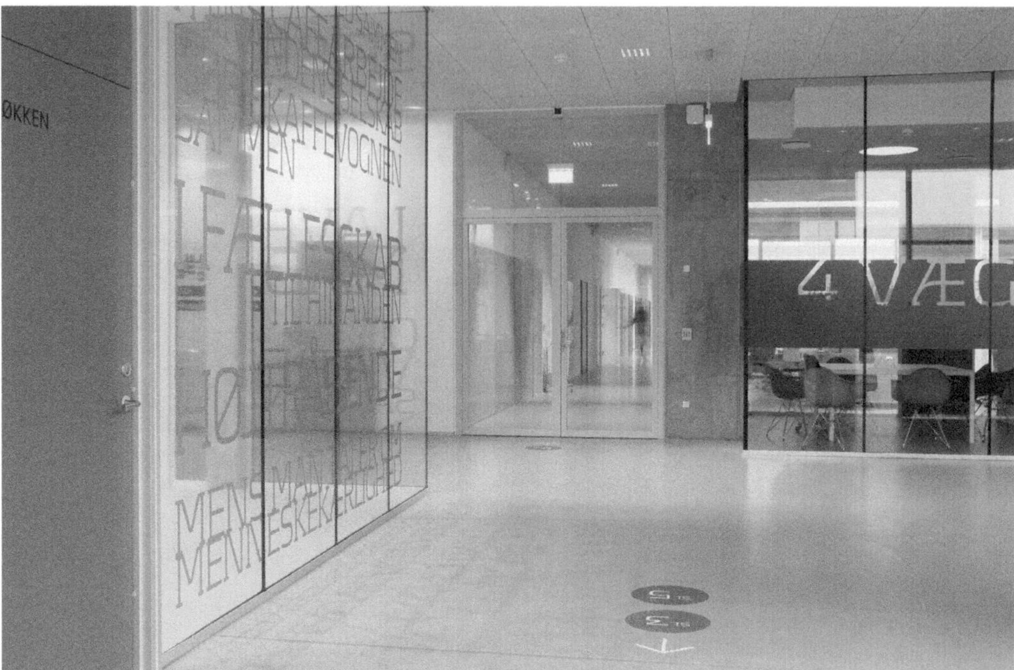

Figure 39.3 Hallways within hospital, showing wayfinding and transparency. Photo by Karlsson Architects/Jens Linde.

The intention was to create natural interaction (Jakobsen et al., 2014) between staff and patients through a series of deliberate design interventions, including the widespread use of glass to promote visibility, and the abundance of formal and informal common areas, establishing what the architects termed a hierarchy of spaces and stimuli. By changing the physical layout of inpatient settings, the hope was also that changes would occur in the work practices that maintain any distinctions between 'them' and 'us'. Perhaps the most salient of these interventions is the nursing station. The inspiration for this aesthetic and spatial organization was derived from modern offices, not psychiatric facilities. As the lead architect explains:

> [...] the whole thing about being able to see and understand what is happening. After all, that's something from our own world, our working life. Even if you're not immersed in it [the activity], you get a sense of what's going on, and who's who, and where you can go [to reach staff]. That concept of transparency was actually taken from office building conference rooms, you might say, and moved down. [...] It [transparency] might be even more important when in doubt about what's real, and who's who, and [wondering about] how close can we get to each other and stuff like that. We get an environment with people, where you can see people, and you can, to the best of your abilities, understand what's going on. (Interview, Lead architect, 2017)

Enabling the opportunity to see people is articulated as a precondition for comprehending what is going on with the hospital spaces thought to mirror the road to recovery. As such, the entire facility is designed to support a particular progression from removal of stimuli to their gradual reintroduction, with design interventions selected down to the choice of furniture based on the philosophy that staff and patients are considered equals. As I have shown elsewhere (Simonsen and Vikkelsø, 2022), when the architecture seeks such equality by creating flexible and open spaces, staff engage in the ongoing work of (re-) establishing social hierarchies. While inspired by the notion of recovery, the building also reflects contemporary technological developments, with LED lighting playing an especially important role in the design due to its ability, not only to reflect the time of day, but also to create spatial conditions by providing variation in lighting. The architecture is designed to function as a subtle facilitator and mediator, *working* towards healing and recovery.

Conclusion: how to study 'healing architecture'?

Although the contention that architectural properties and elements of the built environment can have a positive impact on treatment outcomes and experiences of healing is well-established, the dynamics of these relationships are far from settled (e.g., Andrews and Duff, 2019; Bell et al., 2018; Cummins et al., 2007). Conceptual developments related to green and blue spaces (Foley and Kistemann, 2015), therapeutic landscapes (Marcus and Sachs, 2013), enabling places (Duff, 2012), therapeutic assemblages (Foley, 2011), and healing spaces (DuBose et al., 2018) are part and parcel to developing our understanding of such dynamics, with increasing attention paid to the importance of design approaches as well (Duque et al., 2020; Stevens et al., 2019; Vaughan et al., 2018). These developments are particularly salient for the emerging discussions about the notion of 'healing architecture', particularly in relation to the development of healthcare innovations in the Nordic countries (e.g., Frandsen et al., 2009; Lundin, 2021, 2015). Interestingly, there is no common or operative definition of 'healing architecture' and there is limited knowledge of how 'healing architecture' actually shapes clinical and patient outcomes (Simonsen et al., 2022). Theodore (2017) critically engages with the broader assumptions about the healing effects of architecture, proposing that many of the ills produced by hospital environments are more about everyday practices, which, therefore, may be addressed through staff training rather than design. Indeed, as Theodore (2017, p. 196) contends, "the role of architecture is clearly secondary here to the cultural practice of hospital work." If we are to consider the significance of 'healing architecture', its impact on, and implications for, care practices in psychiatric settings, then, and in following Theodores critical interjection about the importance of hospital work, we should consider the relations between such work and the spatial arrangements afforded by the 'healing architecture' being developed and built. Especially if architecture is increasingly considered proxies for care (Johannessen and Holm, 2022).

The conceptualisation of biopolitical shifts in hospital architecture (Johannessen and Holm, 2021) notwithstanding, we might productively study 'healing architecture' as both a historically determinable phenomenon rooted in the changing spatial formations of psychiatry – as the accomplishment of particular conditions of production – *and* as circumstantial spatial arrangements in specific care settings – as particular conditions of possibility. Scholarship has on the one hand pointed out that architecture and the spatial organisation of care may best be understood in relation to discursive practices, highlighting how forms of medical knowledge are inextricably bound to the design and development of specific buildings (Prior, 1988). On the other hand, recent scholarship in

STS has highlighted the importance of better understanding the implications of particular spatial dispositions by studying specific spatial and material circumstances (d'Hoop, 2020; see also Moser, 2006). Bringing these ideas together enables a complementary analytical perspective, where the historicity of particular spatial forms – where did 'healing architecture' come from? – and the situated local enactment and accomplishment of 'healing' in hospital buildings – how does 'healing architecture' make a difference? – can be studied simultaneously. While my description of such an approach is inspired by Ian Hackings (2004) work on understanding how classifications of people interact with the people classified, it surely also resonates with recent work on 'caring architecture' (Nord and Högström, 2017b), where a relational approach to the study of how architecture makes a difference in practice, is foregrounded.

I have argued elsewhere (Simonsen and Duff, 2021) that care practices recursively build upon and make use of the ordered outcomes of interactions between patients and nurses that the enacted spaces provide, revealing the relational dynamics between architecture and practice. To the extent that any given architecture may be regarded as *healing*, any therapeutic effect may more productively be considered a function of spatial orderings than any simple material causation. The conceptual and empirical tensions between the spatial order of designs and the ongoing spatial orderings of psychiatric care are a productive starting point for better understanding what it is that 'healing architecture' does. By closely following and detailing the situated practical actions taking place within and across 'healing architecture' we may therefore come to better understand how 'healing architecture' actually makes a difference *in practice*.

While I have previously considered the conditions of possibilities in a specific new build, detailing the organisational (Simonsen and Vikkelsø, 2022) and interactional (Simonsen and Duff, 2021, 2020) implications of the 'healing architecture' of inpatient settings, in this chapter I have tried to describe the conditions of production by tracing some of the key ideas about treatment and recovery drawn upon in the development of the Slagelse site by the leading architects and the hospital management. The 'healing architecture' of the Slagelse site is considered a standard within healthcare architecture, offering stakeholders ideas and spatial forms for the development of the future of psychiatry. While understanding the conditions of production are important, describing the ongoing, practical action, *taking place* within and across the so-called 'healing architecture' of modern psychiatric institutions, directs the focus towards the perhaps subtler affordances of the carefully designed material environments, something that is very important in light of the promises of 'healing architecture'. For this reason, and as opposed to much research on evidencebased-design, I propose the less dramatic, but in my view more relevant approach, where considering whether 'healing architecture' indeed affords the production of healing spaces is more about studying the tensions between spatial order and spatial ordering in practice, rather than about identifying the 'healing' qualities of any one architectural property.

References

Adams, A., 2008. *Medicine by Design – The Architect and the Modern Hospital, 1893–1943*. University of Minnesota Press.

Andrews, G.J., Duff, C., 2019. Matter beginning to matter: On posthumanist understandings of the vital emergence of health. *Soc. Sci. Med.* 226, 123–134. https://doi.org/10.1016/j.socsci med.2019.02.045

Astbury, J., 2016. Road to recovery. https://doi.org/10.1136/bjsports-2015-094672

Bell, S.L., Foley, R., Houghton, F., Maddrell, A., Williams, A.M., 2018. From therapeutic landscapes to healthy spaces, places and practices: A scoping review. *Soc. Sci. Med.* 196, 123–130. https://doi.org/10.1016/j.socscimed.2017.11.035

Bromley, E., 2012. Building patient-centeredness: Hospital design as an interpretive act. *Soc. Sci. Med.* 75, 1057–1066. https://doi.org/10.1016/j.socscimed.2012.04.037

Bruun Petersen, T., Poulsen, L.V., Svarrer, S.M., 2013. Psykiatriske hospitaler i et historisk perspektiv, in: aarhus arkitekterne a/s (Ed.), Mentale Rum: Arkitektur – Psykiatri – Samfund. aarhus arkitekterne a/s, pp. 39–45.

Connellan, K., Gaardboe, M., Riggs, D.W., Due, C., Reinschmidt, A., Mustillo, L., 2013. Stressed spaces: Mental health and architecture. *Heal. Environ. Res. Des. J.* 6, 127–168. https://doi.org/10.1177/193758671300600408

Cummins, S., Curtis, S., Diez-Roux, A. V., Macintyre, S., 2007. Understanding and representing "place" in health research: A relational approach. *Soc. Sci. Med.* 65, 1825–1838. https://doi.org/10.1016/j.socscimed.2007.05.036

Curtis, S., Gesler, W.M., Priebe, S., Francis, S., 2009. New spaces of inpatient care for people with mental illness: A complex "rebirth" of the clinic? *Heal. Place* 15, 340–348. https://doi.org/10.1016/j.healthplace.2008.06.007

Curtis, S.E., Gesler, W.M., Fabian, K., Francis, S., Priebe, S., 2007. Therapeutic landscapes in hospital design: A qualitative assessment by staff and service users of the design of a new mental health inpatient unit. *Environ. Plan. C Gov. Policy* 25, 591–610. https://doi.org/10.1068/c1312r

d'Hoop, A., 2020. On the potentialities of spaces of care: Openness, enticement, and variability in a psychiatric Center. *Sci. Technol. Hum. Values* 1–23. https://doi.org/10.1177/0162243920942881

DuBose, J., MacAllister, L., Hadi, K., Sakallaris, B., 2018. Exploring the concept of healing spaces. *Heal. Environ. Res. Des. J.* 11, 43–56. https://doi.org/10.1177/1937586716680567

Duff, C., 2012. Exploring the role of 'enabling places' in promoting recovery from mental illness: A qualitative test of a relational model. *Heal. Place* 18, 1388–1395. https://doi.org/10.1016/j.healthplace.2012.07.003

Duque, M., Vaughan, L., Pink, S., Sumartojo, S., 2020. *Service designing in psychiatric care.* Published in: ServDes.2020 Tensions, Paradoxes and Plurality Conference Proceedings, 2-5th February 2021, Melbourne, Australia Linköping Electronic Conference Proceedings 173:28, pp. 277–287.

Foley, R., 2011. Performing health in place: The holy well as a therapeutic assemblage. *Heal. Place* 17, 470–479. https://doi.org/10.1016/j.healthplace.2010.11.014

Foley, R., Kistemann, T., 2015. Blue space geographies: Enabling health in place. *Heal. Place* 35, 157–165. https://doi.org/10.1016/j.healthplace.2015.07.003

Folmer, M.B., 2014. *Helende arkitektur – Rum og Interaktion.* Helende Arkit. – Rum og Interaktion. Aalborg University.

Foucault, M., 1977. *Discipline & Punish – The Birth of the Prison,* Second Vin. ed. Vintage, New York.

Foucault, M., 1973a. *The Birth of the Clinic – An Archeology of Medical Perception,* Vintage Bo. ed. Vintage, New York.

Foucault, M., 1973b. *Psychiatric Power – Lectures at the collége de France 1973–74,* 2008th ed. Palgrave Macmillan, New York.

Foucault, M., 1961. *Madness & Civilization – A History of Insanity in the Age of Reason,* Vintage Bo. ed. Vintage Books, New York.

Frandsen, A.K., Ryhl, C., Folmer, M.B., Fich, L.B., Øien, T.B., Sørensen, N.L., Mullins, M., 2009. *Helende arkitektur, Institut for Arkitektur og Design.* Aalborg University. https://doi.org/1603-6204

Gesler, W.M., Bell, M., Curtis, S., Hubbard, P., Francis, S., 2004. Therapy by design: Evaluating the UK hospital building program. *Heal. Place* 10, 117–128. https://doi.org/10.1016/S1353-8292(03)00052-2

Gieryn, T.F., 2002. What buildings do. *Theory Soc.* 31, 35–74. https://doi.org/10.1023/A:1014404201290

Goffman, E., 1961. *Asylums – Essays on the Social Situation of Mental Patients and Other Inmates*, Penguin Bo. ed. Penguin Books, London and New York.

Hacking, I., 2004. Between Michel Foucault and Erving Goffman: Between discourse in the abstract and face-to-face interaction. *Econ. Soc.* 33, 277–302. https://doi.org/10.1080/0308514042000225671

Hummelvol, an K., Karlsson, B., Borg, M., 2015. Recovery and person-centredness in mental health services: Roots of the concepts and implications for practice. *Int. Pract. Dev. J.* 5, 1–7. https://doi.org/10.19043/ipdj.5sp.009

Jakobsen, S.F., Petersen, A., Martin, H.M., Knudsen, H., Johansen, K.S., 2014. Psykiatrien Region Sjælland før flytning til det nye psykiatrisygehus Etnografiske beskrivelser af arbejdsgange og kultur. Copenhagen: KORA Det Nationale Institut for Kommuners og Regioners Analyse og Forskning.

Johannessen, R., Holm, I.W., 2022. *Healing Architecture and the Crisis of Care, in: Architectures of Dismantling and Restructuring: Spaces of Danish Welfare 1970–Present*. Zürich: Lars Müller Publishers, pp. 311–339.

Johannessen, R., Holm, I.W., 2021. *Vi bygger for livet – Medikalisering af den danske hospitalsarkitektur*. Kult. Klasse.

Jovanović, N., Campbell, J., Priebe, S., 2019. How to design psychiatric facilities to foster positive social interaction – A systematic review. *Eur. Psychiatry* 60, 49–62. https://doi.org/10.1016/j.eurpsy.2019.04.005

Karlsson Arkitekter/Vilhelm Lauritzen AS, 2015. Den lille bog om psykiatrisygehuset [WWW Document]. Issuu Webpublication. URL https://issuu.com/karlssonarkitekter/docs/karlsson_arkitekter_gaps_2015 (accessed 11.29.18).

Karlsson Arkitekter, n.d. Et fyrtårn for fremtidens psykiatribyggeri [WWW Document]. URL www.karlssonark.com/projekter#/nyt-psykiatrisygehus-i-slagelse/ (accessed 5.6.19).

King, A., 1980. *Buildings and Society – Essays on the Social Development of the Built Environment*. Routledge.

Lawson, B., 2010. Healing architecture. *Arts Health* 2, 95–108. https://doi.org/10.1080/17533010903488517

Lundin, S., 2021. Can healing architecture increase safety in the design of psychiatric wards? *Heal. Environ. Res. Des. J.* 14, 106–117. https://doi.org/10.1177/1937586720971814

Lundin, S., 2015. *Healing Architecture: Evidence, Intuition, Dialogue*. Chalmers University of Technology.

Marcus, C.C., Sachs, N.A., 2013. *Therapeutic Landscapes: An Evidence-Based Approach to Designing Healing Gardens and Restorative Outdoor Spaces*. John Wiley & Sons.

McGrath, L., Reavey, P. (Eds.), 2018. *The Handbook of Mental Health and Space – Community and Clinical Applications*. Routledge. https://doi.org/10.1192/bjp.112.483.211-a

Moser, I., 2006. Disability and the promises of technology: Technology, subjectivity and embodiment within an order of the normal. *Inf. Commun. Soc.* 9, 373–395. https://doi.org/10.1080/13691180600751348

Nord, C., Högström, E., 2017a. Introduction, in: Nord, C., Högström, E. (Eds.), *Caring Architectures – Institutions and Relational Practices*. Cambridge Scholars Publishing, pp. 7–17.

Nord, C., Högström, E. (Eds.), 2017b. *Caring Architecture – Institutions and Relational Practices*. Cambridge Scholars Publishing.

Prior, L., 1988. The architecture of the hospital: A study of spatial organization and medical knowledge. *Source Br. J. Sociol.* 39, 86–113. https://doi.org/10.2307/590995

Quirk, A., Lelliott, P., Seale, C., 2006. The permeable institution: An ethnographic study of three acute psychiatric wards in London. *Soc. Sci. Med.* 63, 2105–2117. https://doi.org/10.1016/j.socscimed.2006.05.021

Reavey, P., Harding, K., Bartle, J., 2017. Design With People in Mind. **Design in Mental Health Network.** https://dimhn.org/wp-content/uploads/2021/05/DWPIM_250x210_24PP_AW_V05_LR-1.pdf

Region Denmark, 2009. *En psykiatri i verdensklasse – Regionernes visioner for en fremtidens psykiatri.* Copenhagen. .

Region Denmark, n.d. *Helende arkitektur – psykiatrisygehuset i Slagelse.* https://god tsygehusbyggeri.dk/inspiration/cases/helende-arkitektur-psykiatrisygehuset-i-slagelse/. Retreived 8.7.24

Region Zealand, 2008. *Psykiatriplan for Region Sjælland.* www.psykiatrienregsj.dk/om-psykiatr ien/noegletal-politikker-og-planer/planer/psykiatriplan. Retrieved 8.7.24

Simonsen, T., Duff, C., 2021. Mutual visibility and interaction: Staff reactions to the 'healing architecture' of psychiatric inpatient wards in Denmark. *Biosocieties 16*, 249–269. https://doi.org/10.1057/s41292-020-00195-4

Simonsen, T., Duff, C., 2020. Healing architecture and psychiatric practice: (Re)ordering work and space in an in-patient ward in Denmark. *Sociol. Heal. Illn.* 42, 379–392. https://doi.org/10.1111/1467-9566.13011

Simonsen, T., Højlund, H., 2018. Rummets grammatik – Helende arkitektur i psykiatrien. *Politik*, 21, 22–42.

Simonsen, T., Sturge, J., Duff, C., 2022. Healing architecture in healthcare: A scoping review. *Heal. Environ. Res. Des. J.*, 15, 1–14. https://doi.org/10.1177/19375867211072513

Simonsen, T., Vikkelsø, S., 2022. Organizational space as sites of contention: Unravelling relations of dis/order in a psychiatric hospital. *Ephemer. Theory Polit. Organ.* 22, 79–105.

Sloterdijk, P., 2017. *The Aesthetic Imperative.* Polity.

Sloterdijk, P., 2016. *Foams: Spheres Volume III: Plural Sphereology.* Semiotext(e), Los Angeles.

Spaulding, W.D., 2016. The Idea of Recovery, in: Singh, N.N., Barber, J.B., Van Sant, S. (Eds.), *Handbook of Recovery in Inpatient Psychiatry.* Springer, pp. 3–38.

Stevens, R., Petermans, A., Vanrie, J., 2019. Design for human flourishing: A novel design approach for a more 'Humane' architecture. *Des. J.* 22, 391–412. https://doi.org/10.1080/14606 925.2019.1612574

Theodore, D., 2017. Decline of the Hospital as a Healing Machine, in: Schrank, S., Ekici, D. (Eds.), *Healing Spaces, Modern Architecture, and the Body.* Routledge, London and New York, pp. 186–202.

Topp, L., Moran, J.E., Andrews, J. (Eds.), 2007. *Madness, Architecture and the Built Environment – Psychiatric Space in Historical Context.* Routledge, New York and London.

Ulrich, R.S., 1984. View through a window may influence recovery from surgery. *Science (80-.).* 224, 420–421. https://doi.org/10.1126/science.6143402

Ulrich, R.S., Berry, L.L., Quan, X., Parish, J.T., 2010. A Conceptual Framework for the Domain of EBD. HERD 4 No 1, 95–114.

Ulrich, R.S., Zimring, C., Zhu, X., Dubose, J., Hyun-bo, S., Young-Seon, C., Xiaobo, Q., Anjali, J., 2008a. A review of the research literature on evidence based healthcare design. *Heal. Environ. Res. Des. J.* 1, 101–165.

Ulrich, R.S., Zimring, C., Zhu, X., DuBose, J., Seo, H.-B., Choi, Y.-S., Quan, X., Joseph, A., 2008b. A review of the research literature on evidence-based design. *Heal. Environ. Res. Des. J.* 1, 61–125. https://doi.org/10.1177/193758670800100306

Vaughan, L., Sumartojo, S., Pink, S., 2018. Patient-Centered Care and the Design of a Psychiatric Care Facility, in: Vaughan, L. (Ed.), *Designing Cultures of Care.* Bloomsbury Publishing, pp. 69–84.

Williams, J., Leamy, M., Bird, V., Harding, C., Larsen, J., Le Boutillier, C., Oades, L., Slade, M., 2012. Measures of the recovery orientation of mental health services: Systematic review. *Soc. Psychiatry Psychiatr. Epidemiol.* 47, 1827–1835. https://doi.org/10.1007/s00127-012-0484-y

Wood, V.J., Curtis, S.E., Gesler, W.M., Spencer, I.H., Close, H.J., Mason, J.M., Reilly, J.G., 2013. Creating "therapeutic landscapes" for mental health carers in inpatient settings: A dynamic perspective on permeability and inclusivity. *Soc. Sci. Med.* 91, 122–129. https://doi.org/10.1016/j.socscimed.2012.09.045

40 Islands as spaces of institutionalised mental health and wellbeing

Robin Kearns and John Connell

Introduction

Islands have a long history of being regarded as spaces of health and specifically mental health. For the seeker of solitude, they can be sites of escape from the clamour of urban life, a quest graphically narrated in Tom Neale's (1966) account of living for many years as the only resident of Suwarrow atoll in the Cook Islands. For others of a less isolationist disposition, islands can be places of inner reset in the company of others. Hence luxury resorts such as the exclusive Turtle Island in Fiji market themselves as curated spaces of restoration (James & Kearns, 2020). Although an island resort is a chosen destination, it invariably has some semi-institutional features (e.g., meal times, conduct rules). However, a resort is ultimately a destination for fee-paying customers. More formalised institutions in which people have been detained for various reasons have also been established on islands for a range of reasons from quarantine to recovery from addiction.

What is the origin of this link between islands, institutions and mental wellbeing? Utopia, the short book written just over five centuries ago by Thomas More, offers clues. It outlines the social and literal contours of an idealised island-state which amplified residents' wellbeing through being both effectively governed and scrupulously planned. Happiness, it argues, is an outcome of an equitable, yet controlled, society and the absence of private property. The influence of More's idealised political satire has been enduring and the source of a dominant trope within the western consciousness: that islands can offer utopian and often managed alternatives to mainland and mainstream societies. Such ideas contribute to the allure of islands and suggest they can offer happiness and well-being – whether idealised or real. While More's vision has had diminished purchase in the contemporary capitalist world of rampant housing markets and commodified mass tourism. Nonetheless the underlying discourse has been durable: islands are still regarded as utopian settings.

This chapter surveys the character of islands as spaces of mental wellbeing, considers islands as both a metaphorical and topographical reality, and examines a case study of Rotoroa, an island offshore from Auckland, New Zealand as a site that has transitioned from a space of enclosure to one of escape. We ask, as part of a long tradition to what extent islands can be 'spaces of wellbeing' (Fleuret and Atkinson 2007) and how they have been both host to, and constructed as, distinctive institutionalised sites.

DOI: 10.4324/9781003345725-45

Islands as spaces of mental wellbeing

Three near-universal aspects of island life are: isolation (evident in the purposeful journey – usually over water – to reach the separate world of the island); boundedness (the distinct physical outline of islands that allows one to picture the island as a whole); and small size relative to 'mainlands' (the potential to know more closely the places and people within the smaller-scale of the island setting) (Royle 2001). Wellbeing, we contend, emerges within the tension between these three characteristics (isolation, boundedness and intimacy) that shape the contours of island life. At its best everyday life on islands is characterised by strong and positive social cohesion, a quality recognised as a strong determinant of mental and social wellbeing (Labonte, 2016). Yet, at its worst, island life can be beset by a sense of social claustrophobia and entrapment, corrosive of mental wellbeing, where divisions and differences are inescapable so that residents must constantly negotiate and maintain 'unnatural emotions' (Lutz 1988).

Two types of wellbeing can be considered in relation to islands. There is the wellness that implies a movement away from a condition of ill-health or impairment (i.e., 'getting well'). This is a conventional concern of medicine: making and keeping people well, but not necessarily having concern for the subtleties and cultural contexts of wellbeing itself (Kearns and Andrews 2010). Second, beyond the discourses of medicine and more placed within the geographies of everyday life, wellbeing is increasingly evoked as a state that is important on an ongoing basis in and of itself.

Arguably, in island contexts that have been historically hard hit by epidemics and often colonised by quarantine functions, health has been too easily medicalised. A place-based understanding of the quest for wellbeing allows us to embrace a wide set of influences at work, many of which are 'enabling resources' (Duff 2011) intrinsic to the character of islands themselves.

However, what of the institutional 'colonisation' of islands? In addition to utopia, a number of other tropes link islands and wellbeing in the public imagination. First is the idea of islands as sanctuaries – literally sites of refuge from pursuit or persecution for human and non-human species (Kearns and Collins 2016). Just as islands have been sites of imprisonment (as was Robben Island, off Cape Town, South Africa, or Alcatraz in San Francisco Bay, USA), so too islands can be places of protection from unhealthy mainland influences. We see this today in the way islands are established as wildlife sanctuaries and refuges for endangered biodiversity. With respect to people, protection can be for the benefit of mainland society in the case of quarantine islands (Bashford 1998). To this extent, remoteness has benefits: the greater the distance from a mainland, the more likely that an island can offer safety to its inhabitants through the intervening waterway serving as a protective moat. While the ill-effects of toxic products and unhealthy behaviours can take hold, the small scale of many island settlements can facilitate a collective will for change. The declaration of Niuean villages as 'smokefree' offers a good example (Kearns and Coleman, 2018) but island populations could also be reactionary. In extremis, Sentinel Islanders (nominally part of India) continue to violently oppose all outsiders.

Yet an island can offer little protection once its protective moat has been breached. Thus the island of Rotuma (a northerly Polynesian outlier within the Fiji group) experienced extreme mortality when measles first arrived in 1911. The cumulative measles-related mortality that year of 12.8 per cent indicates that very limited earlier exposure to only a narrow range of microbes (as well as the genetic homogeneity of isolated island populations) can leave residents liable to deadly outcomes upon initial contact with contagious viruses (Shanks 2011). Similarly, in Samoa, the 1918–1919 influenza epidemic hit hard, with deaths of up to 30 per cent of the men and 22 per cent of women. Beyond the obvious tragedy of such death rates, this extraordinarily sudden and high level of mortality resulted in collective and individual grief, rapid change in political structures and acute labour shortages which all contribute to mental stress (Tomkins 1992). The message from this historical epidemiology is that remoteness is replete with ambivalence: while a watery distance can afford protection, an island's isolation can also generate vulnerability to threats such as infectious diseases from over the horizon, separate island populations from remedies and solutions and, in several Pacific islands, contribute to an emerging 'climate anxiety'.

A second idea that relates to wellbeing is the notion of islands as get-aways (Kearns and Collins 2016). Tourism, however, is commonly associated with more climatically and topographically hospitable islands and at least implicitly promises wellbeing – respite for visitors and employment for residents. For tourists – whether day-trippers to nearby islands or long-stayers on more remote locations – the 'getting away from it all' involves an escape from the stresses of employment, traffic and various other mundane preoccupations: a physical distancing from the 'rat-race', that has been facilitated by working from home during and after the COVID pandemic, and which has accounted for a significant post-COVID rise in island purchases.

Invariably, however, get-aways involve returns and so the act of 'escape' and the memories upon return potentially add to an unrealistic romanticising of islands. This contrived sense of islands as exotic locations that offer enhanced mental and physical health through visitation has been played upon and amplified by 'wellbeing tourism': the marketing of retreats and spas on islands that require a journey and involve payment in return for pampering. By way of example, the rocky and isolated island of Niue in the South Pacific is one of the world's smallest nations in terms of population with only approximately 1,600 residents in 2016. As part of a broader quest to attract visitors, 'Yoga and Wellness Retreats' are offered, enticing participants with advertising that features spectacular landscape images and meditative serenity in close proximity to restful coastal blue spaces. But Niue faces intense competition from islands in Fiji, Bali and elsewhere (Connell 2016).

Increasingly, poorer island nations are promoting tourism explicitly aimed at visitors seeking medical care. In the Caribbean region, for instance, medically-focused health is being seen as a means to diversify the tourism sector and contribute to economic development. The central idea is that patients and their supporters (largely from high-income) seek out high quality but lower cost medical care in less developed countries and combine the journey with a period of vacation and convalescence. Hence returns to the local economy include expenditures on both medicine and tourism. Connell (2013) points out that medical tourism projects in small Caribbean jurisdictions such as the Bahamas, Barbados and the Cayman Islands are developed by overseas corporations and are predominantly oriented to a US market. Ethical issues are raised by the fact that business principles rather than health care imperatives dominate development strategies. Do these initiatives contribute to islands as spaces of mental health? Perhaps the answer is yes to the extent that there is stress-relief in curated convalescence that is entangled in leisure. Further there is another layer of stress-relief with benefits to 'locals' through the generation of foreign exchange and the creation of new employment opportunities.

Medina-Muñoz and Medina-Muñoz (2013) prefer to write of 'wellness tourism': in a sense all travel to holiday destinations could be constructed as such: the quest to be refreshed and find enhancement of mental wellbeing through the novelty of being else-where, often in a more benign climate away from the stresses and strains of everyday life (see Hoffman, 2017). To summarise, much marketing of island destinations plays up to the imperatives of 'getaway', 'unwind' and 'be pampered' within the confined and topographically (as well as imaginatively) defined space of the island. At times, the invo-cation of such tropes can lead to a dissonance between expectation and reality, but it is improbable that hyperbole will be tempered in image or description (Hoffman and Kearns 2013).

Ambivalence, popular culture and wellbeing

The ebb and flow of visitors, including organised 'medical tourists', can be vital to island economies, but can at times be a source of annoyance and service discrimination. Islands are never closed systems, given their connections to 'mainlands' through flows of people, goods and ideas. Nevertheless, where distances are sufficient, these flows may be limited and nuanced. The characteristic of insularity often gives rise to islands being associated with separateness and vulnerability, and island life can be characterised by a "powerful sense of community" (Royle 2001, p. 42). This quality was potently observed among the residents of Ireland's offshore islands whose collective identity was seen to cohere around a positively perceived isolation and an associated sense of belonging, strong feeling of community, secure and regular social interactions, and enduring values (Burholt, Sharf and Walsh 2013). Likewise, on Pitcairn Island, the very isolated Pacific island lying between Rapanui (Easter Isand) and French Polynesia, a measure of solidarity within the tiny population of approximately 70 was ensured by the need for all able-bodied men to assist when a longboat had to be launched. However, as in any community, there are politics of both inclusion and exclusion at work. While islands may enable a sought-after separation from the mainland, they may also impose a strategic distance from other opportunities and resources, and embrace an extreme antipathy to outsiders. This antip-athy is graphically described for a Hebridean island: 'It is a beautiful world of stubborn pride, hatred of difference and fear of change. In many ways it remains feudal, with its own unique honour system that is quick to take offence and slow to pardon' (Calidas 2020: 130).

Ambivalences can be acute when one considers wellbeing in island-like resort settings. Investigating these settings, Minca (2009) argues that the power relations between visitors and workers results in a 'contact zone' in which ideas about class, gender, sexuality and the body, as well as health and wellbeing, must be negotiated. In other words, islands are replete with ambivalence and what on face value may be good for the advance-ment of mental as well as physical wellbeing may, in time or in excess, have negative impacts on people's experience. By way of example, beaches are intrinsic to most 'warm water' islands and offer potential sites of recreation and relaxation. Yet, as Collins and Kearns (2007) argue, it is all too easy to romanticise such places when they invariably also incorporate elements of risk and threats to wellbeing (sunburn, drowning, or even Hepatitis C from contaminated sand).

Notwithstanding these risks, and fuelled by images within tourism and popular cul-ture, islands are coded in the popular imagination as largely happy places. Yet the 'on-the-ground' reality can be abjectly different. The gap between advertising-generated expectations and the actual experience of visitors can be considerable, as revealed in research based on New Zealand's Aotea/Great Barrier Island (Hoffman and Kearns

2013). Moreover, while visitors travel to island resorts in the Pacific and Indian Oceans as well as the Caribbean for mid-winter holidays, seeking respite from everyday stresses, 'locals' can experience very different stresses. In a study set in the Solomon Islands, for instance, Blignault et al. (2009) found high rates of drug use, interpersonal violence and teenage pregnancy. Similarly, closer to a metropolitan centre, Waiheke Island offshore from Auckland, New Zealand, experiences over-tourism to the point that the pleasures of visitors come at the cost and mental stress of residents who experience difficulties finding space on the increasingly unaffordable ferries (Oliver and Kearns, 2023).

Why is there such a drive on the part of travellers to seek out island destinations? Psychotherapeutic research signals how imaging places can be beneficial to mindfulness and how the practice of going to real or imagined 'get-aways' can improve wellbeing (Williams 1998). We can also note links to popular culture. In books including Robinson Crusoe and The Swiss Family Robinson islands are constructed as places replete with treasure, drama and dreams (Connell 2013). But, famously, an island was also the location for William Golding's novel *Lord of the Flies* in which a group of young boys marooned on a deserted island, degenerate in a dystopian manner into a regime of brutality and violence. Multiple tensions, ambivalences and contradictions attend to islandness. We can now examine these dualities further.

Dualities

Dualities are readily apparent on islands: places of community as well as claustrophobia. Just as Tom Neale valued isolation on Suwarrow for his mental wellbeing, and religious orders found places of contemplation on islands like Iona in Scotland, many others have been exiled to islands, and gay populations have historically valued islands like Fire Island (New York) as respite from the disapproving gaze and legal regimes of 'mainstream' society. Even more have abandoned islands as social relationships have strained and choices (e.g., for marriage partners) have declined. And still others, institutionalised to the isolation of islands and cut off from family and 'normality', have failed to thrive.

At the core of the relationship between islands and mental health is that of separation; a notion that cure is more possible in isolated and focused environments. Occasionally separation had positive overtones, in attempts to remove people from the social determinants of ill-health. More frequently, it followed the desire to separate those with mental illness from the wider population and render them 'out of sight, out of mind' (Ramsay, 1990). That was also a motivation for the placement of leprosariums and other hospitals for infectious diseases, especially under colonial regimes, with some 'leper colonies' such as Molokai (Hawaii) acquiring a degree of fame (Dawes, 1984).

Separation, of course, was especially true of the use of islands as prisons where the most 'difficult' prisoners (in any sense – violent criminals, political prisoners, repeat offenders) were most likely to be incarcerated on islands such as Norfolk Island (Australia), Devil's Island (Guyane) or Alcatraz (San Francisco). At such sites, any pretence at rehabilitation could be ignored and prisoners were unlikely to escape. Ironically, perhaps, as many such places have closed in post-colonial times (on economic grounds rather than through new more sensitive regimes of care and detention) many, like Robben Island (Deacon 2003) and Devil's Island (Fuggle 2022), have become tourist destinations (see also our case of Rotoroa island below). In terms of mental health, such transitions might, speculatively, move island-based institutional sites from spaces of mental ill-health to spaces of mental release and spaciousness though the relative freedom of visitation, even if the sites might constitute 'dark tourism' (Stone 2013).

The practice of placing 'illegal' refugees and asylum-seekers on isolated islands has had disastrous consequences in terms of mental health, notably amongst refugees (most of whom were Iranians) forcibly placed by Australia in offshore detention on the Pacific island of Nauru. The NGO, Médecins Sans Frontières/Doctors Without Borders (MSF), provided mental healthcare before being forced to leave by the Nauruan government in 2018. They reported extreme mental health suffering on the island as refugees perceived no hope of achieving freedom and seemingly indefinite detention. Almost a third of MSF's refugee and asylum seeker patients had attempted suicide, while others were diagnosed with the rare psychiatric condition of 'resignation syndrome'. Nauruan nationals also had high levels of severe mental illness; almost half of MSF's Nauruan patients needed treatment for psychosis (MSF 2018).

Other nefarious activities, from islands as military target practice (such as Kahoolawe (Hawaii) and Vieques (Puerto Rico)), bomb testing (Bikini, Marshall Islands and Muroroa, French Polynesia) or simply military bases (Guam, Diego Garcia) have resulted in some populations being forcibly removed followed by grave and ongoing subsequent health problems. Not only were many mental health care problems despatched to islands but a range of 'marginal' practices were also located there: something of the antithesis of the trope of islands as places of wellbeing

While some military practices have faded many island prisons have mostly closed and the extremities of treatment (or neglect) of those with mental health problems are increasingly likely to be undertaken 'within the community'. In most places islands as accompanying institutions for the unwell have had their day. We now therefore turn to a case study of a particular type of island with mental health implications: one where detoxification from alcohol addiction has dominated its recent history, and which also emphasises how the 'value' of islands and the perceived role of separation and isolation has changed over time.

Rotoroa, New Zealand

Belief in the capacity of coastal environments to contribute to restore mental and physical wellbeing has been explored through activities such as walking near to (Wylie 2005) and swimming in (Foley 2015) the ocean. Few studies, however, trace how this understanding has been acted upon in specific places, or how such places – and, in particular, institutionalised island spaces – have changed over time. On Rotoroa Island, 32 km from downtown Auckland, the Salvation Army ran an alcohol treatment facility for almost a century (Kearns, Collins and Conradson, 2014). The island's relative isolation was a key rationale for its entangled mix of therapeutic and carceral roles. For 94 years the island was closed to the general public while used as an addiction recovery facility. Then, with a change in tenure and intent, it was re-opened in 2011 as a philanthropically funded sanctuary of a different sort: a reserve for recreation, remembrance and environmental restoration affirming a wider vision of wellbeing involving the activities of both human and non-human actors.

Over the course of its institutional life, approximately 12,000 men and women, both voluntarily and through court order, spent time on the island over its almost century of operation. It closed in 2005 with the wider move away from isolated institutional forms

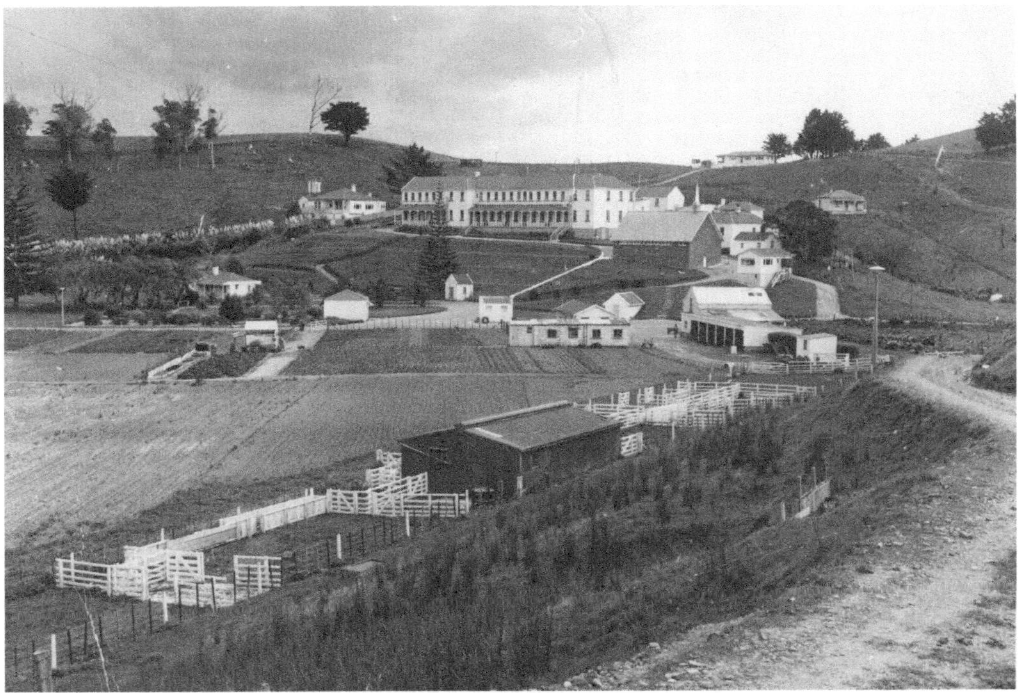

Figure 40.1 Home Bay, Rotoroa Island Alcohol Treatment Facility. Photograph credit: Salvation Army.

of treatment that were both costly and increasingly counter to a public and political disdain for institutional treatment (Kearns et al., 2014).

As with all islands, at Rotoroa, the encircling sea defines it and, in so doing, served to contain and detain those assigned time there. However, the island also offered a space for activities such as swimming and fishing, and through participation in these sea-based activities, had social and symbolic dimensions. From this vantage point, the mental health-enhancing qualities of blue space are a relational outcome, emerging from the intersection of human agency (establishment of the facility), social relations (established routines), and material environments (the chapel and dormitories with sea views as well as the beaches themselves). Through a combination of these related resources, many detainees paradoxically sought to return once they found themselves free from detention and back on the mainland.

With respect to spaces of mental health promotion, water is not only a common feature of spaces of therapeutic intention but also as a potentially salutogenic element in itself (Volker and Kistemann, 2011). One aspect that Rotoroa residents reported, and as displayed in the island's museum, is their engagement with and affinity for the sea. Detainees enjoyed fishing, swimming and walking island's sandy beaches. To others, the watery expanse between island and mainland was felt as a barrier separating the self from other populations and all the opportunities that mainland societies offer in terms of resources and support.

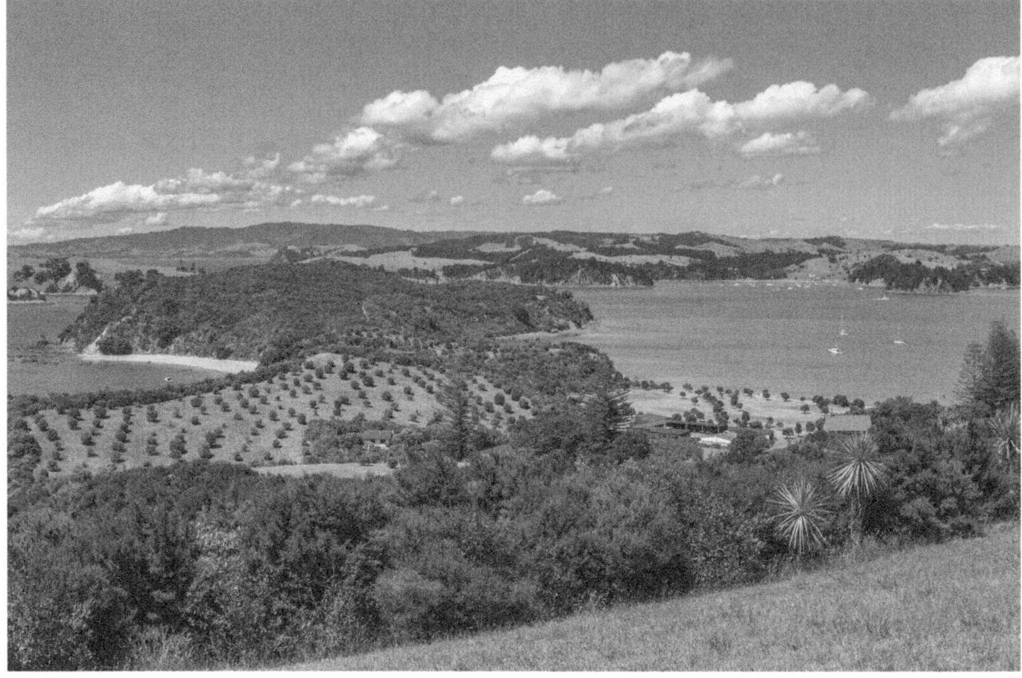

Figure 40.2 Replanted island as biodiversity sanctuary. Photograph by James Gow.

Rotoroa Island's institutional history and role as a space of mental health restoration can be interpreted through engagement with Duff's (2011) idea of 'enabling places' (see Kearns et al, 2014). His notion focuses on the diverse actor-networks that generate resources in place, which in turn enable some places to promote health more than others. In developing this idea, Duff (2011) identifies three categories of enabling resources: social (centred on intimacy, trust and reciprocity), affective (centred on feelings, disposition and action-potential) and material (centred on access to goods, services and the physical environment). In the case of Rotoroa, the authors considered the enabling resources created and experienced by detainees and staff during its time as a site of treatment as well as more recently by recreational visitors who come to experience the island's historical heritage, its rare wildlife and its art installations. This focus on 'enabling' resources emphasises that the restorative benefits of place are not necessarily a function of the setting itself but rather are continually made, and re-made, through the interactions and practices of a diverse set of human and non-human actors. With respect to mental health, therefore, an island setting is always in a state of becoming (following Pred, 1984). The story of Rotoroa is one of the island being reconstituted as a place for a broader vision of wellbeing. Founded in a time of the medicalisation of alcoholism, the island has outlived the ideological acceptability of confined treatment. Now this offshore space has been re-worked and re-imagined as a place where members of the public can enjoy new expressions of recreational wellbeing, and several rare bird species, previously critically endangered, are being conserved and restored to health. With its open access and mix of art, heritage and ecosystem restoration (Kearns, Collins and Wiles, 2016), Rotoroa is arguably a new space of post-institutional positive mental health.

Conclusion

Parallels exist between islands and asylums as spaces for mental health, recovery and sanctuary (the latter increasingly for non-human species). Both have elements of isolation and boundedness with the former having a natural seabound separation from the mainland and the latter being commonly located in rural areas with farmland serving as a buffer from more densely populated spaces (Moon, Kearns and Joseph, 2015). Islands, and the waters that surround and define them, are mutually interdependent, with water self-evidently being the defining topographic character of any island. This brief survey has explored a question that logically flows from this interdependence: how islands, given their encirclement by the sea, contribute to the experience of mental wellbeing. Understanding the structure of care on islands is important; both informal care and organised services are invariably shaped by distance, isolation and absence of economies of scale. Meanwhile, critical consideration of place-based wellbeing brings into view a wider set of 'enabling resources' (Duff 2011) intrinsic to the character of islands themselves and extending into more nuanced and holistic approaches to health and wellbeing.

Our case study of Rotoroa showed the potency of the sea as a salutogenic surrounding and that healthy 'islandness' is created and sustained through enabling encounters, networks and associations involving a gestalt between an island and its institutional context. A final point is the danger in over-attributing salutogenic effects to islands themselves. Doing so risks forgetting dualisms and granting of too much mental health-related agency to the island itself. Rather, just as visitors and 'locals' experience the same island differently, so too do different groups and individuals among the population of permanent residents. One person might experience claustrophobia, preferring to escape from stifling intimacy; another might seek to achieve a delicate balance, living for a time each year on the mainland. Others might instead relish the isolation and closely connected community and wild landscape. In other words, and as our examples indicated, therapeutic experiences of islands and their encircling blue spaces vary according to the relational dynamic between self and place. Experiences of mental wellbeing also change as the places themselves change. Indeed it is a characteristic of many islands that they experienced sequential changes imposed on them by outsiders.

The diversity of islands needs to be acknowledged, along with the difficulty – and risks – in attempting to generalise. Yet, we surely must seek to generalise because the only alternative would be an archipelago of disconnected case studies. The common theme within the field of island studies is the vast and diverse numbers of islands themselves, where islandness varies enormously and is intertwined with mobility and emotion.

Our chapter has asked in what ways do islands, given their encirclement by the sea, contribute to the experience of mental wellbeing for residents as well as visitors? Promotional as well as popular imagery suggests that island settings can be sources of enhanced mental health. We have argued that islands can be not only ordinary but also exceptional spaces for mental wellbeing. Their defined and confined topography has predisposed islands to be places of exile for recovery and restoration, whether chosen or imposed. In the case of imposed detention, the institutional history of islands includes prison and quarantine facilties as well as spaces of surveilled recuperation from conditions of mental ill-health such as alcoholism. To this extent, islands mirror the character of the asylums of old: clearly bounded, challenging to escape from yet replete with health-promoting character. While asylums were mainly rural in location, and hence bestowed with green space, the offshore location of islands grants them a different therapeutic valence: blue space. In the case of Rotoroa Island, we illustrated the ways the sea, sky and outdoors in general was sufficiently appealing that detainnees plotted opportunities to return. Hence we conclude that islands are important as spaces of mental health for both their intrinsic character characteristics and for the ways in which they offer an analogue to the asylum as the quintessential institional space: separate, bounded and a world unto itself.

References

Bashford, A. (1998) Quarantine and the imagining of the Australian nation. *Health*, 2(4), 387–402.

Blignault, J., Bunde-Birouste, A., Ritchie, J., Silove, D., and Zwi, A. (2009) Community perceptions of mental health needs: A qualitative study in the Solomon Islands, *Interntaional Journal of Mental Health Systems*, 3(6), 1–14.

Burholt, V., Sharf, T., and Walsh, K. (2013) Imagery and imaginary of islander identity: Older people and migration in Irish small-island communities. *Journal of Rural Studies*, 31(1), 1–12.

Calidas, T. (2020) *I am an Island*, London: Doubleday.

Collins, D., and Kearns, R. (2007) Ambiguous Landscapes: Sun, Risk and Recreation on New Zealand Beaches. In A. Williams (ed.), *Therapeutic Landscapes*, London, Ashgate, pp. 15–31.

Connell, J. (2016) Fiji: Reflections in the Infinity Pool. In K. Alexeyeff and J. Taylor, (eds.), *Touring Pacific Cultures*, Canberra, ANU Press, pp. 427–438.

Connell, J. (2013). *Islands at Risk?: Environments, Economies & Contemporary Change*. Edward Elgar: Cheltenham, UK & Northhampton, MA, USA

Dawes, G. (1984) *Holy Man: Father Damien of Molokai*, University of Hawai'I Press, *Honolulu*.

Deacon, H. (2003) Patterns of Exclusion on Robben Island. In C. Strange and A. Bashford, (eds.), *Isolation. Places and Practices of Exclusion*, London, Routledge, pp. 153–172.

Duff, C. (2011) Networks, resources and agencies: On the character and production of enabling places. *Health & Place*, 17(1), 149–156.

Fleuret, S., and Atkinson, S. (2007) Wellbeing, health and geography: A critical review and research agenda. *New Zealand Geographer*, 63(2), 106–118.

Foley R. (2015) Swimming in Ireland: Immersions in therapeutic blue space. *Health and Place*, 35, 218–25.

Fuggle, C. (2022) Toxic colonialism: Between sickness and sanctuary on Ilet la Mère, French Guiana. *Island Studies Journal*, 17(1), 26–43.

Hoffman, L. (2017) Pharmaceuticals and tourist spaces: Encountering the medicinal in Cozumel's linguistic landscape. *ACME: An International Journal for Critical Geographies*, 16(1), 59–88.

Hoffman, L., and Kearns, R. (2013) A Necessary Glamorisation? Resident Perspectives on Promotional Literature and Images on Great Barrier Island, New Zealand. In J. Lester and C. Scarles (eds.), *Mediating the Tourist Experience: From Brochures to Virtual Encounters*, Surrey, Ashgate, pp. 57–74.

James, E., and Kearns, R. (2020) Linking therapeutic (is)landscapes, experiences of digitality and the quest for wellbeing. *Wellbeing, Space & Society*, 1, 100010. https://doi.org/10.1016/j.wss.2020.100010

Kearns, R.A., and Andrews, G. (2010) Wellbeing. In S. Smith, R. Pain, S. Marston and J. Jones III (eds.), *Handbook of social geographies*, London, Sage, pp. 309–328.

Kearns, R.A., and Coleman, T.M. (2018) Health and Wellbeing. In G. Baldacchino (ed.), *International Handbook of Island Studies*, Routledge, London, pp. 279–295.

Kearns, R., and Collins, D. (2016) Aotearoa's archipelago: Re-imagining New Zealand's island geographies. *New Zealand Geographer*, 72(3), 165–168.

Kearns, R.A., Collins, D., and Conradson, D. (2014) A healthy island blue space: From space of detention to site of sanctuary. *Health & Place,* 30(1), 107–115.

Kearns, R., Collins, D., and Wiles, J. (2016) The Rotoroa Island and Auckland Zoo Partnership: Connecting heterotopic spaces. *New Zealand Geographer,* 72(3), 192–204.

Labonte, R. (2016) Social Inclusion/Exclusion and Health: Dancing the Dialectic. In D. Raphael (ed.), *Social Determinants of Health: Canadian Perspectives,* 3rd ed., Canadian Scholars' Press, Toronto, pp 253–266.

Lutz, C. A. (1988) *Unnatural emotions: Everyday sentiments on a Micronesian atoll & their challenge to Western theory.* University of Chicago Press. Chicago and London.

Medina-Muñoz, D.R., and Medina-Muñoz, R.D. (2013) Critical issues in health and wellness tourism: An exploratory study of visitors to wellness centres on Gran Canaria. *Current Issues in Tourism,* 16(5), 415–435.

Minca, C. (2009) The island: Work, tourism and the biopolitical. *Tourist Studies,* 9(2), 88–108.

Moon, G., Kearns, R.A., and Joseph, A.E. (2015) *The Afterlives of the Psychiatric Asylum: Recycling Concepts, Sites and Memories,* Ashgate Press, Farnham, UK.

MSF. (2018) Indefinite Despair: The Tragic Mental Health Consequences of offshore processing on Nauru, MSF.

Neale, T. (1966). *An Island to Oneself: Six Years on a Desert Island,* Collins, London.

Oliver, P., and Kearns, R. (2023) Plucking the 'golden goose', alive: The impacts of 'supercity' governance on a small island community. *New Zealand Geographer.* http://dx.dsoi.org/10.1111/nzg.12352

Pred, A. (1984). Place as historically contingent process: Structuration and the time-geography of becoming places. *Annals of the Association of American Geographers,* 74(2), 279–297.

Ramsay, R. (1990). Banished to a Greek Island. *Psychiatric Bulletin,* 14, 134–135.

Royle, S. (2001) *Geography of Islands,* Routledge, London, p. 42.

Shanks, G.D., Lee, S.-E, Howard, A., and Brundage, A.F. (2011). Extreme mortality after first introduction of measles virus to the Polynesian island of Rotuma, 1911. *American Journal of Epidemiology,* 173(10), 1211–1222.

Stone, P. (2013) Dark tourism scholarship: A critical review. *International Journal of Culture, Tourism and Hospitality Research,* 7 (3), 307–318.

Tomkins, S. (1992) The Influenza Epidemic of 1918–19 in Western Samoa, *Journal of Pacific History,* 27(2), 181–197.

Völker, S., and Kistemann, T. (2011) The impact of blue space on human health and well-being – Salutogenetic health effects of inland surface waters: A review. *International Journal of Hygiene and Environmental Health,* 214(6), 449–460.

Williams, A. (1998) Therapeutic landscapes in holistic medicine. *Social Science & Medicine,* 46(9), 1193–1203.

Wylie, J. (2005) A single day's walking: Narrating self and landscape on the South West Coast Path. *Transactions of the Institute of British Geographers,* 30, 234–247.

41 The new institutional landscape for people with mental health problems

Alain Topor, Tore Dag Bøe, Øyvind Hope,
Ottar Ness, and Jan Friesinger

Places, spaces and landscapes

Landscape is a widely used concept in health geography. In the literature, terms such as landscapes (Gesler, 1992), environments (Conradson, 2003), spaces (Kearns and Milligan, 2020) and places (Duff, 2012) occur with different and sometimes overlapping and contradictory meanings and uses. As one example, Gesler's landscapes (1992) might equally be considered as places. Places and landscapes might also be defined as green (forest), blue (sea), yellow (desert), and grey (cities) (Bell et al., 2023), all of them referring to public spaces, environments and places.

Another division in health and places literature is between healing (Gesler, 1992), therapeutic (Bell et al., 2018), enabling (Duff, 2012) or carrying (Knibbe & Horstman, 2019) places. What are the differences between these places, and should not 'non-therapeutic' (Kearns & Milligan, 2020) and even disabling and impairing places, as described in 'atrocity stories' (Hydén, 1995), also be included in these landscapes?

Finally, and regarding the positive effect on people looking for places able to enhance their wellbeing, it could be possible to separate non-programed places being experienced as enabling, from places planned, built and organised to help, offer support or treatment. As Mossabir et al. (2021, p. 10) mentioned: "Studies of marginal groups and communities raise concern about inconsistencies between what is considered as positive for health and wellbeing by those commissioning and designing particular landscapes and those who engage with them". In this contribution, we focus on institutional settings.

Contemporary archeology

Today there is still limited research about the total institutional landscapes developed in different countries, regions and other meaningful administrative geographical units in the wake of the dismantling of mental hospitals. Common to studies in this field, is that they have their starting point in personal landscapes or in specific places in these landscapes. A problem with these perspectives is a lack of knowledge about what are the potential places at the persons' disposal. Such a knowledge would make it possible to explore which parts of the actual landscape are included and excluded from persons' enabling landscapes and how different places interact in the everyday life of persons.

Dear and Wolch (1987) defined the landscape they studied in the aftermath of the downsizing of mental hospitals in California in the 1980's as a "landscape of despair" (p. 254). They also had a vision of what alternatives to this landscape would meet "future

DOI: 10.4324/9781003345725-46

archeologists" (p. 254) looking for the institutional landscapes after the downsizing of mental hospitals. One possibility they mentioned was a "landscape of haunted places" (p. 254); places created in a process of "re-institutionalization" (p. 254); of re-creation of mental hospital-like structures. They also formulated an optimistic vision of "a landscape of caring" (p. 255). "In it, community-based care is the norm: client would have the right to service provision in their own community and communities would have the obligation to look after their own" (p. 255).

We present in this chapter the findings from a contemporary archeological study of the situation forty years since the initiation of the dismantling process of mental hospitals in the Norwegian welfare society.

The crisis of the total institution

Initially, mental hospitals were built as therapeutic landscapes, constituted of a range of places reproducing the different aspects of a normal life, where people, perceived as having lost their mind, were forced to live a totally organised life in a harmonious environment according to a treatment plan. Living in such place would bring back reason to their chaotic soul (Scull, 1984).

Goffman (1961) characterised these "asylums" as total institutions and described how what was planned to be therapeutic in fact produced behaviors that were thought to be symptoms of mental illness. To be forced to participate in the different parts of a normal life, sleep, work, free-time, but with the same persons and according to a central plan made by others for one's best interests was exactly the contrary to what happened outside the hospital's walls in a normal life. It had devastating effects on people (Wing and Brown, 1970).

New places for a de-institutionalized landscape

During the second half of the twentieth century, life in the community became the solution to these inadequacies. It was perceived as offering access to normalised and normalising living conditions. De-hospitalisation gave people who would earlier have been confined into 'total institutions' the possibility to create their own therapeutical landscapes in the community.

"Freedom is therapeutic" was a slogan on the walls of the Trieste mental health hospital before it was closed completely in 1978 (Foot, 2014). However, some professionals and users understood that just opening hospital doors was not enough (Basaglia, 1987). A return to, or a continued life in, the local communities had to be supported through specific structures in these communities. It was necessary to build the "institutions of de-institutionalisation" – different structures that would not reproduce the segregating processes of the old system (Rotelli, 1988, p. 138). The development of such integrating institutions was a condition to transform a mere de-hospitalisation to de-institutionalisation. Thus, in the process of downsizing mental hospitals, places for treatment in many local communities such as clinics and community mental health centre, and places for rehabilitation and for socialisation such as different forms of housing and meeting places were developed. These places were built to replace or complement the mental hospitals (Topor, 2020).

The result of the downsizing of mental hospitals could be seen as the creation of new institutional landscapes in permanent transformation. New places are constantly created,

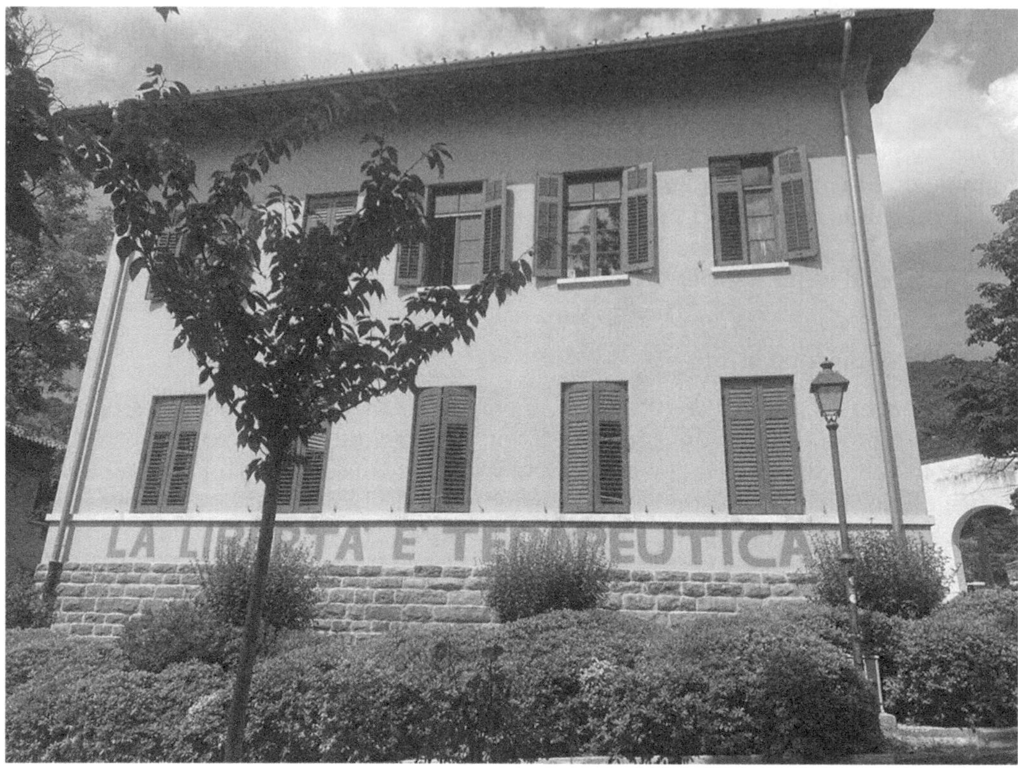

Figure 41.1 "Freedom is therapeutic". Slogan on the wall of Trieste's ex-mental hospital. Photograph by Alain Topor.

merged and closed down resulting in a changing institutional landscape at the disposal of people with mental health problems. This might be reflected in the proliferation of concepts analysing their development in terms of therapeutic (Kearns & Milligan, 2020), enabling (Hope et al., 2023), post-deinstitutionalised (Rosenberg, 2009; Fjellfeldt et al., 2021), post-asylum (Larsen & Topor, 2017; Högström, 2018), new institutional (Topor et al., 2016) landscapes; as well as landscapes of care (Milligan & Wiles, 2010) and of deinstitutionalisation (Wolch & Philo, 2000). Because of the many terms used in different ways in different studies, we introduce our contribution by presenting the main terms we will use in this chapter. Even if sometimes places have been considered as landscapes, we will define a landscape as *an assemblage of places.*

Based on time-geographical studies of service users' movements in time and space, Andersson (2009) divided their daily lives into a person-organised sphere and a community-organised sphere. Places in the community organised sphere will be the focus of this chapter. This does not diminish the importance of public and private places in the person's organised sphere, as their presence in people's construction of their personal enabling landscape can be considered as a major result of the de-institutionalisation of mental health care.

We then divided the *community-organised sphere* into two segments:

Formal health care places:

These places include services created and administrated by municipalities, counties, and states and directed at people with mental health problems, such as Community Mental Health Centres, housing facilities and activity centres. Access to these places is based on a formal evaluation of the persons and their needs.

Voluntary places:

These places, such as some meeting places, are run by voluntary organisations (e.g., religious congregations or users' movements) and directed at people with mental problems. Access to these places is free.

The sum of these institutional places in a delimited geo-administrative area, constitutes what we will call *the total institutional landscape,* in relation to the old institutional landscape, before de-hospitalisation started.

Because people with mental health problems are no longer confined for long periods of their lives in mental hospitals, they have access to natural, public and institutional places and build their own *personal landscapes,* parts of it consisting of places they experience as helping them in their well-being and in a recovery process and thus forming their *personal enabling landscape.* Places in these landscapes may include places from the community organised sphere; thus, a *personal institutional enabling landscape.*

The Norwegian way of de-institutionalisation

Roughly, two different landscapes emerged in the wake of de-hospitalisation; *a landscape of despair* and *a new institutional landscape.*

The neo-liberal turn in some countries starting at the beginning of the 1970s, stopped the development of alternatives, or complementary structures, to downsized mental hospitals. Dismantling mental hospital structures opened instead for tax reductions, a reduced role of the state in the life of citizens and a responsabilisation of the individual for their own fate (Scull, 2022). This policy created an association between de-institutionalisation and abandonment in a "landscape of despair" (Dear & Wolch, 1987), as well as an image of people with severe mental health problems as being dangerous, drug-addicted, homeless and unable to live in the community (Knowles, 2000. Prisons are now described as the biggest mental health institutions in the US (Konrad, 2002).

Thanks to developed and general welfare states, another development was possible in other countries, as in Scandinavia, where the normalisation of 'disabled' people's living conditions, was considered as the basis of de-institutionalising mental health care (Nirje, 1985). People with severe mental health problems were guaranteed a basic income, different housing possibilities, and access to different forms of psychiatric and social support.

Even if a slow dismantling of mental hospitals could be noticed around the 1980s, a turning point in Norway's institutional history was the Norwegian Parliament's adoption of the Escalation Plan for Mental Health in 1998 (Pedersen & Kolstad, 2009). Although new structures (in addition to mental health hospitals) had been created earlier, the Escalation Plan marked an official national turning point. The plan comprised sensible economic state support between 1998 and 2008 for efforts to radically change structures, practices, treatments and laws related to mental health care.

The place of the landscape

Our geographical and administrative locus of interest is Agder; a region in southern Norway, with roughly 300,000 inhabitants on 1 January 2022. Agder is divided into 25 municipalities, but for practical reasons, we chose to focus on five adjacent municipalities (Kristiansand, 113,737; Arendal, 45,509; Grimstad, 24,017; Lillesand, 11,279; Birkenes, 5,342), which together have a total population of around 200,000.

We collected information about the different places/services in the region at a workshop involving around 40 professionals and people with their own experience of mental health problems and mental health services. Subsequently, we contacted colleagues in the mental health field and asked them to add places not mentioned at the workshop, after which we explored the homepages of actual municipalities and mental health services. Finally, this information was supplemented by individual interviews with key figures regarding the development of local health structures. None of the four forms of information gathering involved collecting personal data linked to any real person. We analysed the places according to two aspects; namely organisational affiliation and functions.

A permeable and fluctuant reality

Places are not easy to characterise. As described by Goffman (1961), even total institutions had "free places" (205) (e.g., parts of the parks surrounding the wards that professionals, by tacit agreement, seldom visited) challenging his definition of their totalitarian character. Therefore, characterising and categorising is often committing violence against the complexity of the world. In our case, for example, places built by religious congregations and user's organisations could be categorised in two ways; as part of the person organised sphere but also of the community organised sphere, as most of these places are founded by formal health care. Here, we have chosen to define them as voluntary places in the community organised sphere.

People's homes belong primarily to the person's organised sphere. However, if one lives in supported housing, where staff are present up to 24 hours a day and have access to tenants' private space, we considered these places as part of the community-organised sphere. Studies of supported housings (Andersen et al., 2016; Friesinger et al., 2020) reveal important institutional aspects regarding the regulation of everyday life, although service users have the right to come and go as they please and are not considered to be 'patients'.

Another difficulty is characterising different kinds of mobile teams visiting people in their own homes. These might be teams coming to the homes in crisis situations or visiting people on a regular basis to help them in their daily life and in their contact with authorities. The person's home is the ground for their interventions, and the question arises to what extent these interventions transform private dwellings into institutions. We have chosen to consider the time-limited presence of these teams in people's own homes as insufficient to characterise these homes as part of the community organised sphere, as the professionals cannot determine rules about the person's daily living.

One difficulty with studying mental health problems is the field's permeable borders (Quirk et al., 2006; Curtis et al., 2009). This permeability is inherent to the field. Historically, it also encompassed illnesses such as dementia and the final stages of syphilis. Today this permeability means the inclusion of, for example, drug dependency (including 'dual diagnosis'). Therefore, the reader should keep in mind that all the places presented here are dedicated to people with mental health problems, but that some of them are also open to those with 'dual diagnoses'.

A wide landscape – The community organised sphere in Agder

Landscapes are in constant movement. Therefore, our findings should only be considered as a snapshot of the total institutional landscape in Agder region at a fixed point in time in 2022.

During the data collection process, we collected information about 120 different places established for people with mental health problems. Most of the places in this new institutional landscape are open and situated in the local communities and service users do not necessarily have any contact with in-patient care.

Organisational affiliations

Of the total 120 places, slightly over half are organised by local authorities and slightly less than half by different branches of the voluntary sector, mostly religious congregations and users' organisations.

Over half of the places are located in Kristiansand, the main municipality, with more than half the total population in the study area. This proportion is also found in Arendal, the second largest municipality, which has about a quarter of the population and a quarter of the places.

Function of the places

Regarding the places' function in people's lives, we have also been forced to simplify a complex reality characterised by the hybridisation of functions (Knibbe & Horstman, 2019):

Meeting Places: Sociality; somewhere to go to.

These places' main purpose is to offer a place to be or to go to when leaving one's home when one cannot afford public places such as coffee houses or cinemas, or when one does not want to encounter the gaze of those without experience of mental health problems. Usually, some activities are proposed for visitors, but they are not the main purposes of these places. This type of place accounts for a sixth of the total *number of places and are present in all the municipalities* under discussion.

Activity Places: Places for production and creative activities. These places include goal-directed rehabilitative structures, or places for creative activities, pastimes, and sometimes the production of objects for markets. Even here, different activities might occur in the same place. Activity places are also places for social interaction, but this is not their primary focus.

One third of the places focus on offering diverse activities for visitors. To be active is often seen as an important part of the recovery process, both according to the literature (Doroud et al., 2018) and policy documents in Norway (Norge Helsedirektoratet, 2014).

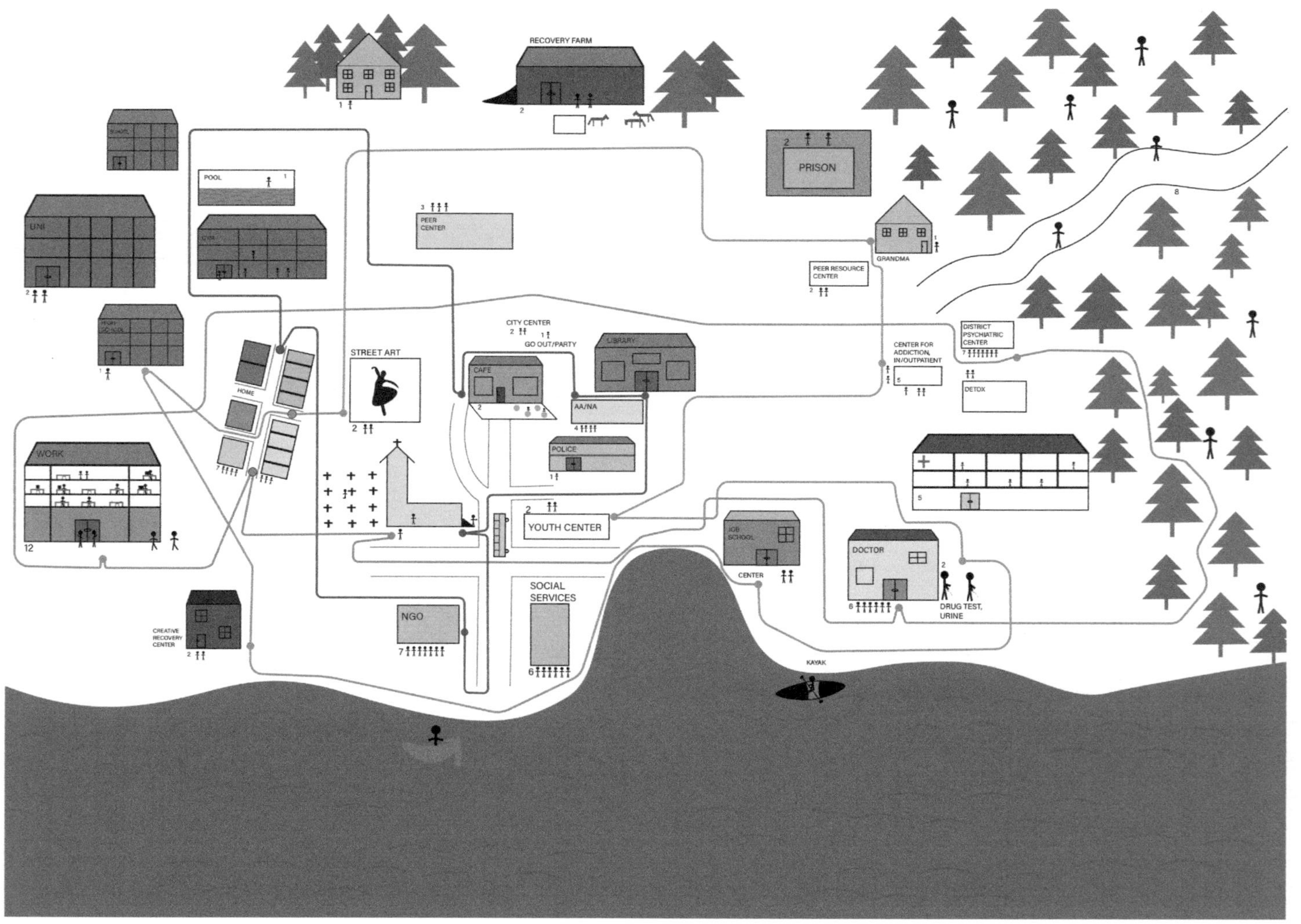

Figure 41.2 The institutional landscape of a town in Agder. (Drawing by Øyvind Hope, 2022).

Table 41.1 The institutional landscape in Agder by Organizational Affiliation and Municipality, 2022

Organisation Type	Kristian-sand	Arendal	Lillesand	Birkenes	Grimstad	Common	Total
Formal health care	30	18	4	3	2	11	68
Volunteer-organised	36	8	2	2	3	1	52
Total	66	26	6	5	5	12	120

Table 41.2 Places in the institutional landscape in Agder by Function and Municipality, 2022

Function	Kristian-sand	Arendal	Lillesand	Birkenes	Grimstad	Common	Total
Meeting places	11	5	3	1	3	0	23
Activity places	24	13	2	2	1	1	43
Housing places	19	5	0	0	0	0	24
Treatment places	9	5	2	1	2	11	30
Total	63	28	7	4	6	12	120

The presence of different places to go to implies an activity in itself: leaving one's home and going to another place to participate in activities or just to meet other people, as one might do in a meeting place.

Housing places:

As a home. As mentioned earlier, here we focus on organised forms of housing. In supported housing, each person has their own flat, but there might also be a common dining room. Staff members are present and have separate spaces. Parts of everyday life are regulated by a set of special rules. Staff members also have the ability to enter the tenants' rooms or flats. However, tenants are able to come and go freely. Certain housing places organise activities such as cooking and eating together, which offers the possibility of socialising.

Supported housing units in Agder represent one fifth of the places in the institutional landscape; they are concentrated in the two largest cities, and we will get back to housing places when we analyse further the new institutional landscape in Agder.

Treatment places:

In-patient stays, medication and psychotherapeutic interventions.

The downsizing of the mental health hospital in Agder has resulted in the spreading and diversification of places for inpatient care, as well as in the creation of psychiatric open care units in the community. Today, inpatient care is available in different places throughout the community, including a mental hospital and six community mental health centres. These centres offer also outpatient care and serve as bases for crisis out-reach teams.

Table 41.2 reflects the proliferation of places directed to different aspects of the life of the persons with mental health problems in the community. These places correspond roughly to Goffman's classical division of what he called "a basic arrangement in modern society"; the spatial division of places where one sleeps, plays and works that was broken in total institutions (1961, p. 17).

A division of labour

The new landscape reflects a division of labour (Table 41.3) between the voluntary sector (which tends to concentrate its efforts on meeting and activity places) and municipalities (which focus their interventions on home-like living environments and the opportunity to leave them and participate in a social life outside the home). As can be expected, treatment remains the monopoly of specialised mental health services.

Mental health services were focused on treatment and were available in 19 places. Municipalities' primary offer was housing, which represented 23 of the total 47 places organised by them. In places organised by the voluntary sector, the focus was on activities (34 places), and social meetings (18 places). Seven of these places were run by user's organisations.

Changes and constancies in 24/7 places

When analysing transformations in the institutional landscape, special attention should be given to living facilities with staff members present up to 24 hours every day.

The number of inpatients in mental health hospital settings in Agder started decreasing around 1990, partly due to the trans-institutionalisation of long-term patients first from the local hospital to former tuberculosis sanatoriums throughout the region. Around 1995–2000, some of these new long-term institutions were transformed into Community Mental Health Centres, while others were closed. These centres combined in- and outpatient care services. During the same period, supported housing was developed in the wake of the Norwegian state's Escalation Plan for Mental Health. Thus, the traditional centralised in-patient institution has been divided in a range of diversified institutionalised living places going from traditional in-patient units to supported housings.

Table 41.4 shows the development of different types of institutional living places (24/7), ranging from hospital care to supported housing.

A clear downsizing of traditional inpatient care in medical surroundings (hospitals and community mental health centres) can be observed in Agder. In 1970, the mental hospital alone had 350 beds. Thirty years later, in 2000, 100 beds remained. Between 2000 and 2020 we can notice a continued reduction in the number of beds in the hospital structure down to 78 beds. In parallel, we can also see a halving of the number of

Table 41.3 Places in the institutional landscape in Agder by Function and Affiliation, 2022

Places	Voluntary	Municipalities	Mental health care	Total
Meeting places	18	5	0	23
Activity places	34	9	0	43
Housing places	1	23	0	24
Treatment places	1	10	19	30
Total	54	47	19	120

Table 41.4 Number of places ("Beds") in different types of institutional living places, 2000–2020

Year	Hospital*	Community mental health centre	Supported housing	Total
2000	100	155	17	272
2020	78	70	258	406

Note. *The number of hospital "beds" are for the whole Agder region.

beds in community mental health centres. This could be interpreted as a sharp reduction of the number of persons in institutionalised forms of living, from 255 in 2000 to 148 in 2020. However, if we also take into account supported housings, which often shows important institutional characteristics (Chow & Priebe, 2013), it could be argued that de-hospitalisation has actually resulted in re-institutionalisation and the augmentation of the number of people living in institutional conditions. The number of people living in supported housing increased from 17 to 258 during the same period.

This means that the total number of people living in institutional settings with staff present up to 24 hours a day has increased from 272 in 2000 to 406 in 2020; i.e. over the period of presumed de-hospitalisation.

However, even in this case, reality is more complex than the numbers show. To some extent, the residents in these institutions might not be the same in 2020 as in 2000. As we earlier mentioned, during this period the administrative border between mental health and addiction problems has become more permeable. Thus, members of both these groups can now be present in the same institutions.

A new institutional landscape

The focus of our contemporary archaeological investigation has been on places built specifically to have a therapeutic and/or supporting capacity for people with mental health problems. In the Agder region, de-hospitalisation has occurred in parallel with the development of a range new structures and services to manage different aspects of daily life in the community. Our findings indicate the presence of a wide community organised sphere that could represent "safe havens… all around Agder", to para-phrase Pinfold (2000). As we also have seen, the mental health hospital still exists, albeit in a reduced form but supplemented with new forms of institutional living arrangements.

Deshospitalisation included a process of trans- and reinstitutionalisation. Still, almost 100 places for social support are disseminated in local communities. The integration of these places could be seen as an aspect of striving to destigmatise mental health problems. People with mental health distress are no longer necessarily removed from their social context and hidden behind walls, far from their homes and social networks. They can still live in their place of origin, maintaining contact with their friends and families and able to access new forms of support and treatment.

Thus, in a welfare country like Norway, de-hospitalisation has not resulted in sys-tematic abandonment and homelessness as in the accounts of Dear & Wolch (1987) and Knowles (2000) from North America. Welfare structures still exist in Agder and new structures are developed. In addition to the community-organised welfare protection net and the presence of mental health services in the community, the volunteer-organised places play an important role, whether financed by state or municipal subsidies or not.

Contradictions and paradoxes in the new total institutional landscape

Considering the multitude of initiatives and structures, a new understanding of the community organised landscape developed for people with mental health problems has become possible. To analyse the new institutional landscape, we propose the formulation of a series of paradoxes or contradictions.

De-hospitalisation and re-institutionalisation: The so-called process of de-institutionalisation has resulted not only in the downsizing of the local mental hospital, but also in the proliferation of mental health institutions with the presence of professionals and with specific architecture and rules for everyday life, in the community or at its fringe (Fjellfeldt et al., 2021). Thus, de-institutionalisation resulted in a certain de-hospitalisation combined with a parallel process of re-institutionalisation.

Separate total institutions and a community spread total institution: The new network of micro institutions replicates Goffman's division between place to work, to sleep and to be in your spare time, not circumscribed behind a wall, but spread in the local communities. In this context, the recurrent emphasis on the necessity of coordinating the efforts of the different actors from the institutional network in terms of recovery plans and other plans reminds us of a part of Goffman's description of the life inside total institutions (Goffman, 1961, p. 17).

Panopticon and panoptisism: Goffmans' understood total institutions as a social order. This social order is still existing. The presence of the new institutional places and of their teams of professionals involved in people's everyday lives (and even their intimate sphere) to offer them help, widens the gaze of mental health professionals. Thus, the network of segregated micro-institutions throughout the community can even be seen as part of system of soft monitoring by the state of parts of the population no longer inside brick-and-mortar institutions but in the community; as a new decentralised form of 'panopticon' (Foucault, 1989); a "panoptisism" (Burnon-Ernst, 2012, p. 2).

Normalisation/socialisation and medicalisation/individualisation: The new institutional landscape targets a population no longer limited to 'madness' or 'severe mental illnesses. The spread of a psychiatric gaze in the community (Högström, 2018) through the presence of a local based network of institutional places reflects, but might also create a need for psychiatric interventions. An extensive part of the population is now said to experience 'mental health' issues. Through the dissemination of psychological and medical models, people tend to interpret their difficulties to adapt to the increasing demands of worklife and of self-fulfilment as well as their difficulties and shortcomings in individualised terms; as the results of imbalances in their brains or of cognitive deficits (Beeker et al., 2021; Topor et al., 2022). Thus, to both get access to an acceptable narrative about their shortcomings and to help from the welfare state, they need to be diagnosed with some kind of mental illness resulting in a psychiatrisation of society (Beeker et al., 2021) and of social phenomena (Mills, 2015). This development has been facilitated by the reduced requirements to obtain diagnoses such as depression, bi-polar and neuropsychiatric disorders (Frances, 2013).

Citizenship and total institutional landscape: When analysing the new institutional landscapes, it should not be forgotten that an important goal of this development was that people previously confined behind the walls of the mental hospitals would gain access to all the places (public, natural and institutional) constituting all citizens' landscapes. Studies reveal the importance of the *person-organised sphere* for those living with mental health problems (Knibbe & Horstman, 2019). Thus, the composition of personal and enabling landscapes might differ from person to person and from time to time. The quantity and diversity of places at people's disposal might also counteract the potential risk inherent in a sparce landscape as the access to few places reduce the possibility to choose different social contexts over time but also at the same time. The role of one place for a specific person is not only due to its intrinsic characteristics but also depends on the presence or absence of other possible places to integrate in that person's enabling landscape. Places might be disabling or not adequate for the needs one might have in a phase of their recovery process. But the availability of different places under different authorities or under no authority at all might be considered as increasing the probability that such a personal enabling landscape could be developed.

General welfare and one's own responsibility: Regarding contemporary history from a social-political point of view, de-hospitalisation occurred in a period when neo-liberal ideas started to guide political decisions. State incursion in people's private life was now

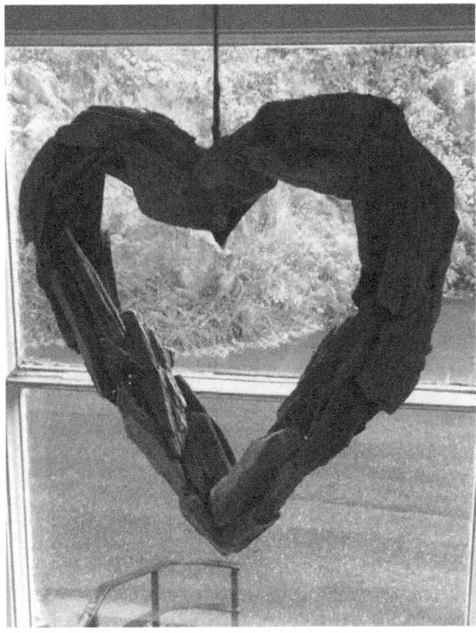

Figure 41.3 Heart in a window. Looking out of a meeting place in a town in Agder. Photograph by Alain Topor.

described as a hinder to their own capacity to take care of themselves (Gerstle, 2022). From this perspective, it means that people should to a greater extent, take responsibility for their own life choices and their consequences and thus become responsible citizens making adequate decisions (Adams, 2019). Landscape of despairs was studied in California, where former governor and later US president Ronald Reagan practiced this policy. Later it has gained a world-wide application. So, what is the future, what are the possible and desirable improvements or alternatives to a new institutional landscape?

Closing reflection: the necessary knowledge about total landscapes

In welfare countries, a new total institutional landscape together with non-institutional settings and a guaranteed basic welfare provision offer a basis for people with mental health problems to develop liveable lives (Hope et al., 2023). As Pinfold (2000, p. 210) stated:

> Service users are not passive players in the rehabilitation landscape, moreover: they are active participants shaping, as well as being shaped by, socio-medical pathways that are negotiated using personal coping mechanisms to sustain everyday equilibrium. Instead of absolute positions, individuals often occupy a (preferred) evolving middle-ground between isolation and integration, between states of dependency and ones of independence.

Without knowledge about the total institutional landscape, we lack the possibility to fully understand the spread of an individualising psychiatric culture in our societies. This knowledge also constitutes a background to understand different persons' construction of their personal enabling landscapes. It offers an opportunity to study what places are seldom or never mentioned by service users as enabling. Finally, it makes it possible to compare different institutional landscapes and critically analyse them and the different policies behind them.

In this chapter we have presented the development of a new institutional landscape made of places directed to people with mental health problems in the community in a region in Norway. Such a landscape is made possible due to the Norwegian state's commitment to general welfare regime that ensures all citizens an acceptable living standard. Thus, citizens, including people leaving in-patient care can remain independent from support from their families and from voluntary organisations. This model is not free from criticism, and but stand in contrast to more neo-liberal oriented countries where the individuals' independence from support from the state is stressed, creating other forms of dependences and abandonment.

Acknowledgement

Figure 41.2 was published previously in Hope, Ø., Ness, O., Friesinger, J.G., Topor, A. & Bøe, T.D. (2023). 'Living needs a landscape': A qualitative study about the role of enabling landscapes for people with mental health and substance abuse problems. *Health & Place*, 84, https://doi.org/10.1016/j.healthplace.2023.103144.

References

Adams, G., Estrada-Villalta, S., & Sullivan, D. (2019). The psychology of neoliberalism and the neoliberalism of psychology. *Journal of Social Issues, 75*(1), 189–216. https://doi.org/10.1111/josi.12305

Andersen, A. J. W., Larsen, I. B., & Topor, A. (2016). Caring through discipline? Analyzing house rules in community mental health services in Norway. *Scandinavian Psychologist, 3.* http://dx.doi.org/10.15714/scandpsychol.3.e1

Andersson, G. (2009). *Vardagsliv och boendestöd – en studie om människor med psykiska funktionshinder* [Doctoral dissertation, Department of Social Work, Stockholm University].

Basaglia, F. (1987). *Psychiatry inside out – Selected writings of Franco Basaglia.* Columbia University Press.

Beeker, T., Mills, C., Bhugra, D., Te Meerman, S., Thoma, S., Heinze, M., & Von Peter, S. (2021). Psychiatrization of society: A conceptual framework and call for transdisciplinary research. *Frontiers in Psychiatry, 12.* https://doi.org/10.3389/fpsyt.2021.645556

Bell, S. L., Foley, R., Houghton, F., Maddrell, A., & Williams, A. M. (2018). From therapeutic landscapes to healthy spaces, places and practices: A scoping review. *Social Science & Medicine, 196*, 123–130. https://doi.org/10.1016/j.socscimed.2017.11.035

Bell, S. L., Hickman, C., & Houghton, F. (2023). From therapeutic landscape to therapeutic 'sensescape' experiences with nature? A scoping review. *Wellbeing, Space and Society, 4.* https://doi.org/10.1016/j.wss.2022.100126

Burnon-Ernst, A. (2012). Deconstructing panopticism into the plural panopticons. In A. Brunon-Ernst (ed.), *Beyond Foucault – New perspectives on Bentham's panopticon.* Routledge: London & New York, pp. 17–41.

Chow, W. S., & Priebe, S. (2013). Understanding psychiatric institutionalization: A conceptual review. *BMC Psychiatry, 13*, 169. https://doi.org/10.1186/1471-244X-13-169

Conradson, D. (2003). Geographies of care: Spaces, practices, experiences. *Social & Cultural Geography, 4*(4), 451–454. https://doi.org/10.1080/1464936032000137894

Curtis, S., Gesler, W., Priebe S., & Francis, S. (2009). New spaces of inpatient care for people with mental illness: A complex 'rebirth' of the clinic? *Health & Place, 15*, 340–348.

Dear, M., & Wolch, J. (1987). *Landscape of despair. From deinstitutionalization to homelessness.* Polity Press.

Doroud, N., Fossey, E., & Fortune, T. (2018). Place for being, doing, becoming and belonging: A meta-synthesis exploring the role of place in mental health recovery, *Health & Place, 52*, 110–120. https://doi.org/10.1016/j.healthplace.2018.05.008

Duff, C. (2012). Exploring the role of 'enabling places' in promoting recovery from mental illness: A qualitative test of a relational model. *Health & Place, 18*, 1388–1395. https://doi.org/10.1016/j.healthplace.2012.07.003

Fjellfeldt, M., Högström, E., Berglund-Snodgrass, L., & and Markström, U. (2021). Fringe or not fringe?: Strategies for localizing supported accommodation in a post-deinstitutional era. *Social Inclusion, 9*, 201–213. https://doi.org/10.17645/si.v9i3.4319

Foot J. (2014). Franco Basaglia and the radical psychiatry movement in Italy, 1961-1978. *Critical and Radical Social Work, 2*(2), 235–249. https://doi.org/10.1332/204986014X14002292074708

Foucault, M. (1960/1989). *Madness and civilization. A story of insanity in the age of reason.* Routledge.

Frances, A. (2013). *Saving normal.* Harper Collins.

Friesinger, J. G., Topor, A., Bøe, T. D., & Larsen, I. B. (2020). Materialities in supported housing for people with mental health problems: A blurry picture of the tenants. *Sociology of Health & Illness, 42*(7), 1742–1758. https://doi.org/10.1111/1467-9566.13162

Gerstle, G. (2022). *The rise and fall of the neoliberal order – America and the world in the free market era.* Oxford University Press.

Gesler, W. M. (1992). Therapeutic landscapes: Medical issues in light of the new cultural geography. *Social Science & Medicine, 34*(7), 735–746. https://doi.org/https://doi.org/10.1016/0277-9536(92)90360-3

Goffman, E. (1961/1976). *Asylums: Essays on the social situation of mental patients and other inmates.* Doubleday & Co.

Högström, E. (2018). 'It used to be here but moved somewhere else': Post-asylum spatialisations – A new urban frontier? *Social & Cultural Geography, 19*(3), 314–335. https://doi.org/10.1080/14649365.2016.1239753

Hope, Ø., Ness, O., Friesinger, J.G., Topor, A., & Bøe, T.D. (2023). 'Living needs a landscape': A qualitative study about the role of enabling landscapes for people with mental health and substance abuse problems. *Health & Place, 84.* https://doi.org/10.1016/j.healthplace.2023.103144

Hydén L. C. (1995). The rhetoric of recovery and change. *Culture, medicine and psychiatry, 19*(1), 73–90. https://doi.org/10.1007/BF01388249

Kearns, R., & Milligan, C. (2020). Placing therapeutic landscape as theoretical development in Health & Place. *Health & Place, 61,* 102224. https://doi.org/https://doi.org/10.1016/j.healthplace.2019.102224

Knibbe, M., & Horstman, K. (2019). The making of new care spaces. How micropublic places mediate inclusion and exclusion in a Dutch city. *Health & Place, 57,* 27–34. https://doi.org/https://doi.org/10.1016/j.healthplace.2019.03.008

Knowles, C. (2000). *Bedlam on the streets.* Routledge.

Konrad, N. (2002). Prisons as new asylums. *Current Opinion in Psychiatry, 15*(6), 583–587. https://journals.lww.com/co-psychiatry/fulltext/2002/11000/prisons_as_new_asylums.4.aspx

Larsen, I. B., & Topor, A. (2017). A place for the heart: A journey in the post-asylum landscape. Metaphors and materiality. *Health & Place, 45,* 145–151. https://doi.org/10.1016/j.healthplace.2017.03.015

Milligan, C., & Wiles, J. (2010). Landscapes of care. *Progress in Human Geography, 34*(6), 736–754. https://doi.org/10.1177/0309132510364556

Mills, C. (2015). The psychiatrization of poverty: Rethinking the mental health-poverty nexus. *Social and Personality Psychology Compass, 9*(5), 213–222. https://doi.org/10.1111/spc3.12168

Mossabir, R., Milligan, C., & Froggatt, K. (2021). Therapeutic landscape experiences of everyday geographies within the wider community: A scoping review. *Social Science & Medicine (1982), 279,* 113980. https://doi.org/10.1016/j.socscimed.2021.113980

Nirje, B. (1985). The basis and logic of the normalization principle. *Australia & New Zealand Journal of Developmental Disabilities, 11*(2), 65–68. https://doi.org/10.3109/13668258509008747

Norge Helsedirektoratet. (2014). *Sammen om mestring: Veileder i lokalt psykisk helsearbeid og rusarbeid for voksne: et verktøy for kommuner og spesialisthelsetjenesten. Helsedirektoratet.* https://helsedirektoratet.no/Lists/Publikasjoner/Attachments/410/Sammen-om-mestring-Veileder-i-lokalt-psykisk-helsearbeid-og-rusarbeid-for-voksne-IS-2076.pdf.pdf

Pedersen, P. B., & Kolstad, A. (2009). De-institutionalisation and trans-institutionalisation – Changing trends of inpatient care in Norwegian mental health institutions 1950-2007. *International Journal of Mental Health Systems, 3*(1), 28. https://doi.org/10.1186/1752-4458-3-28

Pinfold, V. (2000). 'Building up safe havens…All around the world': Users' experiences of living in the community with mental health problems." *Health and Place, 6*(3), 201–212. https://doi:10.1016/S1353-8292(00)00023-X.

Quirk, A., Lelliott, P., & Seale, C. (2006). The permeable institution: An ethnographic study of three acute psychiatric wards in London. *Social Science & Medicine, 63,* 2105–2117.

Rosenberg, D. (2009). *Psychiatric disability in the community: Surveying the social landscape in the post-deinstitutional era* [Doctoral thesis, Umeå University].

Rotelli, F. (1988). L'instituzione inventata, in F. Rotelli (ed.), *Per la normalita – Taccuino di uno psichiatria.* Edizione e.

Scull, A. T. (1984). *Decarceration. Community treatment and the deviant – A radical view*, Polity press.

Scull, A.T. (2022). *Desperate remedies. Psychiatry and the mysteries of mental illness*. Random Penguin House.

Topor, A. (2020). Deinstitutionalisation, welfare state and social engineering: Basaglia in the Swedish context, in T. Burns & J. Foot (eds.), *Basaglia's International Legacy: From Asylum to Community* (pp. 333–346). Oxford University Press.

Topor, A., Andersson, G., Bülow, P., Stefansson, C. G., & Denhov, A. (2016). After the Asylum? The New Institutional Landscape. *Community Mental Health Journal*, 52(6), 731–737. https://doi.org/10.1007/s10597-015-9928-7

Topor A., Boe, T. D., & Larsen, I. B. (2022). The lost social context of recovery: Psychiatrization of a social process. *Frontiers in Sociology, 7*. https://doi.org/10.3389%2Ffsoc.2022.832201

Wing, J.K., & Brown G.W. (1970). *Institutionalism and schizophrenia – A comparative study of three mental hospitals 1960–1968*. Cambridge University Press.

Wolch, J., & Philo, C. (2000). From distributions of deviance to definitions of difference: Past and future mental health geographies. *Health & Place*, 6(3), 137–157. https://doi.org/10.1016/s1353-8292(00)00019-8

42 A new space for 'curing madness'

Circulation of an open-door model between France and Argentina in the early twentieth century

Hervé Guillemain and Fernando Ferrari

Introduction

In the autumn of 2022, we were both walking through *the Hospital Asilo Colonia de Oliva* [the Oliva Psychiatric Colony][1] in Cordoba, Argentina, camera in hand. As in a great 'urbex experiment', (i.e., historian experiments looking for traces of the past in abandoned places; Offenstadt 2022), we grasped the extent of the degradation of the site created at the beginning of the twentieth century. The last patients on the site were nowhere to be seen and – while keeping an eye out for the many stray dogs that roamed the site in packs – we were able to wander easily through the ruins of the hundred-year-old pavilions. This psychiatric institution, which was innovative when it opened at the beginning of the twentieth century, was only a shadow of its former self.

The Open Door system in the history of psychiatry, a reform that sought to create a less restrictive and more humane environment for psychiatric patients by reducing coercive methods, had its origins in the psychiatric reform movement that took place in Europe and North America from mainly in the second half of the nineteenth century onwards (Scull 1981; Porter and Wright 2003). This reform movement was rooted in the asylums crisis which began shortly after they were established. These institutions quickly became overcrowded, attracting criticism fuelled by numerous scandals of abusive internment (Fauvel 2005). In Great Britain, the 'trade in lunacy' was denounced (Porter and Wright 2003), and several European countries were revising their legislation, but in France the law of 1838 seemed impossible to amend due to the aliénists' conservative view. For some rare care givers, this crisis in psychiatric care meant that they had to experiment, in particular by opening institutions (Freeman 2005). The second half of the nineteenth century also saw the emergence of rural colonies in France. In Scotland and Flemish Belgium a 'boarding-out system' was developed, based on foster care for the insane. Shortly before the Great War, the German psychiatrist Gustav Kolb helped to invent 'the free ward', i.e., psychiatric care without internment, which also spread at the same time in France and became widespread during the Great War (Derrien, 2020).

Our focus, in this chapter, is how the reconstruction of the Open-Door model was deployed in Argentina by the Argentinian psychiatrist Domingo Cabred in the early nineteenth century, after having travelled to Europe. In doing so, we resituate this place of care in the wider history of institutional and architectural evolutions of psychiatric care as spaces of mental health and wellbeing. In order to do so, we will establish a cross-reference between Oliva, an Argentinean institution and a few French institutions of the

DOI: 10.4324/9781003345725-47

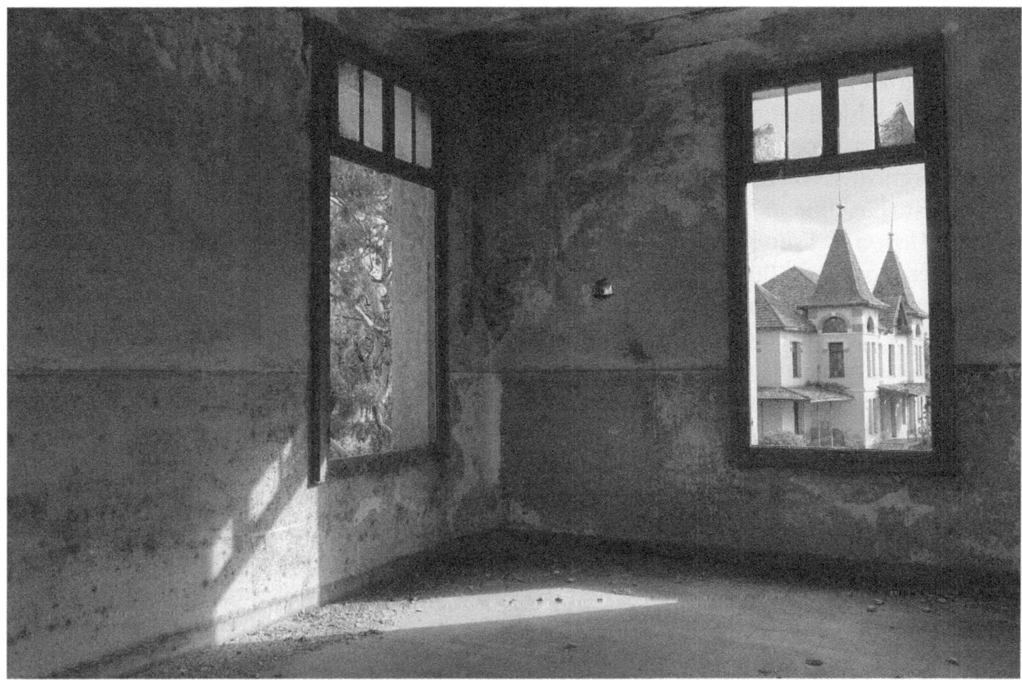

Figure 42.1 View from inside a ward towards one of the many buildings at the now derelict Oliva Psychiatric Colony in Cordoba, Argentina (Photograph by Fernando Ferrari, 2022).

years 1890–1914, comparing the way in which the Open-Door model was generated and applied in both countries.

The birth of a new model of psychiatric space in the early twentieth century and its circulation between France and Argentina

Domingo Cabred, grew from a wealthy bourgeois family in the province of Corrientes and graduated in Buenos Aires as Doctor of Medicine in 1881 (Marquiegui 2020). A few years later, in 1886, he was promoted as sub-director of the *Hospicio de las Mercedes* until 1892, Cabred was very close to Julio Argentino Roca – politician, military man and statesman – who served twice as president of Argentine (1880–1886 and 1898–1904) during two key periods in the formation of the Nation State. Backed by Roca, Cabred travelled to Europe in 1888, where he toured the British clinics and colonies of Argyll, Fife and Kinross, Inverness, Haddington and Perth, as well as the Belgian colony of Gheel and the German colony of Alt Scherbitz, which he took as a model for his project in Argentina.

It is well known that Argentina was always culturally influenced by France (Marquiegui 2020). In fact, every doctor and intellectual usually made a 'consecrating trip' to that country after completing their training. In 1889, Cabred took part in the *International Congress of Mental Medicine* held in Paris, where the first attempt to classify and systematise mental illnesses was made (Caponi 2012). There, Cabred made a brief intervention (Cabred, 1889), from which he was able to interact with renowned figures such as Jean Martin Charcot, Valentin Magnan, Adolphe Quételet, Ernest Kraepelin and Enrico Morselli and Jules Morel. He published an article, *The Progress of Psychiatry*, in 1896 in which he analyses the asylums in Belgium (Morel, 1987). In 1894, Cabred, whose proposal for classification of mental illnesses was considered old and extemporaneous, returned to Argentina and set up a project based on the models being adopted in Europe at that time.

The Hospital Asilo Colonia de Oliva was inaugurated in 1914. One year earlier, the first alternative psychotherapeutic center was opened in France. A little more than a century after the beginnings of modern psychiatry, which historians place around 1800 (Castel 1977), a place of care was opened in France whose design principles – location, architecture, plan and organisation of the psychiatric hospital – were new and, in many ways, comparable to those that were at the origin of the Argentinean institution of Oliva. This place of care was *the Fleury-les-Aubrais Hospital*, located not far from the city of Orléans, itself located about a hundred kilometers south of Paris (Marquis 2013).

To understand the roots of this pioneering work in France, it is necessary to go back half a century, where the notion of 'ideal psychiatric hospital architecture' originated in an old critique of the asylums model by Western alienists in the first half of the nineteenth century (note that 'alienist' is a now outdated term for 'psychatrist'; OED, 2023) . This criticism began to appear publicly during a controversy in 1866 between two men and two representations of the ideal asylum. The first of these two men was Léopold Turck (1797–1887), a republican doctor and representative in the National Assembly, who had been interested in psychiatry for a long time, launched in 1865, a petition against the alienists, accusing asylums of creating mental illness and promoting excess hospital mortality. He was one of the republican doctors who attacked the corporation of alienists, which was linked to the emperor's regime (Turck 1865). Facing him was Maximien Parchappe de Vinay (1800–1866), who responded in a speech to the Société Médico-Psychologique on 27 November 1865 (Parchappe 1865). This doctor, so-called 'general inspector of the service for the insane' since 1848, defended the French-style asylum in the name of the corporation of alienists, whose program had been planned by the French psychiatrist Jean-Etienne Esquirol[2] in the preceding decades.

A political controversy thus arose around psychiatric hospital architecture and the prevailing model of psychiatric care (see Figure 42.2 for a representation of typical asylum architecture prior to the Open-Door era, advanced by Parchappe, 1865).

In his criticism of the models advocated by Parchappe, the Inspector General of Asylums Léopold Turck refers to another model which he considered ideal for the care of the 'insane': that of Gheel, which Domingo Cabred also supported (Maldonado, Pedraza, & Naides, 2002). The reputation of Gheel was built on two things: the dynamism of an ancient healing pilgrimage, and the development of an original, not very medicalised, system of care for the sick by nurses (Fauvel et Dupont, 2018). Numerous study trips by European doctors to this site took place between the 1840s and 1860s. The campaign in favour of such 'family colonies for the insane' like Gheel culminated in 1867. Jules Duval, a utopian socialist close to the Fourierists, defended the open model and that of family colonisation. In particular, Duval promoted Baron Mundy's[3] 'family home for psychiatric care', which was exhibited to the public at the 1867 Paris Universal Exhibition (Mueller 2008). Thus, the global questioning of the system of care for the

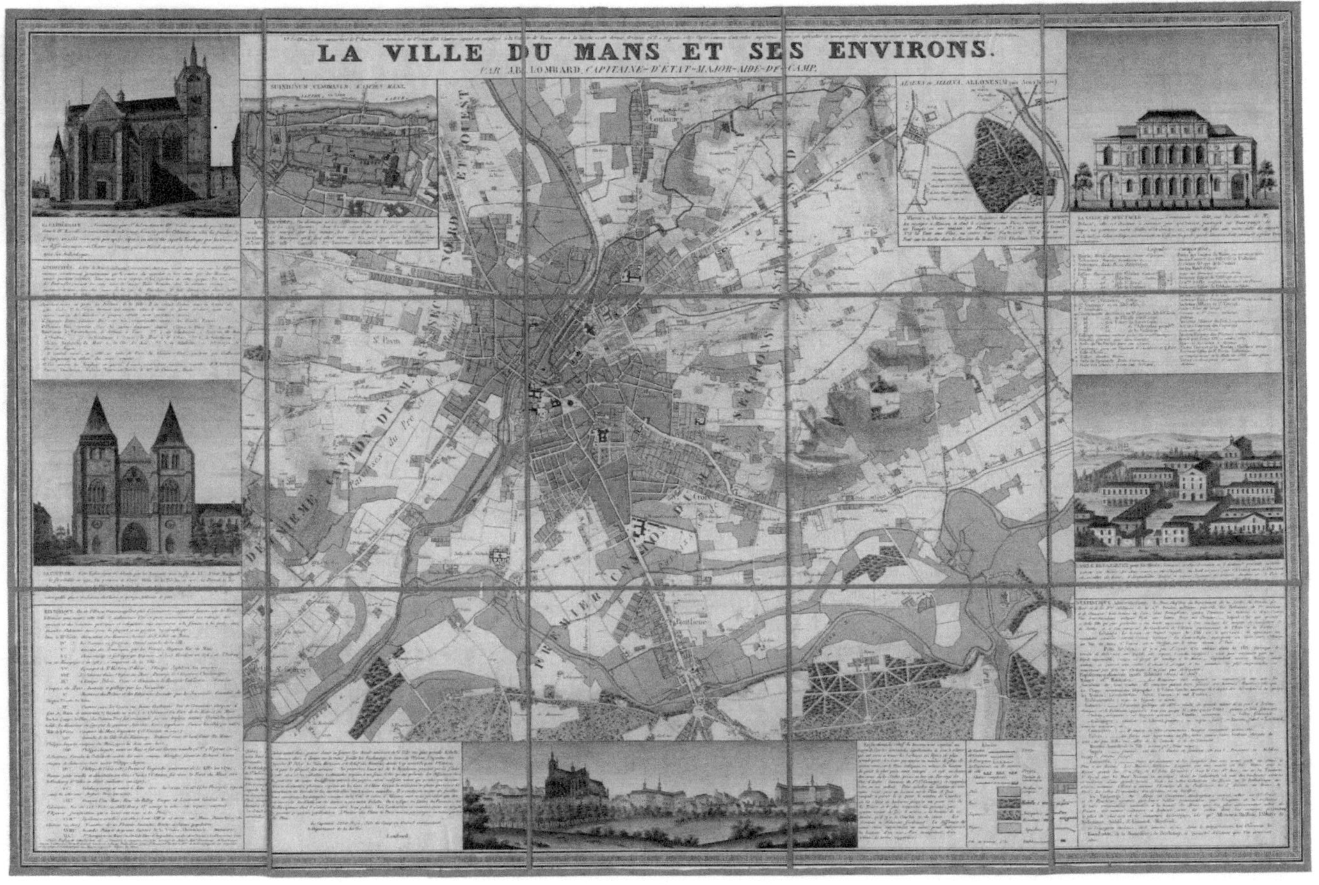

Figure 42.2 *Le Mans asylum* in Lombard's map, 1840. A typical asylum architecture prior to the Open Door era, advanced by Parchappe (1865). Permission: MAINE 4 11544.

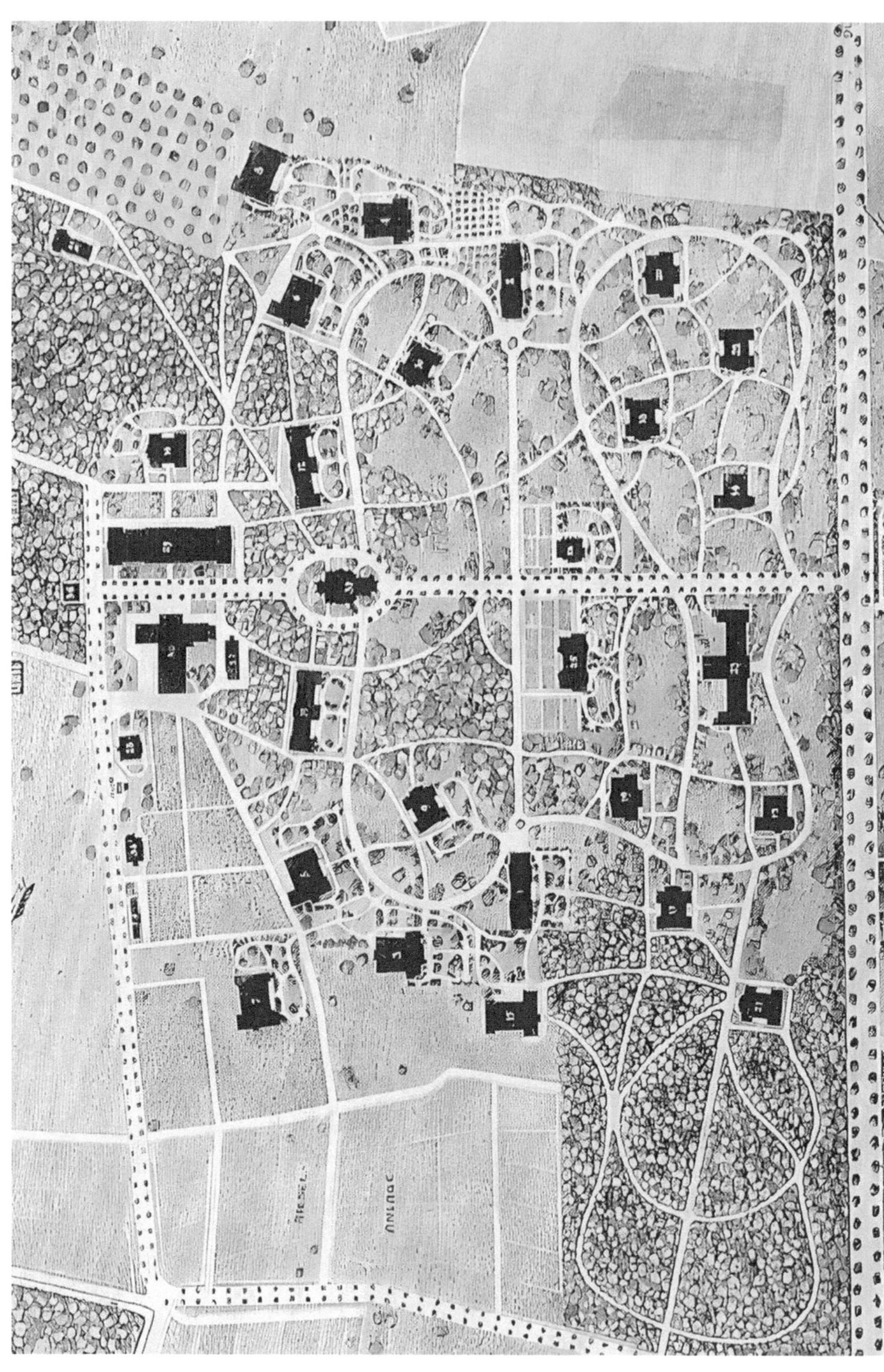

Figure 42.3 The new German model in a French medical investigation. Photo from: Sérieux, 1903.

'insane' involved questioning the psychiatric hospital architecture but also questioning the political order.

In Germany, new psychiatric hospital models (Figure 42.3) were beginning to prefigure what would later be called 'the village hospital' – meaning a hospital with the structure of a small open-door villages In France the following years were marked by a kind of status quo, with the exception of the creation of a few very original family colonies in the centre of France (Derrien 2020). The new public asylums built in the Paris region during the time of Baron Hausmann remained based on the model of large symmetrical buildings (Laget 2004). *The John Bost Hospital* in La Force, an open-door institution for 'epileptics' in south-western France, was an exception, but it was a private Protestant institution influenced partly by the alternatives developed in Great Britain (Figure 42.4).

However, many factors were pushing the authorities to question this French-style asylum model. Firstly, the demographic growth in the number of patients was becoming impressive. It was the case everywhere, in France and also in South America. In Argentina from 1870 to 1910, the national population of 'alienated patients' rose from a total of 4003 to double in 1920, to a total of 8800 patients (Requiere 2000). Asylum internment became a common experience throughout the country. The institutions, subjected to strong pressure and paralysing congestion, increased the number of extensions, but these became difficult in urban areas. Some asylums therefore added rural annexes to make the chronically ill work in peace. New categories of people were admitted to psychiatric hospitals: the elderly, children, 'alcoholics' (the scientific construction of alcoholism in the 1870s made it possible to envisage specific wards) and 'syphilitics' (affected by general paralysis, a disease which often generated a third of the internments). The optimistic period of moral treatment[4] supported by Pinel and Esquirol was followed by a pessimistic period marked by a depressing discourse on incurability and degeneration (Coffin 2003). The question of how to manage an ever-increasing and aging mass of chronically ill people weighed on architectural and institutional thinking. In other words, new models of spatial organisation and architectural design emerged to manage the large numbers of patients, signalling the rise of Open Door asylums. The creation of bigger asylum in rural areas, like Oliva in Argentina, was part of this reflexion. Although the First World War caused a hecatomb among patients in Belgium as well as in France, this demographic pressure was growing until 1914. The period preceding the war was, therefore, logically the one that stimulated the most desire for reform in Europe and also in Argentina.

It was in this context that *the Fleury-les-Aubrais Hospital*, the first psychotherapeutic centre in France, was built in 1913, an equivalent, at least to some extent in architectural terms, of the Oliva asylum (Marquis 2013). This highly original establishment in the history of French psychiatry depended to some extent on the existence of a virgin institutional terrain. The same situation was repeated in the French colonies in North Africa in the 1930s and gave rise to the same institutional and architectural experiments (Von Bueltzingsloewen, 2010). The most radical development was in French Algeria between the two world wars, where psychiatrists had a clean slate of traditional medicine and were free to propose the creation of an institution that differed from the choices made in metropolitan France. The first pavilions of the hospital of Blida in Algeria were opened in 1933 and resembled in many ways those of the Open Door asylums of Fleury and Oliva (Marquis 2022). The layout of the pavilions of the three hospitals is particularly striking, breaking with the symmetry of the old asylums. Furthermore, the pavilions had all plastered façades in white colour. However, where the pavilions of Oliva and Blida

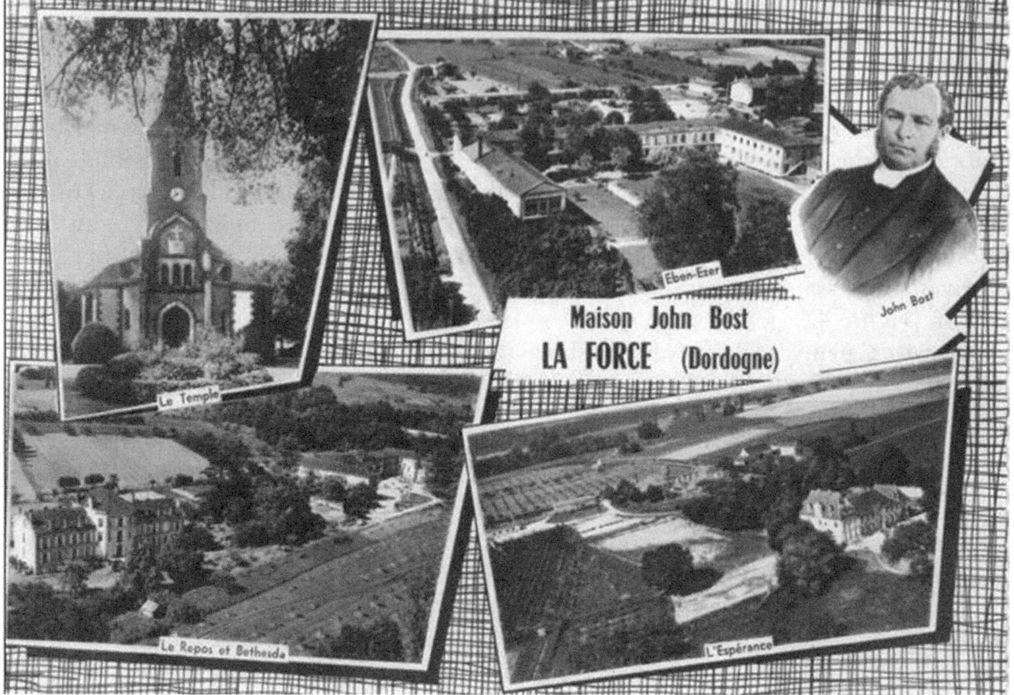

Figure 42.4 A post card showing *John Bost Foundation for Epileptics* in La Force, southwest of France, 19th century. Photo: Private collection.

had gable roofs with overhanging eaves and wooden brackets, those of Fleury were flat and with the sparse ornamentation.

Germany was similarly concerned with the search for an efficient way of separating the acute and chronically ill. In France, this model only really existed in Strasbourg, which, given its history, had developed a Germanic clinical model that would last after the territory was returned to France after 1918. A few experiments were nevertheless attempted in this direction before the Great War, particularly in the north of France. During the Great War, the Fleury hospital became one of the pioneering places for this freer care of the sick, especially soldiers, without internment (Marquis, 2013). Before the better known Edouard Toulouse experiment in Paris in the early 1920s, other places combined institutional and architectural innovation which led to the constitution of a new model that envisaged large, open spaces for the treatment of mental illness (Derrien, 2020).

In the early years of the twentieth century, the French alienist Paul Sérieux, an admirer of Kraepelin's Germanic nosology (he was one of the first to write on dementia praecox), travelled throughout Europe and brought back a large 1000-page report on the best European institutional models (Sérieux 1903). German and Swiss hospitals are presented, some of which were also visited by Cabred. For Cabred, it was necessary to adopt the principles that governed the German reforms: subordination of the plan to medical ideology; segmentation into independent wards; reduction of the number of patients

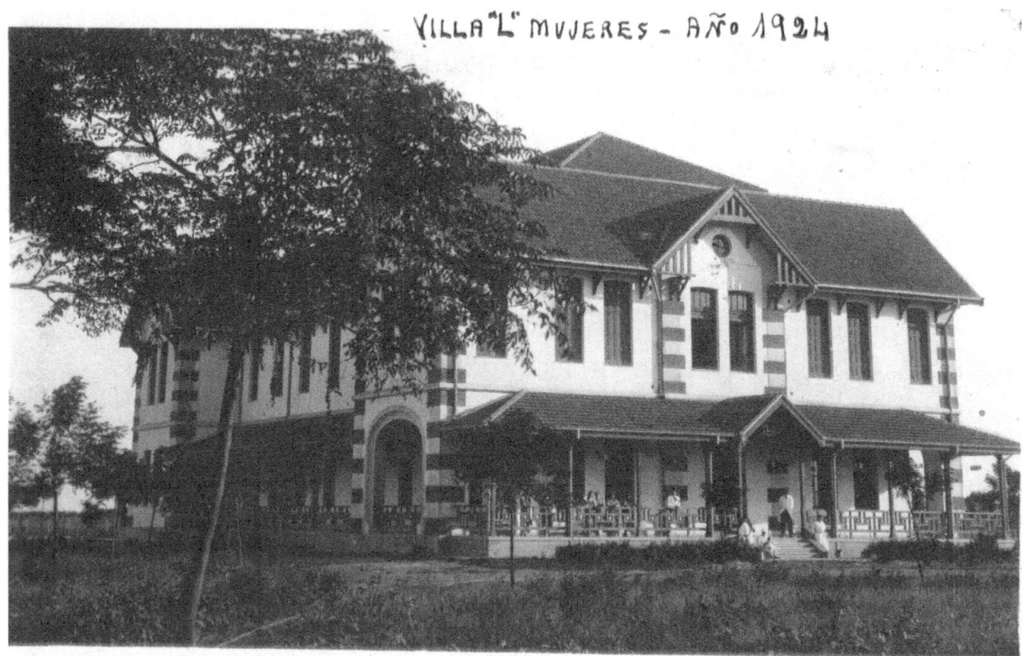

Figure 42.5 Villa L for women at Hospital Colonia de Alienados de Oliva, Argentina. Photo: José Cuenca.

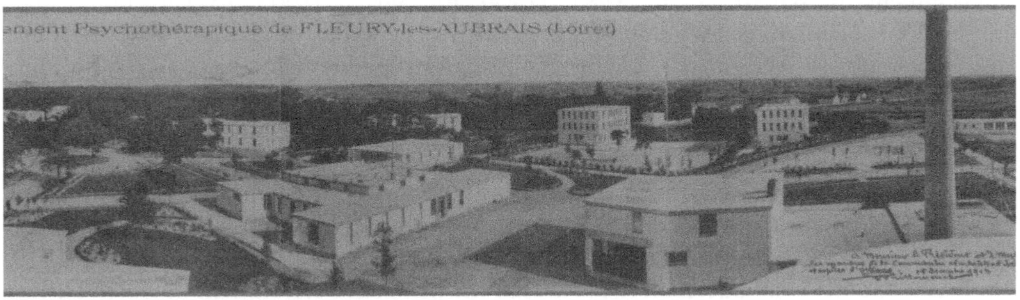

Figure 42.6 Center Fleury-les -Aubrais, France. Photo: Fleury-les-Aubrais Hospital archives.

per ward; differentiation of wards; and development of the colony system for chronic patients (Maldonado et al., 2002). The Open-Door Asylum Colony in Alt Scherbitz (1876) and the Galkhausen Asylum Colony (1900) are for Sérieux the model of modernity: no walls, no covered galleries, no railings and no wolf jumps; maximum differentiation of the wards; division into two parts (colony/central wing); free living in the colony; bedding in the acute hospital; and farm work for the quiet patients (Séreux, 1903). This form of village hospital and German open-door, which inspired the Fleury-les-Aubrais experiment, was very close to the one that was created in Argentina in 1914 according principles mentioned above (see also Cabred in Maldonado et al., 2002, p.159–164).

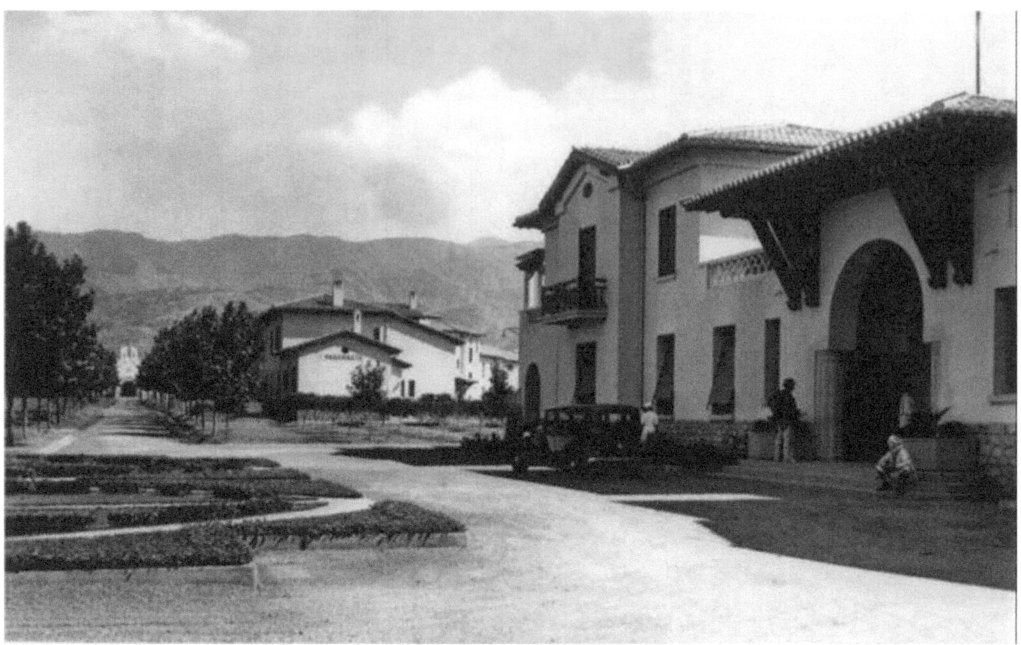

Figure 42.7 Hospital Blida Joinville, Algeria. Photo: Private collection.

The Open Door movement sought to create a more therapeutic and less restrictive environment for patients (Scull 1981, Porter and Wright 2003, Fauvel 2005). These innovations included: i) designing buildings with large windows to allow in natural light and connection to the outside environment, as opposed to the closed, dark buildings that dominated earlier psychiatric hospital architecture, ii) elimination of individual cells and physical restraints for patients, and creation of common rooms and open spaces to allow social interaction and free movement, iii) creation of green areas and gardens so that patients could enjoy contact with nature and engage in outdoor recreational and therapeutic activities, and iv) design of areas for occupational and recreational therapy, such as workshops, libraries, music rooms and sports spaces. Clearly, these architectural innovations were based on the idea that the physical environment in which patients found themselves could significantly affect their emotional and mental well-being. The aim was thus to create a more humane and therapeutic environment that would be conducive to the recovery of the patients.

It is possible to see all these experiments as part of the same reforming moment in modern psychiatry. The psychotherapeutic centre at Fleury-les-Aubrais, like the asylum at Oliva, corresponded in every way to this model, which was based on the absence of walls, the dissemination of the pavilions in the forest, the centrality of a social space (chapel, etc.), and the addition of agricultural and craft work. Like Cabred, the doctor in charge of Fleury, Jean Rayneau, a psychiatrist with an interest in hypnotherapy and balneotherapy, was attracted by the English and German alternative models and was inspired by Paul Sérieux's trip when he was asked by the prefect of the Loiret to think about the creation of a new psychiatric hospital for 1000 patients on more than 200 hectares of forest (Marquis, 2013). Being doctor and director of the institution from 1913 to 1926, he had the power to put the innovations of care into architecture and wanted to change the image of the asylum. In order to do this, he abandoned the term 'asylum' early on (before the generalisation of the term 'psychiatric hospital' in 1937) and adopted the very modern term "psychotherapeutic center" (Marquis, 2013). It can, therefore, be said that there was a Franco-Argentine community of thought and experience at the beginning of the twentieth century when it came to thinking about the ideal hospital for psychiatric care.

The Hospital Asilo Colonia de Oliva: A new psychiatric space for a new population

In the period from 1880 to 1940, a series of political, economic and cultural ideas took shape in Argentina, which led to a series of medical care strategies which resulted in the adoption of European architectural models for psychiatric hospitals. At the beginning of this spatial reorganisation, a project named "Para la creación de asilos y hospitals regionales" [For the creation of asylums and regional hospitals] was presented (Marquiegui, 2020). The secular public health and hygiene apparatus was modelled on European canons. The charity-philanthropy articulation was evident in the political welfare work, and the Argentinean state was entrusted with setting the guidelines for public health intervention. Medical action was linked to the civilising ideals of the new modern state (Vezzetti, 1985). These ideals comprised the centralisation of power to unify the territory and strengthen the state, economic liberalism and openness to international trade, the promotion of education, science and technology, the separation of Church and State, the promotion of secularism, and the stimulation of immigration as a means of development and growth. Throughout this process of transformation of the State apparatus, it began to instrument the regulation of the popular sectors (Vezzetti, 1985). The above-mentioned civilising ideals were linked to the aesthetic, ethical and legal canons of French culture. The figure of the doctor, for example, was given a very important political function in such a way that a series of practical provisions were deployed in various political universes: legal, penal, welfare and pedagogical as a requirement to harmonise the vast problems of disorder, basically urban, in which marginality, madness and crime called for medical-social intervention (Vezzetti, 1985).

These problems were clearly fostered by the complex phenomenon of mass immigration that Argentina had called for in order to promote the economic growth of the country within the framework of the constitution of the recent national state. The Argentine leadership and intelligentsia were deeply concerned about the problems that had brought about a massive call for European immigration. The fantasies of populating Argentina with a more refined strain of workers, far removed from what was believed to be the idleness of the criollo and the Indian, had been undermined by the contingents of poor, alcoholic and insane immigrants who often disembarked from European ships (Ferrari, 2012). Furthermore, not to mention the contingent of trade unionists and communists who tended to disarm the capitalist dreams of the Argentine haute bourgeoisie. It is usual to find within the contingents of alienated patients that many who were communists were labelled with psychiatric pathology (Sozzo, 2015). In the United States, the same processes were accelerating the creation of a new institution at Ellis Island dedicated to sorting migrants according to their health status, their mental health and also their political affiliation (Anbinder 2018).

The corollary of this situation was the constitution of a technological complex where the emergence of specific institutions, hospital services, asylums, penitentiaries and professional associations became visible, which generally had greater economic stimulus in the capital city of Buenos Aires (Sozzo 2015). However, from 1900 onwards, the health system entered a new stage of federalisation that included the constitution of a system deployed in the provinces (Ferrari 2016). It is in this context that the *Hospital Asilo Colonia de Oliva* was founded in Cordoba, Argentina in 1914. But this hospital was not the first to have the characteristic of an open-door hospital. In Buenos Aires, the *Asilo de Alienadas de Lomas* had already been established in 1908, which was the first Open Door hospital in Argentina, founded also by Cabred.

In some ways the open-door model was adopted mechanically. In fact, to this day it is still possible to see that gable roof architecture was unnecessary in the climate of Cordoba, just as the same way we can find a useless space for the skies behind the doors (Ferrari, 2016). This indicates that the displacement of architectural and clinical models could be driven by the appropriation of aesthetic canons that do not always have a pragmatic function and serve to display cultural ideals. Similarly, a form of cultural colonialisation that does not always respond to local conditions can also be observed in these displacements.

The most complex of the problems faced by the Argentine state was the systematic overcrowding of patients with different pathologies ranging from alcoholism, mental alienation and also an important mass of homeless and beggars. One of the reasons for the exponential growth of mentally ill patients was clearly immigration. Thus, for Lucio Meléndez, professor and director of the *Hospicio de las Mercedes*, it was easy to find the profile of the 'crazy immigrant' in the population of the new open-door asylums (Vezzetti, 1985). During the opening year of the *Hospital Asilo Colonia de Alienados* in Oliva, 1,250 patients were admitted. They were mainly from Buenos Aires through the transfer of important contingents of chronically ill patients from the different asylums of Hospicio de las Mercedes y Hospital de Alienadas, and to a lesser extent from the interior of the country. Likewise, the diversity in nationality that can be observed informs us about the large number of immigrants entering the country in that period, mainly from Italy and Spain, and to a lesser extent Russia, France and Uruguay (Soria, 2015).

Conclusion

As we discovered during via our own urban explorations, the *Hospital Asilo Colonia de Alienados* is today a derelict site. Its decline is a sign of the new turning point that occurred at the beginning of this century towards the splitting up of psychiatric care structures, which renders the great historical architectural operations obsolete. The Oliva Hospital, however, is a good observation point for the changeover that occurred between the nineteenth and twentieth centuries in terms of healthcare architecture in Europe and South America. When considering the history of the Open Door asylum, and its circulation between Europe and Argentine, it is possible to see that the model was less about adapting to local needs and more about aspiring to a cultural ideal. By resituating the Hospital Asilo Colonia de Oliva as a place of care in the wider history of institutional and architectural evolutions of psychiatric care, we have highlighted the complex historical, social, cultural, and spatial dynamics of twentieth century institutional reforms in psychiatric care.

Acknowledgements

This chapter contribution was made by the authors within the framework of the ECOS-SUD-MinCyT project.

Notes

1 The term colony refers to a specific psychiatric institution which is located in a rural area. These institutions aimed to provide treatment, care and attention to people with chronic mental illness.
2 Esquirol was a prominent 19th century French physician and psychiatrist who made important contributions to the field of psychiatry: among others, he defined the concept of monomania, folie a deux and moral treatment, as well as founding the first chair of psychiatry in France at the Salpétriere Hospital in Paris.
3 This Austrian doctor visited Gheel in 1859, met the families in the psychiatric colony and adocated for this new model all other Europe. Then he oversaw the construction of a model family home on the Universal exhibition in Paris.
4 Pinel's moral treatment was based on the belief that mental illness was caused by social and environmental factors, and that treatment should focus on improving the moral and emotional condition of patients (Swain 1994). Pinel advocated a more humane and less coercive approach to the treatment of psychiatric patients, and became an advocate for the abolition of the use of chains and individual cells for patients.

References

Anbinder, Tyler. (2018) *La cité des rêves, New York. Une histoire de 400 ans*, Perrin.

Cabred, Domingo. (1889) «Intervención de Domingo Cabred». En *Extraits des procès-verbaux des séances de la Société médico-psychologique*. París: Libraire de L'académie de Médicine, pp. 53–58.

Caponi, S. (2012) «Clasificaciones, acuerdos y negociaciones: Bases de la primera estadística internacional de enfermedades mentales (París, 1889)». *Dynamis* 32, pp. 185–207. https://doi.org/10.4321/S0211-95362012000100009.

Castel, Robert. (1977) *L'Ordre psychiatrique*, Paris, Minuit.

Derrien, Marie. (2020) « Soigner les incurables? L'expérience des colonies familiales et la réforme de l'assistance aux aliénés en France (1892–1939) ». *Revue d'Histoire Moderne et Contemporaine*, no. 67-1, pp. 24–43. https://doi.org/10.3917/rhmc.671.0024.

Fauvel, Aude. (2005) *Témoins aliénés et « bastilles modernes ».une histoire politique, sociale et culturelle des asiles en France (1800–1914)*, Thèse de doctorat, 3 vol., EHESS.

Fauvel, Aude, Dupont, Wannes. (2018) *Gheel, la « ville des fous »: Un mythe séculaire, une pratique méconnue (1860–2010)*. In Guillemain, Hervé (dir.); Klein, Alexandre (dir.); et Thifault, Marie-Claude (dir.), *La fin de l'asile? Histoire de la déshospitalisation psychiatrique dans l'espace francophone au xxe siècle*, Rennes: Presses universitaires de Rennes, pp. 25–37. https://doi.org/10.4000/books.pur.172088.

Ferrari, Fernando José, (2016) *De la locura a la enfermedad mental. Córdoba 1758–1930. Una historia cultural de los discursos y prácticas médicas sobre la locura*, Córdoba, Aletheia Clío.

Ferrari, Fernando José. (2012) Entre el dispositivo psiquiátrico y la disciplina monacal: una historia genealógica de las primeras lecturas de la psicopatología freudiana en Córdoba (1758–1930) [Tesis de doctorado] [Córdoba]_ Facultad de Psicología, Universidad Nacional de Córdoba.

Freeman, Hugh, Gijswijt-Hofstra, Marijke, Oosterhuis, Harry, Vijselaar, Joost (dir.) (2005) *Psychiatric Cultures Compared. Psychiatry and Mental Health Care in the Twentieth Century: Comparisons and Approaches*, Amsterdam, Amsterdam University Press.

Laget, Pierre-Louis (2004) Naissance et évolution du plan pavillonnaire dans les asiles d'aliénés. In: *Livraisons d'histoire de l'architecture*, n°7, 1er semestre, pp. 51–70.

Maldonado, A., Pedraza, G., & Naides, E. (2002) *El asilo Memorias de la vida cotidiana (Oliva, 1914–2001)*, Buenos Aires, Sal Cor.

Marquis, Paul. (2022) *Les fous de Joinville. Une histoire sociale de la psychiatrie dans l'Algérie coloniale (1933-1962)*, Thèse Sciences politiques Paris.

Marquis, Paul. (2013) « Le centre de Fleury-les-Aubrais, un 'service ouvert'? L'asile au défi des troubles psychiques de guerre (1914–1923) », dans BEAUVALLET, Scarlett, DINET, Marie-Claude (dir.), *Lieux et pratiques de santé du Moyen Age à la 1ère Guerre mondiale*, Amiens, Éditions Encrage, avril, pp. 217–235.

Marquiegui, Norberto, Dedier. (2020) «Domingo Cabred, la Comisión Nacional de Asilos y la Colonia de Puertas Abiertas a finales del siglo XIX e inicios del siglo XX». *Revista Cambios y Permanencias* 11, n.º 1 pp. 572–601.

Morel, Jules. (1987): «The progress of psychiatry in 1896», *Journal of Mental Science* 181, n.º 43, pp. 384–387. https://doi.org/10.1192/bjp.43.181.384.

Mueller, Thomas. (2008) « Le placement familial des aliénés en France. Le baron Mundy et l'Exposition universelle de 1867 », *Romantisme*, 141, n.º 3, pp. 37–50.

Offenstadt, Nicolas. (2022) *Urbex. Le phénomène de l'exploration urbaine décrypté*, Albin Michel,

OED (Oxford English Dictionary). online. Retrieved 15 December, 2023. www.oxfordreference.com/display/10.1093/oi/authority.20110803095402645

Parchappe, Maximien. (1865) *Des principes à suivre dans la fondation et la construction des asiles d'aliénés*, Paris : Librarie de Victor Masson.

Porter, Roy & Wright, David (eds.) (2003) *The Confinement of the Insane: International Perspectives, 1800–1965*, Cambridge, Cambridge University Press.

Requiere, M. (2000) *Beneficencia y Asistencia Social: la política manicomial en Buenos Aires. (1880–1940)*. Alcmeon, Revista Argentina de Clínica Neuropsiquiátrica, Año XI, 2, pp.1–22.

Scull, Andrew. (1981) Madhouses, *Mad-Doctors, and Madmen: The Social History of Psychiatry in the Victorian Era*, University of Pennsylvania Press.

Sérieux, Paul.(1903) *L'Assistance des aliénés en France, en Allemagne, en Italie et en Suisse*, Paris, Impr. Municipale.

Soria, Gonzalo. (2015) «Relevamiento, sistematización y descripción de Historias Clínicas en el Archivo del Hospital Dr. Emilio Vidal Aval (1914)».

Sozzo, Máximo. (2015) *Locura y crimen: nacimiento de la intersección entre dispositivo penal y dispositivo psiquiátrico*. Bs. As.: Didot.

Swain, Gladys.(1994) *Dialogue avec l'insensé: essais d'histoire de la psychiatrie*, Gallimard.

Turck, Léopold. (1865) *Pétition au sénat sur le régime des aliénés en France*, Gray, impr. de A. Roux.

Vezetti, Hugo. (1985) *Historia de la locura en Argentina*. Bs. As. Paidós. 1985.

von Bueltzingsloewen, *Isabelle,* (2010) "Quel(s) malade(s) pour quel asile? Le débat sur l'internement psychiatrique dans la France de l'entre-deux-guerres ", In Stéphane Tison, Laurence Guignard et Hervé Guillemain (eds.), *Expériences de la folie. Criminels, soldats, patients en psychiatrie. XIXe-XXe siècle*, PUR.

43 Carceral riskscapes in the institutions of care

Virve Repo

Introduction

Institutions of care are under constant debate and development. Although many have been closed down since de-institutionalisation started globally in the 1970s, they cannot be "magically wished away" (Philo and Parr, 2019, p. 246); thus, many are still operating and much needed in some cases. For example, de-institutionalised care cannot meet the needs of some patients, who benefit much more from the stability and routines of institutions (Ahonen, 2019). Thus, to improve institutional care, there is a need to know more about life inside the institutions by examining them from different viewpoints.

This chapter highlights the connection between care, risk, and the carceral as well as their spatial meaning in institutions by introducing the concept of *carceral riskscape* (Repo, 2020). All these aspects are intertwined, creating manifold spaces and practices that have an influence on the everyday life in the institutions. While the origins of carceral studies was based on prison studies, recent carceral studies have included institutions of care, for example orphanages (Disney, 2015, 2017a, 2017b), secure units for children (Schliehe, 2016), nursing homes and aged care (Repo, 2019b; Loughnan, 2022), gero-psychiatric units (Repo, 2019a, 2020) and acute psychiatric care (Berkhout, Macgillivray and Sheehan, 2021). Recent studies have shown that control in institutions of care may lead to quasi-carceralities (Repo, 2019b) or carceralities (Repo, 2019a; Berkhout, Macgillivray and Sheehan, 2021; Loughnan, 2022) which cause detriment to people living in institutions.

The concept of *riskscape* introduces the idea of spatiality into the research on risk (Lupton, 2006; Müller-Mahn and Everts, 2013; Müller-Mahn, Everts and Stephan, 2018). In this case, the spatiality is connected to the concept by using term "scape". For Salazar (2013, p. 753) "scape refers to both a scene and a 'view', the notion lends itself expediently to analysing the way people experience and understand their world(s), thereby superseding standard geographical thinking in social cultural analysis." Scapes can be called "imagined worlds" constituted through the historical and cultural imagination of groups and individuals from different perspectives (Appadurai, 1990, p.589). Scapes are given meaning and a material shape by human action, thus, they are a result of processes but not the processes themselves (Salazar, 2013). In a way, scape represents a similar imagined world to risks, which also represent something that is imagined, but has not yet happened.

The origin of the concept of riskscape is in the research on environmental hazards (Morello-Frosch, Pastor and Sadd, 2001; Macey, 2010; Frick-Trzebitzky, Baghel and

DOI: 10.4324/9781003345725-48

Bruns, 2017) and the related societal challenges (Morello-Frosch and Lopez, 2006; Morello-Frosch and Shenassa, 2006; Jenerette *et al.*, 2011; Mair, Cutchin and Peek, 2011). The concept of riskscape has also been used in care environments (Gee and Skovdal, 2017) by following the concept of caringscapes (McKie, Gregory and Bowlby, 2002) to emphasise the spatiotemporal perspective, individual experiences and embodied practices in the care environment. Even though risks are strongly related to institutions (Moon, 2000), fewer studies have been conducted in institutional (e.g., psychiatric hospitals) and post-institutional spaces (e.g., outpatient care facilities and community care). The concept of a carceral riskscape draws on carceral geography to explore the spatio-temporalities of the riskscapes in restricted and controlled spaces, and was created to adjust the concept of riskscape into institutional environments (Repo, 2020).

According to the current tendency in human geography, space can be seen as relational, constructed for example through physical frames, social interactions and objects, which are in a relation to space and vice versa (Massey, 2005; Ridell, Kymäläinen and Nyyssönen, 2009; Moran, 2015). Space is under a constant process of being made and is constitutive of as well as constituted by relationships (Massey, 2005). Space and time are strongly linked together, and they exist simultaneously and dynamically through social relations (Massey, 2008). For example, the same space may be experienced as totally different at different times and depending on the people in that space and their relations.

Some of the findings in this chapter are based on my previous studies concerning institutional care in Finland (Repo, 2019a, 2019b, 2020). Thus, they might not be directly adaptable to the context of other countries. Nevertheless, the concept of carceral riskscape can be adapted to (institutional) care as such. In the next part of the chapter I briefly describe the concept of care related to institutions. Then, I will introduce the concept of carceral space and furthermore the concept of risk and how risks relate to institutions. After that, I conceptualise the carceral riskscape and explain the dimensions related to the concept. Finally, I will conclude the chapter by contemplating the meaning of the concept in relation to studies on institutions.

Care in institutions

In institutions, care can be seen as something offered to those who cannot cope by themselves. The aim is either to maintain the quality of life and wellbeing (e.g., care of older individuals) or to support the rehabilitation of a person so that they can continue living outside of that institution (e.g., psychiatric care). Care can be seen as medical treatment in certain spaces, implemented by staff members. Thus, care encompasses for example, the use of drugs, therapeutics, and medical expertise (Parr, 2003). Care is also political because it is linked to such typical questions in a democracy as public resources, equity, justice, obligations, and rights (Brown, 2003).

Scholars have long recognised the significant connection of space and care (Brown, 2003; Conradson, 2003; Milligan, 2003, 2009; Milligan and Wiles, 2010; Green and Lawson, 2011; Brown *et al.*, 2018). For example, physical remoteness effects the availability of care services (Parr and Philo, 2003), but it also matters whether the care is implemented at home, in an institution or in some other space. Thus, care produces particular social spaces (Conradson, 2003), constructed by the social relations between caregiver and caretaker. For example, in the care of older individuals, the new care technologies along with de-institutionalisation and increasing home care blurs the boundaries between private and public as well as institutional and non-institutional spaces (Milligan

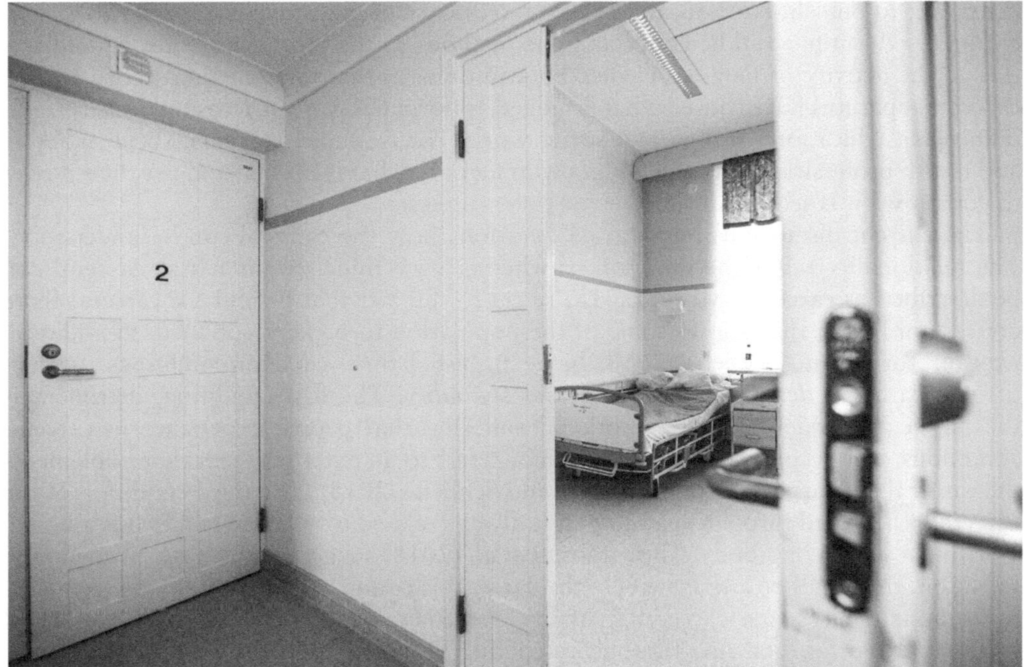

Figure 43.1 Care produces special kind of spaces. Photograph Turun Sanomat/Riitta Salmi.

and Wiles, 2010). The relationship between control and care leads to situations where they cannot easily be separated (Philo, 2017). For example, in Finnish nursing homes, care is sometimes planned with control in mind, and this leads to delicate situations when control is seen as a form of care. Control is often performed in the name of safety, especially related to residents with dementia, but the regulations concerns all residents (Repo, 2019b). Care relationships are dependent on the space where they take place. They are not only about "interpersonal relations but also people-place relationships" (Milligan and Wiles, 2010, p. 738). It should be considered that in institutions, care is seen as a product (Green and Lawson, 2011). Thus, care can be implemented as a routine-like performance (e.g., Milligan and Wiles, 2010) and the possibilities for "careless care", (Repo, 2019b, p.235) are increased. Careless care implies that care is something that is performed without actually having a sense or feeling of care in it. This may lead to control and exclusion, where everything that is not included in the mandatory regime or paid for is excluded (e.g. outdoor activities) or when residents are left alone for protracted periods of time (Repo, 2019b). These actions may lead to "violence that emanates from neglect" (Loughnan, 2022, p. 2) and the development of carceral spaces (Repo, 2019b), which I will elaborate on in the next chapter.

Carceral spaces

For the French philosopher Michel Foucault (1995) a carceral system is something that stretches beyond the actual place of punishment (prison) and influences the whole of society. It not only spread carceral power more widely in society but also legitimates the power to punish. For Foucault (1995) the essence of punishment is similar to that of curing or educating, and he connects these methods to the idea of normalising and further to the activity of judging. Hence, Foucault claims that these methods born from a carceral apparatus have caused what is judged as normal to spread across all society; even influencing education, healing and social work. For example, teachers, social workers and health professionals become judges who identify what is normal and use their power to correct what is seen as deviant.

The current discussions have raised questions how the carceral can be understood. The relationality raises the question of whether everything that is felt as carceral can be described as carceral. Morin (2018) refers to the fact that behind the carceral there are certain logics, that allows some of the population to be kept confined. In addition, Moran, Turner and Schliehe (2018) have suggested three carceral conditions to identify the carceral: *detriment, intention* and *spatiality*. The first condition, detriment is the physical, physiological or emotional suffering that people experience in carceral conditions. The second condition, intention, refers to an external agent that implements the carceral on purpose (Moran, Turner and Schliehe, 2018). The third condition of the carceral is achieved through spatiality; it is always related to space, whether it is a home, a prison, a school or a body. Thus, Moran *et al.* (2018) suggest, if there is detriment and intention, there will be a space where the carceral is conducted. This especially concerns institutional spaces, but carceral spatiality can emerge in many ways: through actual bricks and mortar, but also through restricting mobility (e.g., electronic monitoring). It also manifests in the ways in which the carceral influence people before and after the actual confinement, as a form of stigma for example. Thus, carceral spaces continue to have an influence on people and may expose them to economical and societal risks also outside the institutions. Therefore, risk has important implications related to life inside institutions. Sometimes all these three conditions are not fulfilled. For example, the carceral might not be intentionally created. In institutions of care especially, the carceral may appear due to a lack of resources or arise from control that ignores care. In these cases the space might be called quasi-carceral (Altin and Minca, 2017; Repo, 2019b; Loughnan, 2022). In the following, I explain how risk is seen in this chapter.

Risk

Risk shapes spaces and vice versa (November, 2008). They have an influence on how we make mundane choices, use spaces and how we construct social spaces. Beck (2000) introduces several points related to the concept of risk. He states that when trust in our security and belief in progress ends, a discourse on risk appears. Thus, risk characterises a state between security and destruction (Beck, 2000), where the perception of risk starts to influence thoughts and actions. What harm could occur and how could it be avoided? Such questions allude to something that has not yet happened, thus, the risk itself is considered to be related to the future (Müller-Mahn, Everts and Stephan, 2018). The future starts to determine the present, and "risks become the all-embracing background for perceiving the world, the alarm they provoke creates an atmosphere of powerlessness and paralysis" (Beck, 2000, p. 218). This gives the impression that potential risks have started to rule our lives and thus limit our actions.

Beck (2000) connects risk and risk perception with the logic of control which originated from the control of the state. People are controlled from the top down using the perceptions of risk. These actions of control normally suggest what should *not* be done, not what should be done. Risks are also socially constructed and depend on individual choices (Kasperson, 1992; Beck, 1995; Lupton, 2006; Tierney, 2014; Müller-Mahn, Everts and Stephan, 2018), which suggests that the concept of risk needs to be considered in relation to societies and contexts (Furedi, 2006). That means, that different societies have different perceptions of risks and the means and abilities to cope with them.

Risk can be seen as a dynamic phenomenon that is constantly present in the everyday lives of individuals (Mythen and Walklate, 2006). These everyday challenges are described as the individualisation of risk (Beck, 1995; Lupton, 2006). The individual is responsible for their own fate through the choices they make. In such situations, the potentiality of any harm, damage and loss has to be balanced against the potential gain and benefit (Furedi, 2006; Tierney, 2014). What people consider to be a risk depends on their previous experiences, attitudes, coping skills and social influences (Renn *et al.*, 1992; Müller-Mahn, Everts and Stephan, 2018). The possibility of harm is not seen as equal by all people, but depends on various aspects, such as age, gender, and geographical location. Hence, the perception of risk varies between societies, groups, and even individually. Risk can be understood as being a multiple context as risks are entwined with each other because of causalities (Müller-Mahn and Everts, 2013).

To a great extent risk is a part of the environment of closed institutions such as psychiatric wards and prisons, since people who are thought to be a risk to themselves, to others or to society are confined in these spaces in order to be cured or/and corrected (see also Moon, 2000). However, by entering these spaces of confinement people are entering a setting that is under the influence of different risks and further carceral riskscapes, which I will conceptualise next.

Carceral riskscape

The carceral and risk are interrelated, since risk can lead to carceral actions (e.g. coercive measures) and carceral measures can create risks that cause harm or detriment. What can be considered a risk, varies at different times and in different areas. For example poverty and homelessness may have lead to confinement (Foucault, 2001; Ahonen, 2019) and these aspects are still present in contemporary confinement through for example carceral logics (Morin, 2018; Story, 2019). Spaces of confinement employ both multiple risk assessment methods and practices, for example, in order to decrease violent behaviour (Almvik, Woods and Rasmussen, 2007) various therapeutic measures and techniques are used in challenging situations (Kuivalainen *et al.*, 2017). Furthermore, the carceral and risk interact with each other through spatiality. For example, risks are minimised on the ward by placing risky 'inmates' into specific physical spaces, such as seclusion rooms; however, this might in turn create risks both to the inmates and staff members, if the situation deteriorates into violence.

The risks in the physical environment of carceral spaces are usually well acknowledged and reflected in the design of the wards (for example as a form of locked spaces and unbreakable windows) and surveillance practices (such as camera monitoring and routine searches) (Curtis *et al.*, 2013). However, the spatiality of risk is not limited to physical premises, but is a complicated combination of several other factors, for example, care, control, regulations and human relationships (Parr, 2003). All these aspects have an influence on how risks are perceived and managed in space. For instance, the relations between staff members may have an influence on how the patients are cared for and

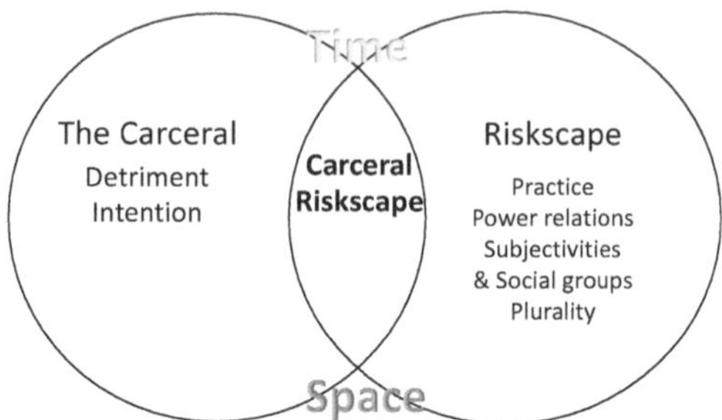

Figure 43.2 The dimensions of carceral riskscape. Figure by the author.

controlled (Repo, 2020). These different spatial aspects are very much linked to temporality, since in closed institutions schedules and surveillance may be linked to a diurnal rhythm (Repo, 2019b; Thorshaug and Brun, 2019).

The concept of carceral riskscape combines the carceral conditions (detriment, intention and spatiality) (Moran, Turner and Schliehe, 2018) and the dimensions of riskscape (practice, power relations, spatiality, social groups and subjectivity, temporality and plurality) (Müller-Mahn, Everts and Stephan, 2018)

In contrast to Müller-Mahn, Everts and Stephan (2018) spatiality and temporality are not discussed here as separate dimensions; this is because of the spatiotemporal features of the carceral and a recognition that all the dimensions are related to space and time. First of all, the connection between time and space is acknowledged, especially in geography, although it is often not easy to separate the two. For example, carceral space affects how the passing of time is experienced (Moran, 2015). In addition, in institutions of care the practices may vary over a 24-hour period (for example during the nightshift), which may also influence how the spaces are used and experienced (Repo, 2019a). For example, night shift carceral practices may be used on a ward due to the lack of resources (Repo, 2019b) or in order to ease the work load of the staff members (Repo, 2019a). In these cases, patients rooms may transformed into carceral spaces, if they are left alone without help (Repo, 2019b) or locked in or overmedicated to keep them calm (Repo, 2019a). Next, I will elaborate on the formation of carceral riskscapes via the four dimensions: practice, power relations, social groups and subjectivity, and plurality.

Practice

The idea of risk is socially and culturally constructed to help us cope with uncertainty and danger. Thus, different social practices are used to avoid risks in everyday life. Riskscapes are constituted through social practices, reflecting what is said and done. One might add that riskscapes also reflect what is unsaid and undone, since ignorance and neglect create riskscapes through exclusion and punitive ignorance (Loughnan, 2022). Practices within carceral spaces, especially in institutions, are strongly linked to the current regime, legal requirements and official regulations. Although such practices are created to reduce risks they do not always succeed, especially if the supervision fails and the subsequent methods used to control and coerce patients become amplified (Repo, 2019a, 2020) Additionally, people can 'do riskscapes' deliberately, for example, by encountering something commonly considered risky (Lundgren, 2018). When implementing laws and regulations, people may also have to instigate riskscapes as a part of care work and be obliged to go into situations they might consider risky. Furthermore, the demands of care work in institutions indicate that staff members may have to use and actualise carceral practices in the form of coercive methods, which are sometimes considered risky both to the patients and to the staff members, if not used safely or correctly (Repo, 2020). The spatiality of the practices can be seen clearly in the case of coercive methods, which are commonly used in specific spaces, such as seclusion or restraint rooms. Furthermore, practices may mutate and develop into policies used beyond carceral spaces. Thus, forms of control and surveillance may be implemented in practices used outside of actual confinement areas, such as, electronic monitoring to make public spaces more secure (Gill, Conlon and Moran, 2013) In addition, the practices may alter the spaces and people that are considered as risky by society. These practices of control that are targeted towards people who are considered to be risky, may influence economical and societal situations and peoples' ability to cope with future risks.

Power relations

Power relations have a considerable effect on everyday life in institutions (Milligan, 2003; Foucault, 2006; Repo, 2019a), as institutional systems depend on hierarchy and strictly appointed power relations. Although power relations are often produced through state policies and structures, they influence the equality of riskscapes at an individual level. For example, the individual features and possibilities to cope with risks differ if you have the power to influence things, or not. For example, people with power may be in a secure position so that they can take risks or transfer the risks to those who have less power (see Repo, 2020).

Power relations are also connected to the architecture and in some cases buildings and spaces support certain spatial practices that may enable the use of power over people living in these spaces (Nord and Högström, 2017) or to shape people, who live in these buildings, which may create similarities between buildings of care and confinement (Olsson and Gren, 2017). Furthermore, power manifests through laws and regimes, sanctioning a small number of people with the ability to make decisions that affect a large number of people (Tierney, 2014). This is particularly relevant in the context of carceral riskscapes where the law strictly defines the hierarchy, the power relations, and the responsibilities. However, power relations are also important between different, legally equal groups inside the institutions, for example the different working groups formed by the staff members of the institution. These groups may define the use of working hours, the use of spaces, and in the worst cases produce carceral riskscapes for other groups through their dominance (Repo, 2020). For example, when staff members use nurses' offices or smoking areas to just 'hangout' and leave the actual care work to their co-workers (Repo, 2020).

This suggests that through inequality in power relations some working groups are more exposed to risks than others. Establishing an unequal workload may influence the well-being of staff members and it has been found that, in some cases, those who try to raise such grievances may become the target of exclusion or bullying practices (Repo, 2020). Furthermore, patients may be at risk of mistreatment if power is targeted or used inappropriately (for example the use of seclusion without proper reasons) (Repo, 2019a).

This idea resonates with Foucault's (2006) perceptions concerning the imbalanced power relations between doctors, nurses and patients inside (psychiatric) institutions.

Subjectivities and social groups

Riskscapes are experienced differently through subjectivity and by social groups. Subjective perceptions of risk influence the formation of riskscapes. Moreover, some of the social groups may have stronger possibilities to influence riskscapes than others. For example, not all riskscapes are similarly significant; the influence of experts and their ideas on risks may dominate political agendas and public perception. Thus, the idea of what is considered a risk is influenced by people who are seen as experts and their opinion is valued more than others. For example, in institutions of care the opinions of senior workers may be valued more than the opinions of junior workers, even if the junior workers may have more current knowledge about new care practices (Repo, 2020).

Social groups of staff members can also form cliques that are in conflict with each other (Emmerson, 2019). In the worst cases, the social groups may cause the bullying or excluding of others, especially whistle-blowers, which then creates a carceral riskscape for these individuals/staff members (Repo, 2020). This has an influence on the risk perception of co-workers regarding trust, since trust in co-workers may diminish the feeling of being at risk (Gee and Skovdal, 2017). Trust has also a spatial meaning since staff members should be able to trust that their co-workers will be in the right place at the right time (Repo, Kymäläinen and Humalisto, 2022). If staff members are constantly in contention with each other, the quality of care is affected. The subjectivities as regards carceral riskscapes mean that risks are evaluated individually and they are not seen in a similar way by all. This may cause collisions as regards working cultures and practices. These subjective perceptions suggest that carceral riskscapes are relative by nature and experienced through individual perceptions.

Plurality

The plurality of riskscapes means that people are constantly under the influence of several riskscapes in the same space. In addition, riskscapes may overlap and cause new risks instead of a reduction of risks. This makes some spaces "hot spots", and riskier than others, suggesting that these overlapping riskscapes accumulate in spatially and temporally (Repo, 2020, p. 125). This kind of accumulation influences people's perception of risk and their ability to cope. The plurality of the riskscapes may extend through physical spaces. For example, the seclusion rooms in psychiatric institutions are considered more risky than other spaces due to the potential violent behaviour of the patient. Thus, seclusion rooms are designed in a special way and special practices, such as coercive methods, are used in the context of seclusion rooms. The plurality of the carceral riskscapes may create groups that are more vulnerable to risks than others. For example, junior staff members may be more at risk of being excluded from the working community, of not obtaining a permanent employment contract or of being bullied. Furthermore, my previous findings (Repo, 2019a) show that patients with dementia are more likely to be exposed to several carceral riskscapes from misconduct, such as rough handling and being heavily medicated to improper care; this is because they might not be able to tell anyone about these events. Thus, they should be situated in the most appropriate kind of care facilities, where staff members have had suitable training and there are sufficient care spaces.

To summarise, a carceral riskscape is a combination of power relations, practices, and the effects of individuals, social groups and pluralities; this may cause some spaces at certain times to be more risky than others. While power relations can be seen as creating relationships between people, they also define the who, how and when of the use of spaces – just as the spaces themselves can define their use and accessibility Thus, power relations are related to relationships between people and space. These dimensions of carceral riskscape actualise how carceral riskscapes are spatiotemporally conducted, and how these scapes are perceived. To conclude this chapter, I will discuss the potentiality of the concept concerning institutional studies.

Conclusion

The concept of riskscape adds a spatial dimension to the concept of risk. The concept of *carceral riskscape* raises the opportunity of utilising spatial studies in relation to carceral spaces and combine the insights from these studies to the studies on riskscapes. Power relations, practices, subjectivities and social groups as well as the plurality of carceral riskscapes increase the inequality inside institutions, and this has a strong influence on everyday life in carceral spaces. These inequalities cause risks and further carceral actions (Repo 2020). While the inequality related to geographical locations has been acknowledged in relation to riskscapes (Mair, Cutchin and Peek, 2011), the multiple spatio-temporalities inside carceral spaces also create inequalities through control and surveillance; since not all the spaces are available for all people at all times. In institutions, the regime defines the use of time, because the diurnal rhythm is usually strictly based on schedules, rules and regulations. Spatial inequalities can also be seen in the way staff members use the spaces with some spaces being territorialised by certain people at certain times. Furthermore, carceral practices may evolve in particular spaces at specified times. These shifting practices may cause different kinds of riskscapes, which are time-related.

There is still considerable potential for further development of the concept. For example, there is the possibility of including a more gender sensitive approach concerning the dimensions of riskscape. In addition, the conceptualisation of the carceral is an ongoing discussion that allows researchers to further contemplate the essence and aspects of detriment, intention and space. Currently, the deliberations around these research questions show a lack of studies that include people with lived experience of institutions.

However, the concept of carceral riskscapes provides a useful means of acknowledging the mechanisms behind inequalities that influence everyday life in spaces of confinement. Acknowledging the mechanisms of inequality is a first step to supporting and consequently improving institutional care and advancing wellbeing in institutions.

Acknowledgements

Parts of this chapter has previously been published in Fennia- the International Journal of Geography (Repo, 2020). I would like to thank Ebba Högström for the valuable comments concerning the manuscript. I would also like to thank JustSpaces research network of Tampere University for their support.

References

Ahonen, K. (2019) 'Suomalainen mielenterveyspolitiikka: Julkisen vallan ohjaus mielenterveyden häiriöön sairastuneiden ihmisoikeuksien turvaamiseksi'.

Almvik, R., Woods, P. and Rasmussen, K. (2007) 'Assessing risk for imminent violence in the elderly: the Broset Violence Checklist', *International Journal of Geriatric Psychiatry*, 22(9), pp. 862–867. Available at: https://doi.org/10.1002/gps.1753.

Altin, R. and Minca, C. (2017) 'The ambivalent camp Mobility and excess in a quasi-carceral Italian asylum seekers hospitality centre', *Carceral Mobilities: Interrogating Movement in Incarceration*, 68, pp. 30–43.

Appadurai, A. (1990) 'Disjuncture and difference in the global cultural economy', *Theory, Culture & Society*, 7, pp. 295–310.

Beck, U. (1995) 'International high-risk society – political-dynamics of global threats', *Internationale Politik*, 50(8), pp. 13–20.

Beck, U. (2000) 'Risk Society revisited: Theory, politics and research programmes', *The Risk Society and Beyond: Critical Issues for Social Theory*. Edited by A. Barbara, U. Beck, and J. van Loon. Sage.

Berkhout, S.G., Macgillivray, L. and Sheehan, K. (2021) *Carceral Politics, Inpatient Psychiatry, and the Pandemic Risk, Madness, and Containment in COVID-19*, International Journal of Critical Diversity Studies, 4(1), pp.74–91.

Brown, M. (2003) 'Hospice and the spatial paradoxes of terminal care', *Environment and Planning A*, 35(5), pp. 833–851. Available at: https://doi.org/10.1068/a35121.

Brown, T. *et al.* (2018) *Health Geographies. A Critical Introduction*. Wiley Blackwell.

Conradson, D. (2003) 'Geographies of care: spaces, practices, experiences', *Social & Cultural Geography*, 4(4), pp. 450–454. Available at: https://doi.org/10.1080/1464936032000137894.

Curtis, S. *et al.* (2013) 'Compassionate containment? Balancing technical safety and therapy in the design of psychiatric wards', *Social Science & Medicine*, 97, pp. 201–209. Available at: https://doi.org/10.1016/j.socscimed.2013.06.015.

Disney, T. (2015) 'Complex spaces of orphan care – a Russian therapeutic children's community', *Childrens Geographies*, 13(1), pp. 30–43. Available at: https://doi.org/10.1080/14733 285.2013.827874.

Disney, T. (2017a) 'Ethnographic perspectives on emotion in a Russian orphanage', *Journal of Social Policy Studies*, 15(3), pp. 407–420. Available at: https://doi.org/10.17323/ 727-0634-2017-15-3-407-420.

Disney, T. (2017b) 'The orphanage as an institution of coercive mobility', *Environment and Planning A*, 49(8), pp. 1905–1921. Available at: https://doi.org/10.1177/0308518x17711181.

Emmerson, P. (2019) 'More-than-therapeutic landscapes', *Area*, Online fir, pp. 1–8. Available at: https://doi.org/10.1111/area.12557.

Foucault, M. (1995) *Discipline and Punish: The Birth of the Prison*. Vintage Books.

Foucault, M. (2001) *Madness and Civilization*. Routledge.

Foucault, M. (2006) *Psychiatric Power. Lectures at the Collegé de France 1973–1974*. Picador.

Frick-Trzebitzky, F., Baghel, R. and Bruns, A. (2017) 'Institutional bricolage and the production of vulnerability to floods in an urbanising delta in Accra', *International Journal of Disaster Risk Reduction*, 26, pp. 57–68. Available at: https://doi.org/10.1016/j.ijdrr.2017.09.030.

Furedi, F. (2006) *Culture of Fear Revisited. Risk-Taking and the Morality of Low Expectation*. Continuum.

Gee, S. and Skovdal, M. (2017) 'Navigating "riskscapes": the experiences of international health care workers responding to the Ebola outbreak in West Africa', *Health & Place*, 45, pp. 173–180. Available at: https://doi.org/10.1016/j.healthplace.2017.03.016.

Gill, N., Conlon, D. and Moran, D. (2013) 'Dialogues across Carceral Space: Migration, Mobility, Space and Agency'. In: Moran, D., Gill, N. & Conlon, D. (Eds.) *Carceral Spaces: Mobility and Agency in Imprisonment and Migrant Detention*. Farnham: Ashgate.

Green, M. and Lawson, V. (2011) 'Recentring care: interrogating the commodification of care', *Social & Cultural Geography*, 12(6), pp. 639–654. Available at: https://doi.org/10.1080/14649 365.2011.601262.

Jenerette, G.D. *et al.* (2011) 'Ecosystem services and urban heat riskscape moderation: water, green spaces, and social inequality in Phoenix, USA', *Ecological Applications*, 21(7), pp. 2637–2651. Available at: https://doi.org/10.1890/10-1493.1.

Kasperson, R.E. (1992) 'The social amplification of risk – progress in developing an integrative framework', *Social Theories of Risk*, pp. 153–178.

Kuivalainen, S. *et al.* (2017) 'De-escalation techniques used, and reasons for seclusion and restraitn, in a forensic psychiatric hospital', *International Journal of Mental Health Nursing*, 26, pp. 513–524. Available at: https://doi.org/10.1111/inm.12389.

Loughnan, C. (2022) 'The scene and the unseen – neglect and death in immigration detention and aged care', *Incarceration*, 3(2), pp. 1–17. Available at: https://doi.org/10.117/2632666322 1103444.

Lundgren, M. (2018) 'Riskscapes: strategies and practices along the Georgian-Abkhazian boundary line and inside Abkhazia', *Journal of Borderlands Studies*, 33(4), pp. 637–654. Available at: https://doi.org/10.1080/08865655.2017.1300778.

Lupton, D. (2006) 'Sociology and Risk', in G. Mythen and S. Walklate (eds) *Beyond the Risk Society*. London: Open University Press, pp. 11–24.

Macey, S.M. (2010) 'A respiratory riskscape for Texas cities: A spatial analysis of air pollution, demographic attributes and deaths from 2000 through 2004', *Geospatial Techniques in Urban Hazard and Disaster Analysis*, 2, pp. 127–155. Available at: https://doi.org/10.1007/978-90-481-2238-7_7.

Mair, C.A., Cutchin, M.P. and Peek, M.K. (2011) 'Allostatic load in an environmental riskscape: the role of stressors and gender', *Health & Place*, 17(4), pp. 978–987. Available at: https://doi.org/10.1016/j.healthplace.2011.03.009.

Massey, D. (2005) *for Space*. Sage.

McKie, L., Gregory, S. and Bowlby, S. (2002) 'Shadow times: the temporal and spatial frameworks and experiences of caring and working', *Sociology-the Journal of the British Sociological Association*, 36(4), pp. 897–924. Available at: https://doi.org/10.1177/0038038 50203600406.

Milligan, C. (2003) 'Location or dis-location? Towards a conceptualization of people and place in the care-giving experience', *Social & Cultural Geography*, 4(4), pp. 455–470. Available at: https://doi.org/10.1080/1464936032000137902.

Milligan, C. (2009) *There's No Place Like Home: Place and Care in an Ageing Society*. Routledge.

Milligan, C. and Wiles, J. (2010) 'Landscapes of care', *Progress in Human Geography*, 34(6), pp. 736–754. Available at: https://doi.org/10.1177/0309132510364556.

Moon, G. (2000) *Risk and Protection: The Discourse of Con®nement in Contemporary Mental Health Policy*, pp. 239–250. Available at: www.elsevier.com/locate/healthplace.

Moran, D. (2015) *Carceral Geography: Spaces and Practices of Incarceration*. Routledge.

Moran, D., Turner, J. and Schliehe, A.K. (2018) 'Conceptualizing the carceral in carceral geography', *Progress in Human Geography*, 42(5), pp. 666–686. Available at: https://doi.org/10.1177/0309132517710352.

Morello-Frosch, R. and Lopez, R. (2006) 'The riskscape and the color line: examining the role of segregation in environmental health disparities', *Environmental Research*, 102(2), pp. 181–196. Available at: https://doi.org/10.1016/j.envres.2006.05.007.

Morello-Frosch, R., Pastor, M. and Sadd, J. (2001) 'Environmental justice and Southern California's "riskscape" – the distribution of air toxics exposures and health risks among diverse communities', *Urban Affairs Review*, 36(4), pp. 551–578. Available at: https://doi.org/10.1177/107808 70122184993.

Morello-Frosch, R. and Shenassa, E.D. (2006) 'The environmental "Riskscape" and social inequality: implications for explaining maternal and child health disparities', *Environmental Health Perspectives*, 114(8), pp. 1150–1153. Available at: https://doi.org/10.1289/ehp.8930.

Morin, K.M. (2018) *Carceral Space, Prisoners and Animals*. Routledge.

Müller-Mahn, D. and Everts, J. (2013) 'Riskscapes. The Spatial Dimensions of Risk', *The Spatial Dimension of Risk. How Geography Shapes the Emergence of Riskscapes*. Edited by D. Müller-Mahn. Routledge.

Müller-Mahn, D., Everts, J. and Stephan, C. (2018) 'Riskscapes revisited – exploring the relationship between risk, space and practice', *Erdkunde*, 72(3), pp. 197–213. Available at: https://doi.org/10.3112/erdkunde.2018.02.09.

Mythen, G. and Walklate, S. (2006) 'Introduction', *Beyond the Risk Society: Critical Reflections on Risk and Human Security*. Edited by G. Mythen and S. Walklate. Open University Press. Available at: https://ebookcentral.proquest.com/lib/kutu/detail.action?docID=316308.

Nord, C. and Högström, E. (2017) 'Introduction', *Caring Architecture. Institutions and Relational Practices*. Edited by C. Nord and E. Högström. Cambridge Scholars Publishing.

November, V. (2008) 'Spatiality of risk', *Environment and Planning A*, 40(7), pp. 1523–1527. Available at: https://doi.org/10.1068/a4194.

Olsson, G. and Gren, M. (2017) 'Commentary I. Between Caring and Architecture', *Caring Architecture. Institutions and Relational Practices*. Edited by C. Nord and E. Högström. Cambridge Scholars Publishing.

Parr, H. (2003) 'Medical geography: care and caring', *Medical Geography*, 27(2), pp. 212–221. Available at: https://doi.org/10.1191/0309132503ph423pr.

Parr, H. and Philo, C. (2003) 'Rural mental health and social geographies of caring', *Social & Cultural Geography*, 4(4), pp. 471–488. Available at: https://doi.org/10.1080/1464936032000137911.

Philo, C. (2017) 'Covertly Entangled Lines', *Caring Architecture. Institutions and Relational Practices*. Edited by C. Nord and E. Högström. Cambridge Scholars Publishing.

Philo, C. and Parr, H. (2019) 'Staying with the trouble of institutions', *Area*, 51(2), pp. 241–248. Available at: https://doi.org/10.1111/area.12531.

Renn, O. *et al.* (1992) 'The social amplification of risk: theoretical foundations and empirical applications', *Journal of Social Issues*, 48(4), pp. 137–160.

Repo, V. (2019a) 'Carceral layers in a geropsychiatric ward in Finland', *Geografiska Annaler: Series B, Human Geography*, 101(3), pp. 187–201. Available at: https://doi.org/10.1080/04353684.2019.1627852.

Repo, V. (2019b) 'Spatial control and care in Finnish nursing homes', *Area*, 51(2), pp. 233–240. Available at: https://doi.org/10.1111/area.12443.

Repo, V. (2020) 'Carceral riskscapes and working in the spaces of mental health care', *Fennia*, 198(1–2), pp. 121–134. Available at: https://doi.org/10.11143/FENNIA.88950.

Repo, V., Kymäläinen, P. and Humalisto, N. (2022) '"You can feel it in the air": the institutional atmosphere of the psychiatric hospital for prisoners', *Health & Place*, 78, p. 102934. Available at: https://doi.org/10.1016/j.healthplace.2022.102934.

Ridell, S., Kymäläinen, P. and Nyyssönen, T. (2009) 'Julkinen tila tänään – kuhinaa lomittuvilla rajapinnoilla', *Julkisen tilan poetiikkaa ja politiikkaa*. Edited by S. Ridell, P. Kymäläinen, and T. Nyyssönen. Tampere University Press.

Salazar, N.B. (2013) 'Scapes', *Theory in Social and Cultural Anthropology: An Encyclopedia*. Edited by R.J. McGee and R.L. Warms. Sage. Available at: https://doi.org/10.4135/9781452276311.n244.

Schliehe, A.K. (2016) 'Locking up children and young people: secure care in Scotland', *Play and Recreation, Health and Wellbeing*, 9, pp. 601–619. Available at: https://doi.org/10.1007/978-981-4585-51-4_19.

Story, B. (2019) *Prison Land. Mapping Carceral Power across Neoliberal America*. University of Minnesota Press.

Thorshaug, R.O. and Brun, C. (2019) 'Temporal injustice and re-orientations in asylum reception centres in Norway: towards critical geographies of architecture in the institution', *Fennia*, 197(2), pp. 232–248. Available at: https://doi.org/10.11143/fennia.84758.
Tierney, K.J. (2014) *The Social Roots of Risk: Producing Disasters, Promoting Resilience. High Reliability and Crisis Management.* Stanford University Press.
Valkonen, J., Rantanen, P., & Lehtonen, M. (Eds.) (2008). *Doreen Massey: Samanaikainen tila.* Tampere: Vastapaino.

44 Writing the Asylum
Archive and creativity in the abandoned space

Gillean McDougall

Introduction

Other people have sustained losses, I remind myself sleepily, thinking of the birds; only grubby Glasgow pigeons, but they are birds, nonetheless, flying in and out of the abandoned space of the East House. Maybe we are like birds, visiting and revisiting the place we know. The absence formed by a wing shaped like a blade. The asylum fenced off like the memories. Dangerous to go in here. Stay out, say the birds, we have it now.

Our short, original flights end up here, in the empty rooms where the words have become dust and the terrible goodwill lingers only in the furniture. The front doors are grand, but in the back, take care not to stumble, not to roll down the hill to the railway line. A train calls in the distance, a bright perfect fourth, but then silence falls again and when the leaves drop from the trees, they make no sound.

(McDougall, 2021, p.105)

These are words from my PhD thesis, inspired by a former Victorian asylum near my home in Glasgow. I am a creative writer, having worked in classical music and broadcasting, and interested in the creative potential of archive as well as writing on and for mental health. As a writer, I have a particular view of the world and a reason for taking it; my experiences serve me in different ways, with the geographies and spaces I inhabit open to scrutiny.

Writing led me from the distress of my father's mental illness, through the fear I would have similar problems, to calm acceptance – I literally wrote my way free. I walked at the former Gartnavel Royal Asylum in Glasgow over the course of a year; this centred me, providing the starting point for my PhD thesis, which was a memoir of that illness. Researching the Gartnavel archives, I understood I could critically and creatively explore historical and contemporary notions of mental health through the framework of the asylum. Others might join me, pushing the boundaries of Gartnavel's diverse terrains to voice asylum experience anew. Through creative work, writers and artists could inhabit and embody the repurposed asylum space.

Sitting high above the streets and buildings around it, the old Gartnavel buildings and their surrounding geography have evocative qualities:

DOI: 10.4324/9781003345725-49

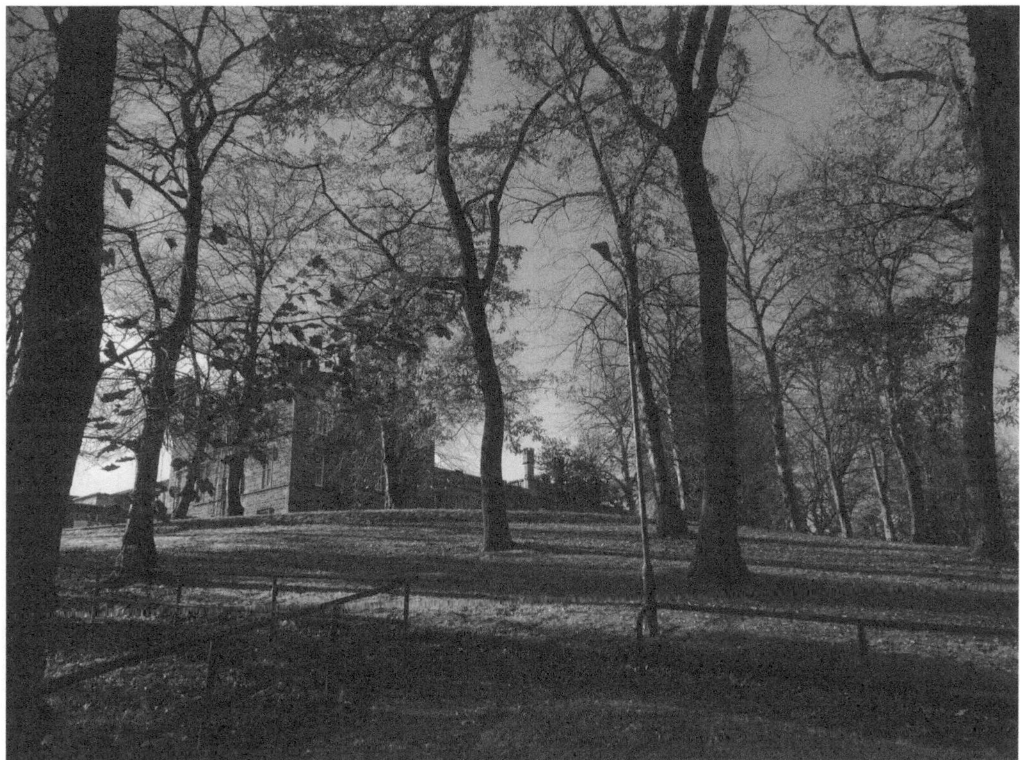

Figure 44.1 Gartnavel Royal Asylum, West House, 2022. Photo: Gillean McDougall.

The vaguely castle-like form, the dark stonework, the tendency to create a black silhouette against the skyline when the sun is in certain directions: all these features combine to create this impression of a dark place cross-coded with scariness and fear.

(Högström and Philo, 2023, p.2)

It is an accurate description of the Victorian part of the site, and the authors go on to discuss the 'dark' and 'light' elements of a site full of contrasts, both direct and implied.

I was seventeen years old when I encountered Gartnavel Royal for the first time in 1972, as a music undergraduate recently arrived at the University of Glasgow. The University's Chapel Choir had a regular commitment to sing on Christmas Day at the Asylum Chapel. I have few memories of the seasonal music and Bible readings in a gloomy little church where the chaplain seemed as mad as the inmates (a congregation made up of 'poor souls' from the Asylum well enough to attend, and some lifeless relatives). Later, we were taken to the Asylum's West House, its unlocked wards revealing rows of old ladies in beds of snowy white linen. They didn't know why we were there, but a male attendant wept at our singing.

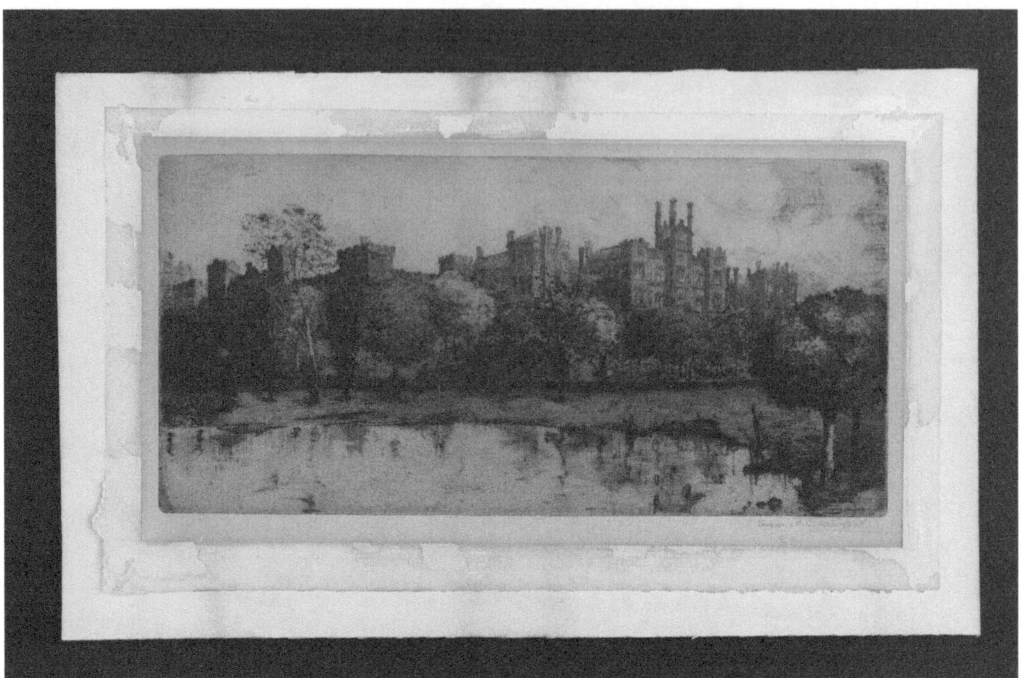

Figure 44.2 Framed etching of hospital by Susan T Crawford (1914) (Permission: Attribution 4.0 International (CC BY 4.0). Source: Wellcome Collection.)

Gartnavel Royal Asylum

Gartnavel is in a busy district, a mix of business and residential development, on the west side of Glasgow. The site occupies some 68 acres (27 hectares) of greenbelt land and was originally farmlands; the name was anglicised from the Gaelic *Gart nan Ubhal*, place of the apple orchards (Snedden, 1993). It sits on Great Western Road, a broad dual carriageway leading out of the city. Gartnavel is a notable local landmark and yet many who visit it are unaware of the historic parts of the site.

An older Town's Hospital in the centre of the city became the Glasgow Asylum for Lunatics in 1814 before the move to the Gartnavel site in 1843. A Royal Charter re-named the Asylum the Glasgow Royal Mental Hospital in 1931, becoming Gartnavel Royal Hospital in 1963 (Greene, 1993). In the 1970s a new General Hospital was built, and more recently other centres for health treatment and research. The old Royal was replaced by a new psychiatric facility in 2008 – the original West House becoming offices for the National Health Service, while East House has fallen into disrepair and is unsafe to enter.

The Asylum functioned as the main facility for the west of Glasgow between 1843 and 2008. Originally, West House accommodated paying patients, and East House those pauper patients dependent on parish support. Funds ran out for the impressive church intended to join the two (and thus spiritually the two communities), so a smaller chapel was built in 1904 (Haley, 1993). A medical infirmary, farm and workshops for routine maintenance and occupational therapy were added, and in the 1930s a nurses' hostel.

Gartnavel's story is one of adaptation, whether in name or medical practices or geographies, and this complexity of identity acquired over centuries is described by Högström and Philo (2020):

> Such spaces often appear to possess simple boundaries, sharply demarcating them from the residences, businesses, thoroughfares and other settings of urban life, but the reality may be different, with borders that are moveable, porous and, we might say, 'fractal,' in that what seems to be a 'straight line' at one scale turns out to be a much more complex, jaggy, twisting 'geometry' at another.
>
> (Högström and Philo, 2020, p. 107)

As I led the contributors in the 'Writing the Asylum' project (Writing the Asylum, 2023) I thought often about Gartnavel's geography and that idea of something moveable and porous, as it seemed very close to the flexibility of the creative process. Fictional characters can be porous too; writers push and explore boundaries, as frequently described in their commentaries for the 'Writing the Asylum' project.

The Gartnavel archive

The Gartnavel archive occupies 88 metres of shelf space at The Mitchell Library and includes Town's Hospital documents from the early 1800s in a collection extending to the early 2000s. Wellcome Collection have facilitated the online display of a partially digitised selection of records from the archive since 2017 (documents covering ECT treatment and patient records after 1914 were not included for reasons of Data Protection and potential patient identification (Wellcome Collection, n.y.).

Little work has been done on the archive since, and no cataloguing beyond basic organisation by year. It is not possible to trace a named patient through initial and subsequent admissions (although some instances have been noted in the handwritten records by individual physicians). While the patients are named on their medical record, the physician attending them is not. Unlike some nineteenth-century UK asylums, patient photographs were not routinely documented at Gartnavel. The small number of photographs in the archive are of nursing groups, concert parties and sports teams drawn from the staff. Extensive records were kept, however, of gardening and farm work.

The potential for archive in creative writing is very great and extends outwards from any historic material:

> The focus on the physical manifestation of archives looms large and can make it feel like archives are located in and about the past, and not only solid but factual – that they aren't ours but rather something that belongs to another time, other people. However, simply, archives can be considered attempts to gather and hold specific moments of time so they may be shared. If that's the case then we all have the ability to create, access and share archives.
>
> (Reeder, 2020, n.p.)

As an idea for a collaborative project started to take shape, I began to approach members of the Glasgow creative community who might be interested in these little-known records. I knew that the Gartnavel archive would provide inspiration as well as ethical challenges in its creative use.

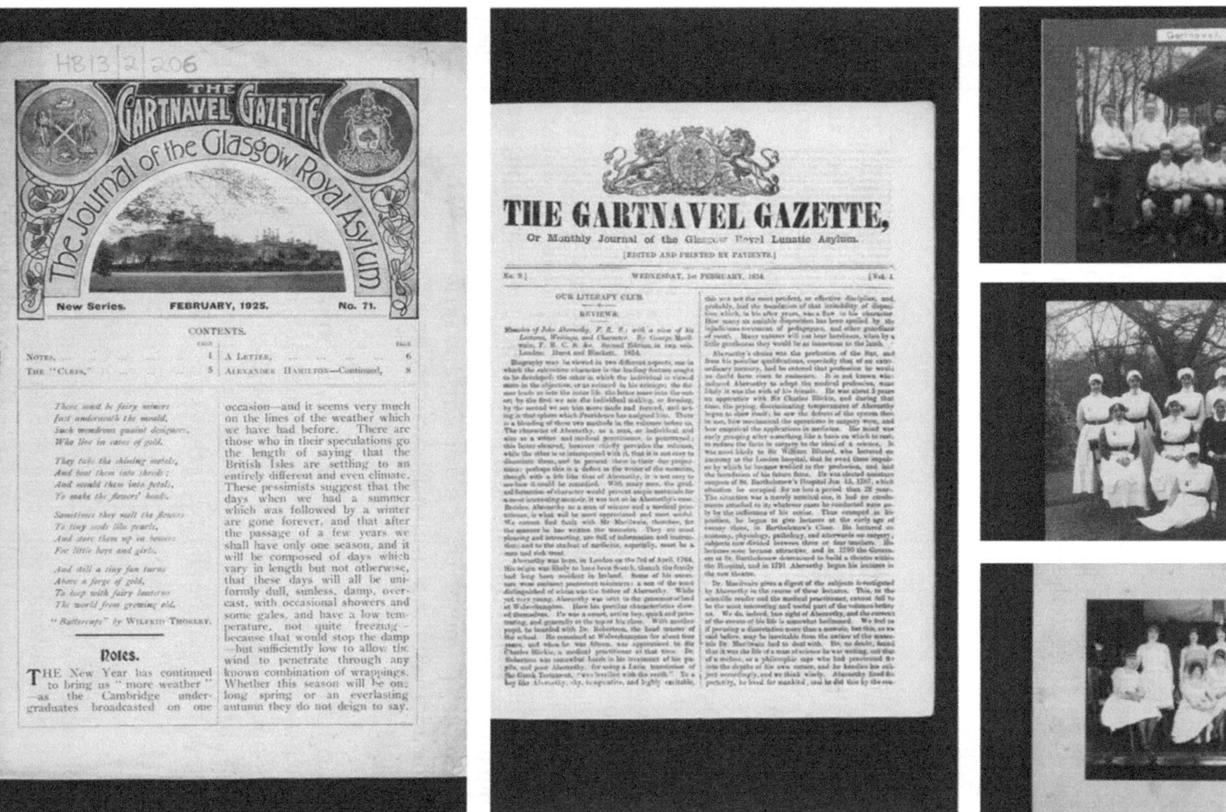

Figure 44.3 Patient magazines and staff group photos from the Gartnavel Royal Asylum archive (Photo 1 and 2: Gartnavel Gazette; Photo 3: Group photograph of Gartnavel FC; Photo 4: Nurses with Matron Brodie; Photo 5: Concert party, all female, in flapper costumes. Source: Wellcome Collection. Provider: NHS/GCC Archives).

Ethics and a mixed experience group

Twenty-eight participants accepted my invitation to join the project. The group includes established creative writers/artists, early career academics and academics with wide experience of creative writing, allowing a wide range of responses and shared insight into different working practices. There's a broad age range and gender balance with representation from LGBT+ and queer communities. Most are based in Glasgow but there are participants from Bangladesh, France, Ireland, South Africa, Sweden and the US. The members of 'Writing the Asylum' volunteered their work for no payment; I am grateful to all those who agreed to take part on this basis and their names appear at the end of this chapter.

In some of our shared discussions it became apparent that there was a divide in language used between our communities. Those who were creative writers in the outside world didn't always understand the academic language sometimes used to describe asylum spaces; their subsequent re-purposing, the role of the patient in the asylum geography. Terms like *geographies, space and place* and *patient embodiment* were unfamiliar to them, although when explained, quickly understood.

I introduced the archive material to the participants very generally before suggesting particular extracts. Sometimes this worked well, and writers/artists ran with the record I'd given them – in other cases the contributor veered off-piste to write about something entirely different yet somehow linked to the places and spaces of mental illness. I was happy with either approach. It sometimes felt that we were walking a delicate line between research and revelation, for so much of Gartnavel's history is unknown, even when the patient records are accessible. At these times, the ethos of collaborative work was important to everyone involved; we were jointly bringing this archive to greater public knowledge.

The work of art therapist Joyce Laing helped to establish a school of important creative work emanating from the asylum and other carceral institutions (like the Gartnavel records, much of Laing's 'Art Extraordinary' collections of 'outsider art' made by asylum patients are held by Greater Glasgow Council) and Laing's significance has been well documented:

> How can their lives be valued, their experiences validated, and their geographies disclosed? (...) The woundedness of these pieces is intimately enfolded into their abandonment, painful reminders of a wider neglect of individuals experiencing mental ill health who have been forgotten and left behind (...) Our wish is not simply to incorporate these spaces and experiences into our geographical dialogues, but to prioritize them, to attune ourselves more fully to the human condition of mental ill health and to trace out its lived geographies.
>
> (McGeachan and Philo, 2023, p.1)

The collaborative project 'Writing the Asylum' sits *outside* the asylum, looking in with empathy to its forgotten stories; the ongoing significance of lives lived within the boundaries is our starting point, too. Present-day writers become mouthpieces for the patient records which inspired them, contributing to lived geographies and giving new voice to individuals who have been silent for too long.

The creative work

The work contributed to the 'Writing the Asylum' project comprises 15 explorations in poetry, 6 short stories, 4 creative non-fiction pieces and 3 responses in image, although these categorisations are loose and participants were encouraged to think in hybrid terms and across boundaries (Writing the Asylum, 2023). Participants added a commentary on their working process. Some explored found objects from the Gartnavel landscape or individual patients; experiments in stitching touch on a noted aspect of asylum history. One writer chose to create fictional archive items, another reflected on the recent suicide of a family member. On the sad news of the death of one participant as the project started, their partner stepped up to take part, bringing an added poignancy to the process.

I've selected five extracts from the project, the first from poet David Ross Linklater. His poem 'Other Side of the Sky' was inspired by an 1895 patient record of a young doctor close to David in age. It's a particularly lively account of a male physician dependent on morphine and cocaine. The Asylum doctors take a dim view, thinking 'his mental state is very distinctly weakened by his indulgence in cocaine. He is not truthful nor does he pretend to be…He does not respect either himself or his profession in his manner of talking to and association with the nurses and attendants' (HB13/5/ 129, 1895).

Doctors view the patient's behaviour as a betrayal of his profession; after many trips home where he resumes his habit, he disappears one day and simply doesn't return. There's a rather sniffy final comment – 'as he has not returned up till the present date his name is today taken off the Books, and he's noted as Discharged Recovered' (HB13/5/ 129, 1895).

In his commentary on the poem, David says 'I was drawn to [this patient's] transcript over the others suggested for two simple reasons: it's intriguing and felt personal enough to explore. Here was a man who spent his life trying to help others but who could not show the same care for himself; a very human trait and all too common. Self-care is often not a priority.'

Other Side of the Sky' (extract)

Who was one form of reality wandering the garden,
a vast absentee
living at the bottom of a well in search of the truth.
Finding strange things there – inheritances of the blood,
the wars in it, each heavy flight of the butterfly.
Who cured the sick but could not turn the tools inward,

lacking application among the lilies of society.
Who was a silhouette in practice
hungering for heaven but inhabiting hells,
and studied under the lamp, that purgatory,
the intimacies of the body and soul
perfect in their inclusion of each other

or who did not fit there at all.

(Linklater, 2023, n.p.)

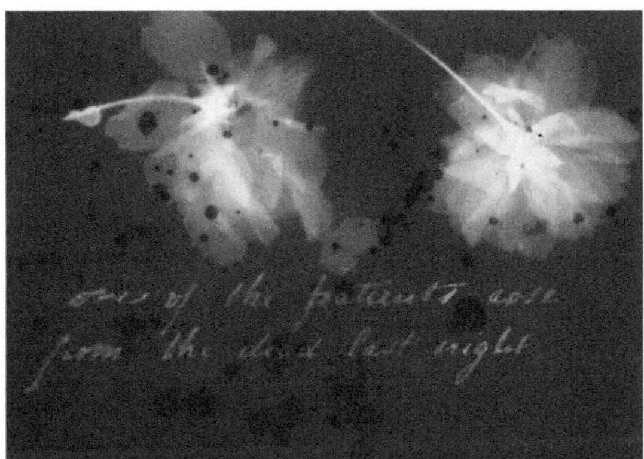

Figure 44.4 Lumen Print: 'one of the patients rose from the dead last night' (2022) (Permission: Claire Quigley).

Summing up his creative process, David adds: 'I wanted the poem to say this: here was a soul who suffered, but who lived and walked the garden and gazed upon the same moon as I do, same as his mother and father did, same as their mother and their father did, and so on all the way back to the ancients. 1895 isn't that long ago in the grand scheme. A flicker. We could have been friends. So this poem is, in my own small way, a tribute or celebration of sorts, a handshake, a strange hello from afar' (Linklater, 2023).

Poet and photographer Claire Quigley took a Gartnavel entry from the 1840s; a female patient who 'raves about religion and imagines visions of Angels and extraordinary influences of the Holy Ghost' (HB13/5/15, 1842a). Claire picked cherry blossom from the Gartnavel grounds, pressing it between dampened light-reactive photo paper and glass then adding acetate sheets printed with the handwritten words from the patient's notes. Left exposed to sunlight, the image emerges, a 'Lumen print' where only the areas hidden from the light remain bright.

In her commentary for the 'Writing the Asylum' website, Claire says 'The Gartnavel motto is 'Reluceat,' meaning 'let there be light again' ('Reluceat 'is the subjunctive form of the verb 'reluceo,' where the subjunctive 'expresses an element of uncertainty, often a wish, desire, doubt or hope').' She goes on to describe the historical Lumen photographic technique, dating from around the time of the patient's admission, as 'an uncertain process, with colours and images dependent on the strength of sunlight, but it produces a picture in which darkness has been replaced by light.'

Another contributor to the project was Sarah Smith, who has used archive extensively in her writing (her historical novel 'Hear No Evil,' published in 2022, is a fictionalised account of the first trial in a Scottish court of a Deaf defendant in 1817). For 'Writing the Asylum,' Sarah was inspired by the archive record of a Gartnavel inmate obsessed by her dead children coming back to life (HB13/5/15, 1842b). Her short story 'Invisible Familiars' goes into the mind of the patient:

Invisible Familiars' (extract)

You are again permitted into the Gallery and enjoy reading and talking there with the other patients. The matron remarks that, when devoid of curses, your cheerfulness and lively conversation is a tonic to those who suffer from melancholia. When you are stricken with a cold and full of catarrh, you take to your bed for three days, alternately shivering and sweating. Mrs Muir comes to your room in the afternoons and reads to you. Sometimes she brings a book of poetry and leaves it for you to take up later if you wish. When the urse comes in the evening to draw down the blind, your children slip from the pages of Tennyson and curl sweetly in your arms…

(Smith, 2023, n.p.)

In her commentary for the 'Writing the Asylum' website, Sarah describes further genealogical research undertaken to furnish more detail on the patient's life. In the story, she protects the patient's identity by giving only first names; the unusual and challenging second person narrative voice gives her further creative mileage, and she says 'I wanted to centre [her] in the reader's mind and allow her more emotional depth than that conveyed by the objective tone and content of the records.'

For another visual essay in 'Writing the Asylum,' artist and feminist writer R. Fraser researched women's experience of asylums and was drawn to a notable tradition of textile art, creating six stitched pieces around a female patient's record. She writes:

It felt like I was channelling her, her feelings, the mania, the exhaustion, the rage, onto the fabric. I tore up an old bedsheet as if she had done this perhaps taken from her hospital bed, and using the transcript, I did stitch work to document her visions, who she believed herself to be and the thoughts she was having. Asemic writing (writing without meaning), formed a large part of it, I wrote down the rage that [she] may have been feeling, then stitched on top of this. I also drew one on paper, words becoming illegible.

(Fraser, R., 2023, n.p.)

When a contributor dropped out, I used their archive extract myself for a short story inspired by photographs of nursing staff and some of my own memories of Gartnavel. It meant a great deal to me to be able to join the group as creative practitioner as well as organiser. An inexperienced nurse in the early years of the twentieth century encounters the temptation of 'the other,' when a new member of the Asylum staff brings his family to live on-site alongside the threat of imminent war:

The Chaplain's Daughter' (extract)

If it was raining, I'd jink inside the wee Chapel with its smell of new wood and candle wax and putty. It hadn't been built long, and the glaziers had just fitted fancy stained glass windows showing St Dorcas and St Luke. Dorcas is patron saint of nurses, but she looked snooty with her flowing robes and Holy Willie phizog. I didn't think I was like her and I didn't feel saintly. A new chaplain had arrived with the building and Mima said some folk had mistaken him for an inmate. He was wandered; bushy white hair standing on end and he never finished a sentence, just let the words drift away.

He came with a wife and a daughter. The wife was stout, and wore a toque hat, always. Straw in good weather, barathea when it rained. And on a Sunday, black fur that looked like Matron's cat Bobby had curled up on her head. They moved into one of the staff cottages and apparently the mother was away much of the time

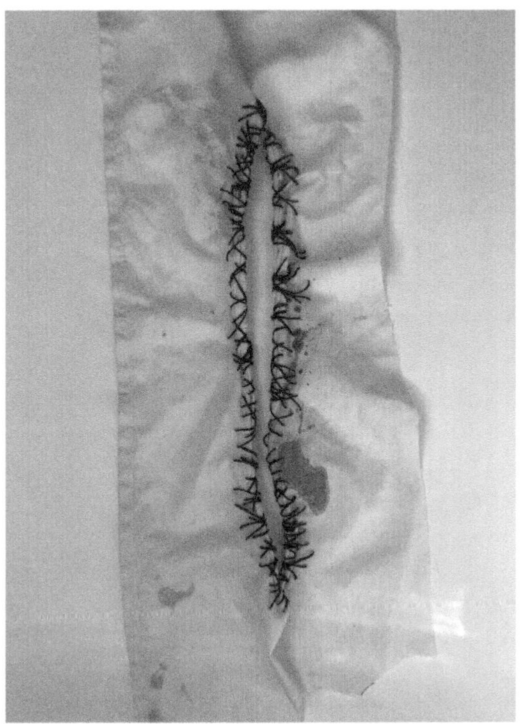

Figure 44.5 Textile piece: 'Cut, Tear, Scratch' by R. Fraser.

Doing Good Works. The girl didn't look like either of them. She was a pretty thing, with fair hair cut in the latest style. The kind of hair that goes curly in the rain. And stylish in her clothes. She was that slim. And kind of English-spoken when I heard her say *yes* and *thank-you* and *how do you do?*

(McDougall, 2023, n.p.)

The commentaries on process are as important as the project's creative contributions, demonstrating the power of the Gartnavel archive at the core of 'Writing the Asylum.' Multiple reflections are possible, shown in the following anonymised extracts, as well as the return time and again to an unknowable, tantalising resource:

Since the ink had faded, the patient notes were difficult to read onscreen, and this becomes the final mystery. What could we, or her doctors, or her family, really know of the affair that had so deranged her? Formally the narrow lines suggest constraint or restraint, both actual and social.

The imaginative space of the written archive acquires greater fabric and resonance when stumbled upon in real life; the written archive opens out into the spatial one:

I discover a heap of abandoned hospital beds in one of the courtyards of West House. The word 'clatter-banes' finds me later. A metallic boneyard, these broken

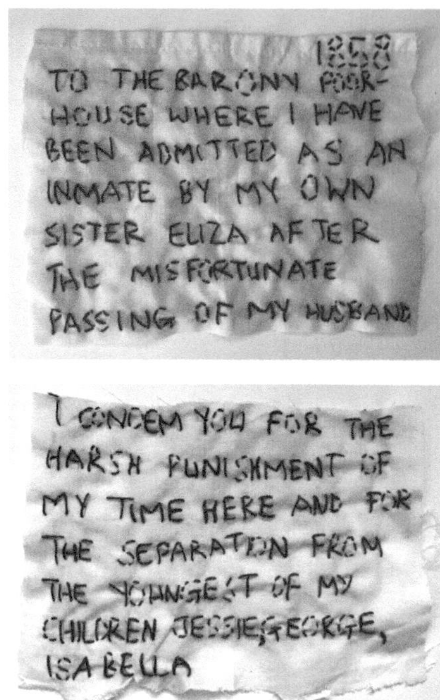

Figure 44.6 Textile piece: 'Sampler I and II, 1858' by R. Fraser.

beds sing for those in the noisy, demonstrative, grief-stricken places – this requiem a quickening between then and now, a throat-song of loss that binds us, three shadowy forms on a cold February afternoon.

Participants acknowledged the significance of the project's invitation to 'visit' – in person, in their reading, in their online explorations – the Asylum's spaces as they developed over time:

I'm interested in the boundaries of madness, where the ill person engages with close family, because I walked that territory with my father. The absence caused by him leaving to have in-patient treatment and then returning. The secrets which could not be spoken [...] How life is changed by mental illness [...] And, I think, a kind of lived sadness that comes with mental ill health. My story started to take shape from my leaning into all those spaces [...] I was thinking about family and liminality. A liminality of light and air and colour, too. Similarly, relationships which do not settle but ebb and flow; give and take. Of uncertainty, and living with it.

The website

With help from the Glasgow web designer Gerard Donnelly of Contribute (www.wecon tribute.co.uk), the 'Writing the Asylum' website launched in April 2023 – (www.writi ngtheasylum.co.uk). It has sections to introduce the Asylum to visitors, information on

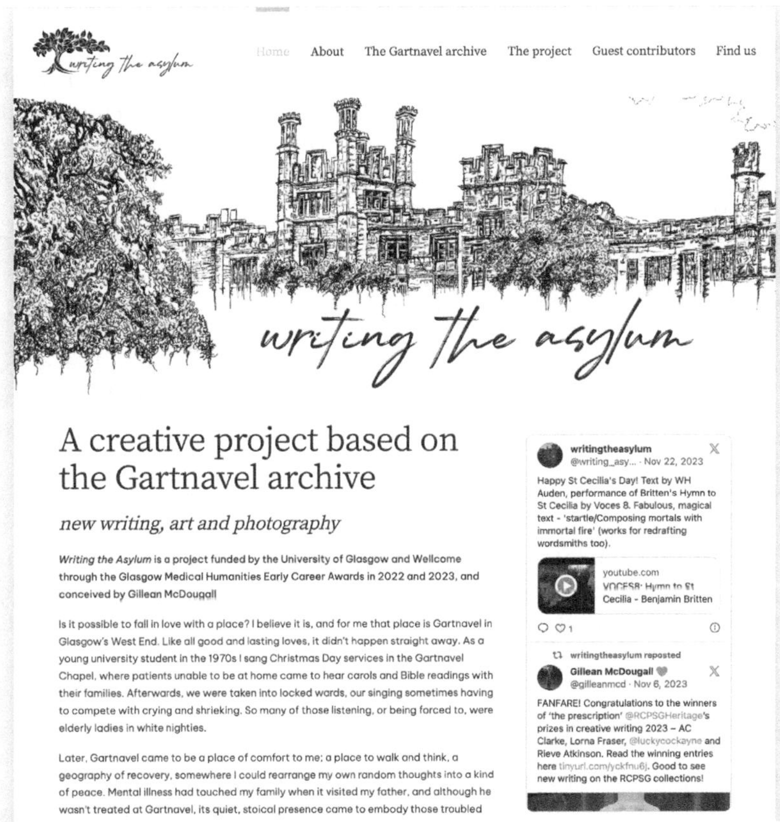

Figure 44.7 'Writing the Asylum' Home Page (2023) (Illustration: Sarah Phelan. Website design: Contribute.)

the archive, and an area where the 28 creative contributions may be accessed via an individual 'tile' for each participant. In addition, resilience in the design allows for future contributions on Gartnavel from other writers.

The website is an economical and wide-reaching way of introducing a forgotten space and its archive to general readership, providing links to the online archive as well as related written sources. The work is of interest to creative communities, encouraging them to see potential in such geographies and archives. Additionally, the project benefits researchers of geographies of mental ill health as well as the wider Gartnavel community.

Conclusion

Gartnavel was known in the nineteenth century as an enlightened and modern geography in the treatment of mental ill health and the study of its history still has much to offer. In the creative reflection of 'Writing the Asylum,' we push that study into unexplored territory, extending existing concepts of creative writing on mental health. Many degrees of engagement are possible, from 'therapeutic' writing to purely 'creative' (these polar points bringing with the need for good practice across the range). The 'viewing' world, rather than the 'writing' one – often within the group of family or friends, employers and neighbours – reacts too, giving further scope to this project.

Many of the contributors' commentaries allude to personal experience of mental ill health. Yet here they are, writers and artists, inspired (compelled?) to memorialise or celebrate that experience in their creative work, walking alongside their own lived stories. And thus the boundary between 'inside' and 'outside' the asylum is all the more blurred, and needfully so.

To close, an extract from my PhD thesis weaves historical patient experience with its archival existence and the geography of Gartnavel, this abandoned and yet still-peopled space:

> From the copperplate lists of garments, pictures begin to appear, and even characters […] on the page, the life of one John Beale. 'Sleeping gown, 6 dress shirts, 2 prs drawers. Suit (black), vests (3), snuff, gloves, nightcap.' And in the final line, 'shroud, coffin, lair.
>
> Two small gatehouses turn by standing into sentry boxes. I'm unsure if they are there to keep the people in, or to keep visitors out. Someone is planting, but they have left the surplus unwatched. Wild overgrowth sits unsupervised, waiting for a weekday or a following wind. No fires burn and the tall chimneys are empty, but the air is full of the smell of smoke. Shroud, coffin, lair. What little space we occupy when all is accounted for. (McDougall, 2021, p. 97 and p. 107)

Taking part in 'Writing the Asylum'

Gregor Addison, Jim Carruth, Martin Cathcart Fródén, AC Clarke, Shehzar Doja, R Fraser, Sally Gales, Dee Heddon, Vicki Husband, Elizabeth Lewis, David Ross Linklater, Gillean McDougall, Cheryl McGeachan, James McGonigal, Mairi Murphy, Sarah Phelan, Claire Quigley, Elizabeth Reeder, Rose Ruane, Finola Scott, Gillian Shirreffs, Sarah Smith, Zoe Strachan, Sheila Templeton, Lynnda Wardle, Nuala Watt, Stephen Watt, Christie Williamson

Acknowledgements

Funding for 'Writing the Asylum' was provided by the University of Glasgow Medical Humanities Network Early Career Foundation Awards scheme (with Wellcome Trust support) in 2022 and 2023.

The original material for the Gartnavel Archive images is held at NHS Greater Glasgow and Clyde Archives, the Mitchell, Library, Glasgow, Scotland. Wellcome Collection have facilitated the online display of this partially digitised archive since 2017 under Licence: Attribution 4.0 International (CC BY 4.0).

References

Fraser, R. (2023) Grace Binning Responds, Available online at: https://writingtheasylum.co.uk/portfolio-items/r-fraser/

Greene, G. (1993) Chapter 1 – Administration and finance. In: Andrews, J., Smith, I. (Eds.), *Let There Be Light Again: A History of Gartnavel Royal Hospital from its Beginnings to the Present Day*. Greater Glasgow Health Board, Glasgow, pp. 1–17.

Haley, D. (1993) Chapter 2: Religion and the chaplaincy. In: Andrews, J., Smith, I. (Eds.), *Let There Be Light Again: A History of Gartnavel Royal Hospital from its Beginnings to the Present Day*. Greater Glasgow Health Board, Glasgow, pp. 18–24.

HB13/5/129 (1895) Patient record for Alexander Peacock, *Records of Gartnavel Royal Hospital*, Glasgow: Wellcome Collection. https://wellcomecollection.org/works/x4n7q4jw/items?canvas= 463HB13/5/15 (1842a) Patient record for Agnes Dow, *Records of Gartnavel Royal Hospital*, Glasgow: Wellcome Collection. https://wellcomecollection.org/works/pk2ufbn

HB13/5/15 (1842b) Patient record for Agnes Simpson, *Records of Gartnavel Royal Hospital*, Glasgow: Wellcome Collection. https://wellcomecollection.org/works/esmg6knh/items?canvas= 130–133/314

Högström, E. and Philo, C. (2023) " 'Let there be light" or life in the dark: Vital geographies of mental healthcare,' *Social Science & Medicine*, 333, 116137.

Högström, E. and Philo, C. (2020) 'Ontological boundaries or contextual borders: The urban ethics of the asylum,' *Urban Planning*, 5(4), pp. 106–120.

Linklater, D.R. (2023) Other Side of the Sky, Available online at: https://writingtheasylum.co.uk/ portfolio-items/david-ross-linklater/?portfolioCats=7

McDougall, G. (2023) The Chaplain's Daughter, Available online at: https://writingtheasylum. co.uk/portfolio-items/gillean-mcdougall/?portfolioCats=7

McDougall, G. (2021), *Madness to Memoir: The Creative Cure*. DFA thesis, University of Glasgow.

McGeachan, C. and Philo, C. (2023) '"Hanging around in their brokenness": On mental Ill-Health geography, asylums and camps, artworks and salvage,' *Annals of the American Association of Geographers*, 113(5), pp. 1224–1242.

Reeder, E. (2020) "Happiness isn't asinine or banal, but active' – Elizabeth Reeder on writing An Archive of Happiness,' Penned in the Margins, November 17 2020. Available at: www.pen nedinthemargins.co.uk/index.php/2020/11/happiness-snt-asinine-or-banal-but-active-interview-with-elizabeth-reeder/

Smith, S. (2023) Invisible Familiars, Available online at: https://writingtheasylum.co.uk/portfolio-items/sarah-smith/?portfolioCats=7

Snedden, A. (1993) Chapter 3: Environment and architecture. In: Andrews, J., Smith, I. (Eds.), *Let There Be Light Again: A History of Gartnavel Royal Hospital from its Beginnings to the Present Day*. Greater Glasgow Health Board, Glasgow, pp. 25–50.

Wellcome Collection (n.y.) Records of Gartnavel Royal Hospital, Glasgow, Scotland, 1811–2002 https://wellcomecollection.org/works/pk2ufbnt

Writing the Asylum (2023) Available online at: www.writingtheasylum.co.uk

45 Mental health geography in the cracks

Between abolition and reform

Ebba Högström and Chris Philo

Introduction

> The intention here is not to contest or pick holes in the demands of activists who have called for the abolition of police and prisons – demands which should be supported wholeheartedly – but to extend the same kind of analysis to the mental health system. While we should welcome the ways in which abolitionist critiques have drawn attention to the structural racism, sexism, and violence which is embedded within the criminal justice system, it is vitally important that these critiques be applied also to mental health services. The alternative is to risk replacing one set of carceral, violent, and racist institutions with another; to permit the continuation of policing by other means.
>
> (Blayney, 2020, n.p.)

Critical scholarship on 'asylum and post-asylum geographies' (Philo, 2000) has been ongoing since at least the early-1980s, but rarely has it attended directly to the problematic of whether the mental health system itself should exist or, conversely, be abolished. Indeed, rarely if ever has it asked the searching question of whether the very object that it studies – organised forms of mental healthcare, usually in some way spatially demarcated – should ideally disappear, potentially leaving it with no work to do any more (except in an historical guise). Our chapter explores this question, recognising that answers to it necessarily acquire complexity and nuance due to the vulnerable, maybe suffering, character of people accessing mental healthcare provisions. Moreover, to anticipate, many geographers researching these provisions, from different conceptual and ethico-political starting-points, have concluded that some version of congregate, place-centred, 'retreat' or 'refuge' – wherein people with mental health problems can share experiences and support, with or without input from mental health professionals – *is* still required.

'Abolitionist' critiques have been trenchant with respect to other forms of institutional facilities, most obviously prisons, as we will elaborate shortly. While rarely framed in an abolitionist vocabulary, equivalent critiques have been levelled at the large, often remote and secretive, mental or psychiatric hospitals that emerged in many parts of the world during the nineteenth century, the Victorian 'lunatic asylums' of so many haunting tales. These critiques – sometimes informed by the radical if fragmented perspective of 'anti-psychiatry' (e.g., Cooper, 1967) – fuelled the scaling-back and eventual closure of many of these institutions from the 1960s onwards, leading the 'asylum geographies' of old to be replaced by a newer palimpsest of 'post-asylum geographies' – comprising smaller-scale

DOI: 10.4324/9781003345725-50

mental health facilities, day centres, group homes, drop-in clinics, and more, spanning public, voluntary and private sectors – where the ideals of 'care in the community' would be realised. In practice such ideals were often far from met, as emphasised by many critical scholars, geographers included, who inquired into such phenomena (e.g., Chesters, 2005; Gleeson & Kearns, 2001), but the basic vision here – a 'deinstitutional' landscape pockmarked by identifiable spaces dedicated to people with mental health problems – remained relatively unquestioned.

For some self-identified 'psychiatric survivors', people who may have endured compulsory psychiatric detention alongside forced medication and other abuses, even this less institutional mental healthcare landscape is seen as problematic. Associated with 'Mad Studies' (Beresford, 2020; Beresford et al., 2020; also Burstow, 2015; Karanikolas, 2022) as an emergent survivor-led academic subfield, the result has been – in shorthand – to extend abolitionist logics from the asylum to psychiatry, wherever it is practised, and, at its most extreme, to *all* varieties of organised mental healthcare, particularly if public and state-run, and even extending to service-user-centred and charitable schemes and projects. For some, then, '[c]losure of repressive institutions, such as mental hospitals and prisons, … [is] a necessary but not sufficient action on the road to abolition' (Ben-Moshe, 2013, p. 84). Such a critique has spawned the kinds of explicitly named abolitionist arguments indicated in the epigraph, including an abolitionist critique of mental health law (Wilson, 2021), inherently hostile to the mental health system in any of its manifestations: 'The most important element in institutional closure is to ensure that people do not end up re-incarcerated in other formats such as group homes or other institutional placements' (ibid., p. 84). The objection is that most prevailing societal arrangements pertaining to mental ill-health and how it is treated – medicalised, psychiatrised, set within punitive benefits regimes, seen as mark of individual weakness and irresponsibility – press down oppressively on the lived and felt realities of living with mental distress, despair and dislocation.

The epigraph reflects a particular conjuncture, in the early-2020s US and UK, when politicians of different stripes, Right and Left, begin to propose that many difficulties apparent within police and penal systems – hinging on the damaged mental health of offenders, likely linked to substance abuse – might best be tackled through the mental health system. The radical wing of such proposals in the US has sometimes invoked abolitionist logics, conjoining an historical account of racism, slavery and the plantation with the demand to 'defund' policing and prisons, notably the 'supermax' prisons with such high proportions of Black and Latinx inmates. Prisons in particular, taken as the logical, highly spatialised progeny of that dismal history, are to be abolished just as slavery was eventually subject to 'abolition'. From a critical mental health studies, maybe Mad Studies, perspective, the mental health system – whether lodged in large asylums or small community care facilities – is beset by much the same fundamental abuses, which means that it too ought to be abolished.

Our purpose with this chapter is to chart in outline these treacherous waters, mapping them back into the writings of both mental health geographers and other scholars ostensibly tackling rather different socio-spatial thematics. To begin, we briefly explain how earlier generations of mental health geographers critiqued both asylum and post-asylum geographies, noting that the latter was critiqued more for its reality than its vision while even being defended against its *own* dismantling in the face of capital-driven urban restructuring. Then, we discuss what has been termed 'abolition geography', showing that, for the likes of Gilmore (2022), the prison is only an element within a more expansive regime of hostile institutional forms – ones predicated on 'racial capitalism' but also damagingly extractive 'ecologies' of all sorts – which potentially includes many sites of mental health intervention. Abolition geography is intimately associated with a growing interest in Black geographies, and we will sketch out the readiness of Black geographies to detect generative 'Black senses of place' even in the depths of what are self-evidently the most abusive of spaces. This move shapes what we argue about certain kinships between the plantation and the asylum, or between 'Black senses of place' and 'Mad senses of place'. Finally, before concluding, we return to more recent incarnations of mental health geography wherein we locate a similar willingness to identify, even within the worst excesses of the total asylum or a fragmenting, austerity-riven post-asylum landscape, what might indeed be termed supportive 'Mad senses of place'. Those Mad places might still be regarded with suspicion by an uncompromising abolitionist standpoint, but they arguably constitute the careful answer that today's mental health geographers may venture in response to the provocation of our opening question.

Earlier mental health geographies: critiquing asylum and post-asylum spaces

Historical geographies of asylums (e.g., Philo, 2004) – heavily influenced by the radical-critical traditions within histories of madness, asylums and psychiatry (e.g., Foucault, 1961, 1975; Scull, 1977; Rothman, 1980) – certainly identify many abuses within institutional settings where historical 'mad people' have unfortunately found themselves, notably when confined to so-called 'regions below', specifically meaning darkened basements but more metaphorically all badly-run 'houses for the insane'. A critical ethos is hence present in such studies, if tempered by appreciating the genuinely humane ambitions of many 'lunacy reformers' – for whom the asylum was to be a curative or at least sheltering establishment – and by noting how advocates of *public* asylums were striving to avoid the abuses endemic to non-specialist spaces (the workhouses) and, crucially, profiteering spaces (the private madhouses).

Those studying more recently established deinstitutional landscapes have been clear on the dangers of large-scale mental hospitals and, if not all that explicitly, appear to have favoured their closure and replacement by smaller-scale community-based facilities. Hence, Dear and Wolch, in their epic 1987 text *Landscapes of Despair* – inspired by founding studies by the Wolperts (1974, 1976) and C.J. Smith (1976, 1977) – echo 'Progressive' era and then post-WWII official and more radical critiques of the asylum, if recognising how radical ideals often nestled alongside the use of drug therapies (pacifying 'mad people') *and* fiscal conservativism within a 'golden consensus' that closed the big institutions and heralded deinstitutional assemblages. What Dear and Wolch then emphasise how the ideal of 'care in the community' was compromised, partly by cost-savings that meant community provisions never appeared in the quantity and quality properly to replace what was lost, but also by a problematic locational politics that – reflecting 'Not-In-My-Backyard' (NIMBY) tendencies – steered post-asylum assemblages into resource-poor, run-down, environmentally unappealing city regions, and hence their pivotal claims about 'service-dependent ghettos' and 'the public city'. In play here was a dramatic translocation, sometimes following an 'inverse care law' (Smith, 1987) allocating resources where they were least needed, causing, as Scull (1977) proposes, mentally unwell people to be uplifted from one set of 'dumps' (the old asylums) and then 'dumped' again in the uncaring, unprepared and under-resourced community.

Even here, though, good, supportive possibilities could arise, not least in an informal shared infrastructure often centring on places made by/for mental health 'clients' themselves (Estroff, 1981), and one of the present authors recalls being particularly struck long ago by a conference paper referencing the humble, yet consequential, community-making qualities of a tiny, cheap café (in a run-down Canadian city neighbourhood) where such clients gathered every day (Kearns, 1986). In sum, this early generation of mental health geographers had abolitionist instincts when it came to the mental hospitals, but also detected the appearance, often quietly and marginally, of 'good places' carved out by mental health clients themselves, sometimes in alliance with open-minded mental health professionals and volunteers.

Abolition geographies and Black geographies

In 2022, a collection of essays appeared that brought together writing from across three decades by Ruth Wilson Gilmore, entitled *Abolition Geography: Essays Towards Liberation*. Gilmore pioneered US-based work on carceral geographies focused on prisons, specifically the massive sites of 'hyper-incarceration' wherein Black and Latinx populations become so disproportionately represented (Gilmore, 2007; Philo and Schliehe, 2024). Her work subsequently enlarged the optic to embrace a wider array of spaces, systems and structures integral to the making of 'unfree' societies hostile to all manner of unwanted 'others' surreptitiously siphoned into situations likely to hasten their premature demise. It is this wider array that becomes the object for her abolitionist calls. 'Abolition geography starts from the homely premise that freedom is a place,' Gilmore (2022:427) states, signalling its task of exposing and opposing all those intersecting processes that produce 'unfreedom' and, concomitantly, 'human sacrifice'. For her, it is less an academic subfield, more a sensibility spanning both critical and utopian registers. It demands a stern look at history, especially at slavery, but also invites a casting forward that should envisage worlds otherwise, propelled by an ambition of realising new, non-carceral, ways of 'free' place-making, 'the undoing of bondage' (ibid., p. 481). In the mental health domain, an almost identical charge is heard for moving beyond just 'protesting against the current circumstances to envisioning a more just and equitable world', one 'enabling us to engage in politics of the future' (Ben-Moshe, 2013, p. 92).

Abolition geographies are intimately associated with work on Black geographies. Authoring a foreword to the 2019 edition of Bobby Wilson's monograph on race and capitalist development in 'America's Johannesburg', Birmingham in Alabama, Gilmore (2019:xi) positions Black geographies as 'a field', 'diasporic consciousness in action', alert to how 'Black people make life' wherein '[t]he socio-spatial character of struggle grounds meaning in the making of place, thanks to a viscerality that feels precise but is always provisional'. The emphasis is a viscerality of feeling, an emotional embodiment of place-making, but one that is uncertain, fragile, always in the shadow of broader oppressions, unfreedoms, prone to place-unmaking. What must be underscored here is the centralising of Black, particularly Afro-American, experience in the crucibles of slave-ship, plantation, ghetto, and prison, all spaces, in one way or another, of confinement, oppression and exploitation (McKittrick, 2006). The deathly 'necropolitics' of these spaces reside in anti-Black violence as a conjoint existential and political-economic struggle over the parameters of life, and such deathliness is what fired both the initial abolitionist cause – to abolish slavery – and an ongoing abolitionist ethos *contra* that wider array of unfreedom, of place-unmaking, on which Gilmore fastens.

Leading Black geographer Katherine McKittrick (2013, p. 7) nonetheless counters any move that *only* sees the above-mentioned necropolitical spaces as 'uninhabitable': 'If some places are rendered lifeless in the broader geographic imagination, what of those inhabiting the lifeless?'. Instead, without remotely wishing to find simple comfort or solace, she identifies 'a political location that fosters more humanely workable, and alternative, geographic practice,' populated by 'differential modes of survival ... – creolisation, the blues, maroonage, revolution, and more' (ibid.: 15, p. 5). Borrowing particularly from the Jamaican essayist Sylvia Wynter (McKittrick, 2015), for whom the *praxis* of being human, in all conceivable situations, remains pivotal, McKittrick (2011, p. 954) offers this reflection: 'It seems to me that many analyses of racial violence leave little room to attend to human life, and consequently disregard narratives that bring into sharp focus practices that politicise place-life and place-death differently.' For her, therefore, 'place-life' can also arise simultaneously in the dreadful sites of 'place-death', and hence one strand of Black geographies critically, carefully, attends to this shimmer of Black life-making. As Wilson's grandfather would shout from his pickup truck: 'Come on. Get in. We're going to march today' (Gilmore, 2019, p. xi).

The plantation and the asylum

McKittrick (2013, p. 2–3) is crystal-clear that the plantation be regarded as an 'ongoing locus of anti-Black violence and death,' a site whose logics of Black exclusion and eradication translocate to other spaces such as the US mass incarceration penal system, abandoned inner-city housing schemes, disappeared suburban settlements of 'freed' slaves, and more. Such lists might also include US lunatic asylums, particularly in the South, which from the nineteenth century onwards became filled with Black patients whose 'race' was associated by many lunacy experts with a natural susceptibility to 'madness'. Indeed, when one historian of lunatic asylums in America's Deep South, Mab Segrest (2020), gets asked in an interview 'how did the asylum resemble a plantation?', she replies:

> Patient exploitation at the Georgia Asylum took the form of 'occupational therapy' that filled the gap from the absence of other resources or treatments for patients. A careful examination of Georgia Asylum annual reports in the last two decades of the nineteenth century showed how moral therapy' gave way to 'occupational therapy', which involved a huge farming operation producing tons of vegetables, plus cows, chickens, and pigs. As far as I can tell, the patients were not getting much of this food. Race and gender shaped work regimes – sewing for white women, laundry for Black women, gardening for white men, growing cotton and other cash crops for Black men.

Much more should ideally be said about the racialisation of the asylum, and of psychiatry more generally in the US and elsewhere, but for what follows such details are less important than the resemblance between asylum and plantation as both terrible spaces that might still, in certain cautious registers, be thought differently.

A prime influence on Black geographies is the Black feminist writer bell hooks, whose concept of 'homeplace' is a valuable additional input for rethinking what occurs in spaces ostensibly devoid of hope. In her well-known essay on 'Homeplace: a site in resistance', hooks (1990; also hooks, 1984) draws on her experience of living in marginal spaces, 'on the wrong side of the tracks' as a child in small-town Kentucky, to encapsulate both the demeaning exclusions wrought by anti-Blackness and what her memories of such spaces – the exclusions but also the sociabilities arising in counterpoint – offer as a resource to sustain thought, self and life in the present. McKittrick notes her debt to hooks, and her own landmark *Demonic Grounds* book (McKittrick, 2006) frequently references both hooks and the 'Homeplace' essay. McKittrick worries that 'geographic investigations of Blackness and Black culture [may] stop at bell hooks,' as if hooks can herself (meta-phorically) stand-in for the actual work required, as well as gently critiquing hooks for 'hemming' herself – and Black feminities/feminisms – into 'margins' forever alienated from 'centres' (McKittrick, 2006, p. 19, pp. 55-56, p. 58). Yet McKittrick's own attempt to inject life into otherwise 'lifeless' Black spaces nonetheless still learns from hooks, if substantially reworking her ideas through diverse Black Studies scholars and the likes of Wynter's 'humanness as praxis' (McKittrick, 2015).

With caution, then, we are now inspired to think laterally about asylum and post-asylum landscapes with their own darkened corners, ones often viewed as obsolete, dehumanising and deadening. Indeed, our chapter now proceeds on the assumption that there *could* be warrant for replacing or, better, pairing hooks's Black 'homeplace' with Mad 'homeplace'. The risks of such a repurposing of these constructions are legion, and some might understandably see here a misappropriation of both hooks and Black geog-raphies, even another form of academic 'extractivism' that quarries the latter for insights relevant to places that are not *necessarily* occupied, forcibly or willingly, by Black people. On that count, though, we draw encouragement from the remark by Camilla Hawthorne (2019, p. 6) that 'Black geographies is not exclusively the study … of Black people, nor does it entail the identification of some sort of reductive, non-relational "Black space.'

Later mental health geographies: uncovering and valuing 'Mad places'

As indicated above, earlier mental health geographers (e.g., Dear & Wolch 1987, Kearns & Taylor, 1989) acknowledged supportive, barely-institutional 'Mad places', albeit ones that had some form of congregate spatial coherence, where people with mental health problems could share lives and worlds. Some more recent mental health geographers took this line further, notably in a body of more ethnographically inspired work arising in the 1990s and early-2000s, typified by Hester Parr's (2008) pioneering work on a rich variety of community spaces, schemes and projects for (and often co-run by) people with mental health problems. Here, broadly accepting if rarely labouring the critique, the likes of Parr oppose the old mental hospitals – the sites for a spatialised 'scripting' of 'the lunatic' or 'mental patient' – and look instead for exciting, affirmative possibilities for re-placing people with mental health problems in everyday communities and scenes of living and working. Even while recognising the limitations on being able to get such people fully working and hence integrated into mainstream political economies, Parr's 'hopeful ontologies' mesh with Vanessa Pinfold's (2000) excavation of people with mental health problems striving to create 'safe havens all over the world' and 'spaces for Mad Pride'. The idea within these works is mapping more-or-less self-organised spaces where quite other ways of supporting 'good days' arise through encounter and collaboration with peers (e.g., when gardening, workworking, filming, or running a café).

This body of inquiry derives impetus from psychiatric survivor critiques and voices, but such a borrowing – also from Mad studies – has arguably become more prominent in a still-more-recent body of mental health geographies endeavour. Elements can be found in Duff (2012), Högström (2018), DeVerteuil (2013), McGeachan (2019), and McGeachan & Philo (2023), as well as in work of the present authors (Högström & Philo, 2020, 2023). The immersive approach characterising many of these works opens towards multiple voices; of people with their own experience of mental ill-health, maybe as employees, family carers, volunteers, and more. A wide range of contextual factors such as provision, policy, stigma, economics, and (lack of) coordination are put in relation to an equally wide range of spatial arrangements which, altogether, problematise 'the institutional'. Hopeful and empowering messages stemming directly from everyday life in the mental healthcare sphere sit side-by-side with critical accounts of mental healthcare conditions (e.g., austerity, neoliberal restructuring, hidden abuses). Stories of sanctuaries, safe heavens, and carceral and disciplining spaces are told, 'good' and 'bad' spaces blend with accounts of 'good' and 'bad' days, and what particularly stands out in this body of work is indeed the survivors' voices.

Jacqueline Liggins's (2016) frontline ethnographic inquiry, for example, hails from someone who had experienced a long period of residential treatment in a (private) mental health facility. The ontological standpoint here places itself clearly on the side of the 'psychiatrised' person, and her work has an explicitly to-one-side relationship with survivor perspectives. It recognises problems with the residential treatment setting, but still underlines how it served as a genuine sanctuary, enabling her and others to create and experience caring/nurturing relationships that give them the possibility of returning to existence in/engagement with wider worlds outside the treatment space. Cast in part as an exercise in 'magic realism', Jenny Laws (2012, 2017) inquires into the 'Mad worlds' and 'Mad work' of service users at day centre drop-in. The survivor perspective engaging her is very much 'in the grain' of experiencing hurt and suffering, but also sometimes the joy and humour of survivor-user worlds. She seeks closeness to how these service users developed shared coping mechanisms, sometimes quite subversively in outdoor spaces.

Another explicitly 'survivor-user' centred inquiry is offered by Ed Kiely (2021, 2022), who digs into how neoliberal austerity demands affective buy-in from mental health policymakers believing that they are doing the right thing by cutting funding for any forms of congregate mental health care/community. Reducing their dependency and encouraging them to seek work/training was seen as a spur to survivor-users re-joining wider society (even if that is a wholly unrealistic option for many). Kiely's account underlines how much one particular day centre mattered as an anchor, a lifeline, for many 'clients', but notes that it closed when the funding was cut but then reopened as a pale shadow of what it was previously able to offer (and in a much less welcoming, homely environment). The narrative here is hence of a much-loved site of place-making being summarily unmade, to be replaced by another place much less conducive to surviving let alone thriving. The simple point is hence that even in recent mental health geographies work clearly inspired by radical-critical perspectives – by Mad Studies, Black studies, abolitionist logics – there remains this poignant openness to the value of Mad place-making, even when it involves mentally unwell individuals congregating together, perhaps depending on one another or others, possibly voicing their own 'vulnerability' and wish to be assisted, maybe seeking in part to shut out the wider (threatening, alienating, destabilising) world, and even when it might invite in 'non-Mad' specialists (perhaps ones aligned in some way with psychiatry, therapy, occupational health, and more).

Alternative Mad place-making

In the initial quote of this chapter, Blayney (2020) spotlights the risk of replacing one oppressive system (police, prisons) with another equally oppressive (the mental health system). He advocates for an array of alternatives for how a mental healthcare system could be organised, which would also require radical transformations in many aspects of society. In the same vein, we would argue that there are so many different species of 'carceral' institutions or 'closed spaces', serving so many different sorts of 'troubled, troubling and troublesome' people (Disney and Schliehe, 2019), that it is arguably wrong to propose a singular, one-size-fits-all abolitionist logic to all such institutions and spaces. Most obviously, it is one thing to be a staunch prison (and broader penal) abolitionist, but another to extend that logic to all mental healthcare spaces given that many persons using these spaces really are 'vulnerable' (even given problems with this notion for suggesting passivity/dependence/victimhood: see Wilson, 2021) and almost certainly do need some kind of place-based – however weakly-demarcated – spaces shared with others who may experience the same psychological troubles and/or may have genuine therapeutic/caring expertise.

Considering what mental health geographers, past and present, have addressed in their inquiries suggests that all of them, to a greater or lesser extent, arrive at – accept and even advocate around – this root principle. Moreover, rather than such a principle being entirely set against abolition, a focus on place-making – on alternative, creative, supportive, caring place-making – lies at the heart of Gilmore's abolition geography and indeed some of the Black geographies' literature, including that inspired by hooks's 'Homeplace'. Careful attention must remain trained on the question of which 'reforms' to the likes of mental health and penal systems *really* do constitute changes that counter abuses in those systems – *contra* those that only serve to sure up the established order of things – in which regard Gilmore and others draw on André Gorz's formulation of 'non-reformist reforms' (Gorz, 1967), meaning reforms that do much more than *just* reform existing systems, and rather work productively/generatively towards a longer-term goal of abolishing abusive systems full stop. Our sense is that many if not all mental health geographers have been operating in this 'non-reformist reform' orbit.

Finally, it might be proposed that geographers are perhaps always destined to proceed in the cracks between outright abolitionist and a quieter 'non-reformist reform' stance precisely because they are so attuned – whatever their exact philosophical or ethico-political standpoints – to the significance of place in the lives of all people, but notably those people who are vulnerable and only-just surviving. They so often do need some kind of anchorage, some form of mooring, to a recognisable, demarcatable place with which they feel affinity and from which they can derive some form of support, care, nurturance, and hope. The 'big bad spaces' arguably do need to be abolished, for all manner of reasons, but a rich ecology of 'small good places' are surely needed in their stead, especially when the evaluation of these sites derives from people with their own experience of such places. Such, perhaps, is the simple but fundamental message deriving from the overall arc of geographical inquiries into spaces of mental (ill)health and well-being/ill-being.

Acknowledgements

The authors would like to thank Sarah Golightly for valuable feedback on this manuscript.

References

Ben-Moshe, L. (2013) The tension between abolition and reform. In: Nagel, M. E. and Nocella II, A. J. (Eds.) *The End of Prisons: Reflections from the Decarceration Movement.* Amsterdam & New York: Brill, 83–92.

Beresford, P. (2020) 'Mad', Mad studies and advancing inclusive resistance. *Disability & Society,* 35(8), 1337–1342.

Beresford, P., Russo, J., and Boxall, K. (Eds.) (2020) *Doing Mad Studies: Critical International Perspectives—An International Handbook.* London: Routledge.

Blayney, S. (2020) The continuation of policing by other means? Extending abolitionist critiques to the mental health system. *New Socialist,* available online at http://newsocialist.org.uk.

Burstow, B. (2015) *Psychiatry and the Business of Madness: An Ethical and Epistemological Accounting.* New York: Palgrave Macmillan.

Chesters, J. (2005) Deinstitutionalisation: An unrealised desire. *Health Sociology Review* 14(3), 272–282.

Cooper, D. (1967). *Psychiatry and Anti-Psychiatry.* London: Tavistock.

Dear, M. J., and Wolch, J. (1987) *Landscapes of Despair: From Deinstitutionalisation to Homelessness.* Oxford: Polity.

DeVerteuil, G. (2013) Where has NIMBY gone in urban social geography? *Social & Cultural Geography,* 14(6), 599–603.

Disney, T., and Schliehe A. (2019) Troubling institutions. *Area,* 51, 194–199.

Duff, C. (2012) Exploring the role of 'enabling places' in promoting recovery from mental illness: A qualitative test of a relational model. *Health & Place,* 18, 1388–1395.

Estroff, S. E. (1981) *Making it Crazy: An Ethnography of Psychiatric Clients in an American Community.* Berkeley: University of California Press.

Foucault, M. (2006 [1961]). *History of Madness.* London and New York: Routledge.

Foucault, M. (1976 [1975]). *Discipline and Punish: The Birth of the Prison.* London: Allen Lane.

Gilmore, R.W. (2007). *Golden Gulag: Prisons, Surplus, Crisis and Opposition in Globalising California.* San Diego: University of California Press.

Gilmore, R.W. (2019). Foreword to the 2019 edition. In: Wilson, B.M. (ed.) *Americas Johannesburg: Industrialisation and Racial Transformation in Birmingham,* Athens, University of Georgia Press, ix–xii.

Gilmore, R.W. (2022). *Abolition Geography: Essays Towards Liberation,* London: Verso.

Gleeson. B. and Kearns, R. (2001) Remoralising landscapes of care. *Environment and Planning D,* 19, 61–80.

Gorz, A. ((1964)1967) *Strategy for Labour: A Radical Proposal.* Boston: Beacon Press.

Hawthorne C. (2019) Black matters are spatial matters: Black geographies for the twenty-first century. *Geography Compass,* 13, e12468.

Högström, E. (2018) 'It used to be here but moved somewhere else': Post-asylum spatialisations – A new urban frontier? *Social & Cultural Geography,* 19(3), 314–335.

Högström, E., and Philo, C. (2023) 'Let there be light' or life in the dark? Vital geographies of mental healthcare. *Social Science & Medicine,* 333, 116–137.

Högström, E., and Philo, C. (2020) Ontological boundaries or contextual borders: The urban ethics of the asylum. *Urban Planning,* 5(4), 106–120.

Hooks, B. (1984). *Feminist Theory: From Centres to Margins.* Boston: South End Press.

Hooks, B. (1990). Homeplace: A site in resistance. In: Hooks, B. (ed.) *Yearning: Race, Gender and Cultural Politics.* Boston, South End Press, 41–49.

Karanikolas, P. (2022) Imagining non-carceral futures with(in) mad studies. In: Beresford, P., and Russo, J. (Eds.) *The Routledge International Handbook of Mad Studies,* Abingdon & New York, Routledge, 217–222.

Kearns, R.A. (1986). Convergence of humanistic and social thought in social geographic practice. In: *Paper read at the Annual Meeting of the Association of American Geographers*, Minneapolis, USA.

Kearns, R.A., and Taylor, S.M. (1989) Daily life experience of people with chronic mental disabilities in Hamilton, Ontario. *Canada's Mental Health*, 37, 1–4.

Kiely, E. (2021) Stasis disguised as motion: Waiting, endurance and the camouflaging of austerity in mental health services. *Transaction Institution British Geography* 46, 717–731.

Kiely, E. (2022). *The Camouflaging of Austerity: Institutional Geographies of Mental Health in Contemporary England*. Unpublished PhD thesis, University of Cambridge (https://doi.org/10.17863/CAM.93789).

Laws, J. (2012) *'Working Through': An Inquiry into Work and Madness*. Unpublished PhD thesis, University of Durham. (http://etheses.dur.ac.uk/3557/).

Laws, J. (2017) Magic at the margins: Towards a magical realist human geography. *Cultural Geographies*, 24, 3–19.

Liggins, J. (2016) A *Place for Healing in Mental Healthcare and Recovery*. Unpublished PhD thesis, University of Auckland (https://researchspace.auckland.ac.nz/handle/2292/29211).

McGeachan, C. (2019) "A prison within a prison"? Examining the enfolding spatialities of care and control in the Barlinnie Special Unit. *Area*, 51, 200–207.

McGeachan, C., and Philo, C. (2023). 'Hanging around in their brokenness': On mental ill-health geography, asylums and camps, artworks and salvage. *Annals of the American Association of Geographers*, 113, 1224–1242.

McKittrick, K. (2006) *Demonic Grounds: Black Women and the Cartographies of Struggle*, Minneapolis: University of Minnesota Press.

McKittrick, K. (2011) On plantations, prisons and a Black sense of place. *Social and Cultural Geography*, 12, 947–963.

McKittrick, K. (2013) 'Plantation futures', Small Axe: A Caribbean. *Journal of Criticism*, 17, 1–15.

McKittrick, K. (ed.) (2015). *Sylvia Wynter: on being human as praxis*. Durham: Duke University Press

Parr, H. (2008) *Mental Health and Social Space: Towards Inclusionary Geographies?* Oxford: Blackwell.

Philo, C. (2000). Post-asylum geographies: An introduction. *Health & Place*, 6, 135–136.

Philo, C. (2004) *The Geographical History of Institutional Provision for the Insane from Medieval Times to the 1860s in England and Wales: The Space Reserved for Insanity*. Lewiston, NY: Edwin Mellen.

Philo, C., and Schliehe, A. (2024) Abolishing carceral geography? In: Stuit, H., Turner, J., and Weegels, J. (Eds.), *Carceral Worlds Legacies, Textures and Futures*. London: Bloomsbury Academic, 221–240.

Pinfold, V. (2000) 'Building up safe havens. All around the world': Users' experiences of living in the community with mental health problems. *Health & Place*, 6, 201–212.

Rothman, D.J. (1980) *Conscience and convenience: the asylum and its alternatives in progressive America*. Boston: Little, Brown.

Scull, A.T. (1977) *Decarceration: Community Treatment and the Deviant*. Englewood Cliffs: Prentice-Hall.

Segrest, M. (2020). *Administrations of Lunacy: Racism and the Haunting of American Psychiatry at the Milledgeville Asylum*. New York: The New Press.

Smith, C.J. (1976) Distance and the location of community mental health facilities: A divergent viewpoint. *Economic Geography*, 52, 181–191.

Smith, C.J. (1977) Geography and Mental Health. Washington, DC: *Association of American Geographers*, Resource Paper Series.

Smith, C.J. (1987) Progress report: Mental health and the fiscal crisis: The prospects for a socially conscious urban geography. *Urban Geography*, 8, 55–64.
Wilson, K. (2021) *Mental Health Law: Abolish or Reform?* Oxford: Oxford Academic.
Wolpert, J. and Wolpert, E. (1974). From asylum to ghetto. *Antipode*, 6, 63–76.
Wolpert, J. (1976) Opening closed spaces. *Annals of the Association of American Geographers*, 66, 1–13.

Index

Theoretical Physics to Face the Challenge of LHC

École de Physique des Houches

Session XCVII, 1–26 August 2011

Theoretical Physics to Face the Challenge of LHC

Edited by

Laurent Baulieu, Karim Benakli, Michael R. Douglas,
Bruno Mansoulié, Eliezer Rabinovici,
and Leticia F. Cugliandolo

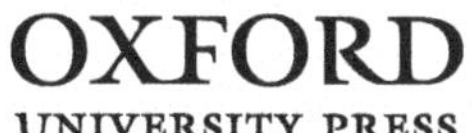

OXFORD

UNIVERSITY PRESS

OXFORD
UNIVERSITY PRESS

Great Clarendon Street, Oxford, OX2 6DP,
United Kingdom

Oxford University Press is a department of the University of Oxford.
It furthers the University's objective of excellence in research, scholarship,
and education by publishing worldwide. Oxford is a registered trade mark of
Oxford University Press in the UK and in certain other countries

© Oxford University Press 2015

The moral rights of the authors have been asserted

First Edition published in 2015

Published in the United States of America by Oxford University Press
198 Madison Avenue, New York, NY 10016, United States of America

British Library Cataloguing in Publication Data
Data available

Library of Congress Control Number: 2014953047

ISBN 978-0-19-872796-5

École de Physique des Houches

Service inter-universitaire commun
à l'Université Joseph Fourier de Grenoble
et à l'Institut National Polytechnique de Grenoble

Subventionné par l'Université Joseph Fourier de Grenoble,
le Centre National de la Recherche Scientifique,
le Commissariat à l'Énergie Atomique

Directeur:

Leticia F. Cugliandolo, Sorbonne Universités, Université Pierre et Marie Curie, Laboratoire de Physique Théorique et Hautes Energies, CNRS UMR 7589, Paris, France

Directeurs scientifiques de la session XCVII:

Laurent Baulieu, Sorbonne Universités, Université Pierre et Marie Curie, Laboratoire de Physique Théorique et Hautes Energies, CNRS UMR 7589, Paris, France

Karim Benakli, Sorbonne Universités, Université Pierre et Marie Curie, Laboratoire de Physique Théorique et Hautes Energies, CNRS UMR 7589, Paris, France

Michael R. Douglas, Department of Physics and Astronomy, Rutgers University, USA

Bruno Mansoulié, Institut de Recherches sur les lois Fondamentales de l'Univers, CEA Saclay, France

Eliezer Rabinovici, Racah Institute of Physics, Hebrew University, Jerusalem, Israel

Leticia F. Cugliandolo, Sorbonne Universités, Université Pierre et Marie Curie, Laboratoire de Physique Théorique et Hautes Energies, CNRS UMR 7589, Paris, France

Previous sessions

XXXIV	1980	Laser plasma interaction
XXXV	1980	Physics of defects
XXXVI	1981	Chaotic behavior of deterministic systems
XXXVII	1981	Gauge theories in high energy physics
XXXVIII	1982	New trends in atomic physics
XXXIX	1982	Recent advances in field theory and statistical mechanics
XL	1983	Relativity, groups and topology
XLI	1983	Birth and infancy of stars
XLII	1984	Cellular and molecular aspects of developmental biology
XLIII	1984	Critical phenomena, random systems, gauge theories
XLIV	1985	Architecture of fundamental interactions at short distances
XLV	1985	Signal processing
XLVI	1986	Chance and matter
XLVII	1986	Astrophysical fluid dynamics
XLVIII	1988	Liquids at interfaces
XLIX	1988	Fields, strings and critical phenomena
L	1988	Oceanographic and geophysical tomography
LI	1989	Liquids, freezing and glass transition
LII	1989	Chaos and quantum physics
LIII	1990	Fundamental systems in quantum optics
LIV	1990	Supernovae
LV	1991	Particles in the nineties
LVI	1991	Strongly interacting fermions and high Tc superconductivity
LVII	1992	Gravitation and quantizations
LVIII	1992	Progress in picture processing
LIX	1993	Computational fluid dynamics
LX	1993	Cosmology and large scale structure
LXI	1994	Mesoscopic quantum physics
LXII	1994	Fluctuating geometries in statistical mechanics and quantum field theory
LXIII	1995	Quantum fluctuations
LXIV	1995	Quantum symmetries
LXV	1996	From cell to brain
LXVI	1996	Trends in nuclear physics, 100 years later
LXVII	1997	Modeling the earths climate and its variability
LXVIII	1997	Probing the Standard Model of particle interactions
LXIX	1998	Topological aspects of low dimensional systems
LXX	1998	Infrared space astronomy, today and tomorrow
LXXI	1999	The primordial universe
LXXII	1999	Coherent atomic matter waves
LXXIII	2000	Atomic clusters and nanoparticles
LXXIV	2000	New trends in turbulence
LXXV	2001	Physics of bio-molecules and cells
LXXVI	2001	Unity from duality: Gravity, gauge theory and strings

LXXVII	2002	Slow relaxations and nonequilibrium dynamics in condensed matter
LXXVIII	2002	Accretion discs, jets and high energy phenomena in astrophysics
LXXIX	2003	Quantum entanglement and information processing
LXXX	2003	Methods and models in neurophysics
LXXXI	2004	Nanophysics: Coherence and transport
LXXXII	2004	Multiple aspects of DNA and RNA
LXXXIII	2005	Mathematical statistical physics
LXXXIV	2005	Particle physics beyond the Standard Model
LXXXV	2006	Complex systems
LXXXVI	2006	Particle physics and cosmology: the fabric of spacetime
LXXXVII	2007	String theory and the real world: from particle physics to astrophysics
LXXXVIII	2007	Dynamos
LXXXIX	2008	Exact methods in low-dimensional statistical physics and quantum computing
XC	2008	Long-range interacting systems
XCI	2009	Ultracold gases and quantum information
XCII	2009	New trends in the physics and mechanics of biological systems
XCIII	2009	Modern perspectives in lattice QCD: quantum field theory and high performance computing
XCIV	2010	Many-body physics with ultra-cold gases
XCV	2010	Quantum theory from small to large scales
XCVI	2011	Quantum machines: measurement control of engineered quantum systems
XCVII	2011	Theoretical physics to face the challenge of LHC
Special Issue	2012	Advanced data assimilation for geosciences

Publishers

- Session VIII: Dunod, Wiley, Methuen
- Sessions IX and X: Herman, Wiley
- Session XI: Gordon and Breach, Presses Universitaires
- Sessions XII–XXV: Gordon and Breach
- Sessions XXVI–LXVIII: North Holland
- Session LXIX–LXXVIII: EDP Sciences, Springer
- Session LXXIX–LXXXVIII: Elsevier
- Session LXXXIX– : Oxford University Press

Preface

Every Les Houches Summer School has its own distinct character. The objective of the August 2011 session "Theoretical physics to face the challenge of LHC" was to describe, to an audience of advanced graduate students and postdoctoral fellows, the areas in high-energy physics in which profound new experimental results are hopefully on the verge of being discovered at LHC at CERN. This was to be done with the expectation that contact with new fundamental theories on the nature of fundamental forces and the structure of spacetime will be made. The students benefited from lectures by, and interacted with, many of the leaders in the field.

The school was held in a summer of tense anticipation. Exciting new results from high-energy colliders were in the air, whether about the long anticipated discovery of the Higgs particle or about a "divine" surprise, evidence for the existence of supersymmetry in nature.

For some years, the community of theorists had split into several components: those doing phenomenology, those dealing with highly theoretical problems, and some trying to explore if it was possible to bridge the two. In this school, we celebrated the reunification of these groups—at least for a few years.

The talks given by experimentalists accurately pointed out how intensively and how precisely the newborn collider has verified all theoretical predictions that were at the frontline of the revolutionary experimental discoveries of the 1970s, 1980s, and 1990s. They detailed many of the ingenious and pioneering techniques developed at CERN for the detection and data analysis of several billions of proton–proton collisions. During the entire period of the school, the students received daily news about the progress of these searches. A trip to the CERN facilities was organized, with visits to the LHC and ATLAS detector control rooms, as well as the CMS detector coordination room and the Cosmic Antimatter Detector control room coordinated with the space laboratory.

The talks given by theoreticians were about many of the attempts to go beyond the Standard Model that yield beautiful new physical insights yet to be observed experimentally.

The students were very active during the talks and had interesting interactions. The organizers and speakers encouraged them to pose unrestricted questions during and after the lectures. In addition, we had a "Wisdom Tree" session during which Michael Douglas, Juan Maldacena, and Bruno Mansoulié shared their thoughts on any subject the students desired. We also held the traditional "Gong Show" in which every participant could speak about his or her work for three minutes. The cocktail of theorists and experimentalists proved to be most interesting.

More precisely, the topics covered in the school were as follows.

In the first morning, Jean Iliopoulos and Luis Alvarez-Gaumé gave an introduction to the school. Jean Iliopoulos recalled the historical path taking us from the Standard

Model to considering possible extensions, and Luis Alvarez-Gaumé summarized the achievements of string theory and the present open problems.

Lyndon Evans reviewed the physics challenges faced in the design of the LHC in order to achieve the desired rate of highest-energy collisions. He shared with the audience the difficult road leading from envisaging how to built a Large Hadron Collider and actually doing it.

Massimo Giovanozzi gave an account of how the accelerator had been commissioned, how the setback caused by a hardware failure was overcome, how the LHC functioned in the Summer of 2011, and what were the plans for its future upgrade.

Dan Green took us from the accelerator to the giant detectors surrounding it. He described the requirements for the detectors and the different choices made in their design.

Bruno Mansoulié guided the audience along the way from the registration of the events in the detectors to their analysis. He explained the difficulties involved in correct identification of the signals.

Yves Sirois and Louis Fayard discussed the available LHC data and their implications for the Higgs boson searches at CMS and ATLAS, respectively, while Karl Jakobs summarized the constraints derived on new physics.

Michelangelo Mangano explained the methods needed to compute the expected backgrounds without whose detailed knowledge one could not extract the new discoveries.

Nima Arkani-Hamed and David Kosower explained new techniques recently developed to perform in a more efficient way the calculations of amplitudes, in particular for the underlying QCD processes.

Gia Dvali described how unitarity is realized in effective field theories in particle physics and its implication for graviton scattering.

Juan Maldacena reviewed our theoretical knowledge on quantum gravity. He described how the amazing correspondence between field theories on the boundary and gravity theories in a bulk with a negative cosmological constant arises. This comes under the umbrella of AdS/CFT. He outlined the state of the art in the field, which is a very concrete realization of the concept of holography.

Jan de Boer went into the details of basic examples of AdS/CFT duality.

Yaron Oz explained how to obtain hydrodynamics equations from the study of black hole solutions and described the emergence of an amazing correspondence between features of gravity and fluids.

Gian Giudice discussed the most popular supersymmetric extension of the Standard Model.

Gerard 't Hooft unveiled his ideas for addressing the black hole physics information paradox. He described several consequences of the spontaneous breaking of a local conformal invariance and how this helps to obtain concrete complementarity maps between different sets of observables in the presence of a black hole.

Zohar Komargodski described the possible definition of a c-function and his proof of the associated a-theorem.

Alex Pomarol described the implementation of electroweak symmetry-breaking mechanisms in different extensions of the Standard Model.

Karim Benakli described in detail the basics of supersymmetry breaking.

Luis Ibáñez reviewed the implementation of the phenomenologically viable super-symmetric extensions of the Standard Model in string theory.

Michael Douglas discussed the problems of classifying the possible models and estimating their frequency in the landscape of string vacua.

Laurent Baulieu explained the use of a twisted supersymmetry algebra in supergravity and its consequences.

Eliezer Rabinovici described his work with José Luis Barbón on various types of big crunches using the AdS/CFT correspondence, and the surprising result that some big crunches can be equivalently described by a nontrivial infrared theory living on a singularity-free de Sitter space.

Gabriele Veneziano summarized some 25 years of work on the transplanckian-energy collisions of particles, strings, and branes. He discussed different regimes in these processes, recovering physical expectations (e.g., gravitational deflection and tidal excitation) at large distance and exposing new phenomena when the string length exceeds the gravitational radius of the collision's energy. He also presented recent attempts to approach the short-distance regime where black hole formation is expected to occur.

Daniel Zwanziger explained formal aspect of the Gribov problem in QCD.

Altogether, it is the general feeling of the organizers, lecturers, and students that the School was a success, striking the right balance between the exciting physics that is currently coming out of LHC, while covering important recent developments in the theory of elementary particles.

More than one of the speakers reminisced on their days as students and postdocs in Les Houches, and were grateful for this chance to return at the moment where LHC is starting to unveil a yet-unknown domain of energy. We were happy to have the chance to maintain such a longstanding tradition, and are confident that our students will make important contributions in the coming era. We hope some of them will have the chance to return as lecturers in their turn.

As organizers, we express our gratitude to the local staff of the Les Houches School for their help, as well as to the funding agencies (CEA, CERN, CNRS, European Science Foundation, IN2P3, and the Les Houches School of Physics) that made possible the organization of this event.

Laurent Baulieu
Karim Benakli
Michael R. Douglas
Bruno Mansoulié
Eliezer Rabinovici
Leticia F. Cugliandolo

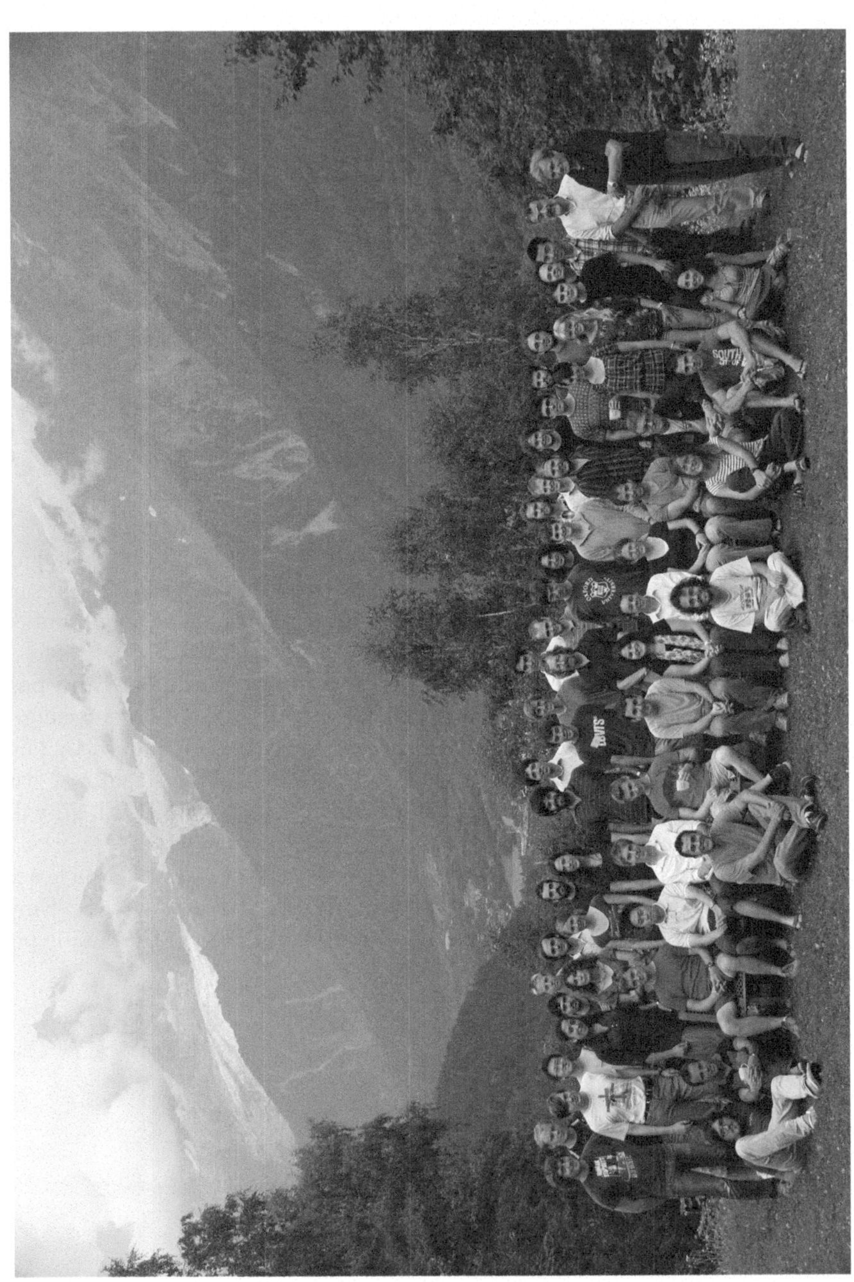

Contents

List of participants

ORGANIZERS

BAULIEU LAURENT
Sorbonne Universités, Université Pierre et Marie Curie, Laboratoire de Physique
Théorique et Hautes Energies, CNRS UMR 7589, Paris, France

BENAKLI KARIM
Sorbonne Universités, Université Pierre et Marie Curie, Laboratoire de Physique
Théorique et Hautes Energies, CNRS UMR 7589, Paris, France

DOUGLAS MICHAEL R.
Department of Physics and Astronomy, Rutgers University, New Jersey, USA

MANSOULIÉ BRUNO
Institut de Recherches sur les Lois Fondamentales de l'Univers, CEA Saclay, France

RABINOVICI ELIEZER
Racah Institute of Physics, Hebrew University, Jerusalem, Israel

CUGLIANDOLO LETICIA F.
Sorbonne Universités, Université Pierre et Marie Curie, Laboratoire de Physique
Théorique et Hautes Energies, CNRS UMR 7589, Paris, France

LECTURERS

ÁLVAREZ-GAUMÉ LUIS
Theory Division, CERN, Geneva Switzerland

ARKANI-HAMED NIMA
Institute for Advanced Studies, Princeton University, New Jersey, USA

BAULIEU LAURENT
Sorbonne Universités, Université Pierre et Marie Curie, Laboratoire de Physique
Théorique et Hautes Energies, CNRS UMR 7589, Paris, France

BENAKLI KARIM
Sorbonne Universités, Université Pierre et Marie Curie, Laboratoire de Physique
Théorique et Hautes Energies, CNRS UMR 7589, Paris, France

DE BOER JAN
Physics Department, University of Amsterdam, The Netherlands

DOUGLAS MICHAEL R.
Department of Physics and Astronomy, Rutgers University, New Jersey, USA

DVALI GIA
Department of Physics, New York University, USA

EVANS LYNDON
Imperial College, London, UK and CERN, Geneva, Switzerland

FAYARD LOUIS
Laboratoire de l'Accélérateur Linéaire, Université de Paris-Sud Orsay, France

GIOVANOZZI MASSIMO
Beams Department, CERN, Geneva, Switzerland

GIUDICE GIAN
Theory Division, CERN, Geneva, Switzerland

GREEN DAN
Fermilab, USA

IBAÑEZ LUIS
Departamento de Física Teórica, and Instituto de Física Teórica, Universidad Autónoma de Madrid, Spain

ILIOPOULOS JEAN
Laboratoire de Physique Théorique, Ecole Normale Supérieure, Paris, France

JAKOBS KARL
Albert-Ludwigs-Universität Freiburg, Germany

KOMARGODSKI ZOHAR
Department of Particle Physics and Astrophysics, Weizmann Institute of Science, Rehovot, Israel

KOSOWER DAVID
Service de Physique Théorique, CEA Saclay, France

MALDACENA JUAN
Institute for Advanced Studies, Princeton University, New Jersey, USA

MANGANO MICHELANGELO
Theory Division, CERN, Geneva, Switzerland

MANSOULIÉ BRUNO
Institut de Recherches sur les Lois Fondamentales de l'Univers, CEA Saclay, France

OZ YARON
Physics Department, Tel Aviv University, Israel

POMAROL ALEX
Departament de Física, Universitat Autònoma de Barcelona, Spain

RABINOVICI ELIEZER
Racah Institute of Physics, Hebrew University, Jerusalem, Israel

SIROIS YVES
École Polytechnique, Paris, France

'T HOOFT GERARD
Physics Department, Utrecht University, The Netherlands

VENEZIANO GABRIELE
Collège de France, Paris, France and Theory Division, CERN, Geneva, Switzerland
ZWANZIGER DANIEL
Physics Department, New York University, USA

PARTICIPANTS

ALBA VASYL
Institute for Theoretical and Experimental Physics, Russian Federation
ALONSO RODRIGO
Departamento de Física Teórica, Univerisdad Autónoma de Madrid, Spain
AL-SAYEGH AMARA
Department of Physics, American University of Beirut, Lebanon
ASSEL BENJAMIN
Laboratoire de Physique Théorique, École Normale Supérieure, Paris, France
AUZZI ROBERTO
High Energy Physics Group, The Hebrew University, Jerusalem, Israel
BARYAKHTAR MASHA
High Energy Theory Group, Stanford University, California, USA
BENTOV YONI
Department of Physics, University of California at Santa Barbara, USA
BERASALUCE-GONZÁLEZ MIKEL
Insituto de Física Teórica, Universidad Autónoma de Madrid, Spain
BESSE ADRIEN
Laboratoire de Physique Théorique, Université de Paris-Sud Orsay, France
BURDA PHILIPP
Institute for Theoretical and Experimental Physics, Russian Federation
CHAPMAN SHIRA
Department of Physics and Astronomy, Tel Aviv University, Israel
CONSTANTINOU YIANNIS
Department of Physics, University of Crete, Greece
DE ADELHART TOOROP REINIER
The National Institute for Nuclear Physics and High Energy Physics, Amsterdam, The Netherlands
FRELLESVIG HJALTE AXEL
Niels Bohr Institute, Copenhagen, Denmark
GIANNUZZI FLORIANA
Dipartimento di Fisica, Università di Bari and INFN, Italy
GUDNASON SVEN BJARKE
High Energy Physics Group, The Hebrew University, Jerusalem, Israel

HEISENBERG LAVINIA
Département de Physique Théorique, Université de Genève, Switzerland

HOWE KIEL
High Energy Theory Group, Stanford University, California, USA

IATRAKIS IOANNIS
Department of Physics, University of Crete, Greece

KHMELNITSKIY ANDREY
Faculty of Physics, Lüdwig Maximilians Universtät, Munich, Germany

KOL URI
Department of Physics and Astronomy, Tel Aviv University, Israel

KUDRNA MATEJ
Academy of Sciences, Czech Republic

LOU HOU KEONG
Department of Physics, Princeton University, New Jersey, USA

MOELLER JAN
Fakultät für Physik, Universität Bielefeld, Germany

NAJJARI SAEREH
Institute of Theoretical Physics, Warsaw University, Poland

NEIMAN YAAKOV
School of Physics and Astronomy, Tel Aviv University, Israel

NOGUEIRA FERNANDO
Department of Physics, University of British Columbia, Canada

ORGOGOZO AXEL
Laboratoire de Physique Théorique et Hautes Enegies, Université Pierre et Marie Curie, Paris, France

PLENCNER DANIEL
Faculty of Physics, Lüdwig Maximilians Universtät, Munich, Germany

POZZOLI VALENTINA
Ecole Polytechnique, Paris, France

REDIGOLO DIEGO
Faculté des Sciences, Université Libre de Bruxelles, Belgium

RETINSKAYA EKATERINA
Skobeltsyn Institute of Nuclear Physics, Moscow State University, Russian Federation

REYS VALENTIN
Laboratoire de Physique Théorique et Hautes Energies, Université Pierre et Marie Curie, Paris, France

ROSEN CHRISTOPHER
Department of Physics, University of Colorado at Boulder, USA

SAFDI BENJAMIN
Physics Department, Princeton University, New Jersey, USA

SALAS HERNÁNDEZ CLARA
Instituto de Física Teórica, Universidad Autńoma de Madrid/CSIC, Spain

SALVIONI ENNIO
CERN–Università di Padova, Italy

SCHMELL CHRISTOPH
Institut für Physik, Johannes Guttenberg Universität-Mainz, Germany

SJORS STEFAN
Department of Physics, Stockholm University, Sweden

STAMOU EMMANUEL
Department of Physics, Technische Universität München, Germany

STEFANIAK TIM
Bethe Center for Theoretical Physics, Universität Bonn, Germany

STORACE STEFANO
Physics Department, New York University, USA

TAN HAI SIONG
Physics Department, University of California at Berkeley, USA

TARONNA MASSIMO
Scuola Normale Superiore, Italy

THAMM ANDREA
CERN, Geneva, Switzerland

TOBIOKA KOHSAKU
Institute for the Physics and Mathematics of the Universe, University of Tokyo, Japan

UBALDI LORENZO
Physikalisches Institut, Universität Bonn, Germany

WALTERS WILLIAM
Mathematical Sciences, University of Liverpool, UK

WITASZCZYK PRZEMEK
Jagiellonian University, Cracow, Poland

ZARO MARCO
Centre for Cosmology, Particle Physics and Phenomenology, Université Catholique de
Louvain, Belgium

1
The Large Hadron Collider

Lyndon EVANS

Imperial College London, UK
and CERN Geneva, Switzerland

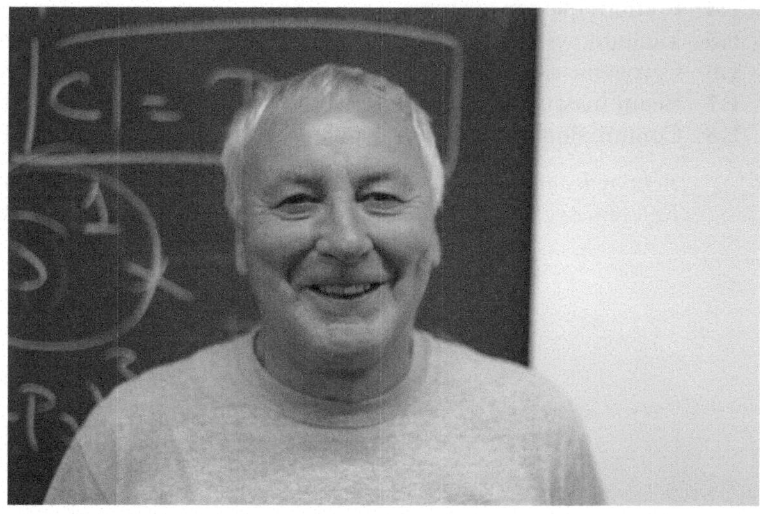

Theoretical Physics to Face the Challenge of LHC. Edited by L. Baulieu, K. Benakli, M. R. Douglas,
B. Mansoulié, E. Rabinovici, and L. F. Cugliandolo. © Oxford University Press 2015.
Published in 2015 by Oxford University Press.

Chapter Contents

The Large Hadron Collider (LHC) is the most complex scientific instrument ever built for particle physics research. It will for the first time give access to the TeV energy scale. To achieve this, a number of technological innovations have been necessary. The two counter-rotating proton beams are guided and focused by superconducting magnets with a novel two-in-one structure to save cost and allow the machine to be installed in an existing tunnel. The very high field of more than 8 T in the dipoles can only be achieved by cooling them below the transition temperature of liquid helium to the superfluid state. More than 80 tons of superfluid helium is needed to cool the whole machine. In its first year of operation, it has been shown to behave in a very reliable and predictable way. Single-bunch currents 30% above the design value have already been achieved, and the luminosity has increased by five orders of magnitude in the first 200 days of operation.

In this chapter, a brief description of the design principles of the major systems is given and some of the results of commissioning and first operation discussed.

1.1　Introduction

The LIIC is a two-ring superconducting hadron accelerator and collider installed in the existing 26.7 km tunnel that was constructed between 1984 and 1989 for the CERN Large Electron Positron (LEP) collider. The LEP tunnel has eight straight sections and eight arcs and lies between 45 and 170 m below the surface on a plane inclined at 1.4%, sloping towards Lake Léman. Approximately 90% of its length is in molasse rock, which has excellent characteristics for this application, and 10% is in limestone under the Jura mountain. There are two transfer tunnels, each approximately 2.5 km in length, linking the LHC to the CERN accelerator complex that acts as injector. Full use has been made of the existing civil engineering structures, but modifications and additions have also been needed. Broadly speaking, the underground and surface structures at Points 1 and 5 for ATLAS and CMS, respectively, are new, while those for ALICE and LHCb, at Points 2 and 8, respectively, were originally built for LEP.

The approval of the LHC project was given by the CERN Council in December 1994. At that time, the plan was to build a machine in two stages, starting with a centre-of-mass energy of 10 TeV, to be upgraded later to 14 TeV. However, during 1995–96, intense negotiations secured substantial contributions to the project from nonmember states, and in December 1996, the CERN Council approved construction of the 14 TeV machine in a single stage.

The LHC design depends on some basic principles linked with the latest technology. Since it is a particle–particle collider, there are two rings with counter-rotating beams, unlike particle–antiparticle colliders, which can have both beams sharing the same ring. The tunnel in the arcs has a finished internal diameter of 3.7 m, which makes it extremely difficult to install two completely separate proton rings. This hard limit on space led to the adoption of the twin-bore magnet design that was proposed by John Blewett at the Brookhaven Laboratory in 1971. At that time, it was known as the "two-in-one" superconducting magnet design [1] and was put forward as a cost-saving measure [2, 3], but in the case of the LHC, the overriding reason for adopting this solution was the lack of space in the tunnel.

In the later part of the twentieth century, it became clear that higher energies could only be reached through better technologies, principally through superconductivity. The first use of superconducting magnets in an operational collider was in the ISR, but always at 4–4.5 K [4]. However, research was moving towards operation at 2 K and lower, to take advantage of the increased temperature margins and the enhanced heat transfer at the solid–liquid interface and in the bulk liquid [5]. The French Tokamak Tore II Supra demonstrated this new technology [6, 7], which was then proposed for the LHC [8] and brought from the preliminary study to the final concept design and validation in six years [9].

In a chapter of this length, it is impossible to describe in detail all the different systems needed to operate the LHC. Instead, we concentrate on the principal new technologies developed for the machine. A detailed description of the machine as built can be found in the LHC Design Report [10], which is in three volumes. This chapter ends with a brief description of commissioning and the first year of operation.

1.2 Main machine layout and performance

1.2.1 Performance goals

The aim of the LHC is to reveal the physics beyond the Standard Model with centre-of-mass collision energies of up to 14 TeV. The number of events per second generated in the LHC collisions is given by

$$N_{\text{event}} = L\sigma_{\text{event}}, \tag{1.1}$$

where σ_{event} is the cross section for the event under study and L the machine luminosity. The machine luminosity depends only on the beam parameters and can be written for a Gaussian beam distribution as

$$L = \frac{N_b^2 n_b f_{\text{rev}} \gamma_{\text{r}}}{4\pi\varepsilon_n\beta^*} F, \tag{1.2}$$

where N_b is the number of particles per bunch, n_b the number of bunches per beam, f_{rev} the revolution frequency, γ_r the relativistic gamma factor, ε_n the normalized transverse beam emittance, β^* the beta function at the collision point, and F the geometric luminosity reduction factor due to the crossing angle at the interaction point (IP). F is given by

$$F = \left[1 + \left(\frac{\theta_c\sigma_z}{2\sigma^*}\right)^2\right]^{-1/2}, \tag{1.3}$$

where θ_c is the full crossing angle at the IP, σ_z the root mean square (RMS) bunch length, and σ^* the transverse RMS beam size at the IP. The expression (1.3) assumes round beams, with $\sigma_z << \beta$, and equal beam parameters for both beams. The exploration of rare events in the LHC collisions therefore requires both high beam energies and high beam intensities.

The LHC has two high-luminosity experiments, ATLAS [11] and CMS [12], both aiming at a peak luminosity of $L = 10^{34}\,\mathrm{cm^{-2}\,s^{-1}}$ for proton operation. There are also two low-luminosity experiments: LHCB [13] for B physics, aiming at a peak luminosity of $L = 10^{32}\,\mathrm{cm^{-2}\,s^{-1}}$, and TOTEM [14] for the detection of protons from elastic scattering at small angles, aiming at a peak luminosity of $L = 2 \times 10^{29}\,\mathrm{cm^{-2}\,s^{-1}}$ with 156 bunches. In addition to the proton beams, the LHC will also be operated with ion beams. The LHC has one dedicated ion experiment, ALICE [15], aiming at a peak luminosity of $L = 10^{27}\,\mathrm{cm^{-2}\,s^{-1}}$ for nominal lead–lead ion operation.

The high beam intensity required for a luminosity of $L = 10^{34}\,\mathrm{cm^{-2}\,s^{-1}}$ excludes the use of antiproton beams, and hence excludes the particle–antiparticle collider configuration of a common vacuum and magnet system for both circulating beams, as used for example in the Tevatron. To collide two counter-rotating proton beams requires opposite magnetic dipole fields in both rings. The LHC is therefore designed as a proton–proton collider with separate magnet fields and vacuum chambers in the main arcs and with common sections only at the insertion regions where the experimental detectors are located. The two beams share an approximately 130-m-long common beam pipe along the interaction regions (IRs).

As already mentioned, there is not enough room for two separate rings of magnets in the LEP/LHC tunnel, and so the LHC uses twin-bore magnets consisting of two sets of coils and beam channels within the same mechanical structure and cryostat. The peak beam energy depends on the integrated dipole field around the storage ring, which implies a peak dipole field of 8.33 T for the 7 TeV energy. This can only be achieved with "affordable" niobium–titanium (NbTi) superconductor by lowering the temperature to 1.9 K, below the phase transition of helium from a normal to a superfluid state.

1.2.2 Performance limitations

Beam–beam limit

When the beams collide, a proton in one beam is affected by the electromagnetic field of the other beam. The maximum particle density per bunch is limited by the nonlinearity of this beam–beam interaction, the strength of which is measured by the linear tune shift, given by

$$\xi = \frac{N_b\, r_p}{4\pi \varepsilon_n}, \tag{1.4}$$

in which $r_p = e^2/(4\pi \varepsilon_0 m_p c^2)$ is the classical proton radius. Experience with existing hadron colliders indicates that the total linear tune shift summed over all IPs should not exceed 0.015. With three proton experiments requiring head-on collisions, this implies that the linear beam–beam tune shift for each IP should satisfy $\xi < 0.005$.

Maximum dipole field and magnet quench limits

The maximum beam energy that can be reached in the LHC is limited by the peak dipole field in the storage ring. The nominal field is 8.33 T, corresponding to an energy of 7 TeV. Operating at this very high field level requires that the magnets be cooled in a bath of superfluid helium at 1.9 K.

Energy stored in the circulating beams and in the magnetic fields

A total beam current of 0.584 A corresponds to a stored energy of approximately 362 MJ. In addition to the energy stored in the circulating beams, the LHC magnet system has a stored electromagnetic energy of approximately 600 MJ, yielding a total stored energy of more than 1 GJ. This stored energy must be absorbed safely at the end of each run or in the case of a malfunction or an emergency. The beam dumping system and the magnet system therefore provide additional limits for the maximum attainable beam energies and intensities.

Heat load

Although synchrotron radiation in hadron storage rings is small compared with that generated in electron rings, it can still impose practical limits on the maximum attainable beam intensities if the radiation has to be absorbed by the cryogenic system. In addition to the synchrotron-radiation heat load, the LHC cryogenic system must absorb the heat deposition from luminosity-induced losses, impedance-induced losses (resistive wall effect), and electron-cloud bombardment.

Field quality and dynamic aperture

Field quality errors compromise the particle stability in the storage ring, and hence loss-free operation requires a high field quality. A characterizing feature of superconducting magnets is the decay of persistent currents and their "snap back" at the beginning of the ramp. Achieving small beam losses therefore requires tight control of the magnetic field errors during magnet production and during machine operation. Assuming fixed limits for the beam losses (set by the quench levels of the superconducting magnets), the accuracy of the field quality correction during operation and its limitation on machine performance can be estimated.

Collective beam instabilities

The interaction of the charged particles in each beam with each other via electromagnetic fields and the conducting boundaries of the vacuum system can result in collective beam instabilities. Generally speaking, the collective effects are a function of the vacuum system geometry and its surface properties. They are usually proportional to the beam currents and can therefore limit the maximum attainable beam intensities.

1.2.3   Lattice layout

The basic layout of the LHC follows the LEP tunnel geometry (see Fig. 1.1). The LHC has eight arcs and eight straight sections. Each straight section is approximately 528 m long and can serve as an experimental or utility insertion. The two high-luminosity

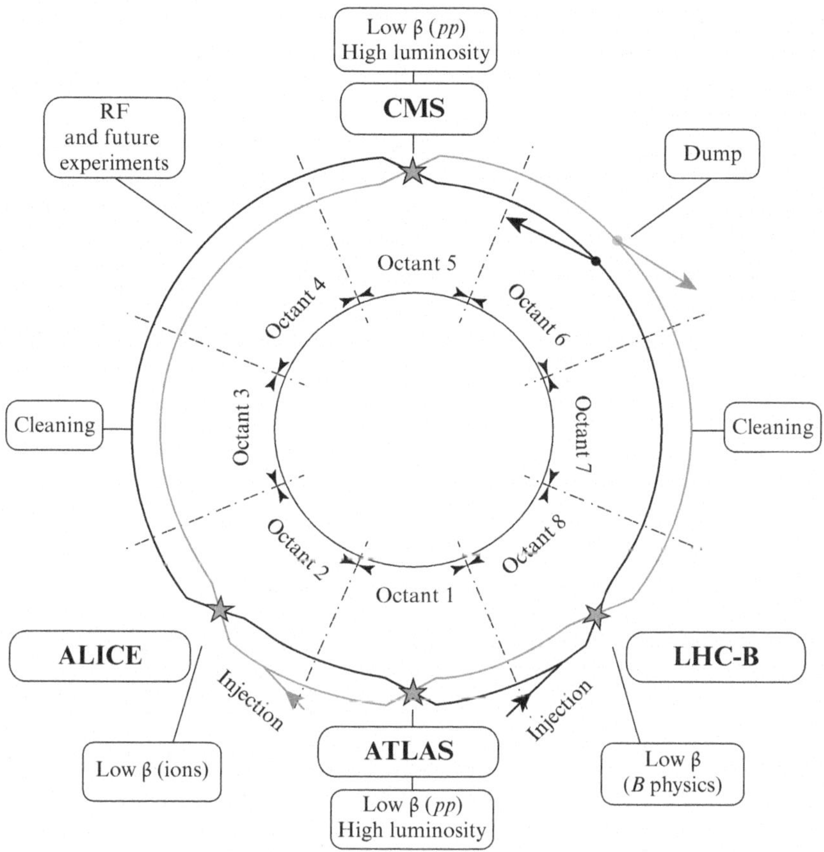

Fig. 1.1 Schematic layout of the LHC (Beam 1 clockwise; Beam 2 anticlockwise).

experimental insertions are located at diametrically opposite straight sections: the AT-LAS experiment is located at Point 1 and the CMS experiment at Point 5. Two more experimental insertions are located at Points 2 and 8, which also include the injection systems for Beams 1 and 2, respectively. The injection kick occurs in the vertical plane, with the two beams arriving at the LHC from below the LHC reference plane. The beams cross from one magnet bore to the other at four locations. The remaining four straight sections do not have beam crossings. Insertions at Points 3 and 7 each contain two collimation systems. The insertion at Point 4 contains two radiofrequency (RF) accelerating systems: one independent system for each LHC beam. The straight section at Point 6 contains the beam dump insertion, where the two beams can be safely extracted from the machine if needed. Each beam features an independent abort system.

The arcs of the LHC lattice are made of 23 regular arc cells. The arc cells are 106.9 m long and are made out of two 53.45-m-long half cells, each of which contains one 5.355-m-long cold mass (6.63-m-long cryostat), a short straight section (SSS) assembly, and three 14.3-m-long dipole magnets. The LHC arc cell has been optimized for a maximum integrated dipole field along the arc with a minimum number of magnet interconnections and with the smallest possible beam envelopes.

The two apertures of Ring 1 and Ring 2 are separated by 194 mm. The two coils in the dipole magnets are powered in series, and all dipole magnets of one arc form one electrical circuit. The quadrupoles of each arc form two electrical circuits: all focusing quadrupoles in Beams 1 and 2 are powered in series, and all defocusing quadrupoles in Beams 1 and 2 are powered in series. The optics of Beam 1 and Beam 2 in the arc cells are therefore strictly coupled via the powering of the main magnetic elements.

A dispersion suppressor (DS) is located at the transition between an LHC arc and a straight section, yielding a total of 16 DS sections. The aim of the DS is threefold:

- Adapt the LHC reference orbit to the geometry of the LEP tunnel.
- Cancel the horizontal dispersion arising in the arc and generated by the separation/recombination dipole magnets and the crossing angle bumps.
- Facilitate matching the insertion optics to the periodic optics of the arc.

1.2.4 High-luminosity insertions (IR1 and IR5)

Interaction regions 1 and 5 house the high-luminosity experiments of the LHC and are identical in terms of hardware and optics, except that the crossing angle is in the vertical plane at Point 1 and in the horizontal plane at Point 5. The small β-function values at the IPs are generated between quadrupole triplets that leave ± 23 m free space about the IP. In this region, the two rings share the same vacuum chamber, the same low-β triplet magnets, and the D1 separation dipole magnets. The remaining matching section and the DS consist of twin-bore magnets with separate beam pipes for each ring. From the IP up to the DS insertion, the layout comprises the following:

- A 31-m-long superconducting low-β triplet assembly, operated at a temperature of 1.9 K and providing a nominal gradient of 205 T/m.
- A pair of separation/recombination dipoles separated by approximately 88 m.
- The D1 dipole located next to the triplet magnets, which has a single bore and consists of six 3.4-m-long conventional warm magnet modules yielding a nominal field of 1.38 T.
- The following D2 dipole, which is a 9.45-m-long twin-bore superconducting dipole magnet, operating at a cryogenic temperature of 4.5 K with a nominal field of 3.8 T. The bore separation in the D2 magnet is 188 mm and is thus slightly smaller than the arc bore separation.
- Four matching quadrupole magnets. The first quadrupole following the separation dipole magnets, Q4, is a wide-aperture magnet operating at a cryogenic temperature of 4.5 K and yielding a nominal gradient of 160 T/m. The remaining three quadrupole magnets are normal-aperture quadrupole magnets, operating at a cryogenic temperature of 1.9 K with a nominal gradient of 200 T/m.

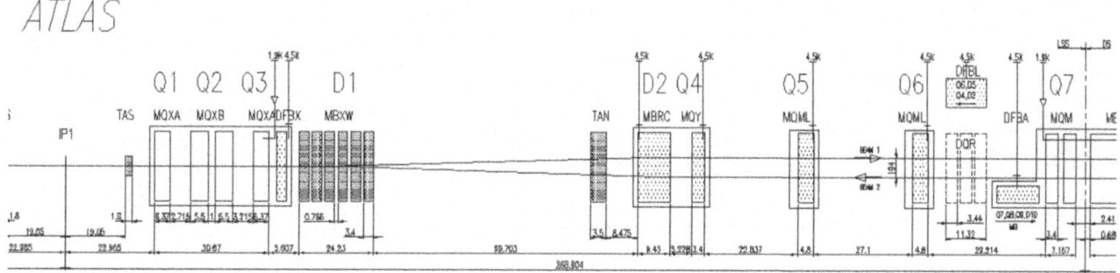

Fig. 1.2 Schematic layout of the right side of IR1 (distances in m).

1.2.5 Medium-luminosity insertion in IR2

The straight section of IR2 (see Fig 1.3) houses the injection elements for Ring 1, as well as the ion beam experiment ALICE. During injection, the optics must satisfy the special constraints imposed by the beam injection for Ring 1, and the geometrical acceptance in the interaction region must be large enough to accommodate both beams in the common part of the ring, with a beam separation of at least 10σ.

1.2.6 Beam-cleaning insertions in IR3 and IR7

The IR3 insertion houses the momentum-cleaning systems (capturing off-momentum particles) of both beams, while IR7 houses the betatron-cleaning systems (to control the beam halo) of both beams. Particles with a large momentum offset are scattered by the primary collimator in IR3 and particles with large betatron amplitudes are scattered by the primary collimator in IR7. In both cases, the scattered particles are absorbed by secondary collimators. Figures 1.4 and 1.5 show the right sides of IR3 and IR7, respectively.

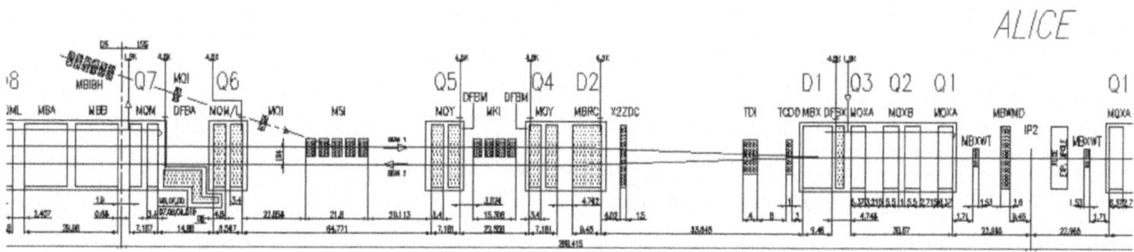

Fig. 1.3 Schematic layout of the matching section on the left side of IR2 (distances in m).

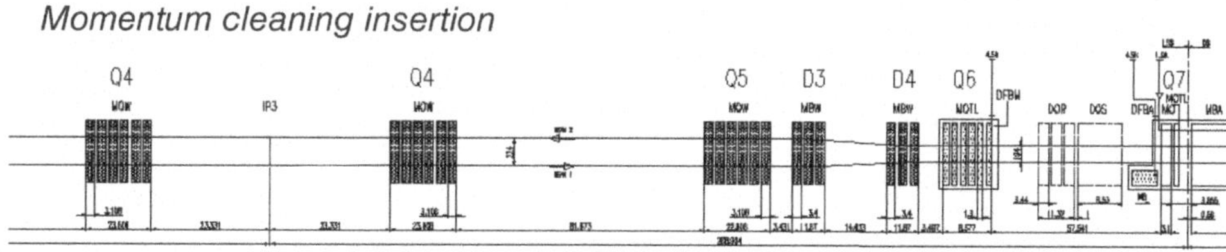

Fig. 1.4 Schematic layout of the matching section on the right side of IR3 (distances in m).

Betatron cleaning insertion

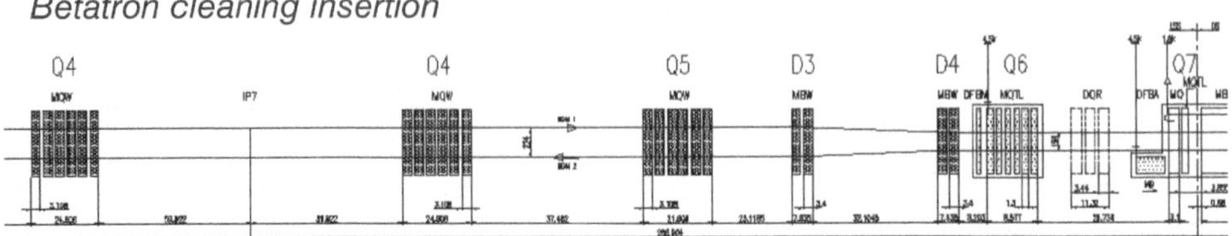

Fig. 1.5 Schematic layout of the matching section on the right side of IR7 (distances in m).

In IR7, the layout of the long straight section between Q7L and Q7R is mirror-symmetric with respect to the IP. This allows a symmetrical installation for the collimators of the two beams and minimizes the space conflicts in the insertion. Starting from Q7 left, the superconducting quadrupole Q6 is followed by a dogleg structure made of two sets of MBW warm single-bore wide-aperture dipole magnets (two warm modules each). The dogleg dipole magnets are labelled D3 and D4 in the LHC sequence, with D3 being the dipole closer to the IP. The primary collimators are located between the D4 and D3 magnets, allowing neutral particles produced in the jaws to point out of the beam line and most charged particles to be swept away. The inter-beam distance between the dogleg assemblies left and right from the IP is 224 mm, i.e. 30 mm larger than in the arc. This increased beam separation allows a substantially higher gradient in the Q4 and Q5 quadrupoles, which are not superconducting because of the heavy irradiation from the collimators. The space between Q5 left and right from the IP is used to house the secondary collimators at appropriate phase advances with respect to the primary collimators.

1.2.7 RF insertion in IR4

IR4 (see Fig. 1.6) houses the RF and feedback systems, as well as some of the LHC beam instrumentation. The RF equipment is installed in the old ALEPH (LEP) cavern, which provides a large space for the power supplies and klystrons. In order to provide the transverse space for two independent RF systems for Beam 1 and Beam 2, the separation must be increased to 420 mm. This is achieved by two pairs of dogleg dipole magnets labelled D3 and D4 in the LHC sequence, with D3 being the dipole magnets closer to the IP. In contrast to IR3 and IR7, the dogleg magnets in IR4 are superconducting, since the radiation levels are low.

RF insertion

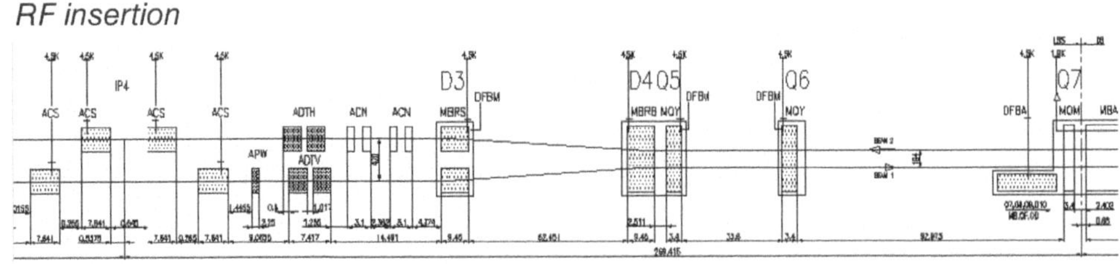

Fig. 1.6 Schematic layout of the matching section on the right side of IR4 (distances in m).

1.2.8 Beam abort insertion in IR6

IR6 (see Fig. 1.7) houses the beam abort systems for Beams 1 and 2. Beam abort from the LHC is done by kicking the circulating beam horizontally into an iron septum magnet, which deflects the beam in the vertical direction away from the machine components to absorbers in a separate tunnel. Each ring has its own system, and both are installed in IR6. To minimize the length of the kicker and of the septum, large drift spaces are provided. Matching the β-functions between the ends of the left and right DS requires only four independently powered quadrupoles. In each DS, up to six quadrupoles can be used for matching. The total of 16 quadrupoles is more than sufficient to match the β-functions and the dispersion and to adjust the phases. There are, however, other constraints to be taken into account concerning apertures inside the insertion.

Special detection devices protect the extraction septum and the LHC machine against losses during the abort process. The TCDS absorber is located in front of the extraction septum and the TCDQ in front of the Q4 quadrupole magnet downstream of the septum magnet.

1.2.9 Medium-luminosity insertion in IR8

IR8 houses the LHCb experiment and the injection elements for Beam 2. The small β-function values at the IP are generated with the help of a triplet quadrupole assembly that leaves ± 23 m of free space around the IP. In this region, the two rings share the same vacuum chamber, the same low-β triplet magnets, and the D1 separation dipole magnet. The remaining matching section and the DS consist of twin-bore magnets with separate beam pipes for each ring. From the IP up to the DS insertion, the layout comprises the following:

- Three warm dipole magnets to compensate the deflection generated by the LHCb spectrometer magnet.
- A 31-m-long superconducting low-β triplet assembly operated at 1.9 K and providing a nominal gradient of 205 T/m.
- A pair of separation/recombination dipole magnets separated by approximately 54 m. The D1 dipole located next to the triplet magnets is a 9.45-m-long single-bore superconducting magnet. The following D2 dipole is a 9.45-m-long

Beam dump insertion

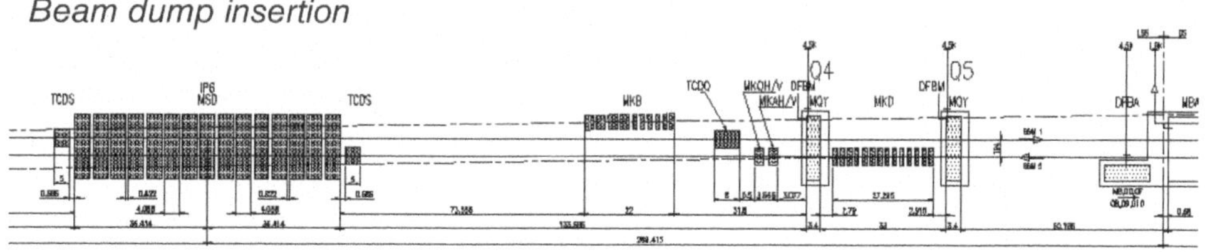

Fig. 1.7 Schematic layout of the matching section on the right side of IR6 (distances in m).

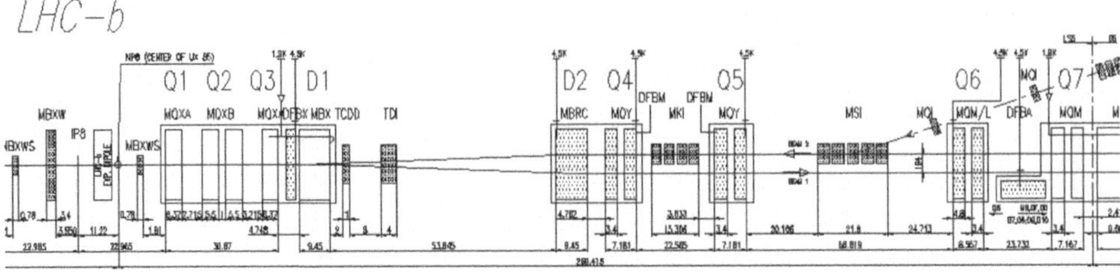

Fig. 1.8 Schematic layout of the matching section on the right side of IR8 (distances in m).

double-bore superconducting dipole magnet. Both magnets are operated at 4.5 K. The bore separation in the D2 magnet is 188 mm, and is thus slightly smaller than the arc bore separation.

- Four matching quadrupole magnets. The first quadrupole following the separation dipole magnets, Q4, is a wide-aperture magnet operating at 4.5 K and yielding a nominal gradient of 160 T/m. The remaining three matching-section quadrupole magnets are normal-aperture quadrupole magnets operating at 1.9 K with a nominal gradient of 200 T/m.
- The injection elements for Beam 2 on the right side of IP8. In order to provide sufficient space for the spectrometer magnet of the LHCb experiment, the beam collision point is shifted by 15 half RF wavelengths (3.5 times the nominal bunch spacing $\approx$ 11.25 m) towards IP7. This shift of the collision point has to be compensated before the beam returns to the DS sections and requires a nonsymmetric magnet layout in the matching section.

1.3 Magnets

1.3.1 Overview

The LHC relies on superconducting magnets that are at the edge of present technology. Other large superconducting accelerators (Tevatron-FNAL, HERA-DESY, and RHIC-BNL) all use classical NbTi superconductors, cooled by supercritical helium at temperatures slightly above 4.2 K, with fields below or around 5 T. The LHC magnet system, while still making use of the well-proven technology based on NbTi Rutherford cables, cools the magnets to a temperature below 2 K, using superfluid helium, and operates at fields above 8 T. Since the electromagnetic forces increase with the square of the field, the structures restraining the conductor motion must be mechanically much stronger than in earlier designs. In addition, space limitations in the tunnel and the need to keep costs down have led to the adoption of the "two-in-one" or "twin-bore" design for almost all of the LHC superconducting magnets. The two-in-one design accommodates the windings for the two beam channels in a common cold mass and cryostat, with magnetic flux circulating in the opposite sense through the two channels.

1.3.2 Superconducting cable

The transverse cross section of the coils in the LHC 56-mm-aperture dipole magnet (Fig. 1.9) shows two layers of different cables distributed in six blocks. The cable used in the inner layer has 28 strands, each having a diameter of 1.065 mm, while the cable in the outer layer is formed from 36 strands, each of 0.825 mm diameter.

The filament size chosen is 7 μm for the strand of the inner layer cable and 6 μm for the strand of the outer layer cable. They are optimized to reduce the effects of the persistent currents on the sextupole field component at injection. The residual errors are corrected by small sextupole and decapole magnets located at the end of each dipole.

1.3.3 Main-dipole cold mass

The LHC ring accommodates 1232 main dipoles: 1104 in the arc and 128 in the DS regions. They all have the same basic design. The geometric and interconnection characteristics have been targeted to be suitable for the DS region, which is more demanding than the arc. The cryodipoles are a critical part of the machine, both from the machine performance point of view and in terms of cost. Figure 1.10 shows the cross section of the cryodipole.

The successful operation of the LHC requires that the main dipole magnets have practically identical characteristics. The relative variations of the integrated field and the field shape imperfections must not exceed $\sim 10^{-4}$, and their reproducibility must be better than 10^{-4} after magnet testing and during magnet operation. The reproducibility of the integrated field strength requires close control of coil diameter and length and of the stacking factor of the laminated magnetic yokes, and possibly fine tuning of the length ratio between the magnetic and nonmagnetic parts of the yoke. The structural stability of the cold mass assembly is achieved by using very rigid collars, and by opposing the electromagnetic forces acting at the interfaces between

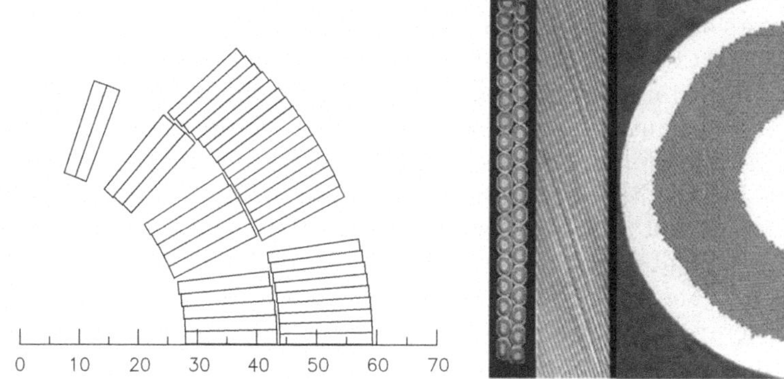

Fig. 1.9 Conductor distribution in the dipole coil cross section (X axis in mm on left). Picture of cables and strand on right.

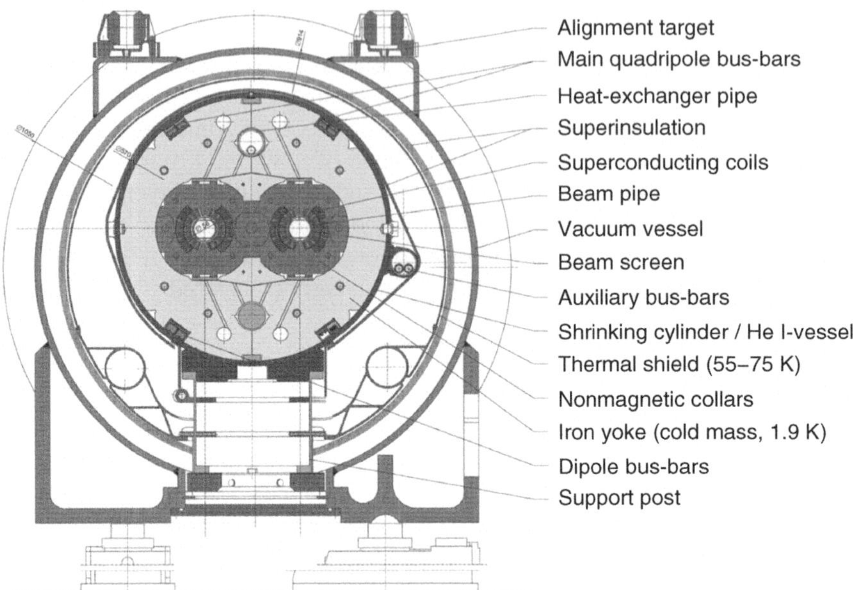

Fig. 1.10 Cross section of cryodipole (lengths in mm).

the collared coils and the magnetic yoke with the forces set up by the shrinking cylinder. A prestress between coils and retaining structure (collars, iron lamination, and shrinking cylinder) is also built in. Because of the larger thermal contraction coefficient of the shrinking cylinder and austenitic steel collars with respect to the yoke steel, the force distribution inside the cold mass changes during cool down from room temperature to 1.9 K.

1.3.4 Dipole cryostat

The vacuum vessel consists of a long cylindrical standard tube with an outer diameter of 914 mm (36 inches) and a wall thickness of 12 mm. It is made from alloyed low-carbon steel. The vessel has stainless steel end flanges for vacuum-tight connection via elastomer seals to adjacent units. Three support regions feature circumferential reinforcement rings. Upper reinforcing angles support alignment fixtures. An ISO-standard flanged port is located azimuthally on the wall of the vessel at one end. In normal operation, the vessel will be under vacuum. In case of a cryogenic leak, the pressure can rise to 0.14 MPa absolute, and a sudden local cooling of the vessel wall to about 230 K may occur. The steel selected for the vacuum vessel wall is tested to demonstrate adequate energy absorption during a standard Charpy test at $-50\,^\circ$C. A front view of the cryodipole is shown in Fig. 1.11.

In the main dipoles, the magnetic field is up in one aperture and down in the other. In straight sections 2 and 8, the beams are separated into two apertures with special superconducting dipoles D1 with a single aperture and D2 with two apertures, where the field direction is identical for both. Such special dipoles are also used in the

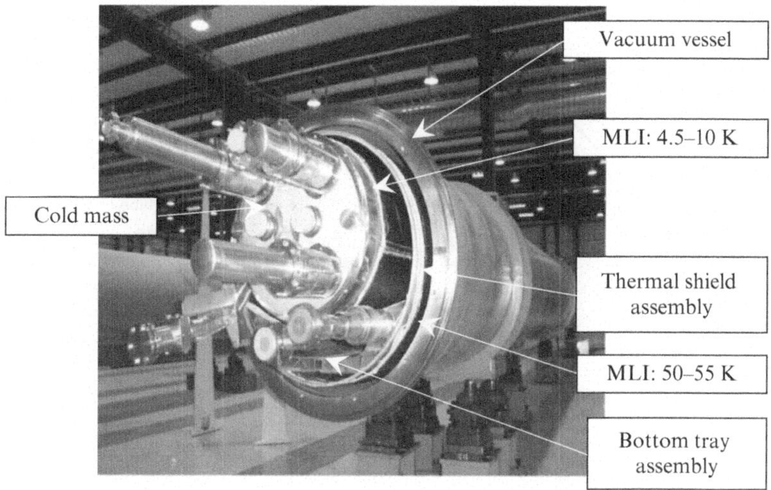

Fig. 1.11 LHC dipole cryomagnet assembly.

RF insertion at Point 4, where the beams are separated further to make way for the cavities. All these special dipoles were designed and built in the USA at Brookhaven Laboratory.

1.3.5 Short straight sections of the arcs

Figure 1.12 shows a perspective view and Fig. 1.13 illustrates the cross section of an SSS. The cold masses of the arc SSSs contain the main quadrupole magnets (MQ) and

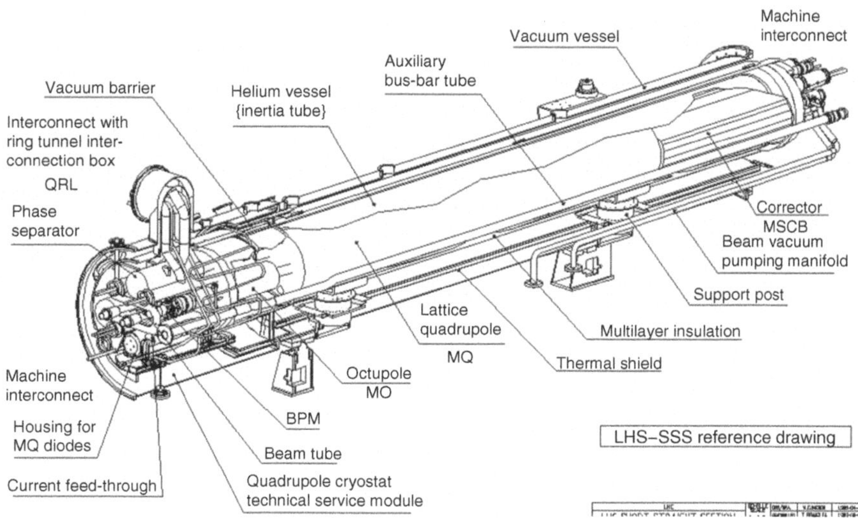

Fig. 1.12 Short straight section (SSS) with jumper.

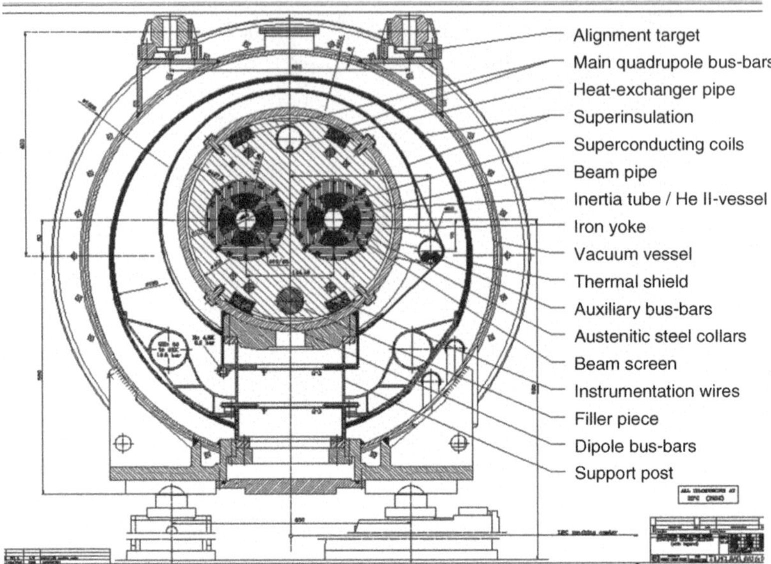

Fig. 1.13   Cross section of SSS at quadrupole cold mass inside cryostat.

various corrector magnets. On the upstream end, these can be octupoles (MO), tuning quadrupoles (MQT), or skew quadrupole correctors (MQS). On the downstream end, the combined sextupole–dipole correctors (MSCB) are installed.

Because of the lower electromagnetic forces than in the dipoles, the two apertures do not need to be combined, but are assembled in separate annular collaring systems.

1.3.6   Insertion magnets

The insertion magnets are superconducting or normally conducting and are used in the eight insertion regions of the LHC. Four of these insertions are dedicated to experiments, while the others are used for major collider systems (one for the RF, two for beam cleaning, and one for beam dumping). The various functions of the insertions are fulfilled by a variety of magnets, most based on the technology of NbTi superconductors cooled by superfluid helium at 1.9 K. A number of standalone magnets in the matching sections and beam separation sections are cooled to 4.5 K, while in the radiation areas, specialized normally conducting magnets are installed.

1.3.7   Matching-section quadrupoles

The tuning of the LHC insertions is provided by the individually powered quadrupoles in the matching and DS sections. The matching sections consist of standalone quadrupoles arranged in four half-cells, but the number and parameters of the magnets are specific for each insertion. Apart from the cleaning insertions, where specialized normally conducting quadrupoles are used in the high-radiation areas, all matching quadrupoles are superconducting magnets. Most of them are cooled to 4.5 K, except the Q7 quadrupoles, which are the first magnets in the continuous arc cryostat and are cooled to 1.9 K.

CERN has developed two superconducting quadrupoles for the matching sections: the MQM quadrupole, featuring a 56-mm-aperture coil, which is also used in the DS sections, and the MQY quadrupole, with an enlarged, 70 mm, coil aperture. Both quadrupoles use narrow cables, so that the nominal current is less than 6 kA, substantially simplifying the warm and cold powering circuits. Each aperture is powered separately, but a common return is used, so that a three-wire bus-bar system is sufficient for full control of the apertures.

In the cleaning insertions IR3 and IR7, each of the matching quadrupoles Q4 and Q5 consists of a group of six normally conducting MQW magnets. This choice is dictated by the high radiation levels due to scattered particles from the collimation system, and therefore the use of superconducting magnets is not possible. It features two apertures in a common yoke (2-in-1), which is atypical for normally conducting quadrupole magnets, but is needed because of transverse space constraints in the tunnel. The two apertures may be powered in series in a standard focusing/defocusing configuration (MQWA), or alternatively in a focusing/focusing configuration (MQWB) to correct asymmetries of the magnet. In a functional group of six magnets, five are configured as MQWA, corrected by one configured as MQWB.

1.3.8 Low-β triplets

The low-β triplet is composed of four single-aperture quadrupoles with a coil aperture of 70 mm. These magnets are cooled with superfluid helium at 1.9 K using an external heat-exchanger system capable of extracting up to 10 W/m of power deposited in the coils by the secondary particles emanating from the proton collisions. Two types of quadrupoles are used in the triplet: 6.6-m-long MQXA magnets designed and developed by KEK, Japan and 5.7-m-long MQXB magnets designed and built by Fermilab, USA. The magnets are powered in series with 7 kA, with an additional inner loop of 5 kA for the MQXB magnets. Together with the orbit correctors MCBX, skew quadrupoles MQSX, and multipole spool pieces supplied by CERN, the low-β quadrupoles are completed in their cold masses and cryostated by Fermilab. The cryogenic feed-boxes (DFBX), providing a link to the cryogenic distribution line and power converters, are designed and built by Lawrence Berkeley National Laboratory, USA. Alongside the LHC main dipoles, the high-gradient wide-aperture low-β quadrupoles are the most demanding magnets in the collider. They must operate reliably at 215 T/m, sustain extremely high heat loads in the coils and high radiation dose during their lifetime, and have a very good field quality within the 63 mm aperture of the cold bore.

1.4 Radiofrequency systems

1.4.1 Introduction

The injected beam is captured, accelerated, and stored using a 400 MHz superconducting cavity system, and the longitudinal injection errors is damped using the same system. This choice defines the maximum allowable machine impedance, in particular for higher-order modes in cavities [16]. Transverse injection errors will be damped by a separate system of electrostatic deflectors that will also ensure subsequent transverse stability against the resistive wall instability [17]. All RF and beam feedback systems are concentrated at Point 4 and extend from the UX45 cavern area into the tunnel on either side.

The beam and machine parameters that are directly relevant to the design of the RF and beam feedback systems are given in Table 1.1. At nominal intensity in the SPS, an emittance of 0.6 eV s has now been achieved, giving a bunch length at 450 GeV of 1.6 ns. The phase variation along the batch due to beam loading is within 125 ps. This emittance is lower than originally assumed, and, as a result, an RF system in the LHC of 400.8 MHz can be used to capture the beam with minimal losses, accelerate,

Table 1.1 The main beam and RF parameters

	UNITS	INJECTION, 450 GeV	COLLISION, 7 TeV
Bunch area (2σ)*	eV s	1.0	2.5
Bunch length (4σ)*	ns	1.71	1.06
Energy spread (2σ)*	10^{-3}	0.88	0.22
Intensity per bunch	10^{11} p	1.15	1.15
Number of bunches		2808	2808
Normalized RMS transverse emittance, V/H	μm	3.75	3.75
Intensity per beam	A	0.582	0.582
Synchrotron radiation loss/turn	keV	—	7
Longitudinal damping time	h	—	13
Intrabeam scattering growth time: H	h	38	80
L	h	30	61
Frequency	MHz	400.789	400.790
Harmonic number		35 640	35 640
RF voltage/beam	MV	8	16
Energy gain/turn (20 min ramp)	keV	485	
RF power supplied during acceleration/beam	kW	~ 275	
Synchrotron frequency	Hz	63.7	23.0
Bucket area	eV s	1.43	7.91
RF (400 MHz) component of beam current	A	0.87	1.05

*The bunch parameters at 450 GeV are an upper limit for the situation after filamentation, $\sim$100 ms after each batch injection. The bunch parameters at injection are described in the text.

and finally store it at top energy. Higher frequencies, while better for producing the short bunches required in store, cannot accommodate the injected bunch length.

There will be some emittance increase at injection, but this will be within the capabilities of the RF system for acceleration and, in particular, will be below the final emittance needed in storage. This final emittance is defined by intrabeam scattering lifetime in the presence of damping due to synchrotron radiation, RF lifetime, and instability threshold considerations. Controlled emittance increase is provided during acceleration by excitation with band-limited noise, the emittance increasing with the square root of the energy to optimize both narrow and broadband instability thresholds [16].

The final emittance at 7 TeV (2.5 eV s) and a maximum bunch length given by luminosity considerations in the experiments lead to a required maximum voltage of 16 MV/beam. There are many advantages in having a separate RF system for each beam. However, the standard distance between beams in the machine, 194 mm, is insufficient. Consequently, the beam separation is increased in the RF region to 420 mm by means of special superconducting dipoles. With the increased separation and also by staggering the cavities longitudinally, the "second" beam can pass outside the cavity. However, it must still pass through the cryostat.

1.4.2 Main 400 MHz RF accelerating system (ACS)

The two independent RF systems must each provide at least 16 MV in coast, while at injection about 8 MV is needed. The frequency of 400 MHz is close to that of LEP, 352 MHz, allowing the same proven technology of niobium-sputtered superconducting cavities to be applied. The present design, using single-cell cavities each with 2 MV accelerating voltage, corresponding to a conservative field strength of 5.5 MV/m, minimizes the power carried by the RF window. A large tuning range is required to compensate the average reactive beam component. Each RF system has eight cavities, with $R/Q = 45\Omega$ and of length $\lambda/2$, grouped by four with a spacing of $3\lambda/2$ in one common cryostat [18]. Each cavity is driven by an individual RF system with klystron, circulator, and load. Complex feedback loops around each cavity allow precise control of the field in each cavity, which is important for the unforgiving high-intensity LHC proton beam.

The use of niobium sputtering on copper for construction of the cavities has the important advantage over solid niobium that susceptibility to quenching is very much reduced. Local heat generated by small surface defects or impurities is quickly conducted away by the copper. During the low-power tests, the 21 cavities produced all reached an accelerating field of twice nominal without quenching. The niobium-sputtered cavities are insensitive to the Earth's magnetic field, and special magnetic shielding, as needed for solid-niobium cavities, is not required. Four cavities, each equipped with their helium tank, tuner, higher-order mode (HOM) couplers, and power coupler, are grouped together in a single cryomodule (see Fig. 1.14). The conception of the cryomodule is itself modular; all cavities are identical and can be installed in any position. If a problem arises with a cavity, it can be replaced. The cavity is tuned by elastic deformation, by pulling on a harness using stainless steel cables that are

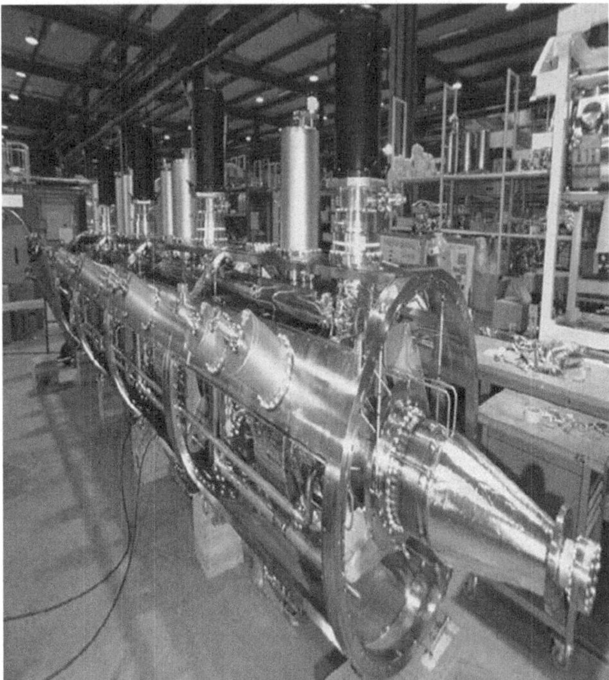

Fig. 1.14   Four-cavity cryomodule during assembly.

wound around a shaft. A stepping motor, fixed to the outside of the cryostat, drives the shaft. The motor therefore works in normal ambient conditions and can be easily accessed for maintenance or repair.

1.5   Vacuum system

1.5.1   Overview

The LHC has three vacuum systems: the insulation vacuum for the cryomagnets, the insulation vacuum for helium distribution (QRL), and the beam vacuum. The insulation vacua before cool down do not have to be better than 10^{-1} mbar, but at cryogenic temperatures, in the absence of any significant leak, the pressure will stabilize at about 10^{-6} mbar. The requirements for the beam vacuum are much more stringent, driven by the required beam lifetime and background at the experiments. Rather than quoting equivalent pressures at room temperature, the requirements at cryogenic temperature are expressed as gas densities normalized to hydrogen, taking into account the ionization cross sections for each gas species. Equivalent hydrogen gas densities should remain below 10^{15} H_2 m^{-3} to ensure the required 100 hour beam lifetime. In the interaction regions around the experiments, the densities will be below 10^{13} H_2 m^{-3} to minimize the background to the experiments. In the room-temperature parts of the beam vacuum system, the pressure should be in the range $10^{-10} - 10^{-11}$ mbar.

A number of dynamic phenomena have to be taken into account in the design of the beam vacuum system. Synchrotron radiation will hit the vacuum chambers, in particular in the arcs, and electron clouds (multipacting) could affect almost the entire ring. Extra care has to be taken during the design and installation to minimize these effects, but conditioning with beam will be required to reach nominal performance.

1.5.2 Beam vacuum requirements

The design of the beam vacuum system takes into account the requirements of 1.9 K operation and the need to shield the cryogenic system from heat sources, as well as the more usual constraints set by vacuum chamber impedances. Four main heat sources have been identified and quantified at nominal intensity and energy:

- synchrotron light radiated by the circulating proton beams (0.2 W/m per beam, with a critical energy of about 44 eV);
- energy loss by nuclear scattering (30 mW/m per beam);
- image currents (0.2 W/m per beam);
- energy dissipated during the development of electron clouds, which will form when the surfaces seen by the beams have a secondary electron yield that is too high.

Intercepting these heat sources at a temperature above 1.9 K has necessitated the introduction of a beam screen. The more classical constraints on the vacuum system design are set by the stability of the beams, which sets the acceptable longitudinal and transverse impedance [19, 20], and by the background conditions in the interaction regions.

The vacuum lifetime is dominated by the nuclear scattering of protons on the residual gas. The cross sections for this interaction at 7 TeV depend on the gas species [21, 22] and are given in Table 1.2, together with the gas density and pressure (at 5 K) compatible with the requested 100 hour lifetime. This number ensures that the contribution of beam–gas collisions to the decay of the beam intensity is small

Table 1.2 Nuclear scattering cross sections at 7 TeV for different gases and corresponding densities and equivalent pressures for a 100 h lifetime

GAS	NUCLEAR SCATTERING CROSS SECTION (cm^2)	GAS DENSITY (m^{-3}) FOR 100 h LIFETIME	PRESSURE (Pa) AT 5 K FOR 100 h LIFETIME
H_2	9.5×10^{-26}	9.8×10^{14}	6.7×10^{-8}
He	1.26×10^{-25}	7.4×10^{14}	5.1×10^{-8}
CH_4	5.66×10^{-25}	1.6×10^{14}	1.1×10^{-8}
H_2O	5.65×10^{-25}	1.6×10^{14}	1.1×10^{-8}
CO	8.54×10^{-25}	1.1×10^{14}	7.5×10^{-9}
CO_2	1.32×10^{-24}	7×10^{13}	4.9×10^{-9}

compared with other loss mechanisms; it also reduces the energy lost by scattered protons in the cryomagnets to below the nominal value of 30 mW/m per beam.

1.5.3 Beam vacuum in the arcs and dispersion suppressors

The two beams are confined in independent vacuum chambers from one end of the continuous cryostat to the other, extending from Q7 in one octant to Q7 in the next octant. Cold bores with an inner diameter of 50 mm, part of the cryomagnets, are connected together by so-called cold interconnects, which compensate for length variations and alignment errors. A beam-position monitor, with an actively cooled body, is mounted on each beam in each SSS (i.e. at each quadrupole). An actively cooled beam screen is inserted into the cold bores of all magnets (see Fig. 1.15). A racetrack shape has been chosen for the beam screen, which optimizes the available aperture while leaving space for the cooling tubes. The nominal horizontal and vertical apertures are 44.04 and 34.28 mm, respectively. Slots, covering a total of 4% of the surface area, are perforated in the flat parts of the beam screen to allow condensing of the gas on surfaces protected from the direct impact of energetic particles (ions, electrons, and photons). The pattern of the slots has been chosen to minimize longitudinal and transverse impedance, and the size has been chosen to keep the RF losses through the holes below 1 mW/m. A thin copper layer (75 μm) on the inner surface of the beam screen provides a low-resistance path for the image current of the beam. A saw-tooth pattern on the inner surface in the plane of bending helps the absorption of synchrotron radiation.

The beam screen is cooled by two stainless steel tubes with an inner diameter of 3.7 mm and a wall thickness of 0.53 mm, allowing the extraction of up to 1.13 W/m in nominal cryogenic conditions. The helium temperature is regulated to 20 K at the output of the cooling circuit at every half-cell, resulting in a temperature of the cooling tubes between 5 and 20 K for nominal cryogenic conditions. The cooling tubes

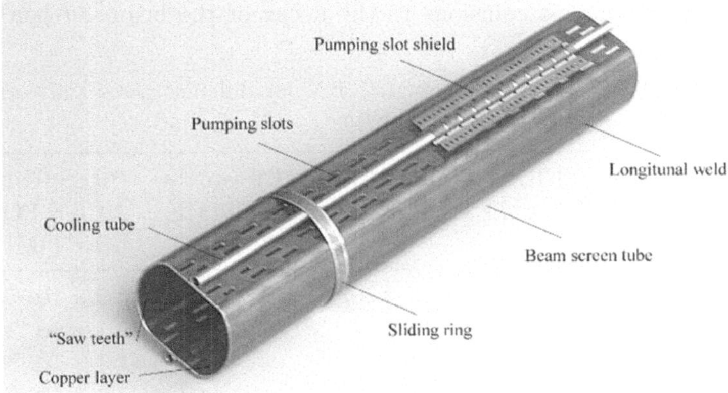

Fig. 1.15 Conceptual design of the LHC beam screen.

are laser-welded onto the beam-screen tube and fitted at each end with adaptor pieces that allow their routing out of the cold bore without any fully penetrating weld between the helium circuit and the beam vacuum. Sliding rings with a bronze layer towards the cold bore are welded onto the beam screen every 750 mm to ease the insertion of the screen into the cold bore tube, to improve the centring, and to provide good thermal insulation. Finally, since the electron clouds can deposit significant power into the cold bore through the pumping slots, the latter are shielded with copper–beryllium shields clipped onto the cooling tubes. The net pumping speed for hydrogen is reduced by a factor of two, which remains acceptable.

Cold interconnects

Beam vacuum interconnects ensure the continuity of the vacuum envelope and of the helium flow, as well as a smooth geometrical transition between beam screens along the 1642 twin-aperture superconducting cryomagnets installed in the continuous cryostat. The physical beam envelope must have a low electrical resistance for image currents and must minimize coupled bunch instabilities. It must also have a low inductance for the longitudinal single-bunch instability. The maximum DC resistance allowed at room temperature for a complete interconnect is 0.1 mΩ. To meet these requirements, a complex interconnect module integrates a shielded bellows to allow thermal expansion, as well as for compensation of mechanical and alignment tolerances between two adjacent beam screens. The shielding of the bellows is achieved by means of a set of sliding contact fingers made out of gold-plated copper–beryllium, which slide on a rhodium-coated copper tube.

1.5.4 Beam vacuum in the insertions

Room-temperature chambers alternate with standalone cryostats in the IRs. The room-temperature part includes beam instrumentation, accelerating cavities, experiments, collimation equipment, and the injection and ejection kickers and septa, as well as some of the dipole and quadrupole magnets where superconducting elements are not used. In these regions, the vacuum systems for the two beams sometimes merge, notably in the four experimental insertions, but also in some special equipment like the injection kickers and some beam stoppers.

Beam screen

The beam screen is only required in the cold bores of the standalone cryostats. It is derived from the arc type, but uses a smaller (0.6 mm) steel thickness and comes in various sizes, to match different cold-bore diameters. The orientation of the beam screen in the cold bore is adapted to the aperture requirements, which means that the flat part with the cooling tubes can be either vertical or horizontal. The saw-tooth structure has been abandoned for these beam screens, since synchrotron radiation hitting the screen in these regions is at most 1/10 as intense as in the arc, and because fitting the saw teeth at the appropriate location of the beam screen would be too expensive.

Room-temperature beam vacuum in the field-free regions

The baseline for the room-temperature beam vacuum system is to use 7-m-long oxygen-free silver-bearing (OFS) copper chambers, with an inner diameter of 80 mm and fitted with standard DN100 Conflat flanges. The thickness of the copper is 2 mm, and the chambers are coated with TiZrV non-evaporable getter (NEG) [23]. After activation at low temperature (200 °C), the getter provides distributed pumping and low outgassing to maintain a low residual gas pressure, as well as a low secondary electron emission yield to avoid electron multipacting. The chambers are connected by means of shielded bellows modules, some of them including pumping and diagnostic ports.

1.6   Cryogenic system

1.6.1   Overview

The superconducting magnet windings in the arcs, the dispersion suppressors, and the inner triplets will be immersed in a pressurized bath of superfluid helium at about 0.13 MPa (1.3 bar) and a maximum temperature of 1.9 K [24]. This allows a sufficient temperature margin for heat transfer across the electrical insulation. As the specific heats of the superconducting alloy and its copper matrix fall rapidly with decreasing temperature, the full benefit in terms of the stability margin of operation at 1.9 K (instead of at the conventional 4.5 K) may only be gained by making effective use of the transport properties of superfluid helium, for which the temperature of 1.9 K also corresponds to a maximum in the effective thermal conductivity. The low bulk viscosity enables the coolant to permeate the heart of the magnet windings. The large specific heat (typically 10^5 times that of the conductor per unit mass, 2×10^3 times per unit volume), combined with the enormous heat conductivity at moderate flux (3000 times that of cryogenic-grade oxygen-free high-thermal conductivity (OFHC) copper, peaking at 1.9 K) can have a powerful stabilizing action on thermal disturbances. To achieve this, the electrical insulation of the conductor must preserve sufficient porosity and provide a thermal percolation path, while still fulfilling its demanding dielectric and mechanical duties.

The cryogenic system must be able to cope with the load variations and a large dynamic range induced by the operation of the accelerator, as well as being able to cool down and fill the huge cold mass of the LHC, 37×10^6 kg, within a maximum delay of 15 days while avoiding thermal differences in the cryomagnet structure higher than 75 K. The cryogenic system must also be able to cope with resistive transitions of the superconducting magnets, which will occasionally occur in the machine, while minimizing loss of cryogen and system perturbations. It must handle the resulting heat release and its consequences, which include fast pressure rises and flow surges. The system must limit the propagation to neighbouring magnets and recover in a time that does not seriously detract from the operational availability of the LHC. A resistive transition extending over one lattice cell should not result in a down time of more than a few hours. It must also be possible to rapidly warm up and cool down limited lengths of the lattice for magnet exchange and repair. Finally, the cryogenic system must be able to handle, without impairing the safety of personnel or equipment, the largest credible incident of the resistive transition of a full sector. The system is designed with some redundancy in its subsystems.

1.6.2 General architecture

The main constraints on the cryogenic system result from the need to install it in the existing LEP tunnel and to re-use LEP facilities, including four refrigerators. The limited number of access points to the underground area is reflected in the architecture of the system. The cooling power required at each temperature level will be produced by eight refrigeration plants and distributed to the adjacent sectors over distances up to 3.3 km. To simplify the magnet string design, the cryogenic headers distributing the cooling power along a machine sector, as well as all remaining active cryogenic components in the tunnel, are contained in a compound cryogenic distribution line (QRL). The QRL runs alongside the cryomagnet strings in the tunnel and feeds each 106.9-m-long lattice cell in parallel via a jumper connection (Fig. 1.16).

The LHC tunnel is inclined at 1.41% with respect to the horizontal, thus giving height differences of up to 120 m across the tunnel diameter. This slope generates hydrostatic heads in the cryogenic headers and could generate flow instabilities in two-phase, liquid–vapour, flow. To avoid these instabilities, all fluids should be transported over large distances in a monophasic state, i.e. in the superheated-vapour or supercritical region of the phase diagram. Local two-phase circulation of saturated liquid can be tolerated over limited lengths, in a controlled direction of circulation. Equipment is installed as much as possible above ground to avoid the need for further excavation, but

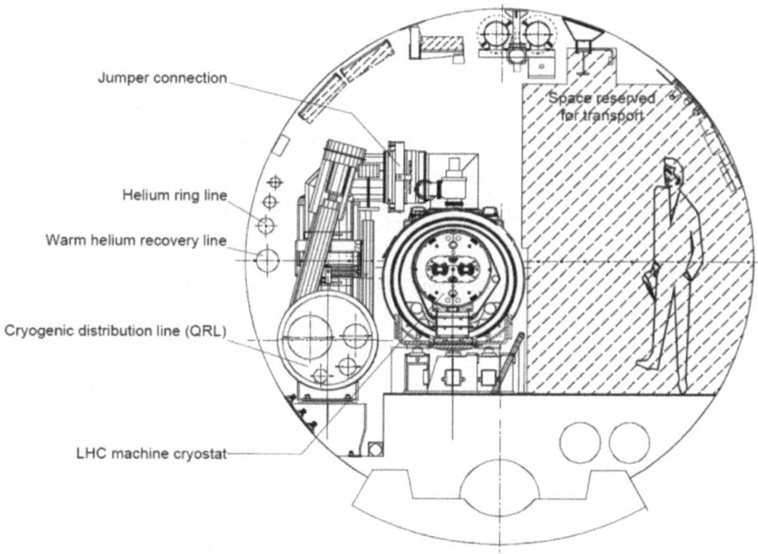

Fig. 1.16 Transverse cross section of the LHC tunnel.

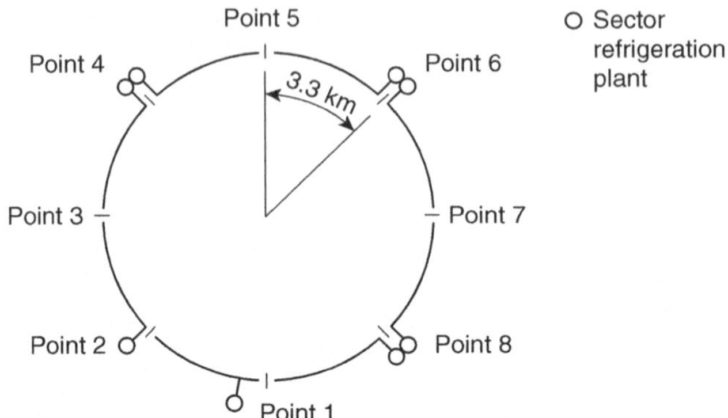

Fig. 1.17 General layout of the cryogenic system.

certain components have to be installed underground near the cryostats. For reasons of safety, the use of nitrogen in the tunnel is forbidden, and the discharge of helium is restricted to small quantities only.

Figure 1.17 shows the general layout of the cryogenic system, with five "cryogenic islands" at access Points 1, 2, 4, 6, and 8, where all refrigeration equipment and ancillary equipment is concentrated. Equipment at ground level includes electrical substations, warm compressors, cryogen storage (helium and liquid nitrogen), cooling towers, and cold boxes. Underground equipment includes lower cold boxes, 1.8 K refrigeration unit boxes, interconnecting lines, and interconnection boxes. Each cryogenic island houses one or two refrigeration plants that feed one or two adjacent tunnel sectors, requiring distribution and recovery of the cooling fluids over distances of 3.3 km underground.

1.6.3 Temperature levels

In view of the high thermodynamic cost of refrigeration at 1.8 K, the thermal design of the LHC cryogenic components aims at intercepting the main heat influx at higher temperatures—hence the multiple-staged temperature levels in the system. The temperature levels are as follows:

- 50–75 K for the thermal shield protecting the cold masses;
- 4.6–20 K for lower-temperature interception and for cooling the beam screens that protect the magnet bores from beam-induced loads;
- 1.9 K quasi-isothermal superfluid helium for cooling the magnet cold masses;
- 4 K at very low pressure for transporting the superheated helium flow coming from the distributed 1.8 K heat-exchanger tubes across the sector length to the 1.8 K refrigeration units;
- 4.5 K normal saturated helium for cooling some insertion region magnets, RF cavities, and the lower sections of the high-temperature superconductor (HTS) current leads;
- 20–300 K cooling for the resistive upper sections of the HTS current leads [4].

To provide these temperature levels, use is made of helium in several thermodynamic states. The cryostats and cryogenic distribution line (QRL) combine several techniques for limiting heat influx, such as low-conduction support posts, insulation vacuum, multilayer reflective insulation wrapping, and low-impedance thermal contacts, all of which have been successfully applied on an industrial scale.

1.7 Beam instrumentation

An accurate and complete set of beam instrumentation is essential for efficient commissioning and operation of the LHC. This instrumentation includes beam-position measurement all around the ring, beam-loss monitors, current and profile measurement, and specialized instrumentation to measure beam properties such as chromaticity and tune.

1.7.1 Beam-position measurement

The majority of the LHC beam-position monitors (BPMs; 860 of the 1032) are of the arc type (see Fig. 1.18), consisting of four 24-mm-diameter button electrode feed-throughs mounted orthogonally in a 48 mm inner-diameter beam pipe. The electrodes are curved to follow the beam-pipe aperture and are retracted by 0.5 mm to protect the buttons from direct synchrotron radiation from the main bending magnets. Each electrode has a capacitance of 7.6 ± 0.6 pF, and is connected to a 50 Ω coaxial, glass-ceramic, ultrahigh-vacuum feedthrough.

The inner triplet BPMs in all interaction regions are equipped with 120 mm, 50 Ω directional stripline couplers (BPMS×), capable of distinguishing between counter-rotating beams in the same beam pipe. The locations of these BPMs (in front of Q1, in the Q2 cryostat, and after Q3) were chosen to be as far as possible from parasitic crossings to optimize the directivity. The 120 mm stripline length was chosen to give a signal similar to the button electrode, thereby allowing the use of the same acquisition electronics as for the arcs. All cold directional couplers use an Ultem dielectric for use in a cryogenic environment, while the warm couplers use a Macor dielectric to allow bake-out to over 200 °C.

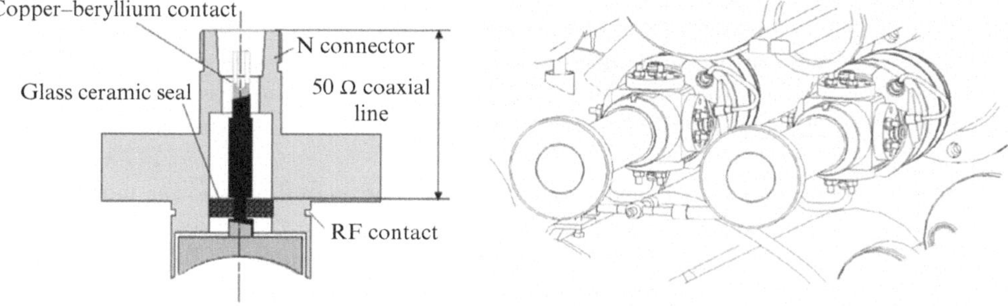

Fig. 1.18 (a) 24 mm button electrode. (b) Mounted beam-position monitor bodies.

The cleaning insertions at Points 3 and 7 are equipped with warm 34-mm-diameter button electrode BPMs (BPMW) fitted either side of the MQWA magnets. The electrodes are an enlarged version of the arc BPM button. The same button electrodes are also used for the cold BPMs in the matching sections either side of the four interaction regions, as well as for the warm BPMs located near the D2 magnets and either side of the transverse damper (ADTV/H). The BPMCs, installed at Point 4, are combined monitors consisting of one BPM using standard 24 mm button electrodes for use by the orbit system and one BPM using 150 mm shorted stripline electrodes for use in the transverse damper system.

1.7.2   Beam-current measurement

Beam-current transformers of two different kinds provide intensity measurements for the beams circulating in the LHC rings, as well as for the transfer lines from the SPS to the LHC, and from the LHC to the dumps. The transformers are all installed in sections where the vacuum chamber is at room temperature and where the beams are separated.

The fast beam-current transformers (FBCTs) are capable of integrating the charge of each LHC bunch. This provides good accuracy for both bunch-to-bunch measurements and average measurements, intended mainly for low-intensity beams, for which the accuracy of the DC current transformers (DCCTs) will be limited. For redundancy, two transformers, with totally separated acquisition chains, will be placed in each ring. These will be located at Point 4. The measurement precision for the pilot beam of 5×10^9 protons in a single bunch is around 5% (worst case 10%), and for the nominal beam below 1%.

The DCCTs are based on the principle of magnetic amplifiers and measure the mean intensity or current of the circulating beam, and they can be used to measure the beam lifetime. Because of their operational importance, two of the devices will be installed in each ring. Currently a resolution of 2 μA can be reached, but 1 μA is targeted, corresponding to 5×10^8 circulating particles.

1.7.3   Beam-loss system

The loss of a very small fraction of the circulating beam may induce a quench of the superconducting magnets or even physical damage to machine components. The detection of lost beam protons allows protection of the equipment against quenches and damage by generating a beam-dump trigger when the losses exceed thresholds. In addition to quench prevention and damage protection, the loss detection allows the observation of local aperture restrictions, orbit distortion, beam oscillations, and particle diffusion.

The loss measurement is based on the detection of secondary shower particles using ionization chambers located outside the magnet cryostats. The secondary particle energy flux depends linearly on the initiating proton parameters. To observe a representative fraction of the secondary particle flux, detectors are placed at likely loss locations. The calibration of the damage and quench level thresholds with respect to the measured secondary particle energy deposition is simulation-based.

1.7.4 Transverse profile measurement

User requirements led to the definition of four functional modes to be mapped on the different types of hardware monitors:

- A single-pass monitor of high sensitivity (pilot beam) with a modest demand on accuracy and few restrictions on the beam blowup due to the traversal.
- A "few-pass monitor" (typically 20 turns) dedicated to the intermediate to nominal intensity range of the injected beam for calibration or matching studies. The blowup per turn should be small compared with the effect to be measured.
- A circulating beam monitor, working over the whole intensity range. No blowup is expected from such a monitor.
- A circulating beam tail monitor optimized to scan low beam densities. In this mode, one may not be able to measure the core of the beam. The measurement should not disturb the tail density significantly.

The monitor types include wire scanners, residual gas ionization monitors and synchrotron light monitors using light from D2-type superconducting dipoles. Synchrotron light monitors are also under development for using light from superconducting undulators in each ring. Point 4 is the default location for all instrumentation.

1.7.5 Tune, chromaticity, and betatron coupling

Reliable measurement of betatron tune and of the related quantities tune spread, chromaticity, and betatron coupling will be essential for all phases of LHC running from commissioning through to ultimate performance luminosity runs. For injection and ramping, the fractional part of the betatron tune must be controlled to ± 0.003, while in collision, the required tolerance shrinks to ± 0.001. With the exception of Schottky scans and the "AC-dipole" excitation outside the tune peak, all tune measurement techniques involve some disturbance to the beam. The resulting emittance increase, while acceptable for some modes of running, has to be strongly limited for full-intensity physics runs. Different tune measurement systems are therefore installed.

General tune measurement system

This uses standard excitation sources (single-kick, chirp, slow swept frequency, and noise). It operates with all filling patterns and bunch intensities and will be commissioned early after LHC start-up. Even with oscillation amplitudes down to 50 μm, a certain amount of emittance increase will result, limiting the frequency at which measurements can be made. It is therefore unsuitable for generating measurements for an online tune feedback system.

High-sensitivity tune-measurement system

The beam is excited by applying a signal of low amplitude and high frequency to a stripline kicker. This frequency is close to half the bunch spacing frequency (40 MHz for the nominal 25 ns bunch spacing). The equivalent oscillation amplitude is a few micrometres or less for a β-function of about 200 m. A notch filter in the transverse feedback loop suppresses the loop gain at this frequency, where instabilities are not expected to be a problem. If the excitation frequency divided by the revolution frequency corresponds to an integer plus the fractional part of the tune, then coherent betatron oscillations of each bunch build up turn by turn (resonant excitation). A batch structure with a bunch every 25 ns "carries" the excitation frequency as sidebands of the bunch spacing harmonics. A beam position pickup is tuned to resonate at one of these frequencies.

1.8   Commissioning and operation

By 10 September 2008, seven of the eight sectors had been successfully commissioned to 5.5 TeV in preparation for a run at 5 TeV. Owing to lack of time, the eighth sector had only been taken to 4 TeV. Beam commissioning started by threading Beam 2, the counterclockwise beam, around the ring, stopping it at each long straight section sequentially to correct the trajectory. In less than an hour, the beam had completed a full turn, witnessed by a second spot on a fluorescent screen intercepting both injected and circulating beams (Fig. 1.19).

Very quickly, a beam circulating for a few hundred turns could be established. Figure 1.20 shows the capture process when the RF cavities are switched on. Each horizontal line on the mountain range display records the bunch intensity every 10 turns. Without the RF, the beam debunches as it should in about 250 turns, or 25 ms. A first attempt was made to capture the beam, but, as can be seen, the injection phase was completely wrong. Adjusting the phase allowed a partial capture, but at a slightly wrong frequency. Finally, adjusting the frequency resulted in a perfect capture.

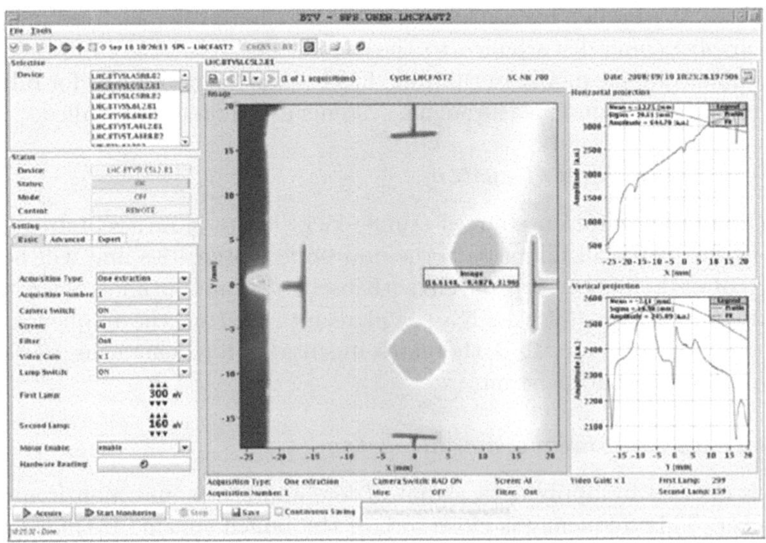

Fig. 1.19   Beam on turns 1 and 2.

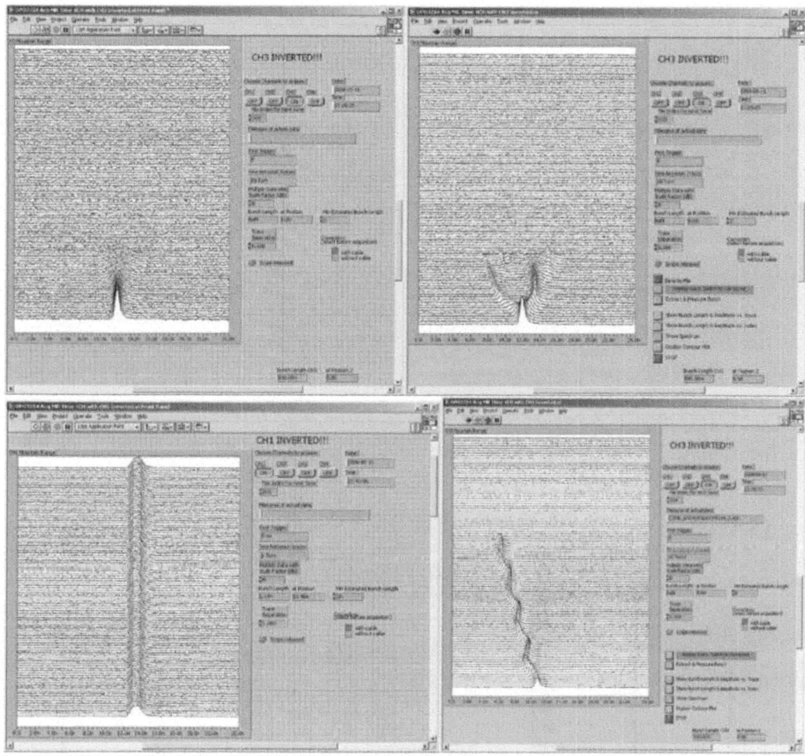

Fig. 1.20 Clockwise from top left: no RF, with debunching in about 250 turns (i.e. roughly 25 ms); first attempt at capture, at exactly the wrong injection phase; capture with corrected injection phase but wrong frequency; capture with optimum injection phasing, correct reference.

The closed orbit could then be corrected. Figure 1.21 shows the first orbit correction, where—remarkably at this early stage—the RMS orbit is less than 2 mm. It can be seen that in the horizontal plane, the mean orbit is displaced radially by about a millimetre, indicative of an energy mismatch of about 10^{-3}.

On 30 March 2010, the first collisions were obtained at a centre-of-mass energy of 7 TeV. Since then, operating time has been split between machine studies and physics data-taking.

In view of the very large stored energy in the beams, particular attention has to be given to the machine protection and collimation systems. More than 120 collimators are arranged in a hierarchy of primary, secondary, and tertiary collimators. Tight control of the orbits in the region of the collimators is achieved with a feedback system.

The collimation system also works very efficiently. Figure 1.22 shows a loss map around the ring obtained by provoking beam loss. The losses are located precisely where they should be, with a factor-of-10 000 difference between the losses on the collimators and those in the cold regions of the machine.

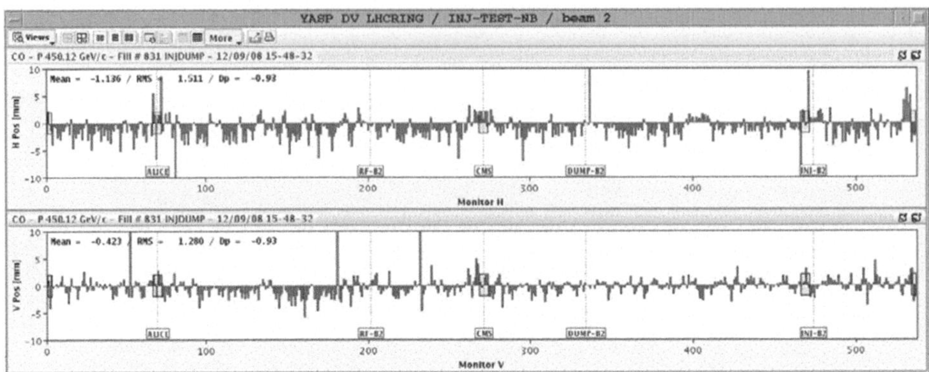

Fig. 1.21 Corrected closed orbit on B2. There is an energy offset of about -0.9 permil due to the capture frequency.

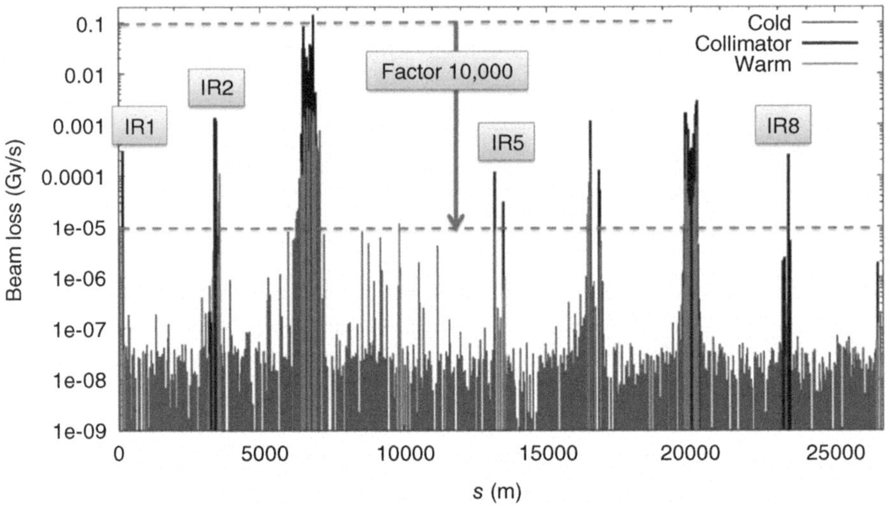

Fig. 1.22 Loss maps for collimation.

The machine performance at this early stage is very impressive. A single-beam lifetime of more than 1000 hours has been observed—an order of magnitude better than expected—proving that the vacuum is considerably better than expected, and also the noise level in the RF system is very low. The nominal bunch intensity of 1.1×10^{11} has been exceeded, and the β^* at the experimental collision points has been squeezed to 2 m. The closed orbit can be kept to better than 1 mm RMS with very good reproducibility. During the 200 days of running in 2010, the luminosity has increased by five orders of magnitude, reaching $2.1 \times 10^{32}\,\mathrm{cm}^{-2}\,\mathrm{s}^{-1}$ with a bunch separation of 150 ns. More than 6 pb^{-1} of integrated luminosity has been produced in each of the two big detectors.

Acknowledgments

The LHC is the most complex scientific instrument ever constructed. It has taken 15 years to build, and many problems have been encountered on the way. These have all been overcome thanks to the resourcefulness and resilience of the people who built it, both inside CERN and in our collaborating laboratories around the world. Now the machine is moving into its operational phase. I am confident that an equally competent team will exploit it to its full potential in the coming years.

References

[1] J. P. Blewett, *200 GeV intersecting storage accelerators*, 8th Int. Conf. on High-Energy Accelerators, CERN, Geneva, 1971, 501–504.

[2] E. J. Bleser, *Superconducting magnets for the CBA project*, Nucl. Instrum. Methods Phys. Res. **A235** (1985) 453–463 (see footnote on p. 435).

[3] *CBA Brookhaven colliding beam accelerator*, Newsletter 2 (Nov. 1982) 27–31.

[4] J. Billan et al., *The eight superconducting quadrupoles for the ISR high-luminosity insertion*, 11th Int. Conf. on High Energy Accelerators, CERN, Geneva, 1980. Birkhäuser, Basel (1980), pp. 848–852.

[5] G. Bon Mardion, G. Claudet, P. Seyfert, and J. Verdier, *Helium II in low-temperature and superconductive magnet engineering*, Adv. Cryo. Eng. **23** (1978) 358–362.

[6] R. Aymar, G. Claudet, C. Deck, R. Duthil, P. Genevey, C. Leloup, J. C. Lottin, J. Parrain, P. Seyfert, A. Torossian, and B. Turck, *Conceptual design of a superconducting tokamak: Torus II Supra*, IEEE Trans. Magn. **MAG15-1** (1979) 542–545.

[7] G. Claudet and R. Aymar, *Tore Supra and helium II cooling of large high-field magnets*, Adv. Cryo. Eng. **35A** (1990) 55–67.

[8] G. Claudet, F. Disdier, P. Lebrun, M. Morpurgo, and P. Weymuth, *Preliminary study of superfluid helium cryogenic system for the Large Hadron Collider*, Proc. ICFA Workshop on Superconducting Magnets and Cryogenics, Brookhaven National Laboratory, USA, 1986, BNL 52006, pp. 270–275.

[9] J. Casas Cubillos, A. Cyvoct, P. Lebrun, M. Marquet, L. Tavian, and R. van Weelderen, *Design concept and first experimental validation of the superfluid helium system for the Large Hadron Collider (LHC) project at CERN*, Cryogenics **32**(ICEC Suppl.) (1992) 118–121.

[10] *The LHC Design Report*, CERN-2004-003 (3 vols.) (June 2004).

[11] *ATLAS Technical Proposal*, CERN/LHCC/94-43, LHCC/P2 (Dec. 1994).

[12] *CMS Technical Proposal*, CERN-LHCC-94-38, LHCC/P2 (Dec. 1994).

[13] *LHCB Technical Proposal*, CERN-LHCC-98-4 (Feb. 1998).

[14] *Total cross section, elastic scattering and diffractive dissociation at the LHC*, CERN/LHCC 99-7 (Mar. 1999).

[15] *ALICE Technical Proposal*, CERN-LHCC-95-71 (Dec. 1995).

[16] E. Shaposhnikova, *Longitudinal beam parameters during acceleration in the LHC*, LHC Project Note 242.

[17] D. Boussard, W. Höfle, and T. Linnecar, *The LHC transverse damper (ADT) performance specification*, SL-Note-99-055.

[18] D. Boussard and T. Linnecar, *The LHC superconducting RF system*, Cryogenic Engineering and International Cryogenic Materials Conf., Montreal, Canada, July 1999, and LHC Project Report 316.

[19] D. Angal-Kalinin and L. Vos, *Coupled bunch instabilities in the LHC*, 8th European Particle Accelerator Conf., Paris, 2002.

[20] D. Brandt and L. Vos, *Resistive wall instability for the LHC: intermediate review*, LHC Project Report 257 (2001).

[21] K. Eggert, K. Honkavaara, and A. Morsh, *Luminosity considerations for the LHC*, LHC Note 263 (1994).

[22] O. Grobner, *The LHC vacuum system*, PAC'97, 1997, Vancouver, Canada.

[23] C. Benvenuti et al., *Vacuum properties of TiZrv non-evaporable getter films for the LHC vacuum system*, Vacuum **60** (2001) 57–65.

[24] P. Lebrun, *Superconductivity and cryogenics for the Large Hadron Collider*, CERN, LHC Project Report 441 (27 Oct. 2000).

2

The LHC machine: from beam commissioning to operation and future upgrades

Massimo GIOVANNOZZI

Beams Department, CERN, Geneva, Switzerland

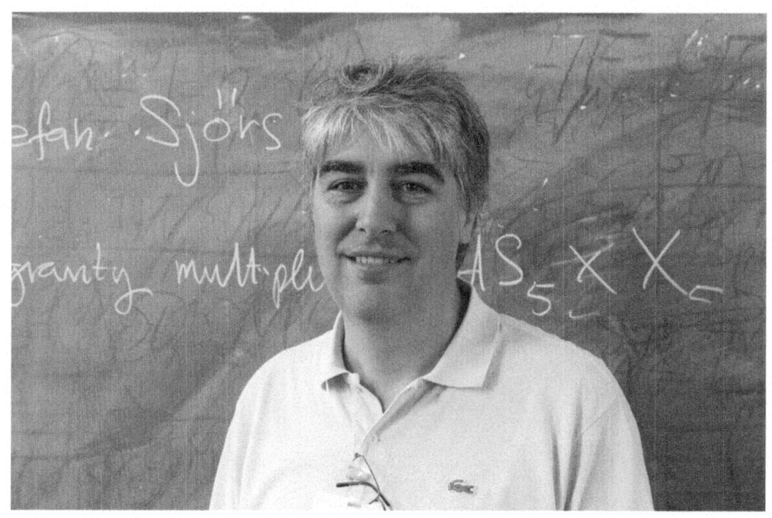

Chapter Contents

This chapter reports on the current status of the CERN Large Hadron Collider. General machine parameters are reviewed and the beam commissioning process is presented, showing the evolution of the performance over recent years. The highlights of the powerful complex of injectors is described, in order to provide a global picture of the impressive performance of CERN's flagship machine, relying on both the astonishing quality of the LHC itself and on the incredible flexibility of the injectors. The focus is on proton physics performance, with emphasis on the different possible scenarios leading to an upgrade of LHC performance. Finally, the future of the machine will be discussed briefly. The main reference on the LHC machine is [1] together with references cited therein. Here, a selection (possibly not complete, owing to the extent of the various topics presented) of additional publications is given for details.

The reader interested in lead ions will find the relevant information in [2–24].

2.1   LHC layout, parameters, and challenges

The LHC in a nutshell is a two-ring, high-energy, high-luminosity, pp collider [1, 25, 26]. The choice of the particles is imposed by the requirement of providing a very high luminosity L defined as

$$L = \frac{N_b^2\, M\, f_{\mathrm{rev}}\, \gamma_r}{4\,\pi\,\epsilon_n\,\beta^*}\, F,\qquad(2.1)$$

where N_b is the number of charges in each bunch, M is the number of bunches in each beam, f_{rev} is the revolution frequency, γ_r is the relativistic γ factor, $\epsilon_n = \beta_r \gamma_r \epsilon$ is the normalized rms beam emittance (β_r being the relativistic β factor), and β^* is the value of the beta function at the collision point. The so-called geometrical factor F takes into account the effect of a crossing angle at the interaction point (IP), which reduces the volume overlap between the two colliding bunches. It is expressed as

$$F = \frac{1}{\sqrt{1 + (\theta_c\, \sigma_z / 2\, \sigma^*)^2}},\qquad(2.2)$$

where θ_c is the value of the crossing angle at the IP, and σ_z and σ^* are the longitudinal and transverse rms beam sizes, respectively. It should be mentioned that (2.1) neglects the so-called hourglass effect, namely the change in volume overlap due to the variation of the beta function over the length of the colliding bunches. Such an effect is small for the LHC.

From the definition of the luminosity, several quantities can be varied in order to maximize L. The bunch charge is certainly one of those. If this approach is followed, then the use of antiprotons is immediately ruled out. These particles need to be produced artificially and this production rate is very low. Furthermore, since they are produced as secondary beams, the natural emittances are in general very large, thus leading to the generation of beams with rather low brightness.[1] To mitigate these

---

[1] The brightness is defined as the number of particles in unit volume of phase space.

drawbacks, complex beam manipulations, such as beam cooling (see [27] and references therein) and beam accumulation [28–34], would be required.

It is worth noting that this complex approach was used for the CERN Super Proton Synchrotron (SPS) at the time of the *pp* collider [35] and for the Fermilab Tevatron [36]. However, both colliders had luminosities much smaller than that required for the LHC.

The use of multibunch beams is another key way to increase L, and is therefore assumed in order to reach the nominal LHC performance.

The need to have a high-energy machine and the fact that its bending radius is imposed by the decision to re-use the tunnel of the former Lepton Positron (LEP) collider [37–39], immediately fixes the value of the magnetic field required to guide the charged particles along the nominal closed orbit. Such a field is beyond the reach of normal-conducting dipoles. Therefore, superconducting magnets had to be considered and are indeed at the heart of the whole machine. A comparison of the geometry of the LEP and LHC machines, including the required bending fields, is shown in Table 2.1.

The choice of the particles, namely protons for both beams, immediately imposes a requirement for two separate magnetic channels. In fact, counter-rotating beams of the same charge require opposite-sign magnetic bending fields, and opposite-sign focusing or defocusing magnetic fields as well. In turn, this choice imposes a challenge to the designers of the superconducting magnets: in order to fit into the limited size of the LEP tunnel, the two superconducting magnets need to share the same cryostat to save space. This leads to the so-called two-in-one design as seen in Fig. 2.1, with deep implications for the crosstalks between the fields in the two apertures and therefore for the technological challenges for the magnet design [40–42].

The LHC ring features an eightfold symmetry with eight arcs and eight long straight sections (LSS), in the middle of which the insertion region (IR) can be located (see Fig. 2.2). Four such IRs house the experiments: ATLAS (IR1), Alice (IR2), CMS (IR5), and LHCb (IR8). The remaining four IRs are dedicated to special machine systems, such as radiofrequency (RF) and beam instrumentation (IR4), beam dump (IR6), and collimation (IR3 for momentum and IR7 for betatron collimation). The experimental IRs 2 and 8 also house the injection systems for Beam 1 (IR2) and Beam 2 (IR8).[2]

As an example, the layout of IR1 is shown in Fig. 2.3. Starting from the left-hand side, the IP is visible, then three quadrupoles (Q1, Q2, and Q3) making the

Table 2.1 An overview of geometry and bending fields required for LEP and LHC

	LEP	LHC
Bending radius (m)	3096.175	2803.95
Momentum (GeV/c)	104	7000
B-field (T)	0.11	8.33

---

[2] Beam 1 is the clockwise beam, and Beam 2 is the counterclockwise beam.

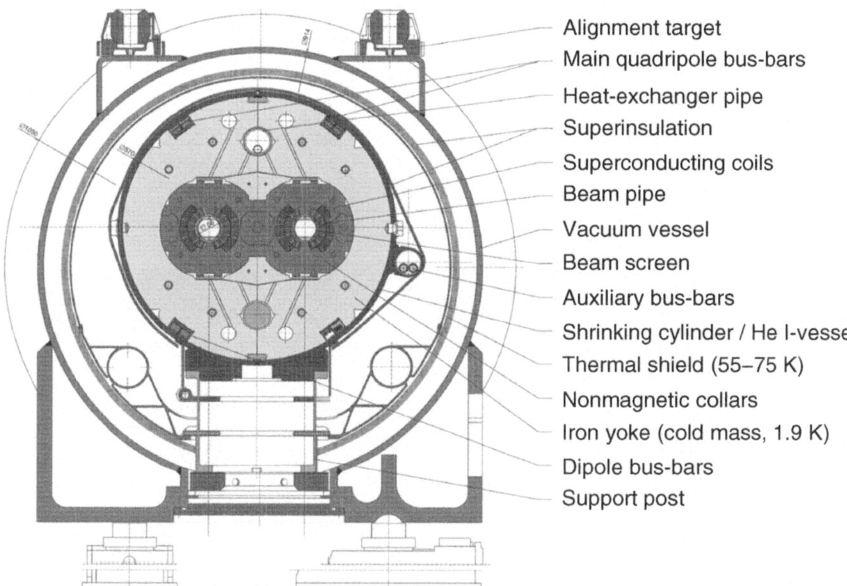

Fig. 2.1 Cross section of an LHC main superconducting dipole (Credit: CERN-LHC-PHO-2001-187).

inner triplet, i.e. the structure that provides the strong focusing required at the IP. Note that Q2 is split into two magnets, while Q1 and Q3 are each a single magnet. Then, moving towards the arc, one encounters the D1 separation dipole. It consists of six normal conducting magnets that start separating in the horizontal plane the two beams travelling in the same beam pipe. The angle imparted by D1 is cancelled by the D2 superconducting separation dipole, which brings the two beams to the nominal horizontal separation of 194 mm characteristics of the arc geometry.

Two absorbers are present in this region: the TAS protects the triplet quadrupoles from the debris generated at the collision point, while the TAN protects the D2 from the neutral particles that are not deflected by the magnets upstream. Finally, three quadrupoles (Q4, Q5, and Q6) provide the transition optics to the elements of the dispersion suppressor, before the continuous cryostat region at the quadrupole Q7.

Correspondingly, the optical parameters for the horizontal and vertical planes as well as the dispersion functions are plotted in Fig. 2.4 for injection (a) and collision (b) energy. For the injection case, β^* (i.e. the value of the beta function at the IP) is 11 m, while in the collision case, it is 0.55 m. Note the huge difference in the value of β_{max} (which is achieved in Q2) for the two configurations. The same layout is used for the other high-luminosity insertion in point 5.

The arcs are made of regular structures, the so-called FODO cells (see Fig. 2.5). Each such structure comprises six main dipoles and two main quadrupoles. This periodic structure provides the necessary bending and focusing strength, based on the principle of alternating gradient or strong focusing [43]. Furthermore, a complex

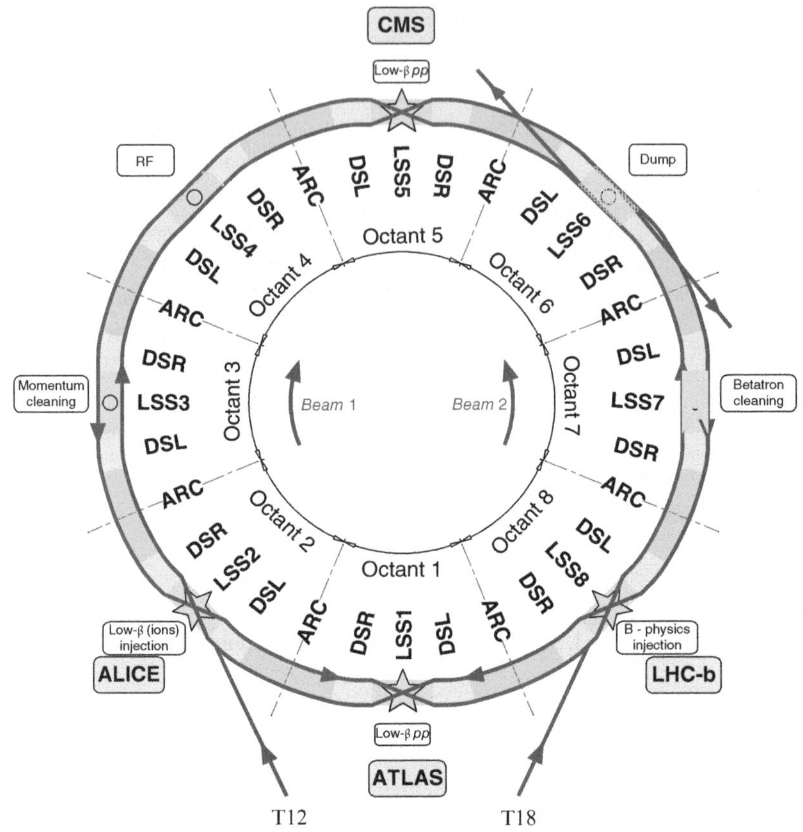

Fig. 2.2 Layout of the LHC ring. (Figure reproduced from [1], © 2004 CERN).

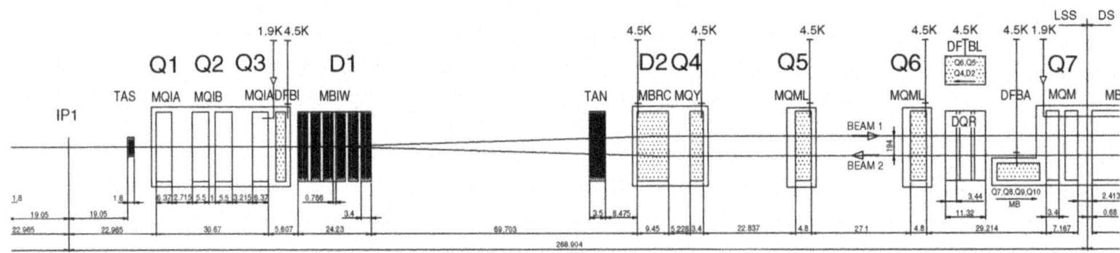

Fig. 2.3 Layout of the LHC high-luminosity IR1. (Figure reproduced from [1], © 2004 CERN).

system of correctors—the so-called spool pieces, which we small corrector magnets (sextupole, octupole, and decapole) installed at the extremities of the main dipoles— have been designed to provide the necessary compensation for the unavoidable field imperfections of the superconducting dipoles. Other sets of correctors are installed close to the main quadrupoles to correct tune (quadrupolar correctors), and linear

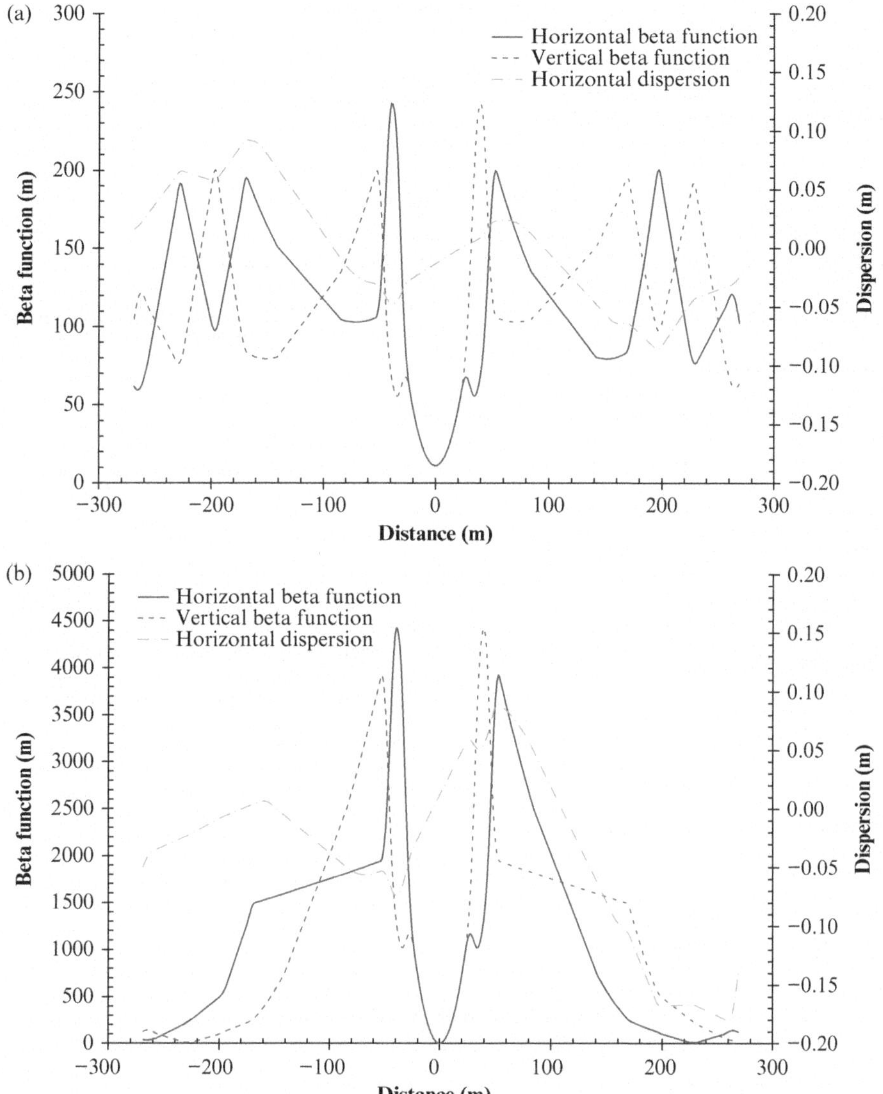

Fig. 2.4 Optical functions at injection (a) and at collision (b). The origin of the horizontal axis is the IP and the distance extends to the Q7 magnet (left/right of the IP).

coupling (skew quadrupolar correctors), and chromaticity (sextupole magnets), and to combat instabilities (octupole magnets).

A summary of the main beam parameters is presented in Table 2.2

The LHC machine is a real technological challenge [1, 44]. The heart of the machine, the system of superconducting magnets, is at the forefront of current technology, given

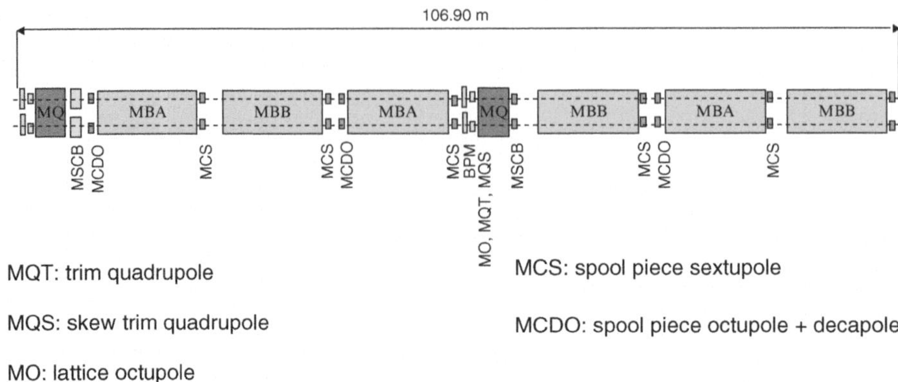

MQT: trim quadrupole

MQS: skew trim quadrupole

MO: lattice octupole

MSCB: sextupole (skew sextupole) + orbit corrector

MCS: spool piece sextupole

MCDO: spool piece octupole + decapole

Fig. 2.5 Layout of the LHC FODO cell. (Figure reproduced from [1], © 2004 CERN).

Table 2.2 Main parameters of the LHC machine

BEAM DATA	INJECTION	COLLISION
Proton energy (GeV)	450	7000
γ_r	479.6	7461
N_b	1.15×10^{11}	
M	2808	
Longitudinal emittance (eV s)	1.0	2.5
$\epsilon_n = \gamma_r \epsilon$ (μm rad)	3.5	3.75
Circulating beam current (A)	0.582	
Stored energy per beam (MJ)	23.3	362
Peak-luminosity-related data		
RMS bunch length (cm)	11.24	7.55
RMS beam size at IP1 and IP5 (μm)	375.2	16.7
Geometric reduction factor F		0.836
Peak luminosity in IP1 and IP5 (cm^{-2} s^{-1})		1.0×10^{34}
Peak luminosity per bunch crossing in IP1 and IP5 (cm^{-2} s^{-1})		3.56×10^{30}

the quality required for use in an accelerator application. Another challenge was the required transfer of the production of the entire ensemble of magnets to industry, as it was not possible to build them at the laboratory [45–47]. The quality assurance process was perfectly transferred to industry, so that the required standards were achieved without any drift in performance during production and with no systematic differences among the various manufacturers.

The superconducting magnets require a powerful cryogenic system, which was the first to be developed on the large scale required for the 27 km ring [48, 49]. The vacuum system, comprising three complete subsystems (for the beam vacuum, for the insulation vacuum of the magnets, and for the vacuum system in the cryogenic line), all reaching an unprecedented scale of complexity, should also be mentioned [50–52].

Last but not least, another key challenge is the machine protection system that is needed to deal with the stored energy in the magnets and in the beams [53–55]. In each main dipole, about 7 MJ are stored in the magnetic field, while the nominal beams store 362 MJ. In case of problems, such as the quench of a magnet or abnormal beam behaviour, the machine protection system is supposed to provide a safe means to dispose of the beam and to manage the resistive transition of the magnets without damaging the machine. For the first time in an accelerator project, fail-safe criteria had to be implemented in the design of several components in order to achieve the required level of protection and performance. The quench protection system (QPS) is a distributed system that provides the necessary protection against magnet quench [56–58], while the LHC beam dumping system (LBDS) [59] is located in IR6 and provides a safe way to dispose of the beams in case of problems.

In addition, the LHC machine is also a challenge in terms of beam physics [1]. A selection of the physical phenomena and processes that affect the proton beams and need to be kept under control to achieve the nominal performance are now briefly reviewed.

To achieve the required performance, tight control of the machine optics is mandatory. Failing this, the machine aperture would not be enough to ensure safe operation with the large values of β_{max} that are generated when β^* is squeezed down. This implies a detailed knowledge of the magnetic properties of the several families of normal and superconducting quadrupoles that control the machine's optics. This information was obtained thanks to a massive programme of magnetic measurements during the production and installation stage of the LHC ring [60, 61]. Further, the knowledge acquired had to be fully used in the control system. To this end, a magnetic model, the so-called field description of the LHC (FiDeL) was developed and successfully implemented during the beam commissioning stage and the ensuing operation [62–68]. In addition, powerful techniques have been developed to measure the machine's optics and perform corrections whenever necessary [69–72]. These techniques were extremely successful in correcting the β beating, i.e., the difference between the nominal and the measured optical parameters, to less than 10% [73], the target value being about 17%, i.e. a factor two better than estimated.

Unlike normally conducting magnets, whose field quality is determined by the pole shape profile, superconducting devices generate a magnetic field by shaping the current distribution. For technical reasons, it is not possible to achieve perfect field quality, and unavoidable perturbations are to be expected. If the usual expansion in multipoles is used,

$$B_y + iB_x = B_{\text{ref}} \sum_{n=1}^{\infty} (b_n + i\, a_n) \left(\frac{x + i\, y}{R_r} \right)^{n-1}, \qquad (2.3)$$

where $n = 1$ stands for a dipole field, a_n, b_n are the skew and normal components, respectively, R_r is a reference radius, and x, y stand for the horizontal and vertical coordinates, respectively, then superconducting dipoles have systematic b_3, b_5, b_7 components and quadrupoles b_6, b_{10}. These components require careful optimization as they introduce nonlinear effects in the beam dynamics, possibly inducing beam losses due to particles that are pushed to high amplitude by these effects. All this was studied in detail in the design phase by analytical estimates and massive numerical simulations. Specifications on the tolerable multipolar components were calculated [74] and imposed at the production level [75–80]. Corrector magnets (the spool pieces) were envisaged to minimize even the residual imperfections further. Finally, at the installation level, when the field quality of each magnet was known, the sorting algorithm devised earlier [81–84] was applied to provide the last optimization of the machine performance [85]. Thanks to these measures, both linear and nonlinear effects are not an issue in the current operational phase of the LHC [86].

The LHC superconducting magnets do not tolerate beam losses, as the lost protons will deposit energy in the magnets, leading to quenches. Therefore, tight control of beam loss is mandatory. Furthermore, the high-amplitude particles, forming the so-called primary halo, must be prevented from generating background problems in the experiments. In addition, passive protection of the machine aperture using the information from the beam loss monitors is necessary. These are the key functions of the powerful collimation system that is installed in the LHC [87–94]. To achieve the required performance, a multistage system was designed, in which a series of collimators of different materials, were used to intercept and absorb protons in the beam halo. In Fig. 2.6, the hierarchy of apertures of the various collimator stages is shown for injection (a) and collision (b) energies.[3]

It is worth pointing out that the aperture hierarchy is essential to ensuring the correct operation of the whole system, which in turn imposes very tight constraints on the machine reproducibility and stability. Furthermore, the choice of material for the collimators faces a dilemma: low-Z materials would be preferred in terms of robustness, but these materials are poor conductors and thus have a negative impact on the machine impedance [95–97]. The opposite occurs for high-Z materials. A tradeoff has been found using different materials for the various type of collimators (primary, secondary, etc.). A staged approach has been selected to profit from incremental improvement of the materials to increase the overall system performance. Two LHC insertions are devoted to the collimation system, with two separate functions: one to intercept particles with large momentum deviation (IR3) and a second to intercept

---

[3] The collimator aperture at top energy will be only a few millimetres.

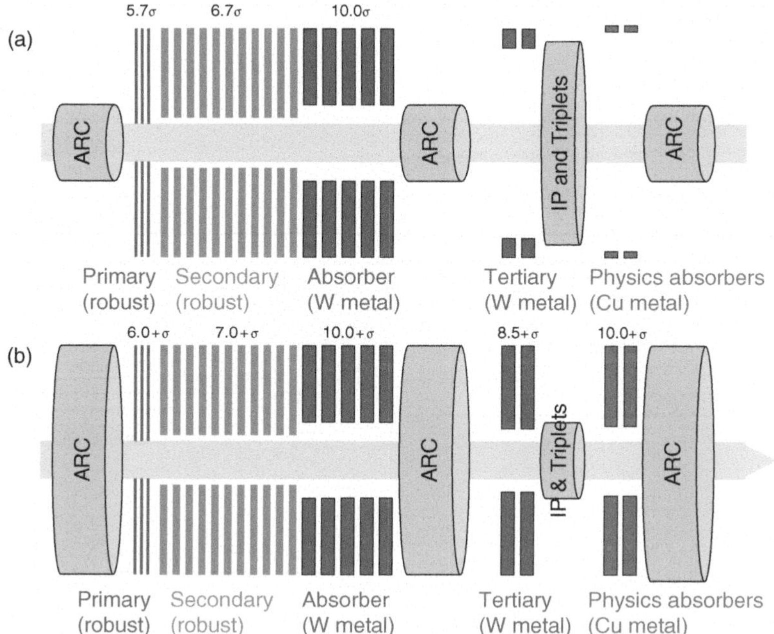

Fig. 2.6 Principle of the collimation system: hierarchy of the collimators aperture at injection (a) and collision (b) energies. (courtesy R. Assmann-CERN).

particles with large betatronic amplitude (IR7). These insertions thus provide the special optics that are required to ensure optimal system performance.

Another subtle effect is that of the so-called electron cloud [98–118]. The circulating proton beams are extracting electrons from the surface of the beam screen. Two different processes are involved: protons hitting the surface can extract electrons (this effect is dominant at lower energies); alternatively, synchrotron radiation can also extract electrons from the beam screen surface (this effect is dominant at higher energies). Furthermore, the subsequent proton bunches can accelerate the extracted electrons, which can then hit the surface and extract even more electrons in an avalanche phenomenon (see Fig. 2.7 (a)), provided that conditions on the bunch spacing are satisfied. The net result is to generate a standing cloud of electrons that reaches a saturation level (Fig. 2.7 (b)). The interaction of the cloud with the proton bunches can lead to strong deformation of the bunch structure (Fig. 2.7 (c)), eventually driving the beam to instability and generating emittance growth and/or beam losses. In both cases, this is detrimental to the luminosity of the LHC.

Mitigation measures had to be studied and implemented. They included the following: special coating of the warm regions with a special non-evaporable getter (NEG) [119] to reduce the secondary emission yield; reduction of the reflectivity of the beam screen surface by means of a sawtooth surface [1, 120]; installation of solenoids around the vacuum chambers to trap the low-energy electrons, preventing

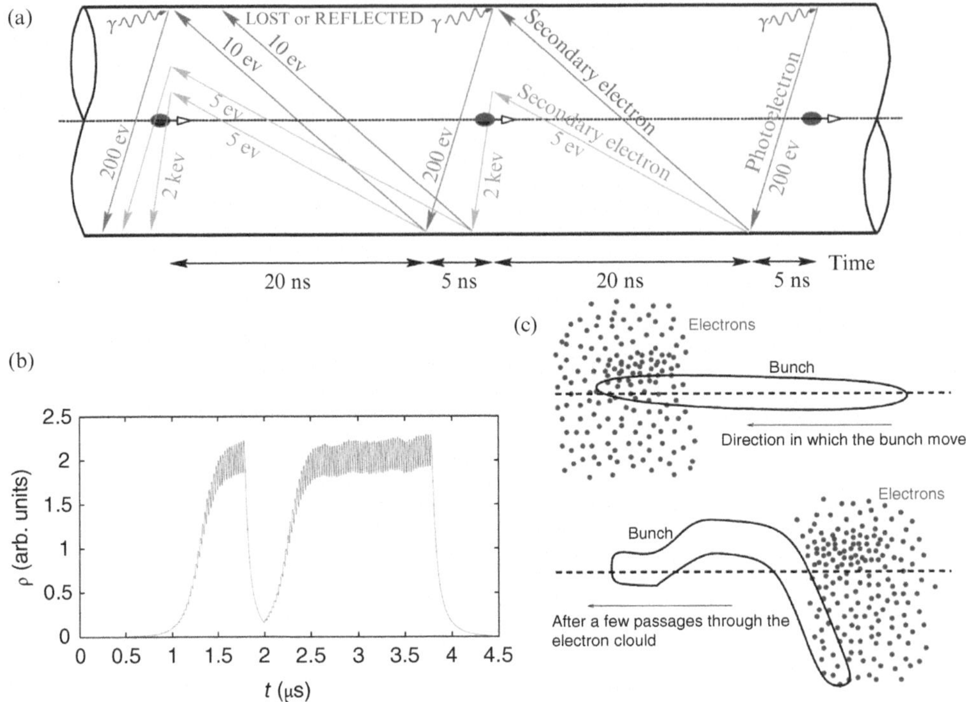

Fig. 2.7 (a) Principle of the electron cloud buildup. (courtesy F. Ruggiero-CERN) (b) Evolution of the electron cloud density due to the passage of two batches of 72 bunches each. (courtesy D. Schulte-CERN) (c) Interaction of the electron cloud with the proton bunch. (courtesy G. Rumolo-CERN).

the development of the avalanche phenomenon [121–126]; surface conditioning of the beam screen in the arcs by means of the cloud itself (beam scrubbing) [100, 118]. In the end, this is the only way of reducing the effect in the LHC arcs, even if it has the drawback of requiring beam time, which will be at the expense of time for the physics programme.

In general, collective effects, arising from the electromagnetic interaction of the beam particles among themselves, with their environment, and with the other beam, will ultimately limit the performance of the LHC [127–150]. Depending on the beam intensity and on the bunch filling pattern, they give rise to parasitic losses, can cause beam instabilities or degrade the beam quality by emittance growth, and can lead to poor lifetimes of all or some specific bunches. Intense efforts have been put into theoretical understanding, implementation of mitigation measures, and stabilization processes with the aim of preventing such harmful effects on beam quality. Currently, the LHC parameters are such that these effects are already appearing, and efforts are being devoted to the observation and the analysis of the detected behaviours with a view to improving machine performance.

2.2 Digression: the chain of proton injectors

The high-brightness proton beam required for the LHC [151] is generated by a chain of accelerators comprising a linac and three synchrotrons. Their performance has been pushed to serve the LHC, and upgrades have been implemented over the years [152, 153]. The travel through the chain of accelerators starts from a hydrogen bottle providing the protons by ionizing the gas. Next, the particles are accelerated by Linac 2 up to a kinetic energy of 50 MeV. Protons are then transferred to the Proton Synchrotron Booster (PSB) [154], which brings them to 1.4 GeV kinetic energy. The extraction energy has been upgraded twice since the construction of this machine, namely from the original value of 800 MeV to 1 GeV and then to 1.4 GeV in order to mitigate space-charge issues for the special beams required by the LHC. The PSB is made of four superimposed rings stacked vertically, as can be seen in Fig. 2.8.

The linac beam has to be deflected in order to fill the four rings. Similarly, the PSB bunches need to be merged back in the vertical plane when extracted towards the Proton Synchrotron (PS) (for a recent account of this machine, see [155] and references therein). This ring accelerates the protons up to 26 GeV total energy and plays a key role in the generation of the longitudinal properties of the bunches for the LHC. In fact, the bunch length and bunch spacing at extraction from the PSB and injection in the PS cannot fulfil the LHC requirements, since these would exceed the space-charge limits tolerable. Therefore, only six bunches are injected, leaving one empty bucket. These bunches, which are much more intense than a single LHC bunch and are also much longer, are then split in the longitudinal plane by means of a complex RF gymnastic [156].[4] At injection, each single bunch is split into three, while at top energy, two double splittings are applied, such that 12 bunches are produced out of one injected bunch (see Fig. 2.9(a)). The spacing is also the nominal, namely 25 ns. The evolution of the longitudinal bunch profile during a triple splitting is shown in Fig. 2.9(b).

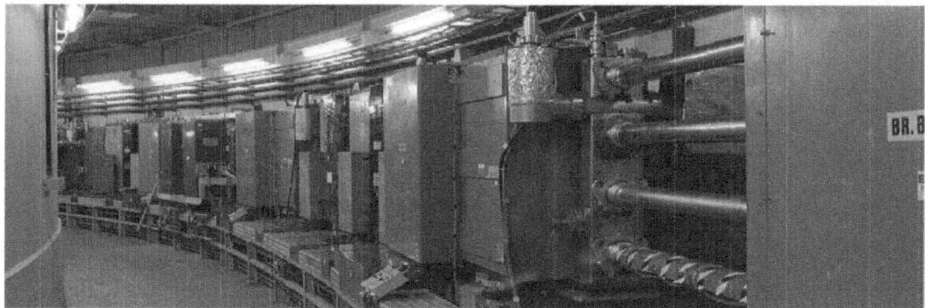

Fig. 2.8 The PS-Booster, showing the four superimposed rings. (Credit: CERN-PHOTO-201405-098).

---

[4] Note that in parallel with the development of these new techniques, another essential tool was developed, namely the tomographic reconstruction of the longitudinal phase space [157, 158], which is currently used in daily operation to monitor the quality of the LHC beams produced by the PS machine.

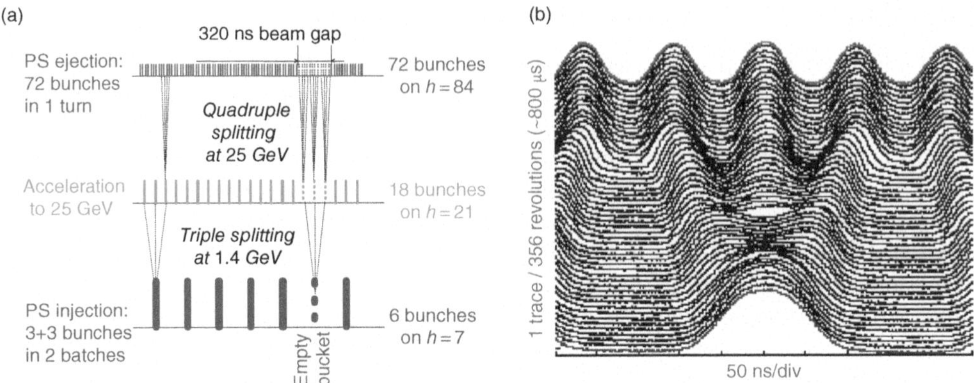

Fig. 2.9 Principle of the longitudinal bunch splitting performed in the PS ring. The sequence of triple and double splittings is shown (a), together with the evolution of the longitudinal profile of one bunch during the triple splitting (b). The various traces represent the time evolution (from bottom to top) of the bunch profile during splitting. (courtesy R. Garoby-CERN).

The traces represent the bunch profile at different times (from bottom to top) and the generation of three bunches out of a single Gaussian is clearly visible. The net result is the production of a batch of 72 bunches. It is clear that by cleverly combining double and triple splitting, it is possible to generate different bunch spacings at extraction from the PS. For instance, the 50 ns bunch spacing variant of the LHC beam, which is currently being used for physics, is derived from the nominal scheme by simply inhibiting the last double splitting at the flat top. The groups of 72 PS bunches are then transferred to the Super Proton Synchrotron (SPS) [159] before the final acceleration towards the LHC injection. The PS batches are injected in the SPS in sequences of two, three, or four, and these will be properly placed in the LHC buckets in order to provide the desired collision schemes in the four LHC experiments.

2.3   Proton beam commissioning and operation

The beam commissioning of the LHC machine started as early as August 2008,[5] even before the rings were completely ready for beam. The first step was a series of injection tests, in which single-bunch beams were transferred from the SPS to the injection lines into the LHC and through the sectors already connected to the injection points and ready to receive beams. These tests were essential to the full preparation for the beam, and allowed a number of crucial tests to be made, such as magnet alignment, mechanical aperture verification, and (what should never be underestimated) polarity tests for the different magnet families [162–175].

The official day for establishing circulating beam was 10 September 2008, and in a few hours both beams were circulating with a good lifetime of a few hours.

---

[5] The hardware commissioning of the rings had already started before that date [160, 161].

Unfortunately, such a bright start was abruptly stopped by the event that occurred on 19 September, which caused severe damage to several magnets in Sector 3–4. A hectic period of analysis to identify the cause and to define the appropriate repair and mitigation measures started, and the machine was back in operation just over a year later [170]. In November 2009, two beams were again circulating in the machine and accelerated to 1.18 TeV, which was at that time a record energy for a particle accelerator.

After the usual winter stop, during which additional tests were performed to permit safe operation at even higher energies, the LHC was restarted, and on 30 March 2009, the first collisions at 3.5 TeV took place. This event marks the beginning of a period of operation intertwined with beam commissioning. The strategy was based on a gradual increase of the beam power, with periods of performance levelling to provide time to study the machine behaviour in the new conditions, before moving on to the next milestone. Also, in order to simplify as much as possible the control of the machine and avoid problems, only one beam parameter was changed at a time. The official goal for the year 2010 was set so as to reach a luminosity of 1×10^{32} cm^{-2} s^{-1} [176–178]. Such a value corresponds to only 1% of the nominal value. Nevertheless, it implies a stored beam energy of 30 MJ, while beforehand the machine was operated with only 0.17 MJ and the Tevatron was operating at 2 MJ level. Initially, the bunch intensity was increased, with only a limited number of bunches, in order to avoid complications due to the needs of the crossing schemes. Also, the value of β^* was reduced, thus leading to an exploration of the uncharted territory of dynamic change of the optics in the experimental insertions.

In the second part of the year, during August/September 2010, it was decided to start the commissioning of bunch trains. A bunch train is a sequence of bunches with a constant bunch spacing and undergoing the same beam–beam effects. This strategy implied that once the potential physical issues were solved for a single bunch train, the addition of more trains would be rather straightforward, thus allowing a faster pace in the improvement of the machine performance. This stage in the beam commissioning is visible in the plateau in Fig. 2.10(a). The performance ramp-up following the successful completion of this phase is impressive and clearly seen in Fig. 2.10(b) in which the evolution of the peak luminosity is plotted for the entire year.

For the year 2011 [179–182], the performance goal was set in terms of the integrated luminosity, namely 1 fb^{-1}. To achieve this result, several improvements had to be implemented. First, the bunch spacing had to be reduced to 50 ns from 150 ns used at the end of 2010. Then the bunch intensity had to be pushed, and, finally, the β^* decreased to 1 m. The machine performance, in terms of turnaround and availability, was such that it was possible to reach the goal for the year by June (see Fig. 2.11(a)). Overall, the total integrated luminosity for 2010 exceeded 5.5 fb^{-1}.

The situation for the year 2012 foresaw a goal of around 15 fb^{-1}, requiring an even smaller β^*, larger intensity per bunch, and, also, a higher collision energy. The evolution of the peak luminosity in the first half of 2012 is shown in Fig. 2.11(b).

All these changes allowed peak luminosities in excess of 0.65×10^{34} cm^{-2} s^{-1} to be reached, as can be seen in Fig. 2.12, where the evolution of the instantaneous luminosity of a typical fill is shown.

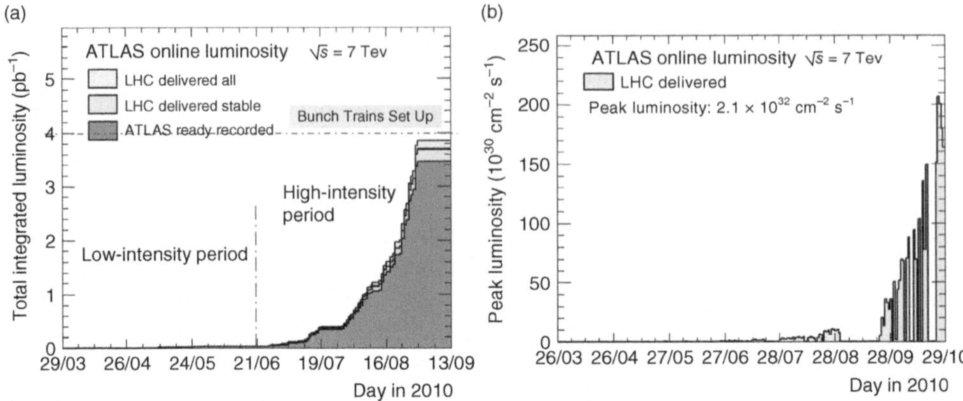

Fig. 2.10 (a) Evolution of the integrated luminosity in the first period of 2010. The flat part of the distribution in August/September corresponds to the setting up of the bunch trains. (b) Overall evolution of the peak intensity in 2010. The goal for 2010 is achieved at the end of the year. The dramatic increase in luminosity due to the introduction of the bunch trains is clearly visible.

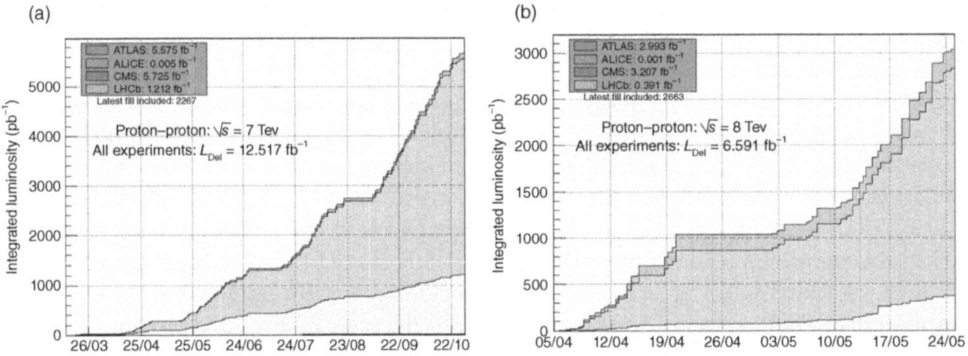

Fig. 2.11 (a) Evolution of the peak luminosity in 2011. The goal for 2011 of 1 fb^{-1} was achieved in June, and the total delivered luminosity reached more than 5.5 fb^{-1} for ATLAS and CMS. (b) Evolution of the peak luminosity for the first part of the year 2012.

For reference, the main beam and optical parameters for the years 2011 and 2012 are listed in Table 2.3, together with the corresponding nominal values. The table indicates that a number of parameters are below the nominal value (e.g. energy, β^*, number of bunches, and factor F), which explains why the nominal value of the luminosity has not yet been achieved. Nevertheless, some other parameters are well beyond their nominal value, as is the case for the beam emittance and the bunch intensity, which explains why the luminosity is already at two-thirds of the nominal value. It should be stressed that the higher bunch charge and smaller emittance are a result of

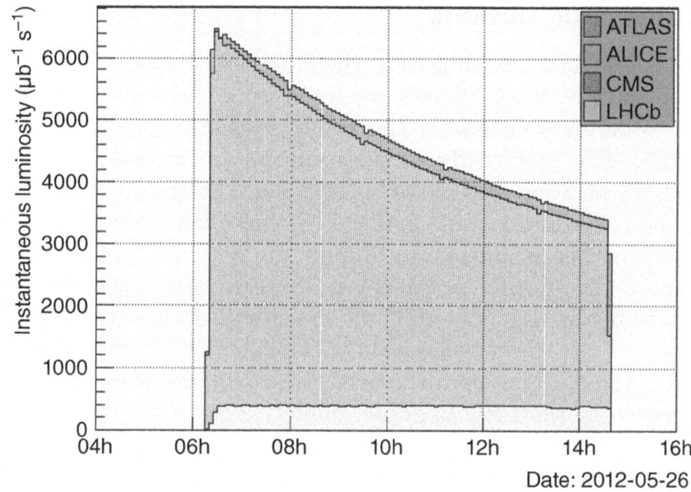

Fig. 2.12 Evolution of the peak luminosity during Fill 2669. During this fill, about 130 pb^{-1} were collected for ATLAS and CMS. The instantaneous luminosity for LHCb does not feature the characteristic decay, because of a levelling procedure applied (see later).

Table 2.3 Main beam and optical parameters of the LHC machine for the nominal case and for the 2011 and 2012 physics runs

	LHC NOMINAL	2011	2012
Proton energy (TeV)	7.0	3.5	4.0
Number of bunches	2808	1380	1380
Bunch spacing (ns)	25	50	50
N_b (10^{11})	1.15	1.4	1.5–1.6
$\epsilon_n = \gamma_r \epsilon$ (μm)	3.75	2.5	2.5
β^* (cm)	55	100	60
Factor F	0.84	0.91	0.81
Peak luminosity (10^{34})	1.0	0.32	0.6–0.7
Number of events/crossing	25	16	32

the gymnastics used to generate the beam in the injectors and, in particular, in the PSB and PS. The flexibility to achieve better-than-nominal beam parameters is available only for the 50 ns bunch spacing, but is almost completely lost for the nominal 25 ns case. The price to pay for the increased bunch charge and very large current peak luminosity is the higher-than-nominal number of events per crossing, which are challenging the experimental apparatus, even if, for the time being, these values are still acceptable.

2.4   Future upgrade options

The complexity of the LHC machine and the long time between the first studies and the construction and operation phases triggered very early questions about possible upgrade options (for an overview of the topic, see [183] and references therein, as well as [184–188]). The first study of these options dates back to 2002 [189]. The rationale behind the strategy presented then is that the triplet magnets have a finite lifetime due to the radiation damage induced by the collision debris. Therefore, rather than simply replacing the magnets, one should aim at improving the overall machine performance. Later on, another argument was taken into account, namely that the nominal LHC parameters might be difficult to achieve. Hence, one of the goals of the upgrade might have been the consolidation of the machine in view of achieving or even slightly surpassing the nominal performance. These considerations led to the definition of a staged approach to the LHC upgrade, namely a so-called Phase 1 upgrade [190], aimed at a modest increase in machine performance (a factor of 2–3 with respect to the nominal in terms of peak luminosity, i.e. $(2-3) \times 10^{34}$ cm^{-2} s^{-1}); then a Phase 2 [191] aiming at a vigorous upgrade (a factor of 10 with respect to the nominal performance, i.e. 10^{35} cm^{-2} s^{-1}). This second upgrade should be carried out in parallel with an upgrade of the experiment detectors.

Additional boundary conditions set for the Phase 1 upgrade consisted of limiting the changes to the machine layout to the strict minimum, i.e. the triplets. The studies performed [192–194] showed that the minimum β^* achievable would be about 30 cm. However, a number of serious limitations, essentially in terms of mechanical aperture leading to beam aperture bottlenecks, arose from the parts of the machine that were not to be upgraded. Furthermore, the smaller-than-nominal β^* called for improved corrections of the chromatic aberrations in order to avoid too strong a dependence of the optical parameters on the momentum offset of the particles. This resulted in an over-constrained optical configuration with hardly any flexibility for realistic operational conditions.

In addition, the strategy based on two upgrades was critically reviewed in light of the experience with previous machines, such as HERA [195, 196] and the Tevatron [197, 198]. In the evaluation of the performance reach, the stop due to the implementation of the upgrade and the following period of beam re-commissioning was compared with the alternative of continuous operation of the existing machine. The outcome of the analysis was that the optimal scenario should envisage only one upgrade of the LHC machine.

Furthermore, in 2010, a critical review of the performance of the LHC injectors was carried out, to identify improvements of the existing machines in terms of continued consolidation and, possibly, some additional upgrade [199], but without considering building new machines as in the standard scenario considered until then (for additional details, see e.g. [200–203]).

Therefore, by mid 2010, the CERN strategy was redefined. Three projects were defined: a high-luminosity LHC upgrade (HL-LHC); an LHC injectors upgrade project (LIU); are a consolidation project to ensure the reliable functioning of the CERN accelerators over a timescale of 25 years.

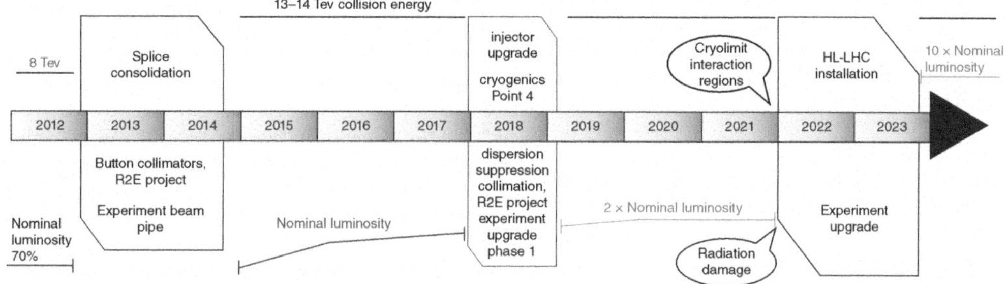

Fig. 2.13 Timeline of the HL-LHC and LIU projects over 10 years as defined in 2010 and reviewed in 2011. (courtesy L. Rossi-CERN).

The timeline of these projects was defined in the framework of a 10-year planning of CERN activities, including periods of long stops for the implementation of the various upgrades approved. The overall scheme is shown in Fig. 2.13, and even if some details might change, and shifts in time are possible, the overall picture is not likely to change.

In this schedule, the installation date for HL-LHC matches very well what is obtained by considerations based on the time required to half the statistical error of the physical results (the so-called halving-time) [183].

The goals of the HL-LHC project are twofold [183]:

- an instantaneous luminosity of 5×10^{34} cm^{-2} s^{-1} with levelling;
- an integrated luminosity of about 250 fb^{-1} per year, reaching 3000 fb^{-1} in 12 years.

Even if the first goal is rather conservative, one should consider that for the first time the performance reach is not specified in terms of peak luminosity, but rather in terms of *levelled* luminosity. This means that the upgrade is based on techniques that allow the luminosity to be kept constant over a period of time, while the intensity is decreasing because of the proton burn-off. This in turn implies that the peak luminosity that is virtually required to reach such a levelled luminosity is much higher. To level the luminosity, there are essentially three possibilities:

- Vary the transverse separation of the beams. This requires precise control of the magnets generating the separation scheme. It is routinely done for the LHCb experiment (see Fig. 2.12).
- Vary the crossing angle. This can be achieved either by controlling the magnets generating the crossing angle or by using the so-called crab cavities [204–211], which are RF devices that provide a transverse kick that varies according to the longitudinal position in the bunch. These devices are part of the baseline of the HL-LHC project because they also restore the head-on collision and hence cancel the effect of the crossing angle affecting the geometrical factor F without altering the beam–beam separation in the common pipe region. Therefore, no additional aperture is needed to accommodate the initial large crossing angle.

Such a large aperture would be required if orbit correctors were to be used instead. A mitigation of this problem can be achieved with transversely elliptical beams, also called *flat beams*.

- Vary β^*. This requires precise control of the optics and orbit, but no additional beam aperture is required with respect to the case of β^* squeezed down to the minimum possible value. It has never been used routinely in any of the colliders built so far.

It is clear that to achieve higher luminosity, the injectors also need to be upgraded. The usual approach consists of reducing β^*, but, unlike Phase 1, the constraint of replacing only the triplets has been removed and the layout of the high-luminosity insertions can now be reviewed. The constraint imposed by the chromatic aberrations remains. To overcome it, a novel optics concept has been developed [212–214] and has notably been already successfully tested in the current machine [215].

In spite of this very encouraging step, many challenges remain, including a few in the domain of beam dynamics, beam–beam, and collective effects in these high-power beams and the collimation system performance.

The technological challenges should not be underestimated. It is planned to build the new triplet quadrupoles using Nb_3Sn superconductors. These devices have never achieved, as yet, the quality required for accelerator applications, which means that a vigorous R&D programme is needed to meet the standards for HL-LHC [216].

Taking advantage of the LHC, as currently operating, an intensive programme of experiments have been planned in order to probe, wherever possible, some of the conditions foreseen for the HL-LHC.

For reference, a list of possible beam parameters for the upgrade are reported in Table 2.4 (see also Refs. [217, 218]). The baseline consists of the 25 ns option, with 50 ns as a backup scenario since, for a given luminosity, the pile-up is doubled for this option. It is worth emphasizing the enormous effect of the geometrical factor F generated by the crossing angle required to control the beam–beam effects. This explains why crab cavities are an essential ingredient for HL-LHC, since they allow efficient use of the protons stored in the machine.

On a longer timescale, two other upgrade scenarios are being considered. One is focused on an energy upgrade of the LHC (HE-LHC) [219–221]. A target energy of 16.5 TeV, corresponding to 20 T main dipole magnets, is the key parameter. At such an energy, the beam dynamics will be dominated by synchrotron radiation, even for protons. This would have a strong impact not only on the dynamics, but also on the cooling system, and synchrotron radiation damage must be seriously considered. It would also require a new LHC injector, delivering protons to the HE-LHC at 1 TeV.

We conclude by mentioning that a second scenario exists, focusing on lepton–proton collisions (LHeC) [222–232], as was done in the HERA machine. Two options have been considered: a ring–ring and a linac–ring. The first envisages a second ring being installed in the LHC tunnel for circulating the electron beam. This option is technically relatively straightforward, even if it requires additional bypasses around the existing experiments for the HL-LHC, together with challenging installation work in the environment of an operating accelerator infrastructure. The second configuration

Table 2.4 Main beam and optical parameters of the nominal LHC and HL-LHC. The peak luminosity for the HL-LHC options has to be considered as the levelled value of the luminosity

	LHC NOMINAL 25 ns	HL-LHC 25 ns	HL-LHC 50 ns
Number of bunches	2808	2808	1404
N_b (10^{11})	1.15	2.0	3.3
Beam current (A)	0.58	1.01	0.83
σ_z (cm)	7.5	7.5	7.5
$\epsilon_n = \gamma_r \epsilon$ $(\mu\mathrm{m})$	3.75	2.5	3.0
β^* (cm)	55	15	15
Factor F	0.84	0.30	0.33
Peak luminosity (10^{34})	1.0	6.0	7.4
Virtual luminosity (10^{34})	1.2	20.0	22.7
Number of events/crossing	25	123	247

foresees the construction of a new linear accelerator for the electron beam acceleration that intersects with the LHC machine in IP2. Several options have been considered for this linear accelerator: pulsed linac, recirculating linac, and energy-recovery linac (ERL) configurations. The energy of the electrons would be 60 GeV for both options. Recently, a panel of experts reviewed both options described in the conceptual design report and stressed that the first is less favourable than the second and will therefore be abandoned.

Acknowledgments

It goes without saying that the achievements reported in this chapter are the result of the joint efforts of several people at CERN and elsewhere. In particular, I would like to express my warm thank yous to all colleagues of the Accelerator Physics Group and of the Operations Group for several discussions and for material used in the preparation of this chapter. My warmest thanks go to E. McIntosh for invaluable comments on the original version of the manuscript.

References

[1] Brüning, O. S., et al. (eds.), "LHC Design Report, v. 1: the LHC Main Ring", CERN-2004-003-V-1, 2004.

[2] Haseroth, H., et al., "Feasibility study concerning a possible layout for a lead-ion injection for the CERN accelerator complex", CERN-PS-87-28-LI, 1987.

[3] Haseroth, H., "Planning and proposals for the CERN heavy ion injector", CERN-PS-88-51-DL, 1988.

[4] Haseroth, H., (ed.), "Concept for a lead-ion accelerating facility at CERN", CERN-90-01, 1990.

[5] Brandt, D., et al., "High intensity options for the CERN heavy ion programme", CERN-PS-90-20-DI, 1990.

[6] Haseroth, H., "A heavy ion injector at CERN", CERN-PS-90-63-DI, 1990.

[7] Haseroth, H., "The CERN heavy ion program", CERN-PS-90-76-DI, 1990.

[8] Warner, D., et al. (eds.), "CERN heavy ion facility design report", CERN 93-01, 1993.

[9] Haseroth, H., "The CERN heavy ion accelerating facility", CERN-PS-95-026, 1995.

[10] Blas, F., et al., "Acceleration of lead ions in the CERN PS booster and the CERN PS", CERN-PS-95-027 HI, 1995.

[11] Haseroth, H., "Pb injector at CERN", CERN-PS-96-051, 1996.

[12] Benedikt, M., et al. (eds.), "LHC Design Report, v. 3: the LHC injector chain", CERN-2004-003-V-3, 2004.

[13] Beuret, A., et al., "The LHC lead injector chain", LHC-Project-Report-776, 2004.

[14] Maury, S., et al., "Ions for LHC: beam physics and engineering challenges", LHC-Project-Report-848, 2005.

[15] Manglunki, D., et al., "Ions for LHC: status of the injector chain", CERN-AB-2007-012, 2007.

[16] Manglunki, D., et al., "Ions for LHC: towards completion of the injector chain", CERN-AB-2008-058, 2008.

[17] Jowett, J., "The LHC as a nucleus–nucleus collider", J. Phys. G: Nucl. Part. Phys. **35**, 104028, 2008.

[18] Bruce, R., et al., "Measurements of heavy ion beam losses from collimation", Phys. Rev. ST Accel. Beams **12**, 011001, 2009.

[19] Bruce, R., et al., "Beam losses from ultra-peripheral nuclear collisions between Pb ions in the Large Hadron Collider and their alleviation", Phys. Rev. ST Accel. Beams **12**, 071002, 2009.

[20] Bruce, R., et al., "Time evolution of the luminosity of colliding heavy-ion beams in BNL Relativistic Heavy Ion Collider and CERN Large Hadron Collider", Phys. Rev. ST Accel. Beams **13**, 091001, 2010.

[21] Manglunki, D., et al., "Ions for LHC: performance of the injector chain", CERN-ATS-2011-050, 2011.

[22] Jowett, J., "Facilities for the energy frontier of nuclear physics", J. Phys. Conf. Ser. **312**, 102017, 2011.

[23] Salgado, C. A., et al. (eds.), "Proton–nucleus collisions at the LHC: scientific opportunities and requirements", J. Phys. G: Nucl. Part. Phys. **39**, 015010, 2012.

[24] Manglunki, D., et al., "Performance of the CERN heavy ion production complex", CERN-ATS-2012-104, 2012.

[25] Evans, L., "The Large Hadron Collider from conception to commissioning: a personal recollection", Rev. Accel. Sci. Technol. **3**, 261, 2010.

[26] Evans, L., "The Large Hadron Collider", Phil. Trans. R. Soc. Loud. **A370**, 831, 2012.

[27] Parkhomchuk, V. V. and Skrinsky, A. N., "Cooling methods for charged particle beams", Rev. Accel. Sci. Technol. **1**, 237, 2008.

[28] Autin, B., et al., "Beam optics studies on the antiproton accumulator", IEEE Trans. Nucl. Sci. **28**, 2055, 1981.

[29] Johnson, R., "Measuring and manipulating an accumulated stack of antiprotons in the CERN antiproton accumulator", IEEE Trans. Nucl. Sci. **30**, 2123, 1983.

[30] Wilson, E. J. N., et al. (eds.), "Design study of an antiproton collector for the antiproton accumulator (ACOL)", CERN-83-10, 1983.

[31] van der Meer, S., "Stochastic cooling and the accumulation of antiprotons", Rev. Mod. Phys. **57**, 689, 1985.

[32] Autin, B., et al., "Performance of the CERN antiproton accumulator complex", CERN-PS-88-43-AR, 1988.

[33] Bharadwaj, V., et al., "Operation of the Fermilab accumulator for medium-energy proton anti-proton physics", in Proceedings of 2nd European Particle Accelerator Conference (ed. Marin P. and Mandrillon, P., Gif-sur-Yvette, France, Editions Frontères), 617, 1991.

[34] Lebedev, V., "Antiproton production and accumulation", in Proceedings of International Workshop on Beam Cooling and Related Topics (COOL07) (ed. Hasse, R.W. and Schaa, V.R.W., Darmstadt, GSI), 255, 2007.

[35] Koziol, H. and Möhl, D., "The CERN antiproton collider programme: accelerators and accumulation rings", Phys. Rep. **403/404**, 91, 2004.

[36] TeVI Group, "Design report Tevatron 1 project", FERMILAB-DESIGN-1984-01, 1984.

[37] The LEP Injector Study Group, "LEP design report, v. 1: the LEP injector chain", CERN-LEP-TH-83-29, CERN-PS-DL-83-31, CERN-SPS-83-26, LAL-RT-83-09,1983.

[38] "LEP design report, v. 2: The LEP main ring", CERN-LEP-84-01, 1984.

[39] Wyss, C., et al. (eds.), "LEP design report, v. 3: LEP2", CERN-AC-96-01-LEP-2, 1996.

[40] Fessia, P., et al., "Selection of the cross-section design for the LHC main dipole", IEEE Trans. Appl. Supercond. **10**, 65, 2000.

[41] Rossi, L., "State-of-the-art superconducting accelerator magnets", IEEE Trans. Appl. Supercond. **12**, 219, 2002.

[42] Tollestrup, A. and Todesco, E., "The development of superconducting magnets for use in particle accelerators: from the Tevatron to the LHC", Rev. Accel. Sci. Technol. **1**, 185, 2008.

[43] Courant, E. D. and Snyder, H. S., "Theory of the alternating-gradient synchrotron", Ann. Phys. (NY) **3**, 1, 1958.

[44] Evans, L. (ed.), "The Large Hadron Collider: A Marvel of Technology", EPFL Press, Lausanne, 2009.

[45] Rossi, L., "The LHC main dipoles and quadrupoles toward series production", IEEE Trans. Appl. Supercond. **13**, 1221, 2003.

[46] Rossi, L., "Experience with LHC magnets from prototyping to large scale industrial production and integration", CERN-LHC-Project-Report-730, 2004.

[47] Savary, F., et al., "Description of the main features of the series production of the LHC main dipole magnets", IEEE Trans. Appl. Supercond. **18**, 220, 2008.

[48] Benda, V., et al., "Conceptual design of the cryogenic system for the Large Hadron Collider (LHC)", LHC-Project-Report-12, 1996.

[49] Claudet, S., et al., "Exergy analysis of the cryogenic helium distribution system for the Large Hadron Collider (LHC)", AIP Conf. Proc. **1218**, 1267, 2010.

[50] Gröbner, O., "Vacuum system for LHC", CERN-AT-94-35-VA, LHC-NOTE-290, 1994.

[51] Gröbner, O., "Overview of the LHC vacuum system", Vacuum **60**, 25, 2001.

[52] Jiménez, J. M., "LHC: The world's largest vacuum systems being operated at CERN", Vacuum **84**, 2, 2009.

[53] Bordry, F., et al., "Machine protection for the LHC: architecture of the beam and powering interlock systems", LHC-Project-Report-521, 2001.

[54] Schmidt, R. and Wenninger, J., "Machine protection issues and strategies for the LHC", LHC-Project-Report-784, 2004.

[55] Assmann, R., et al., "First operational experience with the LHC machine protection system when operating with beam energies beyond the 100 MJ range", CERN-ATS-2012-203, 2012.

[56] Coull, L., et al., "LHC magnet quench protection system", CERN-AT-93-42-MA, LHC-NOTE-251, 1994.

[57] Fernández, A. V. and Rodríguez-Mateos, F., "Reliability of the quench protection system for the LHC superconducting elements", Nucl. Instrum. Methods Phys. Res. **A525**, 439, 2004.

[58] Formenti, F., et al., "Upgrade of the quench protection systems for the superconducting circuits of the LHC Machine at CERN: from concept and design to the first operational experience", CERN-ATS-2010-129, 2010.

[59] Goddard, B., "The LHC injection and beam dumping systems", CERN-LHC-Project-Report-672, 99, 2003.

[60] Walckiers, L., et al., "Towards series measurements of the LHC superconducting dipole magnets", in Proceedings of 17th Particle Accelerator Conference (ed. Comyn, M., et al., IEEE, Piscataway, NJ), 3377, 1998.

[61] Bottura, L., et al., "A strategy for sampling the field quality of the LHC dipoles", CERN-LHC-Project-Report-737, 2004.

[62] Sammut, N., et al., "Mathematical formulation to predict the harmonics of the superconducting Large Hadron Collider magnets", Phys. Rev. ST Accel. Beams **9**, 012402, 2006.

[63] Sammut, N., et al., "Mathematical formulation to predict the harmonics of the superconducting Large Hadron Collider magnets. II. Dynamic field changes and scaling laws", Phys. Rev. ST Accel. Beams **10**, 082802, 2007.

[64] Sammut, N., et al., "Mathematical formulation to predict the harmonics of the superconducting Large Hadron Collider magnets: III. Precycle ramp rate effects and magnet characterization", Phys. Rev. ST Accel. Beams **12**, 102401, 2009.

[65] Bottura, L., et al., "First field test of FiDeL: the magnetic field description for the LHC", CERN-ATS-2009-010, 2010.

[66] Todesco, E., et al., "The magnetic model of the LHC in the early phase of beam commissioning", CERN-ATS-2010-154, 2010.

[67] Deniau, L., et al., "The magnetic model of the LHC during commissioning to higher beam intensities in 2010–2011", CERN-ATS-2011-249, 2011.

[68] Aquilina, N., et al., "Chromaticity decay due to superconducting dipoles on the injection plateau of the Large Hadron Collider", Phys. Rev. ST Accel. Beams **15**, 032401, 2012.

[69] Aiba, M., et al., "First β-beating measurement and optics analysis for the CERN Large Hadron Collider", Phys. Rev. ST Accel. Beams **12**, 081002, 2009.

[70] Aiba, M., et al., "Software package for optics measurement and correction in the LHC", CERN-ATS-2010-092, 2010.

[71] Tomás, R., et al., "CERN Large Hadron Collider optics model, measurements, and corrections", Phys. Rev. ST Accel. Beams **13**, 121004, 2010.

[72] Miyamoto, R., et al., "Accuracy of the LHC optics measurement based on AC Dipoles", CERN-ATS-2011-157, 2011.

[73] Vanbavinckhove, G., et al., "Record low β beating in the LHC", Phys. Rev. ST Accel. Beates **15**, 091001, 2012.

[74] Fartoukh, S. and Brüning, O.S., "Field quality specification for the LHC main dipole magnets", CERN-LHC-Project-Report-501, 2001.

[75] Bottura, L., et al., "Status report on field quality in the main LHC dipoles", CERN-LHC-Project-Report-579, 2002.

[76] Pauletta, S., "Field quality analysis to monitor the industrial series production of the dipole magnets for the Large Hadron Collider", CERN-THESIS-2003-002, 2002.

[77] Scandale, W., et al., "Controlling field quality in magnet production", CERN-LHC-Project-Report-659, 2003.

[78] Todesco, E., et al., "Steering field quality in the main dipole magnets of the Large Hadron Collider", CERN-LHC-Project-Report-704, 2004.

[79] Todesco, E., et al., "Trends in field quality along the production of the LHC dipoles and differences among manufacturers", CERN-LHC-Project-Report-877, 2006.

[80] Hagen, P., et al., "Steering the field quality in the production of the main quadrupoles of the Large Hadron Collider", CERN-LHC-Project-Report-886, 2006.

[81] Fartoukh, S., "LHC installation scenarios and dynamic aperture", CERN-LHC-Project-Report-449, 2000.

[82] Fartoukh, S., "Classification of the LHC main dipoles and installation strategy", CERN-AB-2004-014-ADM, 148, 2004.

[83] Todesco, E., "Selection of the dipoles for the installation in the second sector of the Large Hadron Collider", CERN-LHC-Project-Note-358, 2004.

[84] Fartoukh, S., "Installation strategy for the LHC main dipoles", CERN-LHC-Project-Report-769, 2004.

[85] Bestmann, P., et al., "Magnet acceptance and allocation at the LHC Magnet Evaluation Board", LHC-Project-Report-1058, 2007.

[86] Fartoukh, S. and Giovannozzi, M., "Dynamic aperture computation for the as-built CERN Large Hadron Collider and impact of main dipoles sorting", Nucl. Instrum. Methods **A671**, 10–23, 2012.

[87] Assmann, R. W., et al., "Requirements for the LHC collimation system", CERN-LHC-Project-Report-599, 2002.

[88] Jeanneret, J. B., et al., "Beam loss and collimation at LHC", CERN-LHC-Project-Report-603, 2002.

[89] Assmann, R. W., et al., "Designing and building a collimation system for the high-intensity LHC beam", CERN-LHC-Project-Report-640, 2003.

[90] Assmann, R. W., et al., "Expected performance and beam-based optimization of the LHC collimation system", CERN-LHC-Project-Report-758, 2004.

[91] Assmann, R. W., et al., "Collimation of heavy ion beams in LHC", CERN-LHC-Project-Report-766, 2004.

[92] Assmann, R. W., et al., "The final collimation system for the LHC", CERN-LHC-Project-Report-919, 2006.

[93] Robert-Démolaize, G., "Design and performance optimization of the LHC collimation system", CERN-THESIS-2006-069, 2006.

[94] Assmann, R. W., et al., "Accelerator physics concept for upgraded LHC collimation performance", CERN-ATS-2009-080, 2009.

[95] Burkhardt, H., et al., "Measurements of the LHC collimator impedance with beam in the SPS", CERN-LHC-Project-Report-831, 2005.

[96] Zimmermann, F., et al., "Tune shift induced by nonlinear resistive wall wake field of flat collimator", CERN-AB-2006-070, 2006.

[97] Métral, E., et al., "Transverse impedance of LHC collimators", CERN-LHC-Project-Report-1015, 2007.

[98] Brüning, O.S., "Simulations for the beam-induced electron cloud in the LHC beam screen with magnetic field and image charges", CERN-LHC-Project-Report-158, 1997.

[99] Baglin, V., et al., "Beam-induced electron cloud in the LHC and possible remedies", CERN-LHC-Project-Report-188, 1998.

[100] Brüning, O.S., et al., "Electron cloud and beam scrubbing in the LHC", CERN-LHC-Project-Report-290, 1999.

[101] Ohmi, K. and Zimmermann, F., "Head–tail instability caused by electron clouds in positron storage rings", Phys. Rev. Lett. **85**, 3821, 2000.

[102] Ohmi, K., et al., "Wake-field and fast head-tail instability caused by an electron cloud", Phys. Rev. **E65**, 016502, 2001.

[103] Rumolo, G., et al., "Simulation of the electron-cloud build up and its consequences on heat load, beam stability, and diagnostics", Phys. Rev. ST Accel. Beams **4**, 012801, 2001.

[104] Ohmi, K., et al., "Electron cloud instability in high intensity proton rings", Phys. Rev. ST Accel. Beams **5**, 114402, 2002.

[105] Rumolo, G. and Zimmermann, F., "Electron cloud simulations: beam instabilities and wakefields", Phys. Rev. ST Accel. Beams **5**, 121002, 2002.

[106] Rumolo, G., et al., "Electron cloud effects on beam evolution in a circular accelerator", Phys. Rev. ST Accel. Beams **6**, 081002, 2003.

[107] Zimmermann, F., "Review of single bunch instabilities driven by an electron cloud", Phys. Rev. ST Accel. Beams **7**, 124801, 2004.

[108] Cimino, R., et al., "Can low-energy electrons affect high-energy physics accelerators?", Phys. Rev. Lett. **93**, 014801, 2004.

[109] Benedetto, E., et al., "Simulation study of electron cloud induced instabilities and emittance growth for the CERN Large Hadron Collider proton beam", Phys. Rev. ST Accel. Beams **8**, 124402, 2005.

[110] Benedetto, E., et al., "Incoherent effects of electron clouds in proton storage rings", Phys. Rev. Lett. **97**, 034801, 2006.

[111] Furman, M. A. and Chaplin, V. H., "Update on electron-cloud power deposition for the Large Hadron Collider arc dipoles", Phys. Rev. ST Accel. Beams **9**, 034403, 2006.

[112] Demma, T., et al., "Maps for electron cloud density in Large Hadron Collider dipoles", Phys. Rev. ST Accel. Beams **10**, 114401, 2007.

[113] Rumolo, G., et al., "Dependence of the electron-cloud instability on the beam energy", Phys. Rev. Lett. **100**, 144801, 2008.

[114] Franchetti, G., et al., "Incoherent effect of space charge and electron cloud", Phys. Rev. ST Accel. Beams **12**, 124401, 2009.

[115] Caspers, F., et al., "Beam-induced multipactoring and electron-cloud effects in particle accelerators", CERN-BE-2009-005, 2009.

[116] Li, K. S. B. and Rumolo, G., "Review of beam instabilities in the presence of electron clouds in the LHC", CERN-ATS-2011-095, 2011.

[117] Rumolo, G., et al., "Electron cloud observation in the LHC", CERN-ATS-2011-105, 2011.

[118] Dominguez, O., et al., "Monitoring the progress of LHC electron-cloud scrubbing by benchmarking simulations and pressure-rise observations", CERN-ATS-2012-073, 2012.

[119] Benvenuti, C., et al., "Vacuum properties of TiZrV non-evaporable getter films [for LHC vacuum system]", Vacuum **60**, 57, 2001.

[120] Cimino, R., et al., "Photon reflectivity distributions from the LHC beam screen and their implications on the arc beam vacuum system", CERN-LHC-Project-Report-668, 2004.

[121] Zimmermann, F., et al., "More electron cloud studies for KEKB: long-term evolution, solenoid patterns, and fast blow up", SL-Note-2000-061-AP, 2000.

[122] Cai, Y., et al., "Buildup of electron cloud with different bunch pattern in the presence of solenoid field", SLAC-PUB-9813, 2003.

[123] Cai, Y., et al., "Buildup of electron cloud in the PEP-II particle accelerator in the presence of a solenoid field and with different bunch pattern", SLAC-PUB-10164, 2003.

[124] Novokhatski, A. and Seeman, J., "Simulation of electron cloud multipacting in solenoidal magnetic field", SLAC-PUB-10327, 2005.

[125] Wang, L., et al., "Solenoid effects on an electron cloud", SLAC-PUB-10750, 2005.

[126] Novokhatski, A., et al., "Experimental and simulation studies of electron cloud multipacting in the presence of small solenoidal fields", CERN-2005-001, 2005.

[127] Yokoya, K., et al., "Tune shift of coherent beam-beam oscillations", Part. Accel. **27**, 181, 1990.

[128] Ruggiero, F., "Single-beam collective effects in the LHC", CERN SL/95-09 (AP).

[129] Berg, J. S., "Transverse instabilities in the LHC", CERN-LHC-Project-Report-16, 1996.

[130] Herr, W., "Effects of PACMAN bunches in the LHC", CERN-LHC-Project-Report-39, 1996.

[131] Alexahin, Y., "On the Landau damping and decoherence of transverse dipole oscillations in colliding beams", Part. Accel. **59**, 43, 1996.

[132] Sen, T. and Ellison, J. A.,"Diffusion due to beam–beam interaction and fluctuating fields in hadron colliders", Phys. Rev. Lett. **77**, 1051, 1996.

[133] Ruggiero, F., et al., "Summary of the single-beam collective effects in the LHC", CERN-LHC-Project-Report-120, 1997.

[134] Papaphilippou, Y. and Zimmermann, F., "Weak–strong beam–beam simulations for the Large Hadron Collider", Phys. Rev. ST Accel. Beams **2**, 104001, 1999.

[135] Zorzano, M. P., and Zimmermann, F., "Coherent beam–beam oscillations at the LHC", Phys. Rev. ST Accel. Beams **3**, 044401, 2000.

[136] Shi, J. and Yao, D., "Collective beam–beam effects in hadron colliders", Phys. Rev. E **62**, 1258, 2000.

[137] Grote, H. and Herr, W., "Self-consistent orbits with beam–beam effects in the LHC", CERN-LHC-Project-Report-502, 2001.

[138] Alexahin, Y., et al., "Coherent beam–beam effects in the LHC", CERN-LHC-Project-Report-466, 2001.

[139] Herr, W., et al., "A hybrid fast multipole method applied to beam–beam collisions in the strong-strong regime", Phys. Rev. ST Accel. Beams **4**, 054402, 2001.

[140] Herr, W. and Zorzano, M. P., "Coherent dipole modes for multiple interaction regions", CERN-LHC-Project-Report-461, 2001.

[141] Herr, W., "Beam–beam issues in the LHC and relevant experience from the SPS proton antiproton collider and LEP", CERN-LHC-Project-Report-502, 2001.

[142] Angal-Kalinin, D. and Vos, L., "Coupled bunch instabilities in the LHC", CERN-LHC-Project-Report-585, 2002.

[143] Angal-Kalinin, D., et al., "Intermediate review of single bunch collective effects in the LHC", CERN-LHC-Project-Report-587, 2002.

[144] Muratori, B., "Study of offset collisions and beam adjustment in the LHC using a strong–strong simulation model", CERN-LHC-Project-Report-593, 2002.

[145] Angal-Kalinin, D., "Review of coupled bunch instabilities in the LHC", CERN-LHC-Project-Report-595, 2002.

[146] Alexahin, Y., "A study of the coherent beam–beam effect in the framework of the Vlasov perturbation theory", Nucl. Instrum. Methods. **A380**, 253, 2002.

[147] Papaphilippou, Y. and Zimmermann, F., "Estimates of diffusion due to long-range beam–beam collisions", Phys. Rev. ST Accel. Beams **5**, 074001, 2002.

[148] Herr, W., "Features and implications of different LHC crossing schemes", CERN-LHC-Project-Report-628 (2003).

[149] Jin, L. and Shi, J., "Importance of beam–beam tune spread to collective beam–beam instability in hadron colliders", Phys. Rev. E **69**, 036503, 2004.

[150] Métral, E., et al., "Collective effects in the LHC and its injectors", CERN-ATS-2012-183, 2012.

[151] Benedikt, M., et al., "Performance of the LHC pre-injectors", CERN-PS-2001-011 (DR), 2001.

[152] Benedikt, M., et al. (eds.), "The PS complex as proton pre-injector for the LHC: design and implementation report", CERN-2000-003, 2000.

[153] Collier, P., et al., "The SPS as injector for LHC: conceptual design", CERN-SL-97-007-DI, 1997.

[154] Schindl, K., "The PS Booster as pre-injector for the LHC", CERN-PS-97-011 (DR), 1997.

[155] Gilardoni, S., et al. (eds.), "Fifty years of the CERN Proton Synchrotron, v. 1", CERN-2011-004, 2011.

[156] Garoby, R., "Bunch merging and splitting techniques in the injectors for high energy hadron colliders", in Proceedings of the 17th International Conference on High-Energy Accelerators (ed. Meshkov, I. N., Joint Institute for Nuclear Research, Dubna), 172, 1998.

[157] Hancock, S., et al., "Tomographic measurements of longitudinal phase space density", CERN-PS-99-002-OP, 1999.

[158] Hancock, S., et al., "Longitudinal phase space tomography with space charge", Phys. Rev. ST Accel. Beams **3**, 124202, 2000.

[159] Arduini, G., et al., "The LHC proton beam in the CERN SPS: an update", CERN-LHC-Project-Report-638, 2003.

[160] Bordry, F., "Status of the Large Hadron Collider (LHC)", CERN-LHC-Project-Report-1130, 2008.

[161] Saban, R.I., "LHC Hardware Commissioning Summary", in Proceedings of 11th European Particle Accelerator Conference (ed. Biscari, C. and Petit-Jean-Genaz, C., JACOW, Geneva), 56, 2008.

[162] Lamont, M., et al., "The LHC sector test", CERN-LHC-Project-Report-946, 2006.

[163] Aberle, O., et al., "The LHC injection tests", CERN-LHC-Performance-Note-001, 2008.

[164] Butterworth, A., et al., "Trim magnet polarities, dispersion, and response data in Sector 23", CERN-LHC-Performance-Note-002, 2008.

[165] Fuchsberger, K., et al., "Coupling at injection from tilt mismatch between the LHC and its transfer lines", CERN-LHC-Performance-Note-003, 2008.

[166] Agapov, I., et al., "TI 8 transfer line optics studies", CERN-LHC-Performance-Note-004, 2008.

[167] Calaga, R., et al., "Polarity checks in Sectors 23 & 78", CERN-LHC-Performance-Note-010, 2008.

[168] Uythoven, J., et al., "Beam commissioning of the SPS-to-LHC transfer line TI 2", CERN-LHC-Project-Report-1119, 2008.

[169] Linnecar, T., et al., "Hardware and initial beam commissioning of the LHC RF systems", CERN-LHC-Project-Report-1172, 2008.

[170] Lamont, M., "LHC: status and commissioning plans", arXiv:0906.0347 [physics. acc-ph].

[171] Mertens, V., et al., "Beam commissioning of injection into the LHC", CERN-ATS-2009-012, 2009.

[172] Fartoukh, S., et al., "Linear & nonl. optics checks diring LHC injection tests", CERN-ATS-2009-051, 2009.

[173] Aiba, M., et al., "First beta-beating measurement in the LHC", CERN-ATS-2009-056, 2009.

[174] Lamont, M., et al., "Operational experience with first circulating beam in the LHC", CERN-ATS-2009-061, 2009.

[175] Redaelli, S., et al., "First beam based aperture measurements in the arcs of the CERN Large Hadron Collider", CERN-ATS-2009-064, 2009.

[176] Assmann, R., et al., "Beam parameters and machine performance to be reached in 2010", in Proceedings of Evian 2010 Workshop on LHC Commissioning (ed. Goddard, B., CERN, Geneva), 149, CERN-ATS-2010-028, 2010.

[177] Lamont, M., "Turning on the LHC: commissioning with beam and the outlook for 2010", Nuovo Cim. **C33**, 115, 2011.

[178] Myers, S., "LHC commissioning and first operation", CERN-ATS-2010-123, 2010.

[179] Lamont, M., "The LHC from commissioning to operation", CERN-ATS-2011-186, 2011.

[180] Myers, S., "Large Hadron Collider commissioning and first operation", Phil. Trans. R. Soc. Lond. **A370**, 859, 2012.

[181] Meddahi, M., "Operational schedule 2011 and potential performance", CERN-2011-005, 286, 2011.

[182] Wenninger, J., "Operation of the LHC at high luminosity and high stored energy", CERN-ATS-2012-101, 2012.

[183] Rossi, L., "LHC upgrade plans: options and strategy", CERN-ATS-2011-257, 2011.

[184] Ruggiero, F., et al. (eds.), "2nd CARE-HHH-APD Workshop on Scenarios for the LHC Luminosity Upgrade—LHC-LUMI-05", CERN-2006-008, 2006.

[185] Scandale, W., et al. (eds.), "3rd CARE-HHH-APD Workshop: Towards a Roadmap for the Upgrade of the LHC and GSI Accelerator Complex—LHC-LUMI-06", CERN-2007-002, 2007.

[186] Scandale, W. and Zimmermann, F. (eds.), "CARE-HHH-APD Workshop on Finalizing the Roadmap for the Upgrade of the CERN and GSI Accelerator Complex—BEAM'07", CERN-2008-005, 2008.

[187] Scandale, W. and Zimmermann, F. (eds.), "CARE-HHH-APD Workshop on Interaction Regions for the LHC Upgrade, DAFNE, and SuperB—IR'07", CERN-2008-006, 2008.

[188] Scandale, W. and Zimmermann, F. (eds.), "Final CARE-HHH Workshop on Scenarios for the LHC Upgrade and FAIR - HHH-2008", CERN-2009-004, 2009.

[189] Brüning, O. S., et al., "LHC luminosity and energy upgrade: a feasibility study", CERN-LHC-Project-Report-626, 2002.

[190] Ostojic, R., et al., "Conceptual design of the LHC interaction region upgrade: Phase-I", CERN-LHC-Project-Report-1163, 2008.

[191] Scandale, W. and Zimmermann, F., "LHC Phase-2 upgrade scenarios", CERN-2009-004, 8, 2009.

[192] Fartoukh, S., "LSS magnet aperture requirements for the LHC insertion upgrade, a first estimate", CERN-LHC-Project-Report-1050, 2007.

[193] Fartoukh, S., "Low-beta insertions inducing chromatic aberrations in storage rings and their local and global correction", CERN-sLHC-Project-Report-0020, 2009.

[194] Fartoukh, S., "Optics challenges and solutions for the LHC insertion upgrade Phase I", CERN-sLHC-Project-Report-0038, 2010.

[195] Willeke, F., "HERA status and upgrade plans", in Proceedings of 17th Particle Accelerator Conference (ed. Comyn, M., et al., IEEE, Piscataway, NJ), 51, 1998.

[196] Holzer, B.J., "HERA: lessons learned from the HERA upgrade", CERN-2009-004, 30, 2009.

[197] Marriner, J.P., "TEVATRON luminosity upgrade project", in Proceedings of 6th European Particle Accelerator Conference (ed. Myers, S., et al., Stockholm), 8, 1998.

[198] Shiltsev, V.D., "Achievements and lessons from the Tevatron", in Proceedings of 2nd International Particle Accelerator Conference (ed. Petit-Jean-Genaz, C., Geneva), 903, 2011.

[199] Giovannozzi, M., et al., "Possible improvements to the existing pre-injector complex in the framework of continued consolidation", CERN-ATS-2010-026, 228, 2010.

[200] Benedikt, M., et al., "Preliminary accelerator plans for maximizing the integrated LHC luminosity", CERN-AB-2006-018-PAF, 2006.

[201] Garoby, R., et al., "Comparison of options for the injector of PS2", CERN-AB-2007-014-PAF, 2007.

[202] Baldy, J. L., et al., "Site layout of the proposed new hadrons' injector chain at CERN", CERN-AB-2008-061-PAF, 2008.

[203] Hanke, K., et al., "Study of a rapid cycling synchrotron to replace the CERN PS Booster", CERN-ATS-2011-054, 2011.

[204] Palmer, R.B., "Energy scaling, crab crossing, and the pair problem", SLAC-PUB-4707, 1988.

[205] Oide, K. and Yokoya, Y., "Beam–beam collision scheme for storage-ring colliders", Phys. Rev. **A40**, 315, 1989.

[206] Ohmi, K., "Study of crab cavity option for LHC", CERN-2005-006, 97, 2005.

[207] Calaga, R., et al., "Crab cavity option for LHC IR upgrade", CERN-2007-002, 77, 2007.

[208] Ben-Zvi, I., "LHC crab cavities", CERN-2009-004, 133, 2009.

[209] Calaga, R., et al., "Status of LHC crab cavity simulations and beam studies", CERN-ATS-2009-035, 2009.

[210] De Maria, R. and Fartoukh, S., "Optics and layout for the HL-LHC upgrade project with a local crab cavity scheme", CERN-sLHC-Project-Report-0055, 2011.

[211] De Maria, R. and Fartoukh, S., "A proposal for the optics and layout of the HL-LHC with crab cavities", CERN-ATS-2011-107, 2011.

[212] Fartoukh, S., "Towards the LHC upgrade using the LHC well-characterized technology", CERN-sLHC-Project-Report-0049, 2010.

[213] Fartoukh, S., "Breaching the Phase I optics limitations for the HL-LHC", CERN-sLHC-Project-Report-0053, 2011.

[214] Fartoukh, S., "An achromatic telescopic squeezing (ATS) scheme for the LHC upgrade", CERN-ATS-2011-161, 2011.

[215] Fartoukh, S., "The achromatic telescopic squeezing scheme: basic principles and first demonstration at the LHC", CERN-ATS-2012-080, 2012.

[216] Rossi, L., et al., "Advanced accelerator magnets for upgrading the LHC", CERN-ATS-2012-045, 2012.

[217] Zimmermann, F., "HL-LHC: parameter space, constraints, and possible options", EuCARD-CON-2011-002, 2011.

[218] Brüning, O. S. and Zimmermann, F., "Parameter space for the LHC high-luminosity upgrade", CERN-ATS-2012-070, 2012.

[219] Assmann, R., et al., "First thoughts on a higher-energy LHC", CERN-ATS-2010-177, 2010.

[220] Brüning, O. S., et al., "HE-LHC beam-parameters, optics and beam-dynamics issues", arXiv:1108.1617 [physics. acc-ph].

[221] Todesco, E., et al. (eds.), "EuCARD–AccNet–EuroLumi Workshop: The High-Energy Large Hadron Collider, Matta, Republic of Matta, 14–16 oct 2010", arXiv:1111.7188 [physics. acc-ph].

[222] Klein, M., et al., "Prospects for a Large Hadron Electron Collider (LHeC) at the LHC", CERN-AB-2008-041, 2008.

[223] Zimmermann, F., et al., "Linac–LHC EP collider options", CERN-LHC-Project-Report-1137, 2008.

[224] Zimmermann, F., et al., "The Large Hadron–Electron Collider (LHeC) at the LHC", CERN-ATS-2009-053, 2009.

[225] Zimmermann, F., et al., "Interaction-region design options for a LINAC–ring LHeC", CERN-ATS-2010-043, 2010.

[226] Zimmermann, F., et al., "Designs for a LINAC–ring LHeC", CERN-ATS-2010-045, 2010.

[227] Appleby, R.B., et al., "Interaction region design for a ring ring version of the LHeC study", CERN-ATS-2010-057, 2010.

[228] Zimmermann, F., et al., "RLA and ERL designs for a LINAC-RING LHeC", CERN-ATS-2010-099, 2010.

[229] Fitterer, M., et al., "LHeC lattice design", CERN-ATS-2011-108, 2011.

[230] Abelleira, J., et al., "Final-focus optics for the LHeC electron beam line", CERN-ATS-2012-076, 2012.

[231] Fitterer, M., et al., "Update on LHeC ring–ring optics", CERN-ATS-2012-172, 2012.

[232] Brüning, O.S., et al., "The LHeC project development beyond 2012", CERN-ATS-2012-230, 2012.

3
The LHC detectors and the first CMS data

Dan GREEN

Fermilab, USA

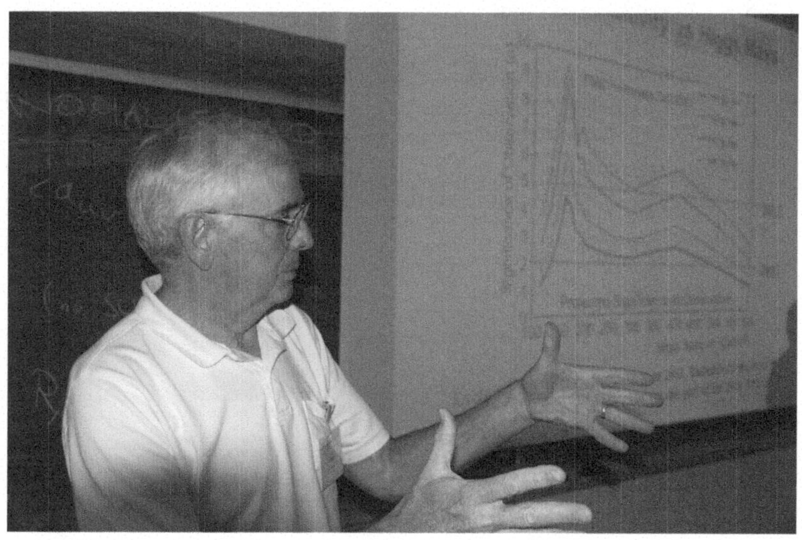

Theoretical Physics to Face the Challenge of LHC. Edited by L. Baulieu, K. Benakli, M. R. Douglas, B. Mansoulié, E. Rabinovici, and L. F. Cugliandolo. © Oxford University Press 2015. Published in 2015 by Oxford University Press.

Chapter Contents

The design of the LHC detectors follows from the requirement of confronting electroweak symmetry breaking (EWSB) in a decisive fashion. The LHC accelerator also meets those requirements. The simple discussion of the subsystems of a "generic" LHC detector presented here explains why the detectors have the parameters they do.

3.1 EWSB and LHC

There are many theoretical speculations, but one thing is certain: WW scattering at a center-of-mass (CM) energy of $\sim$1.8 TeV violates perturbative unitarity. Therefore, one must design the LHC and the LHC detectors to comprehensively study WW scattering at $\sim$1 TeV.

3.2 LHC machine

Given the existing LEP tunnel, 26 km around, one wants to use the most aggressive magnets to achieve the highest-energy pp machine. With only dipoles, a 7 TeV beam requires 5.6 T magnets because of the need for lenses, straight sections, injection, abort and radiofrequency (RF). The LHC magnets are 8.3 T, and such a field requires superfluid helium at 1.8 K (critical current density). Each magnet has 12 kA, $L = 0.1$ h, or 7 MJ/magnet. With 1200 dipoles, this is $\sim$8 GJ which implies the need for quench protection For RF purposes, bunches are short, $\sim$10 cm, separated by $>$7.5 m (25 ns), with a total of $<$3466 bunches (2808 design, and an abort gap is needed). Given 14 TeV pp CM energy ($>$1 TeV parton–parton CM energy), a sufficiently large interaction rate is needed.

The number of protons in a bunch is limited by Coulomb repulsion, depending quadratically on collision rate. The number of bunches is limited by the RF and the bunch length. The revolution frequency is approximately constant. The beam size at the interaction point is limited by the strength of the "low-beta" quadrupoles, their aperture, and the collimation. Putting the factors together, the LHC design luminosity is

$$L \sim 10^{34}\,\mathrm{cm}^{-2}\,\mathrm{s}^{-1}. \tag{3.1}$$

The vector bosons decay to either quark or lepton pairs. However, the enormous backgrounds that exist at the LHC owing to strongly produced QCD processes make the detection of leptonic decays experimentally favored. This explains why LHC detectors tend to focus on lepton detection. The branching ratio for a W to decay to a muon plus neutrino is $\sim$1/9. A crude estimate of the cross section for electroweak $W + W$ production at the LHC with subsequent W decay to muons is

$$\sigma(p + p \to W^+ + W^- \to \mu^+ + \nu_\mu + \mu^- + \bar{\nu}_\mu) \sim \frac{\alpha_W^2}{\hat{s}} B_\mu^2. \tag{3.2}$$

This estimate gives a 5 fb cross section times branching ratio squared for a W-pair mass of 1 TeV. To have sufficient statistical power in studying this process, the LHC should provide 100 fb^{-1}/yr. Taking a running time T of 10^7 s/yr ($\sim$30% of the calendar year), there will be $\sim$790 $W + W$ events produced per year with a mass above 1 TeV that decay into the experimentally favorable final state containing two muons. A similar event sample will be available in the two-electron final state and twice that in the muon-plus-electron final state.

The high luminosity that is required of the LHC because of the need to explore terascale physics means that the detectors will be exposed to high particle rates. Therefore, LHC experiments will require fast, radiation-hard, and finely segmented detectors. It is assumed in what follows that all the detectors can be operated at a speed that can resolve the time between two successive RF bunches: 25 ns at the LHC.

Note that the total inelastic cross section is $\sim$100 mb, as shown in Fig. 3.1. With a luminosity as defined above, the total inelastic reaction rate $R = \sigma L = 10^9\,\mathrm{s}^{-1} = 1\,\mathrm{GHz}$. Each crossing contains $\sim$25 inelastic events at full luminosity. This leads to

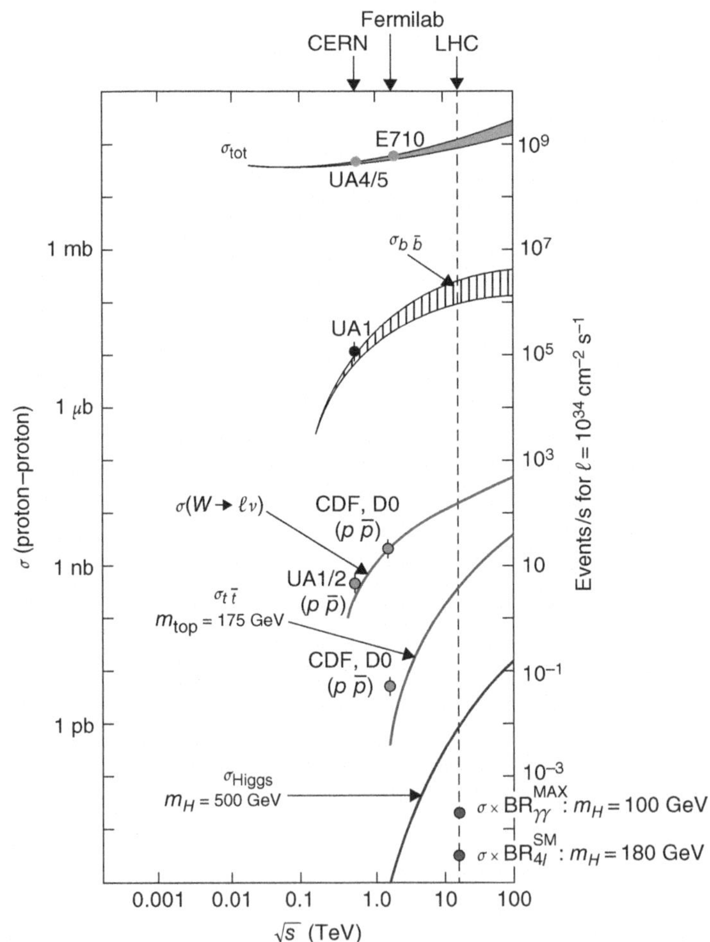

Fig. 3.1 The cross sections for several processes as functions of CM energy.

experimental issues, but the luminosity that is required at the LHC and the size of the inelastic cross section make a "pileup" of $N_I = 25$ inelastic events in each bunch crossing unavoidable.

3.3 Global detector properties

In designing a generic LHC detector, it is crucial to understand what part of phase space the produced particles occupy. Note that single-particle relativistically invariant phase space for a particle of mass M, momentum $\vec{P}$, and energy E is

$$d^4 P\, \delta(P^2 - M^2) = \frac{d\vec{P}}{E} = \pi\, dy\, dP_T^2\,,$$

$$E = M_T \cosh y, \quad M_T^2 = M^2 + P_T^2\,, \tag{3.3}$$

$$y \to \eta = -\log\left(\tan\frac{\theta}{2}\right), \quad P >> M.$$

Therefore, if the produced particles in a typical inelastic reaction are described by single-particle phase space, they can be expected to be found uniformly distributed in rapidity y. The momentum transverse to the proton beam directions is denoted by P_T. For light particles, with $M/P << 1$, the rapidity y can be approximated by the pseudorapidity η. Most of the produced particles are pions, which have a mass of 0.14 GeV, and their mean transverse momentum at the LHC is expected to be ~0.8 GeV. Therefore, the angular variable, the pseudorapidity η, is a good approximation to y in most cases.

Indeed, production data at $\eta \sim 0$ (i.e., near 90° in the $p+p$ CM system) display a roughly uniform distribution. Note also that the density $D = (1/\sigma)(d\sigma/d\eta)$ of particles in the region and the width of that region rise slowly with increasing CM energy. A Monte Carlo example is shown in Fig. 3.2.

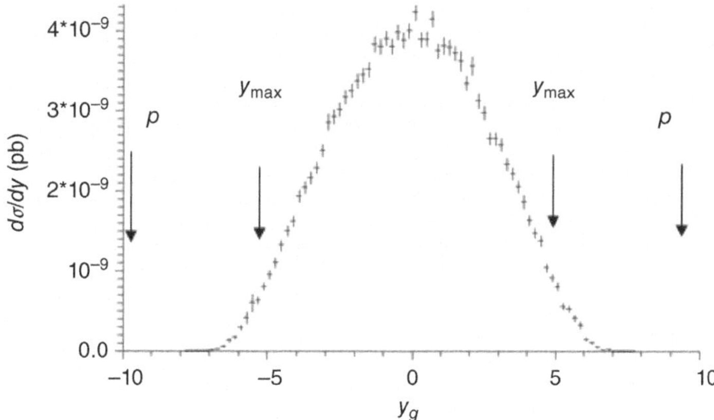

Fig. 3.2 Rapidity distribution of low-transverse-momentum gluon jets at the LHC in the $g + g \to g + g$ reaction.

The kinematic limit for the 7 TeV incident protons is $|y| < 9.6$. Clearly, requiring that the LHC detectors detect most of the produced particles means that a rapidity coverage of $\sim |y| < 5$ is needed. That coverage is sufficient to detect the majority of the particles produced in normal inelastic events.

A generic detector should cover a full rapidity range of 10. The particle density per unit rapidity will be about nine: six charged pions and three neutral pions under the assumption that all produced particles are pions and all charge states of the pions are equally probable. The mean transverse momentum of the pions will be ~ 0.8 GeV. Therefore, in each time-resolved RF bunch crossing, there are 2250 particles in the complete detector coverage. Thus, we have

$$D \sim 9\,\pi/\text{unit of } y: \quad 6\,\pi^\pm + 3\,\pi^0,$$
$$\langle P_T \rangle \sim 0.8\,\text{GeV}, \tag{3.4}$$
$$N_I(2y_{\max})D = 2250\,\text{particles}, \quad 1.8\,\text{TeV total} \sum P_T.$$

The high-mass-scale processes of greatest interest populate phase space somewhat differently. For example, a hypothetical 2 TeV mass recurrence of the Z boson decaying into electrons preferentially appears at small rapidities as shown in Fig. 3.3. Therefore, the generic detector will put more stress on the low-$|y|$ regions of phase space and deploy precision detectors to cover rapidities $|y| < 2.5$. In fact, the more precise generic

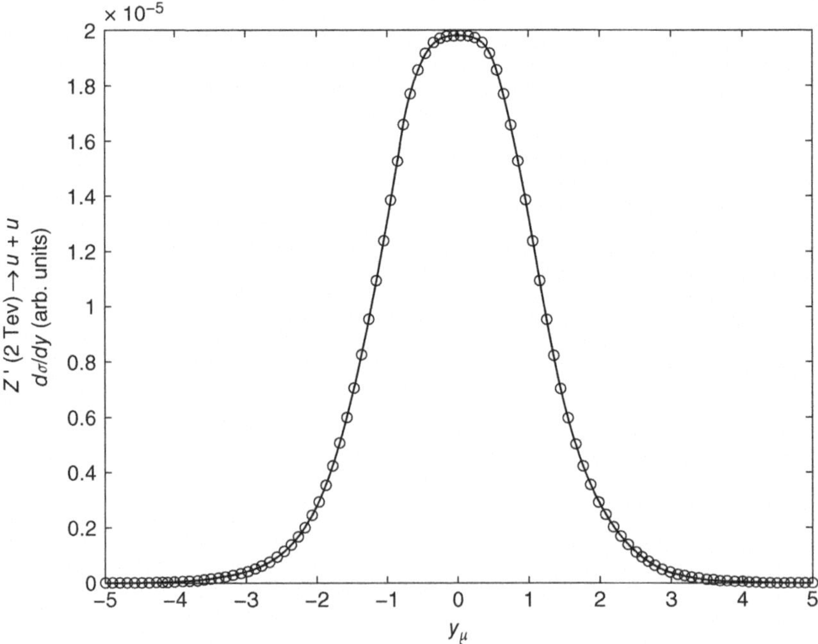

Fig. 3.3 Rapidity distribution for a sequential Z boson with mass 2 TeV.

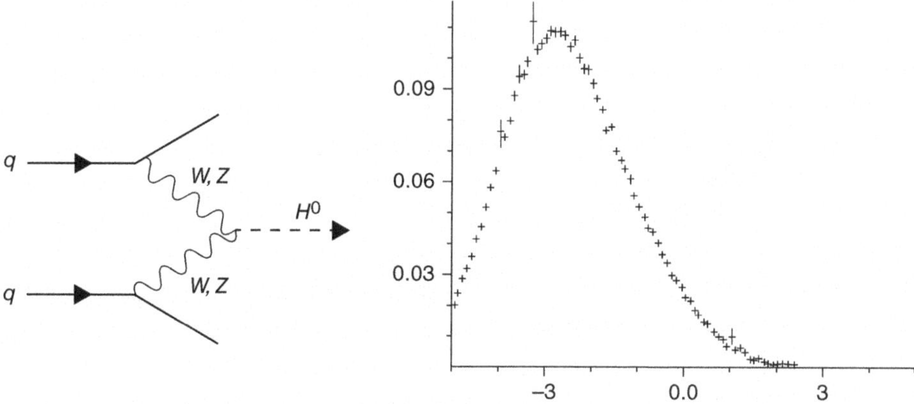

Fig. 3.4 Rapidity distribution of the forward/backward-going "tag" jets in the VBF process.

detectors are limited to the region $|y| < 2.5$ because of their rate limitations and the risk of radiation damage both to the detectors and to the front-end electronics. The larger-$|y|$ region is covered only by radiation-hardened calorimetry.

A study of vector boson fusion (VBF) will allow the isolation of WW, ZZ, and WZ scattering, as illustrated in Fig. 3.4. These measurements may be crucial to the understanding of EWSB. The virtual emission of a W by an initial-state quark in both of the protons will lead to the scattered $W + W$ plus the two quarks recoiling after W emission. This process is a critical component of the LHC physics program because it has a signature that allows experimenters to tag and isolate vector boson scattering.

3.4 The generic detector

The required detector coverage in angle follows from the properties of inelastic events and from the VBF process. The generic detector consists of several subsystems with specific roles in particle detection and identification and is described below. The idea here is simply to observe from the physics requirements what a typical general purpose detector might look like. It is generic in the sense that specific subsystem detector design choices are not made, but rather the general needs of the several detector subsystems are examined. The overall layout of the detector is shown in Fig. 3.5.

The overall coverage in rapidity of 2×5 units has been motivated earlier. This coverage should be "hermetic," which means that all produced particles should be detected and their positions and momenta should be well measured. If this is achieved, then the production of neutrinos may be inferred by vectorially adding all the observed particle transverse momenta in the final state, because the initial state contains almost no transverse momentum. If an imbalance remains, the existence of "missing transverse momentum" (MET) implies that an undetected, noninteracting, neutral stable particle or particles have been produced that carried off the MET.

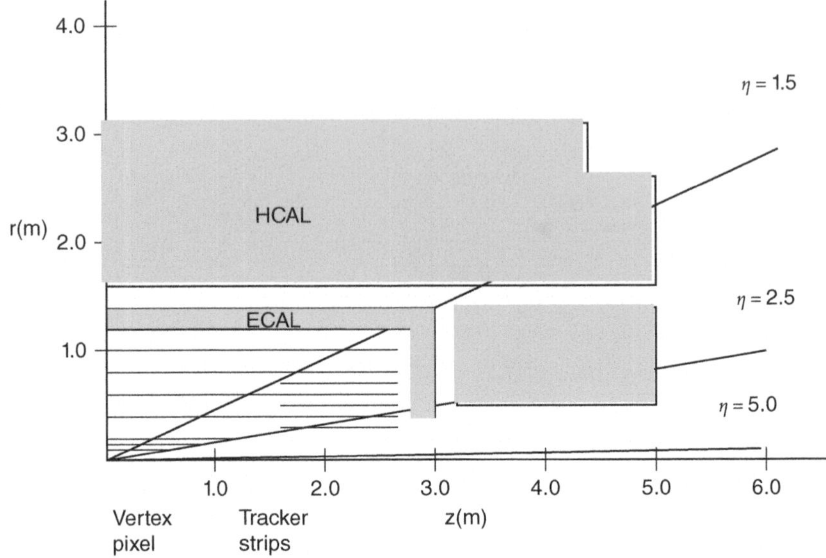

Fig. 3.5 The layout of the generic detector, showing the vertex, tracking, Electromagnetic Calorimeter (ECAL), and Hadronic Calorimeter (HCAL) subsystems.

There are several specific subsystems that are indicated. A general purpose detector, such as those installed at the LHC, aims to measure all the particles of the Standard Model (SM) from each interaction as well as possible. This follows because, whatever form the physics beyond the SM takes, the final-state particles will ultimately decay to the bosons, quarks, gluons, charged leptons, and neutrinos of the SM. The role of the subsystems is shown in Table 3.1.

The detector focuses on the "barrel" or wide-angle region, because heavy new particles are kinematically expected to be produced there (Fig. 3.3). Coverage by the vertex, tracking, and electromagnetic calorimetry is limited to $|y| < 2.5$ because of the fierce radiation field that exists at smaller angles. That field must, however, be confronted because of the high luminosity needed to explore EWSB at the terascale and the need for hermetic coverage (Figs. 3.2 and 3.4).

The size and location of the detector subsystems follow from the physics requirements. The vertex subsystem exists to measure the secondary decay vertices of the heavy quarks and leptons. Therefore, the vertex subsystem is as near to the LHC vacuum beam pipe as is possible. The tracking subsystem is immersed in the magnetic field of a large solenoid (with a uniform field in the z direction). By measuring the trajectory of the charged particles produced in the collisions, the charges, positions, and momenta of all produced charged particles are determined. A radius of 1 m is allocated to the vertex and tracking systems to achieve this objective with sufficient accuracy.

Table 3.1 Particles of the SM detected and identified in detector subsystems

PARTICLES	SIGNATURE	GENERIC SUBSYSTEM
$u, c, t \rightarrow W + b$ $\left.\vphantom{\begin{array}{c}a\\b\end{array}}\right\}$ quarks $\quad$ d, s, b $\quad$ g	Jet of hadrons (λ_0)	Calorimeter ECAL + HCAL
e, γ	Electromagnetic shower(X_0)	Calorimeter ECAL Tracker
ν_e, ν_μ, ν_τ $W \rightarrow \mu + \nu_\mu$	Missing transverse energy (MET)	Calorimeter ECAL+HCAL
$\mu, \tau \rightarrow \mu + \nu_\tau + \bar{\nu}_\mu$ $Z \rightarrow \mu + \mu$	Only ionization (dE/dx)	Muon absorber and detectors Tracker
c, b, τ	Secondary decay vertices	Vertex + Tracker

The size of the calorimetry is dictated by the characteristic distance that is needed to initiate an interaction, either electromagnetic (ECAL) or hadronic (HCAL). These sizes are

$$
\begin{aligned}
(X_0)_{\mathrm{Pb}} &= 0.56\,\mathrm{cm}, \\
(\lambda_0)_{\mathrm{Fe}} &= 16.8\,\mathrm{cm}.
\end{aligned}
\tag{3.5}
$$

The showers in ECAL are fully developed and contained in about 20 radiation lengths X_0. Allowing space for shower sampling and readout, 20 cm in depth is used for ECAL. The HCAL follows in depth with 1.5 m of steel, or 8.9 nuclear absorption lengths λ_0. The focus in angular coverage of all the subsystems is in the "barrel" region, $|\eta| < 1.5$. Coverage by the vertex, tracking, and ECAL subsystems goes only to $|\eta| < 2.5$.

In the region $2.5 < |\eta| < 5.0$, the radiation field at the LHC precludes all but very radiation-resistant calorimetry. This forward calorimeter region is not shown explicitly, but is thought to reside at $z = 10$ m, a large distance that reduces the radiation dose. If it were stationed at $z \sim 3.2$ m, the dose would be ~ 9.8 times larger, and a substantial added radiation resistance would then be required of the specific technology chosen for the calorimetry. This location is indicated in Fig. 3.5.

The high rates of background processes, as shown in Fig. 3.1, imply that the leptons must be measured in robust and redundant systems. For example, muons are measured in the tracking systems and then again in redundant specialized muon systems that have lower rates consisting of fairly pure muons because almost all other SM particles have been absorbed in the thick calorimeters. Electrons are also measured redundantly, in their case using the tracking systems and the electromagnetic calorimeters.

In this way, the generic detector allows for clean lepton identification and measurement even though the cross sections of greatest interest, such as those of Higgs decays, are of order femtobarns or smaller, while the inelastic backgrounds are of order millibarns, a factor of at least 10^{12} larger.

3.5 Vertex subsystem

The subsystem at smallest transverse radius r is the vertex subsystem. It consists of pixels of silicon deployed from radius 10 to 20 cm in three layers in the generic model. The vertex detector is used to efficiently find and identify the secondary decay vertices of the heavy quarks and leptons as shown in Table 3.1. The lifetimes of these particles set the scale for the pixel size:

$$\begin{aligned}
(c\tau)_\tau &= 87 \text{ } \mu\text{m}, \\
(c\tau)_b &\sim 475 \text{ } \mu\text{m}, \\
(c\tau)_c &\sim (123, 312) \text{ } \mu\text{m} \quad (D^0, D^\pm).
\end{aligned}$$

(3.6)

Assuming a pixel size of $\delta z = \delta s = 200$ μm, where s is the distance in the azimuthal direction (on a cylindrical vertex pixel layer) and z is along the beam direction, the vertex detector spatial resolution is sufficient to identify and measure the decay vertices. A CMS result for tagging is shown in Fig. 3.6.

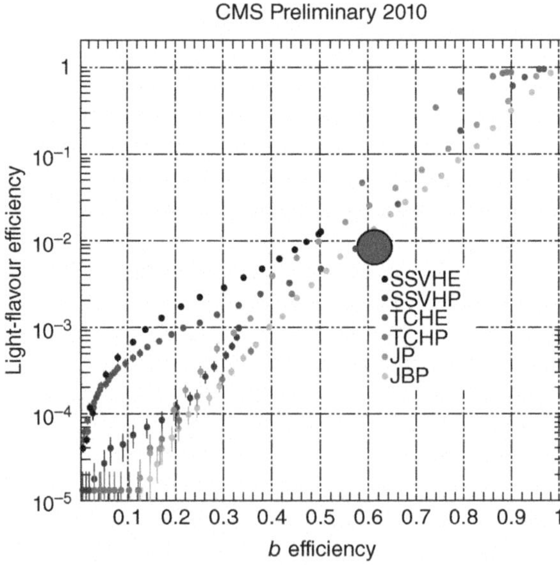

Fig. 3.6 Plot of the CMS b-tag efficiency versus the light-tag efficiency. A typical operating point has 60% b-tag efficiency and 99% light-quark rejection, as indicated by the shaded circle.

Note that analogue readout of the energy deposited in neighboring pixels yields better spatial resolution by interpolation than simple yes/no information. The probability for a pixel to be struck by a charged pion in a single bunch crossing is

$$P_{\text{pix}} \sim D_c N_I \frac{\delta z}{r} \frac{\delta s}{2\pi r}. \tag{3.7}$$

With a density D_c of 6 charged pions per unit of y and $N_I = 25$ inelastic events per bunch crossing at full luminosity, the pixel occupation probability at the innermost layer at a radius $r = 10$ cm is ~ 0.000095. The low occupation probability is achieved at a cost of the independent readout of many silicon pixels. A rough estimate is that, for three layers extending over $|z| < 80$ cm, there are 8000 pixels per layer in z and 4700 pixels in azimuth, for a total of 110 million pixels covering $|\eta| < 2.5$. The sparse occupation of the pixel system makes it an ideal location to start finding track patterns. Indeed, the required high rates at the LHC were what caused ATLAS and CMS to adopt pixel detectors, which was the first time they had been deployed at hadron colliders.

Clearly, there is a tradeoff in radius between the number of pixels and the radiation field. If the vertex system could start at a radius of 5 cm, then the number of pixels would be reduced to 28 million and the radiation would be increased fourfold because of the r^2 behavior of the number of pixels and the $1/r^2$ behavior of the dose. A smaller radius also reduces the position error made in extrapolating from the inner pixel layer to the actual decay vertex, because of multiple scattering in the beam vacuum pipe and the detectors, which limits the accuracy of the angular track measurements.

The radiation field can be approximately evaluated using the number of charged tracks leaving ionization in the silicon detectors, ignoring increases due to secondary interactions of those tracks, to photon conversion, or to their multiple passage through the detectors as a result of particles being curled up in the magnetic field:

$$(\text{Dose})_{\text{pix}} \sim \sigma_I L T D_c \frac{1}{2\pi r^2} \frac{dE_{\text{ion}}}{d(\rho_{\text{Si}} \delta r)}. \tag{3.8}$$

The dose is the energy deposited per weight and 1 Mrad $= 6.2 \times 10^{10}$ GeV/g. The number of inelastic events per second is $\sigma_I L = 10^9$ Hz and the exposure time is taken to be a "year," with $T = 1$ yr defined to be 10^7 s. With a density D_c of 6 charged particles per interaction and vertex detectors at $r = 10$ cm, the charged-particle fluence is 9.5×10^{14} $\pi^\pm$ cm^{-2} yr^{-1}. Each minimum ionizing particle at normal incidence deposits $dE_{\text{ion}}/d(\rho_{\text{Si}} \delta r) = 1.66$ MeV g^{-1} cm^{-2}, or 0.12 MeV in a $\delta r = 300$ μm thick detector. The estimated dose is then 2.5 Mrad/yr for the inner vertex detectors. Clearly, smaller radii will be very challenging.

3.6 Magnet subsystem

The vertex and tracking subsystems are assumed to be immersed in a strong solenoid field. Roughly speaking, the current I flowing through n turns/length of conductor leads to a field $B = \mu_0 n I$. Suppose there were conductors of size 2 cm in z, all stacked by 4 in r for a total of $n = 200$ turns/m. Then, to achieve a field of 5 T, 20.8 kA of current is required. LHC magnets are a large step in stored energy above what has been previously achieved in the Tevatron (CDF and D0) as regards the solenoids used in the detectors. In the generic detector, a field of 5 T is assumed.

3.7 Tracking subsystem

The requirement that the LHC experiments decisively confront EWSB has been seen to imply a complete study of WW scattering at a mass of $\sim$1.0 TeV. In that case, the transverse momentum of the W is $\sim$0.5 TeV and that of the lepton for the two-body W decay is $\sim$0.25 TeV. The radial size of the tracker is then set by the need to measure the lepton momentum well up to this mass scale.

The approximate transverse momentum impulse imparted to a particle of charge e in traversing a transverse distance r in a magnetic field B is

$$(\Delta P_T)_B = erB = 0.3rB, \tag{3.9}$$

where the units are GeV, T, and m, and an electronic charge is assumed. The bend is in the azimuthal direction, and the angle through which the particle is bent, $\Delta\phi_B$, is approximately the impulse divided by the transverse momentum, $(\Delta P_T)_B/P_T$. The error in the inverse transverse momentum is therefore

$$d\left(\frac{1}{P_T}\right) = \frac{dP_T}{P_T^2} = \frac{d(\Delta\phi_B)}{(\Delta P_T)_B} \sim \frac{ds}{er^2 B}, \tag{3.10}$$

where ds is the spatial resolution in the azimuthal direction. Note that the quality factor for the momentum resolution scales as $1/r^2 B$, which argues for a strong magnetic field and a large radius for the cylindrical tracking subsystem.

Assuming a 5 T magnetic field extending over $r = 1$ m, the magnetic impulse is 1.5 GeV. The bend angle is then 6 milliradians for the 0.25 TeV lepton from the W decay. The tracker spatial resolution is estimated by assuming the digital readout of strips of 400 μm width. The root mean square (RMS) resolution is then $ds \sim 400/\sqrt{12}$ μm $= 115$ μm. The momentum will then be measured to 1.9% at 0.25 TeV. Later, it is shown that a 1.2% momentum accuracy is needed in order not to degrade the Z-peak natural width, which implies analogue readout of the tracker detector.

The momentum is measured to 10% accuracy at 1.30 TeV, which makes a sufficiently good measurement at the terascale. A smaller radius or lower-field tracking system would require a more accurate measurement than the ds value quoted above.

At a lower momentum scale, there is another limitation on the measurement accuracy. The multiple-scattering transverse impulse $(\Delta P_T)_{\mathrm{MS}}$ due to scattering in the tracker material compared with the magnetic field impulse sets a limit of

$$\frac{dP_T}{P_T} \sim \frac{(\Delta P_T)_{\mathrm{MS}}}{(\Delta P_T)_B},$$

$$(\Delta P_T)_{\mathrm{MS}} = E_s \sqrt{\sum \frac{L_i}{2X_0}}, \tag{3.11}$$

where the scattering energy $E_s = 21$ MeV, X_0 is the radiation length, and the sum is over all material in the tracker. For a tracker-plus-vertex system having silicon detectors of 400 μm thickness in 11 layers (8 layers in four stations with small-angle stereo in the tracker and 3 vertex layers), the scattering impulse is 3.2 MeV.

There are two terms in the momentum resolution, $dP_T/P_T = cP_T \oplus d$, which are folded in quadrature. There is a term due to measurement error, $c = 0.000078$ GeV^{-1}, (3.10), and a term due to multiple scattering, $d = 0.0021$, (3.11), which limits the low-momentum measurements. The crossover transverse momentum at which the errors are equal is 27 GeV in this example, and the total resolution at this momentum is $\sim 0.3\%$. Clearly, keeping the contribution due to multiple scattering low allows one to improve the momentum measurement accuracy at low momentum, where the fractional momentum resolution is a constant. Incidentally, it should be pointed out that only counting the detectors themselves and ignoring power leads, cooling leads, and other material is very optimistic.

For a complete understanding of the momentum scale and resolution, a detailed understanding of the tracker material throughout the system is needed. One can use photon conversions for probing high-Z materials and nuclear interactions for low-Z material. Results from CMS are shown in Fig. 3.7.

Most of the information provided by the tracker is contained in the measurement of the azimuthal coordinates (the "bend plane"), while the helical paths are less demanding in the z direction. Therefore, to reduce costs, the generic tracking detector is fashioned of silicon strips, 10 cm long in z and 400 μm wide in s. Each of the four stations has a strip layer oriented along z as the long axis and a second at small angle to the first. Using (3.7), the probability for a strip to be occupied ranges from 0.006 to 0.00096 as the strip radius goes from 40 to 100 cm. This level of occupation is sufficiently sparse to allow for robust track pattern recognition and trajectory fitting.

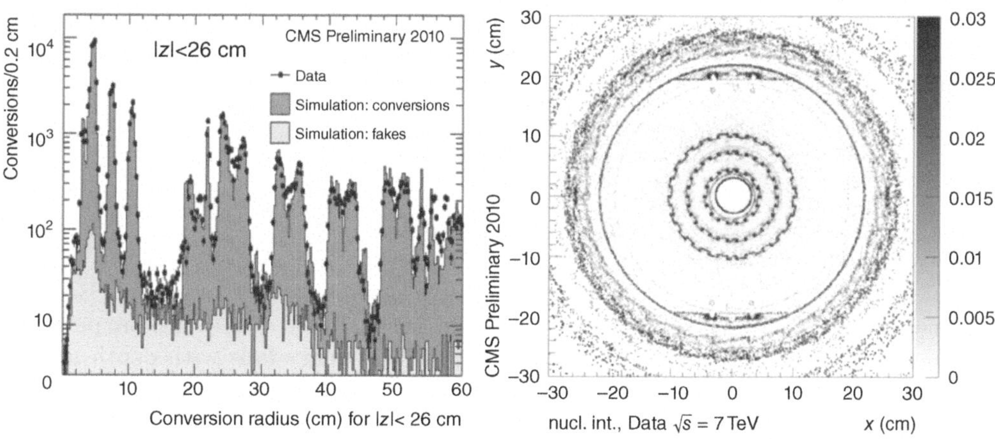

Fig. 3.7 Material in the CMS tracker as determined from photon conversions and hadronic interactions.

The total number of strips in one layer at an average radius of 70 cm is $\sim$52 in z, $|z| < 2.6$ m, times $\sim$11 000 in r. Therefore, in eight layers, there are roughly 4.6 million independent strips to record (and purchase).

3.8   ECAL subsystem

The generic electromagnetic calorimeter has the role of measuring the energy and position of the photons and electrons created in the LHC collisions. It is the first of the calorimeters to be struck by outgoing particles in the generic detector. Calorimeters measure energy by initiating interactions of the incident particles and completely absorbing the resulting energy, which appears as a geometrically growing "shower" of particles. Compared with the tracking and vertex systems, which absorb only the tiny ionization energy deposited in them, the calorimeter readout is "destructive" in that the showering particle is totally absorbed.

The ECAL supplies a redundant measurement of the electrons. The tracking system first measures the electron momentum, charge, position, and direction. The ECAL measures the electron position and energy a second time. The electrons are important in the study of vector boson interactions because they are decay products of the W and Z. Redundancy is needed in order to be able to cleanly study the rare interactions of vector bosons using the final-state electrons in a background of strongly produced neutral pions and the photons resulting from their decay. A figure of merit is set by the sharpness of the Z resonant peak:

$$\Gamma_Z = 2.5\,\text{GeV}, \quad M_Z = 91.2\,\text{GeV},$$

$$\left(\frac{dE}{E}\right)_{\text{ECAL}} < \frac{\Gamma_Z}{2.36 M_Z} = 1.2\%. \tag{3.12}$$

The development of the ECAL shower is parametrized using the depth L in radiation-length units, $t = L/X_0$, and the energy in critical-energy units, $y = E/E_c$. The incident energy is E_0 and $a \sim 1 + (\ln y)/2$. The shower development in depth is then

$$\frac{dE}{dt} = \frac{E_0 b(bt)^{a-1}e^{-bt}}{\Gamma(a)},$$

$$t_{\max} = \frac{a-1}{b}, \quad b \sim 0.5. \tag{3.13}$$

A typical shower profile has a rapid rise owing to the geometric shower growth. Because the energy of the electrons and photons in the shower is shared over ever more particles as the shower grows with depth, the average particle energy falls with depth until a point comes where radiative shower growth stops, at the "shower maximum" at a depth $t_{\max}$ where the average particle energy is near the critical energy. The shower then dies out at greater depths through loss of energy due to ionization and photoelectric absorption. This behavior is due to the geometric growth behavior of the number of particles in the shower:

$$E/E_c \sim N_s \sim 2^{t_{\max}},$$

$$t_{\max} \sim \frac{\ln(E/E_c)}{\ln 2}. \tag{3.14}$$

With fine sampling and a very uniform medium, the stochastic fluctuation of the number N_s of shower particles can largely determine the energy resolution $dE/E \sim 1/\sqrt{N_s} \sim \sqrt{E_c/E}$. For $E = 0.25$ TeV, the number for Pb is 34 245, with a 0.54% fluctuation, which meets the energy resolution requirement. The stochastic coefficient for the energy resolution is estimated to be $a = \sqrt{E_c} = 8.5\%$, where GeV energy units are used.

The transverse shower development is also important, since it defines the requirement for the ECAL tower size and also provides additional particle identification capability. The Molière radius r_M is the radius of a cylinder within which 90% of the shower energy is deposited. In Pb, the radius is $r_M = 1.6\,\mathrm{cm}$, and that sets the tower size. Finer tower segmentation is not called for, since no new information in the dense core of the shower can reasonably be extracted. Particle identification follows from the fact that hadron showers are much wider transversely, with a radius $\sim\lambda_0$.

In the generic detector, the barrel ECAL is at $r_E = 1.2\,\mathrm{m}$ and $|z_E| < 2.8\,\mathrm{m}$, covering the range $|\eta| < 1.5$. The ECAL towers are defined by the Molière radius in lead, $\delta\eta = \delta\phi \sim 2r_M/r_E = 0.027$. The barrel has 175 towers in z and 236 in azimuth. If there are three depth segments read out independently to measure the shower development in depth, then there are a total of 124 000 ECAL readout channels in the barrel alone. An event display of a photon + jet final state in CMS is shown in Fig. 3.8.

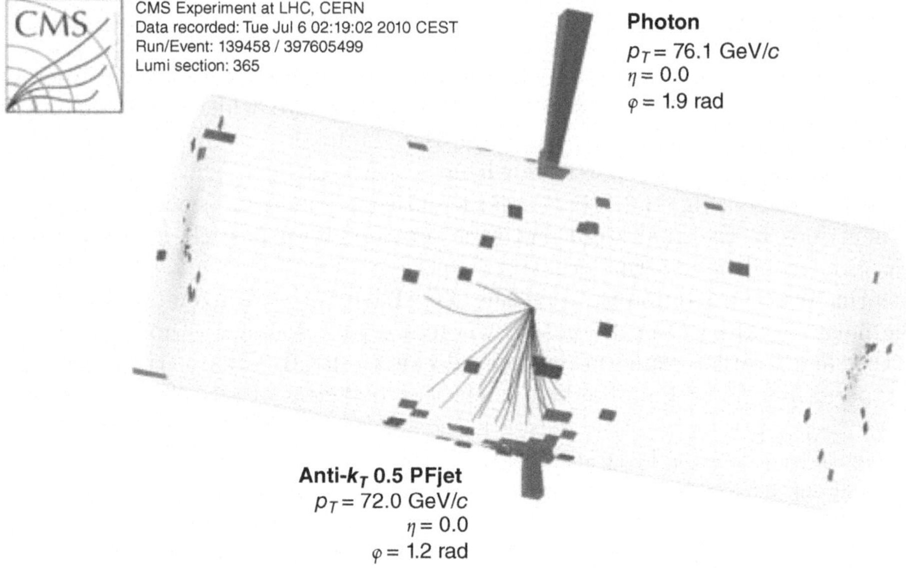

Fig. 3.8 Event display for a CMS candidate event with a photon plus a jet in the final state.

Note that the ECAL towers are displayed summed over 25 contiguous towers, which shows how fine the tower segmentation really is.

The radiation field is severe, since, in contrast to the tracking, the entire particle energy is now absorbed by the medium. The radiation dose in the barrel due solely to neutral-pion absorption by the ECAL medium is

$$(\text{Dose})_{\text{ECAL}} \sim \sigma_I L T D_0 \frac{1}{2\pi r_E^2} \frac{\langle P_T \rangle}{\rho_E \Delta t X_0}. \tag{3.15}$$

With three neutral pions per unit of rapidity, D_0, depositing 0.8 GeV into ECAL with a density ρ_E of Pb over a region $\Delta t X_0$ in depth, $\Delta t \sim 7$, there is a dose of ~ 0.097 Mrad/yr in the ECAL barrel. The dose in the end cap is, however, much higher. Fundamentally, the increase is due to the higher-energy pions in the end cap (at fixed transverse momentum, $E_\gamma = \langle P_T \rangle / \sin\theta$) and the smaller radii covered by the ECAL end cap, which is located at z_E. The dose ratio between the barrel and end cap for ECAL is approximately

$$\frac{(\text{Dose})_{\text{endcap}}}{(\text{Dose})_{\text{barrel}}} \sim \left(\frac{z_E}{r_E}\right)^2 \frac{1}{\theta^3}. \tag{3.16}$$

For the end cap, the minimum angle is at $|\eta_E| = 2.5$, where the dose ratio is about 42, which means that the end-cap ECAL has a yearly dose of about 4 Mrad. This rapid increase of dose with rapidity sets the limit in the generic ECAL on the angular coverage outfitted with precision electromagnetic calorimetry.

3.9   HCAL subsystem

The Hadronic Calorimeter (HCAL) measures the energy of the strongly interacting quarks and gluons by absorbing the jets of particles into which these fundamental particles fragment (Table 3.1). In addition, the "hermetic" calorimetry measures the energy of all the secondary particles within a range of $|y| <, 5$, which is sufficiently complete coverage (Fig. 3.2) that a large missing transverse energy (MET) indicates neutrinos in the final state and thus provides both particle identification and a measurement of the neutrino transverse energy.

In principle, the requirements on the HCAL are very stringent, again being set by the natural width of the W boson, where a dijet resonance is now reconstructed from the quark rather than the leptonic decay of the W. In practice, such precise energy performance, with an implied stochastic coefficient of $\sim 17.4\%$, at an energy of 0.25 TeV, is not attainable. One reason is the small number of particles in a hadronic shower, with the resulting large stochastic fluctuations in that number. The analogue of the critical energy for the ECAL is the threshold energy to make additional secondary pions, $E_{\text{th}} \sim 2m_\pi = 0.28$ GeV. That energy scale leads to an estimate for the number of particles in the hadronic shower of $\sim E/E_{\text{th}}$, which implies a stochastic coefficient of 53%, or 3.35% fractional energy resolution dE/E for $E = 0.25$ TeV, far from the requirement set by the natural resonance width of 1.1%:

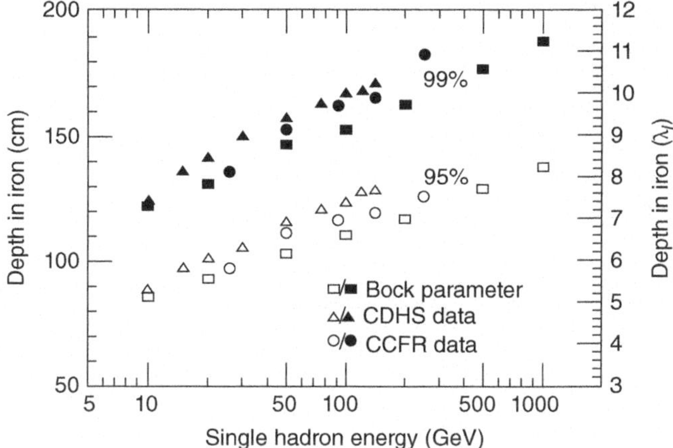

Fig. 3.9 Depth of calorimetry needed to contain a hadronic shower as a function of the energy of the hadron.

$$W^+ \to u + \bar{d}, \; c + \bar{s},$$
$$\Gamma_W / M_W = 2.6\%, \tag{3.17}$$
$$(dE/E)_{\text{HCAL}} \sim 1.1\%.$$

The total depth of the HCAL need not be as deep as that needed to fully contain the ECAL shower, because the hadron calorimetry does not achieve the desired 1.1% precision energy measurement and so leakage of shower energy at the back of the HCAL is not as strictly limited as in the ECAL case. A plot of the depth needed as a function of hadron energy to limit the shower leakage is shown in Fig. 3.9.

The hadronic shower is contained transversely in a cylinder of radius $\sim\lambda_0$. Assuming that overlapping hadronic showers cannot be resolved, a size $\delta z = \delta s = 15$ cm is chosen in the generic HCAL. The generic HCAL begins at radius $r_H = 1.6$ m. The HCAL towers then subtend a rapidity and azimuthal interval

$$\delta\eta = \delta\phi = 0.094 \sim \lambda_0 / r_H. \tag{3.18}$$

The larger transverse tower size leads to a greater probability for an HCAL tower to be occupied by a charged pion, $(D_c = 6)(N_I = 25)(\delta\eta)^2/2\pi = 0.21$. The mean transverse energy in an HCAL tower is then 0.16 GeV $= 0.21 \times 0.8$ GeV. The number of barrel HCAL towers in z is 10 m/0.15 m $= 67$ and in azimuth also 67, or 4490 HCAL readout towers in the barrel. With three depth segments read out independently, there are 13 470 towers in total. Note that the showers in both the ECAL and the HCAL develop longitudinally on the scale of the radiation length, so that a complete knowledge of the hadronic shower should logically have that depth segmentation. However, that level of detail has not been attempted in the LHC calorimeters, although it is planned for in ILC/CLIC calorimetry.

With regard to radiation, the HCAL is at a larger barrel radius than the ECAL, but there are twice as many charged as neutral pions. The hadronic shower energy is more spatially spread out than the electromagnetic shower, where for hadrons the initial interaction point has a mean of one and an RMS of one λ_0. Therefore, the full width of the deposited energy is roughly $\Delta\lambda_0 \sim 2\lambda_0$. Taking the factors together, the dose in the HCAL is about one-third that of ECAL at the same rapidity.

However, the need to cover angles as small as $|y| = 5$ arose from the requirement that the generic detector measure most of the inclusive inelastic pions and also measure the forward jets from the VBF process. This requirement places a large radiation

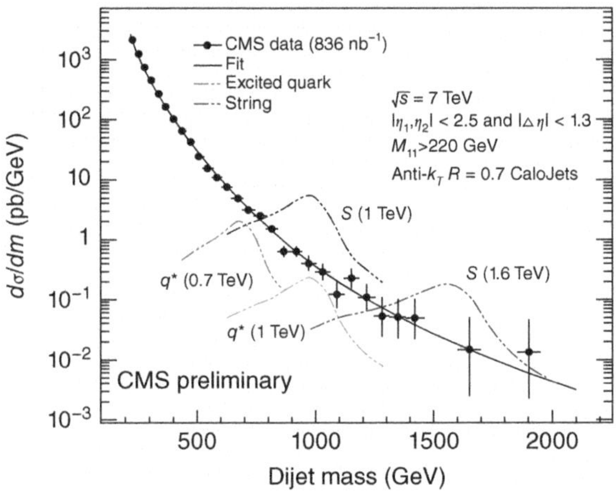

Fig. 3.10   CMS search for dijet resonances from early 2010 data.

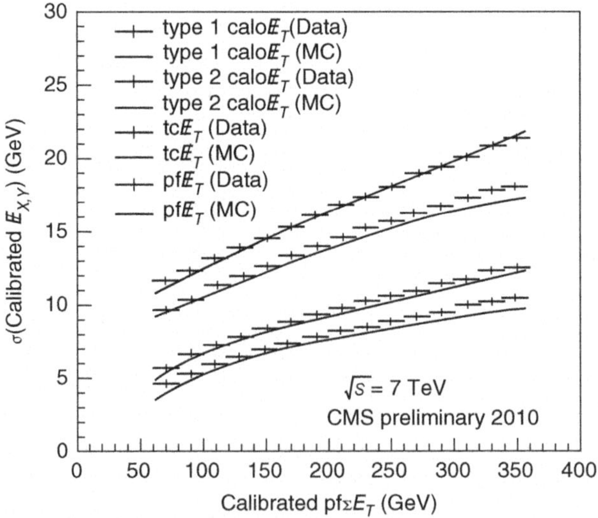

Fig. 3.11   Resolution in missing transverse momentum in CMS for dijet events using pure calorimetry and using "particle flow" combining calorimetry and tracking information.

burden on the forward calorimetry. It covers the range in $|y|$ from 2.5 to 5.0. At $|y| = 4$, the average pion energy is 22 GeV. Secondary particles deposit approximately 77 W of power, which heats the forward calorimetry. The luminosity can be measured in the forward calorimeter with a thermometer!

At $|\eta| = 5$, the polar angle is $0.75°$. At a location $z = 10$ m for the forward calorimetry, the radius in the (x, y) plane is only 13 cm, and a "tower" with the same $\delta\eta$ as the barrel HCAL would have an extent of only 1.2 cm in r and 7.7 cm in azimuth s. Clearly, such fine segmentation, given the physical size of a hadronic shower, is not very useful. Indeed, the pileup probability for a tower of transverse size $\sim \lambda_0$ is quite a bit higher than that for the barrel HCAL. Going to a smaller z, as indicated in Fig. 3.5, only makes the situation worse.

The radiation dose in the forward calorimetry may be roughly estimated to be

$$(\text{Dose})_{\text{forward}} \sim \sigma_I LT D_0 \frac{1}{2\pi z_F^2 \theta^3} \frac{\langle P_T \rangle}{\rho_{\text{forward}} \Delta t X_0} . \tag{3.19}$$

Taking only the most densely deposited neutral energy to be the full radiation dose and the z for the calorimetry, z_F, to be 10 m, and assuming the calorimeter to be made of steel, the dose is approximately 280 Mrad/yr at $|y| = 5$. The size of the dose sets the limit on the calorimetric coverage to $|y| < 5$ because of the need for long-term survivability of the forward calorimetry.

Nevertheless, the HCAL is an indispensable tool for measuring jets in the detector, as indicated in Table 3.1. A spectrum of jet–jet masses and the accompanying limits on new dijet resonances is shown in Fig. 3.10. Even in the first running of the LHC, the HCAL allows an exploration of such resonances at the several TeV mass scales. In Fig. 3.11, the resolution in missing transverse momentum is shown for standalone calorimetry and for the combined use of calorimetry and tracking. Tracking offers better resolution at low momentum than calorimetry alone. This is "particle flow" in the current jargon.

3.10   Muon subsystem

A major physics goal at the LHC is to explore vector boson interactions. Leptonic decays of the bosons are the favored mode, since the lepton backgrounds are low and the leptons can be cleanly and redundantly measured. The muon vector momentum and position are measured first in the tracking system. The muons then deposit only ionization energy in the ECAL and HCAL, while the other final-state particles are almost completely absorbed. In fact, the calorimetry can perform a useful muon identification role if the muons are isolated from other final-state particles by measuring the "minimum ionization particle" ionization energy in the HCAL. Ideally, in the muon system that follows the calorimetry in depth, only muons exist along with noninteracting neutrinos.

Muons at low transverse momentum arise from the decays of inclusively produced pions and kaons. These muons can largely be removed as a background by requiring a good tracker fit to the hypothesis of no decay "kink" in the found track.

For example, in the decay $\pi \to \mu + \nu$, the muon transverse momentum relative to the initial pion direction is only ~ 0.03 GeV. Therefore, a 10 GeV pion that decays in the tracker will have a 3 milliradian "kink" in the full track. In discussing the generic tracker, an angular resolution of 0.12 milliradians was quoted. Therefore, decays can be removed using the tracker up to a few hundred GeV. Since the probability to decay in the tracker falls with increasing momentum, pion and kaon decays are not a major problem at the high momentum scales that are of major interest to the LHC experimenters.

A second source of muons is heavy flavor decay, such as $b \to c + \mu + \nu$, which occurs much more promptly and within or before passage through the vertex detectors. The calculated LHC cross section in leading order for production of a b-quark pair where one b decays into a muon with transverse momentum greater than 10 GeV is $\sigma_\mu \sim 60\mu$b. At the LHC design luminosity, that cross section corresponds to a rate $R_\mu = \sigma_\mu L \sim 0.6$ MHz, which is small with respect to the total inelastic LHC rate of 1 GHz but too large with respect to an acceptable trigger rate.

The requirements for the muon system are similar to those for the tracking system. There should be a good momentum measurement up to ~ 0.25 TeV for the muons. In addition, the system must produce a trigger to reduce the rate of background muons from the heavy flavor decays. The ionization energy loss in the calorimetry provides a lower momentum cutoff for the muons. The generic HCAL contains 1.5 m of steel, which stops all muons with a momentum less than ~ 1.7 GeV. However, that cutoff is not sufficient to reduce the muon rate in the muon system to an acceptable level. Therefore, the muon system must measure the muon transverse momentum accurately, set a threshold value, say 20 GeV, and report it to the trigger system.

In the muon system, nearly all the particles are muons, but they are of low transverse momentum and arise from heavy flavor decays. Since the ionization-range cutoff is in energy, while the intrinsic muon rate is controlled by the transverse momentum, the rates in the forward muon systems are much larger than the rates at wide angles. Beam halo from upstream interactions in the LHC accelerator also makes the forward muon region more difficult. For these reasons, the generic muon system is thought to cover the same limited rapidity range as the tracking system, $|y| < 2.5$.

The steeply falling muon spectrum from heavy flavor decays means that the muon trigger system momentum resolution is very important. Poor resolution lets in a large number of triggers from lower-momentum muons measured to have a higher momentum because of finite resolution, thus increasing the trigger rate.

There is a complication for very-high-momentum muons. At the LHC, their momenta are sufficiently large that radiation is an issue. The muon is a heavy electron, so that it experiences the same forces as the electron but has a much reduced acceleration. Radiation scales as the square of the acceleration, so the critical energy for a muon is much larger, but still finite, compared with the critical energy for an electron; typical values in steel are ~ 300 GeV:

$$(E_c)_\mu \sim (E_c)_e (m_\mu/m_e)^2. \tag{3.20}$$

The particle rates outside the calorimetry are sufficiently low that drift chambers with large drift distances can be used, as opposed to the other subsystems in the generic detector. If the chambers are operated in "air," then the accuracy required is similar to that for the tracker and position resolution, and alignment specifications are stringent. If the chambers are operated in the flux return yoke of the solenoid, then the redundant muon momentum measurement is multiple-scattering-limited. In that case, the fractional momentum error is constant for momenta below which the alignment errors make a negligible contribution:

$$\frac{dP}{P} = \frac{E_s}{\sqrt{2}} \frac{1}{eB\sqrt{LX_0}}. \tag{3.21}$$

For example with $B = 2$ T in steel with an $L = 2$ m return yoke, the muon momentum is measured to 13%. The tracking provides a redundant momentum measurement with $<10\%$ momentum error for muons with momenta <1.3 TeV in comparison. At still higher momenta, the tracker resolution increases as P, so the muon system will improve the tracker muon momentum resolution, provided that good alignment of

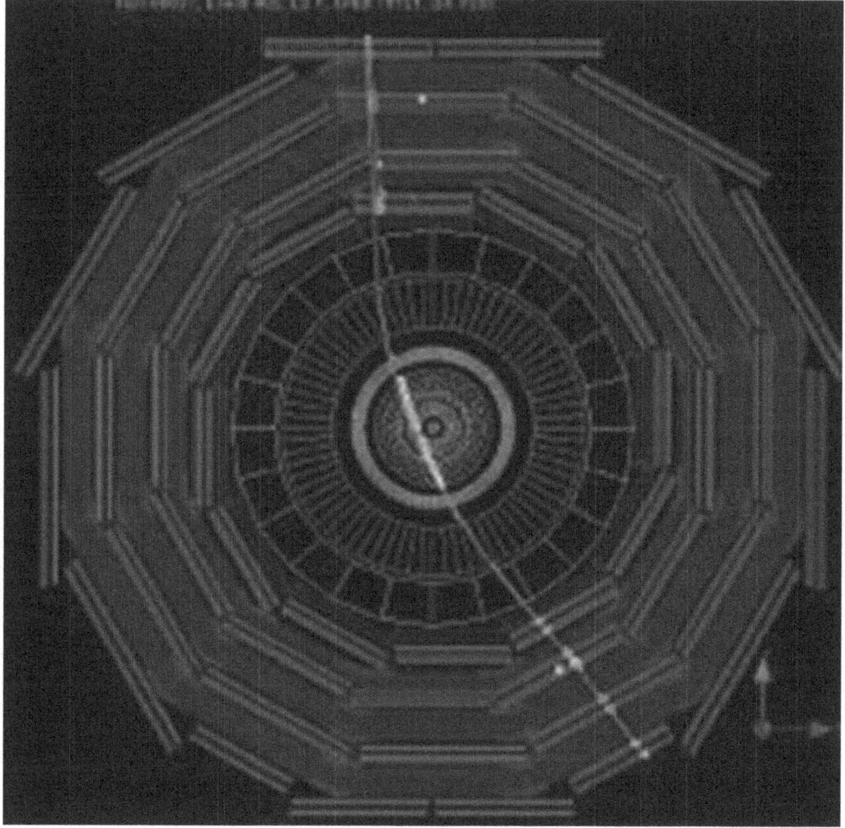

Fig. 3.12 Event display of a cosmic-ray muon in CMS, showing the redundant measurements in the tracking and muon subsystems.

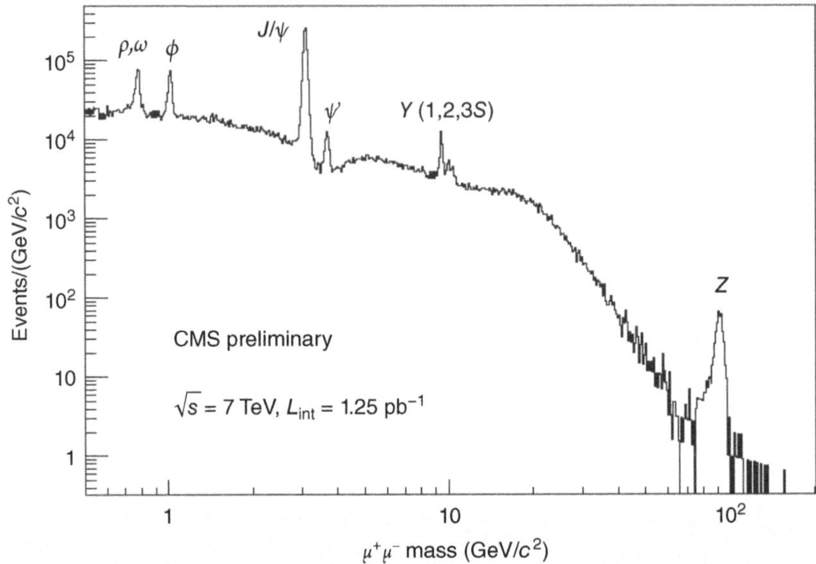

Fig. 3.13   Resonances observed in CMS in the dimuon final state.

the muon chambers can be maintained so that the measurement remains multiple-scattering-dominated.

An event display of a cosmic ray in CMS is shown in Fig. 3.12, where the muon trajectory in both the tracker and the muon subsystem is evident.

Data on dimuon resonances from CMS are shown in Fig. 3.13. The resonances vary from low-mass ones discovered 50 years ago to the Z, found in the 1980s.

3.11   Trigger/DAQ subsystems

The inclusive rate at the LHC design luminosity is 1 GHz. The number of interactions capable of being stored to permanent media is $\sim$100 Hz. Therefore, a reduction in rate by a factor of 10 million is needed. This is accomplished in steps. First, the rate is reduced by "triggering" on leptons and jets above some transverse momentum thresholds. Imposing these thresholds on the events reduces the rate to $\sim$100 kHz. In order to not incur dead time, a front-end "pipeline," which stores all the data until the first-stage trigger decision is made, is provided for each channel of data that is read out. There are $\sim$100 million independent channels of information, mostly analogue, in the generic detector. Typically, after this initial decision, the full event is sent from the detector front ends off the detector by means of digital optical fiber data transmission to a set of digital electronics accessible to the experimenters.

More incisive trigger decisions that reduce the event rate to $\sim$100 Hz are then made. Even after suppression of detector elements with no hits or with signals below some low threshold, the large number of particles per event and the large number of events piling up lead to a typical event size of 1 Mb. Assuming a data-taking run of ~4 months per year, 1000 Petabytes/yr—or about one million DVDs—are stored for offline analysis. The trigger and data acquisition techniques for both ATLAS and CMS are more or less specific to the experiment and thus are not susceptible to a "generic" analysis. In fact, after the first level of triggering, commercial off-the-shelf modules are mostly deployed. Examples are telecommunications switching networks used to assemble the full event using input from the different subsystems and "farms" of commodity PCs that are used for online high-level triggering and for offline analysis.

References

The LHC detectors and accelerator are well documented. ATLAS and CMS are described in [1–4], while the LHC is documented in [5, 6]. A full technical description of the detectors and accelerator is given in [7], and the specific detector choices and capabilities are described in [8].

[1] ATLAS experiment, <http://en.wikipedia.org/wiki/ATLAS_experiment> and links therein.
[2] Compact Muon Solenoid, <http://en.wikipedia.org/wiki/Compact_Muon_Solenoid>.
[3] CMS, <http://public.web.cern.ch/PUBLIC/en/LHC/CMS-en.html>.
[4] ATLAS Experiment, <http://atlas.web.cern.ch/Atlas/index.html>.
[5] The Large Hadron Collider, <http://lhc.web.cern.ch/lhc/>.
[6] LHC Design Report, <http://ab-div.web.cern.ch/ab-div/Publications/LHC-DesignReport.html>.
[7] The CERN Large Hadron Collider: accelerator and experiments, J. Instrum. **3** (2008) SO8001–SO8007.
[8] D. Froidevaux and P. Sphicas, General-purpose detectors for the Large Hadron Collider, Annu. Rev. Nucl. Part. Sci. **56** (2006) 375–440.

4
About the identification of signals at LHC: analysis and statistics

Bruno MANSOULIÉ

CEA IRFU Saclay, France

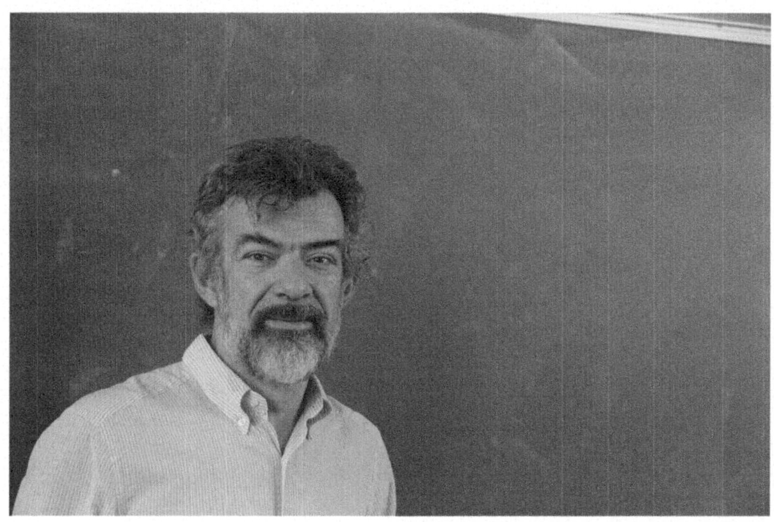

Theoretical Physics to Face the Challenge of LHC. Edited by L. Baulieu, K. Benakli, M. R. Douglas, B. Mansoulié, E. Rabinovici, and L. F. Cugliandolo. © Oxford University Press 2015. Published in 2015 by Oxford University Press.

Chapter Contents

As the vast majority of the students at the 2011 Les Houches Summer School were theoreticians, it was felt appropriate to give them a short guide through a "modern" analysis, typical of the analysis performed on the LHC data. The main ingredients are reviewed: irreducible and reducible backgrounds, background estimates from Monte Carlo or data-driven, signal and control regions, global fit, extraction of limits and signal, and the look-elsewhere effect.

4.1   Introduction

This chapter presents very briefly the main ingredients and steps of the analysis used in the search for the Standard Model Higgs boson decaying into WW $(l, l, \nu\nu)$ in the Atlas experiment, presented during the summer of 2011. This analysis has since been published in [1]. The presentation does not go into the details of the analysis, but rather tries to use it as an example of all analyses at LHC, emphasizing some delicate and important points. Indeed, any given analysis is often a complex construction, involving the classification of the data into several subcategories and the heavy use of Monte Carlo simulations. Most important is the *global modelling* of the whole analysis, used to derive background estimates, include systematic errors of all sorts, and finally extract results from statistical analysis. We then present the statistical aspect of the global search for the Higgs, and in particular we discuss the so-called "look-elsewhere effect".

4.2   Search for the Standard Model Higgs boson decaying into *WW* (in ATLAS)

The search for the Standard Model Higgs boson (SM Higgs) is of course of prime importance at the LHC. Given the Higgs production cross section and decay branching ratios (BRs), the highest sensitivity will be attained for a Higgs with a mass between 130 and 200 GeV, searched for in the WW decay channel where both W bosons decay into a lepton (e, μ) and a neutrino. Figure 4.1 shows the cross section multiplied by BR for the channels that can be considered for a search. WW in $l, l, \nu\nu$ benefits from a large BR of the Higgs to WW, a sizeable BR of the W into leptons (10% each), and a reasonable experimental signature given by the two leptons (ee, $e\mu$, or $\mu\mu$) and the missing transverse energy ($E_{T\mathrm{miss}}$) from the escaping neutrinos.

However, with two neutrinos in the final state, the invariant mass of the final state cannot be reconstructed. Hence, the signal will not show as a narrow mass peak on top of a smooth background continuum, unlike decay modes like $\gamma\gamma$ or $ZZ \to 4l$, but rather as an excess in a broad signal region, i.e. a *counting experiment*. The selection requests two well-identified leptons (e or μ) with transverse momenta p_T larger than 25 and 15 GeV, and $E_{T\mathrm{miss}}$ in excess of 25 or 40 GeV, depending on the supposed Higgs mass. The total cross section is about 200 fb, and after final cuts, it is reduced to 25 fb; i.e. there is a global efficiency for the signal of about 12%.

With the available integrated luminosity ($1\,\mathrm{fb}^{-1}$), the expected number of events is very small (25), and it is very easy to provide much larger numbers of fully

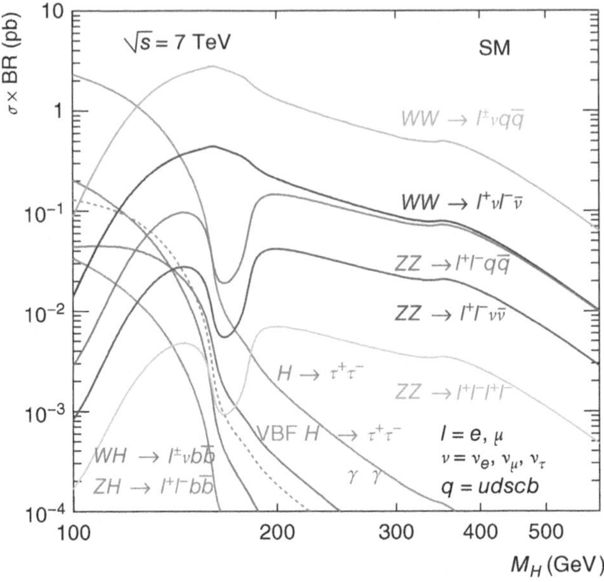

Fig. 4.1 Cross section multiplied by branching ratio for the main Higgs decay modes. (ATLAS Experiment © 2011 CERN).

simulated events. The only question is which theoretical physics to put in. Monte Carlo generators are available based on next-to-leading order (NLO) calculations, and the cross sections are available at next-to-next-to leading order (NNLO) and used for normalization.

4.3 Backgrounds

Despite the good signature offered by two leptons and $E_{T\text{miss}}$, several backgrounds can generate events in the signal region. The diversity of origins of these backgrounds offers a good example of a search for a very small signal among a large number of processes with an enormous range of cross sections. Trivially enough, the total background is the sum of all contributions: $\Sigma\sigma_i \times \epsilon_i$. with σ_i the cross section and ϵ_i the efficiency for each background component i. I would like to emphasize that in this sum, terms of the same order of magnitude can be formed from very different σ_i and ϵ_i.

4.3.1 *WW* continuum

The first background is of course the non-Higgs SM production of W pairs (continuum), followed by the same leptonic decays. Event by event, it is indistinguishable from the signal, and is thus an *irreducible* background. This continuum belongs to the class "small cross-section, large efficiency". Since no mass peak can be expected, the handles to increase the signal-to-background ratio are mostly related to event kinematics, and not to detector performance for particle identification or measurement.

It was noted early that the angular correlation of the charged leptons is different in the Higgs decay and in the continuum process. Indeed, for the scalar Higgs, the W spins are opposite, and from the V–A decay of the W's, the charged leptons tend to go in the same direction. At leading order (LO) and NLO, the continuum comes from quark–antiquark initial states, with no W polarization. Hence the leptons tend to go back to back because of the boost given by the W momenta. At the LHC, this is best seen in the transverse plane, and the $\Delta\phi$ distribution can be used to enrich the signal at small values of $\Delta\phi$. However, it was discovered that at NNLO there is a qualitatively different contribution from the gluon–gluon initial state, and that it induces some W polarization in the same way as that of the Higgs. It is of prime importance to estimate this contribution correctly, as well as the resulting angular distribution.

The Higgs is mostly produced by a gluon–gluon initial state, through a top quark loop. Because of this different initial state, it is more often accompanied by jets than the WW pairs of the continuum. This fact can be best exploited by separating the analysis into subchannels:
$WW + 0$ jet, $WW + 1$ jet, $WW + n(> 1)$ jets.
In this last category, $WW + 2$ jets helps also to select a different process of Higgs production (vector boson fusion), but, with a small event number, this mode was not used at this stage of the search.

This is a general feature of the recent analyses: dividing the analysis into subcategories. Of course, if a category contains a small part of the events but with a much larger signal-to-background ratio (S/B), one would tend to impose cuts that just keep this category. But if the S/B is significantly higher—but not much—one would lose in global significance because of the loss of the information contained in the other events. Dividing into subcategories that have a different S/B allows one to optimize globally the statistical power of the analysis.

In this class of "small cross-section, large efficiency", it is very easy to provide large numbers of simulated events for this background, as for the signal.

4.3.2   Top–antitop

Top quark pair production is a background to many searches at the LHC. The total cross section is large (165 pb), and the final states very diverse. Each top quark decays into a W boson and a b quark, and then the W and b each have a choice of decay modes, hadronic or (semi)leptonic. In this search, the most dangerous contribution to the $WW +$ jets channel comes from the decay chain $t\bar{t} \to WW b\bar{b} \to l\nu l\nu b\bar{b}$. For other analyses that need to identify b-quark jets, the detector has the capability of measuring very precisely the origin of charged tracks in the Inner Detector, and of looking for a secondary vertex, since the b lifetime allows it to fly away from the primary vertex by a few millimetres. In our case, this can be used to veto b quarks. However, the veto efficiency cannot be 100%, giving rise to backgrounds when one or two b-jets are outside the detector acceptance or have not been identified as b's.

For $1\,\mathrm{fb}^{-1}$, about $165\,000$ $t\bar{t}$ pairs have been produced in ATLAS data. If we want to safely simulate the inclusive process, we need at least 10 times more events, to be sure that every decay mode and configuration will be represented in the final Monte Carlo sample after all the analysis cuts. With the present computing systems (i.e. the LHC Grid etc.), it is possible to provide a few millions of simulated events for important processes like $t\bar{t}$. But if we want to trust the simulation to estimate the contribution of this process to the signal region, we need to be sure that the accuracy of the simulation is good to a precision that is typically the ratio of the inclusive cross section of this background to that of the signal: $165\,000/25 =$ order of 10^{-4}. Several factors enter—branching ratios, kinematics, b-jet identification—and it would be hazardous to take blindly the result of the simulation. The method is then to measure as many of these factors as possible in the data themselves: this is called a *data-driven method*. This can be done for example by checking that the *cut flow* is well reproduced in the Monte Carlo events starting from the initial event samples, down to levels of selection where the background still dominates any possible signal. One can also use *control regions*, selecting events with a configuration close to that of the signal but different—for example, inverting one or several of the selection cuts. In the case of the $t\bar{t}$ background, control regions are easily made by inverting the b veto into a b selection. However, one should beware that this method assumes that the ratio of "control-like" to "signal-like" events is again well described in the Monte Carlo simulation. In fact, there is *no rigorous proof* that data-driven methods give the right background estimates. It always requires the analyser (and reader!) physicist's commonsense that there is no strange unnoticed correlation that would make the extrapolation from control region to signal region invalid.

4.3.3 Z bosons

Z bosons are copiously produced at LHC: the cross section is about 30 nb at 7 TeV, and the branching ratio into each lepton species is 3%. The decays into ee or $\mu\mu$ can be efficiently rejected in the HWW analysis by cuts removing pairs with an invariant mass close to the Z mass, and also by requesting a large $E_{T\mathrm{miss}}$. This looks simple, and such well-identified events do not look dangerous. But there are tails in the $E_{T\mathrm{miss}}$ distribution coming from detector effects. $E_{T\mathrm{miss}}$ is obtained by making the vector sum (in the transverse plane) of all calorimetric deposits in the event. But how are these calibrated? Is the calibration the same for a quark jet or a gluon jet or a photon? What is the role of pileup events that add calorimeter energies everywhere? Muons (in particular the muons from Z decay) deposit some ionization energy in the calorimeter. Usually this energy is small and its most probable value can be corrected for. But what about the so-called "catastrophic muon energy losses"? Can we always identify these and take them into account? In some cases, a pileup event deposits energy close to a muon: if we identify it wrongly as muon-induced, this will bias the energy balance and generate spurious $E_{T\mathrm{miss}}$. Etc., etc.

The most dangerous contribution of the Z bosons comes from their decay into $\tau\tau$, which can subsequently decay leptonically. The cross section for these events is still 200 pb. For $1\,\mathrm{fb}^{-1}$, it is possible to simulate these 200 000 events. But are we sure of the correct description of these events by the Monte Carlo simulation to a few parts in 100 000? Indeed, it has been found that the selection of signal-like events is sensitive to the spin correlations between the τ's and to the role of polarization in their subsequent decay. Care should be taken that the Monte Carlo simulation correctly describes these very fine effects.

4.3.4 $W + \text{jets}$

W production corresponds to a very large cross section (about 10 nb). In a significant part of the events, the W is accompanied by one or more jets. The probability that a jet is identified as a lepton is very low: the detectors have been designed for a good lepton identification efficiency with a high jet rejection. Hence this is the typical, dangerous case of a large background submitted to a high rejection.

Generally, these events are rejected by requesting that the leptons be isolated, which is not the case for particles inside jets. One should be aware that this event sample contains different subcategories with very different properties. For example $W + \text{light jets}$ and $W + c$ jets or $W + b$ jets. The probabilities for these jets to fake a lepton are very different: b or c mesons can decay semileptonically into a real lepton. These can be partially rejected by requesting a small track impact parameter. Light jets can fake electrons because γ rays from π^0 decays can convert in the layers of the inner detector, or because a charged pion is very close to one or several γ's, etc. The probability for this to happen depends on the jet energy and location in the detector. Despite all efforts to model jet production and heavy flavour production and decay, and to model the detector very finely, this is a case where the Monte Carlo simulation cannot be used because of the very large numbers involved. It is hardly possible to simulate 10^8 events, and, even if it were, one would not trust the simulation to describe reality to a precision of a few parts in 10^8. Hence the $W + \text{jets}$ background is estimated with data-driven methods. Typically, a control region is defined containing $W + \text{jets}$ events with some selection of jets to make them closer to the signal configuration. The probability that these jets fake a lepton is evaluated on a different sample (QCD jets), and applied to the control region to estimate the contribution to the signal region. Several cross checks are used to control correlations, contribution of special cases, etc.

4.4   Global model of the analysis

4.4.1   The data model

Given the above, the analysis plan has to deal with many separate data samples:

- Nine independent channels:
  - three modes: ee, $e\mu$, $\mu\mu$;
  - for each mode: 0 jet, 1 jet, > 1 jet.
- For each channel:
  - one signal region;
  - two background control regions ($t\bar{t}$, $W + \text{jets}$).

The extraction of a possible Higgs signal consists in a global fit over these 27 data regions. This calculation will try to fit the event content of these regions by using either the expected contributions from the backgrounds only, or the same plus the contributions from a SM Higgs production. The statistical analysis will evaluate if, and by how much, the fit with a Higgs is better than the fit with background only.

This can be compared with another famous analysis: the search for Higgs decaying into two photons. The simplest that can be done is simply to select events with two photons and plot the distribution of their invariant mass. A signal would be seen as a peak on top of a smooth background. This could be considered as a fully data-driven background estimation, with the control regions taken as side bands or a fit to the (data) spectrum. In reality, the two photon analysis is also refined by splitting the sample according to the number of jets, etc., but the principle of searching for a peak above a smooth background remains: it is not necessary to describe in detail this background by simulations and/or data-driven methods. In the WW analysis, the absence of a strong discriminator makes the complicated modelling and fitting necessary. Note the importance of the global model: some backgrounds are estimated directly from the Monte Carlo simulation; others are estimated from control regions in the data themselves.

Table 4.1 Cross sections at the centre-of-mass energy of $\sqrt{s} = 7$ TeV for background processes. $W \to \ell\nu$ and the $Z/\gamma^* \to \ell\ell$ cross sections are single-flavour cross sections

PROCESS	GENERATOR	CROSS SECTION σ (pb) [$\times$ BR]
Inclusive $W \to \ell\nu$	ALPGEN	10.5×10^3
Inclusive $W \to \tau\nu$	PYTHIA	10.5×10^3
Inclusive $Z/\gamma^* \to \ell\ell\,(M_{\ell\ell} > 40\,\mathrm{GeV})$	ALPGEN	10.7×10^2
Inclusive $Z/\gamma^* \to \tau\tau\,(M_{\tau\tau} > 60\,\mathrm{GeV})$	PYTHIA	9.9×10^2
Inclusive $Z/\gamma^* \to \ell\ell\,(10 < M_{\ell\ell} < 40\,\mathrm{GeV})$	ALPGEN	3.9×10^3
Inclusive $Z/\gamma^* \to \tau\tau\,(10 < M_{\ell\ell} < 60\,\mathrm{GeV})$	PYTHIA	4.0×10^3
$t\bar{t}$	MC@NLO	164.6
Single top t-channel	AcerMC	64.2
Single top Wt	AcerMC	15.6
Single top s-channel	MC@NLO	4.6
WZ	MC@NLO	18.0
ZZ	MC@NLO	5.6
$qq/qg \to WW \to \ell\nu\ell\nu(\ell = e, \mu, \tau)$	MC@NLO	4.7
$gg \to WW \to \ell\nu\ell\nu(\ell = e, \mu, \tau)$	gg2WW	0.14
$\gamma W \to \ell\nu(\ell = e, \mu, \tau)$	PYTHIA, MADGRAPH	135.4
$b\bar{b}$ (e filter)	PYTHIA	7.5×10^4
$b\bar{b}$ (μ filter)	PYTHIA	7.7×10^4

The signal efficiency and the amount and efficiency of many backgrounds are evaluated by Monte Carlo simulations. Many event samples are generated, fully simulated by a large program based on GEANT IV, and reconstructed by the same software chain as the data. To give a flavour, Table 4.1 shows the main Monte Carlo data sets that are used [2].

4.4.2 Nuisance parameters

The analysis must of course take into account the possibility of systematic errors in all the quantities measured or estimated. In Table 4.2 shows the main systematic

Table 4.2 Experimental sources of systematic uncertainty per object or event

SOURCE OF UNCERTAINTY	TREATMENT IN ANALYSIS
Jet energy resolution (JER)	$\sim 14\%$
Jet energy scale (JES)	Takes into account close-by jets effect, jet flavour composition uncertainty and event pile-up uncertainty in addition to global JES uncertainty Global JES $< 10\%$ for $p_T > 15$ GeV and $|\eta| < 4.5$ Pile-up uncertainty 2-5% for $|\eta| < 2.1$ and 3–7% for $2.1 < \eta| < 4.5$
Electron selection efficiency	Separate systematics for electron identification, reconstruction, and isolation, added in quadrature Total uncertainty of 2–5%, depending on η and E_T
Electron energy scale	Uncertainty better than 1%, depending on η and E_T
Electron energy resolution	(Small) constant term varied within its uncertainty, 0.6% of the energy at
Muon selection efficiency	0.3–1 % as a function of $|\eta|$ and p_T
Muon momentum scale	η-dependent scale offset in p_T, up to $\sim 0.13\%$
Muon momentum resolution	p_T- and η-dependent resolution smearing functions, $\leq 5\%$
b-tagging efficiency	p_T-dependent scale factor uncertainties, 6–16%
b-tagging mis-tag rate	up to 21 % as a function of p_T
Missing transverse energy	13.2% uncertainty on topological cluster energy Electron and muon p_T changes owing to smearing propagated to MET Effect of out-of-time pileup: $E_{T\text{Miss}}$ smeared by 5 GeV in 1/3 of Monte Carlo events
Luminosity	3.7%

uncertainties [2]. The list of parameters that carry a systematic error is very long, from the integrated luminosity to the jet energy scale and lepton reconstruction efficiency, to cite only a few. Each of these has been determined by separate studies. For example, lepton reconstruction and identification efficiencies are determined from data samples of J/ψ and Z.

These parameters with systematic errors are treated as *nuisance parameters*: in the global fit, they are allowed to vary inside their systematic error. The model describes in detail the impact of each nuisance parameter on the various variables and in turn on the event content of all regions. In this way, with the proper model, correlations are automatically taken into account. For example, a variation of the jet energy scale (JES) is propagated to the measured jet energies, which changes the number of events above a certain energy cut. But it is also propagated to the measurement of $E_{T\mathrm{miss}}$ in which jets enter.

4.5 Statistics

4.5.1 Inferences

At this stage the selection cuts are fixed, the data model is defined (the event content of all data regions is known), and the nuisance parameters are defined and their error margin specified. The objective part of the analysis is complete. The last step is to apply an algorithm to synthesize the information to infer the presence or absence of a Higgs signal. This is usually presented in terms of *statistical significance*, but the reader (and especially young theorists!) should be aware that there is no unique definition of this, and that despite a nice mathematical presentation, *all inference methods* contain some part of arbitrariness and/or subjectivity [3].

In this chapter, 1 will not describe in detail the mathematics used to infer confidence levels: these can be found very clearly explained in [4]. However, in the same spirit as above, I would like to help theorists understand the philosophy behind the maths.

It is well known that there are two main types of methods for inference: Bayesian and deterministic. In Bayesian methods, one makes a hypothesis concerning the distribution of the background, an *a priori* probability (*"prior"*). The data then bring in additional information, and the result, through Bayes' law, can be interpreted in turn as a probability. The question is that the final result depends on the prior. After days of glory during the LEP era, the tendency is now rather in favour of the following, deterministic, method, although Bayesian studies are still in use. In practice, Bayesian results obtained with reasonable priors are very close to the deterministic ones.

In deterministic methods, we build a quantity (a test statistic) that indicates whether the data is more compatible with the background-only hypothesis or with the background-plus-signal hypothesis. This is the method used as a baseline here.

The reference model is the global fit of data to the expected background, fitting also the values of all nuisance parameters within their errors (marginalization of the nuisance parameters). The same fit is then performed adding a signal with strength μ compared with the SM Higgs signal. The likelihood with signal is compared with that without signal, all after marginalization of the nuisance parameters. The test statistic is taken as the ratio of the two likelihoods.

From these fits, we infer answers to two main kinds of questions:

- Concerning *background only*: What is the probability that the background alone has fluctuated up to the level seen in the data?
- Concerning *background and possible signal*, for each mass hypothesis, a statement on a potential signal: What is the signal strength that can be excluded at a given confidence level? (A signal strength μ means that the tested signal is μ times that of the SM Higgs.)

4.5.2 p_0 plot

The first statement is reflected in the p_0 *plot* of Fig. 4.2. Let us first concentrate on the "observed" line. From the definition (probability that the background fluctuates up to the level seen in data), the dips correspond to mass hypotheses where there is some sign of a signal or a signal-like fluctuation. The probability p_0 indicated is the *local* probability, i.e. the probability of a background fluctuation at this precise mass hypothesis. In the plot of Fig. 4.2, we see a broad depression from 110 to 160 GeV, with p_0 around 5%.

Let us now turn to the "expected" line. Given the statistics in the data (number of events) and the possible systematic errors, we would like to know what would the "observed" line be in the presence of a signal. At each mass hypothesis, we can generate a large number of *pseudo-experiments*, each of which represents one occurrence of the real experiment, with the backgrounds and signal of the SM Higgs. In each pseudo-experiment, events are drawn randomly in all regions, with the same

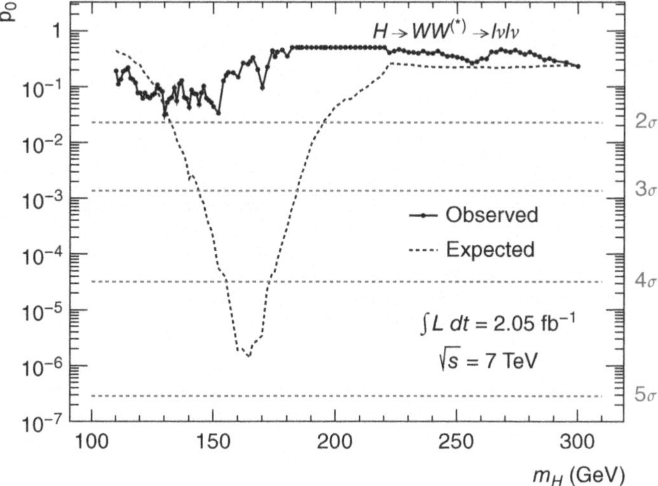

Fig. 4.2 p_0 plot: probability that the background fluctuates more than the data for each mass hypothesis. (ATLAS Experiment © 2011 CERN).

average numbers as that of the data, and a set of values of the nuisance parameters is drawn randomly from their distribution. Then each pseudo-experiment i is analysed as the real experiment, and $p_{0,i}(m)$ is derived for each mass hypothesis. At each mass, we define the "expected" $p_0(m)$ as the median of the $p_{0,i}(m)$ among the pseudo-experiments.

In practice, generating a large number of pseudo-experiments for all mass points, varying all nuisance parameters etc., would be extremely time-consuming computer-wise. One can instead use *asymptotic formulas* that model analytically the fluctuations of the parameters and event numbers. This is what is shown in the plot in Fig. 4.2. We see that the "expected" curve reaches very low values at around 160 GeV. This means that the experiment is very sensitive to a signal in this mass region: in this hypothesis, we would have seen so many events that it would be very improbable to interpret them as a fluctuation of the background. As this is not what is observed, we expect this mass range to be excluded by the actual data. In contrast, the wide dip at low mass is about what we would expect from the presence of a Higgs at 130 GeV, where the "observed" curve meets the "expected" one.

4.5.3 CL_s plot

The second statement is reflected in the famous CL_s plot in Fig. 4.3, also called the "green and yellow bands" plot. For each mass hypothesis, the "observed" line gives the value of μ which can be excluded by the observed data at 95% confidence level (CL). A value of 1 means that the SM Higgs can be excluded (in this channel) at 95% CL. Hence the *exclusion region* is simply the region of the x-axis where the "observed" line is below 1.

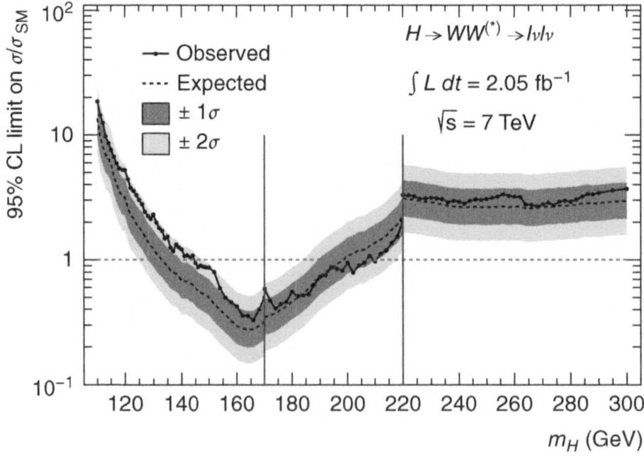

Fig. 4.3 CL_s plot: 95% exclusion level, observed, and expected (median, $\pm 1\sigma$ band, $\pm 2\sigma$ band). The step at 220 GeV is due to the change in analysis cuts at this mass value. (ATLAS Experiment © 2011 CERN).

Now we are interested in knowing if the "observed" line belongs to the class of lines that could normally be expected in the presence of background only, or if it has a distinctive feature (like the presence of a signal). Here again we use the pseudo-experiments, and analyse each of them, i, in the same way as the real one, deriving for each mass hypothesis a 95% CL value $\mu_{95,i}$. From the set of pseudo-experiments, at each mass hypothesis we can derive the median of these $\mu_{95,i}$, which we call the "expected" value, and the percentile values equivalent to $-1\sigma, +1\sigma$ (the dark ("green") band in Fig. 4.3) and $-2\sigma, +2\sigma$ (the light ("yellow") band). With these definitions, one can see directly if the "observed" line behaves as a "normal" experiment or not. If the "observed" line is below the "expected", it means that the actual data enabled one to exclude a *lower* value of μ than expected: presumably there were fewer events observed than expected. This can be interpreted as a downward fluctuation of the background if the background estimate is correct, or as an overestimate of the background. If the "observed" line is above the "expected", it means that the data did not enable one to exclude a value as low as the expected one. Thus can be interpreted as an upward fluctuation of the background, or the presence of a signal, or an underestimate of the background. Again here, we see that the "observed" line is above the "expected" line in a rather wide region between 110 and 160 GeV, at the 1σ or 2σ level. Indeed, the mass resolution of this channel is poor, and the "correlation length" along the x-axis is large.

4.6 Global Higgs analysis

As the Higgs branching ratios vary with mass, some channels are more sensitive than others in different mass ranges. In total, about 12 decay modes can be used, with very different statistical power, depending on the mass hypothesis. At the time of the lecture on which this chapter is based, only one mode (WW) had sensitivity for the SM Higgs in some range, with all the other modes giving a μ_{95} value larger than 1 for all masses. At the time of writing of this chapter, combined analyses have been published by ATLAS and CMS. The discussion here is based on the ATLAS combination published in [5], based on all the 2011 data (almost 5 fb^{-1}).

4.6.1 Global combination

The method for combining different channels is quite similar to the method for combining the information from different data regions in the previous analysis. All signal and control regions are fed into a global model, as well as all nuisance parameters. The fit then tries to adapt the data to background or signal+ background expectations, in each case with marginalization of the nuisance parameters. The resulting p_0 and CL_s plots are shown in Fig. 4.4(a) and (b). A third plot, the $\hat{\mu}$ plot (Fig. 4.4(c)), shows for each mass the best-fit value of the signal strength μ, always relative to the signal of the SM Higgs. The shaded band in this plot is an estimate of the $\pm 1\sigma$ variation that could be expected for the experiment (strictly speaking, this calculation is not exact for the lowest, negative values of $\hat{\mu}$; hence the exact definition of the band is written on the plot).

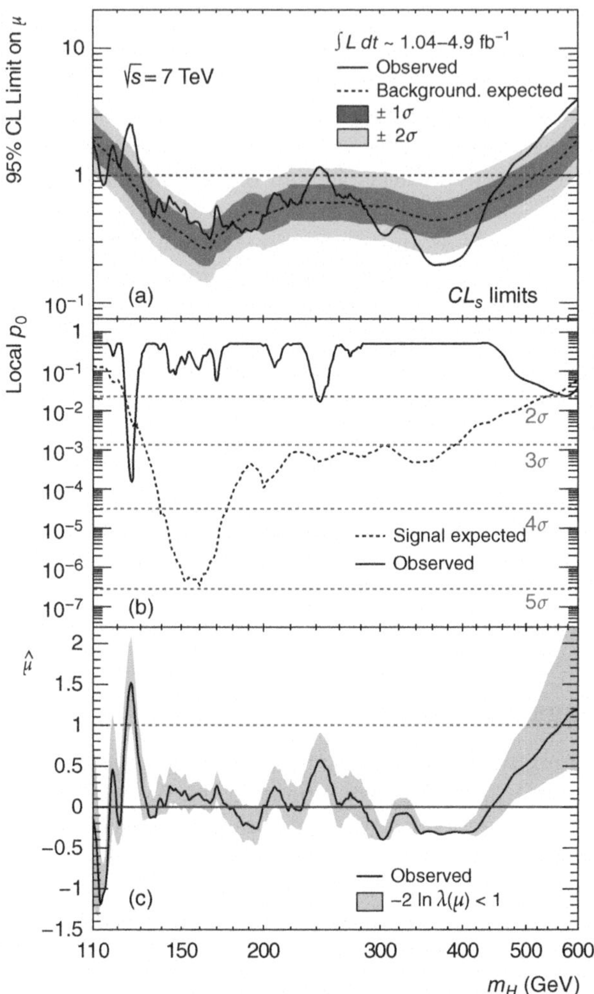

Fig. 4.4 Combined Higgs search: (a) CL_s; (b) p_0; (c) $\hat{\mu}$. (ATLAS Experiment © 2011 CERN).

The plots show asymptotic results, but several points in mass have been cross-checked with a large number of pseudo-experiments, and the differences are reported in [5] (especially so in the vicinity of the apparent excess).

From the CL_s plot, we see that the SM Higgs is excluded at 95% CL in a large mass range 131–468 GeV (the "observed" line is below 1) except for a tiny region at 245 GeV. Note that the line shows a very local dip at 114 GeV, which can be interpreted as a downward fluctuation of the background, but which enables one to exclude the 114.5 GeV value hinted at by LEP data. There is also a large dip around 360 GeV where observed is more than 2σ below expected.

On the p_0 plot, we see some dips corresponding to excesses in the data, that with the lowest p_0 being for a mass hypothesis of 125 GeV with $p_0 = 210^{-4}$, and some other local excesses with higher probability of a background fluctuation. From the $\hat{\mu}$ plot, we see that the signal strength is indeed compatible with zero everywhere except at 125 GeV. The best-fit value is 1.5 at 125 GeV: if it is really due to a 125 GeV Higgs, we have been a bit "lucky", but the 1σ band includes 1, meaning that the number of events is well compatible with a SM Higgs.

Indeed, the three plots display the same features seen from different points of view: exclusion limit, probability of a background fluctuation, best-fit signal strength. In particular, the structure at 125 GeV is the most "signal-like" of the excesses, with a local probability of a background fluctuation of 210^{-4}, i.e. a $3.6\ \sigma$ effect.

4.6.2   Look-elsewhere effect

If one has no a priori preferred mass hypothesis, the interesting question is rather: "What is the probability that the background fluctuates up to the level of the data *anywhere in the explored mass range?*" This probability is obviously larger than any local probability. This is referred to as the *look-elsewhere effect (LEE)*. The LEE has always been considered intuitively, but it is only recently that experiments have tried to quantify it when presenting their results. Consider a histogram of a variable (e.g. an invariant mass) with 10 independent bins, and suppose that the background has a flat distribution. The data consist of 1000 events. For background only, in each bin, the distribution of the content is given by the Poisson law with average 100 (very close to a Gaussian with average 100 and $\sigma=10$). To test the presence of a "signal" in a single bin with content c, we calculate the probability p_c of a background fluctuation beyond c, i.e. the sum of the Poisson probabilities from c to infinity. To translate into "standard deviations", we just recall that in the Gaussian approximation the integral beyond c is the integral of the Gaussian beyond $(c-100)/10$ standard deviations. Now the probability that *any* of the 10 bins had such a fluctuation is obviously $10 \times p_c$, since the bins are independent.

Of course, in a real invariant mass distribution, the bins are not independent. Neighbouring bins are correlated if they are closer than the resolution of the measurement. Roughly speaking, if the resolution is constant over the mass range considered, the number of independent bins is the abscissa range of the histogram Δm divided by the resolution δm. Hence the old rule of thumb to estimate the global probability of a background fluctuation was to take $p_c \times \Delta m/\delta m$. Obviously this naive estimate could not apply in more complicated cases, when the resolution depends on the mass, or in cases like that here where the analysis is based on a fit more complicated than a single-variable histogram. Procedures have been found recently that allow one to calculate a global probability in a consistent way [6]. In the example above of the combined Higgs search, the global probability that a background fluctuation appears anywhere in the mass range with a local p_0 as low as the observed one is 1.4%, corresponding to a 2.2σ effect.

However, it should be noted that just around the corner lies the question of arbitrariness in inferring the presence or absence of a new signal: we know how to quantify the global probability of a background fluctuation in one plot, and even in one analysis. But large experiments make hundreds of plots and dozens of analyses. What is the probability that *any* of these display an excess? First there is the question of *naturalness* of the analysis: was it defined before data-taking? Of course, the best is a blind analysis, or one where we defined the analysis on a first set of data, and just look at a second (independent) set of data without touching anything. Here, for the SM Higgs search, the modes and the analyses are naturally dictated by the SM itself and the analysis is more or less "unique". But for searches beyond the SM, we should keep in mind the number of analyses, as an additional LEE.

4.7 Conclusion

Analyses in large modern particle physics experiments are often quite complex and difficult to comprehend globally. However, a lot of effort has been devoted to standardizing the methods, rationalizing the background and error calculations, systematizing the statistical treatment, and synthesizing the results. The Higgs search is of course of such a importance that all the tools have been refined and utilized to extract as much information as possible from the data, while keeping a safe estimate of the uncertainties.

This chapter has attempted to help young theorists in understanding what is going on in an analysis and what are the delicate points and possible pitfalls, and finally to help them interpret correctly the most usual statistical plots.

References

[1] The ATLAS Collaboration. Search for the Higgs boson in the $H \to WW^{(*)} \to \ell^+\nu\ell^-\bar{\nu}$ decay channel in pp collisions at $\sqrt{s} = 7$ TeV with the ATLAS detector. Phys. Rev. Lett. **108** (2012) 111802 [arXiv:1112.2577 [hep-ex]].

[2] The ATLAS Collaboration. Search for the Standard Model Higgs boson in the $H \to WW^{(*)} \to \ell\nu\ell\nu$ decay mode with the ATLAS detector. ATLAS-CONF-2011-111 (2011).

[3] K. Popper, The Logic of Scientific Discovery, 1934 (as Logik der Forschung, English translation 1959).

[4] G. Cowan, K. Crammer, E. Gross, and O. Vitells. Asymptotic formulae for likelihood-based tests of new physics. Eur. Phys. J. **C71** (2011) 1554 [arXiv 1007.1727v2 [physics. data-anal]], and references within.

[5] The ATLAS Collaboration. Combined search for the Standard Model Higgs boson using up to 4.9 fb^{-1} of pp collision data at $\sqrt{s} = 7$ TeV with the ATLAS detector at the LHC. Phys. Lett. **B710** (2012) 49–66 [arXiv:1202.1408 [hep-ex]].

[6] E. Gross and O. Vitells. Trial factors for the look elsewhere effect in high energy physics. Eur. Phys. J. **C70** (2010) 525–530 [arXiv:1005.1891 [physics. data-anal]].

5
Introduction to the theory of LHC collisions

Michelangelo L. MANGANO

Theory Division CERN, Geneva, Switzerland

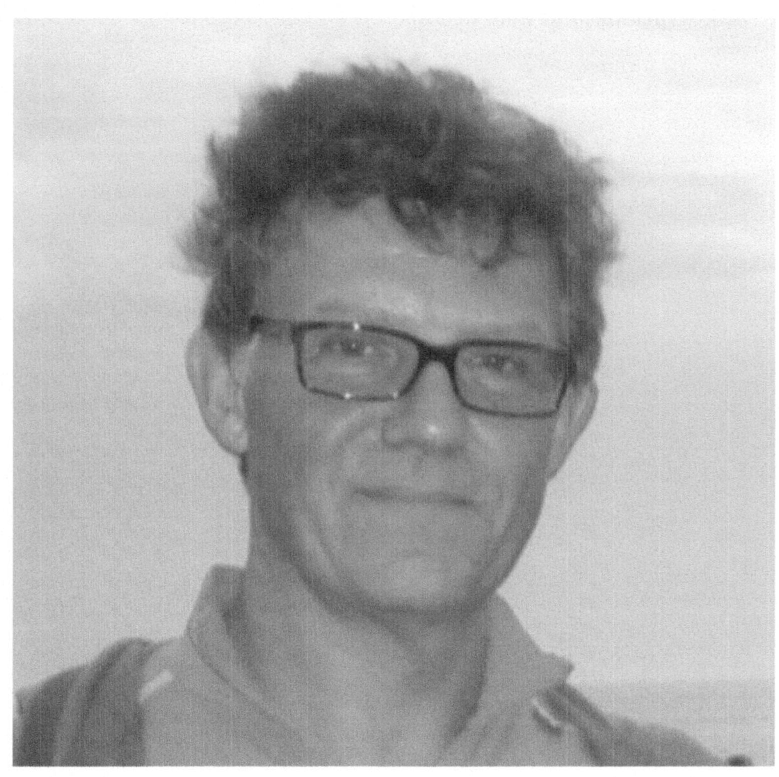

Theoretical Physics to Face the Challenge of LHC. Edited by L. Baulieu, K. Benakli, M. R. Douglas, B. Mansoulié, E. Rabinovici, and L. F. Cugliandolo. © Oxford University Press 2015. Published in 2015 by Oxford University Press.

Chapter Contents

5.1 Introduction

The frontier of high-energy physics is being redefined by the experiments at CERN's Large Hadron Collider (LHC), the proton–proton collider operating at a centre-of-mass energy of 8 TeV (to become $\sim$14 TeV by 2014). The main goal of these experiments is to unveil the nature of electroweak symmetry breaking, via the detection of the Higgs boson and of other new particles associated with possible extensions of the Standard Model (SM). While strong interactions between quarks and gluons—described by quantum chromodynamics (QCD)—have no direct relation to electroweak phenomena, their role in making the LHC physics programme possible cannot be underestimated. The processes leading to the creation of Higgs bosons, and other interesting particles, are all driven by the interactions among quarks and gluons, and it is these interactions that will define the production rate of the new phenomena, as well as of the numerous SM processes that will act as irreducible backgrounds to their detection. A solid and quantitative understanding of the role of strong interactions in LHC physics is therefore essential for full exploitation of the LHC's discovery and measurement potential. Most of the collisions between protons are the result of the complex long-distance QCD dynamics responsible for holding quarks together, and their quantitative description still lacks a robust first-principles understanding. On the other hand, the processes leading to the production of heavy elementary particles arise from the short-distance interactions among the pointlike proton constituents. These *hard* interactions can be described by the perturbative regime of QCD, making it possible to perform quantitative, first-principles predictions.

This chapter will illustrate the basic principles underlying the use of perturbative QCD in predicting the structure of hard processes in high-energy hadronic collisions. The starting point, in Section 5.2, will be a discussion of the factorization formula, which is the basis for the description of all hard processes in terms of universal functions parametrizing the density of quarks and gluons inside the proton. In Section 5.3, I discuss the evolution of the perturbative final states, made of quarks and gluons, toward physical systems made of hadrons. Finally, Section 5.4 collects several applications and examples of comparisons between the theoretical predictions and present data. These will provide a picture of the success of this theoretical framework, giving good confidence on the reliability of its future applications to the study of LHC collisions.

The treatment will be introductory, and the emphasis will be on basic and intuitive physics concepts. Given the large number of papers that have contributed to the development of the field, it is impossible to provide a complete and fair bibliography. I therefore limit my bibliography to some review books and to references to some of the key results discussed here. For an excellent description of the early ideas about quarks and their dynamics, the classic reference is Feynman's book [1]. The emergence of QCD as a theory for strong interactions is nicely reviewed in [2]. For a general, but rather formal, introduction to QCD, see [3]. For a more modern and pedagogical introduction, in the context of an introductory course on field theory, I refer to the excellent book by Peskin and Schroeder [4]. For a general introduction to collider physics, see [5]. For QCD applications to the LEP, Tevatron, and LHC, see [6] and, specifically for the LHC, [7]. Explicit calculations, including the nitty-gritty details of next-to-leading-order (NLO) calculations and renormalization, are given in great detail for several concrete cases of interest in [8]. Many of the ideas used in this review are inspired by the very physical perspective presented in [9]. While I shall be making occasional reference to perturbative calculations and to Monte Carlo generator tools, I shall not provide a systematic review of the state of the art in these very active areas. For recent status reports, see [10, 11].

5.2 QCD and the proton structure at large Q^2

An understanding of the structure of the proton at short distances is one of the key ingredients in predicting cross sections for processes involving hadrons in the initial state. All processes in hadronic collisions, even those intrinsically of electroweak nature such as the production of W/Z bosons or photons, are in fact induced by the quarks and gluons contained inside the hadrons. In this section, I shall introduce some important concepts, such as the notions of partonic densities of the proton and of parton evolution. These are the essential tools used by theorists to predict production rates for hadronic reactions.

We shall limit ourselves to processes where a proton–(anti)proton pair collides at large centre-of-mass energy ($\sqrt{S}$, typically larger than several hundred GeV) and undergoes a very inelastic interaction, with momentum transfers between the participants in excess of several GeV. The outcome of this hard interaction could be the simple scattering at large angle of some of the hadron's elementary constituents, their annihilation into new massive resonances, or a combination of the two. In all cases, the final state consists of a large multiplicity of particles, associated with the evolution of the fragments of the initial hadrons, as well as of the new states produced. As discussed below, the fundamental physical concept that makes the theoretical description of these phenomena possible is 'factorization', namely the ability to isolate separate independent phases of the overall collision. These phases are dominated by different dynamics, and the most appropriate techniques can be applied to describe each of them separately. In particular, factorization allows one to decouple the complexity of the proton structure and of the final-state hadron formation from the elementary nature of the perturbative hard interaction among the partonic constituents.

Figure 5.1 illustrates how this works. As the left proton travels freely before coming into contact with the hadron coming in from the right, its constituent quarks are held together by the constant exchange of virtual gluons (e.g. gluons a and b in the picture). These gluons are mostly soft, because any hard exchange would cause the constituent quarks to fly apart, and a second hard exchange would be necessary to reestablish the balance of momentum and keep the proton together. Gluons of high virtuality (gluon c in the picture) therefore prefer to be reabsorbed by the same quark, within a time inversely proportional to their virtuality, as prescribed by the uncertainty principle. The state of the quark is, however, left unchanged by this process. Altogether, this suggests that the global state of the proton, although defined by a complex set of gluon exchanges between quarks, is nevertheless determined by interactions that have

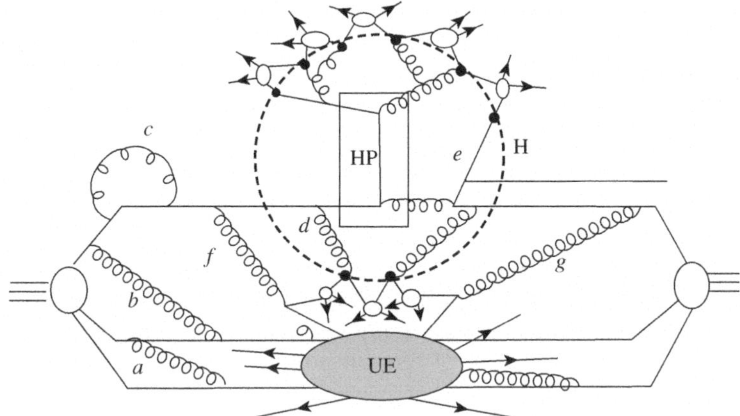

Fig. 5.1 General structure of a hard proton–proton collision.

a timescale of the order of $1/m_p$. When seen in the laboratory frame, where the proton is moving with energy $\sqrt{S}/2$, this time is furthermore Lorentz-dilated by a factor $\gamma = \sqrt{S}/2m_p$. If we disturb a quark with a probe of virtuality $Q\chi m_p$, the time frame for this interaction is so short $(1/Q)$ that the interactions of the quark with the rest of the proton can be neglected. The struck quark cannot negotiate with its partners a coherent response to the external perturbation: it simply does not have the time to communicate to them that it is being kicked away. On this timescale, only gluons with energy of the order of Q can be emitted, something that, to happen coherently over the whole proton, is suppressed by powers of m_p/Q (this suppression characterizes the 'elastic form factor' of the proton). In Fig. 5.1, the hard process is represented by the rectangle labelled HP. In this example a head-on collision with a gluon from the opposite hadron leads to a $qg \rightarrow qg$ scattering with a momentum exchange of the order of Q. This and other possible processes can be calculated from first principles in perturbative QCD, using elementary quarks and gluons as external states.

When the constituent is suddenly deflected, the partons that it had recently radiated cannot be reabsorbed (as happened to gluon c earlier), because the constituent is no longer there waiting for the partons to come back. This is the case, for example, of the gluon d emitted by the quark, and of the quark e from the opposite hadron; the emitted gluon became engaged in the hard interaction. The number of 'liberated' partons will depend on the hard scale Q: the larger the value of Q, the more sudden the deflection of the struck parton, and the fewer the partons that can reconnect before its departure (typically only partons with virtuality larger than Q).

After the hard process, the partons liberated during the evolution before the collision and the partons created by the hard collision will themselves emit radiation. The radiation process, governed by perturbative QCD, continues until a low-virtuality scale is reached (the boundary region labelled with a dotted line H in Fig. 5.1). To describe this perturbative evolution phase, proper care has to be taken to incorporate quantum coherence effects, which in principle connect the probabilities of radiation off different partons in the event. Once the low-virtuality scale is reached, the memory of the hard-process phase has been lost, once again as a result of different timescales in the problem, and the final phase of hadronization takes over. Because of the decoupling from the hard-process phase, the hadronization is assumed to be independent of the initial hard process, and its parametrization, tuned to the observables of some reference process, can then be used in other hard interactions (universality of hadronization). Nearby partons merge into colour-singlet clusters (the grey blobs in Fig. 5.1), which then decay phenomenologically into physical hadrons. To complete the picture, we need to understand the evolution of the fragments of the initial hadrons. As shown in Fig. 5.1, this evolution cannot be entirely independent of what happens in the hard event, because at least colour quantum numbers must be exchanged to guarantee the overall neutrality and conservation of baryon number. In our example, the gluons f and g, emitted early on in the perturbative evolution of the initial state, split into $q\bar{q}$ pairs, which are shared between the hadron fragments (whose overall interaction is represented by the oval labelled UE, for 'underlying event') and the clusters resulting from the evolution of the initial state.

The above ideas are embodied in the following factorization formula, which represents the starting point of any theoretical analysis of cross sections and observables in hadronic collisions:

$$\frac{d\sigma}{dX} = \sum_{j,k} \int_{\hat{X}} f_j(x_1, Q) f_k(x_2, Q) \frac{d\hat{\sigma}_{jk}(Q)}{d\hat{X}} F(\hat{X} \to X; Q), \qquad (5.1)$$

where

- X is some hadronic observable (e.g. the transverse momentum of a pion or the invariant mass of a combination of particles,);
- the sum over j and k extends over the parton types inside the colliding hadrons;
- the function $f_j(x, Q)$ (known as the parton distribution function, PDF) parametrizes the number density of parton type j with momentum fraction x in a proton probed at a scale Q (more later on the meaning of this scale);
- $\hat{X}$ is a parton-level kinematical variable (e.g. the transverse momentum of a parton from the hard scattering);
- $\hat{\sigma}_{jk}$ is the parton-level cross section, differential in the variable $\hat{X}$;
- $F(\hat{X} \to X; Q)$ is a transition function, weighting the probability that the partonic state defining $\hat{X}$ gives rise, after hadronization, to the hadronic observable X.

In the rest of this section, I shall cover the above ideas in some more detail. While I shall not provide you with a rigorous proof of the legitimacy of this approach, I shall try to justify it qualitatively to make it sound at least plausible.

5.2.1 The parton densities and their evolution

As mentioned above, the binding forces responsible for the quark confinement are due to the exchange of rather soft gluons. If a quark were to exchange just a single hard virtual gluon with another quark, the recoil would tend to break the proton apart.

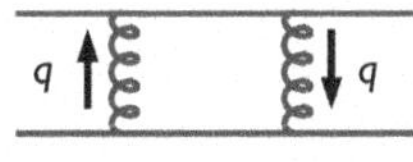

Fig. 5.2 Gluon exchange inside the proton.

It is easy to verify that the exchange of gluons with virtuality larger than Q is then proportional to some large power of m_p/Q, where m_p is the proton mass. Since the gluon coupling constant gets smaller at large Q, exchange of hard gluons is significantly suppressed.[1] Consider in fact the picture in Fig. 5.2. The exchange of two gluons is required to ensure that the momentum exchanged after the first gluon emission is returned to the quark, and the proton maintains its structure. The contributions of hard gluons to this process can be approximated by integrating the loop over large momenta:

$$\int_Q \frac{d^4 q}{q^6} \sim \frac{1}{Q^2}. \tag{5.2}$$

At large Q, this contribution is suppressed by powers of $(m_p/Q)^2$, where the proton mass m_p is included as being the only dimensionful quantity available (one could use here the fundamental scale of QCD, Λ_{QCD}, but numerically this is anyway of the order of a GeV). The interactions keeping the proton together are therefore dominated by soft exchanges, with virtuality Q of the order of m_p. Owing to Heisenberg's uncertainty principle, the typical timescale of these exchanges is of the order of $1/m_p$: this is the time during which fluctuations with virtuality of the order of m_p can survive. In the laboratory system, where the proton travels with energy E, this time is Lorentz-dilated to $\tau \sim \gamma/m_p = E/m_p^2$. If we probe the proton with an off-shell photon, the interaction takes place during the limited lifetime of the virtual photon, which, once more from the uncertainty principle, is given by the inverse of its virtuality. Assuming that the virtuality $Q \gg m_p$, once the photon gets 'inside' the proton and meets a quark, the struck quark has no time to negotiate a coherent response with the other quarks, because the time scale for it to 'talk' to its partners is too long compared with the duration of the interaction with the photon itself. As a result, the struck quark has no option but to interact with the photon as if it were a free particle. Let us look in more detail at what happens during such a process. In Fig. 5.3, we see a proton as it approaches a hard collision with a photon of virtuality Q. Gluons emitted at a scale $q > Q$ have the time to be reabsorbed, since their lifetime is very short. Their contribution to the process can be calculated in perturbative QCD, since the scale is large and in the domain where perturbative calculations are meaningful. Since after being reabsorbed the state of the quark remains the same, their only effect is an overall renormalization of the wavefunction, and they do not affect the quark density. A gluon emitted at a scale $q < Q$, however, has a lifetime longer than the time it takes for the quark to interact with the photon, and by the time it tries to reconnect to its parent

---

[1] The fact that the coupling decreases at large Q plays a fundamental role in this argument. Were this not true, the parton picture could not be used!

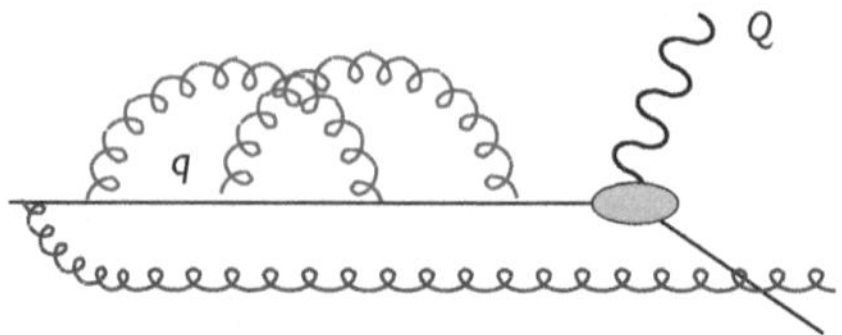

Fig. 5.3 Gluon emission at different scales during the approach to a hard collision.

quark, the quark has been kicked away by the photon, and is no longer there. Since the gluon has taken away some of the quark momentum, the momentum fraction x of the quark as it enters the interaction with the photon is different from the momentum it had before, and therefore its density $f(x)$ is affected. Furthermore, when the scale q is of the order of 1 GeV, the state of the quark is not calculable in perturbative QCD. This state depends on the internal wavefunction of the proton, which perturbative QCD cannot predict. We can, however, say that the wavefunction of the proton, and therefore the state of the 'free' quark, are determined by the dynamics of the soft-gluon exchanges inside the proton itself. Since the timescale of this dynamics is long compared with the timescale of the photon–quark interaction, we can safely argue that the photon sees to good approximation a static snapshot of the proton's inner configuration. In other words, the state of the quark had been prepared long before the photon arrived. This also suggests that the state of the quark will not depend on the precise nature of the external probe, provided the timescale of the hard interaction is very short compared with the time it would take for the quark to readjust itself. As a result, if we could perform some measurement of the quark state using, say, a virtual-photon probe, we could then use this knowledge on the state of the quark to perform predictions for the interaction of the proton with any other probe (e.g. a virtual W or even a gluon from an opposite beam of hadrons). This is the essence of the universality of the parton distributions.

The above picture leads to an important observation. It appears in fact that the distinction between which gluons are reabsorbed and which are not depends on the scale Q of the hard probe. As a result, the parton density $f(x)$ appears to depend on Q. This is illustrated in Fig. 5.4. The gluon emitted at a scale μ has a lifetime short enough to be reabsorbed before a collision with a photon of virtuality $Q < \mu$, but too long for a photon of virtuality $Q > \mu$. When going from μ to Q, therefore, the partonic density $f(x)$ changes. We can easily describe this variation as follows:

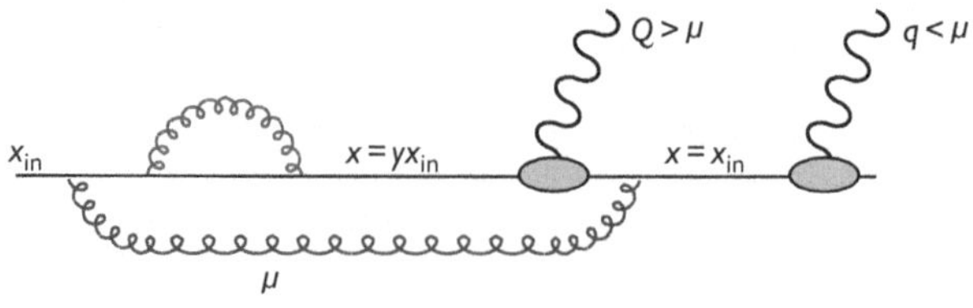

Fig. 5.4 Scale dependence of the gluon emission during a hard collision.

$$f(x, Q) \;=\; f(x, \mu) + \int_x^1 dx_{\mathrm{in}}\, f(x_{\mathrm{in}}, \mu) \int_\mu^Q dq^2 \int_0^1 dy\, P(y, q^2)\, \delta(x - y x_{\mathrm{in}}), \quad (5.3)$$

Here we obtain the density at the scale Q by adding to $f(x)$ at the scale μ (which we label as $f(x, \mu)$) all the quarks with momentum $x_{in} > x$ that retain a proton-momentum fraction $x = y/x_{\mathrm{in}}$ by emitting a gluon. The function $P(y, Q^2)$ describes the 'probability' that the quark emits a gluon at a scale Q, keeping a fraction y of its momentum. This function does not depend on the details of the hard process—it simply describes the radiation of a free quark subject to an interaction with virtuality Q. Since $f(x, Q)$ does not depend upon μ (μ is just used as a reference scale to construct our argument), the total derivative of the right-hand side with respect to μ should vanish, leading to the following equation:

$$\frac{df(x, Q)}{d\mu^2} = 0 \quad \Rightarrow \quad \frac{df(x, \mu)}{d\mu^2} = \int_x^1 \frac{dy}{y}\, f(y, \mu)\, P(x/y, \mu^2). \qquad (5.4)$$

Dimensional analysis and the fact that the gluon emission rate is proportional to the QCD coupling squared allow us to further write

$$P(x, Q^2) \;=\; \frac{\alpha_s}{2\pi} \frac{1}{Q^2}\, P(x), \qquad (5.5)$$

from which the Dokshitzer–Gribov–Lipatov–Altarelli–Parisi (DGLAP) equation follows [12–14]:

$$\frac{df(x, \mu)}{d\log \mu^2} \;=\; \frac{\alpha_s}{2\pi} \int_x^1 \frac{dy}{y}\, f(y, \mu)\, P_{qq}(x/y). \qquad (5.6)$$

The so-called *splitting function* $P_{qq}(x)$ can be calculated in perturbative QCD. The subscript qq is a labelling convention indicating that x refers to the momentum fraction retained by a quark after emission of a gluon.

More generally, one should consider additional processes. For example, one should include cases in which the quark interacting with the photon comes from the splitting of a gluon. This is shown in Fig. 5.5: the diagram (a) is the one we considered above; the diagram (b) corresponds to processes where an emitted gluon has the time to split

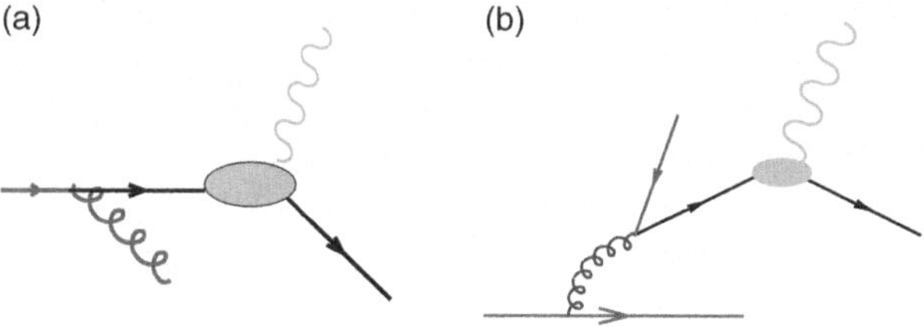

Fig. 5.5 The processes leading to the evolution of the quark density.

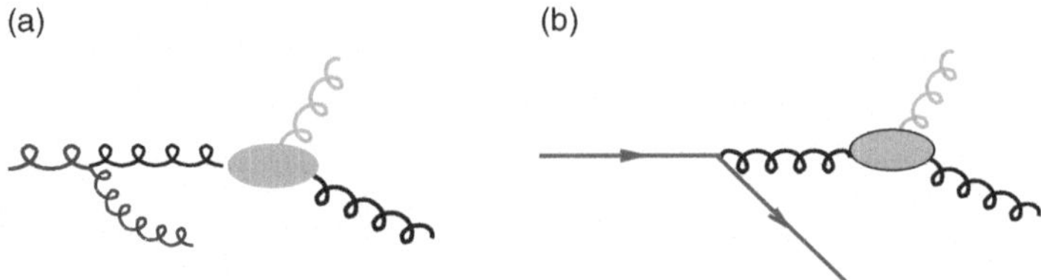

Fig. 5.6 The processes leading to the evolution of the gluon density.

into a $q\bar{q}$ pair, and it is one of these quarks that interacts with the photon. The overall evolution equation, including the effect of gluon splitting, is given by

$$\frac{dq(x,Q)}{dt} = \frac{\alpha_s}{2\pi} \int_x^1 \frac{dy}{y} \left[q(y,Q)\, P_{qq}\left(\frac{x}{y}\right) + g(y,Q)\, P_{qg}\left(\frac{x}{y}\right) \right], \tag{5.7}$$

where $t = \log Q^2$. For external probes that couple to gluons (such as an external gluon, coming, for example, from an incoming proton), we have a similar evolution of the gluon density (see Fig. 5.6):

$$\frac{dg(x,Q)}{dt} = \frac{\alpha_s}{2\pi} \int_x^1 \frac{dy}{y} \left[g(y,Q) P_{gg}\left(\frac{x}{y}\right) + \sum_{q,\bar{q}} q(y,Q)\, P_{gq}\left(\frac{x}{y}\right) \right]. \tag{5.8}$$

At the leading perturbative order (LO), the explicit calculation of the splitting functions $P_{ij}(x)$ (see, e.g. [8]) then gives the following expressions:[2]

$$P_{qq}(x) = P_{gq}(1-x) = C_F \frac{1+x^2}{1-x}, \tag{5.9}$$

$$P_{qg}(x) = \frac{1}{2}\left[x^2 + (1-x)^2 \right], \tag{5.10}$$

$$P_{gg}(x) = 2C_A \left[\frac{1-x}{x} + \frac{x}{1-x} + x(1-x) \right], \tag{5.11}$$

where $C_F = (N_C^2 - 1)/2N_C$ and $C_A = 2N_C$ are the Casimir invariants of the fundamental and adjoint representation of $SU(N_C)$ ($N_C = 3$ for QCD). In the following, we shall derive some general properties of the PDF evolution and give a few concrete examples.

The factorization given by (5.1) cannot of course hold for all phenomena in hadronic collisions. Processes like elastic scattering or generic soft collisions cannot be described in terms of quarks and gluons, since they are driven by the long-distance structure of the proton. Furthermore, modifications to this simple factorization relation can be required to describe processes like hard diffraction. The DGLAP evolution of parton densities, furthermore, requires modifications with respect to what shown here when x

---

[2] The expressions given here are strictly valid only for $x \neq 1$. Slight modifications are required to extend them to $x = 1$.

is so small that $\alpha_s \log(1/x)$ is of order 1, or when the gluon density becomes so large that gluon recombination becomes possible. Since the processes we shall consider in our applications do not cover these cases, we shall not further discuss these aspects in this review.

5.2.2 Example: quantitative evolution of parton densities

A complete solution for the evolved parton densities in x space can only be obtained from a numerical analysis. This work has been done by several groups (for a review see [15, 16]), and is continually being updated [17–21] by including the most up-to-date experimental results used for the determination of the input densities at a fixed scale. Figure 5.7(a) shows the up-quark valence momentum density at various scales Q, as obtained from one of these studies. Note the softening at larger scales and the clear $\log Q^2$ evolution. As Q^2 grows, the valence quarks emit more and more radiation, since they change direction over a shorter amount of time (larger acceleration). They therefore lose more momentum to the emitted gluons, and their spectrum becomes softer. The most likely momentum fraction carried by a valence up quark in the proton goes from $x \sim 20\%$ at $Q = 3$ GeV to $x \lesssim 10\%$ at $Q = 1000$ GeV. Notice finally that the density vanishes at small x.

Figure 5.7(b) shows the gluon momentum density. This grows at small x, with an approximate $g(x) \sim 1/x^{1+\delta}$ behaviour, and $\delta > 0$ slowly increasing at large Q^2. This low-x growth is due to the $1/x$ emission probability for the radiation of gluons, which was discussed Section 5.2.1 and which is represented by the $1/x$ factors in the $P_{gq}(x)$ and $P_{gg}(x)$ splitting functions. As Q^2 grows, we find an increasing number of gluons at small x, as a result of the increased radiation off quarks, as well as off the harder gluons.

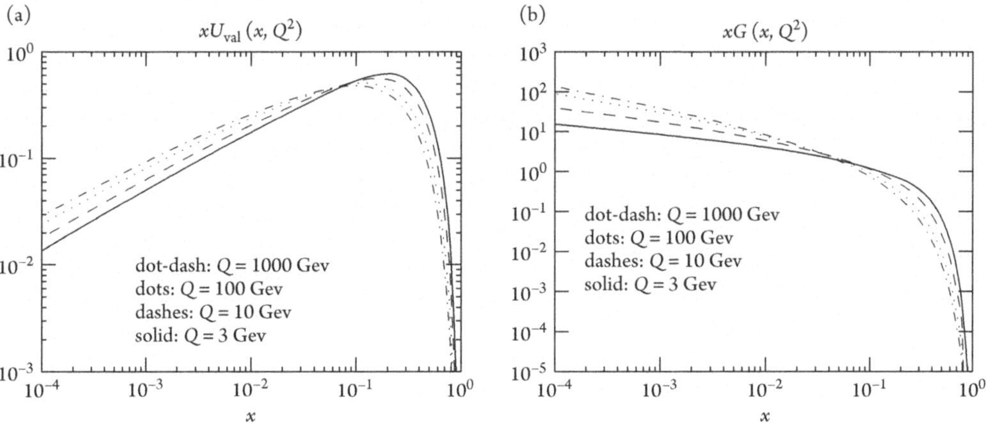

Fig. 5.7 (a) Valence up-quark momentum-density distribution for different scales Q. (b) Gluon momentum-density distribution.

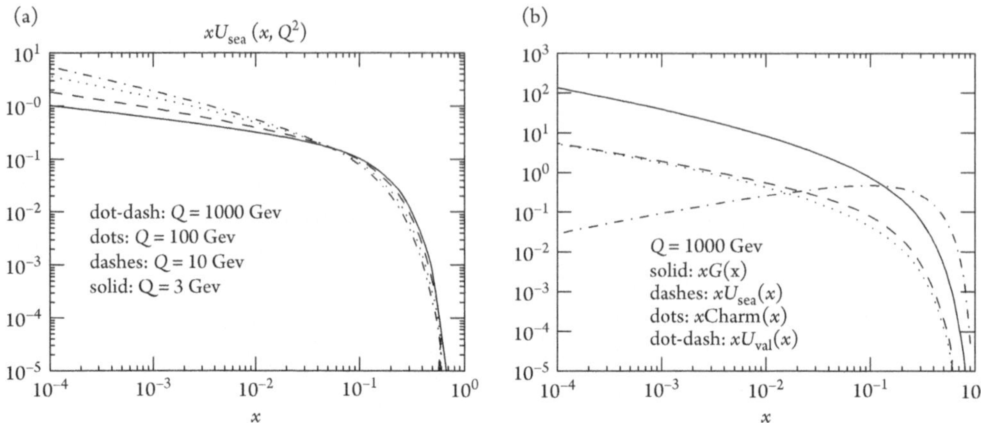

Fig. 5.8 (a) Sea up-quark momentum-density distribution for different scales Q. (b) Momentum-density distribution for several parton species at $Q = 1000$ GeV.

Figure 5.8(a) shows the evolution of the up-quark *sea* momentum density. Shape and evolution match those of the gluon density, a consequence of the fact that sea quarks come from the splitting of gluons. Since the gluon-splitting probability is proportional to α_s, the approximate ratio *sea/gluon* ~ 0.1, which can be obtained by comparing Figs. 5.7 and 5.8, is perfectly justified.

Finally, the momentum densities for gluons, up-sea, charm, and up-valence distributions are shown, for $Q = 1000$ GeV, in Fig. 5.8(b). Note here that u_{sea} and charm are approximately the same at very large Q and small x, as will be discussed in more detail in Section 5.3. The proton momentum is carried mostly by valence quarks and by gluons. The contribution of sea quarks is negligible.

Parton densities are extracted from experimental data. Their determination is therefore subject to the statistical and systematic uncertainties of the experiments and of the theoretical analysis (e.g. the treatment of nonperturbative effects, and the impact of missing higher-order perturbative corrections). Techniques have been introduced recently to take these uncertainties, into account and to evaluate their impact on concrete observables. A summary of such an analysis [22] is given in Fig. 5.9. What is plotted is the uncertainty bands for partonic luminosities[3] corresponding to the gg and $q\bar{q}$ initial-state channels. The partonic flux is given as a function of $\hat{s}$, the partonic CM invariant mass. Obvious features include the growth in uncertainty of the gg density at large mass, corresponding to the lack of data covering the large-x region of the gluon density. Notice, in particular, that the uncertainty bands reported by different groups do not necessarily overlap: this reflects different choices in the input sets of experimental data. In the future, the LHC data will be used in these global fits, leading to an important reduction in the uncertainties.

---

[3] For the definition of parton luminosity see Section 5.4.1.

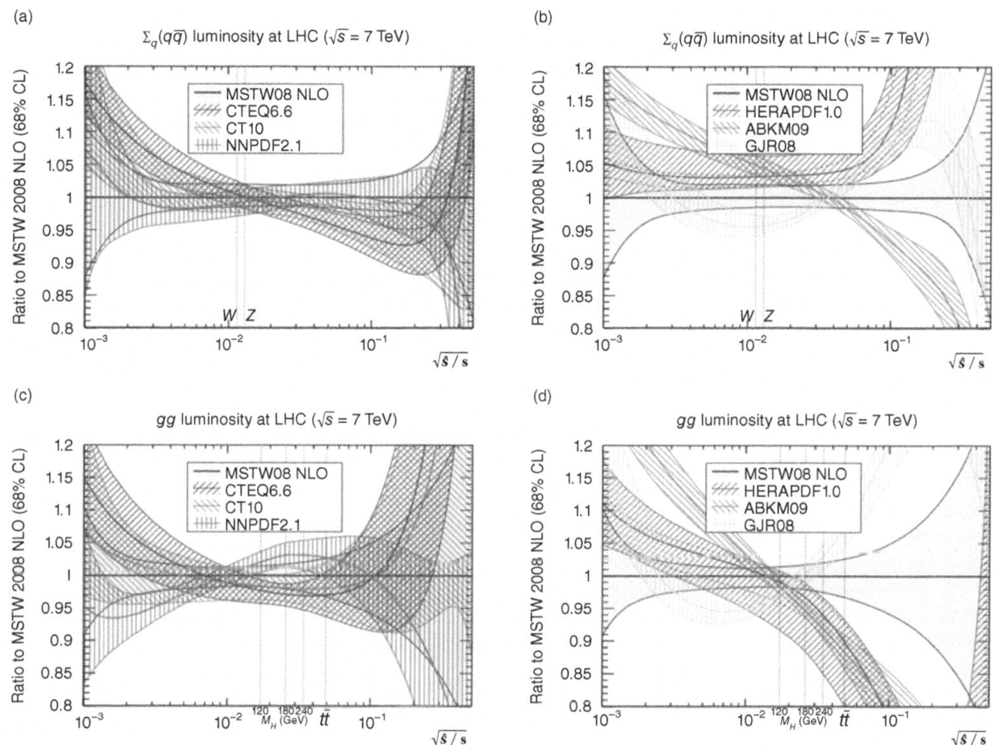

Fig. 5.9 Uncertainty in the parton luminosity functions at the LHC [22].

5.3 The final-state evolution of quarks and gluons

We discussed in Section 5.2 the initial-state evolution of quarks and gluons as the proton approaches the hard collision. We study here how quarks and gluons evolve after emerging from the hard process, and finally transform into hadrons, neutralizing their colours. We start by considering the simplest case, namely e^+e^- collisions, which provide the cleanest environment in which to study applications of QCD at high energy. This is the place where theoretical calculations have today reached their greatest accuracy, and where experimental data are the most precise, especially thanks to the huge statistics accumulated by LEP, LEP2, and SLC. The key process is the annihilation of the e^+e^- pair into a virtual photon or Z^0 boson, which will subsequently decay to a $q\bar{q}$ pair. Therefore, e^+e^- collisions have the big advantage of providing an almost point-like source of quark pairs, so that, in contrast to the case of interactions involving hadrons in the initial state, we at least know very precisely the state of the quarks at the beginning of the interaction process.

Nevertheless, it is by no means obvious that this information is sufficient to predict the properties of the hadronic final state. We know that this final state is clearly not simply a $q\bar{q}$ pair, but some high-multiplicity set of hadrons. For example, as shown in Fig. 5.10, the average multiplicity of charged hadrons in the decay of a Z^0 is

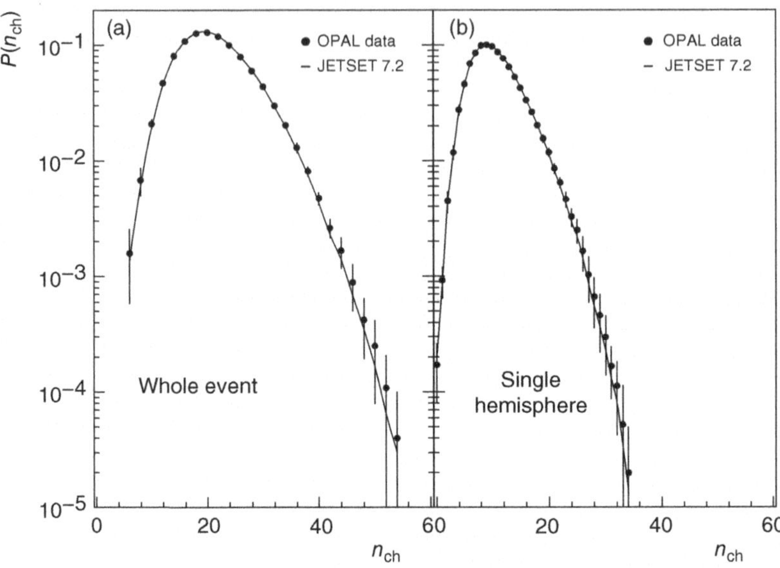

Fig. 5.10 Charged-particle multiplicity distribution in Z^0 decays

approximately 20. It is therefore not obvious that a calculation done using the simple picture $e^+e^- \to q\bar{q}$ has anything to do with reality. For example, one may wonder why we do not need to calculate $\sigma(e^+e^- \to q\bar{q}g \ldots g \ldots)$ for all possible gluon multiplicities to get an accurate estimate of $\sigma(e^+e^- \to \text{hadrons})$. And since in any case the final state is not made of q's and g's, but of π's, K's, ρ's, etc., why would $\sigma(e^+e^- \to q\bar{q}g \ldots g)$ be enough?

The solution to this puzzle lies both in a question of time and energy scales and in the dynamics of QCD. When the $q\bar{q}$ pair is produced, the force binding q and $\bar{q}$ is proportional to $\alpha_s(s)$ ($\sqrt{s}$ being the e^+e^- centre-of-mass energy). Therefore it is weak, and q and $\bar{q}$ behave to good approximation like free particles. The radiation emitted in the first instants after the pair creation is also perturbative, and it will stay so until a time after creation of the order of $(1 \text{ GeV})^{-1}$, when radiation with wavelengths $\gtrsim (1 \text{ GeV})^{-1}$ starts being emitted. At this scale, the coupling constant is large, and nonperturbative phenomena and hadronization start to play a role. However, as we shall show, colour emission during the perturbative evolution organizes itself in such a way as to form colour-neutral, low-mass, parton clusters highly localized in phase space. As a result, the complete colour neutralization (i.e. the hadronization) does not involve long-range interactions between partons far away in phase space. This is very important, because the forces acting among coloured objects at this timescale would be huge. If the perturbative evolution were to separate far apart colour-singlet $q\bar{q}$ pairs, the final-state interactions taking place during the hadronization phase would totally upset the structure of the final state.

In this picture, the identification of the perturbative cross section $\sigma(e^+e^- \to q\bar{q})$ with observable, high-multiplicity hadronic final states is realized by jets, namely collimated streams of hadrons that are the final result of the perturbative and nonperturbative evolution of each quark. The large multiplicity of the final states, shown in Fig. 5.10, corresponds to the many particles that emerge from the collinear emissions of many gluons from each quark. The dynamics of these emissions leads these particles to grossly follow the direction of the primary quark, and the emergent bundle, the jet, inherits the kinematics of the initial quark. This is shown in Fig. 5.11(a). Three-jet events, shown in Fig. 5.11(b), arise from the $O(\alpha_s)$ corrections to the tree-level process, namely to diagrams such as those shown in Fig. 5.12.

An important additional result of this 'pre-confining' evolution, is that the memory of where the local colour-neutral clusters came from is totally lost. So we expect the properties of hadronization to be universal: a model that describes hadronization at a given energy will work equally well at some other energy. Furthermore, so much time has passed since the original $q\bar{q}$ creation that the hadronization phase cannot significantly affect the total hadron production rate. Perturbative corrections due to the emission of the first hard partons should be calculable in perturbation theory, providing a finite, meaningful cross section.

The nature of nonperturbative corrections to this picture can be explored. One can prove, for example, that the leading correction to the total rate $R_{e^+e^-}$ is of order F/s^2, where $F \propto \langle 0|\alpha_s F^a_{\mu\nu} F^{\mu\nu a}|0\rangle$ is the so-called gluon condensate. Since $F = O(1~\text{GeV}^4)$, these nonperturbative corrections are usually very small. For example, they are

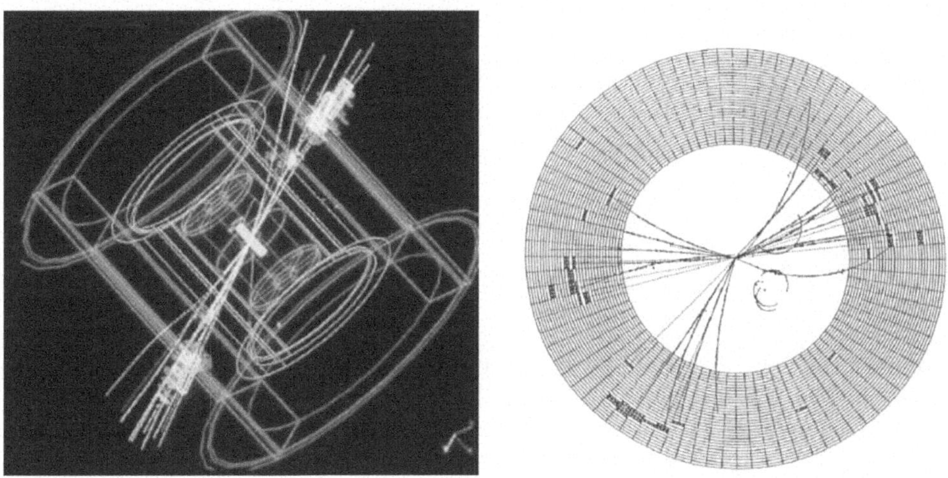

Fig. 5.11 Experimental pictures of 2- and 3-jet final states from e^+e^- collisions.

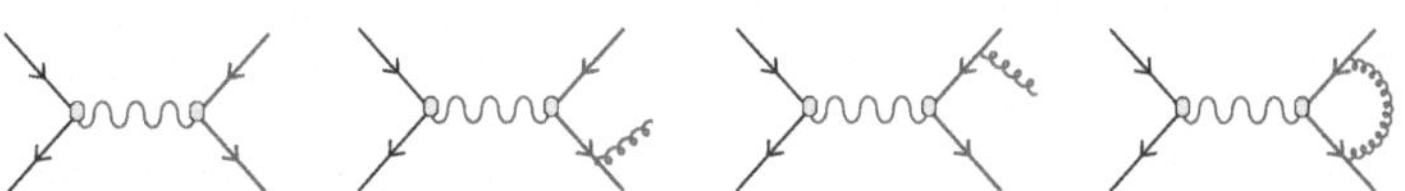

Fig. 5.12 $O(\alpha_s)$ corrections to the tree-level $e^+e^- \to q\bar{q}$ process.

$O(10^{-8})$ at the Z^0 peak. Corrections scaling like Λ^2/s or $\Lambda/\sqrt{s}$ can nevertheless appear in other less inclusive quantities, such as event shapes or fragmentation functions.

We now come back to the perturbative evolution, and shall devote the first part of this section to justifying the picture given above.

5.3.1 Soft-gluon emission

Emission of soft gluons plays a fundamental role in the evolution of the final state [6, 9]. Soft gluons are emitted with large probability, since the emission spectrum behaves like dE/E, typical of bremsstrahlung as familiar in QED. They provide the seed for the bulk of the final-state multiplicity of hadrons. The study of soft-gluon emission is simplified by the simplicity of their couplings. Being soft (i.e. long-wavelength) they are insensitive to the details of the very-short-distance dynamics: they cannot distinguish features of the interactions that take place on timescales shorter than their wavelength. They are also insensitive to the spin of the partons: the only feature to which they are sensitive is the colour charge. To prove this let us consider soft-gluon emission in the $q\bar{q}$ decay of an off-shell photon:

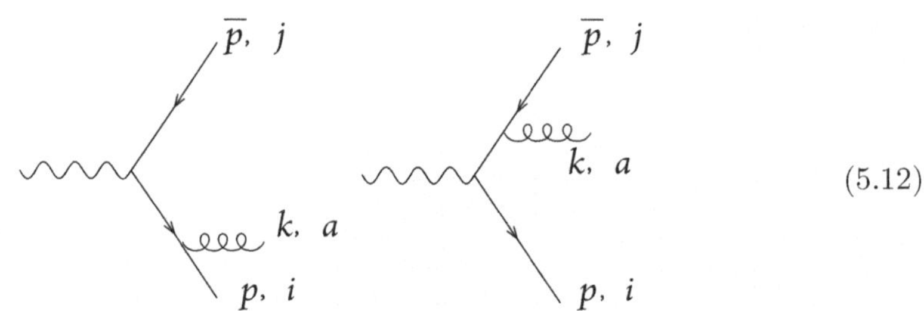

$$(5.12)$$

$$
A_{\text{soft}} = \bar{u}(p)\epsilon(k)(ig)\,\frac{-i}{\not{p}+\not{k}}\,\Gamma^\mu\,v(\bar{p})\,\lambda^a_{ij} + \bar{u}(p)\,\Gamma^\mu\,\frac{i}{\not{\bar{p}}+\not{k}}\,(ig)\epsilon(k)\,v(\bar{p})\,\lambda^a_{ij}
$$

$$
= \left[\frac{g}{2p\cdot k}\,\bar{u}(p)\epsilon(k)\,(\not{p}+\not{k})\Gamma^\mu\,v(\bar{p}) - \frac{g}{2\bar{p}\cdot k}\,\bar{u}(p)\,\Gamma^\mu\,(\not{\bar{p}}+\not{k})\epsilon(k)\,v(\bar{p})\right]\lambda^a_{ij}.
$$

I have used the generic symbol Γ_μ to describe the interaction vertex with the photon to stress the fact that the following manipulations are independent of the specific form of Γ_μ. In particular, Γ_μ can represent an arbitrarily complicated vertex form factor. Neglecting the factors of $\not{k}$ in the numerators (since $k \ll p, \bar{p}$, by definition of soft) and using the Dirac equations, we get

$$
A_{\text{soft}} = g\lambda^a_{ij}\,\left(\frac{p\cdot\epsilon}{p\cdot k} - \frac{\bar{p}\epsilon}{\bar{p}\cdot k}\right)\,A_{\text{Born}}.
\tag{5.13}
$$

We then conclude that soft-gluon emission factorizes into the product of an emission factor and the Born-level amplitude. From this exercise, one can extract general Feynman rules for soft-gluon emission:

$$p, j \quad \longrightarrow \quad p, i \qquad = g\, \lambda_{ij}^a\, 2p^\mu \,. \tag{5.14}$$

An analogous exercise leads to the $g \to gg$ soft-emission rules:

$$c, \nu \quad \longrightarrow \quad b, \rho \quad = ig f^{abc}\, 2p^\mu\, g^{\nu\rho} \,. \tag{5.15}$$

Consider now the 'decay' of a virtual gluon into a quark pair. One more diagram should be added to those considered in the case of the electroweak decay. The fact that the quark pair is no longer in a colour-singlet state makes things a bit more interesting:

$$\stackrel{k\to 0}{=} \left[ig f^{abc}\, \lambda_{ij}^c \left(\frac{Q\epsilon}{Qk} \right) + g(\lambda^b \lambda^a)_{ij} \left(\frac{p\epsilon}{pk} \right) - g\, (\lambda^a \lambda^b)_{ij} \left(\frac{\bar p \epsilon}{pk} \right) \right] A_{\text{Born}}$$

$$= g(\lambda^a \lambda^b)_{ij} \left[\frac{Q\epsilon}{Qk} - \frac{\bar p \epsilon}{pk} \right] + g(\lambda^b \lambda^a)_{ij} \left[\frac{p\epsilon}{pk} - \frac{Q\epsilon}{Qk} \right]. \tag{5.16}$$

The two factors correspond to the two possible ways colour can flow in this process:

$$\tag{5.17}$$

The basis for this representation of the colour flow is the following diagram, which makes explicit the relation between the colours of the quark, antiquark, and gluon entering a QCD vertex:

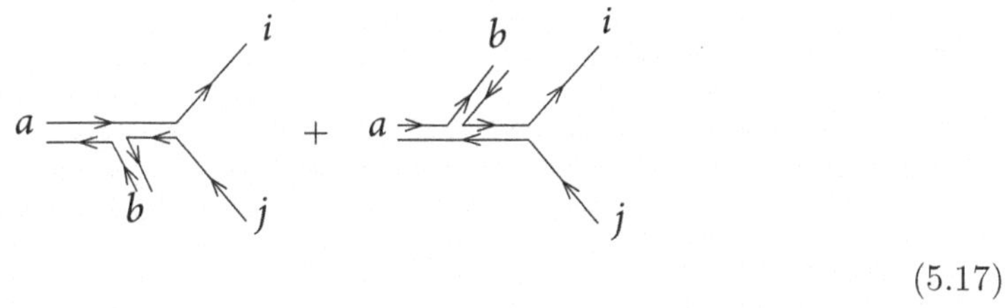

$$\tag{5.18}$$

We can therefore represent the gluon as a double line, with one line carrying the colour inherited from the quark and the other carrying the anticolour inherited from the antiquark. In the first diagram in (5.17), the antiquark (colour label j) is colour-connected to the soft gluon (colour label b), and the quark (colour label i) is connected to the decaying gluon (colour label a). In the second case, the order is reversed. The two emission factors correspond to the emission of the soft gluon from the antiquark and from the quark line, respectively. When squaring the total amplitude and summing over initial and final-state colours, the interference between the two pieces is suppressed by $1/N^2$ relative to the individual squares:

$$\sum_{a,b,i,j} |(\lambda^a \lambda^b)_{ij}|^2 = \sum_{a,b} \text{tr}\left(\lambda^a \lambda^b \lambda^b \lambda^a\right) = \frac{N^2 - 1}{2} C_F = O(N^3), \tag{5.19}$$

$$\sum_{a,b,i,j} (\lambda^a \lambda^b)_{ij}[(\lambda^b \lambda^a)_{ij}]^* = \sum_{a,b} \text{tr}(\lambda^a \lambda^b \lambda^a \lambda^b) = \frac{N^2 - 1}{2} \underbrace{\left(C_F - \frac{C_A}{2}\right)}_{-\frac{1}{2N}} = O(N).$$

$$\tag{5.20}$$

As a result, the emission of a soft gluon can be described, to leading order in $1/N^2$, as the incoherent sum of the emission from the two colour currents. The ability to separate these emissions as incoherent sums is the basic fact that allows a sequential, Markovian description of the parton-shower evolution as implemented in numerical simulations of the hadronic final state of hard collisions. The neglect of subleading $1/N^2$ contributions is therefore an intrinsic approximation of all such approaches.

5.3.2 Angular ordering for soft-gluon emission

The results presented above have important consequences for the perturbative evolution of the quarks. A key property of soft-gluon emission is the so-called *angular ordering* (for an overview of colour coherence and its relation to angular ordering, see [9, 23]). This phenomenon consists in the continuous reduction of the opening angle at which successive soft gluons are emitted by the evolving quark. As a result, this radiation is confined within smaller and smaller cones around the quark direction, and the final state will look like a collimated jet of partons. In addition, the structure of the colour flow during the jet evolution forces the $q\bar{q}$ pairs that are in a colour-singlet state to be close in phase space, thereby achieving the pre-confinement of colour-singlet clusters alluded to at the beginning of this section.

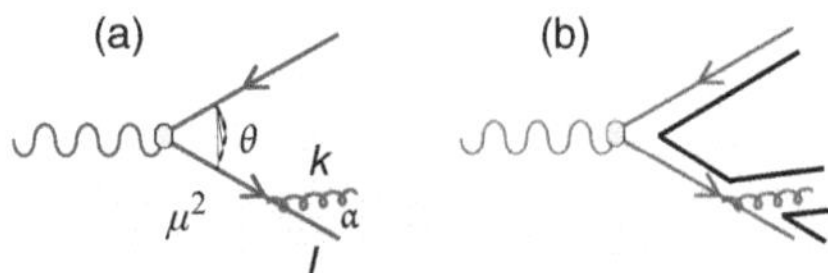

Fig. 5.13 Radiation off $q\bar{q}$ pair produced by an off-shell photon.

A simple derivation of angular ordering, which more directly exhibits its physical origin, can be obtained as follows. Consider Fig. 5.13(a), which shows a Feynman diagram for the emission of a gluon from a quark line. The quark momentum is denoted by l and the gluon momentum by k, the opening angle between the quark and antiquark is denoted by θ, and the angle between the nearest quark and the emitted gluon by α. We shall work in the double-log enhanced soft $k^0 << l^0$ and collinear $\alpha << 1$ region. The internal quark propagator $p = (l + k)$ is off-shell, setting the timescale for the gluon emission:

$$\Delta t \simeq \frac{1}{\Delta E} = \frac{l^0}{(k+l)^2} \quad \rightarrow \quad \Delta t \simeq \frac{1}{k^0 \alpha^2} \, . \tag{5.21}$$

In order to resolve the quarks, the transverse wavelength of the gluon $\lambda_\perp = 1/E_\perp$ must be smaller than the separation between the quarks $b(t) \simeq \theta \, \Delta t$, giving the constraint $1/(\alpha k^0) < \theta \, \Delta t$. Using the results of (5.21) for Δt, we arrive at the angular ordering constraint $\alpha < \theta$. Gluon emissions at an angle smaller than θ can resolve the two individual colour quarks and are allowed; emissions at greater angles do not see the colour charge and are therefore suppressed. In processes involving more partons, the angle θ is defined not by the nearest parton, but by the colour-connected parton (e.g. the parton that forms a colour singlet with the emitting parton). Figure 5.13(b) shows the colour connections for the $q\bar{q}$ event after the gluon has been emitted. Colour lines begin on quarks and end on antiquarks. Because gluons are colour octets, they contain the beginning of one line and the end of another, as we showed in (5.17).

If one repeats now the exercise for emission of one additional gluon, one will find the same angular constraint, but this time applied to the colour lines defined by the previously established *antenna*. As shown in Section 5.3.1, the $q\bar{q}g$ state can be decomposed at the leading order in $1/N$ into two independent emitters, one given by the colour line flowing from the gluon to the quark, the other by the colour line flowing from the antiquark to the gluon. So the emission of the additional gluon will be constrained to take place either within the cone formed by the quark and the gluon or within the cone formed by the gluon and the antiquark. Either way, the emission angle will be smaller than the angle of the first gluon emission. This leads to the concept of angular ordering, with successive emission of soft gluons taking place within cones which get smaller and smaller, as in Fig. 5.14

The fact that colour always flows directly from the emitting parton to the emitted one, the collimation of the jet, and the softening of the radiation emitted at later stages ensure that partons forming a colour-singlet cluster are close in phase space. As a result, hadronization (the nonperturbative process that will bind together colour-singlet parton pairs) takes place locally inside the jet and is not a long-distance phenomenon connecting partons far away in the evolution tree: only pairs of nearby partons are involved. In particular, there is no direct link between the precise nature of the hard process and the hadronization. These two phases are totally decoupled and, as in the case of the partonic densities, one can infer that hadronization factorizes from the hard process and can be described in a universal (i.e. hard-process-independent) fashion.

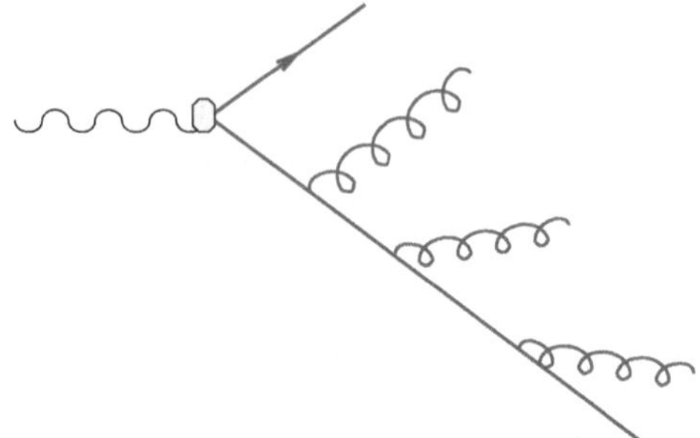

Fig. 5.14 Collimation of soft gluon emission during the jet evolution.

The inclusive properties of jets (e.g. the particle multiplicity, jet mass, and jet broadening) are independent of the hadronization model, up to corrections of order $(\Lambda/\sqrt{s})^n$ (for some integer power n, which depends on the observable), with $\Lambda \lesssim 1$ GeV.

The final picture, in the case of a deep irelastic scattering (DIS) event, therefore appears as in Fig. 5.15. After being deflected by the photon, the struck quark emits the first gluon, which takes away the quark colour and passes on its own anticolour to the escaping quark. This gluon is therefore colour-connected with the last gluon emitted before the hard interaction. As the final-state quark continues its evolution, more and more gluons are emitted, each time leaving their colour behind and transmitting their anticolour to the emerging quark. Angular ordering forces all these gluons to be close in phase space, until the evolution is stopped once the virtuality of the quark becomes of the order of the strong-interaction scale. The colour of the quark is left behind, and when hadronization takes over it is only the nearby colour-connected gluons that are transformed, with a phenomenological model, in hadrons. This mechanism for the transfer of colour across subsequent gluon emissions is similar to what happens when one places a charge near the surface of a dielectric medium. This will become polarized, and a charge will appear on the medium opposite end. The appearance of the charge is the result of a sequence of local charge shifts, whereby neighbouring atoms become polarized, as in Fig. 5.16. Notice that the transfer of colour between the final state jet and the jet associated to the initial state leads to the existence of one colour-singlet

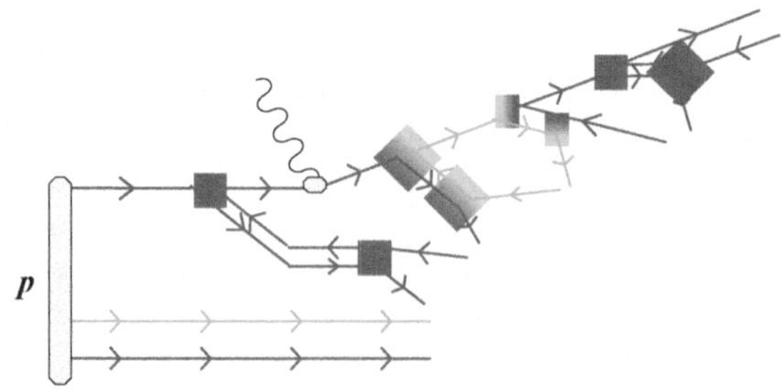

Fig. 5.15 The colour flow diagram for a DIS event.

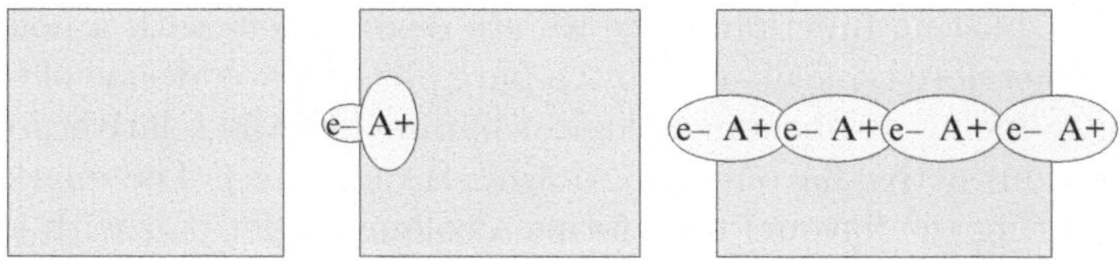

Fig. 5.16 Charge transfer in a dieletric medium, via a sequence of local polarizations.

cluster containing partons from both jets. Therefore, the particles arising from this cluster cannot be associated with either jet: they will be hadrons whose source is a combination of two of the hard partons in the event. This feature will be present in any hard process: it is the unavoidable consequence of the neutralization of the colour of the partons involved in the hard scattering.

5.3.3 Hadronization

The application of perturbation theory to the evolution of a jet, with the sequential emission of partons, governed by QCD splitting probabilities and angular ordering to enforce quantum mechanical quantum coherence, will stop once the scale of the emissions reaches values in the range of 1 GeV. This is called the *infrared cutoff*. The are two reasons why we need to stop the emission of gluons at this scale. To start with, we cannot control with perturbation theory the domain below this scale, where the strong coupling constant α_s becomes very large. Furthermore, we know that the number of physical particles that can be produced inside a jet must be finite, since the lightest object we can produce is a pion, and energy conservation sets a limit to how many pions can be created. This is different from what happens in a QED cascade, where the evolution of an accelerated charge can lead to the emission of an arbitrary number of photons. This is possible because the photon is massless, and can have arbitrarily small energy. The gluons of a QCD cascade, on the contrary, must have enough energy to create pions.

When the perturbative evolution of the jet terminates, we are left with some number of gluons. As shown in Section 5.3.2 and displayed in Fig. 5.15, these gluons are pairwise colour-connected. As two colour-connected gluons travel away from each other, a constant force pulls them together. Phenomenological models (see [6] for a more complete review) are then used to describe how this force determines the evolution of the system from this point on. What I shall describe here is the so-called *cluster model* [24], implemented in the HERWIG Monte Carlo generator [25, 26], but the main qualitative features are shared by other alternatives, such as the Lund string approach [27], implemented in the PYTHIA generator [28, 29].

Most of the hadrons emerging from the evolution of a jet are known to be made of quarks; glueballs, i.e. hadrons made of bound gluons, are expected to exist, but their production is greatly suppressed compared with that of quark-made particles. For this reason, the first step in the description of hadronization is to assume that the force among gluons will rip them apart into a $q\bar{q}$ pair, and that these quarks will act as seeds for the hadron production. The breakup into quarks is not parametrized using the

DGLAP $g \to q\bar{q}$ splitting function, since we are dealing here with a nonperturbative transition. One therefore typically employs a pure phase-space 'decay' of the gluon into the $q\bar{q}$ pair, introducing as phenomenological parameters the relative probabilities of selecting the various active flavours (up, down, strange, etc.). The quark q_i from one gluon (i representing the flavour) then forms a colour-singlet pair with the antiquark $\bar{q}_j$ emerging from the breakup of the neighbouring gluon. This colour-singlet $q_i\bar{q}_j$ pair cannot, however, directly form a hadron, since in general the quarks will still be moving apart, and the invariant mass of the pair will not coincide with the mass of an existing physical state. As they separate subject to a constant force, however, their kinetic energy turns into a linearly rising potential energy. The potential energy accumulated in the system will be able to convert into a new quark–antiquark pair $q_k\bar{q}_k$ once its value exceeds the relevant mass threshold. We are now left with two colour-singlet pairs: $q_i\bar{q}_k$ and $q_k\bar{q}_j$. When converting the potential energy into mass and kinetic energy of the newly produced pair, one can use the freedom in selecting the spatial kinematics of q_k and $\bar{q}_k$ such that both $q_i\bar{q}_k$ and $q_k\bar{q}_j$ invariant masses coincide with some resonance with the proper flavour. The residual energy of the system is then assumed to be entirely kinetic, and the two resonances fly away free. Once again, one can associate phenomenological parameters with the probabilities of selecting flavours k of a given type. Since the pair of flavour indices ik does not specify uniquely a hadron (e.g. a $u\bar{d}$ system could by a π^+ or a ρ^+, as well as many other objects), the model has a further set of rules and/or parameters to select the precise flavour type. For example, a phenomenologically successful description of the π/ρ ratio is obtained by simply assuming a production rate proportional to the number of spin

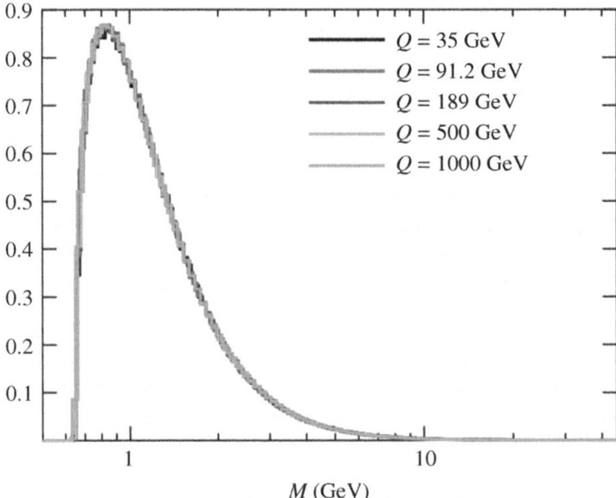

Fig. 5.17 Invariant mass distribution of clusters of colour-singlet quarks after nonperturbative gluon splitting, as obtained with the HERWIG generator [30]. The spectra for final states corresponding to different centre-of-mass energies are normalized to the same area, displaying the energy independence of the shapes.

states (one for the scalar pion, three for the vector rho) and to a Boltzmann factor $\exp(-M/T)$, where M is the resonance mass and T is a universal parameter, to be fitted from data. Furthermore, one can introduce the possibility of converting the potential energy into a diquark–antidiquark pair, namely $(q_k q_\ell)\,(\bar{q}_k \bar{q}_\ell)$. The resulting hadrons $q_i q_k q_\ell$ and $\bar{q}_j \bar{q}_k \bar{q}_\ell$ will be a baryon–antibaryon pair.

The measurement of hadron multiplicities from Z^0 decays is used to tune the few phenomenological parameters of the model, and these parameters can be used to describe hadronization at different energies and in different high-energy hadron-production processes. The internal consistency of this assumption is supported by Fig. 5.17 [30], which shows the invariant mass distribution of clusters of colour-singlet quarks, after the nonperturbative gluon splitting, for e^+e^- collisions at different centre-of-mass energies. All curves are normalized to 1, and they all overlap very accurately. This confirms the validity of the implementation of factorization in the Monte Carlo simulation: higher initial energies provide more room for the perturbative evolution, leading to more splitting and more emitted radiation; but the structure and distribution of colour-singlet clusters at the end of evolution are independent of the initial energy, and the same model of hadronization can be applied.

5.4 Applications

In hadronic collisions, all phenomena are QCD-related. The dynamics is more complex than in e^+e^- or DIS, since both beam and target have a nontrivial partonic structure. As a result, calculations (and experimental analyses) are more complicated. Perturbative corrections to the Born-level amplitudes (leading order, LO) require the calculation of a large number of loop and high-order tree-level diagrams. For example, the first correction to the four LO $gg \to gg$ diagrams for the jet cross section in the purely gluonic channel requires the evaluation of the one-loop insertions in the four LO diagrams, plus the calculation of the 25 LO diagrams for the $gg \to ggg$ process. Next-to-leading-order (NLO) calculations like this are nevertheless available today for most processes with up to two or three final-state partons, and new techniques have emerged recently that are pushing the frontier of NLO results even further (for a recent review, see [10]). Next-to-next-to-leading order (NNLO) results, which require the evaluation of two-loop corrections as well, have so far been completed only for processes with only one final-state particle at the Born level, such as production of massive gauge bosons (W, Z) or of a Higgs boson. For these reasons, the accuracy of QCD calculations in hadronic collisions is typically less than in the case of e^+e^- or DIS processes. Nevertheless, $p\bar{p}$ or pp collider physics is primarily *discovery* physics, rather than precision physics (there are exceptions, such as measurement of the W mass and of the properties of b-hadrons, but these are not QCD-related measurements). As such, knowledge of QCD is essential both for the estimate of the expected signals and for the evaluation of the backgrounds. Tests of QCD in $p\bar{p}$ collisions confirm our understanding of perturbation theory, or, when they fail, point to areas where our approximations need to be improved (see, for example, the theoretical advances prompted by the measurements of ψ production at CDF).

In this section, I shall briefly review some applications to the most commonly studied QCD processes in hadronic collisions: the production of gauge bosons and of jets. More details can be found in [6, 7].

5.4.1 Drell–Yan processes

While the Z boson has recently been studied with great precision by LEP experiments, it was actually discovered, together with the W boson, by the CERN experiments UA1 and UA2 in $p\bar{p}$ collisions. W physics was studied in great detail at LEP2, but the best direct measurements of its mass by a single group still belong to $p\bar{p}$ experiments (CDF and D0 at the Tevatron). Until a new, future, e^+e^- linear collider is built, the monopoly of W studies will remain in the hands of hadron colliders, with the Tevatron, and soon with the start of the LHC experiments.

Precision measurements of W production in hadronic collisions are important for several reasons:

- This is the only process in hadronic collisions that is known to NNLO accuracy.
- The rapidity distribution of the charged leptons from W decays is sensitive to the ratio of the up- and down-quark densities, and can contribute to our understanding of the structure of the proton.
- Deviations from the expected production rates of highly virtual W's ($p\bar{p} \to W^* \to e\nu$) are a possible signal of the existence of new W bosons, and therefore of new gauge interactions. The tail of the invariant mass distribution of the W, furthermore, provides today's most sensitive determination of the W width.

The production rate for the W boson is given by the factorization formula

$$d\sigma(p\bar{p} \to W + X) = \int dx_1 \, dx_2 \sum_{i,j} f_i(x_1, Q) \, f_j(x_2.Q) \, d\hat{\sigma}(ij \to W). \tag{5.22}$$

The partonic cross section $\hat{\sigma}(ij \to W)$ can be easily calculated, giving the following result [5, 6]:

$$\hat{\sigma}(q_i \bar{q}_j \to W) = \pi \, \frac{\sqrt{2}}{3} \, |V_{ij}|^2 \, G_F \, M_W^2 \, \delta(\hat{s} - M_W^2) = A_{ij} \, M_W^2 \, \delta(\hat{s} - M_W^2), \tag{5.23}$$

where $\hat{s}$ is the partonic centre-of-mass energy squared and V_{ij} is an element of the Cabibbo–Kobayashi–Maskawa matrix. The delta function comes from the $2 \to 1$ phase space, which forces the centre-of-mass energy of the initial state to coincide with the W mass. It is useful to introduce the two variables

$$\tau = \frac{\hat{s}}{S_{\mathrm{had}}} \equiv x_1 x_2, \tag{5.24}$$

$$y = \frac{1}{2} \log \left(\frac{E_W + p_W^z}{E_W - p_W^z} \right) \equiv \frac{1}{2} \log \left(\frac{x_1}{x_2} \right), \tag{5.25}$$

where S_{had} is the hadronic centre-of-mass energy squared. The variable y is called the *rapidity*. For slowly moving objects it reduces to the standard velocity, but, in contrast to the velocity, it transforms additively even at high energies under Lorentz boosts along the direction of motion. Written in terms of τ and y, the integration measure over the initial-state parton momenta becomes: $dx_1\, dx_2 = d\tau\, dy$. Using this expression and (5.23) in (5.22), we obtain the following result for the LO total W production cross section:

$$\sigma_{\mathrm{DY}} = \sum_{i,j} \frac{\pi A_{ij}}{M_W^2}\, \tau \int_\tau^1 \frac{dx}{x}\, f_i(x)\, f_j\left(\frac{\tau}{x}\right) \equiv \sum_{i,j} \frac{\pi A_{ij}}{M_W^2} \tau L_{ij}(\tau), \qquad (5.26)$$

where the function $L_{ij}(\tau)$ is usually called the *partonic luminosity*. In the case of $u\bar{d}$ collisions, the overall factor in front of this expression has a value of approximately 6.5 nb. It is interesting to study the partonic luminosity as a function of the hadronic centre-of-mass energy. This can be done by taking a simple approximation for the parton densities. Following the indications of the figures presented in Section 5.3, we shall assume that $f_i(x) \sim 1/x^{1+\delta}$, with $\delta < 1$. Then

$$L(\tau) = \int_\tau^1 \frac{dx}{x} \frac{1}{x^{1+\delta}} \left(\frac{x}{\tau}\right)^{1+\delta} = \frac{1}{\tau^{1+\delta}} \int_\tau^1 \frac{dx}{x} = \frac{1}{\tau^{1+\delta}} \log\left(\frac{1}{\tau}\right) \qquad (5.27)$$

and

$$\sigma_W \sim \tau^{-\delta} \log\left(\frac{1}{\tau}\right) = \left(\frac{S_{\mathrm{had}}}{M_W^2}\right)^\delta \log\left(\frac{S_{\mathrm{had}}}{M_W^2}\right). \qquad (5.28)$$

The Drell–Yan cross section therefore grows at least logarithmically with the hadronic centre-of-mass energy. This is to be compared with the behaviour of the Z production cross section in e^+e^- collisions, which is steeply diminishing for values of s well above the production threshold. The reason for the different behaviour in hadronic collisions is that while the energy of the hadronic initial state grows, it will always be possible to find partons inside the hadrons with the appropriate energy to produce the W directly on shell. The number of partons available for the production of a W increases with the increase in hadronic energy, since the larger the hadron energy, the smaller will be the value of hadron momentum fraction x necessary to produce the W. The increasing number of partons available at smaller and smaller values of x then causes the growth in the total W production cross section.

A comparison between the best available predictions for the production rates of W and Z bosons in hadronic collisions and the LHC experimental data[31] is shown in Fig. 5.18. The experimental uncertainty is already smaller than the spread of the predictions based on different PDF sets, and will therefore add important constraints to improving the knowledge of PDFs.

Since the LHC is a pp collider, the initial state contains more up quarks than down quarks, and therefore the production rates and the distributions of W^+ bosons will be different from those of W^- bosons. For the total rates, this is clearly visible in Fig. 5.18. The rapidity asymmetry between positive and negative leptons produced in $W^\pm$ decays is shown in Fig. 5.19, where the ATLAS data are compared against the predictions of several PDF sets. Once again, the precision of the data strongly constrains the PDFs.

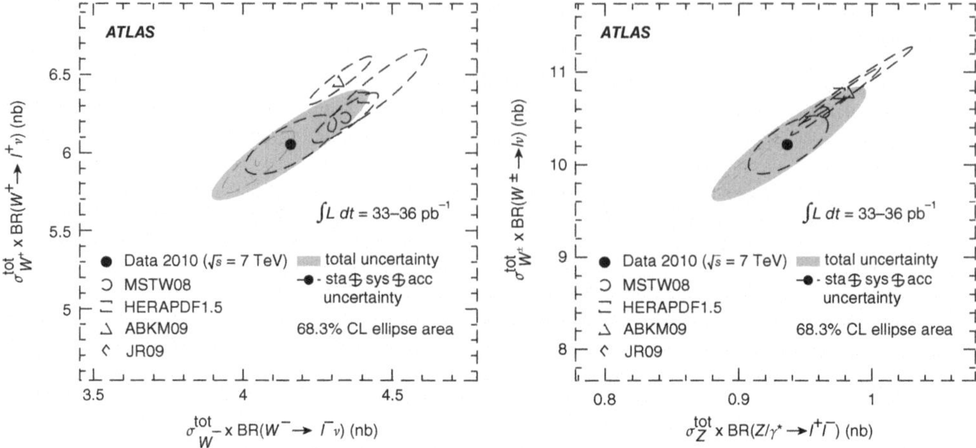

Fig. 5.18 Comparison of W and Z cross sections measured by the ATLAS experiment at the LHC [31] with the predictions of several PDF sets.

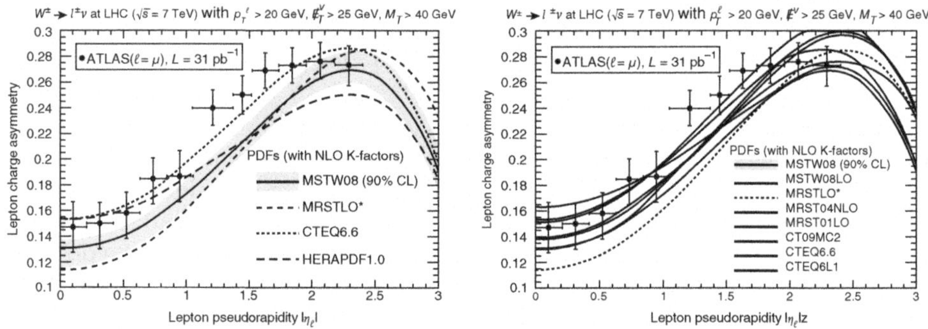

Fig. 5.19 The lepton charge asymmetry at the LHC compared with the predictions of various PDF sets [22].

5.4.2 Jet production

Jet production is the hard process with the largest rate in hadronic collisions. The measurement of highest-energy jets allows one to probe the shortest distances ever reached. The leading mechanisms for jet production are shown in Fig. 5.20.

The two-jet inclusive cross section can be obtained from the formula

$$d\sigma = \sum_{ijkl} dx_1 \, dx_2 \, f_i^{(H_1)}(x_1, \mu) \, f_j^{(H_2)}(x_2, \mu) \, \frac{d\hat{\sigma}_{ij \to k+l}}{d\Phi_2} \, d\Phi_2, \qquad (5.29)$$

which has to be expressed in terms of the rapidity and transverse momentum of the quarks (or jets), in order to make contact with physical reality. The two-particle phase space is given by

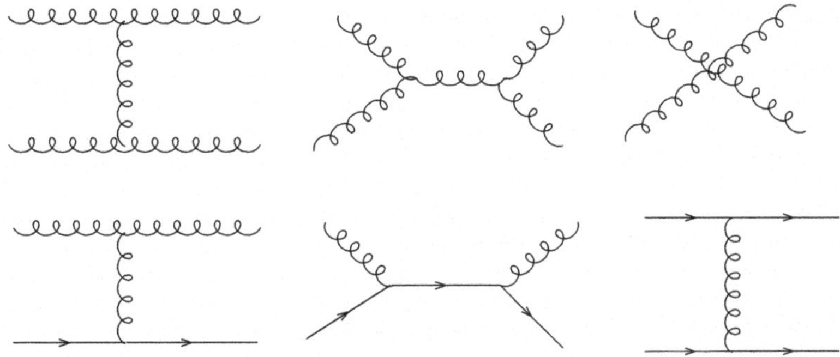

Fig. 5.20 Representative diagrams for the production of jet pairs in hadronic collisions.

$$d\Phi_2 = \frac{d^3k}{2k^0(2\pi)^3}\, 2\pi\, \delta((p_1 + p_2 - k)^2)\,, \tag{5.30}$$

and, in the centre-of-mass frame of the colliding partons, we get

$$d\Phi_2 = \frac{1}{2(2\pi)^2}\, d^2k_T\, dy\, 2\,\delta(\hat{s} - 4(k^0)^2)\,, \tag{5.31}$$

where k_T is the transverse momentum of the final-state partons. Here y is the rapidity of the produced parton in the parton centre-of-mass frame. It is given by

$$y = \frac{y_1 - y_2}{2}\,, \tag{5.32}$$

where y_1 and y_2 are the rapidities of the produced partons in the laboratory frame (in fact, in any frame). We also introduce

$$y_0 = \frac{y_1 + y_2}{2} = \frac{1}{2}\log\frac{x_1}{x_2}\,, \qquad \tau = \frac{\hat{s}}{S_{had}} = x_1\, x_2\,. \tag{5.33}$$

We have

$$dx_1\, dx_2 = dy_0\, d\tau\,. \tag{5.34}$$

We obtain

$$d\sigma = \sum_{ijkl} dy_0\, \frac{1}{S_{\text{had}}}\, f_i^{(H_1)}(x_1,\mu)\, f_j^{(H_2)}(x_2,\mu)\, \frac{d\hat{\sigma}_{ij\to k+l}}{d\Phi_2}\, \frac{1}{2(2\pi)^2}\, 2\, dy\, d^2k_T\,, \tag{5.35}$$

which can also be written as

$$\frac{d\sigma}{dy_1\, dy_2\, d^2k_T} = \frac{1}{S_{\text{had}}\, 2(2\pi)^2}\, \sum_{ijkl} f_i^{(H_1)}(x_1,\mu)\, f_j^{(H_2)}(x_2,\mu)\, \frac{d\hat{\sigma}_{ij\to k+l}}{d\Phi_2}\,. \tag{5.36}$$

The variables x_1 and x_2 can be obtained from y_1, y_2, and k_T by the equations

$$y_0 = \frac{y_1 + y_2}{2}, \tag{5.37}$$

$$y = \frac{y_1 - y_2}{2}, \tag{5.38}$$

$$x_T = \frac{2k_T}{\sqrt{S_{\text{had}}}}, \tag{5.39}$$

$$x_1 = x_T\, e^{y_0}\, \cosh y, \tag{5.40}$$

$$x_2 = x_T\, e^{-y_0}\, \cosh y \,. \tag{5.41}$$

For the partonic variables, we need $\hat{s}$ and the scattering angle θ in the parton centre-of-mass frame, since

$$t = -\frac{\hat{s}}{2}\left(1 - \cos\theta\right), \qquad u = -\frac{\hat{s}}{2}\left(1 + \cos\theta\right). \tag{5.42}$$

Neglecting the parton masses, we can show that the rapidity can also be written as

$$y = -\log\tan\frac{\theta}{2} \equiv \eta, \tag{5.43}$$

with η usually being referred to as pseudorapidity.

The leading-order Born cross sections for parton–parton scattering are reported in Table 5.1.

Table 5.1 Cross sections for light-parton scattering. The notation is $p_1\, p_2 \to k\, l$, $\hat{s} = (p_1 + p_2)^2$, $\hat{t} = (p_1 - k)^2$, $\hat{u} = (p_1 - l)^2$

Process	$\dfrac{d\hat{\sigma}}{d\Phi_2}$
$qq' \to qq'$	$\dfrac{1}{2\hat{s}}\dfrac{4}{9}\dfrac{\hat{s}^2+\hat{u}^2}{\hat{t}^2}$
$qq \to qq$	$\dfrac{1}{2}\dfrac{1}{2\hat{s}}\left[\dfrac{4}{9}\left(\dfrac{\hat{s}^2+\hat{u}^2}{\hat{t}^2} + \dfrac{\hat{s}^2+\hat{t}^2}{\hat{u}^2}\right) - \dfrac{8}{27}\dfrac{\hat{s}^2}{\hat{u}\hat{t}}\right]$
$q\bar{q} \to q'\bar{q}'$	$\dfrac{1}{2\hat{s}}\dfrac{4}{9}\dfrac{\hat{t}^2+\hat{u}^2}{\hat{s}^2}$
$q\bar{q} \to q\bar{q}$	$\dfrac{1}{2\hat{s}}\left[\dfrac{4}{9}\left(\dfrac{\hat{s}^2+\hat{u}^2}{\hat{t}^2} + \dfrac{\hat{t}^2+\hat{u}^2}{\hat{s}^2}\right) - \dfrac{8}{27}\dfrac{\hat{u}^2}{\hat{s}\hat{t}}\right]$
$q\bar{q} \to gg$	$\dfrac{1}{2}\dfrac{1}{2\hat{s}}\left[\dfrac{32}{27}\dfrac{\hat{t}^2+\hat{u}^2}{\hat{t}\hat{u}} - \dfrac{8}{3}\dfrac{\hat{t}^2+\hat{u}^2}{\hat{s}^2}\right]$
$gg \to q\bar{q}$	$\dfrac{1}{2\hat{s}}\left[\dfrac{1}{6}\dfrac{\hat{t}^2+\hat{u}^2}{\hat{t}\hat{u}} - \dfrac{3}{8}\dfrac{\hat{t}^2+\hat{u}^2}{\hat{s}^2}\right]$
$gq \to gq$	$\dfrac{1}{2\hat{s}}\left[-\dfrac{4}{9}\dfrac{\hat{s}^2+\hat{u}^2}{\hat{s}\hat{u}} + \dfrac{\hat{u}^2+\hat{s}^2}{\hat{t}^2}\right]$
$gg \to gg$	$\dfrac{1}{2}\dfrac{1}{2\hat{s}}\dfrac{9}{2}\left(3 - \dfrac{\hat{t}\hat{u}}{\hat{s}^2} - \dfrac{\hat{s}\hat{u}}{\hat{t}^2} - \dfrac{\hat{s}\hat{t}}{\hat{u}^2}\right)$

5.4.3 Comparison of theory and experimental data

Predictions for jet production at colliders are available today at NLO in QCD (see the review in [7]). One of the preferred observables is the inclusive E_T spectrum. The agreement between data and theory at the LHC is excellent, as shown in Fig. 5.21. An accurate comparison of data and theory, should it exhibit discrepancies at the largest values of E_T, could provide evidence for new phenomena, such as the existence of a quark substructure [33]. But how do we know that these discrepancies are not due to poorly known quark or gluon densities at large x? In principle, one could incorporate the jet data into a global fit to the partonic PDFs, and verify whether it is possible to modify them so as to maintain agreement with the other data, and at the same time to also fit satisfactorily the jet data themselves. On the other hand, doing this would prevent us from using the jet spectrum as a probe of new physics. In other words, we might be hiding away a possible signal of new physics by ascribing it to the PDFs. Is it possible to have a complementary determination of the PDF at high x that could constrain the possible PDF systematics of the jet cross section and at the same time leave the high-E_T tail as an independent and usable observable?

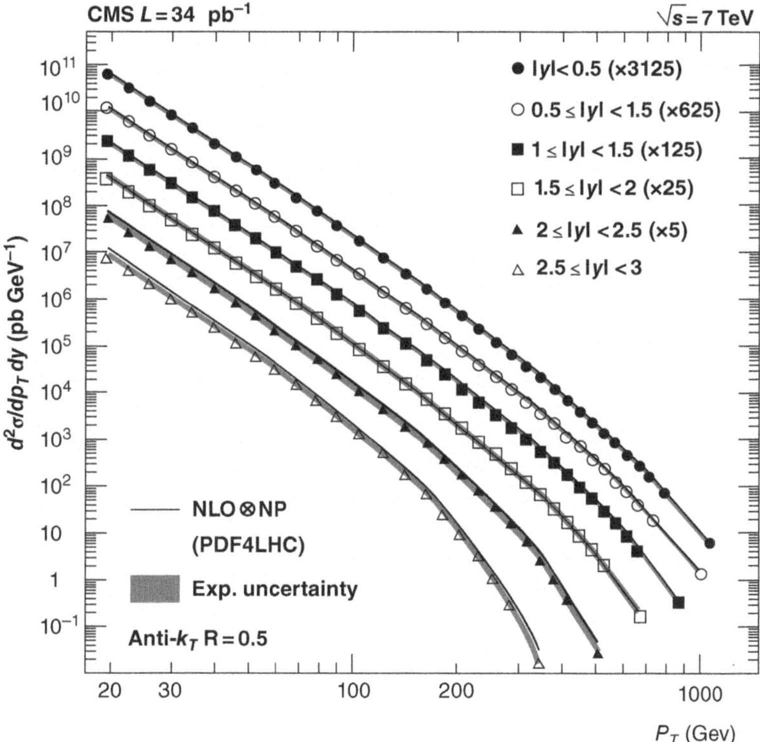

Fig. 5.21 Data versus theory comparison for the inclusive jet spectrum measured by the CMS experiment at the LHC [32].

This is indeed possible, by fully exploiting the kinematics of dijet production and the wide rapidity coverage of the collider detectors. One could in fact consider final states where the dijet system is highly boosted in the forward or backward region. For example, one could consider cases where $x_1 \to 1$ and $x_2 \ll 1$. In this case, the invariant mass of the dijet system would be small (since $M_{jj}^2 = x_1 x_2 S \ll S$), and we know from lower-energy measurements that at this scale jets must behave like pointlike particles, following exactly the QCD-predicted rate. These final states are characterized by having jets at large positive rapidity. One can therefore perform a measurement with forward jets, and use these data to fit the $x_1 \to 1$ behaviour of the quark and gluon PDFs without the risk of washing away possible new-physics effects. At that point, the large-x PDFs thus constrained can be safely applied to the kinematical configurations where both x_1 and x_2 are large, namely the highest-E_T final states, and, if any residual discrepancy between data and theory is observed,

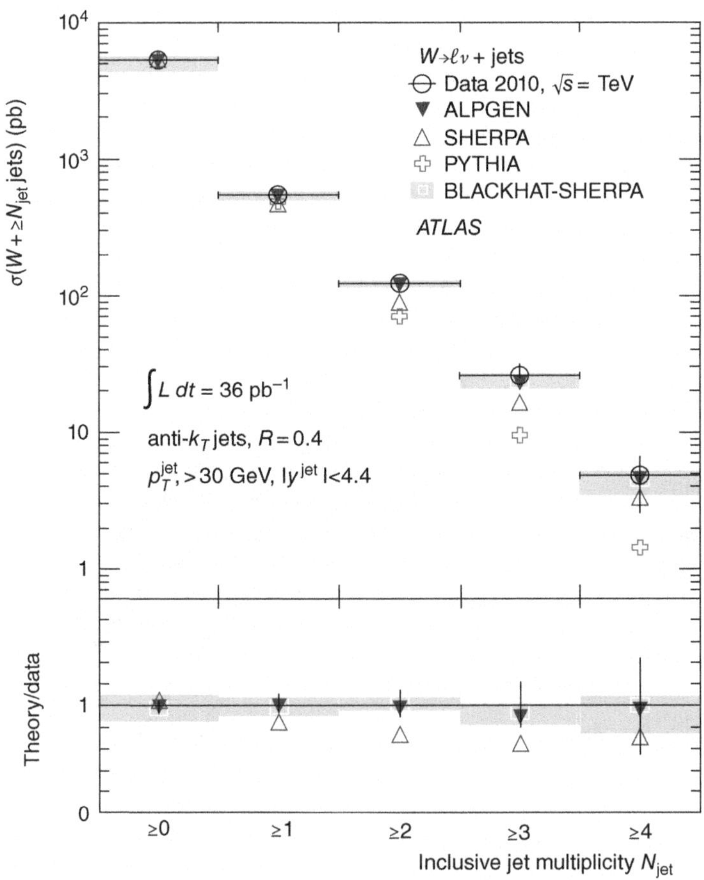

Fig. 5.22 Production rates of W plus multijets, measured by ATLAS at the LHC [35], compared against various theoretical predictions.

infer the possible presence of new physics. The agreement seen in Fig. 5.21 in the data at large rapidity suggests that the PDF parametrizations at large x are reliable. A closer study of correlations among the two leading jets in the events can then lead to strong constraints on the possible composite structure of quarks, as seen for example in the ATLAS study of [34].

Of great phenomenological interest, in particular in the context of the study of backgrounds to the production of top quarks, of the Higgs boson, and of several signals of new physics, is the associated production of W or Z bosons and jets. LHC data and theoretical predictions are so far in very good agreement, as shown in Fig. 5.22. Similar excellent agreement between data and QCD has been observed for a large number of observables, ranging from the inner structure of jets, to the spectra of high-p_T photons, to the production rates of bottom and top quarks.

5.5   Outlook and conclusions

In spite of the intrinsic complexity of the proton, the factorization framework allows a complete, accurate and successful description of the rates and properties of hard processes in hadronic collisions. One of the key ingredients of this formulation is the universality of the phenomenological parametrizations of the various nonperturbative components of the calculations (the partonic densities and the hadronization phase). This universality makes it possible to extract the nonperturbative information from the comparison of data and theory in a set of benchmark measurements, and to apply this knowledge to different observables or to different experimental environments. All the differences will be then accounted for by the purely perturbative part of the evolution.

Many years of experience at the Tevatron collider, at HERA, and at LEP have led to an immense improvement of our understanding, and to the validation, of this framework, and put us today in a solid position to reliably anticipate in quantitative terms the features of LHC final states. LEP, in addition to testing with great accuracy the electroweak interaction sector, has verified at the percent level the predictions of perturbative QCD, from the running of the strong coupling constant, to the description of the perturbative evolution of single quarks and gluons, down to the nonperturbative boundary where strong interactions take over and cause the confinement of partons into hadrons. The description of this transition, relying on the factorization theorem that allows one to consistently separate the perturbative and nonperturbative phases, has been validated by the study of LEP data at various energies, and their comparison with data from lower-energy e^+e^- colliders, allowing the phenomenological parameters introduced to model hadronization to be determined. The factorization theorem supports the use of these parameters for the description of the hadronization transition in other experimental environments. HERA has made it possible to probe with great accuracy the short-distance properties of the proton, with the measurement of its partonic content over a broad range of momentum fractions x. These inputs, from LEP and from HERA, beautifully merge into the tools that have been developed to describe proton–antiproton collisions at the Tevatron, where the agreement between theoretical predictions and data confirms that the key assumptions of the overall approach are robust.

The accuracy of the perturbative input relies on complete higher-order calculations, as well as possible resummations of leading contributions to all orders of perturbation theory. Today's theoretical precision varies from the few-percent level of W and Z inclusive cross sections, which are known to NNLO, to the level of 10% for several processes known to NLO (inclusive jet cross sections, top quark production, and production of pairs of electroweak gauge bosons), up to very crude estimates for the most complex, multijet final states, where uncertainties at the available leading order can be as large as factors of 2 or more. At the LHC, the statistics and systematics for measurements such as the total W, Z, or $t\bar{t}$ cross sections are expected to be reduced to the few-percent level, comparable with the theoretical accuracy. These measurements, and others, will allow us to stress-test our modelling of basic phenomena at the LHC and to validate and improve their reliability, laying the foundations for a successful exploration of the new landscapes that will be uncovered at the energy frontier.

References

[1] R. P. Feynman, Photon–Hadron Interactions (Benjamin, New York, 1972).

[2] D.J. Gross, arXiv:hep-th/9809060; G. 't Hooft, arXiv:hep-th/9808154.

[3] T. Muta, Foundations of QCD (World Scientific, Singapore, 1998).

[4] M. E. Peskin and D. V. Schroeder, An Introduction to Quantum Field Theory (Addison-Wesley, Reading, MA, 1995).

[5] V. Barger and R. J. N. Phillips, Collider Physics (Addison-Wesley, Redwood City, CA, 1997).

[6] R. K. Ellis, W. J. Stirling and B. R. Webber, QCD and Collider Physics (Cambridge University Press, Cambridge, 1996).

[7] J. M. Campbell, J. W. Huston, and W. J. Stirling, Rep. Prog. Phys. **70** (2007) 89 [arXiv:hep-ph/0611148].

[8] R. Field, Applications of Perturbative QCD (Addison-Wesley, Redwood City, CA, 1989).

[9] Yu. L. Dokshitzer, V. A. Khoze, A. H. Mueller, and S. I. Troyan, Basics of Perturbative QCD (Editions Frontières, Gif-sur-Yvette, 1991).

[10] L. J. Dixon, arXiv:0712.3064 [hep-ph].

[11] M. A. Dobbs et al., arXiv:hep-ph/0403045.

[12] V. N. Gribov and L. N. Lipatov, Sov. J. Nucl. Phys. **15** (1972) 438 [Yad. Fiz. **15** (1972) 781].

[13] G. Altarelli and G. Parisi, Nucl. Phys. **B126** (1977) 298.

[14] Y. L. Dokshitzer, Sov. Phys. JETP **46** (1977) 641 [Zh. Eksp. Teor. Fiz. **73** (1977) 1216].

[15] M. Dittmar et al., arXiv:0901.2504 [hep-ph].

[16] H. Jung et al., arXiv:0903.3861 [hep-ph].

[17] P. M. Nadolsky et al., Phys. Rev. **D78** (2008) 013004 [arXiv:0802.0007 [hep-ph]].

[18] A. D. Martin, W. J. Stirling, R. S. Thorne, and G. Watt, arXiv:0901.0002 [hep-ph].

[19] S. Alekhin, K. Melnikov, and F. Petriello, Phys. Rev. **D74** (2006) 054033 [arXiv:hep-ph/0606237].

[20] R. D. Ball et al. [NNPDF Collaboration], Nucl. Phys. **B809** (2009) 1 [Erratum **B816** (2009) 293] [arXiv:0808.1231 [hep-ph]].

[21] B. C. Reisert [ZEUS Collaboration], arXiv:0809.4946 [hep-ex].

[22] G. Watt, JHEP **1109** (2011) 069 [arXiv:1106.5788 [hep-ph]].

[23] Y. L. Dokshitzer, V. A. Khoze, S. I. Troian, and A. H. Mueller, Rev. Mod. Phys. **60**, 373 (1988).

[24] B. R. Webber, Nucl. Phys. **B238** (1984) 492.

[25] G. Marchesini and B. R. Webber, Nucl. Phys. **B310** (1988) 461.

[26] G. Corcella et al., JHEP **0101** (2001) 010 [arXiv:hep-ph/0011363].

[27] B. Andersson, G. Gustafson, G. Ingelman, and T. Sjostrand, Phys. Rep. **97** (1983) 31.

[28] T. Sjostrand, P. Eden, C. Friberg, L. Lonnblad, G. Miu, S. Mrenna, and E. Norrbin, Comput. Phys. Commun. **135** (2001) 238 [arXiv:hep-ph/0010017].

[29] T. Sjostrand, S. Mrenna, and P. Skands, JHEP **0605** (2006) 026 [arXiv:hep-ph/0603175].

[30] S. Gieseke, A. Ribon, M. H. Seymour, P. Stephens, and B. Webber, JHEP **0402** (2004) 005 [arXiv:hep-ph/0311208].

[31] G. Aad et al. [ATLAS Collaboration], Phys. Rev. **D85** (2012) 072004 [arXiv:1109.5141 [hep-ex]].

[32] S. Chatrchyan et al. [CMS Collaboration], Phys. Rev. Lett. **107** (2011) 132001 [arXiv:1106.0208 [hep-ex]].

[33] E. Eichten, K. D. Lane, and M. E. Peskin, Phys. Rev. Lett. **50** (1983) 811.

[34] G. Aad et al. [ATLAS Collaboration], New J. Phys. **13** (2011) 053044 [arXiv:1103.3864 [hep-ex]].

[35] G. Aad et al. [ATLAS Collaboration], Phys. Rev. **D85** (2012) 092002 [arXiv:1201.1276 [hep-ex]].

6
An introduction to the gauge/gravity duality

Juan M. MALDACENA

Institute for Advanced Study, Princeton, New Jersey, USA

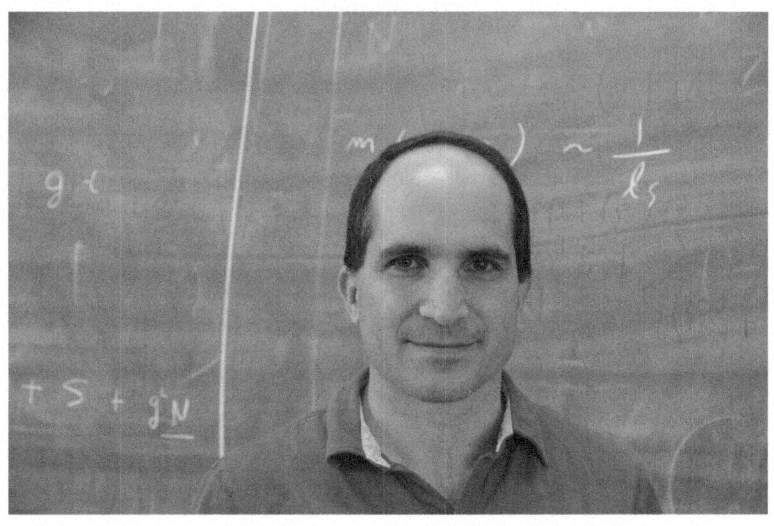

Theoretical Physics to Face the Challenge of LHC. Edited by L. Baulieu, K. Benakli, M. R. Douglas, B. Mansoulié, E. Rabinovici, and L. F. Cugliandolo. © Oxford University Press 2015. Published in 2015 by Oxford University Press.

Chapter Contents

6.1   Introduction to the gauge/gravity duality

In these lectures, we explain the gauge/gravity duality [1–3]. The gauge/gravity duality is an equality between two theories: on one side, we have a quantum field theory in d spacetime dimensions. On the other side, we have a gravity theory on a $(d+1)$-dimensional spacetime that has an asymptotic boundary that is d-dimensional. It is also sometimes called AdS/CFT, because the simplest examples involve anti-de Sitter spaces and conformal field theories. It is often called gauge/string duality. This is because the gravity theories are string theories and the quantum field theories are gauge theories. It is also referred to as "holography" because one is describing a $(d+1)$-dimensional gravity theory in terms of a lower-dimensional system, in a way that is reminiscent of an optical hologram, which stores a three-dimensional image on a two-dimensional photographic plate. It is called a "conjecture," but by now there is a lot of evidence that it is correct. In addition, there are some derivations based on physical arguments.[*]

The simplest example involves an anti-de Sitter spacetime. So, let us start by describing this spacetime in some detail. Anti-de Sitter spacetime AdS is the simplest solution of Einstein's equations with a negative cosmological constant. It is the Lorentzian analog of hyperbolic space, which was historically the first example of a non-Euclidean geometry. In a similar way, AdS/CFT gives the simplest example of a quantum mechanical spacetime.

The metric in AdS can be written as

$$ds^2_{AdS_{d+1}} = L^2 \left[-(r^2+1)\, dt^2 + \frac{dr^2}{r^2+1} + r^2\, d\Omega^2_{d-1} \right], \tag{6.1}$$

where the last term is the metric of a unit sphere, S^{d-1}. L is the radius of curvature. Note that near $r = 0$, AdS looks like flat space. As we go to larger values of r, we see that g_{00} and the metric on the sphere grow. The growth of g_{00} can be viewed as a rising gravitational potential. In fact, a slowly moving massive particle feels a gravitational potential $V \sim \sqrt{-g_{00}}$. If a particle is set at rest at a large value of r, it will execute an oscillatory motion in the r direction, very much like a particle in a harmonic oscillator potential. This gravitational potential confines particles around the origin. A massive particle with finite energy cannot escape to infinity, $r = \infty$. A massless geodesic can go to infinity and back in finite time. One way to see this is to look at the Penrose diagram of AdS. We can factor out a factor of $1 + r^2$ in the metric (6.1), and define a new radial coordinate, x, via $dx = dr/(1 + r^2)$, which now has a finite range. Thus, the Penrose diagram of AdS is a solid cylinder; see Fig. 6.1(a). The vertical direction is time, and the boundary is at $r = \infty$, which is a finite value of x. The S^{d-1} is the spatial section of the surface of the cylinder. The metric in (6.1) has an obvious $\mathbb{R} \times SO(d)$ symmetry. AdS has further symmetries. The full symmetry group is $SO(2, d)$. These symmetries can be made more manifest by viewing AdS as the hyperboloid

[*]Full acknowledgement to Juan Maldacena, The Guage/Gravity Duality, Gary T Horowitz, 2012, © Cambridge University Press 2012, reproduced with permission.

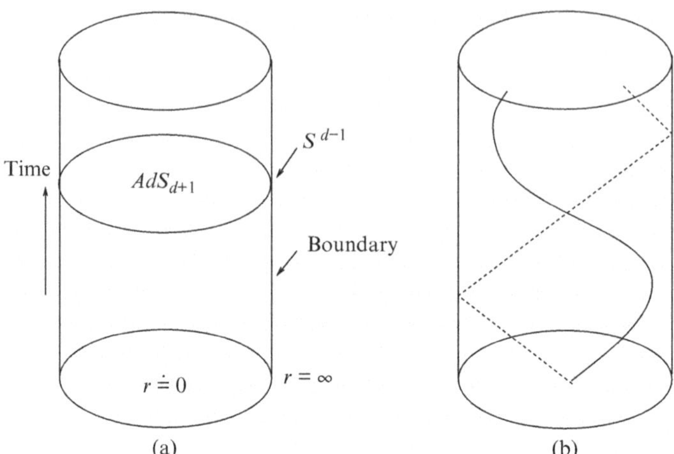

Fig. 6.1 (a) Penrose diagram for anti-de Sitter space. It is a solid cylinder. The vertical direction is time. The boundary contains the time direction and a sphere S^{d-1}, represented here as a circle. (b) A massive geodesic (solid line) and a massless geodesic (dashed line).

$$- Y_{-1}^2 - Y_0^2 + Y_1^2 + \cdots + Y_d^2 = -L^2 \tag{6.2}$$

in $\mathbb{R}^{2,d}$. This description is useful for realizing the symmetries explicitly. However, in this hyperboloid, the time direction, t in (6.1), is compact (it is just the angle in the $[-1,0]$ plane). However, in all physical applications, we want to take this time direction to be noncompact.

These isometries of AdS are very powerful. Let us recall the situation in flat space. If we have a massive geodesic in flat space, we can always boost to a frame where it is at rest. In AdS, it is the same: if we consider the oscillating trajectory of a massive particle, then we can "boost" to a frame where that particle is at rest. Thus, the moving particle does not know that it is moving and, despite appearances, there is no "center" in AdS. The Hamiltonian is part of the symmetry group (as in the Poincaré group) and there are several choices for a Hamiltonian. Once we choose one Hamiltonian, for example the one that shifts t in (6.1), then we choose a "center" and a notion of lowest-energy state, which is a particle sitting at this "center."

In some applications, it is useful to focus on a small patch of the boundary and treat it as $\mathbb{R}^{1,d}$. In fact, there is a choice of coordinates where the AdS metric takes the form

$$ds^2 = L^2 \frac{-dt^2 + d\vec{x}_{d-1}^2 + dz^2}{z^2}. \tag{6.3}$$

Here the boundary is at $z = 0$ and we have slices that display the Poincaré symmetry group in d dimensions (one time and $d-1$ spatial dimensions). In fact, if we take $t \to ix_0$, we get hyperbolic space, now sometimes called Euclidean AdS! In these coordinates, we can also see clearly another isometry that rescales the coordinates $(t, \vec{x}, z) \to \lambda(t, \vec{x}, z)$. These coordinates have a horizon at $z = \infty$ and cover only a portion of (6.1). These coordinates are convenient when we want to consider a CFT living in Minkowski space $\mathbb{R}^{1,d-1}$.

The AdS/CFT relation postulates that all the physics in an asymptotically anti-de Sitter spacetime can be described by a local quantum field theory that lives on the boundary. The boundary is given by $\mathbb{R} \times S^{d-1}$. The isometries of AdS act on the boundary. They send points on the boundary to points on the boundary. This action is simply the action of the conformal group in d dimensions, $SO(2,d)$. Thus, the quantum field theory is a CFT. In fact, the rescaling symmetry of (6.3) translates into a dilatation on the boundary. The boundary theory is thus scale-invariant. It has no dimensionful parameter. Usually theories that are scale-invariant are also conformally invariant. These are theories where the stress–energy–momentum tensor is traceless. The conformal group includes the Poincaré group and the dilatation, as well as "special conformal transformations" that will not be too important for us here. Notice that the conformal symmetry makes sure that we can choose an arbitrary radius for the boundary S^{d-1}, so we can set it to one. In fact, if we have a conformal field theory, the tracelessness of the stress tensor implies that a field theory on a space with a metric $g^b_{\mu\nu}$ or $\omega^2(x)g^b_{\mu\nu}$ is basically the same (up to a well-understood conformal anomaly). Here we are talking about the metric on the boundary, where the field theory lives. This metric is not dynamical, it is fixed.

How can it be that a $(d+1)$-dimensional bulk theory is equivalent to a d-dimensional one? In fact, let us attempt to disprove this. A skeptic would argue as follows. Let us do a simple count of the number of degrees of freedom. Since the bulk has one extra dimension, we seem to have a contradiction. In fact, we could consider the number of degrees of freedom at large energies, in the microcanonical ensemble. To compute it, we can introduce an effective temperature. In a theory with massless fields (or a theory with no scale), we expect the entropy to go like $S \sim V_{d-1}T^{d-1}$. So if the boundary theory is a CFT on $\mathbb{R} \times S^3$, then, for temperatures large compared with the radius of S^3 ($T \gg 1$), we expect the entropy to grow like

$$S \propto c\,T^{d-1}, \tag{6.4}$$

where c is a dimensionless constant that measures the effective number of fields in the theory. For free fields, it can be explicitly computed, as we will do later in an example. On the other hand, from the bulk point of view, it seems that we also have a theory with massless particles, which are the gravitons. We could also have extra fields, but, for the time being, let us include only the gravitons, which give a lower bound to the entropy. The entropy of these gravitons is certainly bigger than the entropy from the region where $r \sim 1$. In that region, which has a volume of order one, we get

$$S_{\text{gas of gravitons}} > T^d, \tag{6.5}$$

because it has d spatial dimensions. For large enough T, we see that (6.5) is bigger than (6.4). So we appear to have a contradiction with the basic claim of AdS/CFT.

However, we are forgetting something essential: it is crucial that the bulk theory contains *gravity*. And gravity gives rise to black holes. And black holes give rise to bounds on entropy. Black holes in AdS have the metric

$$ds^2_{AdS_{d+1}} = L^2 \left[-\left(r^2 + 1 - \frac{2gm}{r^{d-2}} \right) dt^2 + \frac{dr^2}{r^2 + 1 - \frac{2gm}{r^{d-2}}} + r^2 \, d\Omega^2_{d-1} \right], \qquad (6.6)$$

where m is proportional to the mass and g is proportional to the Newton constant in units of the AdS radius,

$$g \propto \frac{G_N^{d+1}}{L^{d-1}}. \qquad (6.7)$$

The gas of gravitons extends up to $r_z \sim T$ and has a mass of the order of $m \sim T^{d+1}$. For large T, we can neglect the 1 in (6.6) when computing the Schwarzschild radius: $r_s^d \sim gm \sim gT^{d+1}$. We see that the Schwarzschild radius is greater than the size of the system for temperatures that are high enough, $T > 1/g$. Thus, the computation in (6.5) breaks down for such high temperatures. At large enough energies, we compute the entropy in terms of the black hole entropy. This entropy grows like the area of the horizon $S \sim r_s^{d-1}/g$. One can see that the Hawking temperature for large black holes is $T \propto r_s$. The entropy of the black hole is $S_{\mathrm{BH}} \sim T^{d-1}/g$. This is now of the expected form, (6.4), with

$$c \propto \frac{1}{g} \propto \frac{L_{AdS}^{d-1}}{G_{N,d+1}}. \qquad (6.8)$$

Thus, AdS/CFT connects the entropy of a black hole with the ordinary thermal entropy of a field theory. This has two very important applications. First, with regard to conceptual issues about the entropy of black holes, it gives a statistical interpretation of black hole entropy. In addition, since it displays the black hole as an ordinary thermal state in a unitary quantum field theory, we see that these black holes are consistent with quantum mechanics and unitary evolution. Second, it allows us to compute the thermal free energy, and other thermal properties, in quantum field theories that have gravity duals.

The number of fields scales like the inverse Newton constant. Notice that g, (6.8), measures the effective gravitational coupling at the AdS scale. It is the dimensionless constant measuring the effective nonlinear interactions among gravitons. Thus, *if we want a weakly coupled bulk theory, we need the field theory to have a large number of fields.* This is a necessary, but not sufficient, condition. One important feature of a weakly coupled theory is the existence of a Fock-space structure in the Hilbert space. Namely, we can talk about a single particle, two particles, etc. Their energies are, up to small corrections, proportional to the sum of the energies of each of the particles. The dual quantum field theory has to have a similar structure. In fact, this structure emerges quite naturally in large-N gauge theories. A large-N gauge theory is a gauge theory based on the gauge group $SU(N)$ (or $U(N)$) with fields in the adjoint representation. In this case, we can form gauge-invariant operators by taking traces of the fundamental fields, such as $\mathrm{Tr}[F_{\mu\nu}F^{\mu\nu}]$, $\mathrm{Tr}[F_{\mu\nu}D_\rho D_\sigma F^{\mu\nu}]$, etc. These are all local operators where the fields are all evaluated at the same point in spacetime. In addition, one could have double-trace operators, such as the product of the two operators we mentioned above. When we act with one such operator on the field theory vacuum, we create a state in the field theory. In a general CFT (even if it does not have a known gravity dual), we have a map between states on the cylinder $\mathbb{R} \times S^{d-1}$ and operators on the plane $\mathbb{R}^d$. The dimension of the operator is equal to the energy of the corresponding state. (The scaling dimension tells us how the operator scales under the scaling transformation that we mentioned after (6.3).) This follows from the fact that we can go to a Euclidean cylinder. The Euclidean cylinder and the plane differ by an overall Weyl transformation of the metric $d(\log r)^2 + d\Omega^2 = r^{-2}(dr^2 + r^2\, d\Omega^2)$. Thus, they are equivalent in a CFT. An operator at the origin of the plane creates a state at fixed r that can be viewed as a state of the field theory on the cylinder; see Fig. 6.2. This state–operator mapping is valid for any CFT. AdS/CFT relates a state of the field theory on the cylinder to a state of the bulk theory in global coordinates (6.1). Since the symmetries on both sides are the same, we can divide the states, or operators, according to their transformation laws under the conformal group. Such representations are characterized by the spin of the operator and its scaling dimension Δ. A simple example is the stress tensor operator $T_{\mu\nu}$. This operator creates a graviton in AdS. The dimension of the stress tensor is d. Single-trace operators are associated with single-particle states in the bulk. Multitrace operators correspond to multiparticle states in the bulk. There exists a general argument, based on a simple analysis of Feynman diagrams, that shows that the dimensions of multitrace operators are the sums of the dimensions of each single-trace component, up to corrections of order $1/N^2$. In fact, the same analysis of Feynman diagrams shows that the large-N limit of general gauge theories gives a string theory [4]. The argument does not specify precisely the kind of string theory we are supposed to get—it only says that we can organize the diagrams in terms of diagrams we can draw on a sphere plus those on the torus, etc. Each time we increase the genus of the surface, we get an additional power of $1/N^2$. This looks like a string theory with a string coupling $g_s \sim 1/N$. The strings we have in the bulk are precisely the strings that are suggested by this argument.

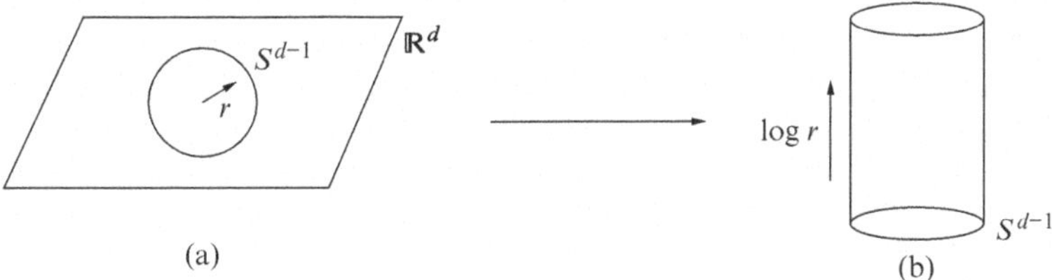

Fig. 6.2 (a) A conformal field theory on the Euclidean plane $\mathbb{R}^d$. We can act with various operators at $r = 0$. These create certain states on S^{d-1}, which are given by performing the path integral of the field theory in the interior of the S^{d-1} with the operators inserted. (b) Because of the Weyl symmetry of the theory, we can rescale the metric and view it as the metric on a cylinder $\mathbb{R} \times S^{d-1}$. States of the theory on this cylinder are in one-to-one correspondence to operators on the plane. This is a general property of CFTs and completely independent of AdS/CFT.

The preceding argument says that the large-N limit is necessary to have a weakly coupled gravity theory. This does not mean that we are restricted to the linearized solutions. In a weakly coupled gravity theory, we can consider full classical nonlinear solutions of the equations, such as the black hole solutions we discussed above. Weak coupling means that we can neglect quantum gravity corrections or loop diagrams.

In string theory, the graviton is the lowest mode of oscillation of a string. The gravitational coupling we discussed above is related to the strength of interaction between strings. However, we have another condition for the validity of the gravity approximation. In gravity, we treat the graviton as a pointlike particle and we ignore all the massive string states. The typical size of the graviton is given by the string length l_s, an additional parameter beyond the Planck scale. In order to ignore the rest of the string states, we need

$$\frac{L_{AdS}}{l_s} \gg 1 \tag{6.9}$$

for gravity to be a good approximation. This condition is simply saying that the typical size of the space should be much bigger than the intrinsic size of the graviton in string theory. This condition is important because in many concrete examples, we have to make sure that this condition is met, otherwise gravity will give the wrong answers, even if we have a large number of fields! If (6.9) is not valid, then we should consider the full string theory in AdS. A salient feature of string theory is that there are massive string states of higher spin $S > 2$. In fact, in a large-N gauge theory, we can easily write down single-trace operators with higher spin, such as $\mathrm{Tr}[F_{\mu\nu} D_+^S F^{\mu\nu}]$, where D_+ is a derivative along a null direction. Such operators have relatively small scaling dimensions at weak coupling, in this case $\Delta = 4+S$. These give rise to particles of spin S whose bulk mass is comparable to the inverse AdS radius. Such light string states render the Einstein gravity approximation invalid. Thus, *in order to trust the gravity approximation, the field theory should necessarily be strongly interacting.* This is a necessary, but not sufficient, condition. The coupling should be strong enough to give a large dimension to all the higher-spin single-trace operators of the theory. Such masses are set by the parameter (6.9). In concrete examples, we find that this quantity, (6.9), is proportional to a positive power of the effective 't Hooft coupling of the theory, $g_{\mathrm{YM}}^2 N$. Here g_{YM} is the coupling constant of the gauge theory. The extra factor of N comes in because color-correlated particles can exchange N gluons, which enhances their interactions at large N. By taking a large value of $g_{\mathrm{YM}}^2 N$, it is possible to give a large dimension to the higher-spin states. We are left with a light graviton, and other lower-spin states. In this case, we expect their interactions to be those of Einstein gravity.

6.2   Scalar field in *AdS*

In order to be more precise about the correspondence between states in AdS and states in the boundary, it is necessary to do the quantum mechanics of a particle in AdS. Equivalently, we quantize the corresponding field in AdS. In this subsection, we consider a massive scalar field in AdS with an action

$$S = \int d^{d+1}x \sqrt{g} \left[(\nabla \phi)^2 + m^2 \phi^2 \right]. \tag{6.10}$$

Let us compute the energy spectrum in *AdS* in global coordinates, (6.1). Let us only focus on the ground state. We expect it to have zero angular momentum. So we make an ansatz for the wavefunction $\phi = e^{-i\omega t} F(r)$, with the boundary condition that $F(r) \to 0$ at infinity. By setting $\nabla^2 \phi - m^2 \phi = 0$, we get an ω-dependent equation for $F(r)$ with two boundary conditions, one at infinity and one at the origin. This is an eigenvalue problem that gives quantized frequencies. It is possible to check that

$$\phi = e^{-i\Delta t} \frac{1}{(1 + r^2)^{\Delta/2}} \tag{6.11}$$

with

$$\Delta = \frac{d}{2} + \sqrt{\frac{d^2}{4} + (mL)^2} \tag{6.12}$$

is a solution of the equation of motion with the right boundary conditions. We identify this solution as the ground state, since it has no oscillations in the radial direction. The energy is $\omega = \Delta$. The energies of all other states differ from this by an integer, $\omega_n = \Delta + n$. This is due to the fact that we can get all the other states from the action of the conformal generators, and thus their energies are determined by the conformal algebra.

We get a wavefunction localized near the center of *AdS*. In the large-mass limit $mL \gg 1$, we see that it becomes sharply localized at $r = 0$, as we expect for a classical particle in *AdS*. For mL of order one, the wavefunction is extended over a region of order one in r, which corresponds to proper distances of order of the *AdS* radius. A particle of zero mass, $m = 0$, has an integer energy $\Delta = d$. The case of the graviton gives an equation that is similar to that of a massless field, and also leads to $\Delta = d$, as expected from the dimension of the stress tensor.

It seems from (6.12) that the dimensions of operators are bounded below by d, which is the dimension of a marginal operator in the field theory. However, there are two effects that allow us to go to lower dimensions. First, there are some allowed "tachyons" in *AdS*. Namely, it is possible for a field to have $-d^2/4 \le (mL)^2 < 0$. In other words, if a field is only slightly tachyonic, it is allowed [5]. The reason that it does not lead to an instability comes from the boundary conditions. These force the field to have some kinetic energy in the radial direction that overwhelms the negative energy of the mass term. In fact, we can check from (6.12) that such states have positive energies. A second fact is that in the range $-d^2/4 \le (mL)^2 < 1 - d^2/4$, we can have a second quantization prescription [6]. To understand this, note that if we choose the other sign for the square root in (6.12), then (6.11) is another solution of the equation of motion. For tachyons, both solutions decay as $r \to \infty$. So we can set boundary conditions that remove any of these. The quantization leading to (6.12) corresponds to removing the solution that decays more slowly as $r \to \infty$.

Let us now do a different computation that will further elucidate the relation between bulk fields and boundary operators. It is convenient to go to Euclidean space and choose the Poincaré coordinates (6.3). We can consider the problem of computing the path integral of this scalar field theory with fixed boundary conditions at the boundary. The quantum gravity problem in AdS contains such a problem: we have to do this for all the fields of the theory, including the graviton.

Let us consider the classical, or semiclassical, contribution to this problem. This is given by finding the classical solution that obeys the boundary condition and evaluating the action for this solution. If we set zero boundary conditions, then the field is zero and the action is zero. If we set nonzero boundary conditions, the classical action gives us something interesting. Since we have translational symmetry along the boundary directions, we go to Fourier space and write $\phi = e^{ikx} f(k, z)$. The wave equation becomes

$$\frac{d^2 f}{dz^2} + (1 - d)\frac{1}{z}\frac{df}{dz} - \left[k^2 + \frac{(mL)^2}{z^2}\right] f = 0. \tag{6.13}$$

Near the boundary, for small z, there are two independent solutions behaving as $f = z^\Delta$, or $f \sim z^{d-\Delta}$. We will put a boundary condition on the largest component of the solution. Since that component of the solution depends on z, we put a boundary condition at $z = \epsilon$ and set the boundary condition to be

$$\phi(x, z)|_{z=\epsilon} = \phi_0(x)\epsilon^{d-\Delta}. \tag{6.14}$$

The solution of (6.13) that decays at $z \to \infty$ is

$$f(k, z) = e^{ikz} z^{d/2} K_\nu(kz) , \qquad \nu = \sqrt{\frac{d^2}{4} + (mL)^2}, \tag{6.15}$$

where K is a Bessel function. In order to satisfy the boundary conditions, we set

$$\phi(k, z) = \phi_0(k)\epsilon^{d-\Delta}\frac{f(k, z)}{f(k, \epsilon)}. \tag{6.16}$$

We now insert this into the action (6.10). We can integrate by parts and use the equations of motion. The computation then reduces to a boundary term. For each Fourier mode, we get [7]

$$S = \phi_0(-\vec{k})\epsilon^{d-\Delta}\frac{1}{\epsilon^d} z d_z \phi(k, z)|_{z=\epsilon} = \phi_0(-k)\phi_0(\vec{k})\epsilon^{d-2\Delta}\frac{z d_z f(k, z)}{f(k, \epsilon)}$$

$$= \phi_0(-k)\phi_0(\vec{k})\left[\epsilon^{-2\nu}\text{Polynomial}[k^2\epsilon^2] - |k|^{2\nu}2^{-2\nu}\frac{\Gamma(-\nu)}{\Gamma(\nu)}2\nu\right]. \tag{6.17}$$

Note that the first term contains divergent terms when $\epsilon \to 0$. These terms are analytic in momentum and, on Fourier transformation, give terms that are local in position space. These terms were to be expected since the boundary conditions we are considering are such that the field grows toward the boundary. From the field theory point of view, these divergences can be viewed as ultraviolet divergences. On the other hand, the last term in (6.17) gives a nonlocal contribution in position space and represents the interesting part of the correlator. Transformed back to position space, this gives

$$S = -\frac{2\nu\Gamma(\Delta)}{\pi^{d/2}\Gamma(\nu)}L^{d-1}\int d^dx\, d^dy\,\frac{\phi_0(x)\phi_0(y)}{|x-y|^{2\Delta}}.$$ (6.18)

The AdS/CFT dictionary states that this computation with fixed boundary conditions is related to the generating function of correlation functions for the corresponding operator in the field theory [2, 3]. In other words, for a field ϕ related to the single-trace operator O, we have the equality

$$Z_{\text{Gravity}}[\phi_0(x)] = Z_{\text{Field Theory}}[\phi_0(x)] = \langle e^{\int d^dx\,\phi_0(x)O(x)}\rangle.$$ (6.19)

The leading approximation to the gravity answer is given by evaluating the classical action and is given by e^{-S}, with S as in (6.18). Correlation functions of operators are then given by

$$\langle O(x_1)\cdots O(x_n)\rangle = \frac{\delta}{\delta\phi_0(x_1)}\cdots\frac{\delta}{\delta\phi_0(x_1)}Z_{\text{Gravity}}[\phi_0(x)].$$ (6.20)

In the quadratic approximation, the gravity answer is given by (6.18), and the correlation functions factorize into products of two-point functions. We can include interactions in the bulk. For example, we can have a ϕ^3 bulk interaction. Then the leading approximation is given by considering the classical, but nonlinear, solution with these boundary conditions and evaluating the corresponding action. This can be computed perturbatively by evaluating Feynman–Witten diagrams in the bulk [3].

For each single-trace operator, we have a corresponding field in the bulk with a certain boundary condition. Among these fields is the graviton, associated with the stress tensor. The generating function of correlation functions of the stress tensor is obtained by considering the field theory on a general boundary geometry $g^b_{\mu\nu}(x)$. At the classical level, we find a solution of Einstein's equations $R_{\mu\nu} \propto g_{\mu\nu}$, with $g^b_{\mu\nu}$ as a boundary condition. We insert this in the action and obtain the quantity $Z_{\text{Gravity}}[g^b_{\mu\nu}(x)] \sim e^{-S_E[g_{\text{cl}}]}$. We can also view this quantity as the Hartle–Hawking wavefunction of the universe in the Euclidean region. As a first step, one can expand Einstein's equations to quadratic order and compute the two-point function. The action for each polarization component is similar to that of a massless scalar field. In this case, the ϵ-dependent factor in (6.14) drops out. So it makes sense to compute the absolute normalization of the two-point function. This two-point function of the stress tensor is another measure of the degrees of freedom of the theory. It is proportional to the overall coefficient in the Einstein action, which is the quantity c introduced earlier, (6.8). In other words, we schematically have $T_{\mu\nu}(x)T_{\sigma\delta}(0) = ct_{\mu\nu\sigma\delta}/|x|^{2d}$, where $t_{\mu\nu\sigma\delta}$ is an x-dependent tensor taking into account the fact that the stress tensor is traceless and conserved. In fact, since the classical gravity action contains c as an overall factor, we conclude that, to leading order in $1/c$, and in the gravity approximation, all stress tensor correlators are proportional to c. They are universal for any field theory that has a gravity dual, for each spacetime dimension. Such correlators are not universal in quantum field theory (except in two dimensions, $d = 2$). The universality arises only in the gravity approximation, and it is removed by higher-derivative corrections to the action. Stringy corrections give rise to these higher-derivative corrections. Similarly, the coefficient that appears in this computation is equal to the coefficient appearing in the computation of the thermal free energy (up to universal constants). Again, this does not hold for general field theories in $d > 2$. It does hold in $d = 2$.

Another interesting case is a gauge field in AdS. This corresponds to a conserved current in the boundary theory. Thus a gauge symmetry in the bulk corresponds to a global symmetry on the boundary. We have an exactly conserved charge in the boundary theory. Because of black holes, the only way to ensure that we have a conserved charge is to have a gauge symmetry in the bulk.

6.3   The $\mathcal{N} = 4$ super Yang–Mills/$AdS_5 \times S^5$ example

The preceding discussion was completely general. To be specific, let us discuss one particular explicit example of a dual pair. We will first discuss the field theory, then the gravity theory. We will show how various objects match on the two sides.

We consider a four-dimensional field theory that is similar to quantum chromo-dynamics. In quantum chromodynamics, we have a gauge field A_μ that is a (traceless) 3×3 matrix in the adjoint representation of $SU(3)$. The action is

$$S = -\frac{1}{4g_{\text{YM}}^2} \int d^4x \, \text{Tr}[F_{\mu\nu} F^{\mu\nu}], \qquad F_{\mu\nu} = [\partial_\mu + A_\mu, \partial_\nu + A_\nu]. \qquad (6.21)$$

We can consider the generalization of this theory to a gauge group $SU(N)$, or $U(N)$, where A_μ is now an $N \times N$ matrix. In QCD, we also have fermions that transform in the fundamental representation. Here we will do something different. We add fermions that transform in the adjoint representation. The reason is that we would like to construct a theory that is supersymmetric. Supersymmetry is a powerful tool to check many of the predictions of the duality. The existence of the duality does not rely on supersymmetry, but it is easier to find a dual pair when we have supersymmetry. Supersymmetry is a symmetry that relates bosons and fermions. In a supersymmetric theory, the bosons and their fermionic partners are in the same representation of the gauge group. If we simply add a Majorana fermion in the adjoint representation, we get an $\mathcal{N} = 1$ supersymmetric theory. This theory is not conformal quantum mechanically—it has a beta function, as in the theory with no fermions. If instead we add four fermions, χ_α, and six scalars, ϕ^I, all in the adjoint, and with special couplings, we get a theory which has maximal supersymmetry, an $\mathcal{N} = 4$ supersymmetric theory [8]. The Lagrangian of this theory is completely determined by supersymmetry and the choice of the gauge group. It has the schematic form

$$S = -\frac{1}{4g_{\text{YM}}^2} \int d^4x \, \text{Tr}\left[F^2 + 2(D_\mu \Phi^I)^2 + \chi \slashed{D} \chi + \chi[\Phi, \chi] - \sum_{IJ}[\Phi^I, \Phi^J]^2 \right]$$

$$+ \frac{\theta}{8\pi^2} \int \text{Tr}[F \wedge F]. \qquad (6.22)$$

We have two constants: the coupling constant $g_{\rm YM}^2$ and the θ angle. All relative coefficients in the Lagrangian are determined by supersymmetry. The fields are all in a single supermultiplet under supersymmetry. This theory is classically and *quantum mechanically* conformally invariant. In other words, its beta function is zero. Thus, unlike QCD, it does not become more weakly coupled as we go to high energies. The coupling is set once and for all. If it is weak, it is weak at all energies; if it is strong, it is strong at all energies. The effective coupling constant is

$$\lambda = g_{\rm YM}^2 N. \tag{6.23}$$

The extra factor of N arises as follows. If we have two fields whose color and anticolor are entangled, or summed over, then there are N gluons that can be exchanged between them that preserve this entanglement. The theory has an $SO(6)$, or $SU(4)$, R-symmetry that rotates the six scalars into each other, and also rotates the fermions. An R-symmetry is a symmetry that does not commute with supersymmetry. This is the case here because bosons and fermions are in different representations of $SU(4)$.

Now let us discuss the gravity theory. It is a string theory, which gives rise to a quantum mechanically consistent gravity theory. Since we started from a supersymmetric gauge theory, we also expect to have a supersymmetric string theory. There are well-known supersymmetric string theories in 10 dimensions. In particular, there is one theory that contains only closed oriented strings, called the type IIB theory. This string theory reduces at long distances to a gravity theory. It is a supergravity theory called, not surprisingly, type IIB supergravity [9]. This is a theory that contains the metric, plus other massless fields required by supersymmetry. In particular, this theory contains a 5-form field strength $F_{\mu_1 \ldots \mu_5}$, completely antisymmetric in the indices. It is also constrained to be self-dual: $F_5 = *F_5$. It is analogous to the 2-form field strength $F_{\mu\nu}$ of electromagnetism. In four dimensions, we can have charged black hole solutions that involve the metric and the electric (or magnetic) 2-form field strength. In particular, the near-horizon solution of an extremal black hole has the geometry $AdS_2 \times S^2$, with a 2-form flux on the AdS_2 (or the S^2) for an electrically (or a magnetically) charged black hole. Something similar arises in 10 dimensions. There is a solution of the equations of the form $AdS_5 \times S^5$ with a 5-form along both the AdS_5 and S^5 directions. We have both electric and magnetic fields owing to the self-duality constraint on F_5. The Dirac quantization condition says that magnetic fluxes on an S^2 are quantized. In the string theory case, the flux on the S^5 is also quantized:

$$\int_{S^5} F_5 \propto N. \tag{6.24}$$

This number is the same as the number of colors of the gauge theory.

The equations of motion of 10-dimensional supergravity that are relevant for us follow from the action

$$S = \frac{1}{(2\pi)^7 l_p^8} \int d^{10}x \, \sqrt{g}(R - F_5^2) \tag{6.25}$$

plus the self-duality constraint $F_5 = *F_5$. The equations of motion relate the radii of AdS_5 and S^5 to N. In fact, we find that both radii are given by $L^4/\ell_p^4 = 4\pi N$. In string theory, we also have the string length, given by $l_s = g_s^{-1/4} l_p$. This sets the string tension $T = (2\pi l_p)^{-1}$. Here g_s determines the interaction strength between strings. It is given by the vacuum expectation value of one of the massless fields of the 10-dimensional theory, $g_s = \langle e^\phi \rangle$. The gravity theory has another massless scalar field χ. This second field is an axion, with a periodicity $\chi \to \chi + 2\pi$. These two fields are associated with the two parameters g_{YM}^2 and θ that we had in the Lagrangian. It is natural to identify θ with the expectation value, or boundary condition, for χ and g_{YM}^2 to the string coupling g_s: $g_{\mathrm{YM}}^2 = 4\pi g_s$. The precise numerical coefficient can be set by the physics of D-branes [10], or by using the S-duality of both theories. After doing this, one can write the AdS_5 and S^5 radii in terms of the Yang–Mills quantities:

$$\frac{L^4}{l_s^4} = 4\pi g_s N = g_{\mathrm{YM}}^2 N = \lambda \,, \qquad \frac{L^4}{l_p^4} = 4\pi N. \tag{6.26}$$

As we discussed in general, in order to have a weakly coupled bulk theory, we need $N \gg 1$. In addition, in order to trust the Einstein gravity approximation, we need a large effective coupling. Thus, we have the following situation:

$$g_{\mathrm{YM}}^2 N \gg 1: \quad \text{gravity is good,} \quad \text{gauge theory is strongly coupled;}$$
$$g_{\mathrm{YM}}^2 N \ll 1: \quad \text{gravity is not good,} \quad \text{gauge theory is weakly coupled.}$$

In these two extreme regimes, it is easy to do computations using one of the two descriptions.

The 't Hooft limit [4], which gives planar diagrams, corresponds to $N \to \infty$ with $g_{\mathrm{YM}}^2 N$ fixed. It is sometimes useful to take the 't Hooft limit first and obtain a free string theory in the bulk and then vary the 't Hooft coupling λ from weak to strong, so that we change the AdS radius in string units. The string is governed by a two-dimensional field theory whose target space is AdS (plus the S^5 and some fermionic dimensions). This two-dimensional field theory is weakly coupled if the AdS radius is large and strongly coupled when the radius is small or the gauge theory is weakly coupled. For values of order one, $g_{\mathrm{YM}}^2 N \sim 1$, it is necessary to use the full string theory description or solve the full planar gauge theory.

The $\mathcal{N} = 4$ super Yang–Mills theory has an S-duality symmetry that exchanges weak and strong coupling. One is tempted to go to strong coupling and then use S-duality in order to get a weakly coupled theory again. This does not work. The bulk theory also has an S-duality symmetry. These two S-duality symmetries are in one-to-one correspondence. So, in order to test whether we can trust the gravity description, first we apply S-duality on both sides to send $g_s < 1$ and then we apply the criterion stated above.

It is interesting to return to the problem of comparing the thermal free energy of the gauge theory and the gravity theory. This time, we keep track of the numerical coefficients. We consider the field theory in $\mathbb{R}^3 \times S_\beta^1$. The free energy at weak coupling is given by the usual formula

$$-\beta F = V \int \frac{d^3 k}{(2\pi)^3} \left[n_{\text{bosons}} \log \frac{1}{(1 - e^{-\beta|\vec{k}|})} + n_{\text{fermions}} \log(1 + e^{-\beta|\vec{k}|}) \right]$$

$$= \frac{\pi^2}{6} V N^2 T^3, \tag{6.27}$$

where $\beta = 1/T$ and we have used $n_{\text{bosons}} = n_{\text{fermions}} = 8N^2$. At strong coupling, we consider the Euclidean black brane solution, with $\tau \sim \tau + \beta$,

$$ds^2 = L^2 \left[\left(1 - \frac{z^4}{z_0^4}\right) \frac{d\tau^2}{z^2} + \frac{dz^2}{z^2 \left(1 - \frac{z^4}{z_0^4}\right)} + \frac{dx^2}{z^2} \right], \tag{6.28}$$

which is simply related to the large-mass limit of (6.6). We can relate $\beta = \pi z_0$ by demanding no singularity at $z = z_0$, as usual. The entropy is given by the usual Bekenstein–Hawking formula [11]

$$S = \frac{\text{Area}}{4G_N} = \frac{L^8 V_{S^5}}{4G_{N,10} z_0^3} = \frac{\pi^2}{2} V N^2 T^3. \tag{6.29}$$

From the entropy, we can simply compute the free energy. We get

$$-\beta F = S/4 = \frac{\pi^2}{8} V N^2 T^3. \tag{6.30}$$

We see that there is a factor of 3/4 difference between (6.30) and (6.27). This does *not* represent a disagreement with AdS/CFT. On the contrary, it is a prediction of how the free energy changes between weak and strong coupling. From general large-N arguments, we expect the free energy to have the form

$$\frac{F(\lambda, N)}{F(\lambda = 0, N)} = f_0(\lambda) + \frac{1}{N^2} f_1(\lambda) + \cdots. \tag{6.31}$$

We expect $f_0(\lambda)$ to go smoothly between $f_0 = 1$ at $\lambda = 0$ and $f_0 = \frac{3}{4}$ at $\lambda \gg 1$. In fact, the leading corrections from both values have been computed and they go in the naively expected direction [12, 13]. In this example, the function f_0 becomes constant at large λ. There are examples where this function goes as $f_0 \sim 1/\sqrt{\lambda}$ for large λ [14, 15].

If we are interested in computing the free energy of super Yang–Mills at strong coupling, we can do it by using the gravity result (6.30).

The existence of the S^5 is related to the $SO(6)$ symmetry of the theory. The Killing vectors generating the S^5 isometries give rise to gauge fields in AdS_5. These are the gauge fields associated with global symmetries that we expected in general. Of course, in other gauge/gravity duality examples, one can also have global symmetries that are not associated with a Kaluza–Klein gauge field.

There are many observables that have a simple geometric description at strong coupling. In fact, the strings (and the branes) of string theory can end on the boundary, and they correspond to various types of operators in the boundary theory. For example, a Wilson loop operator $\mathrm{Tr}[Pe^{\oint_C A}]$ can be computed in terms of a string in the bulk that ends on the boundary along the contour C. At strong coupling, the leading approximation is given just by the area of the surface that ends on this contour. At finite coupling, we need to carry out the worldsheet quantization of this theory. In other words, we need to sum over all surfaces that end on this contour. Certain Wilson loops can be computed exactly using techniques that rely on supersymmetry, confirming the predictions of the duality [16].

The gauge theory contains scalar fields. The potentials for these scalar fields have flat directions. That is, it is possible to give expectation values to the fields in such a way that the vacuum energy continues to be zero. This spontaneously breaks the conformal symmetry. At high energies, the conformal symmetry is restored, but it is broken at low energies. These flat directions correspond to expectation values for the scalar fields that are diagonal matrices. As a simple example, we can set $\Phi^1 = \mathrm{diag}(a, 0, \ldots, 0)$ and all the rest to zero. This breaks the gauge group from $U(N) \to U(1) \times U(N-1)$. In the gravity dual, it correspond to setting a D3-brane at a position $z \sim 1/a$ in the Poincaré coordinates (6.3). One would expect the gravitational potential to push the brane toward the horizon. This force is precisely balanced by an electric repulsion that is provided by the presence of the electric 5-form field strength. The masssless fields living on this D3-brane correspond to the fields in the $U(1)$ factor. The massive W bosons arising from the Higgs mechanism correspond to strings that go from the brane to the horizon. It is interesting that one can find solutions that correspond to general vacuum expectation values. We write

$$ds^2 = f^{-1/2}(-dt^2 + d\vec{x}^2) + f^{1/2}(d\vec{y}^2),$$
$$f = 4\pi \sum_i \frac{l_p^4}{|\vec{y} - \vec{y}_i|^4}. \tag{6.32}$$

Here $\vec{x}$ is a three-dimensional vector and $\vec{y}$ is a six-dimensional vector. The $\vec{y}_i$ are related to the vacuum expectation values of the scalar fields, $\vec{\Phi} = \mathrm{diag}(\vec{y}_1, \vec{y}_2, \ldots, \vec{y}_N)$. This solution looks like a multicentered black brane. In principle, we cannot trust the solution near a single center, since the curvature is very large. However, in situations where we have many coincident centers, we can trust the solution. For example, if we break $U(2N) \to U(N) \times U(N)$ by giving the expectation value $\Phi^1 = \mathrm{diag}(a, \ldots, a, 0, \ldots, 0)$, with N a's, we can trust the solution everywhere. In the ultraviolet, for large $|\vec{y}|$, we have a single AdS geometry, which splits into two AdS throats with smaller radii as we go to lower values of $|\vec{y}|$. This describes the corresponding flow in the gauge theory from the ultraviolet to the infrared, where we have two decoupled CFTs. This is an example of a geometry that is only asymptotically AdS near the boundary but is different in the interior.

It is instructive to consider the solution (6.32) with [17]

$$f = 1 + \frac{4\pi N l_p^4}{|y|^4}. \tag{6.33}$$

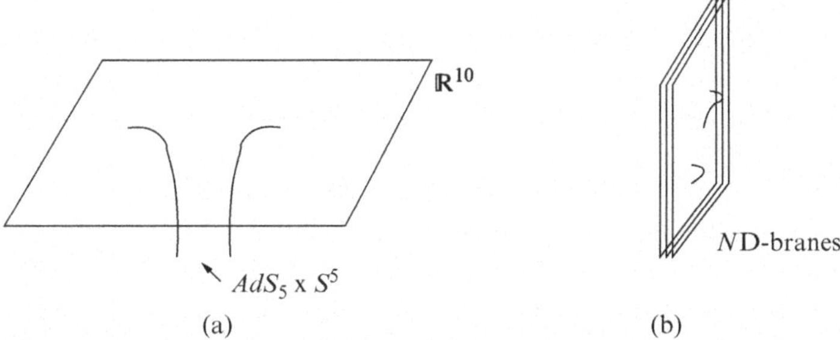

Fig. 6.3 (a) The geometry of the black 3-brane solution (6.32) with (6.33). Far away, we have 10-dimensional flat space. Near the horizon, we have $AdS_5 \times S^5$. (b) The D-brane description. D-brane excitations are described by open strings living on them. They can start and end on any of N D-branes, so we have N^2 of them. At low energies, they give rise to a $U(N)$ gauge theory: $\mathcal{N} = 4$ super Yang–Mills.

This enables us to give a physical derivation of the gauge/gravity duality for this example [1]. This solution goes to 10-dimensional flat space for $|\vec{y}| \gg N^{1/4} l_p$. It represents an extremal black 3-brane; see Fig. 6.3. It is extended along $1 + 3$ of the spacetime dimensions, labeled by t and $\vec{x}$, and it is localized in six of them, labeled by $\vec{y}$. The near-horizon geometry of this black D3-brane is obtained by going to small values of y and dropping the 1 in (6.33). When the string coupling is very small, $g_s N \ll 1$, this system can be described as a set of N D3-branes. D3-branes are solitonic defects that exist in string theory [18]. They are described in terms of an extremely simple string theory construction. This construction tells us that we get $\mathcal{N} = 4$ super Yang–Mills at low energies. In fact, it is easy to understand the scalar fields: they come from the motion of the branes in the six transverse dimensions. We can view the gauge fields as arising from supersymmetry. A system of N identical branes is expected to have an ordinary S_N permutation symmetry. However, for these branes, this symmetry is enlarged into a full $U(N)$ gauge symmetry. Thus, we have two descriptions for the brane: first as a black brane and second as a set of D-branes. We can now take the low-energy limit of each of these descriptions. The low-energy limit of the D-branes gives us the $\mathcal{N} = 4\ U(N)$ super Yang–Mills theory. The low-energy limit on the gravity side corresponds to going very close to the horizon of the black 3-brane. There, the large redshift factor (the fact that $f^{-1/2} \to 0$) gives a very low energy to all the particles living in that near-horizon region. This region is simply $AdS_5 \times S^5$. Assuming that these two descriptions are equivalent, we get the gauge/gravity duality.

6.4   The spectrum of states or operators

In this case, we can construct a complete dictionary between the massless fields in the bulk and operators in the field theory. The massless 10-dimensional fields can be expanded in spherical harmonics on the S^5. In addition, they fill supermultiplets. It is interesting to note that we have 32 supercharges in the bulk theory.

With this large number of supercharges, a generic supermultiplet would contain states with spins greater than two. However, we can have special BPS multiplets with spins only up to two. Thus, all the massless particles of the 10-dimensional theory should be in special BPS multiplets. In 10 flat dimensions, this is only possible if the particles are massless. In $AdS_5 \times S^5$, this is only possible if the AdS energy is fixed in terms of the $SO(6)$ charge. In the field theory, these are in multiplets that contain the operators $\text{Tr}[\Phi^{(I_1}\Phi^{I_2}\cdots\Phi^{I_J)}]$, where the $SO(6)$ indices are symmetrized and the traces extracted. These operators are in the same representation as the spherical harmonics on S^5 with angular momentum J. Their dimension is $\Delta = J$, at all values of the coupling because it is a BPS state. Here we see the power of supersymmetry allowing us to compute these dimensions for all values of the coupling. These operators correspond to a special field in the bulk theory, which is a deformation of the S^5 and the 5-form field strength. The other supergravity fields are related to this one by supersymmetry.

It is interesting to consider the fate of other operators. As we mentioned above, we can consider higher-spin operators. It is simpler to understand the mechanism that gives them a large dimension by considering operators with large charges. Let us consider $Z = \Phi^1 + i\Phi^2$ and the operator $\text{Tr}[Z^J]$. If we now add some derivatives, such as $\text{Tr}[D_+ZZZD_+ZZZ\cdots]$, then at weak coupling the dimension of the operator is the same, independently of the order. As we turn on the coupling, the Hamiltonian, or the dilatation operator, starts moving these derivatives. In some sense, we can view the chain of Z's as defining a lattice. The fact that only planar diagrams contribute implies that the interactions are short-range on this lattice. The range increases as we increase the order in perturbation theory. So the derivatives start moving around, and they gain a kinetic energy that depends on their "momentum" along the chain of Z's. More explicitly, the operators that diagonalize the Hamiltonian (of the dilatation operator) have the schematic form

$$O \sim \sum_l e^{ip^l}\text{Tr}[D_+ZZ^lD_+ZZ^{J-l-2}] + \cdots . \tag{6.34}$$

We have used the cyclicity of the trace to set the first derivative on the first spot. The dots represent extra terms that can appear when l or $J - l - 2$ are small, and are important to precisely quantize the momentum. The momentum p is quantized with an expression of the form $p_n \sim 2\pi n/J + o(1/J^2)$, where the subleading term depends on the extra terms that appear when the two derivatives "cross" each other. A derivative with zero momentum can be pulled out of the trace and act as an ordinary derivative. This is just an element of the conformal group, and it does not give rise to spin, but to ordinary orbital angular momentum in AdS. Thus, in order to get spin, we need derivatives that have some momentum, and thus some kinetic energy. This kinetic energy increases as λ increases. Thus, for large λ, all the states that have nonzero momentum acquire a large energy. This is especially true for a short string (small J), where the momentum has to be relatively large, due to the momentum quantization condition. This was just a qualitative argument. The exact computation of these energies requires considerable technology and it employs a deep "integrability" symmetry of the planar gauge theory, or the corresponding string theory [19]. For the lightest spin-4 state (Konishi multiplet), these energies have been computed for any λ in [20]. They behave as expected and are in complete agreement with AdS/CFT. That is, they go from a value of order one at weak coupling to the strong-coupling answer, which is $\Delta = 2\lambda^{1/4}$. This strong-coupling answer is computed as follows. When the AdS radius is large in string units, the massive string states feel almost as if they were in flat space. The lightest massive string state in flat space has mass $m^2 = 4/l_s^2$ [21]. Using (6.12) and (6.26), this gives $\Delta \sim Lm \sim 2\lambda^{1/4}$.

6.5   The radial direction

One of the crucial elements of the gauge/gravity duality is the emergence of an extra "radial" dimension, the z coordinate in (6.3). Let us discuss this in more detail and in some generality. In ordinary physics, we are used to particles that typically are massive. These particles have a quantum state described by the three spatial positions. Even if they have internal constituents, as protons or atoms do, then (ignoring spin) we can describe the state by simply giving its spatial momentum or position. Of course, its energy is determined by its mass. In a scale-invariant theory, we cannot have massive particles. Naively, we would say that all the particles are massless. On the other hand, these massless particles interact in a nontrivial way and they cannot be viewed as good asymptotic states. This is true even in large-N gauge theories. However, in large-N gauge theories, we have some weakly interacting excitations. These are the objects that are created by acting with single-trace operators on the vacuum. They are characterized by the 4-momentum of the operator. Notice that we have one more component of the momentum, as compared with the case of an ordinary massive particle. For a simple operator, such as $\mathrm{Tr}[F_{\mu\nu}F^{\mu\nu}]$, the state created at zero coupling with a given 4-momentum is a pair of gluons that sum up to the total 4-momentum. As we increase the coupling, we start to produce more and more gluons via a showering process. For these CFT states, we can specify the value of $k^2 = k_\mu k^\mu$ arbitrarily. In the CFT, we can view these as objects that have a position and, in addition, a size. The size is one more continuous variable that we need to specify to characterize the state. This is the reason why we need to give four continuous quantum numbers to specify a state in the four-dimensional CFT. These states are not particles in the CFT—they are particles in AdS. We can say that the size of the state in the CFT is related to the position along the radial direction in AdS; see Fig. 6.4. In the coordinates (6.3), the size is proportional to z. In fact, particles in AdS are a simple way to parametrize the representations of the conformal group. In other words, unitary representations of the conformal group correspond, through a one-to-one mapping, to particles, or fields, in AdS together with a boundary condition. This is a completely general mathematical result. We saw this explicitly above for the case of a scalar field. A representation is characterized by the value of the scaling dimension, which in turn determines the mass of the field.

Now, if this is so general, why don't all theories have gravity duals? Well, to some extent, we can say that they all do. However, the gravity dual could be a strongly coupled theory in the bulk. Large-N theories give weakly coupled string duals.

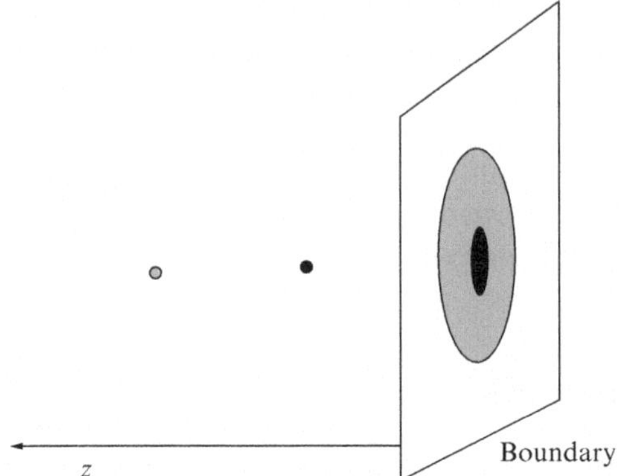

Fig. 6.4 The size/radius correspondence. In the CFT, we have excitations that have a size. We see the same object with two different sizes, related by a dilatation. They correspond to two particles with the same proper size in *AdS* but located at different values of the radial position of *AdS*.

However, they can be highly stringy. We need some additional conditions that ensure an approximate locality of the interactions in the bulk. In particular, we need locality within an *AdS* radius. A necessary condition is that all the higher-spin fields have large anomalous dimensions. It might be that this is a sufficient condition, but it has not been clearly demonstrated from the axioms of CFTs—although, of course, it is expected to hold if we assume bulk locality.

Even though we have focused here on CFTs, the gauge/gravity duality is also valid for nonconformal theories [22–24]. In these cases, the metric has the form $ds^2 = w(z)^2(dx^2 + dz^2)$. As in the conformal case, w increases rapidly when we

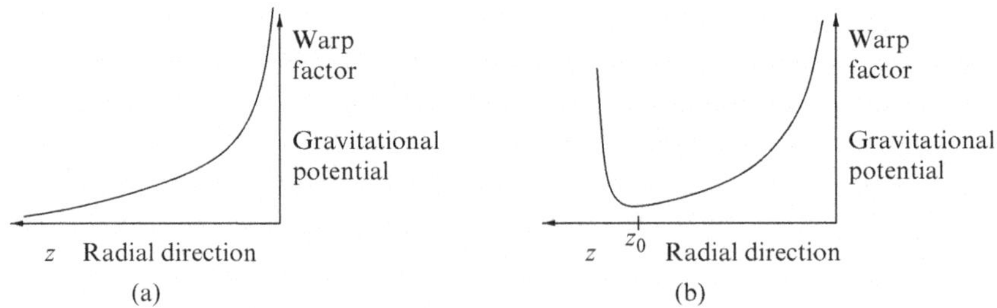

Fig. 6.5 (a) The behavior of the warp factor, or gravitational potential in the *AdS* case. It rises to infinity at the boundary and goes to zero toward the interior. A particle is pushed toward ever larger values of z. In the field theory, this corresponds to an excitation expanding in size. (b) Warp factor in a theory with a mass gap. The warp factor has a minimum, and excitations minimize their energy by sitting at z_0. Typically, the space ends, in smoothly, at $z = z_0$. In the dual field theory, excitations have a preferred size, like the size of a proton in QCD.

approach the boundary. In these cases, the size is also related to the z direction. However, since we do not have a precise scaling symmetry, the physical behavior of boundary objects of different sizes is different. The same happens in the bulk: particles at different positions in the z direction see a geometry with different properties. In some cases, the geometric description fails for small or large z. In particular, this happens when the gauge theory coupling becomes weak in the ultraviolet or infrared [22]. In such cases, the gravity description is a good approximation only for distance (or energy) scales such that the gauge theory coupling is large. One can consider quantum field theories with a mass gap. The corresponding gravity configurations are such that the warp factor has a minimum value at some position z_0. In several cases, one finds that the space ends at z_0 because some other dimensions (similar to the S^5 above) are shrinking smoothly at $z = z_0$. A massive particle minimizes its energy by sitting at z_0. Of course, its wavefunction is concentrated around z_0; see Fig. 6.5. The precise shape of the warp factor has to be computed by solving the bulk equations.

Acknowledgments

I thank G. Horowitz for comments on the draft. This work was supported in part by U.S. Department of Energy Grant DE-FG02-90ER40542.

References

[1] J. M. Maldacena, Adv. Theor. Math. Phys. **2**, 231–252 (1998) [arXiv:hep-th/9711200].

[2] S. S. Gubser, I. R. Klebanov, A. M. Polyakov, Phys. Lett. **B428**, 105–114 (1998) [arXiv:hep-th/9802109].

[3] E. Witten, Adv. Theor. Math. Phys. **2**, 253–291 (1998) [arXiv:hep-th/9802150].

[4] G. 't Hooft, Nucl. Phys. **B72**, 461 (1974).

[5] P. Breitenlohner, D. Z. Freedman, Phys. Lett. **B115**, 197 (1982).

[6] I. R. Klebanov, E. Witten, Nucl. Phys. **B556**, 89–114 (1999) arXiv:hep-th/9905104.

[7] D. Z. Freedman, S. D. Mathur, A. Matusis, L. Rastelli, Nucl. Phys. **B546**, 96–118 (1999) [arXiv:hep-th/9804058].

[8] M. B. Green, J. H. Schwarz, L. Brink, Nucl. Phys. **B198**, 474–492 (1982).

[9] J. H. Schwarz, Nucl. Phys. **B226**, 269 (1983).

[10] J. Polchinski, S. Chaudhuri, C. V. Johnson, [arXiv:hep-th/9602052].

[11] S. S. Gubser, I. R. Klebanov, A. W. Peet, Phys. Rev. **D54**, 3915–3919 (1996) [arXiv:hep-th/9602135].

[12] S. S. Gubser, I. R. Klebanov, A. A. Tseytlin, Nucl. Phys. **B534**, 202–222 (1998) [arXiv:hep-th/9805156].

[13] A. Fotopoulos, T. R. Taylor, Phys. Rev. **D59**, 061701 (1999) [arXiv:hep-th/9811224].

[14] O. Aharony, O. Bergman, D. L. Jafferis, J. Maldacena, JHEP **0810**, 091 (2008) [arXiv:0806.1218 [hep-th]].

[15] N. Drukker, M. Marino, P. Putrov, Commun. Math. Phys. **306**, 511–563 (2011) [arXiv:1007.3837 [hep-th]].

[16] V. Pestun, Commun. Math. Phys. **313**, 71–129 (2012) [arXiv:0712.2824 [hep-th]].

[17] G. T. Horowitz, A. Strominger, Nucl. Phys. **B360**, 197–209 (1991).

[18] J. Polchinski, Phys. Rev. Lett. **75**, 4724–4727 (1995) [arXiv:hep-th/9510017].

[19] N. Beisert et al., Lett. Math. Phys. **99**, 3 (2012) [arXiv:1012.3982 [hep-th]].

[20] N. Gromov, V. Kazakov, P. Vieira, Phys. Rev. Lett. **104**, 211601 (2010) [arXiv:0906.4240 [hep-th]].

[21] J. Polchinski, "String Theory, Vol.I," Cambridge University Press, Cambridge (1998).

[22] N. Itzhaki, J. M. Maldacena, J. Sonnenschein, S. Yankielowicz, Phys. Rev. **D58**, 046004 (1998) [arXiv:hep-th/9802042].

[23] E. Witten, Adv. Theor. Math. Phys. **2**, 505–532 (1998) [arXiv:hep-th/9803131].

[24] I. R. Klebanov, M. J. Strassler, JHEP **0008**, 052 (2000) [arXiv:hep-th/0007191 [hep-th]].

7
Introduction to the AdS/CFT correspondence

Jan de BOER

Institute for Theoretical Physics, University of Amsterdam,
Amsterdam, The Netherlands

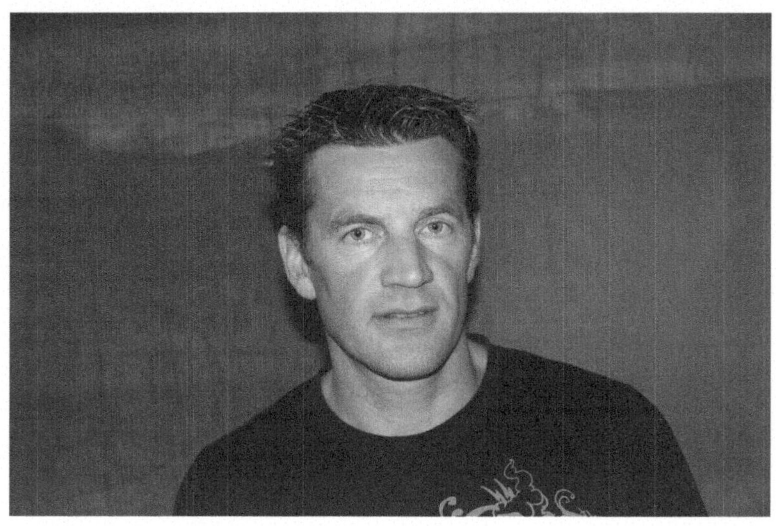

Theoretical Physics to Face the Challenge of LHC. Edited by L. Baulieu, K. Benakli, M. R. Douglas,
B. Mansoulié, E. Rabinovici, and L. F. Cugliandolo. © Oxford University Press 2015.
Published in 2015 by Oxford University Press.

Chapter Contents

7.1 About this chapter

The AdS/CFT correspondence, one of the most exciting discoveries in theoretical physics of the past 15 years, provides a framework to study strongly coupled field theories using weakly coupled gravity, and at the same time gives us a nonperturbative definition of quantum gravity in anti-de Sitter space. A huge number of papers have been written, on the subject, and one can only scratch the surface of the field in an introductory chapter like this. Moreover, this chapter will not give a comprehensive self-contained overview of the material that was covered in the lectures at the Summer School. Rather, it is intended as a summary of the main points, together with some pointers to the literature.

A long list of reviews has been compiled on the String Theory Wiki at ⟨http://www.stringwiki.org/w/index.php?title=The_AdS/CFT_correspondence⟩.

7.2 Introduction

The AdS/CFT correspondence is one of the most significant results that string theory has produced. It refers to the existence of amazing dualities between theories with gravity and theories without gravity, and is also sometimes referred to as the gauge theory/gravity correspondence. The prototype example of such a correspondence, as originally conjectured by Maldacena [1], is the exact equivalence between type IIB string theory compactified on $AdS_5 \times S^5$ and four-dimensional $\mathcal{N} = 4$ supersymmetric Yang-Mills theory. The notation AdS_5 refers to an anti-de Sitter space in five dimensions, and S^5 refers to a five-dimensional sphere. Anti-de Sitter spaces are maximally symmetric solutions of the Einstein equations with a negative cosmological constant. The large symmetry group of five-dimensional anti-de Sitter space matches precisely with the group of conformal symmetries of the $\mathcal{N} = 4$ super Yang–Mills theory, which has long been known to be conformally invariant. The term "AdS/CFT correspondence" has its origin in this particular example, CFT being an abbreviation for conformal field theory. Since then, many other examples of gauge theory/gravity dualities have been found, including ones where string theory is not compactified on an anti-de Sitter space and where the dual field theory is not conformal. Nevertheless, all these dualities are often still referred to as examples of the AdS/CFT correspondence.

At first sight, it is quite startling that a duality between a theory with gravity and a theory without gravity could exist. But what is a consistent theory of gravity anyway? String theory provides a consistent framework to compute finite quantum corrections to classical general relativity, but the full nonperturbative structure of string theory is not very well understood. The AdS/CFT correspondence relates a theory with gravity in d dimensions to a local field theory without gravity in $d - 1$ dimensions. If true, it implies that actual quantum degrees of freedom of gravity cannot resemble the degrees of freedom of a local field theory defined on the same space. That this has to be true follows, among other things, from the existence of black holes, as we briefly review in Section 7.3. If the degrees of freedom in gravity were local, then one could imagine the possibility of arbitrarily large volumes with fixed energy density. However, we know that already in classical gravity this is not true: a fixed energy density in a sufficiently large volume will collapse into a black hole.

In fact, hints of the existence of gauge theory/gravity duality have been around for quite some time, most notably in the case of three dimensions.[1] Gravity in three dimensions can, modulo various subtleties, be described by a Chern–Simons theory [2, 3]. Chern–Simons theory is a topological field theory and when put on a manifold with a boundary reduces to a $(1 + 1)$-dimensional field theory on the boundary [4, 5]. For compact gauge groups, a precise relation between Hilbert spaces and correlation functions can be established. For noncompact gauge groups such as those relevant for $(2 + 1)$-dimensional gravity, there is still an equivalence at the level of the actions, but the precise map between Hilbert spaces and correlation functions is not quite as well understood. Nevertheless, the duality between Chern–Simons theory and two-dimensional conformal field theory has many features in common with the AdS/CFT duality.

It is very hard to directly prove the equivalence between type IIB string theory on $AdS_5 \times S^5$ and four-dimensional $\mathcal{N} = 4$ super Yang–Mills theory. For one thing, as alluded to above, we do not have a good definition of nonperturbative type IIB string theory. Even at string tree level, we do not (yet) know how to solve the theory completely. From this perspective, perhaps a more appropriate perspective is to view $\mathcal{N} = 4$ super Yang–Mills theory as the definition of nonperturbative type IIB string theory on the $AdS_5 \times S^5$ background. This implies in particular that the nonperturbative quantum degrees of freedom of string theory do not resemble those it seems to contain at low energies.

A weaker form of the AdS/CFT correspondence is obtained by restricting to low energies on the string theory side. At low energies, type IIB string theory on $AdS_5 \times S^5$ reduces to type IIB supergravity on $AdS_5 \times S^5$. The corresponding limit on the gauge theory side is one where both N and $g_{\text{YM}}^2 N$ become large, where N is the rank of the $U(N)$ gauge group of the N $= 4$ supersymmetric gauge theory (note that N and $\mathcal{N}$ are different and should not be confused!) and g_{YM}^2 is the gauge coupling constant. The equivalence between type IIB supergravity on $AdS_5 \times S^5$ and $\mathcal{N} = 4$ gauge theory in the large-N, large-$g_{\text{YM}}^2 N$ limit has now been tested in incredibly many ways.

7.3 Why AdS/CFT?

The AdS/CFT correspondence is related to several ideas in physics.

The first idea comes from lattice gauge theory, which in the continuum limit is supposed to yield Yang–Mills theory. For more details, we refer to the book by Polyakov [6]. The basic variables are group-valued variables associated with all the links of a lattice, and the partition function looks roughly like

---

[1] In three or fewer dimensions, gravity has no local propagating degrees of freedom, so perhaps it is not a good example; still, it will turn out that this case has many similarities with the story in dimensions above three.

$$Z \sim \sum_{\{U_i\}} \exp\left[-\beta \sum_{\text{plaq}} \text{Tr}(U_1 U_2 U_3 U_4)\right],$$

where the sum is over all plaquettes (oriented squares in the lattice) and U_1, U_2, U_3, U_4 are the four group variables associated with the side of the square, in order. One can now examine this theory at strong coupling, i.e., small β. The dominant contributions, as follows from group theory, come from surfaces at whose edges one needs to put propagating quarks and antiquarks. A surface contributes $\sim \beta^A$ to the partition function, where A is the surface area. The dominant contributions are therefore minimal-area surfaces, exactly as in string theory.

Not only do we obtain a connection to string theory, but the strings are seen to correspond to $q\bar{q}$ fluxtubes and the area law corresponds to a linear confining potential for the fluxtube, i.e., confinement.

The second idea, namely, that large-N gauge theory might be equivalent to a string theory, is due to 't Hooft[7]. Suppose that one has a theory where the fundamental degrees of freedom M transform in the adjoint representation of a $U(N)$ gauge group, so that under a gauge transformation,

$$M \to U M U^{-1},$$

with $U \in U(N)$. A simple example of such a theory would be a matrix model with action

$$S \sim \frac{1}{g_{YM}^2} \int \text{Tr}\left[(\partial M)^2 + \sum_k c_k M^k\right].$$

The idea is now to study this matrix model in perturbation theory and to keep track of the powers of N that appear. As easy diagrammatic way to do this is to use so-called double-line notation, where a propagator is simply represented by two parallel lines. Each parallel line corresponds to one of the delta functions in

$$\langle M_j^i M_l^k \rangle \sim \delta_l^i \delta_j^k$$

and therefore represents a single index that takes values $1, \ldots, N$. Similarly, one can represent vertices as places where double lines meet each other and are glued together in a cyclic way.

With this double-line notation, the number of factors of N is easily determined, since it is the number of closed single lines in a diagram, because a closed single line represents a single index that is being summed over.

Moreover, it is a classic result of graph theory, basically dating back to Euler, that each double-line graph can be put on a Riemann surface in such a way that no lines cross each other. The genus h (i.e., the number of holes) of this Riemann surface is

$$2 - 2h = \#\text{loops} - \#\text{propagators} + \#\text{vertices}.$$

By reorganizing perturbation theory, keeping track of powers of N and of g_{YM}^2, one then discovers that the perturbative expansion of a large-N gauge theory in $1/N$ and $g_{\mathrm{YM}}^2 N$ can be organized as

$$Z = \sum_{h \geq 0} N^{2-2h} f_h(\lambda), \tag{7.1}$$

where $\lambda \equiv g_{\mathrm{YM}}^2 N$ is the so-called 't Hooft coupling. All of this is explained in detail in the original paper by 't Hooft [7]. This is similar to the loop expansion in string theory,

$$Z = \sum_{g \geq 0} g_s^{2g-2} Z_g, \tag{7.2}$$

with the string coupling g_s equal to $1/N$. Through some peculiar and not completely understood mechanism, Feynman diagrams of the gauge theory are turned into surfaces that represent interacting strings. Feynman diagrams represent skeletons of the Riemann surfaces, and the large-N limit seems to somehow close up the holes in the Riemann surface. A toy example of this phenomenon is discussed, for example, in [8]. Apparently, this is also somehow happening in the AdS/CFT correspondence.

A third important idea that something like AdS/CFT could exist is the invention of the concept of holography [9, 10]. This idea has its origin in the study of the thermodynamics of black holes. It was shown by Bekenstein and Hawking [11] that black holes can be viewed as thermodynamic systems with a temperature and an entropy. The temperature is directly related to the black body radiation emitted by the black hole, whereas the entropy is given by $S = A/4G$, with G the Newton constant and A the area of the horizon of the black hole. With these definitions, Einstein's equations of general relativity are consistent with the laws of thermodynamics. Since in statistical physics entropy is a measure of the number of degrees of freedom of a theory, it is rather surprising to see that the entropy of a black hole is proportional to the area of the horizon. If gravity behaved like a local field theory, one would expect an entropy proportional to the volume. A consistent picture is reached if gravity in d dimensions is somehow equivalent to a local field theory in $d-1$ dimensions. Both have an entropy proportional to the area in d dimensions, which is the same as the volume in $d-1$ dimensions. The analogy between this situation and a hologram, which stores all the information about a three-dimensional object in a two-dimensional picture, led to the use of the name holography in this context. The AdS/CFT correspondence is holographic because it states that quantum gravity in five dimensions (forgetting the compact 5-sphere) is equivalent to a local field theory in four dimensions.

A fourth, incredibly sketchy, idea is the observation that the renormalization group equations in quantum field theory are local equations. Suppose we consider a family of quantum field theories parametrized by an ultraviolet cutoff z. Theories whose cutoffs do not differ too much are quite similar to each other, so one could imagine interpreting z as an extra coordinate and the renormalization group equations as the equations that provide the dynamics in this extra direction. However, this theory with one extra dimension cannot be an ordinary field theory, since that would have too many degrees of freedom. However, as our discussion of the holographic principle shows, the theory with the one extra dimension could be gravitational.

Suppose that this extra theory is indeed gravitational and that the metric takes the form

$$ds^2 = f^2(z)\,dz^2 + g^2(z)(-dt^2 + dx^i\,dx^i). \tag{7.3}$$

This choice respects Poincaré invariance, but has some nontrivial dependence in the z direction. Assume that the coordinates x^i describe a finite volume V. To simplify the discussion, we will also assume the quantum field theory is a conformal field theory, i.e., that it is scale-invariant. Then the entropy of this field theory, with cutoff z_0, scales like $S \sim V z_0^{d-1}$. Let us compare this with the entropy of a black hole in the fiducial metric (7.3), which extends to z_0. That entropy would be proportional to the horizon area at radius z_0, which scales as $g(z_0)^{d-1}V$. This suggests that we should take $g(z) \sim z$. If $g(z) = z$, we see another feature of the metric (7.3), namely, that the second part of the metric is scale-invariant under $t \to \lambda t, x^i \to \lambda x^i, z \to \lambda^{-1}z$, which is precisely how these quantities should scale in a conformal field theory. To make the full metric invariant under this rescaling, we need to choose $f(z) \sim 1/z$. This then finally leads to the metric

$$ds^2 = \frac{dz^2}{z^2} + z^2(-dt^2 + dx^i\,dx^i). \tag{7.4}$$

which happens to be precisely the metric for AdS_{d+1}.

The above is of course not meant as a serious derivation of AdS/CFT, but rather should be viewed as a heuristic motivation.

Many of the arguments above do not rely on conformal invariance and apply to more general quantum field theories, and one may therefore wonder how crucial conformal invariance is. The AdS/CFT correspondence has meanwhile been extended to various other theories, but it appears that generic quantum field theories cannot have a weakly coupled gravitational dual, and even generic scale-invariant quantum field theories will not have weakly coupled gravitational duals. A nice discussion of the very special features that quantum field theories need to have in order to have a weakly coupled gravitational dual can be found in [12].

7.4 Anti-de Sitter space

To describe the correspondence in some more detail, we first need to describe the geometry of anti-de Sitter space in some more detail. Five-dimensional anti-de Sitter space AdS_5 can be described as the five-dimensional manifold

$$-X_0^2 - X_1^2 + X_2^2 + X_3^2 + X_4^2 + X_5^2 = L^2 \tag{7.5}$$

embedded in a six-dimensional space with metric

$$ds^2 = -dX_0^2 - dX_1^2 + dX_2^2 + dX_3^2 + dX_4^2 + dX_5^2.$$

From this way of writing the metric, it is clear that the isometry group of AdS_5 is $SO(2,4)$, which is exactly the conformal group in $3 + 1$ dimensions. By picking a particular parametrization of the solutions of (7.5) in terms of five coordinates, we obtain the metric

$$ds^2 = L^2 \left[dr^2 + e^{2r} (\eta_{\mu\nu} dx^\mu \, dx^\nu) \right]. \tag{7.6}$$

This is exactly the metric we saw before in (7.4), but with z replaced by e^r. The parameter L is just a scale factor. The limit where the radial coordinate r goes to infinity and the exponential factor blows up is called the boundary of anti-de Sitter space. This boundary is the place where the dual field theory lives. One can indeed verify that string theory excitations in anti-de Sitter space extend all the way to the boundary [13]. In this way, one obtains a map from string theory states to states in the field theory living on the boundary. We see that e^r sets the scale of the Minkowski part of the metric, and it turns out that e^r can quite literally also be viewed as a scale of the dual field theory (see, e.g., [14]).

The metric (7.6) is often called planar AdS_5 or Poincaré AdS_5. One can verify that it is geodesically incomplete and does not cover all of (7.5). One can find a different set of coordinates that yields the metric

$$ds^2 = \frac{dr^2}{1 + r^2} - (1 + r^2) \, dt^2 + r^2 \, d\Omega_3^2. \tag{7.7}$$

This metric is called global AdS_5, and it is geodesically complete.

There is an important difference between planar and global AdS_5. The first is dual to a conformal field theory on a plane and the second to a conformal field theory that lives on a "cylinder" $S^3 \times \mathbb{R}$. The most striking difference between the two is that the Hamiltonian for the cylinder has a discrete spectrum, whereas the Hamiltonian for the plane has a continuous spectrum.

To see this in more detail, we notice that the Euclidean cylinder and the Euclidean plane are conformally equivalent to each other:

$$d\tau^2 + d\Omega_3^2 = \frac{1}{u^2} (du^2 + u^2 \, d\Omega_3^2), \tag{7.8}$$

with $\tau = \log u$. Thus, time translations $\tau \to \tau + \text{const}$ act on the plane as rescalings: the Hamiltonian on the cylinder is the same as the dilatation operator on the plane. Because of this, we very often use the eigenvalues of the dilatation operator (called anomalous dimensions) to characterize states and operators on the plane rather than the Hamiltonian on the plane itself.

Another way to see that the spectrum of the Hamiltonian on the plane is continuous is that, by scale invariance, any eigenstate with energy E can be mapped to a different state with energy $\lambda^{-1}E$ by simply rescaling $x^\mu \to \lambda x^\mu$.

7.5 Correlation functions

The AdS/CFT correspondence in the form in which it was proposed in [1] did not yet provide a detailed map between AdS and CFT quantities. Such a map was given in [15, 16] and makes the correspondence much more explicit. To describe it, we first consider the AdS side, and, in particular, we consider a free field with mass m propagating in anti-de Sitter space. The field equation

$$(\Box + m^2)\phi = 0 \tag{7.9}$$

has two linearly independent solutions that behave respectively as

$$e^{-\Delta r} \text{ and } e^{(\Delta - 4)r} \tag{7.10}$$

as $r \to \infty$, where

$$\Delta(\Delta - 4) = m^2. \tag{7.11}$$

Consider now a solution of the supergravity equations of motion with the boundary condition that the fields behave near $r = \infty$ as

$$\phi_i(r, x^\mu) \sim \phi_i^0(r, x^\mu)e^{(\Delta - 4)r}. \tag{7.12}$$

Then the map between AdS and CFT quantities is given by

$$\exp[-\Gamma_{\text{sugra}}(\phi_i)] = \left\langle \exp\left(\int d^4x\, \phi_i^0 O_i \right) \right\rangle, \tag{7.13}$$

where the left-hand side is the supergravity action evaluated on the classical solution given by ϕ_i, and the right-hand side is a generating function for correlation functions in super Yang–Mills theory. Actually, we should really use the full string theory partition function subject to the relevant boundary conditions on the left-hand side, to which the supergravity approximation is only the saddle-point approximation. However, for many applications, the above formula suffices. We also see that there should be an operator O_i in Yang–Mills theory for every field ϕ_i in anti-de Sitter spaces. With some further work, one can show that this operator needs to have conformal dimension Δ_i. Finally, note that we restricted attention to scalar fields in (7.13). The full AdS/CFT correspondence should of course involve all the AdS degrees of freedom, not just the scalar ones. As one can see, to compute a two-point function, one needs to know the Green function of a field in anti-de Sitter space. For a scalar field, the Green function $G(x, y)$ is a function of one variable $d(x, y)$ only, since there is only one $SO(2, 4)$-invariant function that can be made from two coordinates in AdS_5. The resulting Green function is of hypergeometric type and can be solved explicitly; see, e.g., [21] for a detailed discussion. It simplifies dramatically if one of the two points is taken to the boundary of AdS_5: if we choose coordinates on planar AdS_5 of the type

$$ds^2 = \frac{1}{z^2}(dz^2 + \eta_{\mu\nu}\, dx^\mu\, dx^\nu), \tag{7.14}$$

where the boundary is at $z = 0$, then the Green function looks like

$$G(z_1, x_1; z_2, x_2) \sim \left[\frac{(z_2 - z_1)^2 + (x_2 - x_1)^2}{z_1 z_2} \right]^{-\Delta}, \tag{7.15}$$

which is the so-called bulk-boundary propagator [15]. If we take both points to the boundary and strip off some powers of z_1 and z_2, we recognize in (7.15) the two-point function of two operators of conformal weight Δ:

$$\langle O(x_1) O(x_2) \rangle \sim \frac{1}{|x_1 - x_2|^{2\Delta}}. \tag{7.16}$$

We have obviously been quite sketchy; for a more detailed derivation of this two-point function, we refer to the literature.

7.6 Mapping between parameters

To illustrate the fact that the AdS/CFT duality is an example of a strong/weak-coupling duality, we give the relations between the parameters of both theories.

String theory on $AdS_5 \times S^5$ has a dimensionless string coupling constant g_s, which measures the string interaction strength relevant for string splitting and joining, a dimensionful string length l_s, which sets the size of fluctuations of the string worldsheet, and another dimensionful parameter L, the radius of curvature of AdS_5 and S^5 that appears in (7.6).

Four-dimensional $\mathcal{N} = 4$ super Yang–Mills theory with gauge group $U(N)$ has, beside the rank N of the gauge group, a dimensionless coupling constant g_{YM}^2.

The identification of the parameters reads

$$g_s = g_{\mathrm{YM}}^2, \qquad (L/l_s)^4 = 4\pi g_{\mathrm{YM}}^2 N = 4\pi \lambda. \tag{7.17}$$

By comparing the expansions (7.1) and (7.2), we now see that the AdS/CFT correspondence is indeed an example of a weak/strong-coupling duality. Depending on the choice of parameters, either the AdS theory or the CFT provides a weakly coupled description of the system, but never both at the same time. Gauge theory is a good description for small $g_{\mathrm{YM}}^2 N$ and small g_{YM}^2, whereas string theory is good for large $g_{\mathrm{YM}}^2 N$ and small g_{YM}^2. Therefore, the AdS/CFT correspondence can be applied in two directions. We can use string theory to learn about gauge theory, and we can use gauge theory to learn about string theory.

7.7 Derivation of the AdS/CFT correspondence

The derivation of the AdS/CFT correspondence given in [1] crucially involves the notion of D-branes. D-branes are certain extended objects in string theory that were introduced by Polchinski [17]. They are labeled by the number of dimensions of the object, so that a D0-brane is like a particle, a D1-brane is like a string, a D2-brane is like a membrane, etc. There are two ways to think about D-branes. On the one hand, they are solitonic solutions of the equations of motion of low-energy closed string theory. On the other hand, they are objects in open string theory with the property that open strings can end on them. Open strings have a finite tension, and their center of mass cannot be taken arbitrarily far away from the D-brane. As a consequence, the degrees of freedom of the open string can effectively only propagate in a direction parallel to the brane: one says that they are confined to the brane, or that they live on the brane. The open string spectrum can be reproduced directly from the soliton in the closed string description via a collective coordinate quantization.

As a very crude analogy, one can think about two ways to describe a monopole. On the one hand, one can think of it as the 't Hooft–Polyakov monopole, in which case it is an extended soliton solution of the Yang–Mills–Higgs equations of motion. On the other hand, one can view a monopole as a point particle on which magnetic field lines can end. Both descriptions have their advantages, as do the open and closed string descriptions of D-branes.

To derive the AdS/CFT correspondence, one starts with a stack of N D3-branes. This has a description in terms both of open and of closed strings. Next, one takes a suitable low-energy limit of the system, which involves taking $l_s \to 0$. The open string description reduces to $\mathcal{N} = 4\, U(N)$ super Yang–Mills theory, whereas the closed string description reduces to string theory on $AdS_5 \times S^5$. Thus, the AdS/CFT duality arises as a consequence of the duality between open and closed strings. This duality is most easily visualized by thinking of a cylinder. It can be viewed either as the worldsheet of a closed string moving along an interval or, equivalently, as an open string moving along a circle.

Although the above description may sound fairly simple, there are various subtleties in taking the low-energy limit. The closed string description of N D3-branes that extend along the 0123 direction and that are located at $r = 0$ in the remaining 456789 directions with r the radial variable of six-dimensional spherical coordinates reads

$$H^{-1/2}(-dt^2 + dx^i\, dx^i) + H^{1/2}(dr^2 + r^2\, d\Omega_5^2), \tag{7.18}$$

where

$$H = 1 + \frac{4\pi g_s N \ell_s^4}{r^4}. \tag{7.19}$$

The low-energy limit, at the operational level, amounts to simply removing the constant term in H, yielding $AdS_5 \times S^5$.

What is perhaps rather peculiar is that the branes with which we started out were located at $r = 0$. After taking the decoupling limit, however, we often think of the gauge theory as living at $r = \infty$ instead—at least, this is where we insert delta-function sources in order to compute correlation functions of local operators. In the original D-brane description, we computed correlation functions of local operators by inserting sources at $r = 0$ instead—so how does the field theory move from $r = 0$ to $r = \infty$?

It is difficult to explain this in detail here, but if we study scattering of waves in the background (7.18) by solving free field equations, we find that those waves experience an effective potential that has a sharp peak whose distance from the brane is proportional to the frequency ω, while the height is proportional to ω^{-4} [18]. It is the region between the potential barrier and the D-branes that becomes AdS_5. From a closed string, S-matrix point of view, it is more natural to impose boundary conditions somewhere on the barrier as opposed to $r = 0$, and this is why one eventually ends up with delta-function boundary conditions at $r = \infty$. I am not aware of a place in the literature where this is spelled out in great detail, and it could be an interesting exercise to do so.

7.8 Tests of the AdS/CFT correspondence

7.8.1 Spectrum of operators

In order for (7.13) to hold, there should for every gauge-invariant operator in the gauge theory exist a corresponding closed string field on $AdS_5 \times S^5$, whose mass is related to the scaling dimension of the operator according to (7.11).

It is difficult to test this statement in full generality, because we don't know the spectrum of super Yang–Mills theory at strong coupling, nor do we know the string spectrum at strong coupling. However, we do know the spectrum of a subset of the operators of super Yang–Mills theory at strong coupling, namely, the so-called BPS operators.

BPS operators O have the property that the corresponding state $|\psi\rangle = O|0\rangle$ is annihilated by some Hermitian supersymmetry generator Q, which satisfies $Q^2 = \Delta + J$, with J some $U(1)$ generator.[2] If a state $|\psi\rangle$ is annihilated by Q, it obeys

$$0 = |Q|\psi\rangle|^2 = (\Delta + J)||\psi\rangle|^2, \tag{7.20}$$

and therefore $\Delta = -J$. The eigenvalues of J are quantized, and therefore, as long as there is no phase transition at finite coupling constant, the weak- and strong-coupling values of Δ have to be identical.

In 10-dimensional string theory, there are massless and massive fields. The dimensions of the operators corresponding to massive fields scale as $(L/l_s) \sim (g_{\mathrm{YM}}^2 N)^{1/4}$, and vary continuously with the Yang–Mills coupling constant. Such operators therefore cannot be BPS, and it is difficult to compare them with operators in the gauge theory.

Massless fields, on the other hand, have scaling dimensions that are independent of $g_{\mathrm{YM}}^2 N$, and these should therefore correspond to BPS operators. It has been verified [15] that there is indeed a precise match between massless fields in string theory and BPS operators in the gauge theory. A first necessary condition for such a matching to be possible is that the global symmetries match. The space $AdS_5 \times S^5$ has isometry group $SO(2,4) \times SO(6)$, whereas $\mathcal{N} = 4$ super Yang–Mills theory is invariant under the conformal group $SO(2,4)$ and the R-symmetry group $SO(6)$. The bosonic global symmetries therefore do indeed agree. In addition, there are fermionic symmetries

---

[2] The reason why Δ appears is that the Hamiltonian of a conformal field theory has a continuous spectrum when quantized on $\mathbb{R}^4$, but on a cylinder $S^3 \times \mathbb{R}$ it has a discrete spectrum, with eigenvalues given by Δ.

that also agree, and, together with the bosonic symmetries, these form the supergroup $PSU(2,2|4)$. One can verify directly that the massless fields in string theory fall in the same multiplets of $PSU(2,2|4)$ as the BPS operators of super Yang–Mills theory.

A lot of progress has been made in studying the spectrum of operators in $\mathcal{N} = 4$ super Yang–Mills theory for large N but finite values of the 't Hooft coupling. The anomalous dimension operator appears to be one of an infinite series of conserved charges that the theory possesses. In other words, the theory at large N appears to be integrable. An impressive amount of work has been done in order to explore the integrability in detail (see, e.g., [19] for an extensive review). So far, all results that have been obtained strongly support the validity of the AdS/CFT correspondence for large N.

7.8.2 Correlation functions

Correlation functions have been considered in great detail (see e.g. [21] for a review of early work). The results are quite encouraging, although one has to face the same problem as when comparing the spectra of operators; namely, one can only compare quantities that can be computed in the field theory at strong coupling. This originally restricted one to the set of correlation functions that can be compared with those that satisfy nonrenormalization theorems in the field theory, so that the strong-coupling answer is a straightforward extrapolation of the weak-coupling answer. Such correlation functions have been compared with the string theory answer, so far always with success. In addition, the AdS/CFT correspondence has suggested new nonrenormalization theorems, some of which remain to be proven in field theory (but see, e.g., [20]), for extremal correlation functions of the form

$$\langle O_\Delta(x)O_{\Delta_1}(x_1)\ldots O_{\Delta_n}(x_n)\rangle, \tag{7.21}$$

where $\Delta = \sum_i \Delta_i$. More recently, the integrability that has been found, and that we mentioned above, has led to the computation of many more correlation functions for on-shell operators, in other words amplitudes. Once more, we refer the reader to the overview [19] for further details.

7.8.3 Wilson loops

Another interesting quantity to compare is the vacuum expectation value of a Wilson loop,

$$\left\langle \mathrm{Tr}\left(\mathrm{P}\exp\oint_C A_\mu dx^\mu\right)\right\rangle. \tag{7.22}$$

A Wilson loop in field theory can be expanded in terms of local operators, and, together with (7.13), one could in principle use this to determine which computation in supergravity (or string theory) one would have to do to compute this same expectation value. However, it turns out that the string theory calculation has a direct geometric interpretation [22, 23]. A Wilson loop is described by a string worldsheet in *AdS*, which extends all the way to the boundary of *AdS* and approaches there the curve C.

A classically stable string worldsheet is a minimal-area surface, so that the computation of the Wilson loop vacuum expectation value reduces to a minimal-area problem. For a rectangular Wilson loop, one can solve the minimal-area problem and in particular find the quark-quark energy as a function of their separation r:

$$E = -\frac{4\pi^2(2g_{\mathrm{YM}}^2 N)^{1/2}}{\Gamma(\frac{1}{4})^4 r}. \tag{7.23}$$

Interestingly, the 't Hooft coupling $g_{\mathrm{YM}}^2 N$ appears with a fractional power, and therefore this result cannot remain valid at weak coupling, where the answer will be qualitatively different. The result in (7.23) is an example of a nontrivial prediction of the AdS/CFT correspondence.

Wilson loops play a prominent role in computing amplitudes in $\mathcal{N} = 4$ super Yang–Mills theory as well, and are important in many aspects of the underlying integrable structure of the large-N theory. Once more, further details can be found in [19].

It is amusing to notice that the fundamental string in AdS is the same as the QCD string of Yang–Mills theory. In some sense, we have come a full circle toward the original motivation for string theory, namely, as an effective theory for the strong interactions.

7.8.4   Finite temperature

So far, the field theory, $\mathcal{N} = 4$ super Yang–Mills theory, has been a theory at zero temperature, and it has been obtained in the derivation of the AdS/CFT correspondence as the low-energy limit of the degrees of freedom associated with a stack of D3-branes. It turns out that this setup can be generalized to nonzero temperature by employing so-called near-extremal D3-branes. In particular, One can compute the free energy as a function of temperature, using either the field theory or the dual gravitational description. The results are

$$F_{\mathrm{sugra}} = -\frac{\pi^2}{8}N^2 V T^4, \qquad F_{\mathrm{SYM}} = -\frac{\pi^2}{6}N^2 V T^4. \tag{7.24}$$

There is no disagreement, since the first result is valid at strong coupling in the gauge theory and the second at weak coupling. As the coupling varies, one expects a smooth transition between these two results (for a discussion, see, e.g., [24]), but the possibility of a phase transition at a finite value of the coupling has not been ruled out completely.

More generally, we can directly consider a finite-temperature version of the AdS/CFT correspondence, by replacing the boundary geometry $\mathbb{R}^4$ in (7.6) by $S^3 \times S^1$, where the S^1 represents periodic imaginary time, so that the system is indeed at finite temperature [25]. The five-dimensional geometry that solves the string equations of motion and has this boundary is no longer anti-de Sitter space, but a space with a different metric. Actually, there are two different 5-manifolds with conformal boundary $S^3 \times S^1$. One is a finite-temperature version of Euclidean AdS and the other describes a Schwarzschild black hole in AdS.

The finite-temperature version of *AdS* dominates the supergravity path integral at low temperatures. In this geometry, the expectation value of the Wilson loop vanishes, and the center of the gauge group is unbroken, as in a confining phase.

The second solution has a nonzero expectation value for the Wilson loop, and the center is broken, as in a deconfining phase.

Altogether, this provides a tantalizing geometric picture of the confinement/deconfinement transition: it is mapped to a topology-changing process in gravity!

7.8.5   Glueballs and the string tension

So far, successful tests of AdS/CFT have relied heavily on supersymmetry in order to compare answers at weak and strong coupling. Of course, for more realistic applications, it is desirable to consider cases with less or no supersymmetry. One way to break supersymmetry is to consider supersymmetric Yang–Mills at finite temperature and take the $T \to \infty$ limit. Naively, the field theory reduces to some nonsupersymmetric extension of three-dimensional QCD. To test this, one can try to compute quantities in this version of AdS/CFT and compare them with lattice results in three-dimensional QCD. In particular, one can compute glueball masses using field equations in *AdS*, and string tensions using the Wilson loop.

There is considerable disagreement with lattice results. The string theory in question has many additional states with a mass of the order of $T \sim \Lambda_{\mathrm{QCD}}$, which is also the mass scale of the glueballs. At present, no controlled way to remove the cutoff and reach a weak-coupling limit has been found.

The string that appears in the AdS/CFT correspondence yields results that differ from the strong-coupling lattice results, and these in turn differ from the continuum lattice results. For a detailed overview, see [26]. The latter two are separated by a phase transition, but whether there are any such phase transitions in AdS/CFT remains an open problem.

7.9   More on finite temperature

Let us return to D3-branes at finite temperature and derive (7.24) in some more detail. The relevant geometry to describe D3-branes at finite temperature is very similar to that of a black hole, which also has a finite (Hawking) temperature. The usual Schwarzschild solution contains a factor $1 - 2MG/r$, with GM/r being simply the linearized Newton potential. Forces mediated by massless particles in dimension d give rise to a potential that scales like GM/r^{d-3}; it is a great exercise to obtain this qualitative behavior directly from the Feynman diagram for tree-level exchange of a massless particle. For a black hole in d dimensions, we therefore expect to find a factor $1 - 2MG/r^{d-3}$. Since D3-branes have 6 transverse dimensions they should behave like black holes in $6 + 1$ dimensions, and one expects a factor $1 - c/r^4$ for some c. Indeed, the metric for D3-branes at finite temperature, after taking the decoupling limit, reads

$$ds^2 = \frac{1}{z^2}\left[-f(z)dt^2 + dx^i\,dx^i + \frac{dz^2}{f(z)}\right],\tag{7.25}$$

with

$$f(z) = 1 - \frac{z^4}{z_0^4},\tag{7.26}$$

where z_0 is a free parameter related to the temperature of the D3-branes. To find the relation between z_0 and the temperature, we rotate the metric (7.25) to Euclidean signature and introduce a new coordinate $\rho = \sqrt{z_0 - z}$. This Euclidean metric near $\rho = 0$ looks exactly like the two-dimensional plane in polar coordinates, and it is exactly the two-dimensional plane if we make Euclidean time into a periodic variable. We leave it as an exercise to show that its period needs to be πz_0. Therefore, the temperature reads $T = 1/\pi z_0$.

We can now compute the entropy of finite-temperature D3-branes. According to the Bekenstein–Hawking entropy formula, this entropy (per unit area) is equal to

$$S = \frac{R^3}{4G_5 z_0^3},\tag{7.27}$$

where we have reinstated the radius of curvature $R = (4\pi g_s N \ell_s^4)^{1/4}$. In type IIB string theory, the 10-dimensional Newton constant $G_{10} = 8\pi^6 \ell_s^8 g_s^2$, but it is outside the scope of this chapter to review this. The five-dimensional Newton constant is then fixed by reducing the 10-dimensional theory over a 5-sphere of radius R, giving $G_5^{-1} = \pi^3 R^5 G_{10}^{-1}$, where we have used the fact that the volume of a unit 5-sphere is π^3. Putting in all the numbers, we find that the entropy density $S = \frac{1}{2}\pi^2 N^2 T^3$, and, using $dE = T\,dS$, we finally reproduce the energy density given above:

$$E = \frac{3\pi^2}{8} N^2 T^4.\tag{7.28}$$

The weakly coupled computation can be done as follows. Consider a free boson in a box of size L^3. According to standard statistical mechanics, the relevant partition function is

$$Z_B = \prod_{\vec{n}} \frac{1}{1 - e^{-\beta 2\pi|\vec{n}|/L}}.\tag{7.29}$$

The product is over vectors $\vec{n}$ with integer entries that parametrize the wavenumbers of the bosonic field in the box. We next take the log of this expression, write the log of the denominators as a Taylor series, and replace the sum over $\vec{n}$ by an integral since we are interested in the large-volume limit, to obtain

$$\beta F_B = -\frac{L^3}{(2\pi)^3}\int_0^\infty 4\pi n^2\,dn \sum_{l>0} \frac{e^{-\beta l n}}{l}.\tag{7.30}$$

This is easily evaluated using $\zeta(4) = \pi^4/90$, with the result

$$\beta F_B = -\frac{L^3}{\beta^3}\frac{\pi^2}{90}, \tag{7.31}$$

so that the energy $E = \partial_\beta(\beta F)$ becomes

$$E_B = \frac{\pi^2}{30}L^3 T^4. \tag{7.32}$$

For fermions, the result is the almost the same, except that an extra factor $(-1)^{l+1}$ appears on the right-hand side of (7.30), which reduces the result by a factor of 7/8. Now $\mathcal{N} = 4$ super Yang–Mills has $8N^2$ bosonic degrees of freedom: $6N^2$ from the six scalar fields in the adjoint of $U(N)$ and $2N^2$ from the physical polarizations of the $U(N)$ gauge field. Similarly, and by supersymmetry, there are $8N^2$ fermionic degrees of freedom. Including the factor of 7/8, the total energy is therefore equal to $15N^2$ times that of a single boson, and we get

$$E_{\text{free}} = \frac{\pi^2}{2}L^3 T^4. \tag{7.33}$$

The difference between (7.28) and (7.33) is a factor of 3/4, and, when converted into free energies, we recover (7.24).

7.10 Counting black hole entropy

There is a long history of trying to provide a microscopic interpretation of black hole entropy in string theory, starting with [27]. A very important example of such an interpretation is provided by the duality between AdS_3 and two-dimensional CFTs, which underlies the majority of microscopic entropy counting calculations that have been performed to date.

Black holes in AdS_3 are very simple; they look like

$$ds^2 = -(r^2 - M)\,dt^2 + \frac{dr^2}{r^2 - M} + r^2\,d\phi^2. \tag{7.34}$$

The Bekenstein–Hawking entropy of such a black hole is

$$S = \frac{2\pi\sqrt{M}}{4G_3}. \tag{7.35}$$

By AdS_3/CFT_2 duality, this black hole should be dual to a CFT at some finite temperature. As in the case of finite-temperature D3-branes, the temperature is readily obtained by examining the periodicity of imaginary time.

In the case of D3-branes discussed in Section 7.9, there was a mismatch of a factor of 3/4 when comparing the entropy of the weakly coupled field theory and that of the D3-brane system. What makes two-dimensional CFTs very special is that the behavior of the partition function at large temperature is universal and independent of whether the theory is at weak or strong coupling. One can understand this by considering the two-dimensional CFT on a 2-torus with circumferences β and L, which describes a two-dimensional CFT on a circle of size L at finite temperature β. The high-temperature limit is one where $\beta \ll L$. However, there is a priori nothing that tells us that one of the circles of the torus is Euclidean time and the other is space. We might as well interpret the circle of size L as time and the circle of size β as space. Moreover, by scale invariance, the theory will depend only on the ratio of these two quantities.

If we change the interpretation of the two circles, the same torus now describes the CFT—but at a very low temperature. At very low temperature, the theory is dominated by its ground state, and the partition function is easy to evaluate. This high–low temperature duality is also known as modular invariance, and is a very powerful feature of two-dimensional CFTs. The main subtlety in this computation is related to the fact that two-dimensional CFTs on the cylinder have a Casimir energy, which one needs to take into account. In any case, in this way one finds the famous Cardy formula, which states that as a function of the two scaling dimensions[3] Δ and $\bar{\Delta}$, the number of states grows as

$$S = 2\pi \sqrt{c\Delta/6} + 2\pi \sqrt{c\bar{\Delta}/6}, \tag{7.36}$$

where the only property of the entropy that appears is the central charge c, which is a measure of the number of degrees of freedom. Strikingly, this answer does not depend on any coupling constants.

If one translates the M and G_3 in (7.35) into c and $\Delta, \bar{\Delta}$, one finds perfect agreement with (7.36)! Although this computation may not appear to be very profound, the above is an amazing result and a very strong test of AdS/CFT on the one hand and the validity of the microscopic interpretation of the Bekenstein–Hawking entropy formula on the other.

7.11   Concluding remarks

In the past few years, we have seen many applications of AdS/CFT to strongly coupled problems such as QCD and various condensed matter systems. In such applications, we view AdS/CFT as a phenomenological tool that is supposed to address qualitative features only, since it is extremely unlikely that the CFTs that appear in AdS/CFT also appear in nature. For example, AdS/CFT works when the CFT has a very particular strong-coupling and large-N limit where only finitely many degrees of freedom survive at low energies—and systems in nature tend not to have a large N but rather $N = 1$ or $N = 3$ as in QCD.

Still, it is conceivable that some interesting features of strongly coupled systems are captured well by AdS/CFT. Consider, for example, QCD. There are of course many differences between QCD and $\mathcal{N} = 4$ Super Yang–Mills theory (SYM)

---

[3] In fact, $\Delta + \bar{\Delta}$ is the scaling dimension and also the energy as measured by the Hamiltonian on the cylinder, whereas $\Delta - \bar{\Delta}$ is a (half-)integer that measures the spin of the state.

1. QCD is not conformal, although it becomes approximately conformal at high T, whereas $\mathcal{N} = 4$ SYM is exactly conformal.
2. QCD confines below a critical temperature T_c, whereas $\mathcal{N} = 4$ SYM does not.
3. QCD breaks chiral symmetry below T_c, whereas $\mathcal{N} = 4$ SYM does not.
4. QCD does not have supersymmetry, whereas $\mathcal{N} = 4$ SYM does, although this is broken at finite T.
5. QCD is asymptically free, whereas $\mathcal{N} = 4$ SYM must be strongly coupled to be able to use gravity.
6. In QCD, $N = 3$, whereas in AdS/CFT N must be very large. However, various quantities may not depend strongly on N, so this need not be a major problem.
7. In QCD, $N_f \sim N_c$, whereas in $\mathcal{N} = 4$ SYM, we often can only study $N_f \ll N_c$.

There have been various attempts to construct gravity duals that are more realistic representations of QCD, including some that also exhibit confinement. These will not be discussed here, but we would like to mention one situation where AdS/CFT seems to capture some qualitative features of actual QCD dynamics, and where several of the differences we listed above are not that important, namely, a quark–gluon plasma of QCD. In a quark–gluon plasma, QCD is believed to be fairly strongly coupled, and lattice computations suggest that it is also approximately scale-invariant in this regime. This is therefore the regime where QCD looks as similar to a strongly coupled CFT as possible.

Are there interesting quantities that one can compute and compare? One such quantity is the ratio η/s of the shear viscosity divided by the entropy density. This is a quantity that describes a particular feature of a fluid. The term shear viscosity refers to the fact that if one has a fluid between two parallel plates, and keeps one plate at rest while moving the other plate, keeping the distance between the plates fixed, one experiences some resistance. This resistance is the shear viscosity and, as the name suggests it is related to dissipation.

Shear viscosity is one of the parameters that appears in the equations of fluid dynamics. It can be measured experimentally roughly as follows: at the relativistic heavy ion collider in Brookhaven, heavy ions such as gold are collided with each other, leading to production, for a short time, of a quark–gluon plasma. This plasma expands and cools, and eventually hadronizes. By measuring how many particles are emitted in each direction, one can reconstruct part of the time evolution of the plasma, and this turns out to be described well by the equations of fluid mechanics. In particular, one can measure the shear viscosity, which turns out to be a remarkably small number, $\eta/s \sim 0.1$. There is no known fluid for which this quantity is smaller, and the quark–gluon plasma is perhaps the most perfect fluid seen in nature.

One can also compute this quantity using AdS/CFT. According to standard results from linear response theory, the shear viscosity can be extracted from the two-point function of the stress tensor. This two-point function can be computed using standard AdS/CFT techniques, and surprisingly the result for η/s is determined only by the near-horizon physics of the black hole that is dual to the finite-temperature plasma. Moreover, the answer is independent of the details of the theory that lives in AdS and it is given by

$$\frac{\eta}{s} = \frac{1}{4\pi}.$$

(7.37)

This is very close to the number that is measured experimentally, strongly suggesting that finite-temperature $\mathcal{N} = 4$ SYM theory is in the same universality class as the quark–gluon plasma.

We refer the interested reader to [28] for a much more detailed discussion of applications of holography to QCD, and also to the relevant reviews listed on the String Theory Wiki mentioned in Section 7.1 for a discussion of applications to other areas of physics such as condensed matter theory.

Acknowledgments

I would like to thank the organizers of the Les Houches Summer School 2011 for giving me the opportunity to present these lectures and all participants for their enthusiastic participation.

References

[1] J. M. Maldacena, "The large N limit of superconformal field theories and supergravity," Adv. Theor. Math. Phys. **2**, 231 (1998) [Int. J. Theor. Phys. **38**, 1113 (1999)] [arXiv:hep-th/9711200].

[2] E. Witten, "(2+1)-dimensional gravity as an exactly soluble system," Nucl. Phys. B **311**, 46 (1988); "Topology changing amplitudes in (2+1)-dimensional gravity," Nucl. Phys. **B323**, 113 (1989).

[3] A. Achucarro and P. K. Townsend, "A Chern–Simons action for three-dimensional anti-de Sitter supergravity theories," Phys. Lett. **B180**, 89 (1986).

[4] E. Witten, "Quantum field theory and the Jones polynomial," Commun. Math. Phys. **121**, 351 (1989).

[5] S. Elitzur, G. W. Moore, A. Schwimmer, and N. Seiberg, "Remarks on the canonical quantization of the Chern–Simons–Witten theory," Nucl. Phys. **B326**, 108 (1989).

[6] A. M. Polyakov, "Gauge Fields And Strings," Harwood, Chur (1987).

[7] G. 't Hooft, "A planar diagram theory for strong interactions," Nucl. Phys. **B72**, 461 (1974).

[8] H. Ooguri and C. Vafa, "Worldsheet derivation of a large N duality," Nucl. Phys. **B641**, 3 (2002) [arXiv:hep-th/0205297].

[9] G. 't Hooft, "Dimensional reduction in quantum gravity," arXiv:gr-qc/9310026.

[10] L. Susskind, "The world as a hologram," J. Math. Phys. **36**, 6377 (1995) [arXiv:hep-th/9409089].

[11] J. Bekenstein, *"Black Holes And Entropy,"* Phys. Rev. **D7**, 2333 (1973); *"Generalized Second Law of Thermodynamics in black hole physics,"* Phys. Rev. **D9**, 3293 (1974); S. W. Hawking, "Black Holes And Thermodynamics," Phys. Rev. **D13**, 191 (1976).

[12] S. El-Showk and K. Papadodimas, "Emergent spacetime and holographic CFTs," JHEP **1210**, 106 (2012) [arXiv:1101.4163 [hep-th]].

[13] J. de Boer, H. Ooguri, H. Robins, and J. Tannenhauser, "String theory on AdS_3," JHEP **9812**, 026 (1998) [arXiv:hep-th/9812046].

[14] L. Susskind and E. Witten, "The holographic bound in anti-de Sitter space," [arXiv:hep-th/9805114].

[15] E. Witten, "Anti-de Sitter space and holography," Adv. Theor. Math. Phys. **2**, 253 (1998) [arXiv:hep-th/9802150].

[16] S. S. Gubser, I. R. Klebanov and A. M. Polyakov, "Gauge theory correlators from non-critical string theory," Phys. Lett. **B428**, 105 (1998) [arXiv:hep-th/9802109].

[17] J. Polchinski, "Dirichlet-branes and Ramond–Ramond charges," Phys. Rev. Lett. **75**, 4724 (1995) [arXiv:hep-th/9510017].

[18] I. R. Klebanov, "World volume approach to absorption by nondilatonic branes," Nucl. Phys. **B496**, 231 (1997) [arXiv:hep-th/9702076].

[19] N. Beisert et al., "Review of AdS/CFT integrability: an overview," Lett. Math. Phys. **99**, 3 (2012) [arXiv:1012.3982 [hep-th]].

[20] M. Baggio, J. de Boer, and K. Papadodimas, "A non-renormalization theorem for chiral primary 3-point functions," JHEP **1207**, 137 (2012) [arXiv:1203.1036 [hep-th]].

[21] E. D'Hoker and D. Z. Freedman, "Supersymmetric gauge theories and the AdS/CFT correspondence," arXiv:hep-th/0201253.

[22] S. J. Rey and J. Yee, "Macroscopic strings as heavy quarks in large N gauge theory and anti-de Sitter supergravity," Eur. Phys. J. **C22**, 379 (2001) [arXiv:hep-th/9803001].

[23] J. M. Maldacena, "Wilson loops in large N field theories," Phys. Rev. Lett. **80**, 4859 (1998) [arXiv:hep-th/9803002].

[24] I. R. Klebanov, "TASI Lectures: Introduction to the AdS/CFT Correspondence," arXiv:hep-th/0009139.

[25] E. Witten, "Anti-de Sitter space, thermal phase transition, and confinement in gauge theories," Adv. Theor. Math. Phys. **2**, 505 (1998) [arXiv:hep-th/9803131].

[26] M. Caselle, "Lattice gauge theories and the AdS/CFT correspondence," Int. J. Mod. Phys. **A15**, 3901 (2000) [arXiv:hep-th/0003119].

[27] A. Strominger and C. Vafa, "Microscopic origin of the Bekenstein–Hawking entropy," Phys. Lett. **B379**, 99 (1996) [arXiv:hep-th/9601029].

[28] J. Casalderrey-Solana, H. Liu, D. Mateos, K. Rajagopal, and U. A. Wiedemann, "Gauge/String Duality, Hot QCD and Heavy Ion Collisions," Cambridge University Press, Cambridge (2014); an earlier, shorter version of this book is available at arXiv:1101.0618 [hep-th].

8
Hydrodynamics and black holes

Yaron Oz

Raymond and Beverly Sackler Faculty of Exact Sciences
School of Physics and Astronomy,
Tel-Aviv University, Ramat-Aviv, Israel

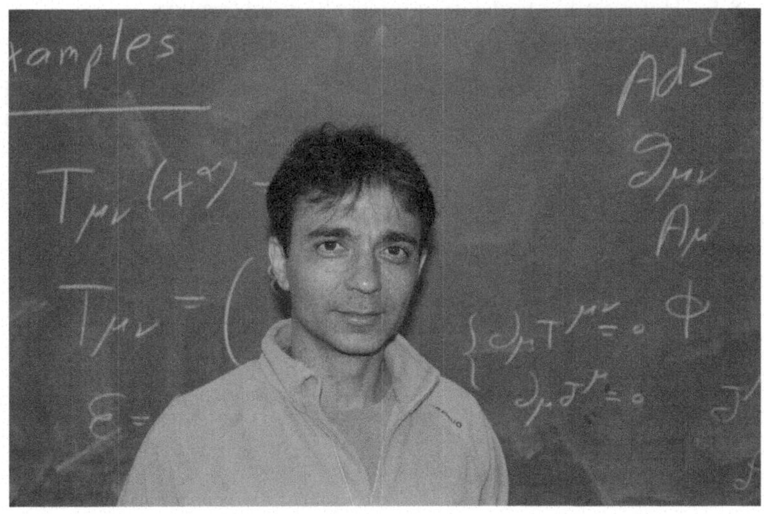

Theoretical Physics to Face the Challenge of LHC. Edited by L. Baulieu, K. Benakli, M. R. Douglas,
B. Mansoulié, E. Rabinovici, and L. F. Cugliandolo. © Oxford University Press 2015.
Published in 2015 by Oxford University Press.

Chapter Contents

8.1   Introduction

According to the Holographic Principle [1], the degrees of freedom of a quantum theory of gravity in a volume of space V are encoded on its boundary A. Thus, the Holographic Principle relates quantum gravity in $d + 1$ spacetime dimensions to quantum field theory without gravity in one lower space dimension. The quantum field theory at the boundary is not necessarily local. In the framework of the AdS/CFT correspondence [2, 3], the quantum theory of gravity is superstring (M-) theory on asymptotically anti-de Sitter (AdS) space, and the theory on the boundary is a local conformal field theory (CFT).

The AdS/CFT correspondence has been generalized in various directions, and there are now a large number of examples of non-AdS/non-CFT relations. Some of the non-CFT theories are QCD-like gauge field theories. Generically, when the field theory is strongly coupled, the gravitational description is weakly coupled; that is, the curved geometry has a small curvature. On the other hand, when the field theory is weakly coupled, the gravitational description is strongly coupled.

A particularly interesting regime of the quantum field theory is the hydrodynamic one, where the theory is in local thermal equilibrium. The AdS/CFT correspondence relates the field theory hydrodynamics to perturbations of black hole (brane) gravitational backgrounds. Indeed, an important experimental framework to which the correspondence has been applied is the description of the QCD plasma produced at RHIC and LHC. This plasma exhibits strong-coupling dynamics, $\alpha_s(T_{\mathrm{RHIC}}) \sim O(1)$. The AdS/CFT correspondence provides a real-time nonperturbative framework, and one typically uses the strong-coupling properties of a CFT plasma as a reference point for describing the strongly coupled QCD plasma. A well-known quantity is the ratio of the shear viscosity η to the entropy density s, which for a generic strongly coupled gauge field theory is low. Indeed, such a low ratio is a generic property of the gravitational description [4]. Hydrodynamic simulations at low shear viscosity to entropy ratio are consistent with RHIC data [5].

In this chapter, we discuss the fluid/gravity correspondence for relativistic and nonrelativistic fluid flows. In Section 8.2, we present the hydrodynamic framework from the field theory point of view. In Section 8.3, we outline the dual gravitational description for relativistic fluids, before turning to consider the nonrelativistic case in Section 8.4. In Section 8.5, we give further details of the fluid/gravity correspondence, discussing the bulk geometry and the dynamics of the black hole horizon.

8.2   Field theory hydrodynamics

In the hydrodynamic regime, the system is in local thermal equilibrium. This is enforced by frequent collisions between the particles. Thus, the hydrodynamic regime is characterized by a short mean free path (correlation length), much smaller than the characteristic scale of variations of the macroscopic fields. Since it is dominated by collisions, an appropriate description is that of a collective fluid-type flow rather than a particle (kinetic theory) one. Hydrodynamics is the theory of this fluid flow.

The postulated effective degrees of freedom in the hydrodynamic regime are charge densities $\rho(\vec{x}, t)$, which may be understood as nonequilibrium thermal averages. The hydrodynamic equations are the conservation laws, which govern the evolution of the charge densities:

$$\partial_t \rho + \partial_i j^i = 0. \tag{8.1}$$

Since the charge densities in the hydrodynamic regime are slowly varying functions, constitutive relations express j^i in terms of ρ and its derivatives. These relations are material-dependent. If we take $j^i = -D\partial^i \rho$ (Fick's law), plug in (8.1), and Fourier transform with respect to the space coordinates $\vec{x}$, we get

$$\rho(\vec{k}, t) = e^{-Dk^2 t} \rho(\vec{k}, t = 0). \tag{8.2}$$

D is called the transport coefficient and depends on the material (microscopic theory). The relation (8.2) is the characteristic behavior of hydrodynamic modes: it has a lifetime $\tau(k) = 1/Dk^2$, which is infinite in the long-wavelength limit $k \to 0$. Indeed, since ρ is a conserved quantity, it cannot disappear locally but can only relax slowly over the entire system.

The dispersion relation for the hydrodynamic mode is $\omega = -iDk^2$. It shows up as a pole in the retarded thermal correlation function of the microscopic theory

$$S(\vec{x}, t) = \langle \rho(\vec{x}, t), \rho(0, 0) \rangle_{\text{eq}}, \tag{8.3}$$

where $\langle ... \rangle_{\text{eq}}$ is the thermal equilibrium average, and we have assumed $\langle \rho(\vec{x}, t) \rangle_{\text{eq}} = 0$. $S(\vec{x}, t)$ describes the fluctuations of the charge density ρ and can be measured experimentally. In the gravitational description of hydrodynamics, the poles of the retarded thermal correlation function correspond to the quasinormal modes of the black hole, which characterize its late time relaxation to equilibrium after a perturbation.

8.3 Relativistic hydrodynamics

We will work in four flat spacetime dimensions with a Lorentzian metric $\eta_{\mu\nu} = \text{diag}(-1, 1, 1, 1)$. We define the hydrodynamic expansion parameter (Knudsen number) Kn as $Kn \equiv l_{\text{cor}}/L \ll 1$, where l_{cor} is the correlation length of the fluid and L is the characteristic scale of variations of the macroscopic fields. The macroscopic fields are the energy density $\epsilon(x)$, the pressure $p(x)$, the charge densities $\rho_a(x)$ and chemical potentials $\mu^a(x)$, the temperature $T(x)$, the entropy density $s(x)$, and finally the local four-velocity field $u^\mu(x) = (\gamma, \gamma\beta^i)$ satisfying $u_\mu u^\mu = -1$. These local fields are not independent. We can choose an independent set, for instance $\epsilon(x)$, $\rho_a(x)$, and $u^\mu(x)$, and determine the other local fields by using the equation of state and the thermodynamic relations

$$d\epsilon = T\,ds + \mu^a\,d\rho_a, \tag{8.4a}$$

$$dp = s\,dT + \rho_a\,d\mu^a. \tag{8.4b}$$

Hydrodynamics is a generalization of thermodynamics, in which the charge densities are upgraded to local currents. The hydrodynamic evolution equations are the conservation laws of these currents:

$$\partial_\mu T^{\mu\nu} = 0, \qquad \partial_\mu J_a^\mu = 0. \tag{8.5}$$

$T^{\mu\nu}$ is the stress–energy tensor, and $J_a^\mu, a = 1, ..., n$, are symmetry currents, which can be abelian such as the electromagnetic charge current or nonabelian such as flavor symmetry currents in QCD. The constitutive relations have the form of series for the stress–energy tensor and the symmetry currents:

$$T^{\mu\nu}(x) = \sum_{l=0}^{\infty} T^{\mu\nu}_{(l)}(x), \qquad J_a^\mu = \sum_{l=0}^{\infty} J^\mu_{a(l)}(x), \tag{8.6}$$

where $T^{\mu\nu}_{(l)}, J^\mu_{a(l)} \sim (Kn)^l$. The expansion in the Knudsen number is a derivative expansion, where l counts the number of derivatives.

One introduces a local entropy current s^μ, whose divergence is required to be non-negative with hyphen order by order in the derivative expansion:

$$\partial_\mu s^\mu \geq 0. \tag{8.7}$$

This local form of the Second Law of Thermodynamics constrains the transport coefficients of the theory. Note, however, that this requirement still lacks a microscopic field theory interpretation.

8.3.1 Ideal hydrodynamics

Keeping only the first term $l = 0$ in the series gives ideal hydrodynamics, which is essentially determined by thermodynamics. We have

$$T^{\mu\nu}_{(0)} = \epsilon u^\mu u^\nu + p P^{\mu\nu}, \tag{8.8a}$$

$$J^\mu_{a(0)} = \rho_a u^\mu, \tag{8.8b}$$

$$s^\mu_{(0)} = s u^\mu, \tag{8.8c}$$

where $P^{\mu\nu} = \eta^{\mu\nu} + u^\mu u^\nu$. There is one less conservation equation than the number of fields $\epsilon, p, \rho_a, u^\mu$, and so one more equation is needed in order to have a complete description of the system. This is called the equation of state, and it allows us to choose a set of independent variables, for instance, ϵ, ρ_a, and u^μ. In CFT hydrodynamics, $T^\mu_\mu = 0$, and the equation of state reads $\epsilon = 3p$. In this case, there is only one dimensionful quantity, the temperature T, and $\epsilon, p \sim T^4$. The ideal conformal fluid stress–energy tensor can be recast, up to an overall constant coefficient, in the form

$$T^{\mu\nu}_{(0)} = T^4(\eta^{\mu\nu} + 4u^\mu u^\nu). \tag{8.9}$$

At the ideal hydrodynamics order, there is no dissipation, and the hydrodynamic conservation laws imply that $\partial_\mu s^\mu_{(0)} = 0$.

8.3.2   Viscous hydrodynamics

First-order dissipative hydrodynamics is obtained by keeping also the $l = 1$ term in the series. When getting out of equilibrium, there is an ambiguity in the definition of the charge densities due to the possibility of adding derivative terms. Fixing this ambiguity requires a choice of frame. In one such frame, the Landau frame, the fluid velocity is an eigenvector of the stress–energy tensor, and the energy density is its eigenvalue: $T^{\mu\nu} u_\nu = -\epsilon u^\mu$. In this frame, the local rest frame of the flow is where the energy density is at rest. The charge density $\rho_a = -u_\mu J_a^\mu$. The first-order stress–energy tensor and the symmetry currents satisfy

$$u_\mu T_{(1)}^{\mu\nu} = 0, \qquad u_\mu J_{a(1)}^\mu = 0. \tag{8.10}$$

They take the forms

$$T_{(1)}^{\mu\nu} = -2\eta\sigma^{\mu\nu} - \zeta(\partial_\alpha u^\alpha)P^{\mu\nu}, \tag{8.11a}$$

$$J_{a(1)}^\mu = -T\sigma_{ab}P^{\mu\nu}\partial_\nu \frac{\mu^b}{T}, \tag{8.11b}$$

where

$$\sigma^{\mu\nu} = P^{\mu\alpha}P^{\nu\beta}\partial_{(\alpha}u_{\beta)} - \frac{1}{3}\partial_\alpha u^\alpha P^{\mu\nu} \tag{8.12}$$

is the shear tensor. There are three types of transport coefficients at this order: the shear viscosity η, the bulk viscosity ζ, and the conductivity matrix σ_{ab}. Note that in the conformal case, $\zeta = 0$. The transport coefficients can be calculated from the retarded Green functions of the microscopic thermal field theory using linear response theory and the Kubo formulas.

The entropy current at this order reads

$$s_{(1)}^\mu = -\frac{\mu^a}{T} J_{a(1)}^\mu. \tag{8.13}$$

It is no longer conserved at the first viscous order, and we have

$$\partial_\mu S^\mu = \frac{\eta}{2T}\sigma_{\mu\nu}\sigma^{\mu\nu} + \frac{\zeta}{T}(\partial_\mu u^\mu)^2 + T\sigma_{ab}P^{\mu\nu}\partial_\mu\frac{\mu^a}{T}\partial_\nu\frac{\mu^b}{T} \geq 0. \tag{8.14}$$

The positivity requirements imposed on the transport coefficients in (8.14) can be verified in the microscopic quantum field theory.

8.3.3   Quantum anomalies and chiral effects

The hydrodynamic description exhibits interesting chiral effects when a global symmetry current J_a^μ of the microscopic theory is anomalous:

$$\partial_\mu J_a^\mu = \frac{1}{8}C_{abc}\epsilon^{\mu\nu\rho\sigma}F_{\mu\nu}^a F_{\rho\sigma}^b. \tag{8.15}$$

C_{abc} is the coefficient of the triangle anomaly of the currents J_a^μ, J_b^μ, and J_c^μ. The form of an anomalous symmetry hydrodynamic current is modified by a term proportional to the vorticity of the fluid,

$$\omega^\mu \equiv \frac{1}{2}\epsilon^{\mu\nu\lambda\rho}u_\nu\partial_\lambda u_\rho. \tag{8.16}$$

This was first discovered in the context of the fluid/gravity correspondence [6].

The global anomalous symmetry hydrodynamic current takes the form

$$j_a^\mu = \rho_a u^\mu + \sigma_a{}^b\left(E_b^\mu - TP^{\mu\nu}\partial_\nu\frac{\mu_b}{T}\right) + \xi_a\omega^\mu + \xi_{ab}^{(B)}B^{b\mu}. \tag{8.17}$$

Here, $E_a^\mu = F_a^{\mu\nu}u_\nu$ and $B^{a\mu} = \frac{1}{2}\epsilon^{\mu\nu\lambda\rho}u_\nu F_{\lambda\rho}^a$, while ρ_a, T, μ_a, and σ_a^b are the charge densities, temperature, chemical potentials, and conductivities of the medium. The anomaly coefficients can be calculated from the requirement that the entropy current must have a positive divergence, $\partial_\mu s^\mu \geq 0$ [7, 8]. They read

$$\xi_a = C_{abc}\mu^b\mu^c + 2\beta_a T^2 - \frac{2\rho_a}{\epsilon + p}\left(\frac{1}{3}C_{bcd}\mu^b\mu^c\mu^d + 2\beta_b\mu^b T^2\right), \tag{8.18a}$$

$$\xi_{ab}^{(B)} = C_{abc}\mu^c - \frac{\rho_a}{\epsilon + p}\left(\frac{1}{2}C_{bcd}\mu^c\mu^d + \beta_b T^2\right). \tag{8.18b}$$

The coefficients β_a are related to the gravitational anomaly [9], that is, to the triangle anomaly diagram of the current J_a^μ and two stress–energy tensors.

There are proposals for detecting experimental signatures of the axial current triangle diagram anomaly in a hydrodynamic description of high-density QCD. At RHIC and LHC, the chemical potentials are small compared with the energy density; hence, $\xi_a = C_{abc}\mu^b\mu^c$ and $\xi_{ab}^{(B)} = C_{abc}\mu^c$. The chiral magnetic effect corresponds to the generation of an electric current in the direction of the magnetic field, $\vec{j} \sim \mu_A\vec{B}$, using C_{abc} of two electric currents and one axial current in (8.17), with μ_A being the axial chemical potential. The chiral vortical effect corresponds to the generation of a baryon number current in the direction of the vorticity vector $\vec{j} \sim \mu_A\mu_B\vec{\omega}$, using C_{abc} of two baryon number currents and one axial current in (8.17), with μ_B being the baryon chemical potential. The chiral magnetic effect and the chiral vortical effect yield charge separation and baryon number separation in the measured spectrum of hadrons [10].

Another possible experimental signature is based on the idea that the axial charge density, in a locally uniform flow of massless fermions, is a measure of the alignment between the fermion spins. When the QCD fluid freezes out and the quarks bind to form hadrons, aligned spins result in spin-excited hadrons. The ratio between spin-excited and low-spin hadron production and its angular distribution may therefore be used as a measurement of the axial charge distribution. An enhancement of spin-excited hadron production along the rotation axis of the collision is predicted [11].

New chiral effects arise in superfluid hydrodynamics [12–14], that is, when there are spontaneously broken symmetries. This is a relevant framework for QCD at high densities and low temperatures. One possible observable effect is the chiral electric effect [13], which is the generation of an electric current perpendicular to the electric field:

$$J^{a\mu}_{\mathrm{CEE}} = c^a{}_{bc}\epsilon^{\mu\nu\rho\sigma} u_\nu \xi^b_\rho E^c_\sigma, \qquad (8.19)$$

compared with the standard electric conductivity term $J^{a\mu}_{\mathrm{Conduct}} = \sigma^{ab} E^\mu_b$. Here, c_{abc} are the transport coefficients proportional to the triangle anomaly diagram coefficient C_{abc}, and ξ^a_μ is the phase gradient of the broken symmetry, which is proportional to the velocity of the superfluid part.

8.4 Nonrelativistic fluid flows

8.4.1 The incompressible Navie–Stokes equations

Consider the equations of relativistic CFT hydrodynamics without charges. At the first viscous order, they take the form

$$u_\nu \partial_\nu T^{\mu\nu} = \partial_\mu u^\mu + 3D \ln T = \frac{1}{2\pi T}\sigma_{\mu\nu}\sigma^{\mu\nu}, \qquad (8.20a)$$

$$P_{\sigma\nu}\partial_\mu T^{\mu\nu} = a_\sigma + P^\mu_\sigma \partial_\mu \ln T = \frac{1}{2\pi T}P^\mu_\sigma(\partial_\alpha \sigma^\alpha_\mu - 3\sigma^\alpha_\mu a_\alpha), \qquad (8.20b)$$

where $D = u^\mu \partial_\mu$, $a_\sigma = Du_\sigma$, and we have used the Einstein gravity relation $\eta/s = 1/4\pi$.

The incompressible Navier–Stokes equations can be obtained in the nonrelativistic limit of relativistic hydrodynamics [15, 16]. We expand $u^\mu = (1 + v^2/2 + \cdots, v^i)$, and $T = T_0(1 + p + \cdots)$, with the scaling $v^i \sim \varepsilon, \partial_i \sim \varepsilon, \partial_t \sim \varepsilon^2$, and $p \sim \varepsilon^2$, where $\varepsilon \sim 1/c$. Equation (8.20a) gives the incompressibility condition $\partial_i v^i = 0$. Equation (8.20b) gives

$$\partial_t v^i + v^j \partial_j v^i = -\partial^i p + \nu \Delta v^i, \qquad (8.21)$$

where $\nu = 1/4\pi T_0$ is the kinematic viscosity.

8.4.2 Turbulent flows

Turbulence refers to a state in which a large number of interacting degrees of freedom deviate far from equilibrium. Most nonrelativistic fluid flows in nature are turbulent. We define the dimensionless Reynolds number

$$R_e = \frac{LV}{\nu}, \qquad (8.22)$$

where L and V are, respectively a characteristic scale and velocity of the flow. Turbulence develops when $R_e \sim 10^3$ or larger. In nature, R_e is generically large since the kinematic viscosity is generically low. For instance, the kinematic viscosity of water at room temperature is $\nu \simeq 10^{-6}\,\mathrm{m}^2\,\mathrm{s}^{-1}$.

Consider a random external force that excites a three-dimensional fluid at a scale L. In general, the statistics of the flow velocity generated by the excitation is not calculable, because of the nonlinear nature of the fluid equations. An important question arises, however: What are the universal characteristics of the flow statistics? In 1941, Kolmogorov suggested that the velocity statistics in the inertial range of turbulence, at a scales r, with

$$\text{viscous scale} \ll r \ll \text{force scale},$$

is scale-invariant. In order to quantify this, we define the velocity difference at distance r as

$$\delta v(r) \equiv [\vec{v}(\vec{r},t) - \vec{v}(0,t)] \cdot \frac{\vec{r}}{|\vec{r}|}. \tag{8.23}$$

Scale invariance means that the probability density function $P(\delta v(r))$ satisfies

$$P(\delta v(r))\delta v(r) = F\left(\frac{\delta v(r)}{r^h}\right), \tag{8.24}$$

where the function F is independent of the force and h is a real number. Thus, the turbulent flow should exhibit a self-similar (fractal) structure. We define the structure functions

$$S_n \equiv \langle [\delta v(r)]^n \rangle. \tag{8.25}$$

S_2 is the energy contained in the fluid modes with wavenumbers larger than $1/r$. The Kolmogorov dimensional scaling argument fixes $h = \frac{1}{3}$ by the requirement for a constant energy flux $[\delta v(r)]^2/[r\delta v(r)]$ in the turbulent (direct) cascade. Note that in the direct cascade, the excitation (force) of the fluid is at a large lengthscales, while the dissipation is at small lengthscales.

The Fourier transform of the energy $E(k)$ has the Kolomogorov scaling

$$E(k) \sim k^{-5/3}. \tag{8.26}$$

However, it is now well established numerically and experimentally that scale invariance is broken in direct cascades, and one expects a multifractal structure in turbulence and a spectrum of anomalous exponents in the structure functions. In particular, the energy spectrum deviates from the Kolmogorov scaling (8.26). There is experimental and numerical evidence that in the inertial range of distance scales, the flows exhibit the behavior $S_n(r) \sim r^{\xi_n}$. Only in the case $n = 3$ does the Kolmogorov scaling $\xi_3 = 1$ agree with the data. The major open problem of turbulence is to calculate the anomalous exponents ξ_n. These anomalous exponents are encoded in the geometry of the black hole horizon [17].

One can distinguish between direct and inverse cascades of the fluid flow. In the inverse cascade (such as in two-dimensional incompressible fluids), turbulence occurs at lengthscales exceeding the force scale, and energy is transferred throughout the scales. Here there is numerical and experimental evidence that turbulence exhibits scale-invariant statistics [18] and perhaps also conformal invariance [19]. In order to describe this structure, the black hole horizon should exhibit statistically a fractal structure.

Note also that the study of the universal structure of turbulence in relativistic flows is only at its beginning and very little is known. It is possible to derive a relativistic scaling relation that reduces to Kolmogorov's relation for S_3 [20]; however, we are still missing even a proper definition of the relativistic higher correlation functions analogous to S_n.

An important issue in the hydrodynamic description is whether, starting with appropriate initial conditions, where the velocity vector field and its derivatives are bounded, the system can evolve such that it will exhibit within a finite time a blowup of the derivatives of the vector field. Physically, such singularities, if present, indicate a breakdown of the effective hydrodynamic description at long distances and imply that some new degrees of freedom are required. The issue of hydrodynamic singularities has an analogue in gravity: Given appropriate Cauchy data, will the evolving spacetime geometry exhibit a naked singularity, i.e., a blowup of curvature invariants and the energy density of matter fields at a point not covered by a horizon? See [21] for a first step in relating the hydrodynamics and gravity singularities using the Penrose inequality [22].

8.5   Holographic hydrodynamics: the fluid/gravity correspondence

8.5.1   Bulk geometry

Consider the five-dimensional Einstein equations with a negative cosmological constant:

$$E_{mn} \equiv R_{mn} + 4g_{mn} = 0. \tag{8.27}$$

These equations have a thermal equilibrium asymptotically AdS solution, the boosted black brane. In Eddington–Finkelstein coordinates, the metric reads

$$g^{(0)}_{mn}\, dx^m\, dx^n = -2u_\mu\, dx^\mu\, dr - r^2 f(br) u_\mu u_\nu\, dx^\mu\, dx^\nu + r^2 P_{\mu\nu}\, dx^\mu\, dx^\nu, \tag{8.28}$$

where $x^m = (r, x^\mu), \mu = 0, ..., 3$, u_μ is the 4-velocity boost vector, $T = 1/\pi b$ is the temperature, and $f(r) = 1 - 1/r^4$. The metric (8.28) is a solution of (8.27) when b and u^μ are constants. It has an event horizon (null hypersurface) with planar topology at $r = b^{-1}$, whose normal is $\ell^m = (\ell^r, \ell^\mu) = (0, u^\mu)$. The Bekenstein–Hawking entropy density $s = (4b^3)^{-1}$ and the normal combine to give the entropy current $S^\mu = (4b^3)^{-1} u^\mu$, where we set $G_N = 1$.

The metric (8.28) is no longer a solution when $b(x^\alpha)$ and $u^\mu(x^\alpha)$ are not constants, and needs to be corrected. We seek a solution of the Einstein equations (8.27) by the method of variation of constants:

$$g_{mn} = g^{(0)}_{mn} + g^{(1)}_{mn} + \cdots, \tag{8.29}$$

where $g^{(1)}_{mn}$ includes first derivatives of $b(x^\alpha)$ and $u^\mu(x^\alpha)$. Imposing AdS asymptotics and regularity at the horizon, we find that the momentum-constraint Einstein equations $E^r_\mu = 0$ give the boundary CFT hydrodynamic equations $\partial_\mu T^{\mu\nu} = 0$ as a series expansion in derivatives [23]. The ratio of the shear viscosity to the entropy density that is calculated from the gravitational background takes the universal value $\eta/s = 1/4\pi$ as a consequence of the requirement that there be no naked singularities.

Consider the metric (8.28) and the timelike boundary $r \to \infty$, where n^m denotes its normal. The boundary stress–energy tensor takes the form [24]

$$T_\mu^\nu \sim \lim_{r\to\infty} r^4 \left(K_\mu^\nu - K\delta_\mu^\nu + 3\delta_\mu^\nu \right), \tag{8.30}$$

where $K_\mu^\nu = \nabla_\mu n^\nu$ is the extrinsic curvature and K is its trace. It is straightforward to check that this is the stress–energy tensor of ideal CFT hydrodynamics. The boundary stress–energy tensor with the derivative corrections (8.29) is the viscous stress–energy tensor of the CFT hydrodynamics.

8.5.2 Horizon dynamics

The CFT hydrodynamic equations can be viewed also as the Gauss–Codazzi equations governing the dynamics of the event horizon [25]. In particular, the null horizon focusing equation is equivalent to the entropy balance law of the hydrodynamic fluid [25, 26]. Here we will discuss the ideal-order CFT hydrodynamics. The viscous case is analyzed in [25].

Geometry of null surfaces

As above, the coordinates of the bulk spacetime are $x^m = (r, x^\mu)$. We now consider x^μ as coordinates on the horizon $\mathcal{H}$ and r as a coordinate transverse to it. We choose $r = 0$ as the location of the horizon. We denote the null normal to the horizon by ℓ^m. In fact, it is both normal and tangent to the horizon and tangent to its null generators. In components, $l^m = (0, \ell^\mu)$. The pullback of the bulk metric g_{mn} into $\mathcal{H}$ is the degenerate horizon metric $\gamma_{\mu\nu}$. Its null directions are the generating light rays of $\mathcal{H}$, i.e., $\gamma_{\mu\nu}\ell^\nu = 0$. The Lie derivative of $\gamma_{\mu\nu}$ along ℓ^μ is the second fundamental form

$$\theta_{\mu\nu} = \frac{1}{2}\mathcal{L}_\ell \gamma_{\mu\nu}. \tag{8.31}$$

We can decompose $\theta_{\mu\nu}$ into a shear tensor $\sigma_{\mu\nu}^{(H)}$ and the expansion θ:

$$\theta_{\mu\nu} = \sigma_{\mu\nu}^{(H)} + \frac{1}{3}\theta\gamma_{\mu\nu}. \tag{8.32}$$

In fact, $\theta_{\mu\nu} = 0$ at the ideal fluid order that we will be working with.

Since $\gamma_{\mu\nu}$ is degenerate, we cannot use it to define an intrinsic connection on the null horizon, as could be done for spacelike or timelike hypersurfaces. The bulk spacetime's connection does induce a notion of parallel transport in $\mathcal{H}$, but only along its null generators. This structure is not fully captured by $\gamma_{\mu\nu}$; instead, it is encoded by the extrinsic curvature $\Theta_\mu{}^\nu$, which is the horizon restriction of $\nabla_m\ell^n$:

$$\Theta_\mu{}^\nu = \nabla_\mu\ell^\nu. \tag{8.33}$$

For a non-null hypersurface, the extrinsic curvature at a point is independent of the induced metric. For null hypersurfaces, this is not so. Indeed, lowering an index of $\Theta_\mu{}^\nu$ with $\gamma_{\mu\nu}$, we get the shear/expansion tensor $\theta_{\mu\nu}$:

$$\Theta_\mu{}^\rho \gamma_{\rho\nu} = \theta_{\mu\nu}. \tag{8.34}$$

This expresses the compatibility of the parallel transport defined by $\Theta_\mu{}^\nu$ with the horizon metric $\gamma_{\mu\nu}$. Contracting $\Theta_\mu{}^\nu$ with ℓ^μ yields the surface gravity κ, which measures the non-affinity of ℓ^μ:

$$\Theta_\mu{}^\nu \ell^\mu = \kappa \ell^\nu. \tag{8.35}$$

At the ideal fluid order, $\Theta_\mu{}^\nu$ can be written as

$$\Theta_\mu{}^\nu = c_\mu \ell^\nu, \qquad c_\mu \ell^\mu = \kappa. \tag{8.36}$$

As we will see, the covector c_μ encodes in its four components all the fluid data, that is, the temperature and the velocity 4-vector.

The null Gauss–Codazzi equations that will give the ideal-order Navier–Stokes equations can be written as

$$c_\mu \partial_\nu S^\nu + 2 S^\nu \partial_{[\nu} c_{\mu]} = 0, \tag{8.37}$$

where we have defined the area entropy current $S^\mu = v\ell^\mu$, and v is a scalar density equal to the horizon area density. S^μ is the gravitational analog of the hydrodynamic entropy current, which we denoted by s^μ.

Hydrodynamic equations

Considering the boosted black brane metric, we can easily check that $c_\mu \sim T u_\mu$ and $S^\nu \sim T^3 u^\mu$. Indeed, the covector c_μ contains all the hydrodynamic information. Plugging these values into the Gauss–Codazzi equations (8.37) and projecting along u^μ, we find the conservation of the entropy current:

$$\partial_\mu(T^3 u^\mu) = \theta = 0. \tag{8.38}$$

This means that the horizon is nonexpanding at the ideal order. Projecting transverse to u^μ, we get the ideal relativistic Euler equation

$$a_\sigma + P_\sigma^\mu \partial_\mu \ln T = 0. \tag{8.39}$$

Bulk viscosity

We can generalize the fluid/gravity correspondence to charged and nonconformal hydrodynamics by including bulk gauge A_μ^a and scalar ϕ_i fields, respectively. Now the bulk viscosity is nonzero. Remarkably, it is possible to derive a simple formula for the ratio of bulk to shear viscosities [27]

$$\frac{\zeta}{\eta} = \sum_i \left(s \frac{d\phi_i^H}{ds} + \rho^a \frac{d\phi_i^H}{d\rho^a} \right)^2, \tag{8.40}$$

where s is the entropy density, ρ^a are the charges associated with the gauge fields A_μ^a, ϕ_i^H are the values of the scalar fields on the horizon, and the derivatives are taken with couplings and mass parameters held fixed.

8.5.3 Outlook

The application of the fluid/gravity correspondence to the study of relativistic and nonrelativistic turbulence is the main open challenge. The universal statistical structure of turbulence is encoded in the geometry of the black hole horizon. Clearly, to describe this, the horizon has to exhibit a fractal structure (in the inverse cascade) and a multifractal structure (in the direct cascade). To see this, one is likely to need to use a random force that will make the horizon a random surface.

Acknowledgments

It is a great pleasure to thank the organizers and participants of the wonderful and stimulating Les Houches Summer School. I would also like to thank my students and collaborators in this ongoing research. This work is supported in part by the ISF Center of Excellence.

References

[1] G. 't Hooft, [arXiv:gr-qc/9310026]; L. Susskind, J. Math. Phys. **36**, 6377 (1995) [arXiv:hep-th/9409089].

[2] J. M. Maldacena, Adv. Theor. Math. Phys. **2**, 231 (1998) [Int. J. Theor. Phys. **38**, 1113 (1999)] [arXiv:hep-th/9711200].

[3] O. Aharony, S. S. Gubser, J. M. Maldacena, H. Ooguri, and Y. Oz, Phys. Rep. **323**, 183 (2000) [arXiv:hep-th/9905111].

[4] G. Policastro, D. T. Son, and A. O. Starinets, Phys. Rev. Lett. **87**, 081601 (2001) [arXiv:hep-th/0104066]; A. Buchel, and J. T. Liu, Phys. Rev. Lett. **93**, 090602 (2004) [arXiv:hep-th/0311175].

[5] M. Luzum, P. Romatschke, Phys. Rev. **C78**, 034915 (2008) [arXiv:0804.4015 [nucl-th]].

[6] J. Erdmenger, M. Haack, M. Kaminski, and A. Yarom, JHEP **0901**, 055 (2009) [arXiv:0809.2488 [hep-th]]; N. Banerjee, J. Bhattacharya, S. Bhattacharyya, S. Dutta, R. Loganayagam, and P. Surowka, arXiv:0809.2596 [hep-th].

[7] D. T. Son and P. Surowka, Phys. Rev. Lett. **103**, 191601 (2009) [arXiv:0906.5044 [hep-th]].

[8] Y. Neiman and Y. Oz, JHEP **1103**, 023 (2011) [arXiv:1011.5107 [hep-th]].

[9] K. Landsteiner, E. Megias, and F. Pena-Benitez, arXiv:1103.5006 [hep-ph]; K. Landsteiner, E. Megias, L. Melgar, and F. Pena-Benitez, arXiv:1107.0368 [hep-th].

[10] D. E. Kharzeev and D. T. Son, arXiv:1010.0038 [hep-ph].

[11] B. Keren-Zur and Y. Oz, JHEP **1006**, 006 (2010) [arXiv:1002.0804 [hep-ph]].

[12] J. Bhattacharya, S. Bhattacharyya, S. Minwalla, and A. Yarom, arXiv:1105.3733 [hep-th].

[13] Y. Neiman and Y. Oz, JHEP **1109**, 011 (2011) [arXiv:1106.3576 [hep-th]]; arXiv:1108.5829 [hep-th].

[14] M. G. Alford, A. Schmitt, K. Rajagopal, and T. Schafer, Rev. Mod. Phys. **80**, 1455 (2008) [arXiv:0709.4635 [hep-ph]].

[15] I. Fouxon and Y. Oz, Phys. Rev. Lett. **101**, 261602 (2008) [arXiv:0809.4512 [hep-th]].

[16] S. Bhattacharyya, S. Minwalla, and S. R. Wadia, JHEP **0908**, 059 (2009) [arXiv:0810.1545 [hep-th]].

[17] C. Eling, I. Fouxon and Y. Oz, arXiv:1004.2632 [hep-th].

[18] P. Tabeling, Phys. Rep. **362**, 1 (2002).

[19] D. Bernard, G. Boffetta, A. Celani, and G. Falkovich, Nature Phys. **2**, 124 (2006) [arXiv:nlin/0602017[nlin.CD]].

[20] I. Fouxon and Y. Oz, Phys. Lett. **B694**, 261 (2010) [arXiv:0909.3574 [hep-th]].

[21] Y. Oz and M. Rabinovich, JHEP **1102**, 070 (2011) [arXiv:1011.5895 [hep-th]].

[22] R. Penrose, Ann. NY. Acad. Sci. **224**, 125 (1973).

[23] S. Bhattacharyya, V. E. Hubeny, S. Minwalla, and M. Rangamani, JHEP **0802**, 045 (2008) [arXiv:0712.2456 [hep-th]].

[24] V. Balasubramanian and P. Kraus, Commun. Math. Phys. **208**, 413 (1999) [arXiv:hep-th/9902121].

[25] C. Eling and Y. Oz, JHEP **1002**, 069 (2010) [arXiv:0906.4999 [hep-th]]; C. Eling, Y. Neiman, and Y. Oz, JHEP **1012**, 086 (2010) [arXiv:1010.1290 [hep-th]]; C. Eling, I. Fouxon, and Y. Oz, Phys. Lett. **B680**, 496 (2009) [arXiv:0905.3638 [hep-th]].

[26] S. Bhattacharyya, V.E. Hubery, R. Loganayagam, G. Mandal, S. Minwalla, T. Morita, M. Rangamani, and H.S. Reall, JHEP **0806**, 055 (2008) [arXiv:0803.2526 [hep-th]].

[27] C. Eling and Y. Oz, JHEP **1106**, 007 (2011) [arXiv:1103.1657 [hep-th]]; arXiv:1107.2134 [hep-th].

9
Supersymmetry

Gian F. Giudice

Theory Division CERN, Geneva, Switzerland

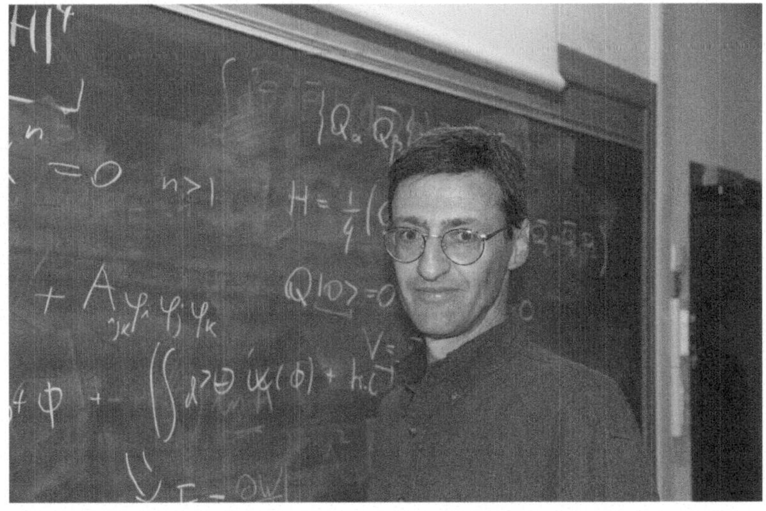

Theoretical Physics to Face the Challenge of LHC. Edited by L. Baulieu, K. Benakli, M. R. Douglas, B. Mansoulié, E. Rabinovici, and L. F. Cugliandolo. © Oxford University Press 2015. Published in 2015 by Oxford University Press.

Chapter Contents

In the lectures at the École de physique des Houches, I presented the motivations for low-energy supersymmetry, the construction of realistic models, the various schemes for generating soft terms (gravity mediation, gauge mediation, anomaly mediation, and gaugino mediation), their collider phenomenology, and their implications for dark matter. The subject is well established and there are excellent reviews and textbooks that fully cover this material. Therefore, rather than documenting the full content of my lectures, I direct readers to appropriate references, where they can find well-organized and exhaustive introductions to supersymmetry.

For some textbooks on supersymmetry, see

- M. Dine, "Supersymmetry and String Theory: Beyond the Standard Model," Cambridge University Press, Cambridge, 2007.
- J. Terning, "Modern Supersymmetry: Dynamics and Duality," Oxford University Press, Oxford, 2006.
- P. Binétruy, "Supersymmetry: Theory, Experiment, and Cosmology," Oxford University Press, Oxford, 2006.
- H. Baer and X. Tata, "Weak Scale Supersymmetry: From Superfields to Scattering Events," Cambridge University Press, Cambridge, 2006.
- M. Drees, R. M. Godbole, and P. Roy, "Theory and Phenomenology of Sparticles: An Account of Four-Dimensional $N = 1$ Supersymmetry in High-Energy Physics," World Scientific, Singapore, 2004.
- N. Polonsky, "Supersymmetry: Structure and Phenomena. Extensions of the Standard Model," Springer-Verlag, Berlin, 2001.
- S. Weinberg, "The Quantum Theory of Fields. Volume III: Supersymmetry," Cambridge University Press, Cambridge, 2000.
- J. Wess and J. Bagger, "Supersymmetry and Supergravity, 2nd edn," Princeton University Press, Princeton, 1992.

For collections of review articles on various topics related to supersymmetry, see

- "Perspectives on Supersymmetry," ed. G. L. Kane, World Scientific, Singapore, 1998.
- "Perspectives on Supersymmetry II," ed. G. L. Kane, World Scientific, Singapore, 2010.

For some reviews on supersymmetry breaking and the various schemes for generating soft terms, see

- Y. Shirman, "TASI 2008 Lectures: Introduction to Supersymmetry and Supersymmetry Breaking," [arXiv:0907.0039 [hep-ph]].
- M. A. Luty, "2004 TASI Lectures on Supersymmetry Breaking," [hep-th/0509029].
- J. Terning, "TASI 2002 Lectures: Nonperturbative Supersymmetry," [hep-th/0306119].
- G. F. Giudice and R. Rattazzi, "Theories with gauge mediated supersymmetry breaking," Phys. Rep. **322** (1999) 419 [hep-ph/9801271].
- J. A. Bagger, "Weak scale supersymmetry: theory and practice" [hep-ph/9604232].

Here, instead, I will present the part of my lectures on more recent results, which cannot be found in standard textbooks. I will focus on the lessons that we have learned from preliminary LHC results on Higgs searches. I will concentrate mostly on the Higgs boson, rather than on new physics, not only because the mechanism of electroweak (EW) symmetry breaking is one of the priorities in the LHC program, but also because we have new data on the Higgs and it is exciting to think about where they lead us.

The phenomenon of EW symmetry breaking had already been established before the LHC. After LEP, we had ample evidence for gauge structure in interactions (including the triple gauge boson couplings γWW and ZWW) and for the existence of longitudinal components of W and Z. Combining this information with knowledge of gauge boson masses, we conclude that propagating particles do not share the full symmetry of interactions, and thus that the EW symmetry is spontaneously broken. This means that every known phenomenon in particle physics (at least before December 13, 2011) can be described by the Lagrangian

$$L = -\frac{1}{4}\mathrm{Tr}\,F_{\mu\nu}F^{\mu\nu} + i\bar{f}\gamma^\mu D_\mu f + \frac{v^2}{4}\mathrm{Tr}\,D_\mu \Sigma^\dagger D^\mu \Sigma - \frac{v}{\sqrt{2}}\bar{f}_L \Sigma \lambda_f f_R + \text{h.c.}, \qquad (9.1)$$

$$\Sigma \equiv \exp\left(\frac{iT^a \pi^a}{v}\right), \qquad (9.2)$$

where π^a are the longitudinal polarizations of W and Z, and $v = 246\,\mathrm{GeV}$. The first two terms in (9.1) describe the kinetic terms and gauge interactions of the Standard Model (SM) particles. The last two terms contain the effect of the longitudinal polarizations and the mass terms that arise when gauge symmetry is realized nonlinearly.

Although the Lagrangian (9.1) was fully satisfying from an experimental point of view, even before December 13 every theorist knew that it could not be the full story. Scattering amplitudes of longitudinal gauge bosons grow like $(E/4\pi v)^2$, signaling loss of perturbative unitarity, and thus the onset of new phenomena, at $E \approx 4\pi v = 3\,\mathrm{TeV}$. One of the goals of the LHC was to discover what the new phenomenon is. It is well known that the simplest option is given by a single real scalar field h, which forms a complete $SU(2)$ doublet together with π^a. So three-quarters of the Higgs had already been found, and the LHC discovered the missing quarter. However, there is no strong motivation, other than simplicity, for choosing a single h, and nature may have good reasons to make different choices. In this respect, hunting for the Higgs is not just looking for the last missing piece of the SM, but it means exploring unknown territory and identifying the nature of the new force responsible for EW breaking, which I will call the *fifth force*.

When we examine the SM, we note that almost all of its open problems originate from Higgs interactions. The flavor problem comes from Yukawa couplings, the hierarchy problem from the Higgs bilinear, the stability problem from the Higgs quartic coupling—and one can add the cosmological constant problem from a constant term in the scalar potential. The crux of these puzzles is that the fifth force is not a gauge force. Therefore, it lacks the properties of uniqueness, robustness against deformations, and predictivity that are characteristic of gauge theories.

In order to discuss what we have learned from Higgs data, I will identify two fundamental questions. The first is: *What is the fifth force?* We want to know if it is weak or strong, if it is a gauge force or associated with a fundamental scalar. The answer to this question will come from precise measurements of Higgs couplings. These measurements will play the role that precision EW data played at the time of LEP. An important difference is that in the case of Higgs couplings, deviations from the SM expectation could be large (not necessarily of one-loop size) and thus show up even at an early stage. Actually, the more natural the Higgs boson is, the more its properties must deviate from the SM. This is because a natural theory must give large corrections to the Higgs two-point function (to cure the hierarchy problem). These large corrections must also modify the Higgs production rate at the LHC and some of its decay channels, as can easily be seen by inserting two gluons (or two photons) in the Feynman diagram of the Higgs two-point function. This expectation is fully confirmed in all the examples of natural theories known to us. So, measuring the Higgs couplings is the way to probe the fifth force and may be the first way for new physics to show up.

The second question is: *Is the Higgs natural?* This is not an idle question. Its importance goes beyond EW symmetry breaking, and its answer will influence the strategy for future directions in particle physics. Naturalness is a concept fully linked to the use of effective field theories (EFTs). EFT is the tool that we use to implement an intuitive notion: separation of scales. In simple words, separation of scales means that we don't need to know the motion of every atom inside the Moon to compute its orbit. Or we don't need to know about quarks to describe physics at the atomic scale. We build a stack of EFTs, one on top of the other, just like a matryoshka doll with one layer inside the other. Each EFT is appropriate to describe a certain energy regime, but it is connected to the next in the sense that free parameters in one layer can be computed in the next layer. One of the most remarkable results of modern physics has been the discovery that at each layer we find simpler physical laws, larger symmetry, and unification of concepts that seemed unrelated in the previous layer. It is amazing that nature works this way, but it is just an empirical fact. We can use the criterion of naturalness in EFT to infer the energy at which the validity of one layer ends and a new layer must set in. Whenever a next layer exists, this procedure gives a reasonable answer, as shown by various examples (electron self-energy, pion mass difference, and neutral kaon mass difference). When applied to the Higgs boson mass, this criterion gives a maximum scale for new physics at about 500 GeV.

Since we have not yet found any new physics at the LHC, one may wonder what is the fate of naturalness. The issue is not yet settled. It is quite possible that new physics is just around the corner. After all, the LHC has entered the territory of naturalness, but the exploration is far from complete. The alternative is that the idea of naturalness does not apply to the Higgs because there is a failure of the EFT approach. After all, dark energy could already be taken as evidence for failure of EFT, since the naturalness of the cosmological constant suggests new physics at around 10^{-3} eV. Holography, gauge/gravity duality, and the AdS/CFT correspondence show that some theories are much richer than can be captured by a single Lagrangian. The best we can do to describe the physical content is to resort to two different Lagrangians, two dual versions. Maybe this is an indication that our theoretical tools are failing, that an EFT Lagrangian is not able to catch all the underlying physics. There could be connections between small and large scales. A numerological curiosity is that if we combine the largest possible scale (the Hubble length $H^{-1} = 10^{26}$ m) with the smallest (the Planck length $M_P^{-1} = 10^{-35}$ m), we can reproduce the scale of the cosmological constant ($\Lambda_{CC} = \sqrt{HM_P} = 5 \times 10^{-3}$ eV) and the weak scale ($\Lambda_{EW} = \sqrt{\Lambda_{CC}M_P} = 5$ TeV). If behind this numerical curiosity there is some theoretical infrared/ultraviolet connection, we will never be able to catch it with an EFT.

Another approach that would invalidate naturalness is the idea of the multiverse. Out of the process of eternal inflation, a multitude of universes are created, each with its own values of the fundamental constants and its own physical laws. Anthropic arguments then select the kind of universe in which we live in, or, in other words, the physical laws that govern nature. It may sound like a crazy idea to some (bordering on science fiction), but at present the multiverse yields the most convincing explanation of the cosmological constant. A lesson from the multiverse is that some of the questions that we thought to be fundamental may actually be just the result of environmental conditions, and carry no more significance than the shapes of continents or the emergence of a particular animal species in Darwinian evolution.

So physics has reached a fork in the road, and the LHC will tell us which path we have to follow. One path follows the road that guided us toward the extraordinary successes of particle physics in the last 100 years or so: a new layer, new symmetry, more unification that bring us closer to a single governing principle of nature. The other path is marked by the failure of naturalness, the collapse of the picture of a multilayered matryoshka doll hiding a single final truth. We have only vague ideas of where this path leads to, and maybe the multiverse is the most concrete construction along this path. It is clear that establishing the fate of Higgs naturalness has far-reaching consequences for particle physics, well beyond the problem of EW breaking.

The LHC will teach us which path we have to follow. The first path is very familiar to particle physicists, and promises new discoveries on the road toward final unification. The other path may mean finding the Higgs and nothing else at the LHC. It will force us to abandon naturalness and EFT, and look for new paradigms in a holistic vision, where nature should be seen as a whole and cannot always be reduced to its smaller components. But physics is a natural science, and we want to find answers with the experimental method. While along the first path there are new phenomena to be studied and the goals are clear, how will we be able to make progress if the second path turns out to be true? This is a difficult question, to which I don't have an answer. However, I want to show how the measured value of the Higgs mass gives us some indirect hints.

For the sake of argument, let me assume that the SM with a single Higgs with mass around 125–126 GeV fully describes physics up to a very large energy scale. In this case, as shown in Fig. 9.1, we learn that our universe is in a very critical condition, at the verge of a cosmic catastrophe. It is a remarkable coincidence that we happen to live just at the boundary between two phases: the ordinary Higgs phase and a region

(a)

(b)

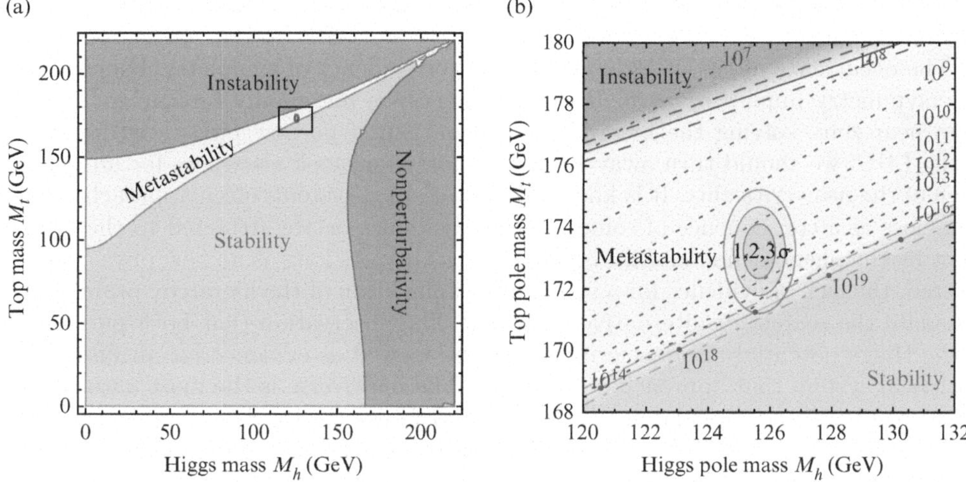

Fig. 9.1 Regions of absolute stability, metastability, and instability of the SM vacuum in the M_t–M_h plane. The frame in (b) zooms in the region of the preferred experimental range of M_h and M_t shown by the rectangular box in (a) (the gray areas in the center denote the allowed regions at 1, 2, and 3σ). The three boundary lines correspond to $\alpha_s(M_Z) = 0.1184 \pm 0.0007$, and the density of the shading indicates the size of the theoretical error. The dotted contour lines show the instability scale Λ in GeV, assuming $\alpha_s(M_Z) = 0.1184$.

where the Higgs field slides to very large values. The condition for absolute stability is

$$M_h \ [\text{GeV}] > 129.4 + 1.4 \left(\frac{M_t \ [\text{GeV}] - 173.1}{0.7} \right) - 0.5 \left(\frac{\alpha_s(M_Z) - 0.1184}{0.0007} \right) \pm 1.0_{\text{th}}.$$

Precise experimental information on the Higgs and top quark masses is needed to ascertain the ultimate fate of the universe and whether we live a stable vacuum or not. The Higgs mass can be measured very precisely at the LHC. The top mass will then become the largest source of uncertainty, and every GeV in M_t counts as a shift of 2 GeV in the Higgs mass. A reduction in the error on the top mass may become the best telescope to peek into the future of our universe.

Also, the hierarchy problem can be interpreted as a sign of near-criticality between two phases. The coefficient m^2 of the Higgs bilinear in the scalar potential is the order parameter that describes the transition between the symmetric phase ($m^2 > 0$) and the broken phase ($m^2 < 0$). In principle, m^2 could take any value between $-M_P^2$ and $+M_P^2$, but quantum corrections push m^2 away from zero toward one of the two endpoints of the allowed range. The hierarchy problem is the observation that in our universe the value of m^2 is approximately zero—in other words, its sits near the boundary between the symmetric and broken phases. Therefore, if the LHC result is confirmed, we must conclude that both m^2 and λ, the two parameters of the Higgs potential, happen to be near critical lines that separate the EW phase from a different (and inhospitable) phase of the SM. Is criticality just a capricious numerical coincidence or is it telling us something deep?

The occurrence of criticality could be the consequence of symmetry. For instance, supersymmetry implies $m^2 = 0$. If supersymmetry is marginally broken, m^2 will remain near zero, solving the hierarchy problem. But if no new physics is discovered at the LHC, we should turn away from symmetry and look elsewhere for an explanation of the near-criticality. It is known that statistical systems often approach critical behaviors as a consequence of some internal dynamics or are attracted to the critical point by the phenomenon of self-organized criticality. As long as no new physics is discovered, the lack of evidence for a symmetry explanation of the hierarchy problem will stimulate the search for alternative solutions. The observation that both parameters in the Higgs potential are quasicritical may be viewed as evidence for an underlying statistical system that approaches criticality. The multiverse is the most natural candidate to play the role of the underlying statistical system for SM parameters. If this vision is correct, it will lead to a new interpretation of our status in the multiverse: our universe is not a special element of the multiverse where the parameters have the peculiarity of allowing for life, but rather it is one of the most common products of the multiverse because it lies near an attractor critical point. In other words, the parameter distribution in the multiverse, instead of being flat or described by simple power laws (as is usually assumed) could be highly peaked around critical lines because of some internal dynamics. Rather than being selected by anthropic reasons,

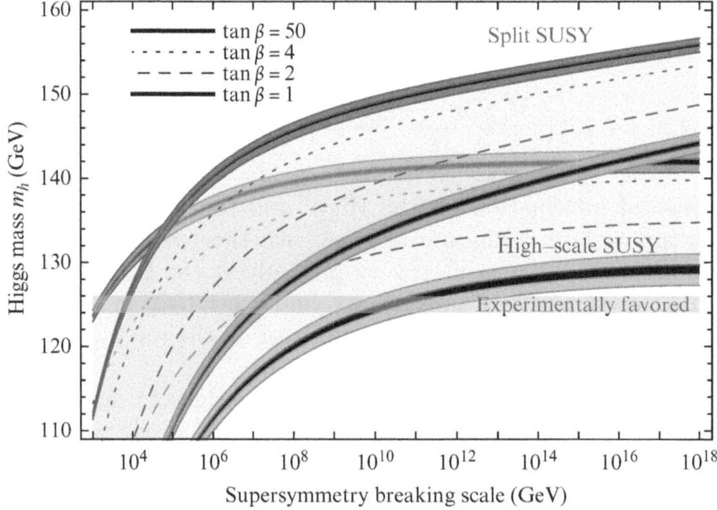

Fig. 9.2 NNLO (next-to-next-to-leading order) prediction for the Higgs mass M_h in high-scale supersymmetry (lower region) and split supersymmetry (upper region) for $\tan\beta = \{1, 2, 4, 50\}$. The thickness of the lower boundary at $\tan\beta = 1$ and of the upper boundary at $\tan\beta = 50$ shows the uncertainty due to the present 1σ error on α_s (dark-coloured band) and on the top quark mass (light-coloured band).

our universe is simply a very generic specimen in the multitude of the multiverse. If you have complained that string theory has made no predictions about our universe, do not rejoice in this. Now the situation may become even worse: the multiverse is making predictions, but about other universes.

What does a Higgs mass of 125–126 GeV tell us about natural theories? A Higgs mass smaller than 120 GeV would have been perfect for natural supersymmetry, while a mass larger than 130 GeV would have excluded the simplest scenarios. If the Higgs mass really is 125 GeV, right in the middle, then it looks like nature wants to tease theoretical physicists. In supersymmetry, a Higgs mass of 125 GeV can be reached— but only for extreme values of the parameters, especially those of the stop squark. Therefore, certain natural setups, where parameters are correlated, are in bad shape (for instance gauge mediation), but the idea of low-energy supersymmetry is not killed. As shown in Fig. 9.2, a Higgs mass of 125 GeV rules out the idea of split supersymmetry with a high scale, say larger than 10^8 GeV. However, it fits very well with split supersymmetry with a low scale. Actually, the simplest model of split supersymmetry, based on anomaly mediation, predicts a hierarchy between scalars and fermions of a one-loop factor and thus looks like a very satisfactory solution.

The indication for a Higgs mass in the range 125–126 GeV is the most exciting result from the LHC so far. It has important consequences for supersymmetry and other theories beyond the SM, but the most puzzling (and surprising) message that we obtained from preliminary LHC data on the Higgs is the apparent near-criticality of the parameters entering the SM Higgs potential.

10
Spontaneous breakdown of local conformal invariance in quantum gravity

Gerard 't HOOFT

Institute for Theoretical Physics and Spinoza Institute, Utrecht University,
Utrecht, The Netherlands

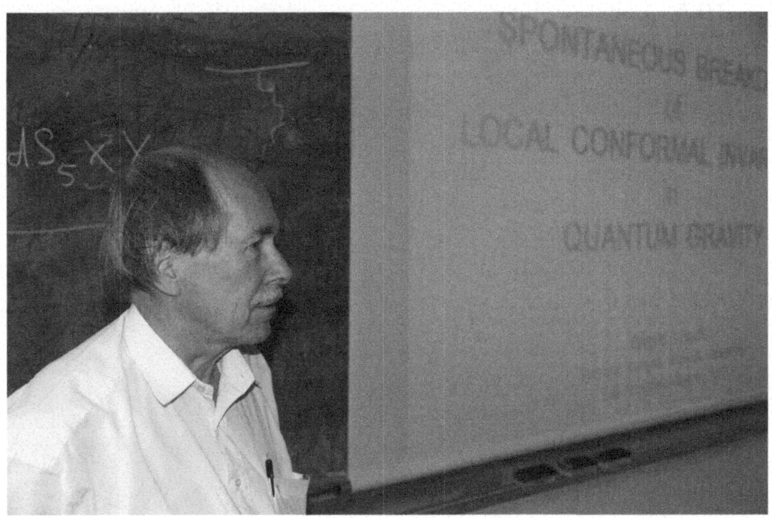

Theoretical Physics to Face the Challenge of LHC. Edited by L. Baulieu, K. Benakli, M. R. Douglas,
B. Mansoulié, E. Rabinovici, and L. F. Cugliandolo. © Oxford University Press 2015.
Published in 2015 by Oxford University Press.

Chapter Contents

10.1 Introductory remarks

This chapter comprises the material discussed in the Les Houches Lectures given by the author in 2011. Part of the text is new, while most of it is based on notes that were sent to the Internet around that time [1, 2]. Some background information is added. We think that the insights obtained here are important and will shed new light on the issues of black hole information, quantum divergences, and symmetry properties of quantum gravity. The key word is local conformal symmetry. Basically, this symmetry has always been there, in a hidden form in canonical quantum gravity, but exploiting it adds interesting twists to what is usually told about the quantum theory of gravity and its divergences.

It is shown that the black hole complementarity principle can be naturally implemented by treating local conformal invariance as an exact, but spontaneously broken, symmetry of quantum gravity. This allows us to describe the black hole either in terms of the imploding particles or entirely in terms of the Hawking particles coming out. These two complementary representations can then be obtained from one another by means of a local conformal transformation—or, in other words, the black hole scattering matrix is equivalent to a local conformal gauge transformation.

Next, one may observe that perturbative canonical quantum gravity, when coupled to a renormalizable model for matter fields, indeed has this conformal symmetry built in, and this symmetry would indeed be exact if the local conformal anomalies were to cancel out. The Einstein–Hilbert action can indeed be regarded as breaking local conformal invariance only dynamically, not explicitly. We show how to disentangle the functional integral over the dilaton component of the metric field from the other integrations over the metric and the matter fields. This turns the remainder of the theory into a trivially conformally invariant system.

When the residual metric is treated as a background, and if this background is taken to be flat, this leads to a novel constraint: in combination with the dilaton contributions, the matter Lagrangian should have a vanishing β function. The zeros of this β function are isolated points in the landscape of quantum field theories, and so we arrive at a denumerable, or perhaps even finite, set of quantum theories for matter, where not only the coupling constants, but also the masses, as well as the cosmological constant, are all fixed, and computable, in terms of the Planck units.

10.2 Conformal symmetry in black holes

It was Hawking's great discovery [3, 4] that, according to quantum field theory placed in a background metric describing a black hole, black holes emit particles with a thermal distribution, where the temperature is given by

$$kT = \frac{1}{8\pi G_N M},\tag{10.1}$$

where k is Boltzmann's constant and G_N is Newton's gravitational constant, and furthermore, $\hbar$ has been normalized to one. This resulted in a an intuitive picture of

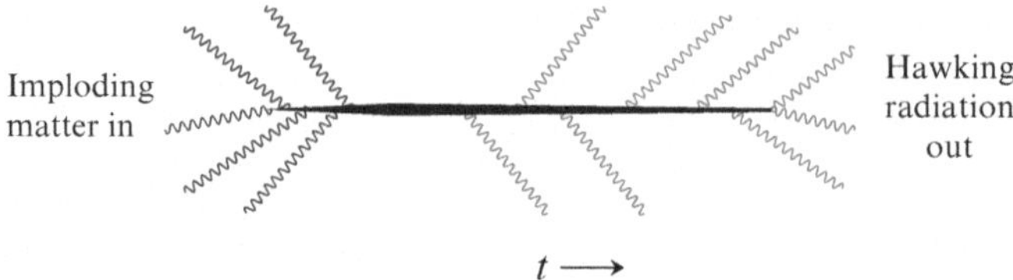

Fig. 10.1 Production and decay of a black hole. Particles enter at the left, while implosion into a black hole takes place, and Hawking particles leave at the right, causing the black hole to end its life in an explosion.

black holes as active, dynamical systems: a black hole on the one hand can be formed by an implosion of material bodies or by heavy collisions of two or more extremely energetic particles, while on the other hand it can decay. In principle, the decay can take place in the same channels as the formation, but in practice the decay is controlled by the laws of statistical physics: every channel is associated with a Boltzmann factor $e^{-E/kT}$, and if the energy E of a state is large while its entropy is small, then decay in that state is strongly suppressed. Figure 10.1 illustrates the situation.

Most descriptions of black holes treat the imploding matter in a way that is very different from the description of the Hawking particles, but what Fig. 10.1 suggests is that one should be able to phrase a theory for black holes that is symmetric under time inversion [5]. Our first step in that direction is to postulate a fundamental principle: the *black hole complementarity* principle [6]. In its most basic form, the principle states the following:

- An observer moving into a black hole can use states inside and outside the black hole to formulate exact rules of the evolution of the entire black hole and its contents.
- An observer outside the black hole can use only the states of the particles outside, but also the particles in the Hawking radiation, to formulate how the evolution of the hole and its surrounding particles proceeds.
- A *mapping* should exist to relate these two complementary descriptions.

A more daring assumption is now added to this:

- *Both observers may use rules that obey the principles of causality and locality.*[1]

Often, this is believed to be impossible, but it is here that we can make progress. Assuming causality and locality means that we can identify light cones, and if any mapping exists between the data of these two different observers, then these light cones must be related. Sets of data that are spacelike-separated as seen by one observer must also be spacelike-separated for the other observer, and the same holds for timelike separations. And so we conclude that our two complementary observers agree about the location of the light cones.

Does this mean that they can both use the same metric tensor $g_{\mu\nu}(\vec{x},t)$? No, because if we write

$$g'_{\mu\nu} = \omega^2(\vec{x},t)\, g_{\mu\nu}, \tag{10.2}$$

then both metrics generate the same light cones. Lightlike vectors x^μ obey $g_{\mu\nu}x^\mu x^\nu = 0$, so factors ω^2 in the metric leave these equations invariant (the square in (10.2) has been put there only for later convenience).

Note that we are not performing further coordinate transformations, so modifications of the metric of the form (10.2) are physically different and nontrivial. Only if ω happened to have the form $C/(x-a)^2$ in flat space would this transformation transform a vacuum into a vacuum; in other cases, spaces with $G_{\mu\nu} = 0$ will transform into spaces with $G_{\mu\nu} \neq 0$. Therefore, particles, and their energy–momentum tensors, are not invariant under such transformations. What we now propose is that these transformations are nevertheless physically significant.

From now on, *local* conformal transformations are defined to be transformations that modify the metric tensor as in (10.2); these do not involve coordinate transformations at all. In contrast, *global* conformal transformations will be defined as an inversion in the spacetime coordinates, with, in addition, possible Poincaré transformations, such that there is an associated local conformal transformation of the form $\omega = C/(x-a)^2$.

In a global conformal transformation, the vacuum is invariant, but for a local one, in general, it is not. We claim that the symmetry (10.2) is *spontaneously broken*, in a way very reminiscent of the Brout–Englert–Higgs mechanism [7].

We also claim that $\omega^2(\vec{x},t)$ is not as easily measurable as one might think. An observer who inspects a region of spacetime might be tempted to use light rays, but then, of course, (s)he measures $g_{\mu\nu}(\vec{x},t)$ *modulo* factors $\omega^2(\vec{x},t)$. Then, one might say, well, let us measure $\omega^2(\vec{x},t)$ by using clocks and measuring rods; these do depend on $\omega^2(\vec{x},t)$. The problem with that, however, is that if we have a vacuum, then this may be well defined, but if we assume that we may be sitting inside a dense medium, then clocks and measuring rods may be strongly affected by the medium in ways that are difficult to control. Once we *know* that we are in a vacuum—but how do we know this?—we can use light signals and leave our clocks and measuring rods at infinity. Well, indeed, if they are at infinity, and we have measured a (more or less) flat $g_{\mu\nu}$, assuming that we are close to a vacuum state, then singular factors C/x^2 can be excluded, and then our measurement becomes unambiguous. As soon as we drop the information that we are close to a vacuum, we lose control over $\omega^2(\vec{x},t)$.

Our two complementary observers may indeed use different values of $\omega^2(\vec{x},t)$ for their description of spacetime. They are not both surrounded by a state that they would call a vacuum, and this may be the cause of a possible disagreement. A slowly decaying black hole may be described by a metric

$$ds^2 = M^2(\tilde{t})\Big(-(1-2/r)\,dt^2 + \frac{dr^2}{1-2/r} + r^2\,d\Omega^2 \Big), \tag{10.3}$$

where $d\Omega$ stands for the angular component, and r and t are scaled by factors $M(\tilde{t})$; the time variable $\tilde{t}$ may be set equal to t or either the advanced or the retarded time variable. Since the mass M varies only very slowly with time, this makes little difference, as the time differences grow only logarithmically with the separation from the horizon. Now, the observer traveling into a black hole at time $t = t_0$ will only see $M(t_0)$, while the outside observer will see him squeezed against the horizon, slowly shrinking to a vanishing size. This is a big disagreement! Clearly, the disagreement can be restricted to a conformal factor $\omega = M(\tilde{t})/M(t_0)$.

The conventional view of what happens at a black hole [8] is illustrated in Fig. 10.2(a). For simplicity, the imploding matter is assumed to be in the form of a thin imploding spherical shell, for which case Einstein's equations are easily solved exactly. The region from which no escape is possible is shaded. Hawking particles are generated near the event horizon. *All* Hawking particles seem to originate from a spot that can be recovered by solving the field equations backward in time. This gives the geometric shape of the "cradle of Hawking's radiation" in the form of a caustic. Only in the case of ideal spherical symmetry is this caustic just a single point.

If we want a time-reversal-symmetric picture, we should include the backreaction of this Hawking radiation. Often, investigators try to argue that this backreaction is absent[9–11], but this is only according to the view of an observer falling into the

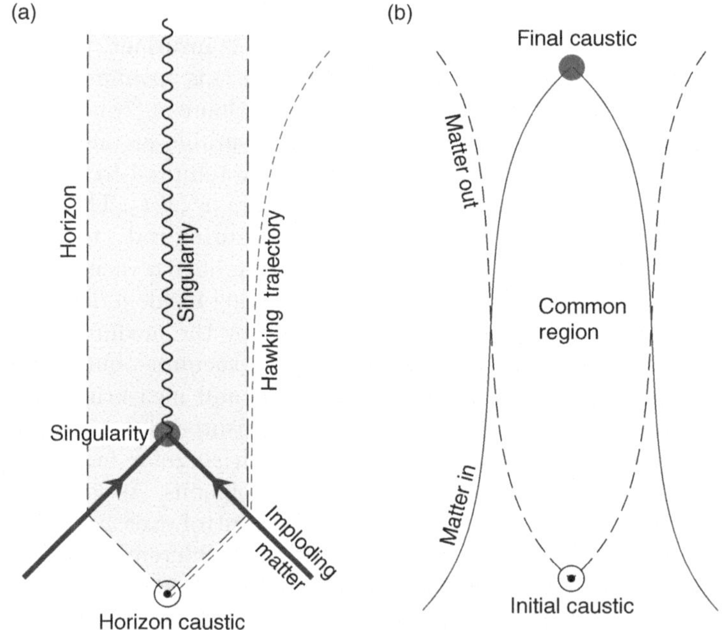

Fig. 10.2 (a) Conventional spacetime picture of a black hole formed by imploding matter. (b) Conformal picture, obtained by stretching the previous picture. Information entering the "common region" may seem to emerge conformally transformed to near the Planck scale, close to the "final caustic." In reality, it is believed, this information leaves the hole much earlier with the Hawking particles.

hole. External observers, of course, do notice the backreaction, simply by noting that the black hole shrinks. This difference, due to the fact that the two observers do not agree about the vacuum state, allows us to draw a time-reversal-symmetric picture as perceived by an outside observer.

Thus, the time-reversal-invariant picture that emerges is as illustrated in Fig. 10.2(b). Here, the lightlike geodesics that all complementary observers agree about are sketched for a black hole that decays in a short amount of time (for macroscopic black holes, the picture must be stretched very far in the time direction). Two things have changed in this second picture. One, the outside observer is given the option either to consider the outgoing matter as visible or invisible Hawking radiation or to consider ingoing matter as visible or invisible Hawking radiation. We postulate that the light cones in all these options remain the same. Since in the standard picture in Fig. 10.2(a), Hawking radiation, optically, appears to originate in a regular region of spacetime, the same must be true for the ingoing matter in the time-reversed picture. Therefore, in that picture, what used to be the onset of a singularity must somehow have been transformed into a regular region of spacetime as well. This regular region has also been transformed into a very tiny region; $\omega(\vec{x}, t)$ there is very small. Note that $M(\tilde{t})$ reached the value zero.

Therefore, the second thing that must have happened here is a local conformal transformation. The singularity has been transformed to be reduced to infinitesimal size. The local conformal transformation is particularly dramatic in an idealized situation sketched in Fig. 10.3. Here, we have taken a special case where the Hawking radiation is emitted in a single shell of matter. Although the probability for this is suppressed by a huge Boltzmann factor, it is not zero, and therefore it is legitimate to consider the transition amplitude from a collapsing shell to an expanding shell of Hawking matter. The light cones then have an internal region in common that is

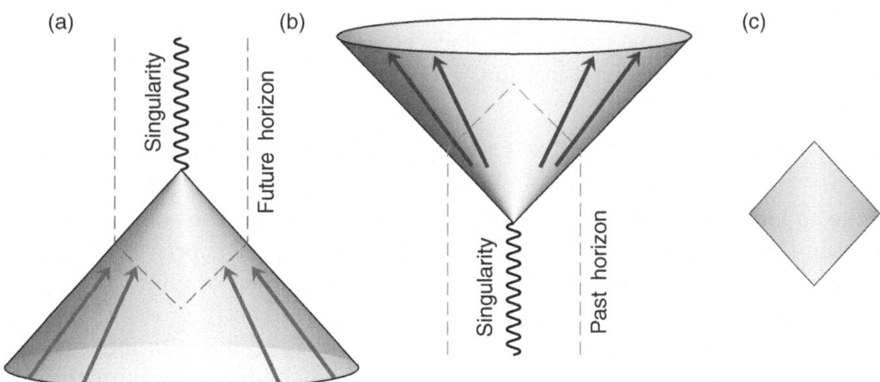

Fig. 10.3 (a) The in-configuration of a black hole. (b) The out-configuration. Dashed lines are the horizons in both pictures. In this case, the ingoing matter and the outgoing matter form a single shell; there is a region at the center that both pictures seem to have in common (c).

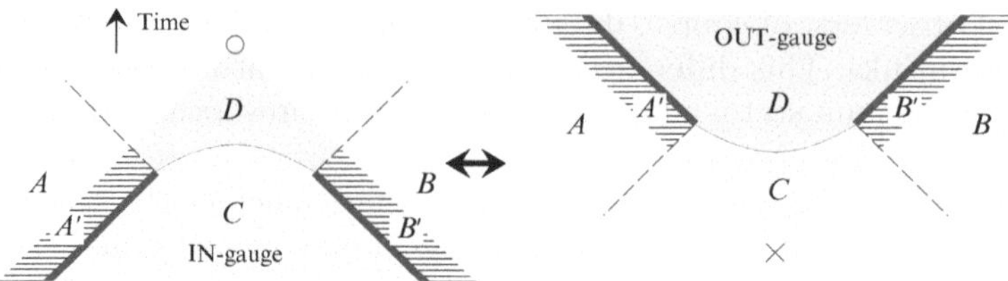

Fig. 10.4 Conformal transformation of the inside region of an imploding black hole ("IN-gauge") to the inside region of an exploding black hole ("OUT-gauge"). The letters show how the various regions are mapped. See text.

vacuum both for the conventional ingoing observer and for an observer who only sees the radiation coming out.

The only conformal transformation that can do the job here is the inversion; see Fig. 10.4. The circle at the left is mapped to the point $t \to \infty$ at the right; the cross at the right is mapped to the point $t \to -\infty$ at the left.

In this figure, the complementary pictures are referred to as the IN-gauge and the OUT-gauge. What this means is that the conformal factor $\omega^2(\vec{x}, t)$ is chosen such that in the IN-gauge, the component T^{++} of the matter energy–momentum tensor is chosen to vanish (ω^2 is then such that $G^{++} = 0$), and in the OUT-gauge, $T^{--} = 0$. Indeed, these are gauge conditions on $\omega(\vec{x}, t)$; the black hole S-matrix is thus seen to coincide with a matrix representing a gauge transformation for the conformal factor. See further Section 10.3.

The letters in the figure show how the various regions are mapped. Regions A and B are not transformed; here, $\omega = 1$. Region $C + D$ is conformally inverted; Eq. (10.4). In the IN-gauge, the backreaction of the ingoing particles, the thick solid lines, is seen to work on the metric. Hawking particles are the dashed lines. In the time-reversed picture, only the outgoing particles are seen to have an effect on the metric; the imploding matter that gave rise to the black hole has now been plutoed to the status of Hawking radiation—reversed in time. The conformal inversion in region $C + D$ is

$$x_{\mathrm{in}}^{\mu} = (-1)^{\delta^{\mu o}} \frac{\varrho^2 x_{\mathrm{out}}^{\mu}}{|(x_{\mathrm{out}})^2|}, \tag{10.4}$$

where the square is of course the Lorentz-invariant square of the coordinate x_{out}. We have chosen the sign here such that the timelike causal order is preserved. All vectors in the relevant region are timelike with respect to the chosen origin.

Figure 10.4 shows the in- and outgoing matter not exactly crossing the singular points of the mapping (the circle and the cross). This is to indicate more clearly the effect of the conformal transformation. In reality, the shaded regions in the picture, regions A' and B', are to be squeezed to become infinitesimally thin, so that the bulk of the matter indeed reaches these singularities; but then the conformal transformation is seen to become highly singular. This is indeed what we expect to be the case; the shells of matter are very close to the shells $x^2 = 0$, which implies that the coefficient ϱ is very small, close to the Planck scale.

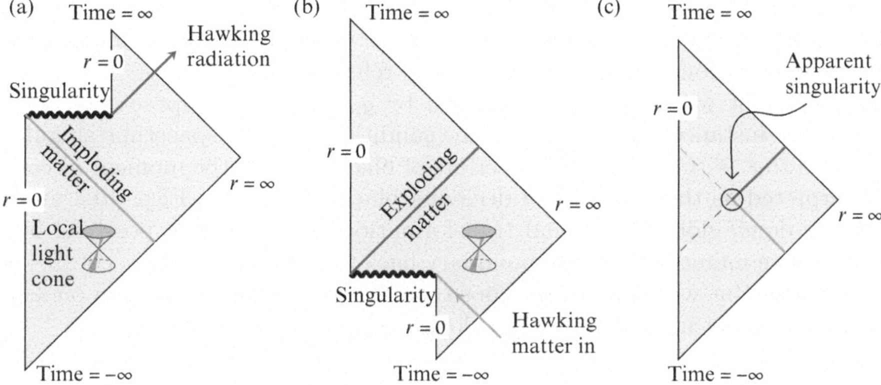

Fig. 10.5 (a) Conventional Penrose diagram for a decaying black hole. (b) Its timereverse. (c) The new Penrose diagram for a decaying black hole is the same as that for Minkowski spacetime. The singularity at the center is only there as seen by a distant observer. Local observers can remove it by choosing appropriate local conformal transformations.

We see *cosmic censorship* [11, 12] at work. In terms of the conventional metric $g_{\mu\nu}$, any naked singularity is hidden behind a horizon. Then, whenever we encounter such a singularity, we can adjust ω in Eq. (10.2) in such a way that a clock shows infinite time when approaching this singularity. Therefore, it now occurs at $t = \infty$. In practical examples, when we apply local conformal transformations, the singularity will also be smeared out so that it effectively disappears, and furthermore also the horizon disappears, as we see in Fig. 10.4.

The *Penrose diagram* [13] for a black hole is usually sketched [8] as shown in Fig. 10.5(a). Its time-reversed form would be as in Fig. 10.5(b). Note, that now, by using conformal transformations, we can replace both of them by the trivial Penrose diagram, that of flat Minkowski spacetime, Fig. 10.5(c). To obtain this Penrose diagram, a nearly singular function $\omega(\vec{x}, t)$ had to be invoked. As we shall see later, such transformations generate highly peaked expressions for the Ricci scalar (which is not conformally invariant). This means that the outside observer decides that some violent explosion took place at the horizon, generating a very large $T^{\mu}_{\ \mu}$ at that point. The local observer, using a different $\omega(\vec{x}, t)$, sees no such singular behavior. We return to this topic in the next section.

10.3 Local conformal invariance and the stress–energy–momentum tensor

The above considerations suggest that the scale factor $\omega(x)$ is ambiguous, yet it is needed to describe clocks and rulers in the macroscopic world, and it is also needed if we wish to compute the Riemann and Ricci curvatures, because they depend on the entire metric $g_{\mu\nu}$, not just $\hat{g}_{\mu\nu}$. Clearly, the world that is familiar to us is not scale-invariant. Without ω, we cannot define distances and we cannot define matter, but we can define the geometry of the light cones, and, if $\hat{g}_{\mu\nu}$ is nontrivial, it should describe some of the physical phenomena that are taking place. It should be possible to write down equations for it without directly referring to ω.

To what extent will $\omega(x)$ be determined by $\hat{g}_{\mu\nu}(x)$, if we impose some physical conditions? For instance, we can impose the condition that the spacetime singularities are all moved to $t \to \infty$, so that the interiors of black holes at the moment of collapse, are re-interpreted as the exteriors of decaying black holes, as in Figs. 10.3 and 10.4. After that is done, global conformal transformations are no longer possible, because they would move infinities from the boundary back to finite points in spacetime, which we do not allow. But we do wish to impose some extra "gauge" condition on $\omega(x)$, to fix its value, allowing us to define what clocks, rulers, and matter are.

A natural thing to impose is that all particles appear to be as light as possible. If we had only noninteracting, massless particles, then $T^\mu_\mu = 0$. Therefore, let us start with what seems to be a natural gauge to choose: the vanishing of the induced Ricci scalar:

$$R(\omega^2 \hat{g}_{\mu\nu}) = 0. \tag{10.5}$$

When $\hat{g}_{\mu\nu}(x)$ is given, we can compute (in four spacetime dimensions)

$$R_{\mu\nu} = \hat{R}_{\mu\nu} + \omega^{-2}(4\,\partial_\mu\omega\,\partial_\nu\omega - \hat{g}_{\mu\nu}\hat{g}^{\alpha\beta}\,\partial_\alpha\omega\,\partial_\beta\omega)$$

$$+ \omega^{-1}(-2D_\mu\,\partial_\nu\omega - \hat{g}_{\mu\nu}\hat{g}^{\alpha\beta}D_\alpha\,\partial_\beta\omega), \tag{10.6}$$

$$\omega^2 R = \hat{R} - 6\,\omega^{-1}\hat{g}^{\mu\nu}D_\mu\partial_\nu\omega. \tag{10.7}$$

Here, we write $R_{\mu\nu}(\omega^2\hat{g}_{\mu\nu}) = R_{\mu\nu}$ and $R_{\mu\nu}(\hat{g}_{\mu\nu}) = \hat{R}_{\mu\nu}$, and similarly for the Ricci scalars. The covariant derivative D_μ treats the field ω as a scalar with respect to the metric $\hat{g}_{\mu\nu}$.

The condition that (10.7) vanishes gives us the equation

$$\hat{g}^{\mu\nu}D_\mu\partial_\nu\omega(x) = \frac{1}{6}\hat{R}\,\omega(x). \tag{10.8}$$

This happens to be a linear equation for $\omega(x)$, which is the reason for having included the square in its definition, in (10.2), since ω is not restricted to be infinitesimal.

Now let $\omega(x)$ obey (10.8) in a region where $\hat{g}_{\mu\nu} = \eta_{\mu\nu}$, so that $\hat{R} = 0$, and consider the Fourier transform $\omega(k)$ of $\omega(x)$, which, at $k \neq 0$, we now take to be infinitesimal. The wavevector k obeys $k^2 = 0$. Let this wavevector be in the $+$ direction. Then, according to (10.6), the only nonvanishing component of the Ricci tensor, and hence also the only nonvanishing component of the stress–energy–momentum tensor, is the $++$ component. Thus, we have shells of massless particles traveling in the x^- direction. Adding all possible Fourier components, we see that in the infinitesimal case, our transition to nontrivial $\omega(x)$ values leads us from the vacuum configuration to the case that massless particles are flying around. As long as $\omega(k)$ at $k \neq 0$ stays infinitesimal, these massless particles are noninteracting.

In the case of an evaporating black hole, these massless particles are the Hawking particles. Our complementarity transformation, the transformation that modifies the values of $\omega(x)$ while keeping (10.8) valid, switches on and off the effects these Hawking particles have on the metric.[1]

Often, it will seem to be more convenient to impose that we have flat spacetime, i.e., $\omega^2 \hat{g}_{\mu\nu} = \eta_{\mu\nu}$ at infinity, rather than imposing $R = 0$ everywhere. In the case of an implosion followed by an evaporating black hole (for simplicity emitting a single shell of matter as in Section 10.2), this would allow us to glue the different conformal regions together, to obtain Fig. 10.6. This then gives us a region of large Ricci scalar curvature near the horizon. Ricci scalar curvature is associated with a large burst of pressure in the matter stress–energy–momentum tensor. This means that an observer who uses this frame sees a large explosion near the horizon that sends the ingoing material back out; that is, the black hole explodes classically. The *local* observer would be wondering what causes this "unnatural" explosion, which, at the very last moment, avoided the formation of a permanent black hole; in our theory, however, the local observer would see no reason to use this function ω, so she would not notice any causality violation. Only the distant, outside observer would use this ω, concluding that, indeed, the black hole is not an eternal one, since it evaporates.

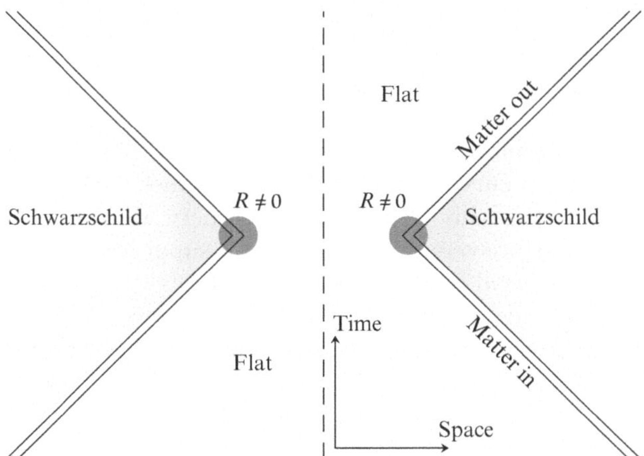

Fig. 10.6 Combining the different conformal frames into one metric for the imploding and subsequently evaporating black hole gives us a region of large Ricci scalar values R near the horizon (here, the two circles). Note that the metric outside the collapsing and evaporating shells is Schwarzschild, while inside the shells it is flat. Demanding ω to be continuous across the shells implies that the r coordinate should be matched there (see [16]).

---

[1] It is often claimed that Hawking particles have little or no effect on the stress–energy–momentum operator on the horizon [9, 10]. This, however, is true only for the expectation values in the states used by the ingoing observer (the Hartle–Hawking states). The outgoing observer uses Boulware states, for which the $T_{\mu\nu}$ diverges [14, 15].

The metric described in Fig. 10.6 is related to the metrics described in [16]. In that paper, care was taken that no conical singularity should arise when ingoing and outgoing shells meet. Here, we do allow this singularity, interpreting it as a region of large R values, which we now demand not to be locally observable.

10.4 Local conformal symmetry in canonical quantum gravity

The Einstein–Hilbert action of the generally covariant theory of gravity reads

$$S^{\text{total}} = \int \mathrm{d}^4 x \sqrt{-g} \left(\frac{1}{16\pi G_N} R + \mathcal{L}^{\text{mat}} \right), \tag{10.9}$$

where the matter lagrangian $\mathcal{L}^{\text{mat}}$ is written in a generally covariant manner using the spacetime metric $g_{\mu\nu}(x)$. In this section, we begin studying the case where $\mathcal{L}^{\text{mat}}$ is globally conformally symmetric, which means that under a spacetime transformation

$$x^{\mu\prime} = C \frac{x^\mu - a^\mu}{(x - a)^2} + b^\mu, \tag{10.10}$$

we have a transformation law for the matter fields such that

$$g_{\mu\nu}(x') = \lambda(x)^2 g_{\mu\nu}(x), \qquad \sqrt{-g(x')}\, \mathcal{L}^{\text{mat}\prime}(x') = \sqrt{-g(x)}\, \mathcal{L}^{\text{mat}}(x), \tag{10.11}$$
$$S^{\text{mat}\prime} = S^{\text{mat}},$$

so that in n dimensions, $\qquad \mathcal{L}^{\text{mat}\prime}(x') = \lambda^n\, \mathcal{L}^{\text{mat}}(x). \tag{10.12}$

For the conformal transformation (10.10) we have $\lambda(x) = C/(x^\mu - a^\mu)^2$, which leaves flat spacetime flat, but for curved background spacetimes, where we drop the condition of flatness, $\lambda(x)$ may be any function of x^μ. There are several examples of such conformally invariant matter systems such as $\mathcal{N} = 4$ super Yang–Mills theory in $n = 4$ spacetime dimensions. We will concentrate on $n = 4$.

We begin by temporarily assuming conformal invariance of the matter fields, only for convenience; later we will see that allowing matter fields to be more general will only slightly modify the picture.

In canonical gravity, the quantum amplitudes are obtained by functionally integrating the exponent of the entire action over all components of the metric tensor at all spacetime points x^μ:

$$\Gamma = \int \mathcal{D}g_{\mu\nu}(x)\, \mathcal{D}\varphi^{\text{mat}}(x)\, e^{iS^{\text{total}}}. \tag{10.13}$$

Although one usually imposes a gauge constraint to reduce the size of function space, this is not formally necessary. In particular, one has to integrate over the common factor $\omega(x)$ of the metric tensor $g_{\mu\nu}(x)$, when we write

$$g_{\mu\nu}(x) \stackrel{\text{def}}{=} \omega^2(x)\, \hat{g}_{\mu\nu}(x), \tag{10.14}$$

where $\hat{g}_{\mu\nu}(x)$ may be subject to some arbitrary constraint concerning its overall factor. For instance, in any coordinate frame, one may impose

$$\det(\hat{g}) = -1, \tag{10.15}$$

besides imposing a gauge condition for each of the $n = 4$ coordinates. The quantity $\hat{g}_{\mu\nu}(x)$ in (10.15) does not transform as an ordinary tensor but as what could be called a "pseudo" tensor, meaning that it scales unconventionally under coordinate transformations with a nontrivial Jacobian. $\omega(x)$ is then a "pseudo" scalar.

The prefix "pseudo" was put in quotation marks here because, usually, *pseudo* means that the object receives an extra minus sign under a parity transformation; it is therefore preferred to use another phrase. For this reason, we replace "pseudo" by *meta*, using the words *metatensor* and *metascalar* to indicate fields that transform as tensors or scalars, but with prefactors containing unconventional powers of the Jacobian of the coordinate transformation.

Rewriting

$$\int \mathcal{D}g_{\mu\nu}(x) = \int \mathcal{D}\omega(x) \int \mathcal{D}\hat{g}_{\mu\nu}(x), \tag{10.16}$$

while imposing a gauge constraint[2] that *only* depends on $\hat{g}_{\mu\nu}$, not on ω, one may consider *first* to integrate over $\omega(x)$ and then over $\hat{g}_{\mu\nu}(x)$ and $\varphi^{\,\mathrm{mat}}(x)$. This has peculiar consequences, as we will see.

In the standard perturbation expansion, the integration order does not matter. Also, if dimensional regularization is employed, the choice of the functional metric in the space of all fields $\omega(x)$ and $\hat{g}_{\mu\nu}(x)$ is unambiguous, since its effects are canceled against all other quartic divergences in the amplitudes (any ambiguity is represented by integrals of the form $\int \mathrm{d}^n k \, \mathrm{Pol}(k)$ that vanish when dimensionally renormalized). $\omega(x)$ acts as a Lagrange multiplier. Again, perturbation expansion tells us how to handle this integral: in general, $\omega(x)$ has to be chosen to lie on a complex contour. The momentum integrations may be carried out in Euclidean (Wick-rotated) spacetime, but, even then, $\omega(x)$ must be integrated along a complex contour, which will later (see Section 10.10) be determined to be

$$\omega(x) = 1 + i\alpha(x), \qquad \alpha \text{ real.} \tag{10.17}$$

If $\omega(x)$ itself had been chosen real, then the Wick-rotated functional integral would diverge exponentially, so that ω would no longer function properly as a Lagrange multiplier.

If there had been no further divergences, one would have expected the following scenario:

- The functional integrand $\omega(x)$ only occurs in the gravitational part of the action, since the matter field is conformally invariant (nonconformal matter does contribute to this integral, but these would be subdominating corrections; see later).

---

[2] A fine choice would be, for instance, $\partial_\mu \hat{g}^{\mu\nu} = 0$. Of course, the usual Faddeev–Popov quantization procedure is assumed.

- After integrating over all scale functions $\omega(x)$, but not yet over $\hat{g}_{\mu\nu}$, the resulting effective action in terms of $\hat{g}_{\mu\nu}$ should be expected to become scale-invariant; i.e. if we were to split $\hat{g}_{\mu\nu}$ again as in (10.14),

$$\hat{g}_{\mu\nu}(x) \stackrel{?}{=} \hat{\omega}^2(x)\hat{\hat{g}}_{\mu\nu}, \tag{10.18}$$

  no further dependence on $\hat{\omega}(x)$ should be expected.
- Therefore, the effective action should now describe a conformally invariant theory, both for gravity and for matter. Because of this, the effective theory might be expected to be renormalizable, or even finite! If any infinities do remain, one might again employ dimensional renormalization to remove them.

However, this expectation is jeopardized by an apparent difficulty: the ω integration is indeed ultraviolet-divergent [17]. In contrast to the usual procedures in perturbation theories, it is not associated with an infinitesimal multiplicative constant (such as the coupling constant in ordinary perturbation theories), and so a renormalization counterterm would actually represent an infinite distortion of the canonical theory. Clearly, renormalization must be carried out with much more care. Later, in Section 10.6, we suggest various scenarios.

First, the main calculation will be carried out, in Section 10.5. Then, the contributions from conformal matter fields are considered, and subsequently the effect of nonconformal matter, by adding mass terms. Finally, we will be in a position to ask questions about renormalization (dimensional or otherwise), and the constraints they may impose on the matter field interactions. We end with some concluding remarks.

In conventional canonical quantum gravity, one may split up the quantum gravity functional integral into an integral over the conformally invariant metric $\hat{g}_{\mu\nu}$ and an integral over the conformal factor $\omega(\vec{x}, t)$. Calculations related to the conformal term in gravity, and their associated anomalies, date back from the early 1970s and have been reviewed, for example, in a nice paper by Duff [18]. In particular, we here focus on footnote 4 in that paper.

First, we go to n spacetime dimensions, in order later to be able to perform dimensional renormalization. For future convenience (see (10.20)), we choose to then replace the parameter ω by $\omega^{2/(n-2)}$, so that (10.14) becomes

$$g_{\mu\nu}(x) = \omega^{4/(n-2)} \, \hat{g}_{\mu\nu}(x). \tag{10.19}$$

In terms of $\hat{g}_{\mu\nu}$ and ω, the Einstein–Hilbert action (10.9) now reads

$$S = \int \mathrm{d}^n x \, \sqrt{-\hat{g}} \left[\frac{1}{16\pi G_N} \left(\omega^2 \hat{R} + \frac{4(n-1)}{n-2} \, \hat{g}^{\mu\nu} \partial_\mu \omega \, \partial_\nu \omega \right) + \mathcal{L}^{\mathrm{mat}}(\hat{g}_{\mu\nu}) \right]. \tag{10.20}$$

This shows that the functional integral over the field $\omega(x)$ is a Gaussian one, which can be performed rigorously: it is a determinant. The conformally invariant matter Lagrangian is independent of ω, although we shall later consider mass terms for matter (this would still allow us to do the functional integral over ω, but for now we wish to avoid the associated complications, assuming that, perhaps, at scales close to the Planck scale the ω dependence of matter might dwindle).

We use the caret ($\hat{\ }$) to indicate all expressions defined by the metatensor $\hat{g}_{\mu\nu}$, such as covariant derivatives, as if it were a true tensor.

Note that, in "Euclidean gravity," the ω integrand has the wrong sign. This is why ω must be chosen to be on the contour (10.17). In practice, it is easiest to do the functional ω integration perturbatively, by writing

$$\hat{g}_{\mu\nu}(x) = \eta_{\mu\nu} + \kappa\, h_{\mu\nu}(x), \qquad \eta_{\mu\nu} = \mathrm{diag}(-1,1,1,1), \qquad \kappa = \sqrt{8\pi G_N}, \qquad (10.21)$$

and expanding in powers of κ (although later we will see that that expansion can sometimes be summed). A factor $\sqrt{-\hat{g}}\, 8(n-1)/16\pi G_N(n-2)$ in (10.20) can be absorbed in the definition of ω.[3] This turns the action (10.20) into

$$S = \int \mathrm{d}^n x \sqrt{-\hat{g}} \left(\tfrac{1}{2}\, \hat{g}^{\mu\nu} \partial_\mu \omega \partial_\nu \omega + \tfrac{1}{2}\, \frac{n-2}{4(n-1)} \hat{R} \omega^2 + \mathcal{L}^{\,\mathrm{mat}}(\hat{g}_{\mu\nu}) \right). \qquad (10.22)$$

Regardless of the ω contour, the ω propagator can be read off from the action (10.22):

$$P^{(\omega)}(k) = -\,\frac{1}{k^2 - i\varepsilon}, \qquad (10.23)$$

where k_μ is the momentum. The $i\varepsilon$ prescription is the one that follows from the conventional perturbative theory. We see that there is a kinetic term (perturbed by a possible nontrivial spacetime dependence of $\hat{g}_{\mu\nu}$), and a direct interaction, "mass" term proportional to the background scalar curvature $\hat{R}$:

$$\frac{n-2}{4(n-1)}\hat{R} \quad \xrightarrow{n\to 4} \quad \frac{1}{6}\hat{R}, \qquad (10.24)$$

The most important diagrams contributing to the effective action for the remaining field $\hat{g}_{\mu\nu}$ are those indicated in Fig. 10.7, which include the terms up to $\mathcal{O}(\kappa^2)$. The "tadpole" (Fig. 10.7(a)), does not contribute if we apply dimensional regularization, since there is no mass term in the single propagator that we have, (10.23). So, in this approximation, we have to deal with the 2-point diagram only.

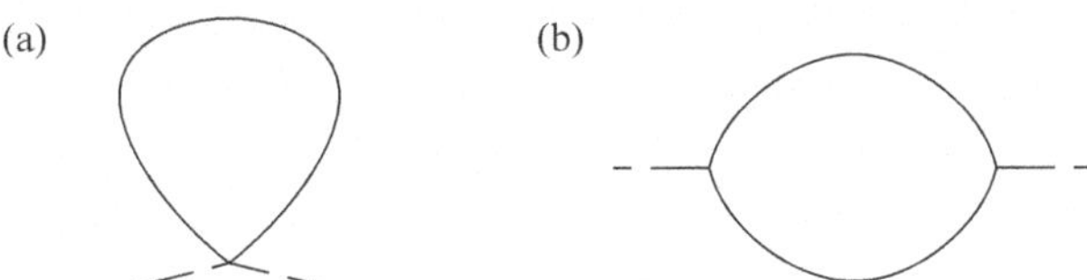

Fig. 10.7 Feynman diagrams for the ω determinant.

---

[3] Note that, therefore, Newton's constant disappears completely (its use in (10.21) is inessential). This a characteristic feature of this approach.

We can compute the integral

$$F(q) \stackrel{\text{def}}{=} \int_{\text{Eucl}} \frac{d^n k}{k^2 (k-q)^2} = \frac{\pi^{\frac{1}{2}n+\frac{3}{2}} 2^{3-n} (q^2)^{\frac{1}{2}n-2}}{\Gamma(\frac{1}{2}n - \frac{1}{2}) \sin \pi(2 - \frac{1}{2}n)}. \tag{10.25}$$

Now we will also need integrals containing extra factors k_μ in the numerator. Therefore, we define

$$\langle k \cdots k \rangle \stackrel{\text{def}}{=} \frac{1}{F(q)} \int_{\text{Eucl}} \frac{d^n k \; k \cdots k}{k^2 (k-q)^2}. \tag{10.26}$$

Then,

$$\langle k_\mu \rangle = \frac{1}{2} q_\mu, \tag{10.27}$$

$$\langle k_\mu k_\nu \rangle = \frac{1}{4(n-1)} (n q_\mu q_\nu - q^2 \delta_{\mu\nu}), \tag{10.28}$$

$$\langle k_\mu k_\nu k_\lambda \rangle = \frac{1}{8(n-1)} \left[(n+2) q_\mu q_\nu q_\lambda - q^2 (\delta_{\mu\nu} q_\lambda + \delta_{\nu\lambda} q_\mu + \delta_{\lambda\mu} q_\nu) \right], \tag{10.29}$$

$$\begin{aligned}
\langle k_\mu k_\nu k_\alpha k_\beta \rangle = \frac{1}{16(n-1)(n+1)} \big[&(n+2)(n+4)\, q_\mu q_\nu q_\alpha q_\beta \\
&- q^2 (n+2)(\delta_{\mu\nu} q_\alpha q_\beta + \text{five terms}) \\
&+ q^4 (\delta_{\mu\nu} \delta_{\alpha\beta} + \delta_{\mu\alpha} \delta_{\nu\beta} + \delta_{\mu\beta} \delta_{\nu\alpha}) \big],
\end{aligned} \tag{10.30}$$

where the five terms are simply the remaining five permutations of the previous term.

These expressions can now be used to compute all diagrams that contribute to the ω determinant, but the calculations are lengthy and not very illuminating. More important are those parts that diverge as $n \to 4$. The expression (10.25) for $F(q)$ diverges at $n \to 4$, so that all integrals in (10.26) diverge similarly. By using general covariance, one can deduce right away that the divergent terms must all combine in such a way that they depend only on the Riemann curvature. Dimensional arguments then suffice to conclude that the coefficients must be local expressions in the squares of the curvature.

The key calculations for the divergent parts were performed in 1973 [19]. There, it was found that a Lagrangian of the form

$$\mathcal{L} = \sqrt{-g} \left[-\tfrac{1}{2} g^{\mu\nu}(x)\, \partial_\mu \varphi \partial_\nu \varphi + \tfrac{1}{2} M(x)\, \varphi^2 \right] \tag{10.31}$$

will generate an effective action, whose divergent part is of the form

$$S^{\text{div}} = \int d^n x \, \Gamma^{\text{div}}(x), \qquad \Gamma^{\text{div}} = \frac{\sqrt{-g}}{8\pi^2 (4-n)} \left[\tfrac{1}{120}(R_{\mu\nu} R^{\mu\nu} - \tfrac{1}{3} R^2) + \tfrac{1}{4}(M + \tfrac{1}{6} R)^2 \right] \tag{10.32}$$

(we use here a slightly modified notation, implying, among others, a sign switch in the definition of the Ricci curvature, and a minus sign as [19] calculated the Lagrangian $\mathcal{L} + \Delta\mathcal{L}$, $\Delta\mathcal{L} = -\Gamma^{\text{div}}$ needed to obtain a finite theory).

In our case, we see that, in the Lagrangian (10.22) (with the dynamical part of ω imaginary),

$$M = -\frac{1}{6}\hat{R}, \qquad \Gamma^{\text{div}} = \frac{\sqrt{-\hat{g}}}{960\pi^2(4-n)}\left(\hat{R}_{\mu\nu}\hat{R}^{\mu\nu} - \frac{1}{3}\hat{R}^2\right), \tag{10.33}$$

since the second term in (10.32) cancels out exactly. Indeed, it had to cancel out, as we will see shortly.

To see what the divergence here means, we use the fact that the mass dependence of a divergent integral typically takes the form

$$C(n)m^{n-4}\Gamma(2 - \tfrac{1}{2}n) \to \frac{C}{4-n}\left[1 + (n-4)\log\left(\frac{m}{\Lambda}\right)\right] \to C\left(\log\Lambda + \frac{1}{4-n}\right) + \text{ finite},$$

where m stands for a mass or an external momentum k, and Λ is some reference mass, such as an ultraviolet cutoff. Thus, the divergent expression $1/(4-n)$ generally plays the same role as the logarithm of an ultraviolet cutoff Λ.

10.5 Local conformal invariance and the Weyl curvature

We consider an effective theory that not only has general covariance,

$$\hat{g}_{\mu\nu} \to \hat{g}_{\mu\nu} + \hat{D}_\mu u_\nu + \hat{D}_\nu u_\mu, \tag{10.34}$$

where $u_\mu(x)$ are the generators of infinitesimal coordinate transformations and $\hat{D}_\mu$ is the covariant derivative with respect to $\hat{g}_{\mu\nu}$, but now also has a new kind of gauge invariance, namely, local conformal invariance, which we write in infinitesimal notation, for convenience:

$$\hat{g}_{\mu\nu} \to \hat{g}_{\mu\nu} + \lambda(x)\hat{g}_{\mu\nu}. \tag{10.35}$$

Note that this transformation is quite distinct from scale transformations in the coordinate frame, which of course belong to (10.34) and as such are always an invariance of the usual theory. In short, we now have a theory with a five-dimensional local gauge group. Theories of this sort have been studied in detail [20, 21].

The Riemann tensor $\hat{R}^\alpha{}_{\beta\mu\nu}$ transforms as a decent tensor under the coordinate transformations (10.34), but it is not invariant (or even covariant) under the local scale transformation (10.35). Now, in four spacetime dimensions, we can split up the 20 independent components of the Riemann tensor into the 10-component Ricci tensor

$$\hat{R}_{\mu\nu} = \hat{R}^\alpha{}_{\mu\alpha\nu} \tag{10.36}$$

and the components orthogonal to that, called the Weyl tensor [13, 22],

$$\begin{aligned}
\hat{W}_{\mu\nu\alpha\beta} = {}& \hat{R}_{\mu\nu\alpha\beta} \\
& + \frac{1}{2}\left(-g_{\mu\alpha}\hat{R}_{\nu\beta} + g_{\mu\beta}\hat{R}_{\nu\alpha} + g_{\nu\alpha}\hat{R}_{\mu\beta} - g_{\nu\beta}\hat{R}_{\mu\alpha}\right) \\
& + \frac{1}{6}(g_{\mu\alpha}g_{\nu\beta} - g_{\nu\alpha}g_{\mu\beta})\hat{R},
\end{aligned} \tag{10.37}$$

which has the remaining 10 independent components. The Weyl tensor has been defined in such a way that it is traceless in every respect; all contractions of two indices yield zero.

The transformation rules under coordinate transformations, (10.34), are as usual; all these curvature fields transform as tensors. To see how they transform under (10.35), first note how the connection fields transform:

$$\hat{\Gamma}_{\alpha\mu\nu} \to (1+\lambda)\hat{\Gamma}_{\alpha\mu\nu} + \tfrac{1}{2}\left(\hat{g}_{\alpha\nu}\partial_\mu\lambda + \hat{g}_{\alpha\mu}\partial_\nu\lambda - \hat{g}_{\mu\nu}\partial_\alpha\lambda\right) + \mathcal{O}(\lambda^2), \tag{10.38}$$

from which we derive

$$\hat{R}_{\alpha\beta\mu\nu} \to (1+\lambda)\hat{R}_{\alpha\beta\mu\nu} + \tfrac{1}{2}\left(\hat{g}_{\alpha\nu}\hat{D}_\beta\partial_\mu\lambda - \hat{g}_{\alpha\mu}\hat{D}_\beta\partial_\nu\lambda - \hat{g}_{\beta\nu}\hat{D}_\alpha\partial_\mu\lambda + \hat{g}_{\beta\mu}\hat{D}_\alpha\partial_\nu\lambda\right). \tag{10.39}$$

From this, we find how the Ricci tensor transforms:

$$\hat{R}_{\mu\nu} \to \hat{R}_{\mu\nu} - \hat{D}_\mu\partial_\nu\lambda - \tfrac{1}{2}\hat{g}_{\mu\nu}\hat{D}^2\lambda, \qquad \hat{R} \to \hat{R}(1-\lambda) - 3\hat{D}^2\lambda. \tag{10.40}$$

The Weyl tensor (10.37), being the traceless part, is easily found to be invariant (apart from the canonical term):

$$\hat{W}_{\alpha\beta\mu\nu} \to (1+\lambda)\hat{W}_{\alpha\beta\mu\nu}. \tag{10.41}$$

Since the inverse $\hat{g}^{\mu\nu}$ and the determinant $\hat{g}$ of the metric transform as

$$\hat{g}^{\mu\nu} \to (1-\lambda)\hat{g}^{\mu\nu}, \qquad \hat{g} \to (1+4\lambda)\hat{g}, \tag{10.42}$$

we establish that exactly the Weyl tensor squared yields an action that is totally invariant under local scale transformations in four spacetime dimensions (remember that $\hat{g}^{\mu\nu}$ is used to contract the indices):

$$\mathcal{L} = C\sqrt{-\hat{g}}\,\hat{W}_{\alpha\beta\mu\nu}\hat{W}^{\alpha\beta\mu\nu} = C\sqrt{-\hat{g}}(\hat{R}_{\alpha\beta\mu\nu}\hat{R}^{\alpha\beta\mu\nu} - 2\hat{R}_{\mu\nu}\hat{R}^{\mu\nu} + \tfrac{1}{3}\hat{R}^2). \tag{10.43}$$

Now the integral of

$$\tfrac{1}{4}\varepsilon^{\mu\nu\alpha\beta}\varepsilon^{\kappa\lambda\gamma\delta}\hat{R}_{\mu\nu\kappa\lambda}\hat{R}_{\alpha\beta\gamma\delta} = \hat{R}_{\mu\nu\kappa\lambda}\hat{R}^{\mu\nu\kappa\lambda} - 4\hat{R}_{\mu\nu}\hat{R}^{\mu\nu} + \hat{R}^2 \tag{10.44}$$

is a topological invariant (related to the topological invariant $\tfrac{1}{4}\varepsilon^{\alpha\beta\gamma\delta}F_{\alpha\beta}F_{\gamma\delta}$ in Yang–Mills theory). Therefore, (10.43) can be further reduced to

$$\mathcal{L} = 2C\sqrt{-\hat{g}}(\hat{R}_{\mu\nu}^2 - \tfrac{1}{3}\hat{R}^2), \tag{10.45}$$

to serve as our locally conformally invariant Lagrangian.

The constant C may be any dimensionless parameter. Note that according to (10.40), neither the Ricci tensor nor the Ricci scalar are invariant; therefore, they are locally unobservable at this stage of the theory. Clearly, in view of Einstein's equation, *matter*, and in particular its stress–energy–momentum tensor, are locally unobservable in the same sense. This will have to be remedied at a later stage, where we must work on redefining what matter is at scales much larger than the Planck scale.

Thus, we have verified that, indeed, the action (10.33) is the only expression that we could have expected there (apart from its overall constant), since we integrated out the scale component of the original metric $g_{\mu\nu}$. Demanding locality immediately leads to this expression. The anomaly is the one called 'type B' in [26]. Type A has the form of the Gauss–Bonnet term (10.44), which we ignore as long as we work in a topologically flat spacetime. The *finite* part of the one-loop amplitudes must contain logarithmic expressions, as described in [23].

In fact, gravity theories with this action as a starting point have been studied extensively [20], and the suspicion has been expressed that such theories might be unitary, in spite of the higher time derivatives in the action. Model calculations show [21] that unitarity can be regained if one modifies the Hermiticity condition, which is equivalent to modifying the boundary conditions of functional amplitudes in the complex plane. Effectively then, the fields become complex, and their operators non-Hermitian. The question whether such procedures are acceptable is strongly debated. Note that we have sound physical reasons for the contour rotation (10.17), which is why similar contour rotations as carried out in refs [20, 21] are difficult to dismiss first hand, and we give the cited work the benefit of the doubt. Before following such a route further, we would have to understand the underlying physics.

In (10.33), we arrived at the conformal action with an essentially infinite coefficient in front. Before deciding what to do with this infinity, and to obtain more insight in the underlying physics, let us study the classical equations that correspond to this action.

To this end, consider an infinitesimal variation $h_{\mu\nu}$ on the metric: $\hat{g}_{\mu\nu} \to \hat{g}_{\mu\nu} + \delta\hat{g}_{\mu\nu}$, $\delta\hat{g}_{\mu\nu} = h_{\mu\nu}$. The infinitesimal changes in the Ricci tensor and scalar are

$$\delta\hat{R}_{\mu\nu} = \tfrac{1}{2}\left(\hat{D}_\alpha\hat{D}_\mu h^\alpha_\nu + \hat{D}_\alpha\hat{D}_\nu h^\alpha_\mu - D^2 h_{\mu\nu} - \hat{D}_\mu\partial_\nu h^\alpha_\alpha\right), \tag{10.46}$$

$$\delta\hat{R} = -h^{\alpha\beta}\hat{R}_{\alpha\beta} + \hat{D}_\alpha\hat{D}_\beta h^{\alpha\beta} - \hat{D}^2 h^\alpha_\alpha. \tag{10.47}$$

Using the Bianchi identity

$$D_\mu R^\mu_\nu = \tfrac{1}{2}\partial_\nu R, \tag{10.48}$$

the variation of the Weyl action (10.43), (10.45) is then found to be

$$\delta S = -2C \int \mathrm{d}^n x \sqrt{-\hat{g}}\, h^{\alpha\beta} \Box^R_{\alpha\beta},$$

with

$$\Box^R_{\alpha\beta} = \hat{D}^2\hat{R}_{\alpha\beta} - \frac{1}{3}\hat{D}_\alpha\hat{D}_\beta\hat{R} - \frac{1}{6}g_{\alpha\beta}\hat{D}^2\hat{R} - 2\hat{R}^\mu_\alpha\hat{R}_{\mu\beta} + 2\hat{R}^{\mu\nu}\hat{R}_{\alpha\mu\beta\nu} - \frac{2}{3}\hat{R}\hat{R}_{\alpha\beta}. \tag{10.49}$$

The classical equations of motion for the Ricci tensor as they follow from the Weyl action are therefore

$$\Box^R_{\alpha\beta} = 0. \tag{10.50}$$

To see their most salient features, let us linearize in $\hat{R}_{\mu\nu}$ and ignore connection terms.

We get

$$\hat{R}_{\mu\nu} - \frac{1}{6}\hat{R}\delta_{\mu\nu} \overset{\text{def}}{=} S_{\mu\nu}, \qquad \partial_\mu S_{\mu\nu} = \partial_\nu S_{\alpha\alpha}, \quad \partial^2 S_{\mu\nu} - \partial_\mu\partial_\nu S_{\alpha\alpha} = 0. \tag{10.51}$$

Defining $\lambda(x)$ by the equation

$$\partial^2\lambda \overset{\text{def}}{=} -S_{\alpha\alpha}, \tag{10.52}$$

we find that the solution $S_{\mu\nu}$ of (10.51) can be written as

$$S_{\mu\nu} = -\partial_\mu\partial_\nu\lambda + A_{\mu\nu}, \quad \text{with} \quad \partial^2 A_{\mu\nu} = 0, \ A_{\alpha\alpha} = 0, \ \partial_\mu A_{\mu\nu} = 0. \tag{10.53}$$

From (10.40), we notice that the free function $\lambda(x)$ corresponds to the local scale degree of freedom (10.35), while the equation for the remainder $A_{\mu\nu}$ tells us that the Einstein tensor, after the scale transformation $\lambda(x)$, can always be made to obey the d'Alembert equation $\partial^2 G_{\mu\nu} = 0$, which is basically the field equation for the stress–energy–momentum tensor that corresponds to massless particles.[4] Thus, it is not true that the Weyl action gives equations that are equivalent to Einstein's equations, but rather that they lead to Einstein equations with only massless matter as their source.

10.6 The divergent effective conformal action

Let us finally address our real problem, the divergence of the effective action (10.33) as $n \to 4$. This really spoils the beautiful program we outlined at the beginning of Section 10.5. One can imagine five possible resolutions of this problem.

10.6.1 Option A1: Cancelation against divergences due to matter

Besides scalar matter fields, one may have Dirac spinors and/or gauge fields that also propagate in the conformal metric $\hat{g}_{\mu\nu}(\vec{x}, t)$. These also lead to divergences. Ignoring interactions between these matter fields, one indeed finds that these fields contribute to the divergence in the effective action (10.33) as well. In fact, all these divergences take the same form of the Weyl action (10.45), and they each just add to the overall coefficient. So, with a bit of luck, one might hope that all these coefficients added up might give zero. That would certainly solve our problem. It would be unlikely that the finite parts of the effective action would also completely cancel out, so we would end up with a perfectly conformally invariant effective theory.

A curious problem would have to be addressed, which is that the effective action scales as the fourth power of the momenta of the conformal $\hat{g}_{\mu\nu}$ fields, so there should be considerable concern that unitarity is lost. One might hope that unitarity can be saved by observing that the theory is still based on a perfectly canonical theory where we started off with the action (10.9).

---

[4] Not quite, of course. The statement only holds when these particles form classical superpositions of plane waves such as an arbitrary function of $x - t$.

Unfortunately, this approach is ruled out for a very simple reason: the matter fields can never cancel out the divergence because they all contribute with the same sign! This is a rather elaborate calculation, of a kind already carried out in the early 1970s [24, 25]. As we are only interested in the part due to the action of scalar, spinor, and vector fields on a conformal background metric $\hat{g}_{\mu\nu}$, we recapitulate the result of this calculation: it is found that, if the matter fields consist of N_0 elementary scalar fields, $N_{1/2}$ elementary Majorana spinor fields (or $\frac{1}{2}N_{1/2}$ complex Dirac fields), and N_1 real Maxwell or Yang–Mills fields (their mutual interactions are ignored), then the total coefficient C in front of the divergent effective action

$$S^{\text{eff}} = C \int \mathrm{d}^n x \, \frac{\sqrt{-\hat{g}}}{8\pi^2(4-n)} \left(\hat{R}^{\mu\nu}\hat{R}_{\mu\nu} - \frac{1}{3}\hat{R}^2 \right) \tag{10.54}$$

is

$$C = \frac{1}{120}(1 + N_0) + \frac{1}{40}N_{1/2} + \frac{1}{10}N_1. \tag{10.55}$$

Here, the first 1 is the effect of the metascalar component ω of gravity itself. All contributions clearly add up with the same sign. This, in fact, could have been expected from simple unitarity arguments, but as such arguments famously failed when the one-loop β functions for different particle types were considered, it is preferred to do the calculation explicitly. In any case, option A1 is excluded.

10.6.2 Option A2: Add the effects of gravitinos and the gravitational field itself

Gravitinos have spin $\frac{3}{2}$ and the gravitational field has spin 2. Why shouldn't we add these [26, 27] to the anomalies in (10.55)? Indeed, the contribution of gravitinos to this particular anomaly is known to be $-\frac{233}{720}N_{3/2}$, so wouldn't this solve the problem? The problem with this is that supergravity is not power-counting renormalizable, so it must be handled differently. Second, it comes with the spin-2 contributions, claimed to be $+\frac{53}{45}N_2$.

10.6.3 Option B: Make the integral finite with a local counterterm, of the same form as (10.54), but with opposite sign

This is the option most physicists who are experienced in renormalization would certainly consider as the most reasonable one. However, a combination of two observations casts serious doubts on the viability of this option. First, in conventional theories where renormalization is carried out, this is happening in the context of a perturbation expansion. The expression that has to be subtracted has a coefficient in front that behaves as

$$\frac{g^\alpha}{(4-n)^\beta}, \tag{10.56}$$

where g is a coupling strength, and the power α is usually greater than the power β. If we agree to stick to the limit where *first* g is sent to zero and *then* n is sent to 4, the total coefficient will still be infinitesimal, and as such not cause any violation of unitarity, even if it does not have the canonical form. This is exactly the reason why the consideration of noncanonical renormalization terms is considered acceptable when perturbative gravity is considered, as long as the external momenta of in- and outgoing particles are kept much smaller than the Planck value.

Here, however, Newton's constant has been eliminated, so there is no coupling constant that makes our counterterm small, and of course we consider all values of the momenta. The Weyl action is quadratic in the Riemann curvature $R^\alpha_{\beta\mu\nu}$ and therefore quartic in the momenta. As stated when we were considering option A, one might hope that the original expression we found can be made compatible with unitarity because it itself follows from the canonical action (10.9). The counterterm itself cannot be reconciled with unitarity (assuming that the curvature operators have to be Hermitian; see Section 10.5). In fact, not only does it generate a propagator of the form $1/(k^2 - i\varepsilon)^2$, which at large values of k^2 is very similar to the difference of two propagators, $1/(k^2 - i\varepsilon) - 1/(k^2 + m^2 - i\varepsilon)$, where the second would describe a particle with indefinite metric, but also the combination with the total action would leave a remainder of the form

$$\frac{1}{4-n}[(k^2)^{n/2} - \mu^{n-4}(k^2)^2] \;\to\; (k^2)^2 \log(k^2/\mu^2), \tag{10.57}$$

where μ is a quantity with the dimension of a mass that defines the subtraction point. The effective propagator would take a form such as

$$\frac{1}{(k^2 + m^2 - i\varepsilon)^2 \, \log(k^2/\mu^2)}, \tag{10.58}$$

which develops yet another pole, at $k^2 \approx \mu^2$. This is a Landau ghost, describing something like a tachyonic particle, violating most of the principles that one would like to obey in quantizing gravity. All these objections against accepting a noncanonical renormalization counterterm are not totally exclusive [28], but they are sufficient reason to search for better resolutions. For sure, one would have to address the problems, and as yet this seems to be beyond our capacities.

10.6.4   Option C

If one follows what actually happens in conventional, perturbative gravity, one might be very much tempted to conclude that it is incomplete: one has to include the contribution of the $\hat{g}_{\mu\nu}$ field itself to the infinity! Only in this way would one obtain the complete renormalization group equations for the coefficient C in the action (10.54). What is more, in some supergravity theories, the *conformal anomaly* then indeed cancels out to zero. [27].[5] However, arguing this way would not at all be in line with the entire approach advocated here: *first* integrate over the ω field and *only then* over the fields $\hat{g}_{\mu\nu}$. We here discuss only the integral over ω, with perhaps in addition the matter fields, and this should provide us with the effective action for $\hat{g}_{\mu\nu}$. If that is no

---

[5] I thank M. Duff for this observation.

longer conformally invariant, we have a problem. Treating C as a freely adjustable, running parameter, even if it turns out not to run anymore, would be a serious threat to unitarity, and would bring us back to perturbative gravity as a whole, with its well-known difficulties. In addition, an important point then comes up: how does the *measure* of the $\hat{g}_{\mu\nu}$ integral scale? Not only might this also be impossible to reconcile with conformal invariance, but also it might be difficult (if not impossible) to calculate: the measure is only well defined if one fixes the gauge à la Faddeev–Popov, and this we wish to avoid, at this stage. We neither wish to integrate over $\hat{g}_{\mu\nu}$, nor fix the gauge there. In conclusion therefore, we dismiss option C as well.

Therefore, yet another option may have to be considered.

10.6.5   Option D: No counterterm is added at all. We accept an infinite coefficient in front of the Weyl action

To see the consequences of such an assumption, just consider the case that the coefficient $K = C/(4 - n)$ is simply very large. In the standard formulation of the functional integral, this means that the quantum fluctuations of the fields are to be given coefficients going as $1/\sqrt{K}$. The *classical* field values can take larger values, but they would act as a background for the quantized fields, and not take part in the interactions themselves. In the limit $K \to \infty$, the quantum fluctuations would vanish, and only the classical parts would remain. In short, this proposal would turn the $\hat{g}_{\mu\nu}$ components of the metric into classical fields!

There are important problems with this proposal as well: classical fields will not react upon the presence of the other, quantized, fields such as the matter fields. Therefore, there is no backreaction of the metric. This proposal, then, should be ruled out because it violates the action = reaction principle in physics. Furthermore, the reader may already have been wondering about gravitons. They are mainly described by the parts of $\hat{g}_{\mu\nu}$ that are spacelike, traceless, and orthogonal to the momentum. If we were to insist that $\hat{g}_{\mu\nu}$ is classical, would this mean that gravitons are classical? It is possible to construct a gedanken experiment with a device that rotates gravitons into photons; this device would contain a large stretch of very strong, transverse magnetic fields. Turning photons into gravitons and back, it would enable us to do quantum interference experiments with gravitons. This then would be a direct falsification of our theory. However, the suspected classical behavior of gravitons comes about because of their interactions with the logarithmically divergent background fluctuations. If the usual renormalization counterterm of the form (10.54) is denied to them, this interaction will be infinite. The magnetic fields in our graviton–photon transformer may exhibit fluctuations that are fundamentally impossible to control; gravitons might still undergo interference, but their typical quantum features, such as entanglement, might disappear.

Yet, there may be a different way to look at option D. In previous publications [29], the author has speculated about the necessity to view quantum mechanics as an *emergent* feature of Nature's dynamical laws. "Primordial quantization" is the procedure where we start with classical mechanical equations for evolving physical variables, after which we attach basis elements of Hilbert space to each of the possible configurations of the classical variables. Subsequently, the evolution is re-expressed in terms of an effective Hamiltonian, and further transformations in this Hilbert space might lead to a description of the world as we know it. This idea is reason enough to investigate this last option further.

There is one big advantage from a technical point of view. Since $\hat{g}_{\mu\nu}$ is now considered to be classical, there is no unitarity problem. All other fields, both the metascalar field ω (the "dilaton") and the matter fields, are described by renormalizable Lagrangians, so that no obvious contradictions arise at this point.

How bad is it that the action = reaction principle appears to be violated? The metric metatensor does allow for a source in the form of an energy–momentum tensor, as described in (10.50)–(10.53). This, however, would be an unquantized source. We get a contradiction if sources are described that evolve quantum mechanically: the background metric cannot react. In practice, this would mean that we could just as well mandate that

$$\hat{g}_{\mu\nu} = \eta_{\mu\nu}; \tag{10.59}$$

in other words, we would live in a flat background where only the metascalar component of the metric evolves quantum mechanically.[6]

Could a nontrivial metric tensor $\hat{g}_{\mu\nu}$ be *emergent*? This means that it is taken either to be classical or totally flat beyond the Planck scale, but it gets renormalized by dilaton and matter fields at much lower scales. This may be the best compromise between the various options considered. Spacetime is demanded to be conformally flat at scales beyond the Planck scale, but virtual matter and dilaton fluctuations generate the $\hat{g}_{\mu\nu}$ as we experience it today. A problem with this argument, unfortunately, is that it is difficult to imagine how dilaton fluctuations could generate a nontrivial effective metric. This is because, regardless of the values chosen for $\omega(x)$, the light cones will be those determined by $\hat{g}_{\mu\nu}$ alone, so that there is no "renormalization" of the speed of light at all. We therefore prefer the following view.

Consider a tunable choice for a renormalization counterterm in the form of the Weyl action (10.54), described by a subtraction point μ. If μ were chosen to be at low frequencies, so at large distance scales, then the Landau ghost (10.58) would be at low values of k^2 and therefore almost certainly ruin unitarity of the amplitudes. Only if μ were chosen as far as possible in the ultraviolet would this ghost stay invisible at most physical lengthscales, so the further away we push the subtraction point, the better, but perhaps the limit $\mu \to \infty$ must be taken with more caution.

Suppose μ is very large (of order $e^{10^{20}}$ for instance), but not infinite? In this case, the graviton propagator (10.58) would stay very small, so that violation of unitarity would be suppressed by factors such as 10^{-20}. The graviton propagator would become quartic at energies beyond $M_{\text{Planck}} \times 10^{-20}$, implying that the gravitational force is effectively screened at distances smaller than the Standard Model mass scale, which ˙has not yet been tested experimentally.

A more mainstream standpoint would be the following.

---

[6] This idea goes back to, among others, Nordström [30].

10.6.6 Option E: The action (10.9) no longer properly describes the situation at scales close to the Planck scale

At $|k| \approx M_{\text{Planck}}$, we no longer integrate over $\omega(k)$, which has two consequences: a natural cutoff at the Planck scale and a breakdown of conformal invariance. Indeed, this would have given the badly needed scale dependence to obtain a standard interpretation of the amplitudes computed this way. Note that, in our effective action (10.67) below, all dependence on Newton's constant has been hidden in an effective quartic interaction term for the ϕ field. That could have been augmented with a "natural" quartic interaction already present in the matter Lagrangian, so we would have lost all explicit references to Newton's constant. Now, with the explicit breakdown of conformal invariance, we get Newton's constant back.

Adopting this standpoint, it is also easy to see how a subtraction point wandering to infinity, as described in option D, could lead to a classical theory for $\hat{g}_{\mu\nu}$. It simply corresponds to the classical limit. Letting the subtraction point go to infinity is tantamount to forcing M_{Planck} to infinity, in which limit, of course, gravity is classical. Only if we were to embrace option D fully, would we insist that the physical scale is not determined by M_{Planck} this way but by adopting some gauge convention at a boundary at infinity. This is the procedure demanded by black hole complementarity.

The price paid for option E is that we lose the fundamental advantages of exact conformal invariance, which are a calculable and practically renormalizable effective interaction and a perfect starting point for a conformally invariant treatment of the black hole correspondence principle as was advocated in Section 10.2. The idea advocated in this chapter is *not* to follow option E representing what would presumably be one of the mainstream lines of thought. With option E, we would have ended up with just another parametrization of nonrenormalizable, perturbative, quantum gravity. Instead, we are searching for an extension of the canonical action (10.9) that is such that the equivalent of the ω integration can be carried out completely.

10.7 Nonconformal matter

To generalize to nonconformal matter fields, the easiest case to consider is a scalar field $\phi(x)$. Conformally invariant scalar fields are described by the action

$$\mathcal{L}_{\text{conf}}^{\phi} = -\tfrac{1}{2}\sqrt{-g}(g^{\mu\nu}\partial_\mu\phi\,\partial_\nu\phi + \frac{1}{6}R\phi^2), \tag{10.60}$$

where the second term is a well-known necessity for complete conformal invariance. Indeed, substituting the splitting (10.14), we find that the field $\phi(x)$ must be written as $\omega^{-1}\hat{\phi}(x)$, and then

$$\sqrt{-g}\,R = \omega^2\left[\sqrt{-\hat{g}}\hat{R} - 6\partial_\mu\left(\sqrt{-\hat{g}}\,\hat{g}^{\mu\nu}\frac{1}{\omega}\partial_\nu\omega\right) - 6\sqrt{-\hat{g}}\,\hat{g}^{\mu\nu}\frac{\partial_\mu\omega}{\omega}\frac{\partial_\nu\omega}{\omega}\right], \tag{10.61}$$

$$\sqrt{-g}\,g^{\mu\nu}\partial_\mu\phi\,\partial_\nu\phi = \sqrt{-\hat{g}}\,\hat{g}^{\mu\nu}\left(\partial_\mu\hat{\phi} - \frac{\partial_\mu\omega}{\omega}\hat{\phi}\right)\left(\partial_\nu\hat{\phi} - \frac{\partial_\nu\omega}{\omega}\hat{\phi}\right), \tag{10.62}$$

$$\mathcal{L}^\phi_{\text{conf}} = -\frac{1}{2}\sqrt{-\hat{g}}\left(\hat{g}^{\mu\nu}\partial_\mu\hat{\phi}\partial_\nu\hat{\phi} + \frac{1}{6}\hat{R}\hat{\phi}^2\right) + \text{derivative.} \tag{10.63}$$

The extra term with the Ricci scalar is in fact the same as the insertion (10.24) in (10.22). Inserting this as our matter Lagrangian leaves everything in Sections 10.4 and 10.5 unaltered.

Now, however, we introduce a mass term:

$$\mathcal{L}^{\phi,\text{mass}} = \mathcal{L}^\phi_{\text{conf}} - \tfrac{1}{2}\sqrt{-g}\,m^2\phi^2. \tag{10.64}$$

After the split (10.14), this turns into

$$\mathcal{L}^{\phi,\text{mass}} = \mathcal{L}^\phi_{\text{conf}} - \tfrac{1}{2}\sqrt{-\hat{g}}\,m^2\omega^2\hat{\phi}^2. \tag{10.65}$$

Thus, an extra term proportional to ω^2 arises in (10.22). But, as it is merely quadratic in ω, we can still integrate this functional integral exactly.[7] At $n \to 4$, and remembering that we had scaled out a factor $6/\kappa^2$ in going from (10.20) to (10.22), the quantity M in Eq. (10.31) is now replaced by

$$M = -\frac{1}{6}\hat{R} + \frac{1}{6}\kappa^2 m^2\hat{\phi}^2, \tag{10.66}$$

and plugging this into the divergence equation (10.32) replaces (10.33) by

$$\Gamma^{\text{div}} = \frac{\sqrt{-\hat{g}}}{8\pi^2(4-n)}\left[\frac{1}{120}(\hat{R}_{\mu\nu}\hat{R}^{\mu\nu} - \frac{1}{3}\hat{R}^2) + \frac{1}{144}(\kappa^2 m^2\hat{\phi}^2)^2\right], \tag{10.67}$$

where $\kappa^2 = 8\pi G_N$. Indeed, the extra term is a quartic interaction term and as such again conformally invariant. $\kappa^2 m^2$ is a dimensionless parameter and, usually, it is quite small.

The two terms in Eq. (10.67) have to be treated in quite a different way. As was explained in Section 10.5, the first term would require a noncanonical counterterm, which we hesitate to add just like that, so it presents real problems that will have to be addressed.

This difficulty does not play any role for the second term. Its divergent part can be renormalized in the usual way by adding a counterterm representing a quartic self-interaction of the scalar field. There will be more subtle complications due to the fact that renormalization of these nongravitational interaction terms in turn often (but not always) destroys scale invariance. As for the matter fields, we return to their contributions in Sections 10.8–10.10.

It is important to conclude from the discussion this section that nonconformal matter does not affect the formal local conformal invariance of the effective action after integration over the metascalar ω field. Also, the nonconformal parts, such as the mass terms, do not have any effect on the dangerously divergent term in this effective action.

---

[7] Note that a cosmological constant would add a term $C\Lambda\omega^4$ to the action, so that the ω integration can then no longer be done exactly. Therefore, for the time being, we omit the cosmological constant.

In Sections, 10.4–10.6, it was argued that the functional integral in canonical quantum gravity,

$$\int \mathcal{D}g_{\mu\nu}\, \mathcal{D}\phi^{\,\mathrm{mat}}\, e^{i[S^{\mathrm{EH}}(g_{\mu\nu})+S^{\mathrm{mat}}(g_{\mu\nu},\phi^{\,\mathrm{mat}})]}, \tag{10.68}$$

where S^{EH} is the Einstein–Hilbert action and S^{mat} is the action of the matter fields, here abbreviated as $\phi^{\,\mathrm{mat}}$, should be considered to be taken in two steps,

$$g_{\mu\nu} \equiv \omega^2 \hat{g}_{\mu\nu}, \quad \det(\hat{g}_{\mu\nu}) = -1, \quad \int \mathcal{D}g_{\mu\nu} = \int \mathcal{D}\hat{g}_{\mu\nu} \int \mathcal{D}\omega, \tag{10.69}$$

and the integral over the dilaton field ω should be taken together with the integrations over the matter fields $\phi^{\,\mathrm{mat}}$.

Rewriting the Einstein–Hilbert action (including a possible cosmological constant) in terms of ω and $\hat{g}_{\mu\nu}$, one finds, in four dimensions,

$$S^{\mathrm{EH}} = \int \mathrm{d}^4 x\, \frac{1}{2\kappa^2}(\hat{R}\,\omega^2 + 6\,\hat{g}^{\mu\nu}\partial_\mu\omega\partial_\nu\omega - 2\Lambda\omega^4), \tag{10.70}$$

where $\kappa^2 = 8\pi G_N$, and $\hat{R}$ is the Ricci scalar associated with $\hat{g}_{\mu\nu}$. Now, let us include those parts of the matter Lagrangian that do not seem to be conformally invariant (though we intend to show that, in our formalism, all interactions are locally conformally invariant). It is convenient to split the Lagrangian of the matter fields into conformally invariant kinetic parts, mass terms, and interaction terms. In a simplified notation (later we will be more precise), we have

$$\phi^{\,\mathrm{mat}} = \{A_\mu(x), \psi(x), \bar{\psi}(x), \varphi(x)\}, \tag{10.71}$$

$$\mathcal{L}^{\mathrm{kin}} = -\frac{1}{4}\hat{g}^{\mu\alpha}\hat{g}^{\nu\beta}F_{\mu\nu}F_{\alpha\beta} - \frac{1}{2}\,\hat{g}^{\mu\nu}\partial_\mu\varphi\,\partial_\nu\varphi - \frac{1}{12}\hat{R}\varphi^2 - \bar{\psi}\gamma^\mu\hat{D}_\mu\psi, \tag{10.72}$$

$$\mathcal{L}^{\mathrm{mass}} = -\frac{1}{2}\,m_s^2\omega^2\varphi^2 - \bar{\psi}\,\omega m_d\,\psi. \tag{10.73}$$

Here, $F_{\mu\nu} = \partial_\mu A_\nu - \partial_\nu A_\mu$; the kinetic term for the Dirac fields is shorthand for the corresponding expression using a vierbein field $\hat{e}_\mu^a$ for the metric $\hat{g}_{\mu\nu}$ with its associated connection field. m_s stands for the scalar masses and m_d for the Dirac masses. The term $\frac{1}{12}\hat{R}\varphi^2$ could be removed by a field redefinition, but is kept here for convenience, making the scalar Lagrangian conformally invariant.

Interaction between the matter fields must now be written in the form

$$\mathcal{L}^{\mathrm{int}} = -\frac{1}{4!}\lambda\varphi^4 - \bar{\psi}y_i\varphi_i\psi - \frac{1}{3!}g_3\varphi^3\omega, \tag{10.74}$$

where the Yukawa couplings y_i could be matrices in the indices labeling the fermion species, and λ and g_3 could be 4- and 3-index tensors in the scalar field indices.

If we now rescale the ω field,

$$\omega(x) = \frac{\kappa}{\sqrt{6}}\,\tilde{\omega}(x), \tag{10.75}$$

we notice two things. First, the action for the $\tilde{\omega}$ field is now nearly identical to the kinetic term for the φ field, both having the same conformal dimension,

$$\mathcal{L}^{\mathrm{EH}} = \frac{1}{2}\,\hat{g}^{\mu\nu}\partial_\mu\tilde{\omega}\,\partial_\nu\tilde{\omega} + \frac{1}{12}\hat{R}\tilde{\omega}^2 - \frac{1}{36}\kappa^2\Lambda\omega^4, \tag{10.76}$$

and, second, the mass terms turn into *conformally invariant quartic coupling terms* between matter fields and the $\tilde{\omega}$ field,

$$\mathcal{L}^{\mathrm{mass}} = -\tfrac{1}{2}\,\tilde{\kappa}^2 m_s^2\,\tilde{\omega}^2\varphi^2 - \tilde{\kappa}m_d\,\bar{\psi}\,\tilde{\omega}\,\psi, \tag{10.77}$$

where $\tilde{\kappa} = \kappa/\sqrt{6} = \sqrt{\tfrac{4}{3}\pi G_N}$ has the dimension of an inverse mass. Also, the scalar 3-field coupling, which originally was not conformally invariant, now turns into a conformally invariant 4-field coupling (see (10.74)),

$$-\frac{1}{3!}\tilde{\kappa}g_3\varphi^3\tilde{\omega}, \tag{10.78}$$

and a new quartic interaction term for the $\tilde{\omega}$ field is generated by the cosmological constant,

$$-\frac{1}{6}\tilde{\kappa}^2\Lambda\,\tilde{\omega}^4. \tag{10.79}$$

It is important to observe that the Lagrangian (10.76) for the dilaton field $\tilde{\omega}$ has an overall sign opposite to that of ordinary scalar fields φ. For any other field theory, this would be disastrous because it would violate causality. Here, however, the unconventional sign is a necessary consequence of the canonical structure of the theory. Since it is an overall sign, it has no net effect on the Feynman rules; this we will exploit by rotating the field in the complex plane,

$$\tilde{\omega}(x) \equiv i\eta(x), \tag{10.80}$$

so that the new field $\eta(x)$ will be indistinguishable from other scalar fields, with one important exception: the conformal interaction terms from the original scalar mass terms m_s and the Dirac mass terms m_d in (10.77), as well as the interaction from the original 3-field interaction, (10.78), acquire unconventional factors -1 or i.

Another important thing to observe is that there is no term at all in the Lagrangian that could serve as a kinetic term for the $\hat{g}_{\mu\nu}$ field.[8] Any such kinetic terms should arise solely from higher-order effects due to the interactions with the matter fields. Naturally, since the entire Lagrangian is now conformally invariant, we should expect the effective Lagrangian for $\hat{g}_{\mu\nu}$ to be conformally invariant as well. It is emphasized in Section 10.4 however that, as is well known [18], this conformal invariance is mutilated by conformal anomalies.

---

[8] Of course, this term reappears if one substitutes $\eta = -i + \mathcal{O}(\kappa\tilde{\eta})$, where $\tilde{\eta}$ is a small oscillating field, by expanding $\hat{R}$.

In our present approach, we now propose to postpone any attempts to describe the functional integrals over $\hat{g}_{\mu\nu}$. Not only do we have anomalies there, but also there are difficulties with unitarity and Landau ghosts.[9] As was explained in Section 10.4, the effective interactions with matter and dilaton fields generate an action for $\hat{g}_{\mu\nu}$ that largely coincides with the familiar conformally invariant action obtained from the square of the Weyl curvature, *but with an infinite numerical coefficient*, which would have to be renormalized. The difficulties associated with that are sufficient reason for us now to postpone this sector of the theory entirely.

At first sight, one may well find logical objections to such a procedure: why not also first integrate over $\hat{g}_{\mu\nu}$ before examining whether the amplitudes obtained obey conformal constraints? We argue, however, that the $\hat{g}_{\mu\nu}$ integration is very different from the rest; $\hat{g}_{\mu\nu}$ determines the location of the local light cones, so that it determines the causal relationships between points in spacetime. It may well be that quantum interference of states with light cones at different places will require treatments that differ in essential ways from the standard functional integral.

In any case, it is worth investigating what happens if we follow this procedure. The implications are quite remarkable, as we will show.

10.8 Renormalization with matter present

Let us assume that the matter fields ϕ^{mat} consist of Yang–Mills fields A_μ^a, Dirac fields $\bar{\psi}$, ψ, and scalar fields φ, the latter three sets being in some (reducible or irreducible, chiral or nonchiral) representation of the local Yang–Mills gauge group. For brevity, we will write complex scalar fields as pairs of real fields, and if Weyl or Majorana fermions occur, the Dirac fields can be replaced by pairs of these.[10] Let us rewrite the Lagrangian for matter interacting with gravity more precisely than in the previous section:

$$\mathcal{L}(\hat{g}_{\mu\nu}, \eta, \phi^{\text{mat}}) = -\frac{1}{4}G_{\mu\nu}^a G_{\mu\nu}^a - \bar{\psi}\,\hat{\gamma}^\mu \hat{D}_\mu\,\psi - \frac{1}{2}\,\hat{g}^{\mu\nu}(D_\mu\varphi\, D_\nu\varphi + \partial_\mu\eta\,\partial_\nu\eta)$$

$$- \frac{1}{12}\hat{R}(\varphi^2 + \eta^2) - V_4(\varphi) - iV_3(\varphi)\eta + \frac{1}{2}\tilde{\kappa}^2 m_i^2 \eta^2 \varphi_i^2 - \tilde{\Lambda}\eta^4$$

$$- \bar{\psi}(y_i\varphi_i + iy_i^5\gamma^5\varphi_i + i\tilde{\kappa}m_d\eta)\psi, \tag{10.81}$$

where $G_{\mu\nu}$ is the (non-Abelian) Yang–Mills curvature, and D_μ and $\hat{D}_\mu$ are covariant derivatives containing the Yang–Mills fields; $\hat{\gamma}_\mu$ and $\hat{D}_\mu$ also contain the vierbein fields and connection fields associated with $\hat{g}_{\mu\nu}$; the Yukawa couplings y_i, y_i^5, and fermion mass terms m_d are matrices in terms of the fermion indices. The scalar self-interactions $V_3(\varphi)$ and $V_4(\varphi)$ must be third- and fourth-degree polynomials in the fields φ_i:

---

[9] In [20, 21] claims are made that unitarity can be restored. This, however, requires the integration contours to be rotated in the complex plane such that $\hat{g}_{\mu\nu}$ becomes complex. Such approaches are interesting and may well serve as good starting points for generating promising theories, but they will not be pursued here.

[10] A single Weyl or Majorana fermion then counts as half a Dirac field.

$$V_4(\varphi) = \frac{1}{4!}\lambda\varphi^4 = \frac{1}{4!}\lambda^{ijk\ell}\varphi_i\varphi_j\varphi_k\varphi_\ell, \tag{10.82}$$

$$V_3(\varphi) = \frac{1}{3!}\tilde{g}_3^{ijk}\varphi_i\varphi_j\varphi_k, \qquad \tilde{g}_3 = \tilde{\kappa}g_3. \tag{10.83}$$

In (10.81), like m_d, the $m_i^2\delta_{ij}$ are also mass matrices, in general. Furthermore, $\tilde{\Lambda}$ stands for $\frac{1}{6}\tilde{\kappa}^2\Lambda$. Of course, all terms in (10.81) must be fully invariant under the Yang–Mills gauge rotations. They must also be free of Adler–Bell–Jackiw anomalies [31].

Now that the dilaton field η has been included, the entire Lagrangian has been made conformally invariant. It is so by construction, and no violations of conformal invariance should be expected. This invites us to consider the β functions of the theory. Can we conclude at this point that the β functions should all vanish?

Let us not be too hasty. In the standard canonical theory, matter fields and their interactions are renormalized. Let us consider dimensional renormalization, and the associated anomalous behavior under scaling. In $4 - \varepsilon$ dimensions, where ε is infinitesimal, the scalar field dimensions are those of a mass raised to the power $1 - \varepsilon/2$, so that the couplings λ have dimension ε. This means that in most of the terms in the Lagrangian (10.81), the integral powers of η will receive extra factors of the form $\eta^{\pm\varepsilon}$ or $\eta^{\pm\varepsilon/2}$, which will then restore exact conformal invariance at all values for ε. If we follow standard procedures, we accept that η is close to $-i$, so that singularities at $\eta \to 0$ or $\eta \to \infty$ are not considered to be of any significance. Indeed, the limit $\eta \to 0$ may be seen to be the small-distance limit. This is the limit where gravity goes wrong anyway, so why bother?

However, now one could consider an extra condition on the theory. Let us assume that the causal structure, that is, the location of the light cones, is determined by $\hat{g}_{\mu\nu}$ and that there exist dynamical laws for $\hat{g}_{\mu\nu}$. This was seen to be a very useful starting point for a better understanding of black hole complementarity, as was shown in the preceding sections. The laws determining the scale $\omega(x)$ should be considered to be dynamical laws, and the canonical theory of gravity itself would support this: formally, the functional integral over the η fields is exactly the same as that for other scalar fields.

In view of the above, we do think it is worthwhile to pursue the idea that the η field must be handled just as any other scalar component of the matter fields; but then all fractional powers, in the $\varepsilon \to 0$ limit, which would lead to $\log \eta$ terms, must clearly be excluded. Renormalization must be done in such a way that no traces of logarithms are left behind. Certainly then, a scale transformation, which should be identical to a transformation where the fields η are scaled, should not be associated with anomalies. Implicitly, this also means that the region $\eta \to 0$ is now assumed to be regular. This is the small-distance region, so that our theory does indeed say something nontrivial about small distances. This is why our theory leads to new predictions that eventually should be testable. Predictions follow from the demand that all β functions of the conformal "theory" (10.81) must vanish.

Note that one set of terms is absent from (10.81): the terms linear in φ and hence cubic in η. This, of course, follows from the fact that, usually, no terms linear in the scalar fields are needed in the standard matter Lagrangians; such terms can easily be removed by translations of the fields: $\varphi_i \to \varphi_i + a_i$ for some constants a_i. Thus, the classical Lagrangian is stationary when the fields vanish: $\varphi = 0$ is a classical solution. In our present notation, this observation is equivalent to the observation that fields may be freely transformed into one another without modifying the physics. One such transformation is a rotation of one of the scalar fields, say φ_1, with the η fields:

$$\left.\begin{aligned}
\varphi_1 &\to \varphi_1 \cosh\alpha_1 + i\eta \sinh\alpha_1, \\
\eta &\to \eta \cosh\alpha_1 - i\varphi_1 \sinh\alpha_1,
\end{aligned}\right\} \tag{10.84}$$

where α_1 stands for the original shift of the field φ_1. The transformation is taken to be a hyperbolic rotation because the "kinetic term" $-\frac{1}{2}\left(\partial\eta^2 + \partial\varphi^2\right) = \frac{1}{2}\left(\partial\tilde{\omega}^2 - \partial\varphi^2\right)$ in (10.81) has to be invariant.

In most cases, these transformations need not be considered, since terms linear in φ will in general not be gauge-invariant.

Notice also that the Yang–Mills fields are not directly coupled to the η field. In the "classical limit," $\eta \to -i$, we can see why this is so. Since not η but $\tilde{\omega}$ is real, the invariant quantity is $\varphi^2 - \omega^2$. Rotating φ fields with η fields would therefore be a noncompact transformation, and Yang–Mills theories with noncompact Lie groups usually do not work. There is food for thought here, but we will not yet pursue this line.

When constructing a complete theory, the next step should be to consider just any configuration of $\hat{g}_{\mu\nu}(\vec{x}, t)$, formulate the renormalized theory in this background, and finally consider functional integrals over $\hat{g}_{\mu\nu}$. Unfortunately, this is still too difficult. In a nontrivial $\hat{g}_{\mu\nu}$ background, there will be anomalies depending on the derivatives of $\hat{g}_{\mu\nu}$; there are divergences [2] proportional to the Weyl curvature squared, which can be seen to correspond to the field combination $\hat{R}_{\mu\nu}^2 - \frac{1}{3}\hat{R}^2$, and subtracting those leads to new conformal anomalies [18]. It was suggested in Section 10.6, option D, to keep the conformal infinity, which would turn gravitons into "classical" particles, or, more precisely, particles that cannot interfere quantum mechanically. To avoid further complications, we now look at the case when $\hat{g}_{\mu\nu}(\vec{x}, t) = \eta_{\mu\nu}$, or spacetime is basically flat, although we do keep the field $\eta(\vec{x}, t)$.

10.9   The β functions

Thus, we return to a theory to which all known quantum field theory procedures can be applied, the only new thing being the presence of an extra, gauge-neutral, spinless field η, and the perfect local scale invariance of the theory.

We have arrived at the Lagrangian (10.81), and we wish to impose on it the condition that all its β functions vanish, since conformal invariance has to be kept. As the theory is renormalizable, the number of β functions is always exactly equal to the number of freely adjustable parameters. In other words, we have exactly as many equations as there are freely adjustable unknown variables, so that *all coupling constants, all mass terms, and also the cosmological constant* should be completely fixed by the equations $\beta_i = 0$. They are at the stationary points. Masses come in the combination $\tilde{\kappa}\, m_i$ and the cosmological constant in the combination $\tilde{\kappa}^2\Lambda$, so all dimensionful parameters of the theory will be fixed in terms of Planck units.

In principle, there is no reason to expect that any of these fixed points should be extremely close to any of the axes, are not exactly on top of them. Neither masses nor the cosmological constant can be expected to be unnaturally small, at this stage of the theory. In other words, as yet, no resolution of the hierarchy problem is in sight: why are many of the physical mass terms 40 orders of magnitude smaller than the Planck mass, and the cosmological constant more than 120 orders of magnitude? We have no answer to that in this paper, but we will show that the equations are quite complex, and exotic solutions cannot be excluded.

The existence of infinitely many solutions cannot be excluded. This is because one can still adjust the composition and the rank(s) of the Yang–Mills gauge group, as well as one's choice of the scalar and (chiral) spinor representations.[11] These form infinite, discrete sets. However, many choices turn out not to have any nontrivial, physically acceptable fixed point at all: the interaction potential terms $V(\varphi)$ must be real and properly bounded, for instance. Searches for fixed points then automatically lead to vanishing values of some or more of the coupling parameters, which means that the symmetries and representations have not been chosen correctly.

Every advantage has its disadvantage. Since all parameters of the theory will be fixed, we cannot apply perturbation theory. However, we can make judicious choices of the scalar and spinor representations in such a way that the existence of a fixed point for the gauge coupling to these fields can be made virtually certain. The β function for $SU(N)$ gauge theories with N_f fermions and N_s complex scalars in the elementary representation is

$$16\pi^2 \,\beta(g) = -a\,g^3 - b\,g^5 + \mathcal{O}(g^7), \tag{10.85}$$

$$a = \frac{11}{3}N - \frac{2}{3}N_f - \frac{1}{6}N_s, \tag{10.86}$$

$$b = \mathcal{O}(N^2,\ N\,N_f,\ N\,N_s). \tag{10.87}$$

Choosing one scalar extra, or one missing, we can have a as small as $a = \pm\frac{1}{6}$, while a quick inspection of the literature [33, 34] reveals that, in that case, b may still have either sign,

$$b = \pm\mathcal{O}(N^2), \tag{10.88}$$

depending on further details, such as the ratio of fermions and scalars, the presence of other representations, and the values of the Yukawa couplings. Choosing the sign of a opposite to that of b, one then expects that a fixed point can be found at

$$g^2 = -b/a = \mathcal{O}(1/N^2). \tag{10.89}$$

This, we presume, is close enough to zero that the following procedure may be assumed to be reliable. Let there be ν physical constants, the νth being the gauge coupling g, which is determined by (10.89). If we take all other coupling parameters

---

[11] which of course must be free of Adler–Bell–Jackiw anomalies [31, 32].

to be of order g or g^2, then the β-function equations are reliably given by the one-loop expressions only, which we will give below. Now these are $\nu - 1$ equations for the $\nu - 1$ remaining coupling parameters, and they are now inhomogeneous equations, since the one coupling, g^2, is already fixed. All we have to do now is find physically acceptable solutions. We have already seen that nonabelian Yang–Mills fields are mandatory; we will quickly discover that, beside the η fields, both fermions and other scalar matter fields are indispensable to find any nontrivial solutions.

One trivial, yet interesting, solution must be mentioned: $\mathcal{N} = 4$ super Yang–Mills. We take its Lagrangian, and add to that the η field while postulating that this η field does not couple to the $\mathcal{N} = 4$ matter fields at all. Then indeed, all β functions vanish [35]. However, since the η field is not allowed to couple, the physical masses are all strictly zero, which disqualifies the theory physically. Note, however, that the cosmological constant is also rigorously zero. Perhaps the procedure described above can be applied by slightly modifying the representations in this theory, so that a solution with masses close to zero, and in particular a cosmological constant extremely close to zero, emerges.

The one-loop β functions are generated by an algebra [36], in which one simply has to plug the Casimir operators of the Yang–Mills Lie group, the types of the representations, the quartic scalar couplings and the fermionic couplings. If we take the scalar fields φ_i and η together as σ_i, the generic Lagrangian can be written as

$$\mathcal{L} = -\frac{1}{4}G^a_{\mu\nu}G^a_{\mu\nu} - \frac{1}{2}(D_\mu\sigma_i)^2 - V(\sigma) - \bar{\psi}\big[\gamma D - (S_i + i\gamma^5 P_i)\sigma_i\big]\psi, \qquad (10.90)$$

where σ_i and $\bar{\psi}$, ψ are in general in reducible representations of the gauge group, D_μ is the gauge-covariant derivative, $V(\sigma)$ is a gauge-invariant quartic scalar potential, and S_i and P_i are matrices in terms of the fermion flavor indices. Everything must be gauge-invariant and the theory must be anomaly-free [31, 32].

The covariant derivatives contain the Hermitean representation matrices T^a_{ij}, $U^{L\,a}_{\alpha\beta}$, and $U^{R\,a}_{\alpha\beta}$:

$$D_\mu\sigma_i \equiv \partial_\mu\sigma_i + iT^a_{ij}A^a_\mu\sigma_j, \qquad (10.91)$$

$$D_\mu\psi_\alpha \equiv \partial_\mu\psi_\alpha + i(U^{L\,a}_{\alpha\beta}P^L + U^{R\,a}_{\alpha\beta}P^R)A^a_\mu\psi_\beta, \qquad P^{L,R} \equiv \frac{1}{2}(1 \pm \gamma^5), \qquad (10.92)$$

The gauge coupling constant(s) g are assumed to be included in these matrices T and U. The operators P^L and P^R are projection operators for the left- and right-handed chiral fermions.

The group structure constants f^{abc} are also assumed to include a factor g, and they are defined by

$$[T^a, T^b] = if^{abc}T^c, \qquad [U^{L\,a}, U^{L\,b}] = if^{abc}U^{L\,c}, \qquad [U^{R\,a}, U^{R\,b}] = if^{abc}U^{R\,c}. \qquad (10.93)$$

Casimir operators C_g, C_s, and C_f will be defined as

$$f^{apq}f^{bpq} = C^{ab}_g, \qquad \mathrm{Tr}\,(T^aT^b) = C^{ab}_s, \qquad \mathrm{Tr}\,(U^{L\,a}U^{L\,b} + U^{R\,a}U^{R\,b}) = C^{ab}_f. \qquad (10.94)$$

All β functions are given by writing down how the entire Lagrangian (10.90) runs as a function of the scale μ [36]:

$$\frac{\mu \partial}{\partial \mu} \mathcal{L} = \beta(\mathcal{L}) = \frac{1}{8\pi^2} \Delta \mathcal{L}, \tag{10.95}$$

$$\Delta \mathcal{L} = -\frac{1}{4} G^a_{\mu\nu} G^b_{\mu\nu} \left(\frac{11}{3} C^{ab}_g - \frac{1}{6} C^{ab}_s - \frac{2}{3} C^{ab}_f \right) - \Delta V - \bar{\psi}(\Delta S_i + i\gamma^5 \Delta P_i)\delta_i \psi. \tag{10.96}$$

Here,

$$\Delta V = \frac{1}{4} V^2_{ij} - \frac{3}{2} V_i (T^2 \sigma)_i + \frac{3}{4} (\delta T^a T^b \sigma)^2$$
$$+ \sigma_i V_j \,\text{Tr}\, (S_i S_j + P_i P_j) - \text{Tr}\, (S^2 + P^2)^2 + \text{Tr}\, [S, P]^2, \tag{10.97}$$

where

$$V_i = \partial V(\sigma)/\partial \sigma^i, \quad V_{ij} = \partial^2 V(\sigma)/\partial \sigma_i \partial \sigma_j .$$

It is convenient to define the complex matrices W_i as

$$W_i = S_i + iP_i. \tag{10.98}$$

Then,

$$\Delta W_i = \frac{1}{4} W_k W^*_k W_i + \frac{1}{4} W_i W^*_k K_k + W_k W^*_i W_k$$
$$- \frac{3}{2}(U^R)^2 W_i - \frac{3}{2} W_i (U^L)^2 + W_k \,\text{Tr}\, (S_k S_i + P_k P_i). \tag{10.99}$$

If we now write the collection of scalars as $\{\sigma_i = \varphi_i,\ \sigma_0 = \eta\}$, taking due notice of the factors i in all terms odd in η, we can apply this algebra to compute all β functions of the Lagrangian (10.81).

The values of the various β functions depend strongly on the choice of the gauge group, the representations, the scalar potential function, and the algebra for the Yukawa terms, and there are very many possible choices to make. However, the signs of most terms are fixed by the algebra (10.96)–(10.99). By observing these signs in the equation ($\Delta \mathcal{L} = 0$), we can determine which are the most essential algebraic constraints they impose on possible solutions. As we will see, they are severely restrictive.

10.10 Adding the dilaton field to the algebra for the β functions

Consider the dilaton field η added to the Lagrangian, as in (10.81). This requires extending the indices i, j, ... in the Lagrangian (10.90) to include a value 0 referring to the η field. The unusual thing is now that the terms odd in η are purely imaginary, while all terms in (10.81) are of dimension 4. Let us split off this special component. In (10.90), we then write

$$V(\sigma) = \tilde{L}\eta^4 - \tfrac{1}{2} m^2_i \eta^2 \varphi^2_i + iV_3(\varphi)\eta + V_4(\varphi), \tag{10.100}$$

$$S_0 = im_d, \quad P_0 = 0, \quad S_i = y_i, \quad P_i = y^5_i. \tag{10.101}$$

Here, m_d is the fermionic mass matrix, y_i are matrices representing the scalar Yukawa couplings, and y^5_i are the pseudoscalar Yukawa coupling matrices. $m^2_i \delta_{ij}$ is the scalar mass matrix, which is allowed to have negative eigenvalues, so we allow the Higgs mechanism to take place. We henceforth choose modified Planck units by setting $\tilde{\kappa}^2 = \frac{4}{3}\pi G_N = 1$.

Note that in the Standard Model, there is no gauge-invariant Dirac mass matrix and no gauge-invariant cubic scalar interaction, so there m_d and V_3 are zero, but we will need to be more general.

We write $W = S + iP$, and now $\tilde{W} = S - iP$. The algebra (10.96)–(10.99) is then found to become

$$\Delta V(\sigma) \;=\; \Delta V^0(\varphi) \tag{a}$$

$$-\frac{1}{2}V_{3i}^2 - V_3\varphi_i \,\mathrm{Tr}\ (m_d y_i) + \frac{1}{4}(m_i^2\varphi_i^2)^2 \tag{b}$$

$$+i\eta\left(-\frac{3}{2}V_{3i}(T^2\varphi)_i + \frac{1}{2}V_{3ij}V_{4ij} + \varphi_i V_{3j}\,\mathrm{Tr}\ (y_i y_j + y_i^5 y_j^5) + V_{4i}\,\mathrm{Tr}\ (m_d y_i)\right.$$

$$-4\,\mathrm{Tr}\ (m_d(y_i\varphi_i)^3) + 2\,\mathrm{Tr}\ ([m_d, y_i^5\varphi_i][y_j\varphi_j, y_k^5\varphi_k]) - 2\,\mathrm{Tr}\ [(y_i^5\varphi_i)^2(m_d y_j + y_j m_d)\varphi_j]$$

$$\left.-2V_{3i}m_i^2\varphi_i - V_3\,\mathrm{Tr}\ m_d^2 - m_j^2\varphi_j^2\varphi_i\,\mathrm{Tr}\ (m_d y_i)\right) \tag{c}$$

$$+\eta^2\left(-\frac{1}{4}V_{3ij}^2 - V_{3i}\,\mathrm{Tr}\ (m_d y_i) - \frac{1}{2}m_i^2 V_{4ii}^2 + 2\,\mathrm{Tr}\ ((m_d\, y_i\varphi_i)^2) + 4\,\mathrm{Tr}\ (m_d^2(y_i\varphi_i)^2)\right.$$

$$+2\,\mathrm{Tr}\ (m_d^2(y_i^5\varphi_i)^2) - \mathrm{Tr}\ ([m_d, y_i^5\varphi_i]^2) - m_j^2\varphi_i\varphi_j\,\mathrm{Tr}\ (y_i y_j + y_i^5 y_j^5) + \frac{3}{2}m_i^2\varphi_i(T^2\varphi)_i$$

$$\left.+2m_i^4\varphi_i^2 + \mathrm{Tr}\ (m_d^2)m_i^2\varphi_i^2 - 6\tilde{\Lambda}m_i^2\varphi_i^2\right) \tag{d}$$

$$+i\eta^3\left(-\frac{1}{2}m_i^2 V_{3ii} - m_i^2\varphi_i\,\mathrm{Tr}\ (m_d y_i) + 4\,\mathrm{Tr}\ (m_d^3 y_i\varphi_i) + 4\tilde{\Lambda}\varphi_i\,\mathrm{Tr}\ (m_d y_i)\right) \tag{e}$$

$$+\eta^4\left(36\tilde{\Lambda}^2 - 4\tilde{\Lambda}\,\mathrm{Tr}\ (m_d^2) + \frac{1}{4}\sum_i m_i^4 - \mathrm{Tr}\ (m_d^4)\right), \tag{f}$$

$$\tag{10.102}$$

where $V_{3i} = \partial V_3/\partial\varphi_i$, etc. and we apply the following summation convention: double indices are summed over starting with 1, except the index in the scalar mass matrix m_i^2, which is only summed over if it occurs twice elsewhere as well, or if this is explicitly indicated. ΔV^0 is the expression that we already had, in (10.97).

The β coefficients for the Yukawa couplings follow from adding the index 0 to (10.99):

$$\Delta W_i = \Delta W_i^0 - \frac{1}{4}(m_d^2\, W_i + W_i\, m_d^2) + m_d\tilde{W}_i\, m_d - m_d\,\mathrm{Tr}\ (m_d\, S_i)$$

$$\tag{10.103}$$

$$-i\Delta W_0 = \Delta m_d = -\frac{3}{2}m_d^3 - m_d\,\mathrm{Tr}\ (m_d^2) + \frac{1}{4}(y_k^2 + y_k^{5\,2})m_d + \frac{1}{4}m_d(y_k^2 + y_k^{5\,2})$$

$$+ y_k\, m_d\, y_k - y_k^5\, m_d\, y_k^5 + y_k\,\mathrm{Tr}\ (y_k\, m_d) + i\gamma^5 y_k^5\,\mathrm{Tr}\ (y_k\, m_d),$$

$$\tag{10.104}$$

where ΔW_i^0 stands for the standard β function for the corresponding dimension-4 interaction terms.

Before demanding that the β functions all vanish, we observe that we can still allow for an infinitesimal field transformation of the form (10.84) in the original Lagrangian. This adds to the counterterms:

$$\delta V(\sigma) = i\alpha_i \left(\eta \frac{\partial V(\sigma)}{\partial \varphi_i} - \varphi_i \frac{\partial V(\sigma)}{\partial \eta} \right)$$

$$= \alpha_i V_3 \varphi_i + i\eta\, \alpha_i \left(V_{4i} + m_j^2 \varphi_j^2 \varphi_i \right)$$

$$+ \eta^2 \alpha_i \left(-V_{3i} \right) + i\eta^3 \alpha_i \left(-m_i^2 \varphi_i - 4\tilde{\Lambda}\varphi_i \right), \tag{10.105}$$

and a similar rotation in the Yukawa couplings. This can be used to eliminate the term (e) in (10.102) by adjusting α_i; it corresponds to a field shift in the nongravitational case. In most cases, however, such as in the Standard Model, the terms in (e) are forced to vanish anyhow owing to gauge invariance. In a similar way, an infinitesimal chiral rotation among the fermions can be used to eliminate the last term in (10.104).

Thus, after the term (e) has been made to vanish by hand, the demand that all β functions vanish, for all values of η, applies in particular to the terms (a)–(d) and (f) in (10.102) and to (10.103) and (10.104).

We have already assumed that the nonabelian Yang–Mills field coupling(s) g have a small but nonvanishing fixed point. Through the effects of the group matrices T^a, U^{La}, and U^{Ra}, the coupling(s) g determine the values of the other parameters, by as many coupled nonlinear equations as there are unknowns. It follows that in this theory, we *must* have nonabelian Yang–Mills fields. In contrast, abelian $U(1)$ components are not allowed, since these do not have fixed points close to the origin.

Next, let us consider the requirement that the term (f) in (10.102) vanishes:

$$36\tilde{\Lambda}^2 = \mathrm{Tr}\ (m_d^4) + 4\tilde{\Lambda}\,\mathrm{Tr}\ (m_d^2) - \frac{1}{4}\sum_i m_i^4. \tag{10.106}$$

The right-hand side of this equation resembles a supertrace. Since its sign must be positive, we read off right away that there *must* be fermions. If, furthermore, we like to have a very small or vanishing cosmological constant Λ, we clearly need that the sum of the fourth power of the Dirac fields (approximately) equals the sum of the fourth powers of the masses of the real scalar particles divided by 4.

Can we do without the scalar fields φ_i? Equation (10.106) would have a solution, although the cosmological constant would come out fairly large. However, now there is only one more equation to consider: (10.104), with all Yukawa couplings y_i and y_i^5 replaced by 0. That gives

$$\frac{3}{2}m_d^3 + m_d\,\mathrm{Tr}\ (m_d^2) \stackrel{?}{=} 0. \tag{10.107}$$

Whenever m_d has a real, nonvanishing eigenvalue, this would imply that the trace of m_d^2 is negative, an impossible demand. Therefore, our theory also *must* have scalars φ_i, beside the dilaton field η.

It appears that in today's particle models, not only the cosmological constant $\tilde{\Lambda}$ but also the mass terms are quite small, in the units chosen, which are our modified Planck units. Also, if there is a triple scalar coupling $V_3(\varphi)$, it appears to be small as well. This is the hierarchy problem, for which we cannot offer any solution other than suggesting that we may have to choose a very complex group structure—as in the landscape scenarios often proposed in superstring theories. Perhaps the small numbers in our present theory are all related.

If the masses are indeed all small, then the only large terms in our equations are those that say how the coupling constants and masses run with scale. Our theory suggests that they might stop running at some scale; in any case, a light Higgs particle indeed follows from the demand that the Higgs self-coupling is near an ultraviolet fixed point.

The author has not (yet) succeeded in finding a physically interesting prototype model with a nontrivial fixed point; this is a very complex, but interesting, technical problem. Let us briefly set out a strategy.

We search for a solution where all mass terms, and of course also the cosmological constant, are small. Start with a theory that has nearly, but not quite, a set of β functions that vanish at one loop. Assume that it has a fixed point near the origin. It is known that (10.96)–(10.99) allow this. For simplicity, let us assume that there are no triple scalar couplings, $V_3 = 0$, and no gauge-invariant scalars, so that the terms (c) and (e) in (10.102) are forbidden by gauge invariance. If we deviate slightly from the fixed point, then the term (b) dictates that we must be at a point where the β function for the scalar self-couplings is negative. This gives us a first guess for m_i^4, the absolute values of the scalar masses, but not the signs of m_i^2.

Knowing the approximate values of the Yukawa couplings y_k and y_k^5 allows us to fix the Dirac mass matrix m_d using (10.104). Since we want these masses to be small, we must assume that the pseudoscalar Yukawa couplings largely cancel against the scalar ones in this equation. Then, (10.103) can be obeyed by moving slightly away from the original fixed point in that direction.

The only remaining equation is then the vanishing of the term (d), the running of the scalar mass-squared terms. Knowing V_{4ii}^2 and $\mathrm{Tr}\,(m_d^2)$, and assuming that m_i^4 is very small, then gives us an equation for m_i^2. Notice that its sign is still free, so that there is some freedom here. Various further attempts to refine this procedure may well lead to interesting models with fixed points. We do note that, apparently, relatively large pseudoscalar Yukawa couplings y_i^5 are wanted. Also, we are talking about primary, gauge-invariant Dirac masses, which have to be there because of the term (f) is (10.102), while they do not occur in the presently known Standard Model.

10.11 Discussion

Consider a large region of spacetime, filled with light particles scattered here and there. Suppose we ask what this state looks like after a very large Lorentz boost. This question is significant for instance if we consider the neighborhood of a black hole horizon: a (large) time boost for an external observer corresponds to a (large) Lorentz boost for a local observer. A problem with that is that light particles in one frame transform to extremely energetic ones in the boosted frame. Their energies may become so large that the ensuing backreaction upon the metric may no longer be ignored. As we saw in Section 10.3, the effects on the spacetime metric due to light particles moving nearly with the speed of light can be efficiently represented by a conformal factor in the metric.[12] This means that large Lorentz transformations may work as usual only on spaces with a $\hat{g}_{\mu\nu}$ metric, but generate delicate gravitational corrections in the scale function $\omega(x)$. This may be seen as a different way to phrase our motivation for claiming that $\omega(x)$ should be considered as locally unobservable, in particular when black hole horizons are considered. This way, the Lorentz group can be kept as a perfect symmetry near the Planck scale, but only for the $\hat{g}_{\mu\nu}$ part of the metric.

Our theory avoids the need to treat spacetime as "emergent" [37, 38]. Rather, we concentrate upon the demands of causality and locality. The light cones therefore come first, and the scale function ω is of secondary importance.

Describing matter in a $\hat{g}_{\mu\nu}$ metric will still be possible as long as we restrict ourselves to conformally invariant field theories, which may perhaps be not such a bad constraint when describing physics at the Planck scale. Of course, that leaves us the question of where Nature's mass terms come from, but an even more urgent problem is to find the equations for the gravitational field itself, considering the fact that Newton's constant G_N is not scale-invariant at all. The Einstein–Hilbert action is not scale-invariant. Here, we cannot use the Riemann curvature or its Ricci components, but the Weyl component is independent of ω, so that may somehow have to be used.

We suspect that, eventually, scales enter into our world in the following way. Information is now strictly limited to move along the light cones, since only lightlike geodesics are well defined, not the timelike or spacelike ones. It is generally believed that the amount of information moving around in Nature is limited to exactly one bit in each surface element of size $4 \ln 2$ squared Planck lengths. Turning this observation around, one might assume that, whatever the equations are, they define information to flow around. The density of this information flow may well define the Planck length locally, and with that all scales in Nature. Obviously, this leaves us with the problem of defining what exactly information is, and how it links with the equations of motion. The notion of information might not be observer-independent, since the scale factor ω isn't. Quantum mechanics will probably require that all these bits of information form distinct elements of a basis for Hilbert space, as described in [39, 40].

Our theory derives constraints from the fact that matter fields interact with gravity. The basic assumption could be called a new version of relativity: the scalar matter fields should not be fundamentally different from the dilaton field $\eta(\vec{x}, t)$. Since there are no singular interactions when a scalar field tends to zero, there is no reason to

---

[12] The configurations described in Section 10.3 are actually limited to superpositions of flat shells of massless matter; this would leave a problem for massless particles that are pointlike. In a quantum theory, this happens to be not such a bad restriction, if we assume that the particles form plane waves, but we will not expand further on this issue here.

expect any singularity when $\eta(\vec{x}, t)$ tends to zero at some point in spacetime. Standard gravity theory does have singularities there: this domain refers to the short-distance behavior of gravity, which is usually considered to be "not understood." What if the short-distance behavior of gravity and matter fields is determined by simply demanding the absence of a singularity? Matter and dilaton then join smoothly together in a perfectly conformally invariant theory. This, however, only works if all β functions of this theory vanish: its coupling parameters must be at a fixed point. There are only discrete sets of such fixed points. Many theories have no fixed point at all in the domain where physical constants are real and positive—that is, stable. Searching for nontrivial fixed points will be an interesting and important exercise.

Indeed, *all* physical parameters, including the cosmological constant, will be fixed and calculable in terms of the Planck units. This may be a blessing and a curse at the same time. It is a blessing because it removes all dimensionless freely adjustable real numbers from our theory; everything is calculable, using techniques known today; there is a strictly discrete set of models, where the only freedom we have is the choice of gauge groups and representations. It is difficult to tell how many solutions there are—the number is probably infinite.

This result is also a curse, because the values these numbers have in the real world is a strange mix indeed: the range of absolute values covers some 122 orders of magnitude:

$$\tilde{\Lambda} = \mathcal{O}(10^{-122}), \qquad \mu_{\text{Higgs}}^2 \approx 3 \times 10^{-36}. \tag{10.108}$$

The question where these various hierarchies of very large, or small, numbers come from is a great mystery called the "hierarchy problem." In our theory, these hierarchies will be difficult to explain, but we do emphasize that the equations are highly complex, and possibly theories with large gauge groups and representations have the potential to generate such numbers.

Our theory is a "top-down" theory, meaning that it explains masses and couplings at or near the Planck domain. It will be difficult to formulate any firm predictions about physics at energies as low as the TeV domain. Perhaps we should expect large regions on a logarithmic scale with an apparently unnatural scaling behavior. There is in principle no supersymmetry, although the mathematics of supersymmetry will be very helpful for constructing the first nontrivial models.

What is missing furthermore is an acceptable description of the dynamics of the remaining parts $\hat{g}_{\mu\nu}$ of the metric field. In option D in Section 10.6, it was suggested that this dynamics may be non-quantum mechanical, although this does raise the question of how $\hat{g}_{\mu\nu}$ can backreact on the presence of quantum matter. Standard quantum mechanics possibly does not apply to $\hat{g}_{\mu\nu}$ because the notion of energy is absent in a conformal theory, and consequently the use of a Hamiltonian may become problematic. A Hamiltonian can only be defined after coordinates and conformal factor have been chosen, while this is something one might prefer not to do. The author believes that quantum mechanics itself will have to be carefully reformulated before we can really address this problem.

Our theory indeed is complex. We have found that the presence of non-Abelian Yang–Mills fields, scalar fields, and spinor fields is required, while $U(1)$ gauge fields are forbidden (at least at weak coupling, since the β function for the charges here is known to be positive). Because of this, one "prediction" stands out: there will be magnetic monopoles, although presumably their masses will be of the order of the Planck mass.

There is one other firm prediction: the constants of nature will indeed be truly constant. Attempts to experimentally observe variations in constants such as the fine structure constant or the proton–electron mass ratio, with time, or position in distant galaxies, are predicted to yield negative results.

10.12 Conclusions

Our research was inspired by recent ideas about black holes (Section 10.2). There, it was concluded that an effective theory of gravity should exist where the metascalar component either does not exist at all or is integrated out. This would enable us to understand the black hole complementarity principle, and, indeed, turn black holes effectively indistinguishable from ordinary matter at tiny scales. A big advantage of such constructions would be that, because of the formal absence of black holes, we would be allowed to limit ourselves to topologically trivial, continuous spacetimes for a meaningful and accurate, nonperturbative description of all interactions. This is why we searched for a formalism where the metascalar ω is integrated out first.

Let us briefly summarize here how the present formulation can be used to resolve the issue of an apparent clash between unitarity and locality in an evaporating black hole. An observer going into the hole does not explicitly observe the Hawking particles going out. (S)he passes the event horizon at Schwarzschild time $t \to \infty$, and from his/her point of view, the black hole at that time is still there. For the external observer, however, the black hole has disappeared at $t \to \infty$. Owing to the backreaction of the Hawking particles, energy (and possibly charge and angular momentum) has been drained out of the hole. Thus, the two observers appear to disagree about the total stress–energy–momentum tensor carried by the Hawking radiation. Now, this stress–energy–momentum tensor was constructed in such a way that it had to be covariant under coordinate transformations, but this covariance only applies to *changes* made in the stress–energy–momentum when creation and/or annihilation operators act on it. About these covariant changes, the two observers do not disagree. It is the *background subtraction* that is different, because the two observers do not agree about the vacuum state. This shift in the background's source of gravity can be neatly accommodated by a change in the conformal factor $\omega(x)$ in the metric seen by the two observers.

This we see particularly clearly in Rindler space. Here, we can generate a modification of the background stress–energy–momentum by postulating an infinitesimal shift of the parameter $\lambda(x)$ in (10.40) and (10.53). It implies a shift in the Einstein tensor $G_{\mu\nu}$ (and thus in the tensor $T_{\mu\nu}$) of the form

$$G_{\mu\nu} \to G_{\mu\nu} - D_\mu \partial_\nu \lambda + g_{\mu\nu} D^2 \lambda. \tag{10.109}$$

If now the transformation λ is chosen to depend only on the lightcone coordinate x^-, then

$$G_{--} \to G_{--} - \partial_-^2 \lambda, \tag{10.110}$$

while the other components do not shift. Thus we see how a modification only in the energy and momentum of the vacuum in the x^+ direction (obtained by integrating G_{--} over x^-) is realized by a scale modification $\lambda(x^-)$.

In a black hole, we choose to modify the pure Schwarzschild metric, as experienced by an ingoing observer, by multiplying the entire metric with a function $\omega^2(t)$ that decreases very slowly from 1 to 0 as Schwarzschild time t runs to infinity. This then gives the metric of a gradually shrinking black hole as seen by the distant observer. Where ω has a nonvanishing time derivative, this metric generates a nonvanishing Einstein tensor, and hence a nonvanishing background stress–energy–momentum. This is the stress–energy–momentum of the Hawking particles.

Calculating this stress–energy–momentum yields an apparently disturbing surprise: it does not vanish at spacelike infinity. The reason for this has not yet been completely worked out, but presumably lies in the fact that the two observers disagree not only about the particles emerging from the black hole, but also about the particles going in, and indeed an infinite cloud of thermal radiation filling the entire universe around the black hole.

All of this is a sufficient reason to suspect that the conformal (metascalar) factor $\omega(x)$ must be declared to be locally unobservable. It is fixed only if we know the global spacetime and after choosing our coordinate frame, with its associated vacuum state. If we did not specify that state, we would not have a specified ω. In "ordinary" physics, quantum fields are usually described in a flat background. Then the choice for ω is unique. Curiously, it immediately fixes for us the sizes, masses, and lifetimes of all elementary particles. This may sound mysterious, until we realize that sizes and lifetimes are measured by using light rays, and then it is always assumed that these light rays move in a flat background. When this background is not flat, because $\hat{g}_{\mu\nu}$ is nontrivial, then sizes and time stretches become ambiguous. We now believe that this ambiguity is a very deep and fundamental one in physics.

Although this could in principle lead to a beautiful theory, we do hit a real obstacle, which is, of course, that gravity is not renormalizable. This "disease" still plagues our present approach, unless we turn to rather drastic assumptions. The usual idea that one should just add renormalization counterterms wherever needed is found to be objectionable. So, we turn to ideas related to the "primitive quantization" proposal of [29]. Indeed, this quantization procedure assumes a basically classical set of equations of motion as a starting point, so the idea would fit beautifully.

Of course, many other questions are left unanswered. Quite conceivably, further research might turn up more alternative options for a cure to our difficulties. One of these, of course, is superstring theory. Superstring theory often leads one to avoid asking certain questions at all, but eventually the black hole complementarity principle will have to be considered, just as the question of the structure of Nature's degrees of freedom at distance and energy scales beyond the Planck scale.

Acknowledgments

The author thanks C. Kounnas and C. Bachas at the ENS in Paris, S. Giddings [41, 42], R. Bousso, C. Taubes, M. Duff, and P. Mannheim for discussions, and P. van Nieuwenhuizen for his clarifications concerning the one-loop pole terms.

References

[1] G. 't Hooft, *Quantum Gravity without space-time singularities or horizons*, Proceedings of Erice School of Subnuclear Physics 2009: The Most Unexpected at LHC and the Status of High Energy Frontier, ed. A. Zichichi, World Scientific, Singapore (2012) [arXiv:0909.3426,[gr-qc]].

[2] G. 't Hooft, *Probing the small distance structure of canonical quantum gravity using the conformal group*, arXiv:1009.0669v2 [gr-qc].

[3] S. W. Hawking, *Particle creation by black holes*, Commun. Math. Phys. **43** (1975) 199, Erratum ibid. **46** (1976) 206, J. B. Hartle and S. W. Hawking, *Path integral derivation of black hole radiance*, Phys. Rev. **D13** (1976) 2188.

[4] G. 't Hooft, *The scattering matrix approach for the quantum black hole: an overview*, J. Mod. Phys. **A11** (1996) 4623. [arXiv:gr-qc/9607022].

[5] G. 't Hooft, *On the quantum structure of a black hole*, Nucl. Phys. **B256** (1985) 727; *The black hole interpretation of string theory*, Nucl. Phys. **B335** (1990) 138.

[6] L. Susskind, L. Thorlacius, and J. Uglum, *The stretched horizon and black hole Complementarity*, Phys. Rev. **D48** (1993) 3743 [arXiv:hep-th/9306069 [hep-th]]; see also G. 't Hooft, *The black hole horizon as a quantum surface*, Physica Scripta **T36** (1991) 247.

[7] F. Englert and R. Brout, *Broken symmetry and the Mass of gauge vector resons*, Phys. Rev. Lett. **13** (1964)321; P.W. Higgs, *Broken symmetries, Massless particles and gauge fields*, Phys. Lett. **12** (1964) 132; *Broken symmetries and the Masses of gauge bosons*, Phys. Rev. Lett. **13** (1964) 508; *Spontaneous symmetry breakdown without massless bosons* Phys. Rev. **145** (1966) 1156; see also A. A. Migdal and A. M. Polyakov, *Spontaneous breakdown of strong interaction symmetry and thev absence of massless particles*, Sov. Physics JETP **24** (1967) 91.

[8] W. G. Unruh, *Notes on black hole evaporation*, Phys. Rev. **D14** (1976) 870; S. W. Hawking, *Breakdown of predictability in gravitational collapse*, Phys. Rev. **D14** (1976) 2460; *The unpredictability of quantum gravity*, Commun. Math. Phys. **87** (1982) 395; D.N. Page, *Is black-hole evapetation predictable?* Phys. Rev. Lett. **44** (1980) 301;
R. Haag, H. Narnhofer, and U. Stein, *On quantum field theory in gravitational background* Commun. Math. Phys. **94** (1984) 219;
R. Sorkin, *Toward a proof of entropy increase in the presence of quantum black holes*, Phys. Rev. Lett. **56** (1986) 1885; L. Boarbelli, R.K. Koul, J. Lee, and R.D. Sorkin, *Quantum serve of entropy for blank holes*, Phys. Rev. **D34** (1986) 373;
P. Mitra, *Black hole entropy*, invited talk delivered at XVIII IAGRG Conference, Madras, February 1996 [hep-th/9603184].

[9] K. W. Howard, *Vacuum $\langle T_\mu^\nu \rangle$ in Schwarzschild space-time*, Phys. Rev. **D30** (1984) 2532.

[10] K. W. Howard and P. Candelas, *Quantum stress tensor in Schwarzschild space-time*, Phys. Rev. Lett. **53** (1984) 403.

[11] R.M. Wald, *Gravitational collapse and cosmic censorship*, Black Holes, Gravitational Radiction and the Universe, eds. B. R. Iyer and B. Bhawal, Springer-Verlag, Berlin (1998), p.69. [arXiv:gr-qc/9710068].

[12] R. Penrose, *The question of cosmic censorship*, Black Holes and Relativistic Stars, ed. R. M. Wald, University of Chicogo Press, Chicago (1988), Chap.5.

[13] S.W. Hawking and G.F.R. Ellis, The Large Scale Structure of Space-Time, Cambridge: Cambridge Univsity Press, Cambridge (1973).

[14] B. P. Jensen, J. G. McLaughlin, and A. C. Ottewill, *Anisotropy of the quantum thermal state in Schwarzschild spacetime*, Phys. Rev. **D45** (1992) 3002.

[15] M. Visser, *Gravitational vacuum polarization II: Energy conditions in the Boulware vacuum*, Phys. Rev. **D54** (1996) 5116 [arXiv:gr-qc/9604008].

[16] T. Dray and G. 't Hooft, *The effect of spherical shells of matter on the Schwarzschild black hole*, Commun. Math. Phys. **99** (1985) 613.

[17] D. M. Capper and M. J. Duff, *Conformal anomalies and the renormalizability problem in quantum gravity*, Phys. Lett. **A53** (1975) 361.

[18] M. J. Duff, *Twenty Years of the Weyl Anomaly*, talk given at the Salamfest, ICTP, Trieste, March 1993 [arXiv:hep-th/9308075].

[19] G. 't Hooft and M. Veltman, *One loop divergences in the theory of gravitation*, Ann. Inst. Henri Poincaré, **20** (1974) 69.

[20] P. D. Mannheim and D. Kazanas, *Exact vacuum solution to conformal Weyl gravity and galactic rotation curves*, Astrophys. J. **342**, (1989) 635; D. Kazanas and P. D. Mannheim, *General structure of the gravitational equations of motion in conformal Weyl gravity*, Astrophys. J. Suppl. **76** (1991) 431; P. D. Mannheim, *Alternatives to dark matter and dark energy*, Prog. Part. Nucl. Phys. **56** (2006) 340, [astro-ph/0505266]; *Intrinsically quantum-mechanical gravity and the cosmological constant problem*, arXiv:1005.5108 [hep-th]; G.U. Varieschi, *A kinematical approach to conformal cosmology*, Gen. Rel. Grav. **42** (2010) 929, [arXiv:0809.4729[gr-qc]].

[21] C.M. Bender and P.D. Mannheim, *No-ghost theorem for the fourth-order derivative Pais–Uhlenbeck oscillator model*, Phys. Rev. Lett. **100** (2008), 110402 [arXiv:0706.0207 [hep-th]]; *Exactly solvable PT-symmetric Hamiltonian having no Hermitian counterpart*, Phys. Rev. **D78**, (2008) 025022 [arXiv:0804.4190 [hep-th]].

[22] H. Weyl, *Reine Infinitesimalgeometrie*, Math. Z. **2** (1918) 384.

[23] S. Deser, *Closed form effective conformal anomaly actions in $D \geq 4$*, Phys. Lett. **B479** (2000) 315, [arXiv:hep-th/9911129].

[24] S. Deser and P. van Nieuwenhuizen, *One-loop divergences of quantized Einstein–Maxwell fields*, Phys. Rev. **D10** (1974) 401.

[25] S. Deser and P. van Nieuwenhuizen, *Nonrenormalizability of the quantized Einstein–Maxwell system*, Phys. Rev. Lett. **32**, (1973) 245; *Nonrenormalizability of the quantized Dirac–Einstein system*, Phys. Rev. **D10** (1974) 411; P. van

Nieuwenhuiozen and J. A. M.Vermaseren, *One loop divergences in the quantum theory of supergravity*, Phys. Lett. **B65** 263 (1976).

[26] S. Deser and A. Schwimmer, *Geometric classification of conformal anomalies in arbitrary dimensions*, Phys. Lett. **B309** (1993) 279, [arXiv:hep-th/9302047].

[27] E. S. Fradkin and A. A. Tseytlin, *Conformal anomaly in Weyl theory and anomaly free superconformal theories*, Phys. Lett. **B134** (1984) 187.

[28] B. Hasslacher and E. Mottola, *Asymptotically free quantum gravity and black holes*, Phys. Lett. **B99**, (1981) 221.

[29] G. 't Hooft, *Entangled quantum states in a local deterministic theory*, presented at 2nd Vienna Symposium on the Foundations of Modern Physics, June 2009, ITP-UU-09/77, SPIN-09/30 [arXiv:0908.3408,[quart-ph].]

[30] G. Nordström, *Relativitätsprinzip und Gravitation*, Phys. Z. **13**, 1126 (1912); F. Ravndal, *Scalar gravitation and extra dimensions*, invited talk at Gunnar Nordström Symposium on Theoretical Physics, Helsinki, August 27–30, 2003 [arXiv:gr-qc/0405030].

[31] S. L. Adler, *Axial-vector vertex in spinor electrodynamics*, Phys. Rev. **177** (1969) 2426; J.S. Bell and R. Jackiw, *A PCAC puzzle: $\pi^0 \to \gamma\gamma$ in the σ-Model*, Nuovo Cim. **A60** (1969) 47.

[32] S. L. Adler and W. A. Bardeen, *Absence of higher-order corrections in the anomalons axial-vector divergence equation*, Phys. Rev. **182** (1969) 1517; W.A. Bardeen, Phys. Rev. **184** (1969) 1848.

[33] D. R. T. Jones, *Two-loop diagrams in Yang–Mills theory*, Nucl. Phys. **B75** (1974) 531; W. E. Caswell, *Asymptotic behavior of non-Abelian gauge theories to two-loop order*, Phys. Rev. Lett. **33** (1974) 244; R. van Damme, *Most general two-loop counterterm for fermion-free gauge theories with scalar fields*, Phys. Lett. **B110** (1982) 239; *2-loop renormalization of the gauge coupling and the scalar potential for an arbitrary renormalizable field theory*, Nucl. Phys. **B227** (1983) 317.

[34] A. G. M. Pickering, J. A. Gracey, and D. R. T. Jones, *Three loop gauge beta-function for the most general single gauge-coupling theory*, arXiv:hep-ph/0104247.

[35] L. Brink, J. H. Schwarz, and J. Scherk, *Supersymmetric Yang–Mills Theories*, ERDA Research and Development Report, CALT-68-574 (1976); M. Sohnius, *Introducing supersymmetry*, Phys. Rep. **128** (1985) 39.

[36] G. 't Hooft, *An algorithm for the poles at dimension 4 in the dimensional regularization procedure.* Nucl. Phys. **B62** 444 (1973); *The birth of asymptotic freedom*, Nucl. Phys. **B254** (1985) 11; *The conceptual basis of quantum field theory*, Handbook of the Philosophy of Science. Philosophy of Physics, eds. J. Butterfield and J. Earman, Elsevier, Amsterdam (2007), p. 661.

[37] S. Liberati, M. Visser, and S. Weinfurtner, *Naturalness in emergent spacetime*, Phys. Rev. Lett. **96** (2006) 151301 [arXiv:gr-qc/0512139].

[38] T. Konopka, F. Markopoulou, and S. Severini, *Quantum graphity: a model of emergent locality*, arXiv:0801.0861v2 [hep-th].

[39] G. 't Hooft, *Emergent quantum mechanics and emergent symmetries*, presented at PASCOS 13, Imperial College, London, July 6, 2007; ITP-UU-07/39, SPIN-07/27 [arXiv:0707.4568 [hep-th]].

[40] G. 't Hooft, *Entangled quantum states in a local deterministic theory*, presented at 2nd Vienna Symposium on the Foundations of Modern Physics, June 2009, ITP-UU-09/77, SPIN-09/30 [arXiv:0908.3408[quant-ph]].

[41] S. B. Giddings, *Black hole information, unitarity, and nonlocality*, Phys. Rev. **D74** (2006) 106005 [arXiv:hep-th/0605196].

[42] S. B. Giddings, D. Marolf, and J. B. Hartle, *Observables in effective gravity*, Phys. Rev. **D74** (2006) 064018 [arXiv:hep-th/0512200].

11
Renormalization group flows and anomalies

Zohar KOMARGODSKI

Department of Particle Physics and Astrophysics,
Weizmann Institute of Science, Rehovot, Israel

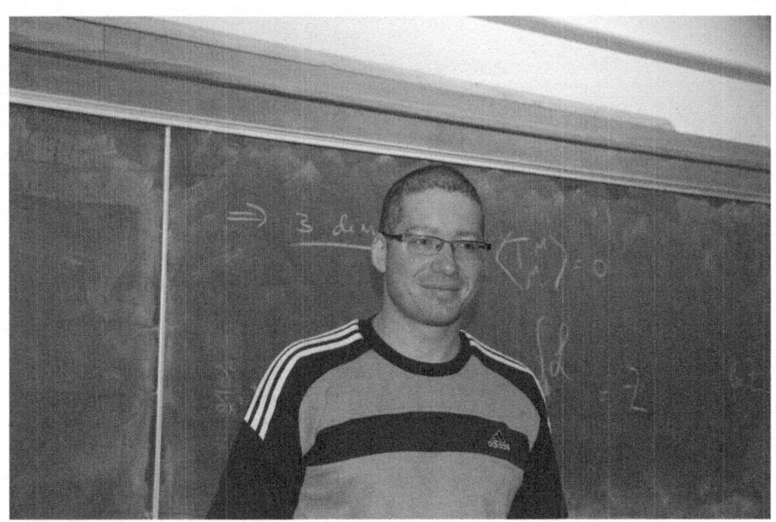

Theoretical Physics to Face the Challenge of LHC. Edited by L. Baulieu, K. Benakli, M. R. Douglas,
B. Mansoulié, E. Rabinovici, and L. F. Cugliandolo. © Oxford University Press 2015.
Published in 2015 by Oxford University Press.

Chapter Contents

This chapter is a brief summary of lectures given at the 2011 Les Houches School "Theoretical Physics to face the Challenge of LHC." Similar lectures were delivered at the 29th Jerusalem Winter School in Theoretical Physics. The aim of the lectures was to review various aspects of renormalization group flows and anomalies.

11.1 Two-dimensional models

We consider Euclidean two-dimensional theories that enjoy the isometry group of $\mathbb{R}^2$. Namely, the theories are invariant under translations and rotations in the two space directions. If the theory is local, it enjoys an energy–momentum tensor operator $T_{\mu\nu}$ that is symmetric and conserved: $T_{\mu\nu} = T_{\nu\mu}$ and $\partial^\mu T_{\mu\nu} = 0$. These equations should be interpreted as operator equations; namely, they must hold in all correlation functions except, perhaps, at coincident points. Here we will study theories where, if possible, these equations hold in fact also at coincident points. In other words, we study theories where there is no local gravitational anomaly. See [1] for some basic facts about theories violating this assumption.

We can study two-point correlation functions of this operator. This correlation function is highly constrained by symmetry and conservation. It takes the following most general form in momentum space:

$$
\begin{aligned}
\langle T_{\mu\nu}(q)T_{\rho\sigma}(-q)\rangle = {} & \frac{1}{2}\left[\left(q_\mu q_\rho - q^2 \eta_{\mu\rho}\right)\left(q_\nu q_\sigma - q^2 \eta_{\nu\sigma}\right) + \rho \leftrightarrow \sigma \right] f(q^2) \\
& + \left(q_\mu q_\nu - q^2 \eta_{\mu\nu}\right)\left(q_\rho q_\sigma - q^2 \eta_{\rho\sigma}\right) g(q^2).
\end{aligned}
\tag{11.1}
$$

The most general two-point function is therefore fixed by two unknown functions of the momentum squared. (Note that above we have stripped out the trivial delta function enforcing momentum conservation.)

Now let us make a further assumption, that the theory is scale-invariant (but not necessarily conformally invariant). This allows us to fix the two functions f and g up to a constant:[1]

$$
f(q^2) = \frac{b}{q^2}, \qquad g(q^2) = \frac{d}{q^2}.
\tag{11.2}
$$

We can now calculate the two-point function $\langle T^\mu_\mu(q)T^\mu_\mu(-q)\rangle$:

$$
\langle T^\mu_\mu(q)T^\mu_\mu(-q)\rangle = (b+d)q^2.
\tag{11.3}
$$

Transforming back to position space, this means that $\langle T^\mu_\mu(x)T^\mu_\mu(0)\rangle \sim (b+d)\Box\delta^{(2)}(x)$. In particular, at separated points, the correlation function vanishes. This means that the trace itself is a vanishing operator: $T^\mu_\mu = 0$ (since it creates nothing from the vacuum, it must be a trivial operator).

---

[1] A logarithm is disallowed since it violates scale invariance. (The rescaling of the momentum would not produce a local term.)

The operator equation

$$T_\mu^\mu = 0 \tag{11.4}$$

is precisely the condition for having the full conformal symmetry of $\mathbb{R}^2$, $SO(3,1)$, present. The equation (11.4) is satisfied by all correlation functions at separated points, but it may fail at coincident points. We have already seen this phenomenon in (11.3). Such contact terms signal an anomaly of $SO(3,1)$. Other than this potential anomaly, (11.4) means that $SO(3,1)$ is a perfectly good symmetry of the theory. Therefore, we see that scale-invariant theories are necessarily conformally invariant in two dimensions [2].[2]

More generally, we find

$$\langle T_\rho^\rho(q) T_{\mu\nu}(-q) \rangle = -(b+d)(q_\mu q_\nu - q^2 \eta_{\mu\nu}), \tag{11.5}$$

which is again a polynomial in momentum and hence a contact term in position space, consistently with (11.4). One may wonder at this point whether there exist quantum field theories for which these contact terms are absent because $b+d=0$. Consider the correlation function $\langle T_{11} T_{11} \rangle$. This has support at separated points. It is proportional to $b+d$. Therefore, in unitary theories, it follows from reflection positivity that

$$b+d > 0. \tag{11.6}$$

So far, we have seen that scale-invariant theories in fact enjoy $SO(3,1)$ symmetry, but the symmetry is afflicted with various contact terms such as (11.5). To see clearly the physical meaning of this anomaly, we can couple the theory to some ambient curved space (there is no dynamics associated with the curved space, it is just a background field). This is done to linear order via $\sim \int d^2x\, T^{\mu\nu} h_{\mu\nu}$, where $h_{\mu\nu}$ is the linearized metric $g_{\mu\nu} = \eta_{\mu\nu} + h_{\mu\nu}$. Hence, in the presence of a background metric that deviates only slightly from flat space,

$$\langle T_\mu^\mu(0) \rangle_{g_{\mu\nu}} \sim \int d^2x \langle T_\mu^\mu(0) T^{\rho\sigma}(x) \rangle h_{\rho\sigma}(x) \sim (b+d) \int d^2x \left[\partial^\rho \partial^\sigma \delta^2(x) - \eta^{\rho\sigma} \Box \delta^2(x) \right] h_{\rho\sigma}$$

$$\sim (b+d)(\partial^\rho \partial^\sigma - \eta^{\rho\sigma} \Box) h_{\rho\sigma}. \tag{11.7}$$

The final object $(\partial^\rho \partial^\sigma - \eta^{\rho\sigma}\Box) h_{\rho\sigma}$ is identified with the linearized Ricci scalar. In principle, if we had analyzed three-point functions of the energy–momentum tensor and so forth, we would have eventually constructed the entire series expansion of the Ricci scalar. Therefore, the expectation value of the trace of the energy–momentum tensor is proportional to the Ricci scalar of the ambient space. This is the famous two-dimensional trace anomaly. It is conventional to denote the anomaly by c (and not by $b+d$ as we have done so far). The usual normalization is

$$T = -\frac{c}{24\pi} R. \tag{11.8}$$

---

[2] Some technical assumptions implicit in the argument above are spelled out in [2].

c is also referred to as the "central charge," but we will not emphasize this algebraic interpretation here. Our argument (11.6) translates to $c > 0$.

Using (11.8), we can present another useful interpretation of c. Consider a two-dimensional conformal field theory compactified on a two-sphere $\mathbb{S}^2$ of radius a:

$$ds^2 = \frac{4a^2}{(1+|x|^2)^2} \sum_{i=1}^{2} (dx_i)^2, \qquad |x|^2 = \sum_{i=1}^{2} (x_i)^2. \tag{11.9}$$

The Ricci scalar $R = 2/a^2$. Because of the anomaly (11.8), the partition function

$$Z_{\mathbb{S}^2} = \int [d\Phi] e^{-\int_{\mathbb{S}^2} \mathcal{L}(\Phi)} \tag{11.10}$$

depends on a. (If the theory had been conformal without any anomalies, we would have expected the partition function to be independent of the radius of the sphere.) We find that

$$\frac{d}{d\log a} \log Z_{\mathbb{S}^2} = -\int_{\mathbb{S}^2} \sqrt{g}\langle T \rangle = \frac{c}{24\pi} \int_{\mathbb{S}^2} \sqrt{g} R = \frac{c}{24\pi} \frac{2}{a^2} \text{Vol}(\mathbb{S}^2) = \frac{c}{3}. \tag{11.11}$$

Thus, the logarithmic derivative of the partition function yields the c anomaly. This particular interpretation of c will turn out to be very useful later.

We will now consider non-scale-invariant theories, i.e., theories where there is some conformal field theory at short distances, CFT_{UV}, and some other conformal field theory (that could be trivial) at long distances, CFT_{IR}. Let us study the correlation functions of the stress tensor in such a case, following [3]. To avoid having to discuss contact terms (which were very important above), we switch to position space. We begin by rewriting (11.1) in position space.

In terms of the complex coordinate $z = x^1 + ix^2$, the conservation equations are $\partial_{\bar{z}} T_{zz} = -\partial_z T$ and $\partial_z T_{\bar{z}\bar{z}} = -\partial_{\bar{z}} T$, where T stands for the trace of the energy–momentum tensor. We can parametrize the most general two-point functions consistent with the isometries of $\mathbb{R}^2$:

$$\langle T_{zz}(z) T_{zz}(0) \rangle = \frac{F(z\bar{z}, M)}{z^4},$$

$$\langle T(z) T_{zz}(0) \rangle = \frac{G(z\bar{z}, M)}{z^3 \bar{z}}, \tag{11.12}$$

$$\langle T(z) T(0) \rangle = \frac{H(z\bar{z}, M)}{z^2 \bar{z}^2}.$$

Here, M stands for some generic mass scale of the theory. As we have seen in our analysis above, (11.1), we know that the conservation equation should bring down the number of independent functions to two. Indeed, we find the relations $\dot{F} = -\dot{G} + 3G$ and $\dot{H} - 2H = -\dot{G} + G$, where $\dot{X} \equiv |z^2| dX/d|z|^2$, leaving two real undermined functions (remember that G and F are complex).

Using these relations, we find that the combination $C \equiv F - 2G - 3H$ satisfies the following differential equation:

$$\dot{C} = -6H. \tag{11.13}$$

However, since H is positive-definite, this equation means that C decreases monotonically as we increase the distance. Let us now identify C at very short and very long distances. At very short and very long distances, it is described by the appropriate quantities in the corresponding conformal field theories. As we have explained above, in conformal field theory, G and H are contact terms and hence can be neglected as long we do not let the operators collide. On the other hand, $F \sim c$. (It is easy to verify that F is sensitive only to the combination $b + d$ as defined in (11.2). Hence, it is only sensitive to c.)

This shows that C is a monotonically decreasing function that starts from c_{UV} and flows to c_{IR}. Since the anomalies c_{UV} and c_{IR} are defined inherently in the corresponding conformal field theories, this means that the space of two-dimensional conformed field theories admits a natural foliation, and the renormalization group flow can proceed in only one direction in this foliation. No cycles of the renormalization group are allowed.

One can think of c as a measure of degrees of freedom of the theory. In simple renormalization group flows, it is easy to understand that c should decrease, since we merely integrate out some massive particles. However, there are many highly nontrivial renormalization group flows where there are emergent degrees of freedom, and the result that

$$c_{\mathrm{UV}} > c_{\mathrm{IR}} \tag{11.14}$$

is a strong constraint on the allowed emergent degrees of freedom.

We can integrate (11.13) to obtain a certain sum rule:

$$c_{\mathrm{UV}} - c_{\mathrm{IR}} \sim \int d\log|z^2| H \sim \int d^2z\,|z^2|\langle T(z)T(0)\rangle > 0. \tag{11.15}$$

Since c can also be understood as the path integral over the 2-sphere, the inequality (11.14) can also be interpreted as a statement about the partition function of the massive theory on $\mathbb{S}^2$.

11.2 Higher-dimensional models

Having understood the two-dimensional case, the main question that comes to mind is whether there exists a function in three and higher dimensions satisfying something similar to (11.14). The problem consists of identifying a candidate quantity that could satisfy such an inequality and then proving that it indeed does so.

There are various ways to define quantities in higher-dimensional field theories that share some common features with c. For example, in conformal theories in two dimensions, c is equivalent to the free energy density of the system, divided by the appropriate power of the temperature. One could define a similar object in higher-dimensional field theories. However, one quickly finds that it is not monotonic [4]. This already shows that such inequalities are quite delicate, and they fail if one chooses to measure the number of effective degrees of freedom in the wrong way (albeit a very intuitive and seemingly natural way).

11.2.1 Three-dimensional models

Progress with the problem of identifying a candidate quantity generalizing (11.14) has happened quite recently [5, 6]. The conjecture arose independently from studies in AdS/CFT and from studies of $\mathcal{N} = 2$ supersymmetric three-dimensional theories.

Any conformal field theory on $\mathbb{R}^3$ can be canonically mapped to a theory on the curved space $\mathbb{S}^3$. This is because $\mathbb{S}^3$ is stereographically equivalent to flat space (thus, the metric on $\mathbb{S}^3$ is conformal to $\mathbb{R}^3$). In three dimensions, there are no trace anomalies, and hence the partition function over $\mathbb{S}^3$ has no logarithms of the radius. (This should be contrasted with the situation in two dimensions, (11.11).)

Consider

$$Z_{\mathbb{S}^3} = \int [d\Phi] e^{-\int_{\mathbb{S}^3} \mathcal{L}(\Phi)}. \tag{11.16}$$

This is generally divergent and takes the form (for a 3-sphere of radius a)

$$\log Z_{\mathbb{S}^3} = c_1 (\Lambda a)^3 + c_2 (\Lambda a) + F. \tag{11.17}$$

Terms with inverse powers of Λ are dropped since they are not part of the continuum theory. Since this is a conformal field theory, Λ is the only scale (of course, a fictitious scale!). The constants c_1 and c_2 are nonuniversal and can be removed with the counterterms $\int \sqrt{g}$ and $\int \sqrt{g}R$. However, no counterterm can remove F.[3]

Imagine a three-dimensional flow from some $\mathrm{CFT}_{\mathrm{UV}}$ to some $\mathrm{CFT}_{\mathrm{IR}}$. We can (in principle) then compute F_{UV} and F_{IR} via the procedure above. The conjecture is

$$F_{\mathrm{UV}} > F_{\mathrm{IR}}. \tag{11.18}$$

Let us outline the computation of F with simple examples. Take a free massless scalar $\mathcal{L} = \frac{1}{2}(\partial\Phi)^2$. To put it in a curved background while preserving conformal invariance (more precisely, Weyl invariance), we write in d dimensions

$$S = \frac{1}{2} \int d^3x \sqrt{g} \left((\nabla \Phi)^2 + \frac{d-2}{4(d-1)} R[g]\phi^2 \right). \tag{11.19}$$

This coupling to the Ricci scalar is necessary to preserve Weyl invariance. Weyl invariance means that the action is invariant under rescaling the metric by any function.

---

[3] More precisely, one can have the gravitational Chern–Simons term, but this cannot affect the real part of F. We disregard the imaginary part of F in our discussion.

We achieve this by accompanying the action on the metric with some action on the fields. For the action above, Weyl invariance means that the action is invariant under

$$g \to e^{2\sigma} g, \qquad \phi \to e^{-\frac{1}{2}(d-2)\sigma} \phi. \tag{11.20}$$

We can now compute the partition function on the 3-sphere by diagonalizing the corresponding differential operator $-\log Z_{\mathbb{S}^3} = \frac{1}{2}\log\det\left(-\nabla^2 + \frac{1}{8}R\right)$. The Ricci scalar is related to the radius in three dimensions via $R = 6/a^2$. The eigenfunctions are of course well known. The eigenvalues are

$$\lambda_n = \frac{1}{a^2}\left(n + \frac{3}{2}\right)\left(n + \frac{1}{2}\right),$$

and their respective multiplicities are

$$m_n = (n+1)^2.$$

The free energy on the 3-sphere due to a single conformally coupled scalar is therefore

$$-\log Z_{\mathbb{S}^3} = \frac{1}{2}\sum_{n=0}^{\infty} m_n \left[-2\log(\mu_0 a) + \log\left(n + \frac{3}{2}\right) + \log\left(n - \frac{1}{2}\right)\right]. \tag{11.21}$$

We have inserted an arbitrary scale μ_0 to soak up the dependence on the radius of the sphere. Since there are no anomalies in three dimensions, we expect that there will be no dependence on μ_0 eventually.

This sum clearly diverges and needs to be regulated. We choose to regulate it using the zeta function. We find that with this regulator, $\sum_{n=0} m_n = \zeta(-2) = 0$, and therefore a logarithmic dependence on the radius is absent, as anticipated. We are left with

$$F_{\text{scalar}} = -\frac{1}{2}\frac{d}{ds}\left[2\zeta\left(s - 2, \frac{1}{2}\right) + \frac{1}{2}\zeta\left(s, \frac{1}{2}\right)\right] = \frac{1}{16}\left(2\log 2 - \frac{3\zeta(3)}{\pi^2}\right) \approx 0.0638.$$

We can perform a similar computation for a free massless Dirac fermion field, and we find

$$F_{\text{fermion}} = \frac{\log 2}{4} + \frac{3\zeta(3)}{8\pi^2} \approx 0.219.$$

The absolute value of the partition function of a massless Majorana fermion is just one-half of the result above. We see that the counting of degrees of freedom is quite nontrivial.

An interesting fact is that a nonzero contribution to F arises also from *topological* degrees of freedom. This has to be contrasted with the situation in two dimensions, where c was defined through a local correlation function and hence was oblivious to topological matter. For example, let us take Chern–Simons theory associated with some gauge group G:

$$S = \frac{k}{4\pi}\int_M \text{Tr}\left(A \wedge dA + \frac{2}{3}A \wedge A \wedge A\right), \tag{11.22}$$

where k is called the level. This theory has no propagating degrees of freedom. Indeed, the equation of motion is

$$0 = F = dA + A \wedge A,$$

which means that the curvature of the gauge field vanishes everywhere. Such gauge fields are called flat connections. The space of flat connections on the manifold M is fixed completely by topological properties of the manifold.

The partition function of Chen–Simons theory on the 3-sphere has been discussed in [7]. In particular, for $U(1)$ Chen–Simons theory the answer is $\frac{1}{2}\log k$, while for $U(N)$ it is

$$F_{\mathrm{CS}}(k, N) = \frac{N}{2}\log(k + N) - \sum_{j=1}^{N-1}(N - j)\log\left(2\sin\frac{\pi j}{k + N}\right). \tag{11.23}$$

We see that the contribution from a topological sector can in fact be arbitrarily large as we take the level k to be large.

Let us now check the inequality (11.18) in a simple flow. We can start from the conformal field theory described by $U(1)_k$ Chen–Simons theory coupled to N_f Dirac fermions of charge 1. This is a conformal field theory because the Lagrangian has no coupling constant that can run. (The Chen–Simons coefficient is discrete because it is topological in nature.) This conformal field theory is weakly coupled when $k \gg 1$. Hence, the F coefficient is

$$F_{\mathrm{UV}} \approx \frac{1}{2}\log k + N_f\left(\frac{\log 2}{4} + \frac{3\zeta(3)}{8\pi^2}\right).$$

Let us now deform this by a mass term. The fermions disappear, but there is a pure Chen–Simons term in the infrared with a shifted level $k \pm N_f/2$, where the sign depends on the sign of the mass term. Hence,

$$F_{\mathrm{IR}} \approx \frac{1}{2}\log\left(k \pm N_f/2\right),$$

and we can convince ourselves that in the regime where our analysis is valid,

$$F_{\mathrm{UV}} > F_{\mathrm{IR}}$$

holds true.

There are many more complicated examples that have been checked, all of which are consistent with the conjecture. In particular, a rather general argument for renormalization group flows in $\mathcal{N} = 2$ theories can be devised [8, 9].

There is not yet a conventional field-theoretic proof of this inequality (11.18), but an ingenious construction relating (11.18) with the entanglement entropy has been given [10]. There, the inequality follows from some inequalities satisfied by the density matrix. Various issues with this construction are discussed in [11].

11.2.2 Four-dimensional models

We saw that in two dimensions, the natural monotonic property of the renormalization group evolution was tightly related to the trace anomaly in two dimensions. In three dimensions, the main role was played by the 3-sphere partition function (there are no trace anomalies in three dimensions).

In four dimensions, there are two trace anomalies, and the monotonic property of flows is concerned again with these anomalies. The anomalous correlation function is now

$$\langle T_{\mu\nu}(q)T_{\rho\sigma}(p)T_{\gamma\delta}(-q-p)\rangle.$$

And again, as in our analysis in two dimensions, there are contact terms that are necessarily inconsistent with $T^\mu_\mu = 0$. In four dimensions, it turns out that there are two independent trace anomalies. Introducing a background metric field, we have

$$T^\mu_\mu = aE_4 - cW^2, \tag{11.24}$$

where $E_4 = R^2_{\mu\nu\rho\sigma} - 4R^2_{\mu\nu} + R^2$ is the Euler density and $W^2_{\mu\nu\rho\sigma} = R^2_{\mu\nu\rho\sigma} - 2R^2_{\mu\nu} + \frac{1}{3}R^2$ is the Weyl tensor squared. These are called the a- and c-anomalies, respectively.

It was conjectured in [12] (and shortly after studied extensively in perturbation theory in [13, 14]) that if the conformal field theory in the ultraviolet, CFT_{UV}, is deformed and flows to some CFT_{IR}, then

$$a_{\text{UV}} > a_{\text{IR}}. \tag{11.25}$$

The four-dimensional c-anomaly does not satisfy such an inequality (this can be seen by investigating simple examples), and also the free energy density divided by the appropriate power of the temperature does not satisfy such an inequality.

In two and three dimensions, we have seen that the quantities satisfying inequalities like (11.14) and (11.18) are computable from the partition functions on $\mathbb{S}^2$ and $\mathbb{S}^3$, respectively. Similarly, in four dimensions, since the 4-sphere is conformally flat, the partition function on $\mathbb{S}^4$ selects only the a-anomaly. Indeed,

$$\partial_{\log r} \log Z_{\mathbb{S}^4} = -\int_{\mathbb{S}^4} \sqrt{g}\langle T^\mu_\mu\rangle = -a\int_{\mathbb{S}^4} \sqrt{g}E_4 = -64\pi^2 a.$$

In this formula, r stands for the radius of $\mathbb{S}^4$. Real scalars contribute to the anomalies $(a, c) = [90(8\pi)^2]^{-1}(1, 3)$, a Weyl fermion $(a, c) = [90(8\pi)^2]^{-1}(11/2, 9)$, and a $U(1)$ gauge field $(a, c) = [90(8\pi)^2]^{-1}(62, 36)$.

We will now present an argument for (11.25), but first it is useful to repeat the two-dimensional story from a new point of view. The main idea is to promote various coupling constants to background fields [15, 16].

Two-dimensional models revisited

Imagine any renormalizable quantum field theory (in any number of dimensions) and set all the mass parameters to zero. The extended symmetry includes the full conformal group. If the number of spacetime dimensions is even, then the conformal group has trace anomalies. If the number of spacetime dimensions is of the form $4k + 2$, then there may also be gravitational anomalies. We will continue to ignore gravitational anomalies here.

Upon introducing the mass terms, one violates conformal symmetry *explicitly.* Thus, in general, the conformal symmetry is violated both by trace anomalies and by an operatorial violation of the equation $T^\mu_\mu = 0$ in flat spacetime. The latter violation can always be removed by letting the coupling constants transform. Indeed, let us replace every mass scale M (either in the Lagrangian or associated with some cutoff) by $Me^{-\tau(x)}$, where $\tau(x)$ is some background field (i.e., a function of spacetime). Then the conformal symmetry of the Lagrangian is restored if we accompany the ordinary conformal transformation of the fields by a transformation of τ. To linear order, $\tau(x)$ always appears in the Lagrangian as $\sim \int d^d x\, \tau T^\mu_\mu$. Setting $\tau = 0$, we are back to the original theory, but we can also let τ be some general function of spacetime. The variation of the path integral under such a conformal transformation that also acts on $\tau(x)$ is thus fixed by the anomaly of the conformal theory in the ultraviolet. This idea allows us to study some questions about general renormalization group flows using the constraints of conformal symmetry. We will sometimes refer to τ as the dilaton.

Consider integrating out all the high-energy modes and flow to the deep infrared. Since we do not integrate out the massless particles, the dependence on τ is regular and local. As we have explained, the dependence on τ is tightly constrained by the conformal symmetry. Since in even dimensions the conformal group has trace anomalies, these must be reproduced by the low-energy theory. The conformal field theory at long distances, $\mathrm{CFT_{IR}}$, contributes to the trace anomalies, but to match to the defining ultraviolet theory, the τ functional has to compensate precisely for the difference between the anomalies of the conformal field theory at short distances, $\mathrm{CFT_{UV}}$, and the conformal field theory at long distances, $\mathrm{CFT_{IR}}$.

Let us see how these ideas are borne out in two-dimensional renormalization group flows. Let us study the constraints imposed by conformal symmetry on action functionals of τ (which is a background field). An easy way to analyze these constraints is to introduce a fiducial metric $g_{\mu\nu}$ into the system. Weyl transformations act on the dilaton and metric according to $\tau \to \tau + \sigma$ and $g_{\mu\nu} \to e^{2\sigma} g_{\mu\nu}$. If the Lagrangian for the dilaton and metric is Weyl-invariant, then on setting the metric to be flat, one finds a conformally invariant theory for the dilaton. Hence, the task is to classify local diffeomorphism (diff) $\times$ Weyl-invariant Lagrangians for the dilaton and metric background fields.

It is convenient to define $\hat{g}_{\mu\nu} = e^{-2\tau} g_{\mu\nu}$, which is Weyl-invariant. At the level of two derivatives, there is only one diff $\times$ Weyl-invariant term: $\int \sqrt{\hat{g}}\hat{R}$. However, this is a topological term, and so it is insensitive to local changes of $\tau(x)$. Therefore, if one starts from a diff$\times$Weyl-invariant theory, on setting $g_{\mu\nu} = \eta_{\mu\nu}$, the term $\int d^2 x\, (\partial\tau)^2$ is absent because there is no appropriate local term that could generate it.

The key is to recall that unitary two-dimensional theories have a trace anomaly

$$T^\mu_\mu = -\frac{c}{24\pi} R. \tag{11.26}$$

We must therefore allow the Lagrangian to break Weyl invariance, such that the Weyl variation of the action is consistent with (11.26). The action functional that reproduces the two-dimensional trace anomaly is

$$S_{\text{WZ}}[\tau, g_{\mu\nu}] = \frac{c}{24\pi} \int \sqrt{g}\,\left[\tau R + (\partial\tau)^2\right]. \tag{11.27}$$

We see that even though the anomaly itself disappears in flat space, (11.26), there is a two-derivative term for τ that survives even after the metric is taken to be flat. This is of course the familiar Wess–Zumino term for the two-dimensional conformal group.

Let us consider now some general two-dimensional renormalization group flow from a conformal field theory in the ultraviolet (with central charge c_{UV}) and one in the infrared (with central change c_{IR}). We replace every mass scale according to $M \to Me^{-\tau(x)}$. We also couple the theory to some background metric. Under a simultaneous Weyl transformation of the dynamical fields and the background field $\tau(x)$, the theory is noninvariant only because of the anomaly $\delta_\sigma S = \frac{1}{24}c_{\text{UV}} \int d^2x \sqrt{g}\sigma R$. Since this is a property of the full quantum theory, it must be reproduced at all scales. An immediate consequence of this idea is that also in the deep infrared the effective action should reproduce the transformation $\delta_\sigma S = \frac{1}{24}c_{\text{UV}} \int d^2x \sqrt{g}\sigma R$. At long distances, we obtain a contribution c_{IR} to the anomaly from CFT_{IR}; hence, the rest of the anomaly must come from an explicit Wess–Zumino functional (11.27) with coefficient $c_{\text{UV}} - c_{\text{IR}}$. In particular, setting the background metric to be flat, we conclude that the low-energy theory must contain a term

$$\frac{c_{\text{UV}} - c_{\text{IR}}}{24\pi} \int d^2x\,(\partial\tau)^2. \tag{11.28}$$

Note that the coefficient of this term is universally proportional to the difference between the anomalies and does not depend on the details of the flow. Higher-derivative terms for the dilaton can be generated from local diff×Weyl-invariant terms, and there is no a priori reason for them to be universal (i.e., they may depend on the details of the flow, and not just on the conformal field theories at short and long distances).

Zamolodchikov's theorem that we reviewed in Section 11.1 follows directly from (11.28). Indeed, from reflection positivity, we must have that the coefficient of the term (11.28) is positive, and thus the inequality is established.

We can be more explicit. The coupling of τ to matter must take the form $\tau T^\mu_\mu + \cdots$, where the corrections have more τ's. To extract the two-point function of τ with two derivatives, we must use the insertion τT^μ_μ twice. (Terms containing τ^2 can be lowered once, but they do not contribute to the two-derivative term in the effective action of τ.) As a consequence, we find that

$$\langle e^{\int \tau T^\mu_\mu d^2x}\rangle = \cdots + \frac{1}{2} \int\int \tau(x)\tau(y)\langle T^\mu_\mu(x)T^\mu_\mu(y)\rangle\,d^2x\,d^2y + \cdots$$

$$= \cdots + \frac{1}{4} \int \tau(x)\partial_\rho\partial_\sigma\tau(x)\left(\int (y-x)^\rho(y-x)^\sigma \langle T^\mu_\mu(x)T^\mu_\mu(y)\rangle\,d^2y\right) d^2x + \cdots. \tag{11.29}$$

In the final line of this equation, we have concentrated entirely on the two-derivative term. It follows from translation invariance that the y integral is independent of x:

$$\int (y-x)^\rho (y-x)^\sigma \langle T^\mu_\mu(x) T^\mu_\mu(y) \rangle \, d^2 y = \frac{1}{2} \eta^{\rho\sigma} \int y^2 \langle T^\mu_\mu(0) T^\mu_\mu(y) \rangle \, d^2 y. \tag{11.30}$$

To summarize, we find the following contribution to the dilaton effective action at two derivatives:

$$\frac{1}{8} \int d^2 x \, \tau \Box \tau \int d^2 y \, y^2 \langle T(y) T(0) \rangle. \tag{11.31}$$

According to (11.28), the expected coefficient of $\tau \Box \tau$ is $(c_{\mathrm{UV}} - c_{\mathrm{IR}})/24\pi$, and so, by comparing, we obtain

$$\Delta c = 3\pi \int d^2 y \, y^2 \langle T(y) T(0) \rangle. \tag{11.32}$$

As we have already mentioned, $\Delta c > 0$ follows from reflection positivity (which is a property of unitary theories). Equation (11.32) precisely agrees with the classic results about two-dimensional flows.

Back to four dimensions

We start by classifying local diff×Weyl-invariant functionals of τ and a background metric $g_{\mu\nu}$. Again, we demand invariance under $g_{\mu\nu} \longrightarrow e^{2\sigma} g_{\mu\nu}$ and $\tau \longrightarrow \tau + \sigma$. We will often denote $\hat{g} = e^{-2\tau} g_{\mu\nu}$. The combination $\hat{g}$ transforms as a metric under diffeomorphisms and is Weyl-invariant.

The most general theory up to (and including) two derivatives is

$$f^2 \int d^4 x \, \sqrt{-\det \hat{g}} \left(\Lambda + \frac{1}{6} \hat{R} \right), \tag{11.33}$$

where we have defined $\hat{R} = \hat{g}^{\mu\nu} R_{\mu\nu}[\hat{g}]$. Since we are ultimately interested in the flat-space theory, let us evaluate the kinetic term with $g_{\mu\nu} = \eta_{\mu\nu}$. Using integration by parts, we get

$$S = f^2 \int d^4 x \, e^{-2\tau} (\partial \tau)^2. \tag{11.34}$$

We can use the field redefinition $\Psi = 1 - e^{-\tau}$ to rewrite this as

$$S = f^2 \int d^4 x \, \Psi \Box \Psi. \tag{11.35}$$

We can also study terms in the effective action with more derivatives. With four derivatives, there are three independent (dimensionless) coefficients:

$$\int d^4 x \, \sqrt{-\hat{g}} \left(\kappa_1 \hat{R}^2 + \kappa_2 \hat{R}^2_{\mu\nu} + \kappa_3 \hat{R}^2_{\mu\nu\rho\sigma} \right). \tag{11.36}$$

It is implicit that indices are raised and lowered with $\hat{g}$. Recall the expressions for the Euler density $\sqrt{-g}E_4$ and the Weyl tensor squared: $E_4 = R^2_{\mu\nu\rho\sigma} - 4R^2_{\mu\nu} + R^2$ and $W^2_{\mu\nu\rho\sigma} = R^2_{\mu\nu\rho\sigma} - 2R^2_{\mu\nu} + \frac{1}{3}R^2$ We can thus choose instead of the basis of local terms (11.36) a different parametrization

$$\int d^4x \, \sqrt{-\hat{g}} \left(\kappa'_1 \hat{R}^2 + \kappa'_2 \hat{E}_4 + \kappa'_3 \hat{W}^2_{\mu\nu\rho\sigma} \right). \tag{11.37}$$

We immediately see that the κ'_2 term is a total derivative. If we set $g_{\mu\nu} = \eta_{\mu\nu}$, then $\hat{g}_{\mu\nu} = e^{-2\tau}\eta_{\mu\nu}$ is conformal to the flat metric, and hence also the κ'_3 term does not play any role as far as the dilaton interactions in flat space are concerned. Consequently, terms in the flat-space limit arise solely from $\hat{R}^2$. A straightforward calculation yields

$$\int d^4x \, \sqrt{-\hat{g}}\hat{R}^2 \bigg|_{g_{\mu\nu}=\eta_{\mu\nu}} = 36 \int d^4x \, \left[\Box\,\tau - (\partial\tau)^2 \right]^2 \sim \int d^4x \, \frac{1}{(1-\Psi)^2} \, (\Box\Psi)^2 . \tag{11.38}$$

So far, we have only discussed diff×Weyl-invariant terms in four dimensions, but from the two-dimensional re-derivation of the c-theorem we have shown above, we anticipate that the anomalous functional will play a key role.

The most general anomalous variation one needs to consider takes the form $\delta_\sigma S_{\text{anomaly}} = \int d^4x \, \sqrt{-g}\sigma \left(cW^2_{\mu\nu\rho\sigma} - aE_4 \right)$. The question is then how to write a functional S_{anomaly} that reproduces this anomaly. (Note that S_{anomaly} is only defined modulo diff×Weyl-invariant terms.) Without the field τ, one must resort to nonlocal expressions, but in the presence of the dilaton, one has a local action.

It is a little tedious to compute this local action, but the procedure is straightforward in principle. We first replace σ on the right-hand side of the anomalous variation with τ:

$$S_{\text{anomaly}} = \int d^4x \, \sqrt{-g}\tau \left(cW^2_{\mu\nu\rho\sigma} - aE_4 \right) + \cdots . \tag{11.39}$$

While the variation of this includes the sought-after terms, as the $\cdots$ indicate, this cannot be the whole answer, because the object in parentheses is not Weyl-invariant. Hence, we need to keep fixing this expression with more factors of τ until the procedure terminates. Note that $\sqrt{-g}W^2_{\mu\nu\rho\sigma}$, being the square of the Weyl tensor, is Weyl-invariant, and hence we do not need to add any fixes proportional to the c-anomaly This makes the c-anomaly "abelian" in some sense.

The "nonabelian" structure coming from the Weyl variation of E_4 is the key to our construction. The a-anomaly is therefore quite distinct algebraically from the c-anomaly.

The final expression for S_{anomaly} is (see [17], where the anomaly functional was presented in a form identical to what we use in this note)

$$S_{\text{anomaly}} = -a \int d^4x \, \sqrt{-g} \left[\tau E_4 + 4\left(R^{\mu\nu} - \frac{1}{2}g^{\mu\nu}R \right)\partial_\mu\tau\partial_\nu\tau - 4(\partial\tau)^2\Box\tau + 2(\partial\tau)^4 \right]$$
$$+ c \int d^4x \, \sqrt{-g}\tau W^2_{\mu\nu\rho\sigma} . \tag{11.40}$$

Note that even when the metric is flat, self-interactions of the dilaton survive. This is analogous to what happens with the Wess–Zumino term in pion physics when the background gauge fields are set to zero, and this is also what we saw in two dimensions.

Setting the background metric to be flat, we thus find that the non-anomalous terms in the dilaton-generating functional are

$$\int d^4x \left\{ \alpha_1 e^{-4\tau} + \alpha_2 (\partial e^{-\tau})^2 + \alpha_3 \left[\Box\tau - (\partial\tau)^2 \right]^2 \right\}, \tag{11.41}$$

where α_i are some real coefficients.

The a-anomaly has a Wess–Zumino term, leading to the additional contribution

$$S_{\mathrm{WZ}} = 2(a_{\mathrm{UV}} - a_{\mathrm{IR}}) \int d^4x \left[2(\partial\tau)^2 \Box\tau - (\partial\tau)^4 \right]. \tag{11.42}$$

The coefficient is universal because the total anomaly has to match (as we have explained in detail in the case of two dimensions).

We see that if we knew the four-derivative terms for the dilaton, we could extract $a_{\mathrm{UV}} - a_{\mathrm{IR}}$. A clean way of separating this anomaly term from the rest is achieved by rewriting it with the variable $\Psi = 1 - e^{-\tau}$. Then the terms in (11.41) become

$$\int d^4x \left(\alpha_1 \Psi^4 + \alpha_2 (\partial\Psi)^2 + \frac{\alpha_3}{(1-\Psi)^2} (\Box\Psi)^2 \right), \tag{11.43}$$

while the Wess–Zumino term (11.42) is

$$S_{\mathrm{WZ}} = 2(a_{\mathrm{UV}} - a_{\mathrm{IR}}) \int d^4x \left(\frac{2(\partial\Psi)^2 \Box\Psi}{(1-\Psi)^3} + \frac{(\partial\Psi)^4}{(1-\Psi)^4} \right). \tag{11.44}$$

We see that if we consider background fields Ψ that are null ($\Box\Psi = 0$), then α_3 disappears and only the last term in (11.44) remains. Therefore, by computing the partition function of the quantum field theory in the presence of four null insertions of Ψ, we can extract $a_{\mathrm{UV}} - a_{\mathrm{IR}}$ directly.

Indeed, consider all the diagrams with four insertions of a background Ψ with momenta k_i, such that $\sum_i k_i = 0$ and $k_i^2 = 0$. Expanding this amplitude $\mathcal{A}$ to fourth order in the momenta k_i, we find that the momentum dependence takes the form $s^2 + t^2 + u^2$ with $s = 2k_1 \cdot k_2$, $t = 2k_1 \cdot k_3$, $u = 2k_1 \cdot k_4$. Our effective action analysis shows that the coefficient of $s^2 + t^2 + u^2$ is directly proportional to $a_{\mathrm{UV}} - a_{\mathrm{IR}}$.

In fact, we can even specialize to the so-called forward kinematics, choosing $k_1 = -k_3$ and $k_2 = -k_4$. Then the amplitude is only a function of $s = 2k_1 \cdot k_2$. It is possible to extract $a_{\mathrm{UV}} - a_{\mathrm{IR}}$ from the s^2 term in the expansion of the amplitude around $s = 0$. Continuing s to the complex plane, there is a branch cut for positive s (corresponding to physical states in the s-channel) and negative s (corresponding to physical states in the u-channel). There is a crossing symmetry $s \leftrightarrow -s$, so these branch cuts are identical.

To calculate the imaginary part associated with the branch cut, we utilize the optical theorem. The imaginary part is manifestly positive-definite. Using Cauchy's theorem, we can relate the low-energy coefficient of s^2, $a_{\mathrm{UV}} - a_{\mathrm{IR}}$, to an integral over the branch cut. Fixing all the coefficients, we find

$$a_{\mathrm{UV}} - a_{\mathrm{IR}} = \frac{1}{4\pi} \int_{s>0} \frac{\mathrm{Im}\,\mathcal{A}(s)}{s^3}. \tag{11.45}$$

As explained, the imaginary part $\mathrm{Im}\,A(s)$ can be evaluated by means of the optical theorem, and it is manifestly positive. Since the integral converges by power counting (and thus no subtractions are needed), we conclude

$$a_{\mathrm{UV}} > a_{\mathrm{IR}}. \tag{11.46}$$

Note the difference between the ways in which positivity is established in two and four dimensions. In two dimensions, one invokes reflection positivity of a two-point function (reflection positivity is best understood in *Euclidean* space). In four dimensions, the Wess–Zumino term involves four dilatons, so the natural positivity constraint comes from the forward kinematics (and hence it is inherently *Minkowskian*).

Let us say a few words about the physical relevance of $a_{\mathrm{UV}} > a_{\mathrm{IR}}$. Such an inequality severely constrains the dynamics of quantum field theory, and in favorable cases can be used to establish that some symmetries must be broken or that some symmetries must be unbroken. In a similar fashion, if a system naively admits several possible dynamical scenarios, one can use $a_{\mathrm{UV}} > a_{\mathrm{IR}}$ as an additional handle.

References

[1] L. Alvarez-Gaume and E. Witten, "Gravitational anomalies," Nucl. Phys. **B234** (1984) 269.

[2] J. Polchinski, "Scale and conformal invariance in quantum field theory," Nucl. Phys. **B303** (1988) 226.

[3] A. B. Zamolodchikov, "Irreversibility of the flux of the renormalization group in a 2D field theory," JETP Lett. **43** (1986) 730 [Pisma Zh. Eksp. Teor. Fiz. **43** (1986) 565].

[4] T. Appelquist, A. G. Cohen, and M. Schmaltz, "A new constraint on strongly coupled gauge theories," Phys. Rev. **D60** (1999) 045003 [arXiv:hep-th/9901109].

[5] R. C. Myers and A. Sinha, "Holographic c-theorems in arbitrary dimensions," JHEP **1101** (2011) 125 [arXiv:1011.5819 [hep-th]].

[6] D. L. Jafferis, I. R. Klebanov, S. S. Pufu, and B. R. Safdi, "Towards the F-theorem: $\mathcal{N} = 2$ field theories on the three-sphere," JHEP **1106** (2011) 102 [arXiv:1103.1181 [hep-th]].

[7] E. Witten, "Quantum field theory and the Jones polynomial," Commun. Math. Phys. **121** (1989) 351.

[8] D. L. Jafferis, "The exact superconformal R-symmetry extremizes Z," JHEP **1205** (2012) 159 [arXiv:1012.3210 [hep-th]].

[9] C. Closset, T. T. Dumitrescu, G. Festuccia, Z. Komargodski, and N. Seiberg, "Contact terms, unitarity, and F-maximization in three-dimensional superconformal theories," JHEP **1210** (2012) 053[arXiv:1205.4142 [hep-th]].

[10] H. Casini and M. Huerta, "On the RG running of the entanglement entropy of a circle," Phys. Rev. **D85** (2012) 125016 [arXiv:1202.5650 [hep-th]].

[11] I. R. Klebanov, T. Nishioka, S. S. Pufu, and B. R. Safdi, "Is renormalized entanglement entropy stationary at RG fixed points?" JHEP **1210** (2012) 058 [arXiv:1207.3360 [hep-th]].

[12] J. L. Cardy, "Is there a c theorem in four-dimensions?" Phys. Lett. **B215** etc (1988) 749.

[13] H. Osborn, "Derivation of a four-dimensional c theorem," Phys. Lett. **B222** (1989) 97.

[14] I. Jack and H. Osborn, "Analogs for the c theorem for four-dimensional renormalizable field theories," Nucl. Phys. **B343** (1990) 647.

[15] Z. Komargodski and A. Schwimmer, "On renormalization group flows in four dimensions," JHEP **1112** (2011) 099 [arXiv:1107.3987 [hep-th]].

[16] Z. Komargodski, "The constraints of conformal symmetry on RG flows," JHEP **1207** (2012) 069 [arXiv:1112.4538 [hep-th]].

[17] A. Schwimmer and S. Theisen, "Spontaneous breaking of conformal invariance and trace anomaly matching," Nucl. Phys. **B847** (2011) 590 [arXiv:1011.0696 [hep-th]].

12
Models of electroweak symmetry breaking

Alex POMAROL

Departament de Física,
Universitat Autònoma de Barcelona,
Bellaterra, Barcelona, Espanya

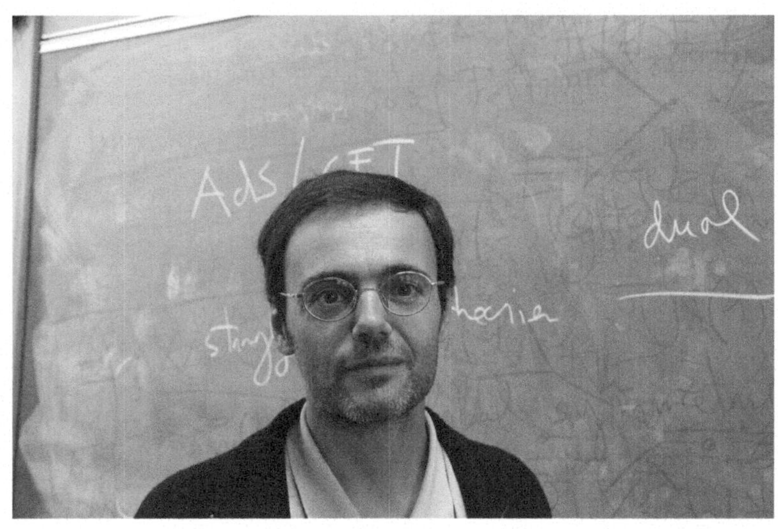

Theoretical Physics to Face the Challenge of LHC. Edited by L. Baulieu, K. Benakli, M. R. Douglas,
B. Mansoulié, E. Rabinovici, and L. F. Cugliandolo. © Oxford University Press 2015.
Published in 2015 by Oxford University Press.

Chapter Contents

12.1 Introduction

Although the Higgs mechanism is a simple and economical way to break the electroweak gauge symmetry of the Standard Model (SM) and at the same cure the bad high-energy behavior of the $W_L W_L$ scattering amplitudes, there is an expensive prize to pay, namely, the hierarchy problem. For this reason, it is interesting to look for other ways to break the electroweak symmetry and unitarize the $W_L W_L$ scattering amplitudes. An example can be found in QCD, where pion–pion scattering is unitarized by the additional resonances that arise from the $SU(3)_c$ strong dynamics. A replica of QCD at energies $\sim$ TeV that breaks the electroweak symmetry can then be an alternative to the Higgs mechanism. This is the so-called technicolor (TC) model [1]. In TC, there is no Higgs particle and the SM scattering amplitudes are unitarized, as in QCD, by infinite heavy resonances. One of the main obstacles to implementing this approach has arisen from electroweak precision tests (EWPT), which have disfavored this type of models. The reason is as follows. Without a Higgs, we expect the new particles responsible for unitarizing the SM amplitudes to have a mass at about 1 TeV. These same resonances give large tree-level contributions to the electroweak observables.

There have been two different approaches to overcoming this problem. One assumes that either (1) there are extra contributions to the electroweak observables that make the model consistent with the experimental data or (2) the strong sector does not break the electroweak symmetry but just delivers a composite pseudo-Goldstone boson (PGB) to be identified with the Higgs. This Higgs gets a potential at the one-loop level and triggers electroweak symmetry breaking (EWSB) at lower energies.

In the first case, the Higgsless approach, the EWPT are satisfied thanks to additional contributions to the electroweak observables that can come from extra scalars or fermions of the TC model, or from vertex corrections. As we will see, the cancellations needed to pass the EWPT are not large, making this possibility not so inconceivable.

In the second case, the Higgs plays the role of *partly* unitarizing the SM scattering amplitudes. Compared with theories without a Higgs, the scale at which new dynamics is needed can be delayed, and therefore the extra resonances that ultimately unitarize the SM amplitudes can be heavier. In this case, the EWPT will be under control. This is the approach of the composite Higgs models, first considered by Georgi and Kaplan [2]. In these theories, a light Higgs arises as a PGB of a strongly interacting theory, in a very similar way as pions do in QCD.

Although these scenarios offer an interesting completion of the SM, the difficulty is performing calculations in strongly coupled theories has been a deterrent against their fully exploration. Nevertheless, the situation has changed in the last few years. Inspired by the AdS/CFT correspondence [3], a new approach to building realistic and predictive Higgsless and composite Higgs models has been developed. The AdS/CFT correspondence states that weakly coupled five-dimensional (5D) theories in anti-de Sitter space (AdS) have a 4D holographic description in terms of strongly coupled conformal field theories (CFT). This correspondence gives a definite prescription for how to construct 5D theories that have the same physical behavior and symmetries as the desired strongly coupled 4D theory. This has allowed the construction of concrete

Higgsless [4] and composite Higgs [5, 6] models that not only are consistent with the experimental constraints, but also make clear predictions for the physics at the LHC. We will briefly discuss them in Section 12.7.

12.2   The original technicolor model: achievements and pitfalls

Technicolor models [1] of EWSB consist of a new strong gauge sector, $SU(N)$ or $SO(N)$, that is assumed to confine at a low scale $\mu_{\mathrm{IR}} \sim$ TeV. In addition, the model contains (at least) two flavors of techniquarks $T_L^{u,d}$ and $T_R^{u,d}$ transforming in the fundamental representation of the strong group and as ordinary quarks under the electroweak group. As in QCD, this implies that the strong sector has a global $G = SU(2)_L \times SU(2)_R \times U(1)_X$ symmetry under which $T_L^{u,d}$ transforms as a $(\mathbf{2},\mathbf{1})_{1/6}$ and $T_R^{u,d}$ transforms as a $(\mathbf{1},\mathbf{2})_{1/6}$ (the hypercharge is given by $Y = 2(T_3^R + X)$). Assuming that the TC-quarks form a condensate, $\langle \bar{T}_L T_R \rangle \sim \mu_{IR}^3$, the global symmetry of the strong sector G is broken down to $H = SU(2)_V \times U(1)_X$. The electroweak symmetry is then broken, giving masses to the corresponding SM gauge bosons. Fermion masses are assumed to arise from higher-dimensional operators such as $\bar{q}_L u_R \bar{T}_R T_L / M^2$ that can be induced from an extended heavy gauge sector (ETC). After the TC-quark condensation, SM fermions acquire masses $m_u \sim \mu_{\mathrm{IR}}^3 / M^2$.

If the number of colors N of the TC group is large enough, the strong sector can be described by an infinite number of resonances [7]. The masses and couplings of the resonances depend on the model. Nevertheless, as in QCD, we can expect vector resonances transforming as a triplet of $SU(2)_V$; the TC-rho of mass $m_\rho \sim \mu_{IR}$. In order to see the implications of these resonances on the SM observables, it is useful to write the low-energy Lagrangian of the SM fields obtained after integrating out the strong sector (the equivalent of the QCD chiral Lagrangian). It is convenient to express this Lagrangian in an $SU(2)_L \times SU(2)_R \times U(1)_X$-symmetric way. To do so, we promote the elementary SM fields to fill complete representations of $SU(2)_L \times SU(2)_R \times U(1)_X$. For the bosonic sector, this means introducing extra nondynamical vectors, i.e., spurions, to complete the corresponding adjoint representations W_μ^L, W_μ^R, and B_μ. With the Goldstone multiplet U parametrizing the coset $SU(2)_L \times SU(2)_R / SU(2)_V$, the bosonic low-energy Lagrangian is given by

$$\mathcal{L}_{\mathrm{eff}} = f^2 \Big[\frac{1}{4} |D_\mu U|^2 + \frac{c_S}{m_\rho^2} \mathrm{Tr}[W_{\mu\nu}^L U W^{R\,\mu\nu} U^\dagger] + \cdots \Big], \tag{12.1}$$

where $D_\mu U = \partial_\mu U + i W_\mu^L U - i U W_\mu^R$ and f is the analog of the pion decay constant that scales as $f \sim \sqrt{N}/(4\pi) \times m_\rho$ [7]. In (12.1), we have omitted terms of order $(DU)^4$ that do not contribute to the SM gauge boson self-energies, and terms of order $f^2 D^2 / m_\rho^4$ that are subleading for physics at energies below m_ρ. The coefficient c_S is of order one and in QCD takes the value $c_S = L_{10} m_\rho^2 / f^2 \simeq -0.4$. The mass of the SM W arises from the kinetic term of U, which gives $M_W^2 = g^2 f^2 / 4$, from which we can deduce

$$f = v \simeq 246~\mathrm{GeV} \quad \text{and} \quad m_\rho \simeq 2 \sqrt{\frac{3}{N}}~\mathrm{TeV}. \tag{12.2}$$

We also obtain $M_W^2 = M_Z^2 \cos^2 \theta_W$ owing to the $SU(2)_V$ symmetry, which corresponds to a custodial symmetry.

12.3 Flavor-changing neutral currents and the top mass

If the SM fermion masses arise from an ETC sector that generates the operators $\bar{q}_L^i u_R^j \bar{T}_R T_L / M^2$, then this sector will also generate flavor-changing neutral currents (FCNC) of order $\bar{q}_L^i u_R^j \bar{q}_L^k u_R^l / M^2$ that are larger than experimentally allowed. Also, the top mass is too large to be generated from a higher-dimensional operator. Solutions to these problems have been proposed (see, e.g., [8] and references therein). Nevertheless, most of the solutions cannot successfully pass EWPT.

12.4 Electroweak precision tests

The most important corrections to the electroweak observables coming from TC-like models are universal corrections to the SM gauge boson self-energies, $\Pi_{ij}(p)$, and nonuniversal corrections to $Z b \bar{b}$, $\delta g_b / g_b$. The universal corrections to the SM gauge bosons can be parametrized by four quantities: $\widehat{S}$, $\widehat{T}$, W, and Y [9]. The first two, the most relevant ones for TC models [10], are defined as

$$\widehat{S} = g^2 \Pi'_{W_3 B}(0), \quad \widehat{T} = \frac{g^2}{M_W^2} \left[\Pi_{W_3 W_3}(0) - \Pi_{W^+ W^-}(0) \right]. \tag{12.3}$$

Since $\widehat{T}$ is protected by the custodial symmetry, the Lagrangian (12.1) only generates $\widehat{S}$. We have

$$\widehat{S} = -g^2 c_S \frac{f^2}{m_\rho^2} \simeq 2.3 \times 10^{-3} \left(\frac{N}{3} \right), \tag{12.4}$$

where we have extracted the result from QCD. Extra contributions to $\widehat{S}$, beyond those of the SM, are constrained by the experimental data as shown in Fig. 12.1. They must be smaller than[1] $\widehat{S} \lesssim 2 \cdot 10^{-3}$ at 99% CL. We see that the contribution (12.4) is at the edge of the allowed value. Models with $N > 3$ or with an extra generation of TC-quarks, needed for realistic constructions (ETC models), are therefore ruled out. The bound $\widehat{S} \lesssim 2 \times 10^{-3}$ can be saturated only if $\widehat{T}$ receive extra positive contributions $\sim 5 \times 10^{-3}$ beyond those of the SM. Although the custodial $SU(2)_V$ symmetry of the TC models guarantees the vanishing of the TC contributions to the $\widehat{T}$ parameter, one-loop contributions involving both the top and the TC sector are nonzero. Nevertheless, in strongly interacting theories, we cannot reliably calculate these contributions and know whether they give the right amount to $\widehat{T}$.

As we said before, the generation of a top mass around the experimental value is difficult to achieve in TC models and requires new strong dynamics beyond the original sector [8]. Even if a large enough top mass is generated, an extra difficulty arises from $Z b \bar{b}$. On dimensional grounds, assuming that $t_{L,R}$ couples with equal strength to the

---

[1] Since TC models do not have a Higgs, we are taking the result of [9] for $M_h \simeq 1$ TeV.

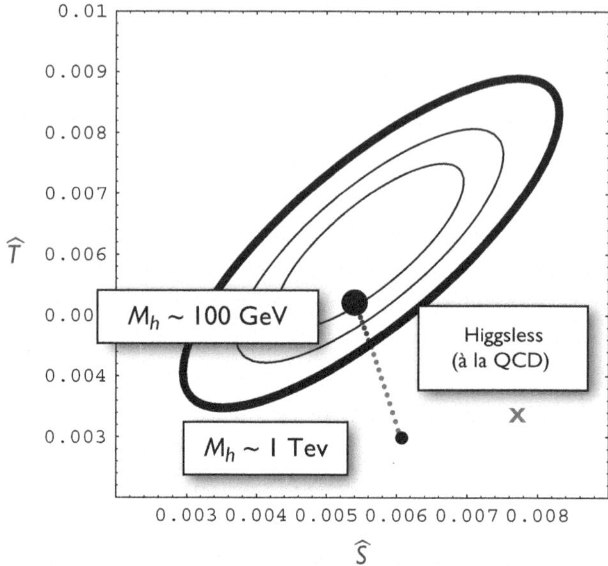

Fig. 12.1 Experimental constraints at 68%, 95%, and 99% CL on the $\widehat{S}$ and $\widehat{T}$ parameters following [9], and the SM prediction as a function of the Higgs mass.

TC sector responsible for EWSB, we have the estimate $\delta g_b/g_b \sim m_t/m_\rho \gtrsim 0.07$, which overwhelms the experimental bound $|\delta g_b/g_b| \lesssim 5 \times 10^{-3}$. Similar conclusions are reached even if $t_{L,R}$ couples with different strength to the TC sector [5], unless the custodial symmetry is preserved by the b_L coupling [11].

Realistic extradimensional Higgsless models can be constructed in which the above problems can be overcome, although this requires extra new assumptions and some adjustments of the parameters of the model [12].

12.5 Composite PGB Higgs

By enlarging the group G, while keeping qualitatively the same properties as the Higgsless models described above, we are driven to a different scenario in which the strong sector, instead of breaking the electroweak symmetry, contains a light Higgs in its spectrum that will be responsible for EWSB. The minimal model consists of a strong sector with the symmetry-breaking pattern [5]

$$SO(5) \to SO(4). \tag{12.5}$$

It contains four Goldstone bosons parametrized by the $SO(5)/SO(4)$ coset:

$$\Sigma = \langle \Sigma \rangle e^{\Pi/f}, \qquad \langle \Sigma \rangle = (0,0,0,0,1), \qquad \Pi = \begin{pmatrix} 0_4 & h_a \\ -h_a^T & 0 \end{pmatrix}, \tag{12.6}$$

where h_a $(a = 1, ..., 4)$ is a real 4-component vector, which transforms as a doublet under $SU(2)_L \in SO(4)$. This is identified with the Higgs. Instead of following the TC idea for fermion masses described before, we can assume, inspired by extradimensional models [5], that the SM fermion couples linearly to fermionic resonances of the strong sector. This can lead to correct fermion masses without severe FCNC problems.

The low-energy theory for the PGB Higgs, written in an $SO(5)$-invariant way, is given by

$$\mathcal{L}_{\text{eff}} = f^2 \left[\frac{1}{2} \left(D_\mu \Sigma \right) \left(D^\mu \Sigma \right)^T + \frac{c_S}{m_\rho^2} \Sigma F_{\mu\nu} F^{\mu\nu} \Sigma^T + V(\Sigma) + \dots \right], \tag{12.7}$$

where $F_{\mu\nu}$ is the field strength of the $SO(5)$ gauge bosons (only the SM bosons must be considered dynamical). From the kinetic term of Σ, we obtain $M_W^2 = g^2(s_h\,f)^2/4$ together with $M_W^2 = M_Z^2 \cos^2 \theta_W$, where we have defined $s_h \equiv \sin h/f$, with $h = \sqrt{h_a^2}$. This implies

$$v = s_h f \simeq 246 \text{ GeV}. \tag{12.8}$$

In this model, the contribution to $\widehat{S}$ has an extra suppression factor v^2/f^2 compared with (12.4), and then for $v \ll f$ one can satisfy the experimental constraint. Also, $\delta g_b/g_b$ can be under control owing to the custodial symmetry [11]. The exact value of v/f comes from minimizing the Higgs potential $V(h)$ that arises at the loop level from SM couplings to the strong sector that break the global $SO(5)$ symmetry. The dominant contribution comes at one-loop level from the elementary $SU(2)_L$ gauge bosons and the top quark. In the model of [6], the potential is given approximately by

$$V(h) \simeq \alpha\, s_h^2 - \beta\, s_h^2 c_h^2, \tag{12.9}$$

where α and β are constants induced at the one-loop level. For $\alpha < \beta$ and $\beta \geqslant 0$, the electroweak symmetry is broken, and, if $\beta > |\alpha|$, the minimum of the potential is at

$$s_h = \sqrt{\frac{\beta - \alpha}{2\beta}}. \tag{12.10}$$

To have $s_h < 1$ as required, we need $\alpha \sim \beta$, which can be accomplished in certain regions of the parameter space of the models. The physical Higgs mass is given by

$$M_h^2 \simeq \frac{8\beta s_h^2 c_h^2}{f^2}. \tag{12.11}$$

Since β arises from one-loop effects, the Higgs is light. In the extradimensional composite Higgs models [6], one obtains $f \gtrsim 500$ GeV, $m_\rho \gtrsim 2.5$ TeV, and $M_h \sim 100$–200 GeV.

12.6 Little Higgs

In the last few years, similar ideas based on the Higgs as a PGB have also been put forward under the name of little Higgs (LH) models [13]. In these models, however, the gauge and fermion sector is extended in order to guarantee that Higgs mass corrections arise at the two-loop level instead of one-loop, allowing for a better insensitivity of the electroweak scale to the strong sector scale m_ρ.

12.7 The AdS/CFT correspondence, Higgsless and composite Higgs models

The AdS/CFT correspondence relates 5D theories of gravity in AdS to 4D strongly coupled conformal field theories [3]. In the case of a slice of AdS, a similar correspondence can also be formulated. The boundary at $y = \pi R$ corresponds to an ultraviolet cutoff in the 4D CFT and to the gauging of certain global symmetries. For example, in the case we are considering where gravity and the SM gauge bosons live in the bulk, the corresponding 4D CFT will have the Poincaré group gauged (giving rise to gravity) and also the SM group $SU(3) \times SU(2)_L \times U(1)_Y$ (giving rise to the SM gauge bosons). Matter localized on the boundary at $y = \pi R$ corresponds to elementary fields external to the CFT that interact only via gravity and gauge interactions. On the other hand, the boundary at $y = 0$ corresponds in the dual theory to an infrared cutoff of the CFT. In other words, it corresponds to breaking the conformal symmetry at the TeV scale. The Kaluza–Klein (KK) states of the 5D theory correspond to the bound states of the strongly coupled CFT. Although the CFT picture is useful for understanding some qualitative aspects of the theory, it is practically useless for obtaining quantitative predictions, since the theory is strongly coupled. In this sense, the 5D gravitational theory in a slice of AdS represents a very useful tool, since it allows one to calculate the particle spectrum, which would otherwise be unknown from the CFT side.

Following the AdS/CFT correspondence, we can design 5D models with the properties of the strongly coupled models discussed before. For example, Higgsless models [4] consist of gauge theories in Randall–Sundrum spaces with the following symmetry pattern:

$$\text{boundary at } y = 0: \qquad SU(2)_V \times U(1)_X \times SU(3)_c,$$

$$\text{5D bulk:} \qquad SU(2)_L \times SU(2)_R \times U(1)_X \times SU(3)_c, \qquad (12.12)$$

$$\text{boundary at } y = \pi R: \qquad SU(2)_L \times U(1)_Y \times SU(3)_c.$$

For composite PGB Higgs models, we have [5, 6] the following:

$$\text{boundary at } y = 0: \qquad O(4) \times U(1)_X \times SU(3)_c,$$

$$\text{5D bulk:} \qquad SO(5) \times U(1)_X \times SU(3)_c, \qquad (12.13)$$

$$\text{boundary at } y = \pi R: \qquad SU(2)_L \times U(1)_Y \times SU(3)_c.$$

In these models, the lightest KK states are the partners of the top with SM quantum numbers $(\mathbf{3},\mathbf{2})_{7/3,1/3}$ and $(\mathbf{3},\mathbf{1})_{4/3}$. The spectrum is shown in Fig. 12.2. Gauge boson and graviton KK states are heavier, around 2.5 and 4 TeV, respectively.

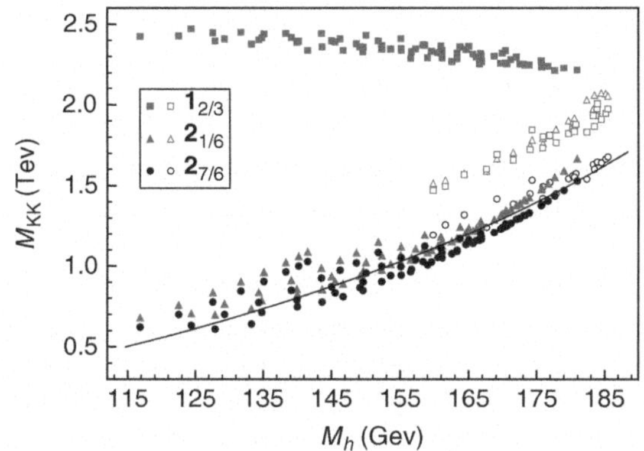

Fig. 12.2 KK fermion masses versus Higgs mass in the model of [6]. All fermion KK states are color triplets under the strong group. The quantum numbers under $SU(2)_L \times U(1)_Y$ is also given. We can see that the normalization of hypercharge in [6] is different from ours; it's necessary to multiply by 2 to get the hypercharges as defined here.

12.8   LHC phenomenology

12.8.1   Heavy resonances at the LHC

The universal feature of strongly coupled theories of EWSB or their extradimensional analogs is the presence of vector resonances, triplets under $SU(2)_V$, with masses in the range 0.5–2.5 TeV; they are the TC-rho or KK states of the W_μ. They can be produced either by $q\bar{q}$ Drell–Yan scattering or via weak boson fusion. These vector resonances will mostly decay into pairs of longitudinally polarized weak bosons (or, if possible, to a weak boson plus a Higgs), and to pairs of tops and bottoms. Studies at the LHC have been devoted to a very light TC-rho, $m_\rho \lesssim 600$ GeV, that will be able to be seen for an integrated luminosity of 4 fb^{-1} (see, e.g., [14]).

In extradimensional Higgsless and composite Higgs models, one also expects heavy gluon resonances. Their dominant production mechanism at the LHC is through $u\bar{u}$ or $d\bar{d}$ annihilation, decaying mostly into top pairs. The signal will be then a bump in the invariant $t\bar{t}$ mass distribution. For an integrated luminosity of 100 fb^{-1}, the reach of the gluon resonances can be up to masses of 4 TeV [15].

The most promising way to unravel some composite Higgs model is by detecting heavy fermions with electric charge 5/3 ($q_{5/3}^*$) [6]. These states are expected to be lighter than vector resonances (see Fig. 12.2). For not-too-large values of its mass $m_{q_{5/3}^*}$, roughly below 1 TeV, these new particles will be mostly produced in pairs, via QCD interactions,

$$q\bar{q}, gg \rightarrow q_{5/3}^* \, \bar{q}_{5/3}^* \,, \tag{12.14}$$

with a cross section completely determined in terms of $m_{q_{5/3}^*}$. Once produced, $q_{5/3}^*$ will mostly decay to a (longitudinally polarized) W^+ plus a top quark. The final state of the process (12.14) consists then mostly of four W's and two b-jets:

$$q_{5/3}^* \, \bar{q}_{5/3}^* \to W^+ t \, W^- \bar{t} \to W^+ W^+ b \, W^- W^- \bar{b}. \tag{12.15}$$

Using same-sign dilepton final states, we could discover these particles for masses of 500 GeV or 1 TeV for an integrated luminosity of 100 pb^{-1} on 20 fb^{-1}, respectively [16]. For increasing values of $m_{q_{5/3}^*}$ the cross section for pair production quickly drops, and single production might become more important; masses up to 1.5 TeV could be reached at the LHC [17].

Beside $q_{5/3}^*$, certain composite models and LH models also predict states of electric charge 2/3 or $-1/3$ that could also be produced in pairs via QCD interactions or singly via bW or tW fusion [18, 19]. They will decay to an SM top or bottom quark plus a longitudinally polarized W or Z, or a Higgs. When kinematically allowed, a heavier resonance will also decay to a lighter one accompanied by a W_{long}, Z_{long}, or h. Decay chains could lead to extremely characteristic final states. For example, in one of the models of [6], the KK with charge 2/3 is predicted to be generally heavier than $q_{5/3}^*$. If pair-produced, they can decay to $q_{5/3}^*$, leading to a spectacular six W's plus two b-jets final state:

$$q_{2/3}^* \, \bar{q}_{2/3}^* \to W^- q_{5/3}^* \, W^+ \bar{q}_{5/3}^* \to W^- W^+ W^+ b \, W^+ W^- W^- \bar{b}. \tag{12.16}$$

In conclusion, our brief discussion shows that there are characteristic signatures predicted by these models that will distinguish them from other extensions of the SM. While certainly challenging, these signals will be extremely spectacular, and will provide an indication of a new strong dynamics responsible for EWSB.

12.8.2 Experimental tests of a composite Higgs

As an alternative to the detection of heavy resonances, the composite Higgs scenario can also be tested by measuring the couplings of the Higgs and seeing differences from those of a SM pointlike Higgs. For small values of $\xi \equiv v^2/f^2$, as needed to satisfy the constraint on $\widehat{S}$, we can expand the low-energy Lagrangian in powers of h/f and obtain in this way the following dimension-6 effective Lagrangian involving the Higgs doublet H:

$$\mathcal{L}_{\text{SILH}} = \frac{c_H}{2f^2} \partial^\mu \left(H^\dagger H \right) \partial_\mu \left(H^\dagger H \right) + \frac{c_T}{2f^2} \left(H^\dagger \overleftrightarrow{D^\mu} H \right) \left(H^\dagger \overleftrightarrow{D}_\mu H \right)$$
$$- \frac{c_6 \lambda}{f^2} \left(H^\dagger H \right)^3 + \left(\frac{c_y y_f}{f^2} H^\dagger H \bar{\psi}_L H \psi_R + \text{h.c.} \right). \tag{12.17}$$

This equation will be referred as the strongly interacting light Higgs (SILH) Lagrangian [20]. We have neglected operators suppressed by $1/m_\rho^2$ that are subleading versus those of (12.17) by a factor $f^2/m_\rho^2 \sim N/(16\pi^2)$, or operators that do not respect the global symmetry G and therefore are only induced at the one-loop level with extra suppression factors—see [20]. The coefficients c_H, c_T, c_6, and c_y are constants of order one that depend on the particular models. In 5D composite Higgs models, they take, at tree level, the values [20] $c_H = 1$, $c_T = 0$, $c_y = 1$ (respectively 0), and $c_6 = 0$ (respectively 1) for the model of [6] (respectively [5]). Only the coefficient c_T is highly constrained by the experimental data, since it contributes to the $\widehat{T}$ parameter. Nevertheless, all models with an approximate custodial symmetry give a small contribution to c_T. The other operators can only be tested in Higgs physics. They modify the Higgs decay widths according to

$$\Gamma\left(h \to f\bar{f}\right)_{\mathrm{SILH}} = \Gamma\left(h \to f\bar{f}\right)_{\mathrm{SM}}\left[1 - \xi\left(2c_y + c_H\right)\right],$$

$$\Gamma\left(h \to WW\right)_{\mathrm{SILH}} = \Gamma(h \to WW^{(*)})_{\mathrm{SM}}\left[1 - \xi c_H\right],$$

$$\Gamma\left(h \to ZZ\right)_{\mathrm{SILH}} = \Gamma(h \to ZZ^{(*)})_{\mathrm{SM}}\left[1 - \xi c_H\right],$$

$$\Gamma\left(h \to gg\right)_{\mathrm{SILH}} = \Gamma\left(h \to gg\right)_{\mathrm{SM}}\left[1 - \xi\,\mathrm{Re}\left(2c_y + c_H\right)\right], \tag{12.18}$$

$$\Gamma\left(h \to \gamma\gamma\right)_{\mathrm{SILH}} = \Gamma\left(h \to \gamma\gamma\right)_{\mathrm{SM}}\left[1 - \xi\,\mathrm{Re}\left(\frac{2c_y + c_H}{1 + J_\gamma/I_\gamma} + \frac{c_H}{1 + I_\gamma/J_\gamma}\right)\right],$$

$$\Gamma\left(h \to \gamma Z\right)_{\mathrm{SILH}} = \Gamma\left(h \to \gamma Z\right)_{\mathrm{SM}}\left[1 - \xi\,\mathrm{Re}\left(\frac{2c_y + c_H}{1 + J_Z/I_Z} + \frac{c_H}{1 + I_Z/J_Z}\right)\right].$$

The loop functions I and J are given in [20]. Notice that the contribution from c_H is universal for all Higgs couplings and therefore it does not affect the Higgs branching ratios, but only the total decay width and the production cross section. Measurement of the Higgs decay width at the LHC is very difficult and can only be reasonably done for a rather heavy Higgs, well above the two-gauge-boson threshold, which is not the case for a composite Higgs. However, for a light Higgs, LHC experiments can measure the product $\sigma_h \times \mathrm{BR}_h$ in many different channels: production through gluon, gauge boson fusion, and top-strahlung; on decay into b, τ, γ, and (virtual) weak gauge bosons. In Fig. 12.3, we show the prediction in the case of a 5D composite Higgs for the relative deviation from the SM expectation in the main channels for Higgs

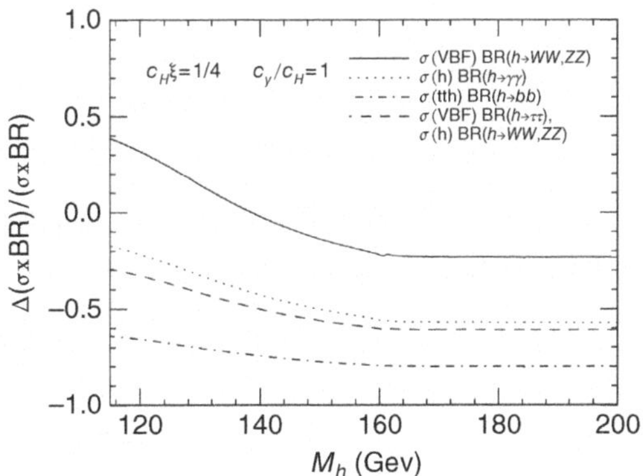

Fig. 12.3 Deviations from the SM predictions of Higgs production cross sections σ and decay branching ratios BR defined as $\Delta(\sigma\mathrm{BR})/(\sigma\mathrm{BR}) = (\sigma\mathrm{BR})_{\mathrm{SILH}}/(\sigma\mathrm{BR})_{\mathrm{SM}} - 1$. The predictions are shown for some of the main Higgs discovery channels at the LHC with production via vector boson fusion (VBF), gluon fusion (h), and top-strahlung (tth).

discovery at the LHC. At the LHC with about 300 fb^{-1}, it will be possible to measure the product of Higgs production rate with branching ratio in the various channels with 20–40% precision [21]. This will translate into a sensitivity on $|c_H\xi|$ and $|c_y\xi|$ up to 0.2–0.4, at the edge of the theoretical predictions. Since the Higgs coupling determinations at the LHC will be limited by statistics, they can benefit from a luminosity upgrade, such as the SLHC. At a linear collider, such as the ILC, precisions on $\sigma_h \times \mathrm{BR}_h$ can reach the percent level [22], providing a very sensitive probe on the scale f.

Deviations from the SM predictions of Higgs production and decay rates could be a hint of models with strong dynamics. Nevertheless, they do not unambiguously imply the existence of a new strong interaction. The most characteristic signals of the SILH Lagrangian have to be found in the very high-energy regime. Indeed, a peculiarity of the SILH Lagrangian is that, in spite of a light Higgs, longitudinal gauge boson scattering amplitudes grow with energy, and the corresponding interaction can become sizable. Indeed, the extra Higgs kinetic term proportional to $c_H\xi$ in (12.17) prevents Higgs exchange diagrams from accomplishing the exact cancellation, present in the SM, of the terms growing with energy in the amplitudes. Therefore, although the Higgs is light, we obtain strong WW scattering at high energies. Using the equivalence theorem [23], it is easy to derive the following high-energy limit of the scattering amplitudes for longitudinal gauge bosons:

$$A\left(Z_L^0 Z_L^0 \to W_L^+ W_L^-\right) = A\left(W_L^+ W_L^- \to Z_L^0 Z_L^0\right) = -A\left(W_L^\pm W_L^\pm \to W_L^\pm W_L^\pm\right),$$

$$A\left(W_L^\pm W_L^\pm \to W_L^\pm W_L^\pm\right) = -\frac{c_H s}{f^2}, \tag{12.19}$$

$$A\left(W^\pm Z_L^0 \to W^\pm Z_L^0\right) = \frac{c_H t}{f^2}, \quad A\left(W_L^+ W_L^- \to W_L^+ W_L^-\right) = \frac{c_H(s+t)}{f^2}, \tag{12.20}$$

$$A\left(Z_L^0 Z_L^0 \to Z_L^0 Z_L^0\right) = 0. \tag{12.21}$$

This result is correct to leading order in s/f^2, and to all orders in ξ in the limit $g_{\mathrm{SM}} = 0$, when the σ-model is exact. The absence of corrections in ξ follows from the nonlinear symmetry of the σ-model, corresponding to the action of the generator T_h, associated with the neutral Higgs, under which v shifts. Therefore, we expect that corrections can arise only at $\mathcal{O}(s/m_\rho^2)$. The growth with energy of the amplitudes in (12.19)–(12.21) is strictly valid only up to the maximum energy of our effective theory, namely m_ρ. The behavior above m_ρ depends on the specific model realization. In the case of the little Higgs, we expect the amplitudes to continue to grow with s up to the cutoff scale Λ. In 5D models, such as the holographic Goldstone, the growth of the elastic amplitude is softened by KK exchange, but the inelastic channel dominates, and strong coupling is reached at a scale $\sim 4\pi m_\rho/g_\rho$. Note that the results in (12.19)–(12.21) are exactly proportional to the scattering amplitudes obtained in a Higgsless SM [23]. Therefore, in theories with an SILH, the cross section at the LHC for producing longitudinal gauge bosons with large invariant masses can be written as

$$\sigma\left(pp \to V_L V_L' X\right)_{c_H} = \left(c_H\xi\right)^2 \sigma\left(pp \to V_L V_L' X\right)_H, \tag{12.22}$$

where $\sigma(pp \to V_L V'_L X)_{\not{H}}$ is the cross section in the SM without Higgs, at the leading order in $s/(4\pi v)^2$. With about 200 fb^{-1} of integrated luminosity, it should be possible to identify the signal of a Higgsless SM with about 30–50% accuracy. This corresponds to a sensitivity up to $c_H \xi \simeq 0.5$–0.7.

In the SILH framework, the Higgs is viewed as a pseudo-Goldstone boson, and therefore its properties are directly related to those of the exact (eaten) Goldstones, corresponding to the longitudinal gauge bosons. Thus, a generic prediction of SILH is that the strong gauge boson scattering is accompanied by strong production of Higgs pairs. Indeed, we find that as a consequence of the $O(4)$ symmetry of the H multiplet, the amplitudes for Higgs pair production grow with the center-of-mass energy as (12.19):

$$A\left(Z_L^0 Z_L^0 \to hh\right) = A\left(W_L^+ W_L^- \to hh\right) = \frac{c_H s}{f^2}. \tag{12.23}$$

Note that scattering amplitudes involving longitudinal gauge bosons and a single Higgs vanish. This is a consequence of the Z_2^4 parity embedded in the $O(4)$ symmetry of the operator $O_H = (\partial_\mu |H|^2)^2$, under which each Goldstone changes sign. Nonvanishing amplitudes necessarily involve an even number of each species of Goldstones.

Using (12.19), (12.20) and (12.23), we can relate the Higgs pair production rate at the LHC to the longitudinal gauge boson cross sections:

$$2\sigma_{\delta,M}\left(pp \to hhX\right)_{c_H} = \sigma_{\delta,M}\left(pp \to W_L^+ W_L^- X\right)_{c_H}$$
$$+ \frac{1}{6}\left(9 - \tanh^2 \frac{\delta}{2}\right)\sigma_{\delta,M}\left(pp \to Z_L^0 Z_L^0 X\right)_{c_H}. \tag{12.24}$$

Here, all cross sections $\sigma_{\delta,M}$ are computed with a cut on the pseudorapidity separation between the two final-state particles (a boost-invariant quantity) of $|\Delta\eta| < \delta$, and with a cut on the two-particle invariant mass $\hat{s} > M^2$. The sum rule in (12.24) is a characteristic of SILH. However, the signal from Higgs-pair production at the LHC is not so prominent. It was suggested that, for a light Higgs, this process is best studied in the channel $b\bar{b}\gamma\gamma$, but the small branching ratio of $h \to \gamma\gamma$ makes the SILH rate unobservable. However, in SILH, one can take advantage of the growth of the cross section with energy. Although we do not perform a detailed study here, it may be possible that with sufficient luminosity, the signal of $b\bar{b}b\bar{b}$ with high invariant masses could be distinguished from the SM background. Note however that because of the high boost of the Higgs boson, the b jets are often not well separated. The case in which the Higgs decays to two real W's appears more promising for detection. The cleanest channel is the one with two like-sign leptons, where $hh \to \ell^\pm \ell^\pm \nu\nu$ jets.

For order-unity coefficients c_i, we have described the SILH in terms of the two parameters m_ρ and g_ρ. An alternative description can be given in terms of two mass scales. These can be chosen as $4\pi f$, the scale at which the σ-model would become fully strongly interacting in the absence of new resonances, and m_ρ, the scale at which new states appear. An upper bound on m_ρ is obtained from the theoretical naive dimensional analysis (NDA) requirement $m_\rho < 4\pi f$, while a lower bound on m_ρ comes from the experimental constraint on the $\widehat{S}$ parameter.

Searches at the LHC, and possibly at the ILC, will probe unexplored regions of the $4\pi f$–m_ρ space. Precise measurements of Higgs production and decay rates at the LHC will be able to explore values of $4\pi f$ up to 5–7 TeV, mostly testing the existence of c_H and c_y. These measurements can be improved with a luminosity upgrade of the LHC. Higgs-physics studies at a linear collider could reach a sensitivity on $4\pi f$ up to about 30 TeV. Analyses of strong gauge boson scattering and double-Higgs production at the LHC can be sensitive to values of $4\pi f$ up to about 4 TeV. These studies are complementary to Higgs precision measurements, since they test only the coefficient c_H and probe processes highly characteristic of a strong electroweak-breaking sector with a light Higgs boson.

On the other side, the parameter m_ρ can be probed at colliders by studying pair production of longitudinal gauge bosons and Higgs, by testing triple gauge vertices, or, more directly, by producing the new resonances. For fixed m_ρ, resonance production at the LHC will overwhelm the indirect signal of longitudinal gauge boson and Higgs production at large $4\pi f$ (small g_ρ). However, at low $4\pi f$ (large g_ρ), resonance searches become less effective in constraining the parameter m_ρ, and the indirect signal gains importance. While the search for new resonances is most favorable at the LHC, precise measurements of triple gauge vertices at the ILC can test m_ρ up to 6–8 TeV. With complementary information from collider data, we will explore a large portion of the interesting region of the $4\pi f$–m_ρ plane, testing the composite nature of the Higgs.

Note added

On July 4, 2012, a scalar with the properties of the SM Higgs was discovered at the LHC with a mass around 125 GeV. This rules out technicolor theories that are Higgsless models. However, it is consistent with composite Higgs models where a light Higgs is present in the spectrum.

References

[1] S. Weinberg, Phys. Rev. **D13** (1976) 974; Phys. Rev. **D19** (1979) 1277; L. Susskind, Phys. Rev. **D20** (1979) 2619.

[2] D. B. Kaplan and H. Georgi, Phys. Lett. **136B** (1984) 183; H. Georgi and D. B. Kaplan, Phys. Lett. **B145** (1984) 216.

[3] J. M. Maldacena, Adv. Theor. Math. Phys. **2** (1998) 231; S. S. Gubser, I. R. Klebanov and A. M. Polyakov, Phys. Lett. **B428** (1998) 105; E. Witten, Adv. Theor. Math. Phys. **2** (1998) 253.

[4] C. Csaki, C. Grojean, L. Pilo, and J. Terning, Phys. Rev. Lett. **92** (2004) 101802; G. Burdman and Y. Nomura, Phys. Rev. **D69**, 115013 (2004); R. Barbieri, A. Pomarol, and R. Rattazzi, Phys. Lett. **B591** (2004) 141.

[5] K. Agashe, R. Contino, and A. Pomarol, Nucl. Phys. **B719** (2005) 165.

[6] R. Contino, L. Da Rold, and A. Pomarol, Phys. Rev. **D75**, 055014 (2007).

[7] G. 't Hooft, Nucl. Phys. **B72** (1974) 461; E. Witten, Nucl. Phys. **B160** (1979) 57.

[8] K. Lane, arXiv:hep-ph/0202255.

[9] R. Barbieri, A. Pomarol, R. Rattazzi, and A. Strumia, Nucl. Phys. **B703** (2004) 127.

[10] M. E. Peskin and T. Takeuchi, Phys. Rev. Lett. **65**, 964 (1990); Phys. Rev. **D46**, 381 (1992).

[11] K. Agashe, R. Contino, L. Da Rold, and A. Pomarol, Phys. Lett. **B641** (2006) 62.

[12] G. Cacciapaglia, C. Csaki, G. Marandella, and J. Terniry, Phys. Rev. **D75** (2007) 015003.

[13] N. Arkani-Hamed, A. G. Cohen, and H. Georgi, Phys. Lett. **B513** (2001) 232–240; N. Arkani-Hamed, A. G. Cohen, T. Gregoire, and J. G. Wacker, JHEP **0208** (2002) 020.

[14] G. L. Bayatian et al. [CMS Collaboration], J. Phys. **G34** (2007) 995–1579.

[15] K. Agashe, A. Belyaev, T. Krupovnickas, G. Perez, and J. Virzi, Phys. Rev. **D77** (2008) 015003.

[16] R. Contino and G. Servant, JHEP **0806** (2008) 026; J. A. Aguilar-Saavedra, JHEP **0911** (2009) 030.

[17] J. Mrazek and A. Wulzer, Phys. Rev. **D81** (2010) 075006.

[18] T. Han, H. E. Logan, B. McElrath, and L.-T. Wany, Phys. Rev. **D67** (2003) 095004; M. Perelstein, M. E. Peskin, and A. Pierce, Phys. Rev. **D69** (2004) 075002.

[19] G. Azuelos et al., Eur. Phys. J. **C39S2** (2005) 13.

[20] G. F. Giudice, C. Grojean, A. Pomarol, and R. Rattazzi, JHEP **0706** (2007) 045.

[21] M. Dührssen, ATL-PHYS-2003-030.

[22] J. A. Aguilar-Saavedra et al. [ECFA/DESY LC Physics Working Group], arXiv:hep-ph/0106315.

[23] M. S. Chanowitz and M. K. Gaillard, Nucl. Phys. **B261** (1985) 379.

13
String phenomenology

Luis IBÁÑEZ

Departamento de Física Teórica and Instituto de Física Teórica UAM-CSIC,
Universidad Autónoma de Madrid, Cantoblanco, Madrid, Spain

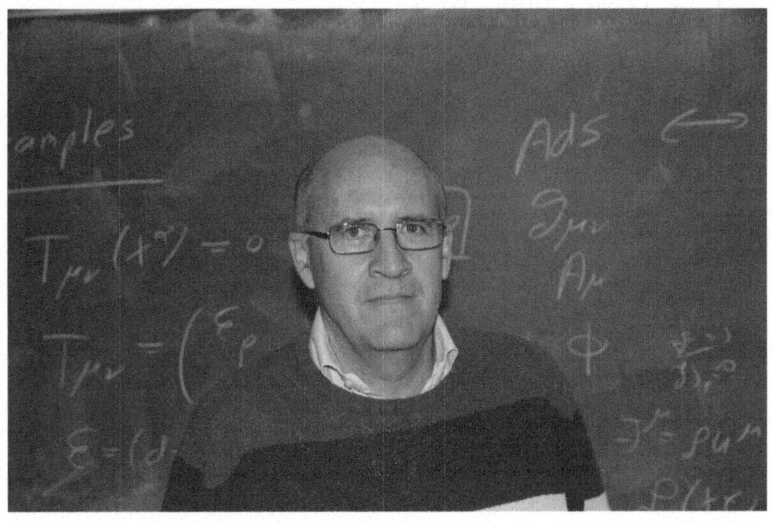

Theoretical Physics to Face the Challenge of LHC. Edited by L. Baulieu, K. Benakli, M. R. Douglas,
B. Mansoulié, E. Rabinovici, and L. F. Cugliandolo. © Oxford University Press 2015.
Published in 2015 by Oxford University Press.

Chapter Contents

This chapter is based on lectures given at the Les Houches Summer School in 2011, in which I reviewed a number of topics in the field of string phenomenology, focusing on orientifold/F-theory models yielding semirealistic low-energy physics. The emphasis was on the extraction of the low-energy effective action and the possible test of specific models at the LHC. The chapter is a brief summary of some of the main topics covered in the lectures, updated where appropriate.

13.1 Branes and chirality

String theory (ST) is the most serious candidate for a consistent theory of quantum gravity coupled to matter. In fact, ST actually predicts the very existence of gravity, since a massless spin-2 particle, the graviton, appears automatically in the spectrum of closed string theories. Furthermore, ST has also allowed us to improve our understanding of the origin of black hole degrees of freedom and provides for explicit realizations of *holography* through the AdS/CFT correspondence. Remarkably, not only is ST a theory of quantum gravity, but it also incorporates all the essential ingredients of the Standard Model (SM) of particle physics: gauge interactions, chiral fermions, Yukawa couplings,... It is thus a strong candidate to provide us with a unified theory of all interactions, including the SM and gravitation. In the last 25 years, enormous progress has been obtained in the understanding of the space of four-dimensional (4d) string vacua [1]. From the point of view of unification, the main objective is to understand how the SM may be obtained as a low-energy limit of string theory. We would like to understand how the SM gauge group, the three quark/lepton generations, chirality, Yukawa couplings, CP violation, neutrino masses, Higgs sector, etc. may appear from an underlying string theory. The first step in that direction is learning which compactifications lead to a chiral spectrum of massless fermions at low energies. There are essentially five large classes of such chiral 4d string vacua, symbolized by the five vertices of the pentagon in Fig. 13.1.

These include three large classes of type II *orientifolds* (IIA with O6 orientifold planes, and IIB with O3/O7 or O9/O5 orientifold planes). In addition, there are the

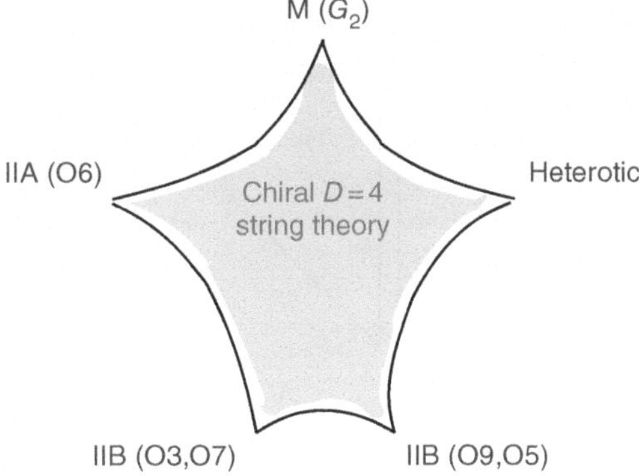

Fig. 13.1 The five large classes of 4d chiral string compactifications.

well-studied heterotic vacua in Calabi–Yau (CY) manifolds. Finally, there are less studied (and difficult to handle) vacua obtained from the 11d M-theory compactified on manifolds of G_2 holonomy. Different dualities connect these different corners, so the different classes of vacua should be considered as five different corners of a single underlying class of theories. It is impossible to overview all these different classes of theories, so we will concentrate on the case of the type II orientifolds whose potential for the construction of realistic SM-like compactifications has been explored in the last 15 years.

The essential objects in chiral type II orientifolds are Dp-branes, nonperturbative solitonic states of string theory that extend over $p + 1$ space $+$ time dimensions. For our purposes, Dp-branes may be considered as subspaces of the 10d space of type II string theory in which open strings are allowed to start and end. They are charged under antisymmetric tensors of the Ramond–Ramond (RR) sector of type II theory with $p + 1$ indices. Since in type IIA (IIB), the massless RR tensors have an odd (even) number of indices, there are Dp-branes with p even (odd) for type IIA (IIB) string theory. We will be interested in Dp-branes large enough to contain the standard Minkowski space inside, so that the relevant Dp-branes will be D4, D6, D8 in type IIA and D3, D5, D7, D9 in type IIB. In compactified theories, Gauss's theorem will force the vanishing of the overall RR charges with respect to these antisymmetric fields. This leads to the so-called *tadpole* cancellation conditions, which turn out to also ensure cancellation of gauge and gravitational anomalies in the theory.

In the worldvolume of Dp-branes, there live (are localized) gauge and charged matter degrees of freedom. In a single Dp-brane lives a $U(1)$ gauge boson, and M such branes located in the same place in transverse dimensions contain an enhanced $U(M)$ gauge symmetry with $\mathcal{N} = 4$ SUSY in flat space (Fig. 13.2). The corresponding spectrum is obviously nonchiral and insufficient to yield realistic physics. In order to obtain chirality, additional ingredients must be present. In the case of type IIA models with the six extra dimensions compactified in a CY manifold, chiral fermions appear at the intersection of pairs of D6-branes, as we will describe later. In the case of type

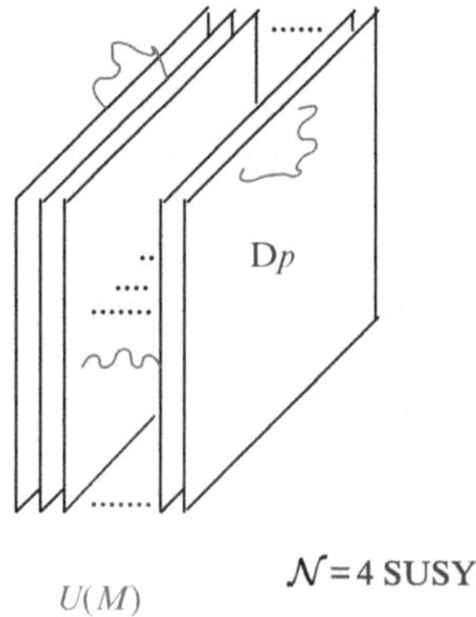

Fig. 13.2 Open strings ending on a stack of M parallel Dp-branes give rise to a $U(M)$, $\mathcal{N} = 4$ gauge theory.

IIB models, chiral fermions may appear at the worldvolume of D7 or D9 branes in the presence of magnetic fluxes in the compact directions. Alternatively, chirality may appear if the geometry is singular, like, for example, the case of D3-branes on $\mathbf{Z}_N$ orbifold singularities.

The other crucial ingredients in perturbative type II models are Op-*orientifolds*. These are geometrically analogous to Dp-branes, with the crucial difference that they are not dynamical and do not contain any field degrees of freedom in their worldvolume. They are, however, charged under the RR antisymmetric fields, and also they have *negative* tension compared with their Dp-brane counterparts. It is precisely these two properties that make the presence of orientifold planes useful, since their negative tension and RR charges may be used to cancel the positive contribution of Dp-branes, allowing the construction of type II vacua with zero vacuum energy (Minkowski) and overall vanishing RR charges in a compact space.

Another important property of type IIA and IIB vacua is mirror symmetry. This is a symmetry that exchanges IIA and IIB compactifications by exchanging the respective underlying CY space with its mirror. For each CY manifold, one can find a mirror manifold in which the Kähler and complex structure moduli are exchanged. In simple examples (such as tori and orbifolds thereof), one can show that mirror symmetry is a particular example of *T-duality*. The action of T-duality in these toroidal/orbifold settings (to be discussed below) is nontrivial and exchanges Neumann and Dirichlet open string boundary conditions. An odd number of T-dualities along 1-cycles exchanges type IIA and IIB theories, and the dimensionalities of Dp-branes change accordingly. Thus, for example, three T-dualities on type IIB D9-branes on $\mathbf{T}^6$ change them into $D6$-branes wrapping a 3-cycle in $\mathbf{T}^6$.

The basic rules for D-brane model building are as follows (for reviews, see, e.g., [2]). One starts with type II theory compactified on a CY (in some simple examples, one may consider $\mathbf{T}^6$ tori or orbifolds). One then considers possible distributions of Dp-branes containing Minkowski space and preserving $\mathcal{N} = 1$ SUSY in 4d. The branes wrap subspaces (cycles) or are located at specific regions inside the CY. The configuration so far has positive energy and RR charges and is untenable if one wants to obtain Minkowski vacua. To achieve that, appropriate Op-orientifold planes will be required to cancel both the positive vacuum energy and the overall RR charges. This will require the construction of a CY orientifold. Finally, the brane distribution is so chosen that the massless sector resembles as much as possible the SM or the Minimal Supersymmetric Standard Model (MSSM). If the brane distribution respects the same $\mathcal{N} = 1$ SUSY in 4d, the theory will be perturbatively stable.

In the above enterprise, two approaches are possible:

- *Global models.* One insists on having a complete globally consistent CY compactification, with all RR tadpoles canceling.
- *Local models.* One considers local sets of lower-dimensional Dp-branes ($p \leq 7$) that are localized on some region of the CY and reproduce the SM or MSSM physics there. One does not care at this stage about global aspects of the compactification and assumes that eventually the configuration may be embedded inside a fully consistent global compact model.

The latter is often called the *bottom-up* approach [3], since one first constructs the local (bottom) model with the idea that eventually one may embed it in some global model. Note that this philosophy is not applicable to heterotic or type I vacua, since in those strings the SM fields live in the bulk six dimensions of the CY.

13.2 Type II orientifolds: intersections and magnetic fluxes

In type IIA compactifications, in principle, we have D4-, D6-, and D8-branes, big enough to contain Minkowski space $\mathbf{M}_4$. They can span $\mathbf{M}_4$ and wrap respectively 1-, 3-, and 5-cycles in the CY. However, since CY manifolds do not have nontrivial 1- or 5-cycles, in IIA orientifolds only D6-branes are relevant for our purposes. It is easy to see that a pair of intersecting branes, $D6_a$, $D6_b$ give rise to chiral fermions at their intersection from open strings starting in one and ending on the other brane (see Fig. 13.3). The mass formula for the fields at an intersection in flat space is given (in bosonized formulation) by

$$M_{ab}^2 = N_{\mathrm{osc}} + \frac{(r + r_\theta)^2}{2} - \frac{1}{2} + \sum_{i=1}^{3} \frac{1}{2}|\theta_i|(1 - |\theta_i|), \qquad (13.1)$$

where $r_\theta = (\theta_1, \theta_2, \theta_3, 0)$ and r belongs to the $SO(8)$ lattice ($r_i = \mathbf{Z}, \mathbf{Z} + \frac{1}{2}$ for NS, RR sectors, respectively, with $\sum_i r_i = $ odd). The reader can check that the state $r + r_\theta = (-\frac{1}{2} + \theta_1, -\frac{1}{2} + \theta_2, -\frac{1}{2} + \theta_3, +\frac{1}{2})$ is massless for any value of the angles, so there is always a massless fermion at the intersection. If there are N $D6_a$ and M $D6_b$ intersecting stacks of branes, the fermion transforms in the bifundamental $(\mathbf{N}, \overline{\mathbf{M}})$. There are also three scalars (e.g., $r + r_\theta = (-1 + \theta_1, \theta_2, \theta_3, 0)$) with mass-squared that may be positive, zero, or negative, depending on the values of the angles. Tachyons are avoided for large ranges of the intersecting angles. On the other hand, for particular choices of the angles, there is a massless scalar, the partner of the chiral fermion, signaling the presence of an $\mathcal{N} = 1$ SUSY, at least at the local level.

To construct 4d models, one compactifies type IIA string theory down to four dimensions on a CY manifold. The resulting theory has $\mathcal{N} = 2$ SUSY and is not yet

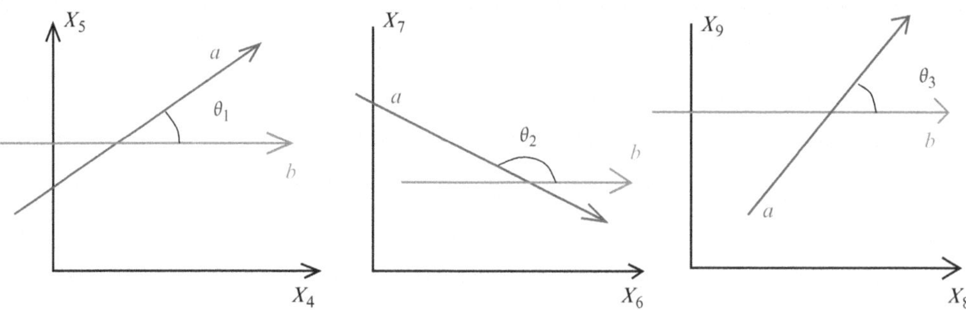

Fig. 13.3 Open strings between $D6_a$ and $D6_b$ branes intersecting at angles yield massless chiral fermions. Here $X_5, \ldots, X_9$ are local coordinates for the compact space.

suitable for realistic model building. One then constructs an orientifold by modding the theory by $\Omega\mathcal{R}$, where Ω is the worldsheet parity operation and $\mathcal{R}$ is a $\mathbf{Z}_2$ antiholomorphic involution on the CY with $\mathcal{R}J = -J$ and $\mathcal{R}\Omega_3 = \overline{\Omega}_3$ (J and Ω_3 are the Kähler 2-form and the holomorphic 3-form characteristic of CY manifolds). The resulting theory now has $\mathcal{N} = 1$ SUSY in 4d, and the submanifolds left fixed under the $\mathcal{R}$ operation are orientifold O6-planes carrying C_7 RR antisymmetric field charge. To flesh out these proceses, let us consider the simplified (yet phenomenologically interesting) case of a $\mathbf{T}^6$ orientifold compactification [4].

Consider type IIA string theory compactified in a factorized torus $\mathbf{T}^6 = \mathbf{T}^2 \times \mathbf{T}^2 \times \mathbf{T}^2$. D6-branes are assumed to wrap $\mathbf{M}_4$ and a 3-cycle that is the direct product of three 1-cycles, one per $\mathbf{T}^2$ (see Fig. 13.4). These cycles are described by integers (n_a^i, m_a^i), $i = 1, 2, 3$ indicating the number of times $n_a^i(m_a^i)$ the D6$_a$ brane wraps around the horizontal(vertical) directions. For each stack of N_a D6$_a$-branes there is a $U(N_a)$ gauge group. Furthermore at the intersection of two stacks of branes D6$_a$, D6$_b$ the exchange of open strings gives rise to massless chiral fermions in bifundamental $(\mathbf{N}_a, \overline{\mathbf{N}}_b)$ representations. Their multiplicity is given by their intersection number

$$I_{ab} = I_{ab}^1 \times I_{ab}^2 \times I_{ab}^3 = (n_a^1 m_b^1 - m_a^1 n_b^1)(n_a^2 m_b^2 - m_a^2 n_b^2)(n_a^3 m_b^3 - m_a^3 n_b^3), \quad (13.2)$$

which is, $2 \times 2 \times 1 = 4$ in the example of Fig. 13.4. We now construct an orientifold by modding out the theory by the worldsheet operator $\Omega(\tau, \sigma) = (\tau, -\sigma)$ acting on the worldsheet coordinates. Simultaneously, we act with a reflection on the three coordinates $R(X_i) = -X_i$, $i = 5, 7, 9$. This geometrical reflection leaves invariant the space defined by $X_5 = X_7 = X_9 = 0$ in which the O6-orientifold lives. In addition, the orientifold projection on invariant states may modify the gauge group of the branes if the latter wrap a 3-cycle that is left invariant by the orientifold. Depending on the details of the projection, one may get $Sp(N)$ or $O(N)$ groups. On the other hand, if the 3-cycle wrapped by the D6-brane stack is not invariant, one must add in the background extra

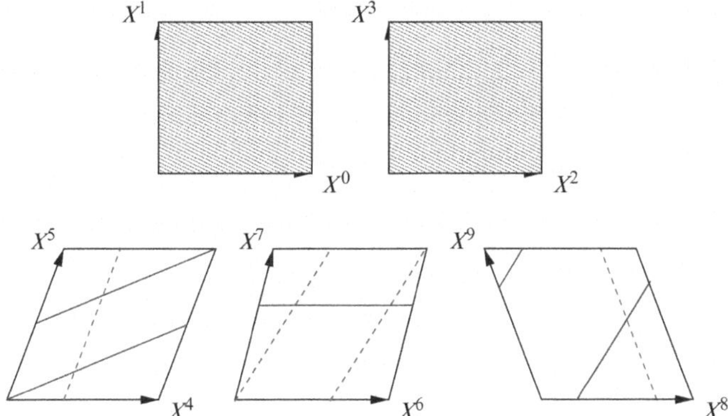

Fig. 13.4 D6-branes wrap 1-cycles in each of the three $\mathbf{T}^2$ and intersect at angles. Chiral bifundamental fermions are localized at the intersections.

Table 13.1 Wrapping numbers of D6-branes in an MSSM-like configuration

N_α	(n_i^1, m_i^1)	(n_i^2, m_i^2)	(n_i^3, m_i^3)
$N_a = 3 + 1$	$(1, 0)$	$(3, 1)$	$(3, -1)$
$N_b = 1$	$(0, 1)$	$(1, 0)$	$(0, -1)$
$N_c = 1$	$(0, 1)$	$(0, -1)$	$(1, 0)$

mirror D6*-branes siting on the reflected 3-cycle with wrapping numbers $(n^i, -m^i)$. Then the configuration is also invariant, but the gauge group $U(N)$ remains.

It is easy to find choices of D6-branes with appropriate wrapping numbers (n^i, m^i) yielding a semirealistic chiral massless spectrum. Let as consider three stacks D6$_a$, D6$_b$, D6$_c$ of branes on rectangular $\mathbf{T}^2$ tori with multiplicities and wrapping numbers as in Table 13.1 [5]. The D6$_b$ and D6$_c$ branes are assumed to be located at $X_7 = 0$ and $X_9 = 0$, respectively, so that the orientifold projection yields an $Sp(1) \simeq SU(2)$ gauge group for both of them. On the other hand, the $3 + 1$ D6$_a$ branes in Table 13.1 should be suplemented by their mirrors with wrapping numbers flipped as $(n_a^i, m_a^i) \rightarrow (n_a, -m_a^i)$, and the gauge group is $U(3) \times U(1)$. The complete gauge group is then $U(3) \times SU(2) \times SU(2) \times U(1)$, but one linear combination of the two $U(1)$'s is anomalous and becomes massive through a generalized Green–Schwarz mechanism. All in all, one obtains the gauge group of the minimal left–right-symmetric extension of the MSSM. The reader may check using (13.2) that these are three generations of quarks and leptons, with three right-handed neutrinos. Furthermore, if the branes D6$_b$ and D6$_c$ sit on top of each other in the first $\mathbf{T}^2$, there is one minimal set of Higgs fields. Choosing $R_x^2/R_y^2 = R_x^3/R_y^3$ for the radii in the second and third tori, one can see that $\theta_2 + \theta_3 = 0$ and there is one unbroken $\mathcal{N} = 1$ SUSY.

The above example is a *good local model*, but it is globally inconsistent. The reason is that, as it stands, it gives rise to RR tadpoles, and the overall charge with respect to the C^7 RR forms does not vanish as it should in a compact space. It is easy to show that those conditions in this toroidal setting are

$$\sum_a N_a n_a^1 n_a^2 n_a^3 = 16, \quad \sum_a N_a n_a^1 m_a^2 m_a^3 = 0 \ (+ \text{ permutations}), \tag{13.3}$$

and plugging in the wrapping numbers from Table 13.1 shows that they are not obeyed. It is, however, easy to constract a $\mathbf{Z}_2 \times \mathbf{Z}_2$ orbifold variation of this model with some additional D6-branes and orientifold planes that is supersymmetric and obeys the corresponding tadpole conditions [6].

This model is remarkably simple, and its chiral sector gets quite close to a phenomenologically interesting model, the L–R extension of the MSSM. It still has the shortcoming that, like most toroidal/orbifold models, the massless spectrum includes additional adjoint chiral multiplets of the SM gauge group. The vacuum expectation values of these adjoints parametrize the freedom to translate in parallel the positions of the branes in any of these models. The latter is a characteristic of toroidal compactifications and is in general absent in more general CY orientifolds.

A second class of interesting type II compactifications comprises type IIB orientifolds. Now the internal orientifold geometric involution acts like $RJ = J$, $R\Omega_3 = -\Omega_3$. In the toroidal setting, these may be obtained as T-duals of type IIA intersecting brane models. Indeed, upon an odd number of T-dualities along the six circles in the $\mathbf{T}^6$, a D6-brane may transform into a D9-, D7-, D5-, or D3-brane, depending on the particular T-duality transformation. If the original D6-, brane is rotated with respect to the orientifold plane, the resulting IIB Dp-branes will in general contain a magnetic flux turned on in their worldvolume. Indeed, higher-dimensional type IIB branes in SUSY configurations (unlike the D6-branes in type IIA) may contain magnetic flux backgrounds. They in turn induce lower-dimensional Dp-brane charge and also chirality. Let us consider [7] the case of N_a D9-branes wrapped m_a^i times on the ith $\mathbf{T}^2$ and with n_a^i units of $U(1)_a$ quantized magnetic flux:

$$m_a^i \frac{1}{2\pi} \int_{\mathbf{T}_i^2} F_a^i = n_a^i. \tag{13.4}$$

Interestingly enough, the (n_a^i, m_a^i) D6 wrapping numbers are mapped under T-duality into the magnetic integers defined above. In addition, the relative angle θ_{ab}^i of D6$_a$–D6$_b$ branes in the ith torus is mapped into the difference

$$\theta_{ab}^i = \arctan F_b^i - \arctan F_a^i, \quad F_a^i = \frac{n_a^i}{m_a^i R_{xi} R_{yi}}. \tag{13.5}$$

In the presence of a magnetic flux F in a IIB brane wrapping $\mathbf{T}^2$, the open string boundary conditions are modified as

$$\partial_\sigma X - F\partial_\tau Y = 0, \quad \partial_\sigma Y + F\partial_\tau X = 0. \tag{13.6}$$

In particular, by varying F, one interpolates between Neumann and Dirichlet boundary conditions and, for example, at formally infinite flux, they are purely Dirichlet. Thus, adding fluxes on a higher-dimensional brane induces RR charge corresponding to lower-dimensional branes. For example, D9-branes with flux numbers $(1,0)(n_a^2, m_a^2)(n_a^3, m_a^3)$ are equivalent to D7^1-branes that are localized on the first $\mathbf{T}^2$ and wrap the remaining $\mathbf{T}^2 \times \mathbf{T}^2$. On the other hand, D9-branes with flux numbers $(1,0)(1,0)(1,0)$ (formally infinite flux in the three $\mathbf{T}^2$'s) are equivalent to D3-branes. Note in particular that the semirealistic model with intersecting D6-branes as in Table 13.1 are mapped into a set of three stacks of D7$_a^1$, D7$_b^2$, D7$_c^3$ that overlap pairwise on a $\mathbf{T}^2$. Chirality arises in this type IIB mirror from the mismatch between L- and R-handed fermions induced by the finite flux in the second and third tori.

This view of the orientifolds in terms of type IIB D7-branes overlapping on 2d spaces ($\mathbf{T}^2$ in the toroidal example) is particularly interesting because it admits a straightforward generalization to type IIB CY orientifolds, at least in the large-compact-volume approximation in which Kaluza–Klein field theory techniques are available. In contrast, the mirror class of models of type IIA orientifolds with intersecting D6-branes is more difficult to generalize to curved CY spaces, since the mathematical definition of BPS D6-branes in curved space (wrapping so-called special Lagrangian 3-cycles) is more difficult to analyze. A further argument for concentrating on type IIB orientifolds with D7/D3-branes is that in the last 10 years we have learnt a great deal about how the addition of type IIB closed string antisymmetric field fluxes can fix most or all the moduli. The equivalent analysis for type IIA or heterotic vacua is at present far less developed.

One generic problem in both IIA and IIB cases is the *top quark problem* in models with a unified gauge symmetry such as $SU(5)$. The point is that in perturbative orientifolds, the GUT symmetry is actually $U(5)$ and the quantum numbers of a GUT generation are $\bar{\mathbf{5}}_{-1} + \mathbf{10}_2$, with Higgs multiplets $\mathbf{5}_1 + \bar{\mathbf{5}}_{-1}$. It is then clear that D-quark/lepton Yukawas are allowed by the $U(1)$ symmetry, but the U-quark couplings from $\mathbf{10}_2\mathbf{10}_2\mathbf{5}_1$ are perturbatively forbidden. This $U(1)$ symmetry is in fact anomalous and massive, but still remains as a perturbative global symmetry in the effective action. Instanton effects may violate it, but one expects the corresponding nonperturbative contributions to be small and to be relevant at most only for the lightest generations, not the top quark. Thus insisting on unification of SM groups in perturbative orientifolds gives rise to a *top quark problem*.

13.3 Local F-theory GUTs

F-theory [8] may be considered as a geometric nonperturbative formulation of type IIB orientifolds. From the model-building point of view, its interest is twofold: (1) it provides a solution to the top quark problem of perturbative type II orientifolds with a GUT symmetry and (2) moduli fixing induced by closed string antisymmetric fluxes is relatively well understood. In loose terms, one could say that it combines advantages from the heterotic and type IIB vacua.

An important massless field of 10d type IIB string theory is the complexified dilaton field $\tau = e^{-\phi} + iC_0$. The dilaton ϕ controls the perturbative loop expansion and C_0 is a RR scalar. The 10d theory has an $SL(2, \mathbf{Z})$ symmetry under which τ is the modular parameter. The symmetry is generated by the transformations $\tau \to 1/\tau$ and $\tau \to \tau + i$ and is clearly nonperturbative (e.g., it exchanges strong and weak coupling by inverting the dilaton). F-theory provides a geometrization of this symmetry by adding two (auxiliary) extra dimensions with $\mathbf{T}^2$ geometry and identifying the complex structure of this $\mathbf{T}^2$ with the type IIB τ field. The resulting geometric construction is 12-dimensional, and one obtains $\mathcal{N} = 1$ 4d vacua by compactifying the theory on a complex 4-fold CY X_4 that is an *elliptic fibration* over a six-dimensional base B_3; i.e., locally one has $X_4 \simeq \mathbf{T}^2 \times B_3$. The theory contains 7-branes that appear at points in the base B_3 at which the fibration becomes singular, corresponding to 4-cycles wrapped by the 7-brane. As in the case of perturbative D7-branes, there is a gauge group associated with these branes. However, unlike the perturbative case, the possible gauge groups include the exceptional ones E_6, E_7, and E_8. This is an important property, since, as we will see momentarily, it allows for the existence of an $SU(5)$ GUT symmetry with a large top Yukawa. A particularly interesting type of F-theory constructions comprises those involving a GUT symmetry such as $SU(5)$ and termed F-theory GUTs (for reviews, see [9]). These are motivated by the apparent unification of coupling constants in the MSSM. Such constructions are a nonperturbative generalization of the type IIB models with intersecting (and magnetized) D7 branes that we discussed in Section 13.2. There is a 7-brane wrapping a 4-cycle S inside B_3, yielding an $SU(5)$ gauge symmetry. As in the bottom-up approach mentioned above, one can decouple the local dynamics associated with the $SU(5)$ brane from the global aspects of the B_3 compact space. Chiral matter again appears at the intersection of pairs of 7-branes, *matter curves* in the F-theory language, corresponding to an enhanced degree of the singularity. These 7-branes are, however, nonperturbative and cannot simply be described in terms of perturbative open strings. A visual intuition of the appearance of matter fields in an $SU(5)$ F-theory GUT is shown in Fig. 13.5. At the matter curves, the symmetry is locally enhanced to $SU(6)$ or $SO(10)$. Recalling the adjoint branchings

$$
\begin{aligned}
SU(6) &\longrightarrow SU(5) \times U(1), \\
\mathbf{35} &\longrightarrow \mathbf{24}_0 + \mathbf{1}_0 + [\mathbf{5}_1 + \text{c.c.}],
\end{aligned}
\tag{13.7}
$$

$$
\begin{aligned}
SO(10) &\longrightarrow SU(5) \times U(1)', \\
\mathbf{45} &\longrightarrow \mathbf{24}_0 + \mathbf{1}_0 + [\mathbf{10}_4 + \text{c.c.}],
\end{aligned}
\tag{13.8}
$$

one sees that in the matter curve associated with the 5-plet, the symmetry is enhanced to $SU(6)$, whereas in that related to the 10-plets, the symmetry is enhanced to $SO(10)$. As in the perturbative magnetized IIB orientifolds, in order to get chiral fermions there must be in general nonvanishing fluxes along the $U(1)$ and $U(1)'$ symmetries. A third matter curve with an enhanced $SU(6)'$ symmetry is also required to obtain Higgs 5-plets. Yukawa couplings appear at the intersection of the Higgs matter curve with the fermion matter curves, as illustrated in Fig. 13.6. At the intersection point, the symmetry is further enhanced to $SO(12)$ in the case of the $\mathbf{10} \times \bar{\mathbf{5}} \times \bar{\mathbf{5}}_H$ couplings and to E_6 in the case of the U-quark couplings. One may now understand why there are

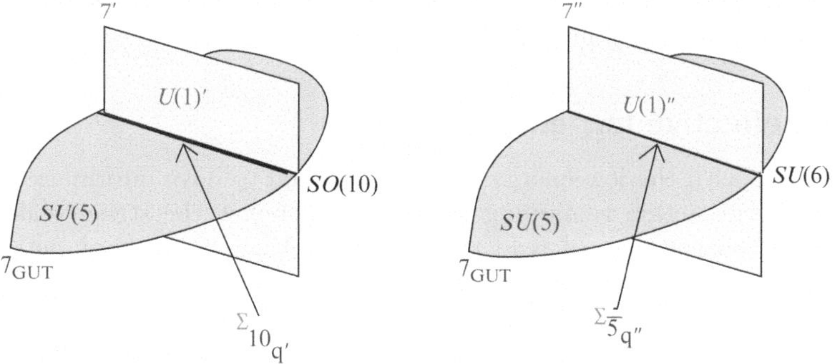

Fig. 13.5 The $SU(5)$ matter fields live at matter curves corresponding to the intersection of the bulk $SU(5)$ brane with $U(1)$ branes. At the matter curves, the symmetry is enhanced to $SU(6)$ and $SO(10)$, respectively, for the multiplets $\mathbf{10}$ and $\bar{\mathbf{5}}$.

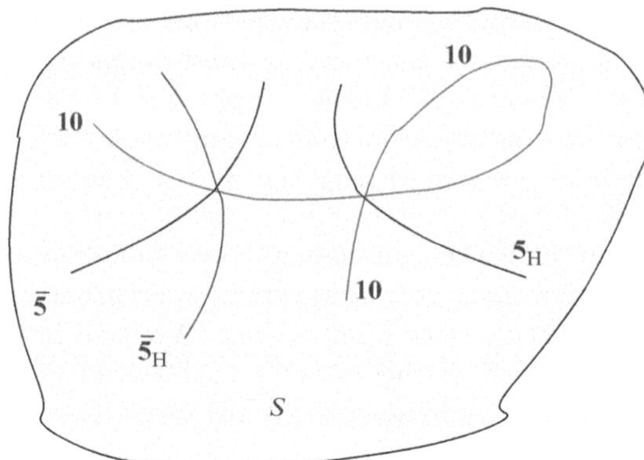

Fig. 13.6 Matter curves generically intersect at points of further enhanced symmetry at which the $\mathbf{10} \times \bar{\mathbf{5}} \times \bar{\mathbf{5}}_H$ and $\mathbf{10} \times \mathbf{10} \times \mathbf{5}_H$ Yukawa couplings localize.

U-quark Yuyawa couplings in F-theory by looking at the branching of E_6 adjoint into $SU(5) \times U(1) \times U(1)'$:

$$E_6 \longrightarrow SU(5) \times U(1) \times U(1)',$$

$$\mathbf{78} \longrightarrow \text{adjoints} \; + \; [(\mathbf{10}, -1, -3) + (\mathbf{10}, 4, 0) + (\mathbf{5}, -3, 3) + (\mathbf{1}, 5, 3) + \text{h.c.}]. \tag{13.9}$$

We now see that one can form a $\mathbf{10} \times \mathbf{10} \times \mathbf{5}$ coupling, which is indeed allowed by the $U(1)$ symmetries. We will come back to the issue of Yukawa couplings in F-theory local GUTs in the Section 13.4.

To make the final contact with SM physics, the $SU(5)$ symmetry must be broken down to $SU(3) \times SU(2) \times U(1)$. In these constructions, there are no massless adjoints to make that breaking, and discrete Wilson lines are also not available. Still, one can make such a breaking by the addition of an additional flux F_Y along the hypercharge direction of the $SU(5)$, which has the same symmetry-breaking effect as an adjoint Higgs. Interestingly enough, this hypercharge flux may also be used to obtain doublet–triplet splitting of the Higgs multiplets $\mathbf{5}_H + \bar{\mathbf{5}}_H$.

13.4 The effective low-energy action

To make contact with the low-energy physics, we need to have information about the effective low-energy action remaining at scales well below the string scale. Here, we will concentrate on the case of field theories with $\mathcal{N} = 1$ supersymmetry, which is assumed to be broken later at scales of order the electroweak (EW) scale. In this case, the action is determined by the Kähler potential K, gauge kinetic functions f_a, and the superpotential W, which we will discuss in turn. For definiteness, we will concentrate on the case of the effective action for type IIB orientifolds, whose general features are also expected to apply to the F-theory case.

In the massless sector of an $\mathcal{N} = 1$ compactification, there are charged fields from the open string sector (to be identified with the SM fields) and closed string fields giving rise to singlet chiral multiplets, the moduli. Among the latter, there is the complex dilaton $S = e^{-\phi} + iC_0$, which is just the dimensional reduction of the complex dilaton τ mentioned above. In addition, there are h_{11} Kähler moduli T^i and h_{21}^- complex structure moduli U^j (the minus means the number of $(2,1)$-forms that are odd under the orientifold projection). The Kähler moduli parametrize the volume of the manifold and also of all the 4-cycles $\Sigma_4^{(i)}$ of the specific CY. The complex structure fields U^j, on the other hand, parametrize the deformations of the CY manifolds and are associated with the 3-cycles $\Sigma_3^{(j)}$ in the CY. Specifically, one has [10] (in the simplest $h_{11}^- = 0$ case)

$$T^i = e^{-\phi}\mathrm{Vol}(\Sigma_4^{(i)}) + iC_4^{(i)}, \qquad U^j = \int_{\Sigma_3^{(j)}} \Omega_3, \tag{13.10}$$

where $\mathrm{Vol}(\Sigma_4^{(i)})$ is the volume of the 3-cycle $\Sigma_4^{(i)}$ and the $C_4^{(i)}$ are 4d zero modes of the RR 4-form C_4 on the 4-cycles. The $\mathcal{N} = 1$ supergravity Kähler potential associated with the moduli in type IIB orientifold compactifications may be written as [10]

$$K_{\mathrm{IIB}} = -\log(S + S^*) - 2\,\log[e^{-3\phi/2}\,\mathrm{Vol}(CY)] - \log\left(-i\int \Omega_3 \wedge \overline{\Omega}_3\right), \tag{13.11}$$

where $\mathrm{Vol}(CY)$ is the volume of the CY manifold. In the toroidal case with rectangular $\mathbf{T}^6 = \mathbf{T}^2 \times \mathbf{T}^2 \times \mathbf{T}^2$, the Kähler potential takes the simple form

$$K_{\mathrm{IIB}} = -\log(S + S^*) - \sum_{i=1}^{3}\log(U_i + U_i^*) - \sum_{i=1}^{3}\log(T_i + T_i^*), \tag{13.12}$$

where $T_i = e^{-\phi}R_x^j R_y^j R_x^k R_y^k - iC_4$, with $i \neq j \neq k \neq i$ and $U_i = R_y^i/R_x^i$. This is the familiar no-scale structure that also appears in heterotic $\mathcal{N} = 1$ vacua.

Concerning the action for the charged matter fields Φ_a on the 7-branes, the corresponding Kähler metrics, gauge kinetic functions, and superpotential are themselves functions of the moduli. One can write for the general form of the supergravity Kähler potential an expression (to leading order in a matter field expansion)

$$K(M, M^*, \Phi_a, \Phi_a^*) = K_{\mathrm{IIB}}(M, M^*) + \sum_{ab} K_{ab}(M, M^*)\Phi_a\Phi_b^*$$
$$+ \log|W(M) + W_Y(M, \Phi_a)|^2, \tag{13.13}$$

where M collectively denotes the moduli S, T^i, U^j, $W(M)$ is the superpotential of the moduli, and $W_Y(M, \Phi_a)$ is he Yukawa coupling superpotential of the SM fields. We have already discussed the first term in (13.13), and we will discuss the remaining terms in what follows.

13.4.1 The Kähler metrics

Equation (13.13) includes the kinetic term for the matter fields, which is controlled by the Kähler metric K_{ab}, which is a function of the moduli. This dependence on the moduli is dictated by the geometric origin of the field. It has been computed at the classical level for some simple cases (mostly toroidal/orbifold orientifolds), either by dimensional redaction from the underlying 10d theory or by using explicit string correlators. We are particularly interested in the Kähler metrics of fields living at intersecting 7-branes, since those are the ones that are associated with the MSSM fields in semirealistic IIB or F-theory compactifications. In the case of type IIB toroidal/orbifold orientifolds, the matter fields associated with a pair of intersecting $D7^i$–$D7^j$ branes has a metric (neglecting magnetic fluxes for the moment) [11]

$$K_{ab}^{ij} = \delta_{ab} \, \frac{1}{u_i^{1/2} u_j^{1/2} t_k^{1/2} s^{1/2}}, \quad i \neq j \neq k \neq i, \tag{13.14}$$

where $t_i = T_i + T_i^*, u_i = U_i + U_i^*$, and $s = S + S^*$. We thus see that the metrics of matter fields at intersections scale like $K_{ab} \simeq t^{-1/2}$ with the Kähler moduli.

Toroidal orientifolds/orbifolds, however, are very special in some ways. We would rather like to see to what extent this type of Kähler metric generalizes to more general IIB CY orientifolds. In particular D7-branes wrap 4-tori whose volumes are directly related to the overall volume of the compact manifold. One would rather like to obtain information about the Kähler metric when the 7-branes wrap a local 4-cycle whose volume is not directly connected to the overall volume of the CY. An example of this is provided by the *Swiss cheese* type of compactifications discussed in [12]. In this more general setting, one assumes that the SM fields are localized at D7-branes wrapping *small* cycles in a CY whose overall volume is controlled by a large modulus t_b (see fig.(13.7) so $\mathrm{Vol}(CY) = t_b^{3/2} - h(t_i)$, where h is a homogeneous function of the *small* Kähler moduli t_i of degree $\frac{3}{2}$. The simplest example of this is provided by the CY manifold $\mathbf{P}_{[1,1,1,6,9]}^4$, which has only two Kähler moduli t_b and t, with a Kähler potential of the form

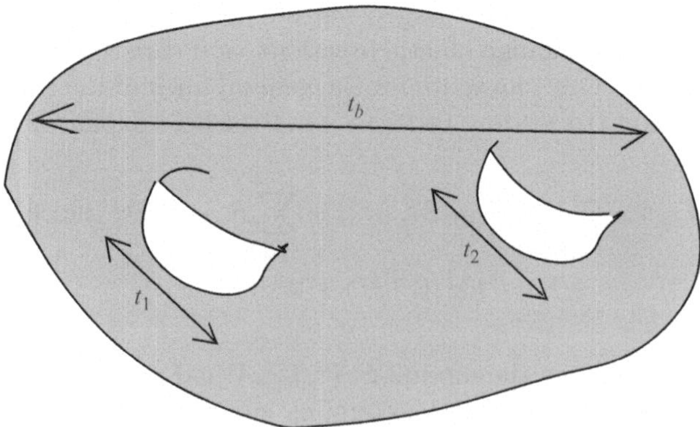

Fig. 13.7 CY manifold with a Swiss cheese structure.

$$K_{\text{IIB}} = -2 \log(t_b^{3/2} - t^{3/2}). \tag{13.15}$$

Here we will assume $t_b \gg t$ and take both large so that the supergravity approximation is still valid. In the F-theory context, the analogue of these moduli t and t_b would correspond to the size of the 4-fold S and the 6-fold B_3, respectively. Focusing only on the Kähler moduli dependence of the metrics, we can write a large-volume ansatz for the Kähler metrics of charged matter fields at the intersections [13]:

$$K_\alpha = \frac{t^{1-\xi_\alpha}}{t_b}, \tag{13.16}$$

with ξ_α to be fixed. We can compute ξ_α by studying the behavior with respect to a scaling of t in the effective action. In particular, in $\mathcal{N} = 1$ supergravity, the physical (i.e., with normalized kinetic terms) Yukawa coupling $\hat{Y}_{\alpha\beta\gamma}$ among three chiral fields is related to the holomorphic Yukawa coupling $Y^{(0)}_{\alpha\beta\gamma}$ by

$$\hat{Y}_{\alpha\beta\gamma} = e^{K/2} \frac{Y^{(0)}_{\alpha\beta\gamma}}{(K_\alpha K_\beta K_\gamma)^{1/2}}. \tag{13.17}$$

On the other hand, it is well known that the perturbative holomorphic Yukawa couplings in type IIB string theory are independent of Kähler moduli. Then, using (13.15) and (13.16), we find a scaling of the physical Yukawa coupling:

$$\hat{Y}_{\alpha\beta\gamma} \simeq t^{(\xi_\alpha + \xi_\beta + \xi_\gamma - 3)/2}. \tag{13.18}$$

The dependence on t_b drops at leading order in t/t_b, as expected for a model whose physics is essentially localized on the 4-cycle parametrized by t. On the other hand, we can alternatively compute the scaling behavior of the physical Yukawa coupling in terms of its computation as an overlap integral of the respective wavefunctions in S (see below) so that

$$\hat{Y}_{\alpha\beta\gamma} \simeq \int \Psi_\alpha \Psi_\beta \Psi_\gamma, \quad \int |\Psi_\alpha|^2 = 1. \tag{13.19}$$

For fields localized at intersecting branes, the above normalization integrals are essentially 2d, so the wavefunctions should scale like $t^{-1/4}$. On the other hand, the overlap integral for the Yukawa coupling is essentially pointlike, so that it scales like $\hat{Y} \simeq t^{-3/4}$. Comparing this with (13.18), we conclude that all $\xi_\alpha = \frac{1}{2}$, and hence the matter metrics of fields at intersecting branes have a metric with a local Kähler modulus dependence of the form

$$K_\alpha = \frac{t^{1/2}}{t_b}. \tag{13.20}$$

Note that setting $t_b \simeq t$ reproduces the Kähler modulus dependence $t^{-1/2}$ of toroidal models, (13.14).

13.4.2 The gauge kinetic function

The gauge kinetic function for the gauge group living on the D7-worldvolume may be extracted by expanding the Dirac–Born–Infeld (DBI) action of the D7-brane to second order in the gauge field strength F_a. We obtain the general expression [1]

$$f_a^{\mathrm{D7}} = \frac{(\alpha')^{-2}}{(2\pi)^5} \left[e^{-\phi} \int_{\Sigma_4^a} \mathrm{Re}\left(e^{J+i2\pi\alpha' F_a}\right) + i \int_{\Sigma_4^a} \sum_k C_{2k}\, e^{2\pi\alpha' F_a} \right], \qquad (13.21)$$

where J is the Kähler 2-form and the second piece performs a formal sum over all RR C_{2k} forms contributing to the integral. On expanding the exponential, the first term produces the volume of the 4-fold Σ_4^a wrapped by the D7 and the second term is proportional to C_4. Taking (13.10) into account, we see that the gauge kinetic function is proportional to the Kähler modulus T_a, i.e.,

$$f_a = T_a. \qquad (13.22)$$

The subsequent terms in the expansion describe contributions from the worldvolume gauge magnetic flux, which will be subleading for large volume $t_a = \mathrm{Re}\, T_a$. In particular, since $\int_{\Sigma_2} F_a = n$, with n an integer for quantized gauge fluxes, we can estimate the flux density as $F_a \simeq n(\mathrm{Re}\, S/\mathrm{Re}\, T_a)^{1/2}$. The leading flux correction to the gauge kinetic function then has the form

$$\mathrm{Re}\, f_a \simeq\ = \mathrm{Re}\, T_a(1 + |F_a|^2) \ \simeq\ \mathrm{Re}\, T_a\left(1 + \frac{n^2 \,\mathrm{Re}\, S}{\mathrm{Re}\, T_a}\right), \qquad (13.23)$$

which indeed will be subleading in the large t_a limit.

13.4.3   The superpotential

As indicated in (13.13), there will be a superpotential for the moduli $W(M)$ and a second superpotential $W(M, \Phi_\alpha)$ involving (moduli-dependent) Yukawa couplings. In the absence of closed string antisymmetric fluxes, the perturbative superpotential of the moduli vanishes: $W_{\mathrm{pert}}(M) = 0$. However, in the presence of type IIB NS (RR) 3-form fluxes H_3 (F_3), there is an induced effective superpotential involving the complex dilaton S and the complex structure moduli U^j given by [14]

$$W_{\mathrm{flux}}(S, U^j) = \int_{CY} (F_3 - iSH_3) \wedge \Omega_3, \qquad (13.24)$$

where Ω_3 is the CY holomorphic 3-form, which may be expanded in terms of the complex structure moduli U^j in the CY. This superpotential depends only on S and the U^j, and its minimization can give rise easily to the fixing of all these moduli. Furthermore, since generic CY manifolds have of the order of a hundred U^j fields or more, and the fluxes F_3 and H_3 also have a range of possible quantized values, at a minimum there may be accidental cancelations such that there is a very tiny value for $\langle W_{\mathrm{flux}} \rangle = W_0$. Such tiny values would be needed to understand the smallness of the SUSY breaking scale compared with a large string scale M_s not much below the Planck scale.

The above fluxes are unable to fix the values of the Kähler moduli. However, in specific compactifications, there are nonperturbative effects that induce superpotential terms involving the Kähler moduli. Examples of such nonperturbative effects are instanton effects induced by Euclidean D3-instantons and gaugino condensation on D7-branes wrapping appropriate 4-cycles in the CY. Such effects have typically an exponentially suppressed behavior of the form $W\mathrm{np} \simeq \sum_a \exp(-B_a T_a)$ for some constants B_a. These effects combined with those induced by fluxes W_{flux} have the potential to fix all the moduli of specific CY orientifold compactifications [12, 15]. Although a detailed example with all the required properties, including a realistic model and nonvanishing (but very small) cosmological constant, is still lacking, it seems very likely that those ingredients have the potential to fix all moduli.

Of more direct phenomenological interest are the Yukawa couplings involving SM quarks and leptons to Higgs scalars. As we have already mentioned, Yukawa couplings among Dp-brane matter fields in type IIB compactification arise from the overlap integral of the wavefunction in the extra dimensions of the three participant fields. Consider the case of D9-branes to simplify the discussion (recall that the case of D7-branes may be described in terms of D9-branes with appropriate fluxes). Suppose we have initially a $D = 10$ type IIB orientifold with D9 branes and a gauge group $U(n)$. In the field theory limit, our action will be 10d super Yang–Mills,

$$L = -\frac{1}{4}\,\mathrm{Tr}\left(F^{MN}F_{MN}\right) + \frac{i}{2}\,\mathrm{Tr}\left(\bar{\Psi}\Gamma^M D_M \Psi\right). \tag{13.25}$$

We then compactify the theory on some CY manifold and turn on magnetic fluxes that may break the gauge group to an SM-like gauge group. The 10d fields can then be expanded à la Kaluza–Klein (KK):

$$\Psi(x^\mu, y^m) = \sum_k \chi_{(k)}(x^\mu) \otimes \psi_{(k)}(y^m), \, A_n(x^\mu, y^m) = \sum_k \varphi_{(k)}(x^\mu) \otimes \phi_{(k),n}(y^m),$$

where x^μ and y^m are 4d and internal coordinates, respectively. The 4d massless spectrum may be chiral and $\mathcal{N} = 1$ supersymmetric with judicious choice of magnetic fluxes. The 4d Yukawa coupling between these matter fields arise from KK reduction of the cubic coupling $A \times \Psi \times \Psi$ from the 10d Lagrangian in (13.25). As illustrated in Fig. 13.8, the Yukawa coupling coefficients are obtained from the overlap integrals

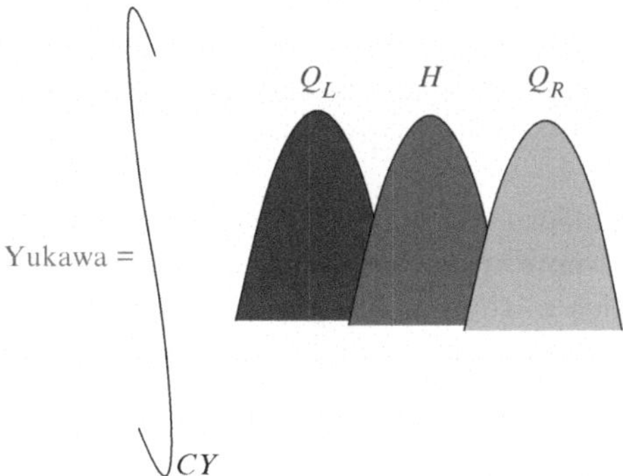

Fig. 13.8 Pictorial representation of the computation of Yukawa coupling constants as overlap integrals of zero modes.

$$Y_{ijk} = \frac{g}{2} \int_{CY} \psi_i^{\alpha\dagger} \, \Gamma^m \, \psi_j^\beta \, \phi_{k\,m}^\gamma f_{\alpha\beta\gamma}, \tag{13.26}$$

where g is the 10d gauge coupling, α, β, γ are $U(n)$ gauge indices, and $f_{\alpha\beta\gamma}$ are $U(n)$ structure constants; also, ψ and ϕ are fermionic and bosonic zero modes, respectively, and i, j, k label the different zero modes in a given charge sector, i.e., the families in semirealistic models. The Yukawa couplings are thus obtained as overlap integrals of the three zero-mode wavefunctions in the CY.

In order to compute the Yukawa coupling constants, we thus need to know the explicit form of the wavefunctions on compact dimensions of the involved matter fields, quarks, leptons, and Higgs multiplets in a realistic model. However, such wavefunctions are only accessible to explicit computation for simple models such as toroidal compactifications or orbifolds thereof. Indeed, this computation has been worked out for general toroidal/orbifold models [16]. The wavefunctions turn out to be proportional to Jacobi θ-functions with a Gaussian profile, and the holomorphic Yukawa couplings also turn out to be proportional to products of Jacobi θ-functions (one per $\mathbf{T}^2$ factor), depending only on the complex structure moduli U^j and the open string moduli (Wilson line degrees of freedom). As an example, the semirealistic model in Table 13.1 has holomorphic Yukawa couplings with the structure

$$\begin{aligned}
Y_{ij}{}^U &\sim \vartheta \begin{bmatrix} \frac{1}{3}i \\ 0 \end{bmatrix} \left(3J^{(2)}\right) \times \vartheta \begin{bmatrix} \frac{1}{3}j \\ 0 \end{bmatrix} \left(3J^{(3)}\right), \\[2mm]
Y_{ij*}{}^D &\sim \vartheta \begin{bmatrix} \frac{1}{3}i \\ 0 \end{bmatrix} \left(3J^{(2)}\right) \times \vartheta \begin{bmatrix} \frac{1}{3}j^* \\ 0 \end{bmatrix} \left(3J^{(3)}\right),
\end{aligned} \tag{13.27}$$

where ϑ is a Jacobi θ-function, $J^{(i)}$ are the Kähler forms of the ith torus, and i, j, and j^* are family indices for the Q, U, and D SM chiral multiplets, respectively. These expressions yield proportional expressions for U- and D-quark Yukawa couplings, but they differ if one takes into account the generic possibility (in tori) of Wilson line backgrounds along the $\mathbf{T}^6$ circles. However, because of the factorized structure of the family dependence, only one quark/lepton generation acquires a mass. The corresponding Yukawa coupling is of the order of the gauge coupling constant. This may be considered as a good first approximation to the observed quark/lepton mass spectrum, and one expects further corrections to give rise to the Yukawa couplings of the lighter generations.

The computation of Yukawa couplings in general curved CY manifolds is more difficult, although it becomes more tractable within the context of the *bottom-up* approach mentioned above. The idea is that in models in which the SM fields are localized in brane intersections, Yukawa couplings appear at points in the CY in which three such intersections (corresponding to SM and Higgs fields) meet. We already saw that in the F-theory context in Fig. 13.5. Thus, for example, the Yukawa coupling $\mathbf{10} \times \bar{\mathbf{5}} \times \bar{\mathbf{5}}_H$ in an $SU(5)$ F-theory GUT is localized at a point of triple intersection of the three matter curves. The Yukawa coupling now has the schematic form $\int_S \psi_i \psi_j \phi_H$, in which the integral, extended over the 4-fold S, is dominated by the intersection region. In such a situation, to compute the Yukawa coupling, we only need to know the wavefunctions *in the neighborhood* of the intersection point [17]. These local wavefunctions may be obtained by solving the Dirac and Klein–Gordon equations at the local level. Interestingly, it is again found that only one (the third) generation gets a nonvanishing Yukawa coupling, which is also of the order of the gauge coupling constant. It has been found, however, that instanton corrections induced by distant 7-branes wrapping other 4-cycles in compact spaces in general induce the required Yukawa couplings for the lighter generations [18, 19].

Instanton effects not only give rise to superpotentials for the Kähler moduli and induce the Yukawa couplings of the lighter generations. They may also give rise to interesting terms in the SM superpotential that are forbidden in perturbation theory. In particular, in brane models of SM physics there are typically extra $U(1)$ gauged symmetries beyond those of the SM. A classical example is $U(1)_{B-L}$ which often appears gauged in many string constructions, including right-handed neutrinos. This symmetry is anomaly-free, but there are often in addition $U(1)$'s with triangle anomalies that are canceled by the 4d version of the Green–Schwarz mechanism. All anomalous $U(1)$'s become massive by combining with the imaginary part of the Kähler (complex structure) moduli in type IIB (IIA) orientifolds. But, in addition, anomaly-free gauge symmetries such as $U(1)_{B-L}$ may also become massive in this way. This happens because, for example, in type IIB, some $\text{Im}\, T_i$ transform under the corresponding gauge $U(1)_a$ symmetries as $\text{Im}\, T_i \to \text{Im}\, T_i + q_i^a \Lambda_a$, with Λ_a the gauge parameter. This has interesting consequences for instanton physics [20]. In a type IIB orientifold, some instanton configurations correspond to Euclidean D3-branes wrapping the compact dimensions (so that they are localized in Minkowski space, as instantons should be). If they intersect the D7-branes where the SM fields live, there appear charged zero modes (from open string exchange) contributing to instanton-induced transitions. This is why this class of stringy instantons are often called *charged* instantons. In particular, if the D3-brane wraps a 4-cycle with Kähler modulus M (some linear combination of the T_i's), nonperturbative operators of the general form

$$e^{-M}\Phi_{q_1}...\Phi_{q_n}, \quad \sum_i q_i \neq 0 \tag{13.28}$$

may appear [20]. These operators are gauge-invariant because the sum of the charges of the Φ chiral fields is compensated by the shift in $\text{Im}\, M$ induced by the gauge transformation. An example of this is the generation of right-handed neutrino masses in MSSM-like orientifolds with a massive $U(1)_{B-L}$ induced by a Green–Schwarz mechanism. In this case, the operator has the form $e^{-M}\nu_R\nu_R$, and the noninvariance of the bilinear under $U(1)_{B-L}$ is compensated by a shift of the $\text{Im}\, M$. The mass is of order $e^{-\text{Re}\, M}M_s$, which may be in the right phenomenological ballpark 10^{12}–$10^{14}\,\text{GeV}$ for $M_s \simeq 10^{16}\,\text{GeV}$ and $\text{Re}\, M \simeq 100$. This type of *charged* instantons could also be important for the generation of other phenomenologically relevant terms, such as the MSSM μ-term.

13.5 String model building and the LHC

With the LHC in operation, an important issue is trying to make contact between an underlying string theory and experimental data. Of course, it would be really exciting if the string scale M_s were within reach of the LHC. We could perhaps observe some string or KK excitation as resonances in LHC data. On the other hand, a large string scale $M_s \simeq 10^{16}\,\text{GeV}$ seems to be favored if one sticks to a SUSY version of the SM such as the MSSM, in which gauge couplings nicely unify at a scale of order $10^{16}\,\text{GeV}$. So it is important to see whether specific classes of string compactifications may lead to low-energy predictions for SUSY breaking parameters.

We have seen that in certain large classes of type II models, there is information about the structure of the low-energy effective action. In particular, in type IIB orientifolds (or their F-theory extension) with SM fields localized at intersecting D7-branes (or matter curves in F-theory GUTs), one can compute the dependence on the local Kähler modulus of the gauge kinetic function (13.22) and also of the Kähler metric (13.20). If an MSSM-like model is constructed in such a setting, one can obtain specific expressions for SUSY-breaking soft terms, assuming Kähler moduli dominance in SUSY breaking, i.e., nonvanishing auxiliary fields $F_t \neq 0$. This is a reasonable assumption within type IIB/F-theory, since in type IIB orientifolds, such nonvanishing auxiliary fields correspond to the presence of nonvanishing antisymmetric RR and NS imaginary self-dual $(0,3)$ fluxes [21], which are known to solve the classical equations of motion [22]. As we mentioned above, such closed string fluxes are generically present in compactifications with fixed moduli. Using standard $\mathcal{N} = 1$ supergravity formulae and the above information on the effective action, one obtains soft terms with the constrained MSSM (CMSSM) structure but with the additional relationships [23]

$$M \;=\; \sqrt{2}m \;=\; -\frac{2}{3}A \;=\; -B, \qquad (13.29)$$

where M is the universal gaugino mass, m the universal scalar mass, A the trilinear scalar parameter, and B the Higgs bilinear parameter. Here one assumes the presence of an explicit μ-term in the low-energy Lagrangian, so that altogether there are only two free parameters: M and μ. The universality of soft terms may be understood if an underlying GUT structure exists as in F-theory GUTs. As we have mentioned, magnetic flux backgrounds are generically present on the worldvolume of the underlying 7-branes in order to get a chiral spectrum. In the presence of magnetic fluxes, the gauge kinetic functions (see (13.23)) and the Kähler metrics may acquire small corrections to (13.22) and (13.20), i.e.,

$$f \;=\; T\left(1 \,+\, a\frac{S}{T}\right), \qquad K_\alpha \;=\; \frac{t^{1/2}}{t_b}\left(1 \,+\, \frac{c_\alpha}{t^{1/2}}\right), \qquad (13.30)$$

where a and c_α are constants and S is the complex dilaton field. These corrections are suppressed in the large-t limit, corresponding to the physical weak coupling. In this limit, one may also neglect the correction to f compared with that coming from K_α. One then finds corrected soft terms of the form

$$m_{\tilde{f}}^2 \;=\; \frac{1}{2}|M|^2\left(1 - \frac{3}{2}\rho_f\right), \qquad (13.31)$$

$$m_H^2 \;=\; \frac{1}{2}|M|^2\left(1 - \frac{3}{2}\rho_H\right), \qquad (13.32)$$

$$A = -\frac{1}{2}M(3 - \rho_H - 2\rho_f),\qquad(13.33)$$

$$B = -M(1 - \rho_H),\qquad(13.34)$$

where $\rho_\alpha = c_\alpha/t^{1/2}$ and the subscripts f and H refer to fluxes through the fermion matter curves and the Higgs curve, respectively. Note that in order of magnitude, one numerically expects $\rho_{H,f} \simeq 1/t^{1/2} \simeq \alpha_{GUT}^{1/2} \simeq 0.2$. The above soft terms apply at the string/unification scale $M_s \simeq 10^{16}$ GeV. To get the low-energy physics around the EW scale, one has to run down the soft parameters according to the renormalization group equations (RGE). Then one has to check that the boundary conditions are consistent with radiative EW symmetry breaking (REWSB) and with present low-energy phenomenological constraints. One may in addition impose the condition that the lightest neutralino is stable and provides the dark matter in the universe. The resulting scheme is extremely constrained [24]. In particular, setting the fermion flux correction to zero for simplicity, one has a theory with three free parameters (M, μ, and ρ_H) and two constraints (REWSB and dark matter), or, equivalently, lines in the planes of any pair of parameters or SUSY masses. As an example Fig. 13.9 shows

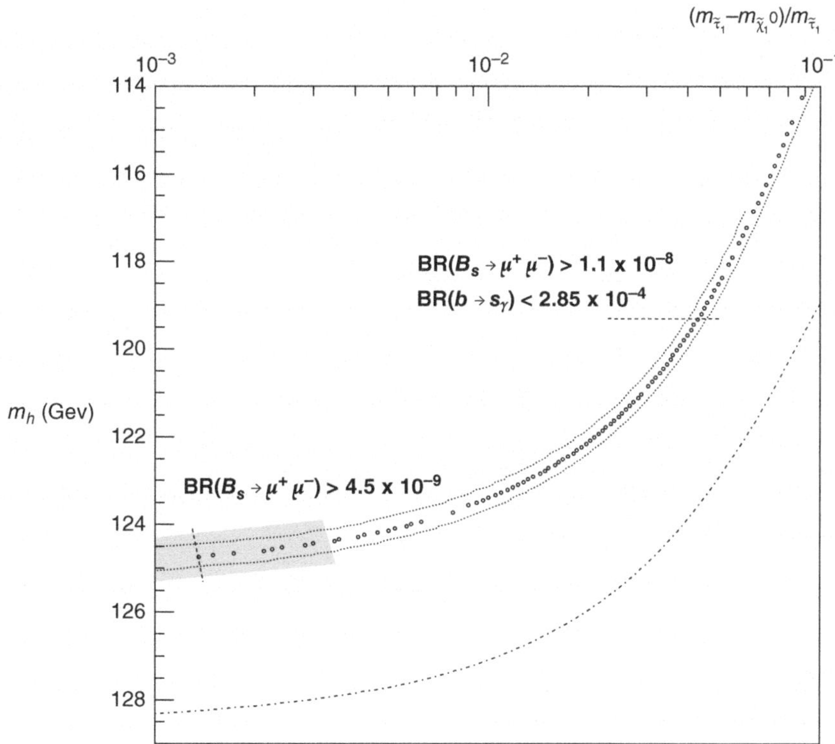

Fig. 13.9 Normalized mass difference $(m_{\tilde{\tau}_1} - m_{\tilde{\chi}_1^0})/m_{\tilde{\tau}_1}$ as a function of the lightest Higgs mass m_h in the modulus dominance scheme. Appropriate REWSB, neutralino dark matter, and BR($B_s \rightarrow \mu^+\mu^-$) limits are only consistent for a Higgs mass in the 125 GeV region. (From [24]).

the normalized mass difference $(m_{\tilde{\tau}_1} - m_{\chi_1^0})/m_{\tilde{\tau}_1}$ as a function of the lightest Higgs mass m_h [24]. Dots correspond to points fulfilling the central value in the result from WMAP for the neutralino relic density and dotted lines denote the upper and lower limits after including the 2σ uncertainty. The dot–dashed line represents points with a critical matter density $\Omega_{\mathrm{matter}} = 1$. The vertical line corresponds to the 2σ limit on the branching ratio $\mathrm{BR}(b \to s\gamma)$ and the upper bound on $\mathrm{BR}(B_s \to \mu^+\mu^-)$ from [25] and the recent LHCb result [26]. The gray area indicates the points compatible with the latter constraint when the 2σ error associated with the SM prediction is included. As is obvious from the figure, the dark matter condition is fulfilled thanks to a stau–neutralino coannihilation mechanism. Interestingly enough, the recent constraint on $\mathrm{BR}(B_s \to \mu^+\mu^-)$ from LHCb forces the Higgs mass to a region around $125\,\mathrm{GeV}$, consistent with the hints of a Higgs particle in that range as measured at CMS and ATLAS. Fixing the mass of any SUSY particle fixes the rest of the spectrum. In particular, with a lightest Higgs mass around $125\,\mathrm{GeV}$, gluinos have a mass around $3\,\mathrm{TeV}$, the first- and second-generation squarks around 2.7–$2.8\,\mathrm{TeV}$, and the lightest stop around $2\,\mathrm{TeV}$. The lightest slepton is a stau with mass around $600\,\mathrm{GeV}$, almost degenerate with the lightest neutralinos. The existence of gluinos and squarks of these masses can be tested at LHC running at $14\,\mathrm{TeV}$ and $30\,\mathrm{fb}^{-1}$ integrated luminosity.

It is remarkable that a lightest MSSM Higgs mass as heavy as $125\,\mathrm{GeV}$ is possible in this scheme. In most SUSY schemes (including minimal gauge and anomaly mediation models and the CMSSM with squarks that are not superheavy), the lightest Higgs mass is typically around $115\,\mathrm{GeV}$ or so (see, e.g., [27]). In this scheme, a relatively heavy Higgs appears because the soft terms in (13.34) predict a large A-parameter with $A \simeq -2m$, giving rise to a large stop mixing parameter and hence a big one-loop correction to the Higgs mass. In addition, the dark matter and REWSB conditions require a large $\tan\beta \simeq 40$, pushing the tree-level Higgs mass to its maximum value. This large $\tan\beta$ and stop mixing parameters imply that, as it stands, this simple scheme may soon be ruled out if LHCb finds no deviation from the SM value for $\mathrm{BR}(B_s \to \mu^+\mu^-)$. On the other hand, a Next-to-Minimal supersymmetric SM (NMSSM) version of the same model, also viable in type IIB/F-theory schemes, would remain consistent, as would R-parity violation, since it would avoid the dark matter overabundance problem. This shows how the LHC results may provide important constraints on the possible compactifications and SUSY-breaking schemes within string theory; see, e.g., [28] for other-string-derived approaches.

References

[1] L.E. Ibáñez and A. Uranga, *String Theory and Particle Physics: An Introduction to String Phenomenology.* Cambridge University Press, Cambridge (2012).

[2] F. Marchesano, "Progress in D-brane model building," arXiv:hep-th/0702094; A. M. Uranga, "Chiral four-dimensional string compactifications with intersecting D-branes," Class. Quant. Grav. **20** (2003) S373 [arXiv:hep-th/0301032]; R. Blumenhagen, M. Cvetic, P. Langacker, and G. Shiu, "Toward realistic

intersecting D-brane models," Annu Rev. Nucl. Part. Sci. **55** (2005) 71 [arXiv:hep-th/0502005]; F. G. Marchesano, "Intersecting D-brane models," [arXiv:hep-th/0307252]; D. Cremades, L. E. Ibáñez, and F. Marchesano, "More about the standard model at intersecting branes," arXiv:hep-ph/0212048.

[3] G. Aldazabal, L. E. Ibáñez, F. Quevedo, and A. M. Uranga, "D-branes at singularities: a bottom-up approach to the string embedding of the standard model," JHEP **0008**, 002 (2000) [arXiv:hep-th/0005067].

[4] R. Blumenhagen, L. Goerlich, B. Kors, and D. Lust, "Asymmetric orbifolds, noncommutative geometry and type I string vacua," Nucl. Phys. **B582** (2000) 44–64. [hep-th/0003024]; G. Aldazabal, S. Franco, L. E. Ibáñez, R. Rabadán, and A. M. Uranga, "$D = 4$ chiral string compactifications from intersecting branes," J. Math. Phys. **42** (2001) 3103–3126. [hep-th/0011073]; "Intersecting brane worlds," JHEP **0102** (2001) 047 [hep-ph/0011132].

[5] D. Cremades, L. E. Ibáñez, and F. Marchesano, "Yukawa couplings in intersecting D-brane models," JHEP **0307** (2003) 038 [hep-th/0302105].

[6] M. Cvetic G. Shiu, and A. M. Uranga, "Chiral four-dimensional $N = 1$ supersymmetric type IIA orientifolds from intersecting D6 branes," Nucl. Phys. **B615** (2002) 3–32 [arXiv:hep-th/0107166]; F. Marchesano and G. Shiu, "Building MSSM flux vacua," JHEP **0411** (2004) 041 [arXiv:hep-th/0409132]; "MSSM vacua from flux compactifications," Phys.Rev. **D71** (2005) 011701 [arXiv:hep-th/0408059].

[7] C. Bachas, "A way to break supersymmetry," arXiv:hep-th/9503030; C. Angelantonj I. Antoniadis, E. Dudas, and A. Sagnotti, "Type I strings on magnetised orbifolds and brane transmutation," Phys. Lett. **B489** (2000) 223 [arXiv:hep-th/0007090]; R. Blumenhagen, B. Kors, and D. Lust, "Type I strings with F- and B-flux," JHEP **0102** (2001) 30 [arXiv:hep-th/0012156].

[8] C. Vafa, "Evidence for F-theory," Nucl. Phys. **B469** (1996) 403 [arXiv:hep-th/9602022]; D. R. Morrison and C. Vafa, "Compactifications of F-theory on Calabi–Yau threefolds – I," Nucl. Phys. **B473** (1996) 74 [arXiv:hep-th/9602114]; "Compactifications of F-theory on Calabi–Yau threefolds – II," Nucl. Phys. **B476** (1996) 437 [arXiv:hep-th/9603161].

[9] M. Wijnholt, "F-theory and unification," Fortsch. Phys. **58** (2010) 846; J. J. Heckman, "Particle physics implications of F-theory," arXiv:1001.0577 [hep-th]; T. Weigand, "Lectures on F-theory compactifications and model building," Class. Quant. Grav. **27**, 214004 (2010) [arXiv:1009.3497 [hep-th]].

[10] H. Jockers and J. Louis, "The effective action of D7-branes in $N = 1$ Calabi–Yau orientifolds," Nucl. Phys. B **705**, 167 (2005) [arXiv:hep-th/0409098].

[11] L. E. Ibáñez, C. Muñoz, and S. Rigolin, "Aspects of type I string phenomenology," Nucl. Phys. **B553** (1999) 43 [arXiv:hep-th/9812397]; D. Lust, P. Mayr, R. Richter, and S. Stieberger, "Scattering of gauge, matter, and moduli fields from intersecting branes," Nucl. Phys. **B696** (2004) 205 [arXiv:hep-th/0404134]; B. Kors and P. Nath, "Effective action and soft supersymmetry breaking for intersecting D-brane models," Nucl. Phys. **B681** (2004) 77 [arXiv:hep-th/0309167].

[12] V. Balasubramanian, P. Berglund, J. P. Conlon, and F. Quevedo, "Systematics of moduli stabilisation in Calabi–Yau flux compactifications," JHEP **0503**

(2005) 007 [arXiv:hep-th/0502058]; J. P. Conlon, F. Quevedo, and K. Suruliz, "Large-volume flux compactifications: Moduli spectrum and D3/D7 soft super-symmetry breaking," JHEP **0508** (2005) 007 [arXiv:hep-th/0505076].

[13] J. P. Conlon, D. Cremades, and F. Quevedo, "Kähler potentials of chiral matter fields for Calabi–Yau string compactifications," JHEP **0701** (2007) 022 [arXiv:hep-th/0609180].

[14] S. Gukov, C. Vafa, and E. Witten, "CFT's from Calabi–Yau four-folds," Nucl. Phys. **B584** (2000) 69 [arXiv:hep-th/9906070].

[15] S. Kachru, R. Kallosh, A. Linde, and S.P. Trivedi, "De Sitter vacua in string theory," Phys. Rev. **D68** (2003) 046005 [arXiv:hep-th/0301240].

[16] D. Cremades, L. E. Ibáñez, and F. Marchesano, "Computing Yukawa couplings from magnetized extra dimensions," JHEP **0405** (2004) 079 [arXiv:hep-th/0404229].

[17] A. Font and L. E. Ibáñez, "Yukawa structure from $U(1)$ fluxes in F-theory grand unification," JHEP **0902**, 016 (2009) [arXiv:0811.2157 [hep-th]]; J. J. Heckman and C. Vafa, "Flavor hierarchy from F-theory," Nucl. Phys. **B837** (2010) 137 [arXiv:0811.2417 [hep-th]]; A. Font and L. E. Ibáñez, "Matter wave functions and Yukawa couplings in F-theory grand unification," JHEP **0909**, 036 (2009) [arXiv:0907.4895 [hep-th]]; G. K. Leontaris and G. G. Ross, "Yukawa couplings and fermion mass structure in F-theory GUTs," JHEP **1102** (2011) 108 [arXiv:1009.6000 [hep-th]].

[18] F. Marchesano and L. Martucci, "Non-perturbative effects on seven-brane Yukawa couplings," Phys. Rev. Lett. **104**, 231601 (2010) [arXiv:0910.5496 [hep-th]].

[19] S. Cecotti, M. C. N. Cheng, J. J. Heckman, and C. Vafa, "Yukawa couplings in F-theory and non-commutative geometry," arXiv:0910.0477 [hep-th]; J. P. Conlon and E. Palti, "Aspects of flavour and supersymmetry in F-theory GUTs," JHEP **1001**, 029 (2010) [arXiv:0910.2413 [hep-th]]; L. Aparicio, A. Font, L. E. Ibáñez, and F. Marchesand, "Flux and instanton effects in local F-theory models and hierarchical fermion masses," JHEP **1108** (2011) 152 [arXiv:1104.2609 [hep-th]]; P.G. Camara, E. Dudas, and E. Palti, "Massive wave functions, proton decay and FCNCs in local F-theory GUTs," JHEP **1112** (2011) 112 [arXiv:1110.2206 [hep-th]].

[20] R. Blumenhagen, M. Cvetic, and T. Weigand, "Spacetime instanton corrections in 4D string vacua: the seesaw mechanism for D-brane models," Nucl. Phys. **B771** (2007) 113–142 [arXiv:hep-th/0609191]; L. E. Ibáñez, and A. M. Uranga, "Neutrino Majorana masses from string theory instanton effects," JHEP **0703** (2007) 052 [arXiv:hep-th/0609213]; B. Florea, S. Kachru, J. McGreevy, and N. Saulina, "Stringy Instantons and Quiver Gauge Theories," JHEP **0705** (2007) 024 [arXiv:hep-th/0610003].

[21] P. G. Cámara, L. E. Ibáñez, and A. M. Uranga, "Flux induced SUSY breaking soft terms," Nucl. Phys. **B689** (2004) 195 [arXiv:hep-th/0311241]; D. Lust, S. Reffert, and S. Stieberger, "Flux-induced soft supersymmetry breaking in chiral type IIB orientifolds with D3/D7-branes," Nucl. Phys. **B706** (2005) 3 [arXiv:hep-th/0406492]; P. G. Cámara, L. E. Ibáñez, and A. M. Uranga, "Flux-induced SUSY-breaking soft terms on D7–D3 brane systems," Nucl. Phys. **B708** (2005)

268 [arXiv:hep-th/0408036]; D. Lust, S. Reffert, and S. Stieberger, "MSSM with soft SUSY breaking terms from D7-branes with fluxes," Nucl. Phys. **B727** (2005) 264 [arXiv:hep-th/0410074]; M. Grana, T. W. Grimm, H. Jockers and J. Louis, "Soft supersymmetry breaking in Calabi–Yau orientifolds with D-branes and fluxes," Nucl. Phys. **B690** (2004) 21 [arXiv:hep-th/0312232].

[22] S. B. Giddings, S. Kachru, and J. Polchinski, "Hierarchies from fluxes in string compactifications," Phys. Rev. **D66** (2002) 106006 [arXiv:hep-th/0105097].

[23] L. Aparicio, D. G. Cerdeño, and L. E. Ibáñez, "Modulus-dominated SUSY-breaking soft terms in F-theory and their test at LHC," JHEP **0807** (2008) 099 [arXiv:0805.2943 [hep-th]].

[24] L. Aparicio, D. G. Cerdeño, and L. E. Ibáñez, "A 119–125 GeV Higgs from a string derived slice of the CMSSM," arXiv:1202.0822 [hep-ph].

[25] "Search for the rare decay $B_s^0 \to \mu^+\mu^-$ at the LHC with the CMS and LHCb experiments," The CMS and LHCb collborations, LHCb-CONF-2011-047, CMS-PAS-BPH-11-019 (8 August 2011).

[26] R. Aaij et al. [LHCb Collaboration], "Strong constraints on the rare decays $B_s \to \mu^+\mu^-$ and $B^0 \to \mu^+\mu^-$," arXiv:1203.4493 [hep-ex].

[27] H. Baer, V. Barger, and A. Mustafayev, "Implications of a 125 GeV Higgs scalar for LHC SUSY and neutralino dark matter searches," arXiv:1112.3017 [hep-ph]; L. J. Hall, D. Pinner, and J. T. Ruderman, "A natural SUSY Higgs near 126 GeV," arXiv:1112.2703 [hep-ph]; A. Arbey, M. Battaglia, A. Djouadi, F. Mahmoudi, and J. Quevillon, "Implications of a 125 GeV Higgs for supersymmetric models," Phys. Lett. **B708** (2012) 162 [arXiv:1112.3028 [hep-ph]]; S. Akula, B. Altunkaynak, D. Feldman, P. Nath, and G. Peim, "Higgs boson mass predictions in SUGRA unification, recent LHC-7 results, and dark matter," arXiv:1112.3645 [hep-ph]: J. Ellis and K. Olive, "Revisiting the Higgs mass and dark matter in the CMSSM," arXiv:1202.3262[hep-ph].

[28] B. C. Allanach, A. Brignole, and L. E. Ibáñez, "Phenomenology of a fluxed MSSM," JHEP **0505** (2005) 030 [hep-ph/0502151]; K. Choi, A. Falkowski, H. P. Nilles, and M. Olechowski, "Soft supersymmetry breaking in KKLT flux compactification," Nucl. Phys. **B718** (2005) 113 [arXiv:hep-th/0503216]; K. Choi and H. P. Nilles, "The gaugino code," JHEP **0704** (2007) 006 [arXiv:hep-ph/0702146]; J. P. Conlon, S. S. Abdussalam, F. Quevedo, and K. Suruliz, "Soft SUSY breaking terms for chiral matter in IIB string compactifications," JHEP **0701** (2007) 032 [arXiv:hep-th/0610129]; J. P. Conlon, C. H. Kom, K. Suruliz, B. C. Allanach, and F. Quevedo, "Sparticle spectra and LHC signatures for large volume string compactifications," JHEP **0708** (2007) 061 [arXiv:0704.3403 [hep-ph]]; R. Blumenhagen, J. P. Conlon, S. Krippendorf, S. Moster, and F. Quevedo, "SUSY breaking in local string/F-theory models," JHEP **0909** (2009) 007 [arXiv:0906.3297 [hep-th]]; J. J. Heckman, G. L. Kane, J. Shao, and C. Vafa, "The footprint of F-theory at the LHC," JHEP **0910** (2009) 039 [arXiv:0903.3609 [hep-ph]]; B. S. Acharya, K. Bobkov, G. L. Kane, J. Shao, and P. Kumar, "The G_2-MSSM: an M theory motivated model of particle physics," Phys. Rev. **D78** (2008) 065038 [arXiv:0801.0478 [hep-ph]]; G. Kane, P. Kumar, R. Lu, and B. Zheng,

"Higgs mass prediction for realistic string/M theory vacua," arXiv:1112.1059 [hep-ph]; S. P. de Alwis, "Classical and quantum SUSY breaking effects in IIB local models," JHEP **1003** (2010) 078 [arXiv:0912.2950 [hep-th]]; T. Li, J. A. Maxin, D. V. Nanopoulos, and J. W. Walker, "A Higgs mass shift to 125 GeV and a multi-jet supersymmetry signal: miracle of the flippons at the $\sqrt{s} = 7$ TeV LHC," arXiv:1112.3024 [hep-ph].

14
The string landscape and low-energy supersymmetry

Michael R. DOUGLAS

Simons Center for Geometry and Physics, Stony Brook University,
Stony Brook, New York, USA

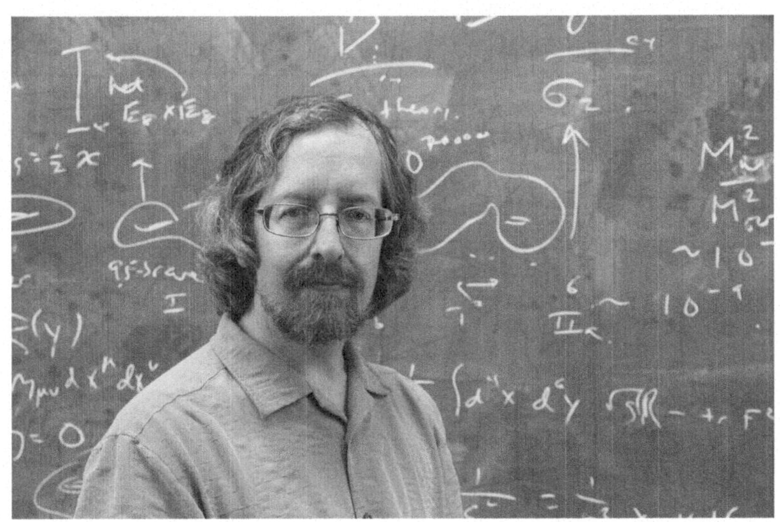

Theoretical Physics to Face the Challenge of LHC. Edited by L. Baulieu, K. Benakli, M. R. Douglas,
B. Mansoulié, E. Rabinovici, and L. F. Cugliandolo. © Oxford University Press 2015.
Published in 2015 by Oxford University Press.

Chapter Contents

We briefly survey our present understanding of the string landscape, and use it to discuss the chances that we will see low-energy supersymmetry at the LHC.

14.1   The goal of fundamental physics

Particle physics is entering a new era. The LHC has finished its first scientific phase at 8 TeV, and the Higgs boson has finally been discovered, with a mass of 125 GeV. This landmark discovery, to which many of the lecturers and participants at this school have contributed, should inspire all particle physicists, theorists, and experimentalists to think about our field in new ways.*

Although the Higgs boson is a signature prediction of the Standard Model, it will be some time before we know whether the real Higgs boson has exactly the properties that the Standard Model predicts. It is not easy to measure the details of interactions in a hadron collider, and many interesting decay modes are rare. There might be additional particles in the Higgs sector, even with masses below 125 GeV.

Of course, many physicists have argued over the years that the Standard Model must be incomplete on theoretical grounds, and that there are many reasons to expect non-Standard Model physics at or just above the electroweak scale. This was a primary motivation to build the LHC, but so far it has given us no clear evidence for any non-Standard Model physics. In particular, colored gauginos, a signature of low-energy supersymmetry, have been excluded below about 900 GeV. Of course, they may be just around the corner, waiting to be discovered in the first 14 TeV runs. But we have no guarantees; we it may simply require many years of data taking and subtle analysis to uncover superpartners that have only electroweak interactions, or conversely to exclude them at these energies.

By now it is almost a truism that string theory makes no definite predictions for LHC physics, only suggestions for rather implausible scenarios such as black hole creation, whose nondiscovery would not falsify the theory. This is not literally true, since there are potential discoveries that would give strong evidence against string theory,[1] but at present there is no reason to expect them.

Even if we find no "smoking gun" that speaks directly for or against the theory, there is a program that could someday lead to falsifiable predictions. It is to understand the landscape of string vacua, and derive a probability measure on the set of vacua based on quantum cosmology. From this, we can infer the probabilities that each of the various possibilities for beyond the Standard Model, cosmological, and other fundamental physics would come out of string theory. If future discoveries and (to some extent) present data come out as highly unlikely by this measure, we have evidence against string theory under the assumed scenario for quantum cosmology. This evidence might or might not be conclusive, but it would be the best we could do with the information to hand.

---

*The string landscape and low energy supersymmetry', by Michael R. Douglas in Strings, Gauge Fields, and the Geometry Behind: The Legacy of Maximilian Kreuzer edited by Anton Rebhan, Ludmil Katzarkov, Johanna Knapp, © 2013 World Scientific.

[1] This includes time-varying α [1] and probably faster-than-light neutrinos.

This program is only being pursued by a few groups today and would require major advances in our understanding of both string theory and quantum cosmology before convincing predictions could be made. My guess at present is that twenty years or more will be needed, taking us beyond the LHC era. Even then, it is likely that such predictions would depend on hypotheses about quantum cosmology that could not be directly tested and might admit alternatives. It is entirely reasonable that skeptics of the landscape should reject this entire direction and look for other ways to understand string theory, or for other theories of quantum gravity. At present, we do not know enough to be confident that they are wrong. Nevertheless, the evidence at hand leads me to think that they are wrong and that this difficult path must be explored.

In this chapter, I will briefly outline this program and how I see it proceeding. Although it is clearly a long-term project, I am going to go out on a limb and argue that

- String/M theory will predict that our universe has supersymmetry, broken at the $30 - 100$ TeV scale. If it is broken at the lower values, we may see gluinos at LHC, while if it is broken at the higher values, it will be very hard to see any evidence for supersymmetry.

This is a somewhat pessimistic claim that far outruns our ability to actually make predictions from string theory. Nevertheless, I am going to set out the argument, fully realizing that many of the assumptions as well as the supporting evidence might not stand the test of time. Indeed, we should all hope that this is wrong!

To begin, we have to make the case that a fundamental theory should allow us to make any predictions of this scope. This is not at all obvious. Certainly most major scientific discoveries were not anticipated in any detail. However, the record in particle physics is far better, with examples including the positron, neutrinos, the charm quark, the third generation of quarks and leptons, the W and Z bosons, and as it now appears, the Higgs boson. The framework of quantum field theory is highly constraining, and this record of success is the evidence.

Of course, quantum field theory is only constraining within certain limits. For example, there is no good argument that favors three generations of quarks and leptons over four. There are many other consistent extensions of the Standard Model that we might imagine discovering. Even the basic structure of the Standard Model, its gauge group and matter representation content, admits consistent variations. As things stand, it is entirely reasonable to claim that this structure was a choice that could not have been predicted a priori, and equally that the existence of as yet undiscovered matter cannot be excluded a priori.

Quantum gravity is hoped to be more constraining, although there is no consensus yet on whether or why this is true. In the case of string/M-theory, we can benefit from over 25 years of work on string compactification. It is clear that there are several different constructions based on the different perturbative limits and compactification manifolds: heterotic on a Calabi–Yau manifold, F-theory, type II with branes, M-theory on G_2 manifolds. Each involves many choices that lead to different outcomes for low-energy physics, and for this reason one cannot make definite predictions.

There is even an extreme point of view that (in some still vague sense) "all" consistent low-energy theories can be realized as string compactifications. This idea can lead in various directions: one can hope that consistency will turn out to be a more powerful constraint in quantum gravity than it was in quantum field theory [2]. On the other hand, this does not seem to be the case in six spacetime dimensions[3]. And so far, in four dimensions, no-go results are surprisingly rare.

While there are too many compactifications to study individually, one can hope that a particular construction or class of compactification would lead to some generic predictions. If the broad structure of the Standard Model or some beyond the Standard Model scenario came out this way, one might hypothesize that that construction was preferred, and look for top-down explanations for this. However, no construction seems especially preferred at this point. For example, it is simple to get grand unification out of the $E_8 \times E_8$ heterotic string. On the other hand, this construction does not naturally lead to three generations of matter; even if we grant that the number of generations must be consistent with asymptotic freedom, most choices of Calabi–Yau manifold and bundle have other numbers of generations. Can one do better? There are brane constructions that relate this "three" to the number of extra (complex) dimensions, but these do not realize grand unification. Which is better?

It seems that any attempt to narrow down the possibilities will involve this type of weighing of different factors, and this is a strong motivation to systematize this weighing and make it more objective. While this would seem a very open-ended problem, in the context of string compactification there is a natural way to do it—namely, to count the vacua of different types, and regard high-multiplicity vacua as favored or "more natural." This includes the considerations of tuning made in traditional naturalness arguments, and extends them to discrete and even qualitative features such as numbers of generations or comparison of different supersymmetry-breaking mechanisms. The basic outlines of such an approach are set out in [4]. And have led so far to a few general results that we will survey below. One can imagine continuing this study along formal, top-down lines to develop a quantitative picture of the landscape.

While this sort of information seems necessary to proceed further, by itself it is not going to lead to convincing predictions. I like the analogy to the study of solutions of the Schrödinger equation governing electrons and nuclei, better known as chemistry [5]. The landscape of chemical molecules is very complicated, but one could imagine deducing it *ab initio* and working out a list of long-lived metastable compounds and their properties. However, in any real world situation (both on Earth and in astronomy), the number density of the various molecules is very far from uniform, or from being a Boltzmann distribution. One needs some information about the processes that created the local environment, be it the surface of the Earth, the interior of a star, or whatever, to make any *ab initio* estimate of this number density. Conversely, we see in astrophysics that fairly simple models can sometimes lead to useful estimates. One can then make statements about "typical molecules," meaning typical for that local environment, on purely theoretical grounds.

While one cannot push this analogy very far, I think it confirms the point that we need some information about the processes that created our vacuum as one of the many possibilities within the landscape, to estimate a measure and make believable predictions. Doing this is a primary goal of quantum cosmology and has been discussed for over 30 years. The first question is whether one needs the microscopic details of quantum gravity to do this, or whether general features of quantum gravity suffice. There is a strong argument, based on the phenomenon of eternal inflation, that the latter is true, so that one can ask the relevant questions and set up a framework to answer them without having a microscopic formulation. Of course, their answers might depend on microscopic details; for example, one needs to know which pairs of vacua are connected by tunneling processes, and this depends on the structure of configuration space. Anyways, these general arguments are well reviewed in [6–8], while some of the most recent developments are discussed in [9, 10].

Quantum cosmology is a contentious subject in which I am not an expert. However, within the eternal inflation paradigm, starting from a variety of precise definitions for the measure factor and using the presence of many exponentially small numbers in the problem, one obtains a fairly simple working definition, the "master" or "dominant" vacuum ansatz [11–13]. This states that the a priori measure is overwhelmingly dominated by the longest-lived metastable de Sitter vacuum. The measure for other vacua is given by the tunneling rate from this "master" vacuum, which to a good approximation is that of the single fastest chain of tunneling events.

Although the measure is dominated by the master vacuum, it is a priori likely (and we will argue) that observers cannot exist in this vacuum—it is not "anthropically allowed." While there are many objections to anthropic postselection, they have been well addressed in the literature, and we will not discuss them here. Nevertheless, we must take a position on what anthropic postselection should mean in practice. The philosophically correct definition that a vacuum admit observers is impossible to work with, while simpler proxies such as entropy production [14] have not yet been developed in the detail we need for particle physics.

In practice, the anthropically allowed vacua will be those that realize the Standard Model gauge group, and the first family of quarks and leptons, with parameters roughly the ones we observe. It is not obvious that even these are all anthropically selected; for example, it is argued is [15] that one does not even need the weak interactions![2] Conversely, while the precise values of quark masses are not usually considered to be selected, given the plethora of fine tunings in chemistry, it might well be that life and the existence of observers is much more dependent on the specific values of these parameters than as first appears.

Besides these questions of detail, any definition of anthropic selection suffers from the objection that it is time-dependent and would be different in 1912 or 2112 than in 2012. While this is so, we would reply that all we can do in the end is to test competing theories with the evidence to hand, and one can try out all the variations on this theme in order to do this. It is quite reasonable to expect our evidence to improve with time, and perhaps our understanding of the anthropic constraints will improve as well.

---

[2] Even granting this point, the need to get several quarks and leptons with similar small nonzero masses is far more easily met by a chiral theory such as the Standard Model than a vector-like weakless theory.

Granting that the master vacuum is not anthropically allowed, the measure we are interested in is thus the "distance" in this precise sense (defined using tunneling rates) from the master vacuum, restricted to the anthropically allowed vacua. Clearly it is important to find the master vacuum, and one might jump to the conclusion that string theory predicts that we live in a vacuum similar to the master vacuum. However, because of the anthropic constraint, whether this is so depends on details of the tunneling rates. The main constraint is that one needs to reach a large enough set of vacua to solve the cosmological constant problem. The more tunneling events required to do this, and the more distinct the vacua they connect, the more disparate a set of vacua will fall into this category, and the weaker the predictions such an analysis will lead to. Somewhat counterintuitively, if the master vacuum admits many discrete variations, then there are more nearby vacua, and one does not need to go so far to solve the cosmological constant problem. If this set of vacua includes anthropically allowed vacua, then these will be favored and one can imagine getting fairly definite predictions.

One can already make some guesses about where to look for the master vacuum in the string landscape, as we will describe. Continuing in this speculative vein, we will argue that this favors "local models" of the Standard Model degrees of freedom, and supersymmetry breaking driven by dynamics elsewhere in the extra dimensions, gravitationally mediated to the Standard Model. This is a much-discussed class of models and, as we discuss in Section 14.3, there is a key difficulty in that their ability to solve the hierarchy problem is limited by the cosmological moduli problem, which seems to require supersymmetry breaking at or above about 30 TeV. Still, compared with the GUT or Planck scales, this is a huge advantage, and thus we predict low-energy supersymmetry but with superpartners around this scale.

The argument that we have just given is not purely top-down and is closely related to the familiar arguments that if low-energy supersymmetry were the solution to the hierarchy problem, then we should see superpartners in the current LHC runs. My phenomenology is rather sketchy, and there are many other scenarios that would need to be considered to make a convincing argument. But the point here is to illustrate the claim that with some additional input from the string theory landscape, allowing us to compare the relative likelihood of different tuned features, we could make such arguments precise.

14.2 Low-energy supersymmetry and current constraints

Most arguments for "beyond the Standard Model" physics are based on its potential for solving the hierarchy problem, the large ratio between the electroweak scale $M_{\mathrm{EW}} \sim 100\,\mathrm{GeV}$ and higher scales such as $M_{\mathrm{Planck}} \sim 10^{19}\,\mathrm{GeV}$ or $M_{\mathrm{GUT}} \sim 10^{16}\,\mathrm{GeV}$. Low-energy supersymmetry is a much-studied scenario with various circumstantial arguments in its favor. Theoretically, it is highly constraining and leads to many generic predictions, most importantly the gauge couplings of superpartners. This is why LHC already gives us strong lower bounds on the masses of colored superpartners, especially the gluino.

If there is a 125 GeV Higgs, this turns out to put interesting constraints on supersymmetric models. Recent discussions of this include [16–18], the talk [19] and [20], which reviews a line of work that has influenced my thoughts on these questions.

A broad-brush analysis of the hierarchy problem can be found in [21]. Its solution by low-energy supersymmetry can be understood by restricting attention to a few fields, most importantly the top quark and its scalar partner the "stop." In general terms, top quark loops give a quadratically divergent contribution to the Higgs mass, which is cut off by stop loops. This leads to the rough estimate

$$\delta M_{H1}^2 \sim 0.15 M_{\mathrm{ST}}^2 \log \frac{\Lambda_{\mathrm{SUSY}}}{M_{\mathrm{ST}}}, \tag{14.1}$$

where M_{H1} is the mass of the Higgs that couples to the top, $\Lambda_{\mathrm{SUSY}} \equiv M_{3/2}$ is the supersymmetry-breaking scale, and M_{ST}^2 is the average stop mass squared.

The strongest sense in which supersymmetry could solve the hierarchy problem would be to ask not just that M_H comes out small in our vacuum, but that it comes out small in a wide variety of vacua similar to ours; in other words, all contributions to M_H are of the same order so that no fine tuning is required. This is called a natural solution, and from (14.1) it requires

$$M_{\mathrm{ST}} \sim M_H$$

in a fairly strong sense (for example [22] estimates $M_{\mathrm{ST}} \lesssim 400\,\mathrm{GeV}$), Although this might sound as if it is already ruled out, the stop cross section is quite a bit smaller than that of the gluino, and there are even scenarios in which the lightest stop is hard to find because it is nearly degenerate with the top.

While $\Lambda_{\mathrm{SUSY}} \sim M_{\mathrm{EW}}$ as well, there are many different types of supersymmetry breaking, and this does not in itself require the gluino to be light. But one can get a much stronger constraint by assuming that M_{ST} is naturally low as well, as it gets mass renormalization from gluon and gluino loops. Assuming that there are no other colored particles involved, this leads to an upper bound on the gluino mass [22]:

$$M_{\tilde{g}} \lesssim 2 M_{\mathrm{ST}}.$$

Thus, LHC appears to be on the verge of ruling out a wide variety of natural models similar to the Minimal Supersymmetric Standard Model (MSSM).

These low bounds on the masses of superpartners in natural models were already problematic before LHC for a variety of reasons, but most importantly because of the difficulty of matching precision measurements in the Standard Model. The longest-standing problem here is the absence of flavor-changing processes other than those mediated directly by the weak interactions, which translates into lower bounds for the scale of much new physics of $\Lambda \gtrsim 10\text{--}100\,\mathrm{TeV}$!

Assuming the superpartners are not found below $1\,\mathrm{TeV}$, a reasonable response is to give up on naturalness and accept some tuning of the Higgs mass. The cleanest such scenario is to grant the standard structure of low-energy supersymmetry, but push it all up to the $10\text{--}100\,\mathrm{TeV}$ scale. Thus, all of the superpartners and the Higgs bosons would a priori lie in the range $0.1\text{--}1$ times Λ_{SUSY}, but we then postulate an additional $10^{-4}\text{--}10^{-6}$ fine tuning of one of the Higgs boson masses. At first sight, this has the problem that we lose the WIMP as a candidate dark matter particle. However, because the gauginos have R-charge and the scalars do not, it is natural for them to acquire a lower mass after supersymmetry breaking.

In a bit more detail, one very generally expects irrelevant interactions between the supersymmetry-breaking sector and the Standard Model sector to produce soft masses for all the scalars of order $\Lambda_{\mathrm{SUSY}} = M_{3/2}$. In the original supergravity models, this scale was set to M_{EW}, but this leads to many lighter particles and by now has been ruled out. One way to try to fix this is gauge mediation, in which other interactions provide larger soft masses. As far as the Standard Model is concerned, this may be good, but it suffers from the cosmological moduli and gravitino problems we will discuss in Section 14.3. One can instead try to work with $\Lambda_{\mathrm{SUSY}} \gg M_{\mathrm{EW}}$, and argue that the naive expectations for the soft masses are incorrect. There are many ideas for this, such as sequestering [23] (see [24] for a recent string theory discussion), focus point models [25], intersection point models [26], and others. Clearly it would be important if a generic mechanism could be found, but as yet none of these have found general acceptance. Thus, we accept the generic result $M_0 \sim \Lambda_{\mathrm{SUSY}}$ for scalar masses. However, the gaugino soft masses have other sources and, as we will discuss below, can be smaller.

The extreme version of this scenario is split supersymmetry [27, 28], in which the scalars can be arbitrarily heavy while all fermionic superpartners are light. In any case, although M_H is tuned, it is essentially determined by the quartic Higgs coupling and the Higgs vacuum expectation value, which we know from M_Z. If the underlying model is the MSSM, then, since the quartic Higgs coupling comes from a D-term, it is determined by the gauge couplings and we get a fairly direct prediction for the Higgs mass. As is well known, at tree level, there is a bound $M_H^2 \leq M_Z^2$, and one must call on (14.1) just to satisfy the LEP bound $M_H > 113\,\mathrm{GeV}$. There has been much recent discussion of the difficulty of getting $M_H \sim 125\,\mathrm{GeV}$ to come out of the MSSM in a natural way [16–19].

If M_H is fine-tuned, the loop contribution (14.1) is no longer directly measurable. However, there is a similar-looking constraint coming from the running of the quartic Higgs coupling, of the general form[3]

$$M_H^2 \sim M_Z^2 \cos^2 2\beta + \frac{3g^2 M_{\mathrm{top}}^4}{16\pi^2 \sin^2 \beta M_W^2} \log \frac{\Lambda_{SUSY}}{M_{\mathrm{top}}}. \tag{14.2}$$

In fact, for $M_H = 125\,\mathrm{GeV}$, this turns out to predict $\Lambda_{\mathrm{SUSY}} \sim 100\,\mathrm{TeV}$. This prediction is not robust; for example, by postulating another scalar that couples to the Higgses through the superpotential (the next-to-minimal supersymmetric Standard Model, NMSSM), or an extra $U(1)$, one can change the relation between the Higgs quartic coupling and the gauge coupling. Such modifications will affect the Higgs branching ratios, so this alternative will be tested at LHC in the coming years.

---

[3] This is a bit simplified, and the precise expression depends on ones' assumptions, see, e.g., [11, 17]. The main difference with (14.1) is that one has put in the observed electroweak parameters and thus accepted the possibility of tuning.

Within this scenario, the key question for LHC physics is whether we will see the gauginos. There are many models, such as anomaly mediation [23, 29, 30], in which the expected gaugino mass is

$$M_\chi \sim \frac{\beta(g)}{2g^2} \Lambda_{\mathrm{SUSY}}. \tag{14.3}$$

where $\beta(g)$ is the exact beta function. This prefactor is of order 10^{-2} for the neutralinos, so we again have a dark matter candidate if $\Lambda_{\mathrm{SUSY}} \sim 100\,\mathrm{TeV}$. For the gluino, it is $\sim 1/40$, and thus we are right at the edge of detection at LHC-14. With $\Lambda_{\mathrm{SUSY}} \sim 30\,\mathrm{TeV}$, we would have gluino mass $M_3 \sim 750\,\mathrm{GeV}$, which should be seen very soon.

Note that there are other string compactifications with large gaugino masses.[4] The relevant contribution is $F^a \partial_a f$, where F^a is an F-term and f is a gauge kinetic term. Thus, gaugino masses will be large if the supersymmetry breaking F-terms are in fields, such as the heterotic string dilaton, whose expectation values strongly affect the observed gauge couplings. This is a question about the supersymmetry-breaking sector that must be addressed top-down; in Section 14.6, we will suggest that small masses are preferred.

It would be very valuable from this point of view to know the lower limit on Λ_{SUSY} in these scenarios, as, all other things being equal, it seems reasonable by naturalness to expect the lower limit (we will discuss stringy naturalness later).

14.3 The gravitino and moduli problems

It has been known for a long time that light, weakly coupled scalars can be problematic for inflationary cosmology [31]. Because of quantum fluctuations, on the exit from inflation they start out displaced from any minimum of the potential, leading to possible "overshoot" of the desired minimum, and to excess entropy and/or energy.

In string/M-theory compactification, moduli of the extra-dimensional metric and other fields very generally lead after supersymmetry breaking to scalar fields with gravitational strength coupling and mass $M \sim \Lambda_{\mathrm{SUSY}}$, making this problem very relevant [32, 33]. For $M \sim 1\,\mathrm{TeV}$, such particles will decay around $T \sim M_{\mathrm{Planck}}^2/M^3 \sim 10^3\,\mathrm{s}$. This is very bad, since it spoils the predictions for abundances of light nuclei based on big bang nucleosynthesis, which takes place during the period $0.1\,s \lesssim T \lesssim 100\,\mathrm{s}$. One needs such particles to be either much lighter or much heavier, so that they decay at $T \ll 0.1\,\mathrm{s}$. One can also increase their couplings so that their decay reheats the universe well above the scale of nucleosynthesis—see [34] for a recent proposal of this type. There is a closely related constraint from gravitino decay [35], which can also be solved this way.

Although not proven, it is quite generally stated that this constraint forces the moduli masses to satisfy

$$M_{\mathrm{moduli}} \gtrsim 30\,\mathrm{TeV}. \tag{14.4}$$

---

[4] I thank Bobby Acharya, Gordy Kane, and Gary Shiu for discussions on this point.

This may not a priori require $\Lambda_{\text{SUSY}} \gtrsim 30\,\text{TeV}$, since there are other ways to lift moduli masses. For example, fluxes can give masses to moduli while preserving supersymmetry [4, 36]. On the other hand, the structure of the $\mathcal{N} = 1$ supergravity potential makes it generic to have at least one scalar with $M \lesssim M_{3/2}$, as shown in [37, 38]. This is a scalar partner of the goldstino, and it need not have gravitational strength interactions, but if supersymmetry breaking takes place in a hidden sector, this will often lead to a constraint. In addition, the gravitino has $M = M_{3/2}$ by definition. If one is going to call on reheating or other physics to solve these problems, it is simplest and probably most generic for the problematic particles to be associated with a single energy scale.

These various considerations all suggest that

$$\Lambda_{\text{SUSY}} = M_{3/2} \gtrsim 30\,\text{TeV}. \tag{14.5}$$

This is an extremely strong constraint that very much disfavors the natural solutions to the hierarchy problem and is independent of the arguments we gave in Section 14.2. This is widely recognized, and therefore there has been a major effort to search for generic ways out, or at least loopholes to this bound. On the other hand, even if there are loopholes, the bound still might be generic. In the context of the string landscape, the correct attitude would then be to accept it as preferred, also allowing the vacua (and cosmological histories) that realize the loophole, but weighting them by appropriate tuning factors. We will begin this discussion below.

Perhaps the main reason that (14.5) has not been more widely accepted is that there is no direct evidence at this point for the significance of the energy scale 30–100 TeV. This is of course related to the lack of direct evidence for supersymmetry, so perhaps we should not be too bothered by it, but we should ask for some more fundamental reason why $\Lambda_{\text{SUSY}} \sim 30\text{--}100$ TeV should be preferred. Later, we are going to argue this from stringy naturalness, essentially that Λ_{SUSY} should take the lowest possible value consistent with anthropic constraints.

A weaker but more general claim, less dependent on anthropic constraints, is that the cosmological moduli problem will always favor a "little hierarchy" between the mass scale of "normal" matter and the supersymmetry-breaking scale. Let us start from a more general statement of the problem—namely, that important cosmological physics (in our universe, big bang nucleosynthesis) takes place at a temperature just below the mass of normal matter, and thus moduli (and the gravitino) must decay well before this happens and/or reheat the universe above this temperature. Thus, we have

$$T_{\text{reheat}} > c M_{\text{matter}}, \tag{14.6}$$

with a constant $c \sim 10^{-3}\text{--}10^{-1}$. Given $T_{\text{reheat}} \sim \Lambda_{\text{SUSY}}/M_{\text{Planck}}^{1/2}$, this implies

$$\Lambda_{\text{SUSY}}^3 > c M_{\text{Planck}} M_{\text{matter}}^2 \tag{14.7}$$

and the large hierarchy $M_{\text{Planck}} \gg M_{\text{matter}}$ forces $\Lambda_{\text{SUSY}} \gg M_{\text{matter}}$, but only as the one-third power of $M_{\text{Planck}}/M_{\text{matter}}$ and suppressed by the constant c.

An even more broadbrush way of arguing would be to say that inflationary cosmology is already difficult enough to make work at each of the relevant scales (the matter/big brag nucleosynthesis scale, the electroweak scale, and now the supersymmetry-breaking scale) that one should expect at least little hierarchies between these various scales just to simplify the problem. Whether this simplicity is of the type that Occam would have favored, or whether it has any relevance for stringy naturalness, remains unclear.

14.4   The set of string vacua

The broad features of string compactification are described in [4] and many other reviews. We start with a choice of string theory or M-theory, of compactification manifold, and of the topological class of additional features such as branes, orientifolds, and fluxes. We then argue that the corresponding supergravity or string/M-theory equations have solutions, by combining mathematical existence theorems (*e.g.*, for a Ricci-flat metric on a Calabi–Yau manifold), perturbative and semiclassical computations of corrections to supergravity, and general arguments about the structure of four-dimensional effective field theory.

Perhaps the most fundamental distinction is whether we grant that our vacuum breaks $\mathcal{N} = 1$ supersymmetry at the compactification (or "high") scale or whether we can think of it as described by a four-dimensional $\mathcal{N} = 1$ supersymmetric effective field theory, with supersymmetry breaking at a lower scale. Almost all work makes the second assumption, largely because there are no effective techniques to control the more general problem, nor is there independent evidence (say from duality arguments) that many high-scale vacua exist. Early work suggesting that such vacua were simply the large-Λ_{SUSY} limit of the usual supersymmetric vacua [39, 40] was quickly refuted by a more careful analysis of supersymmetry breaking [38].

A heuristic and probably correct argument that this type of nonsupersymmetric vacuum is very rare is that stability is very difficult to achieve without supersymmetry– recently this has been shown in a precise sense for random supergravity potentials [41]. There are many versions of this question, some analogous and some dual, such as the existence of Ricci-flat metrics without special holonomy and the existence of interacting conformal field theories without supersymmetry. We will assume that metastable nonsupersymmetric vacua are not common enough to outweigh their disadvantages; of course, if a large set of them were to be discovered, this would further weaken the case for low-energy supersymmetry.

Another context in which nonsupersymmetric vacua might be very important is for the theory of inflation. A natural guess for the scale of observed inflation is the GUT scale, in other words the compactification scale. The requirement of near-stability is still very constraining, however, and almost all work on this problem assumes broken $\mathcal{N} = 1$ supersymmetry as well. Since the inflationary trajectory must end up in a metastable vacuum, it is hard to see how it could be very different from this vacuum anyways.

Granting the need for four-dimensional $\mathcal{N} = 1$ "low-scale" supersymmetry (here meaning compared with the string-theoretic scales), each of the five 10-dimensional string theories as well as 11-dimensional supergravity have a preferred extra-dimensional geometry that leads there. While some theories (such as type I and $SO(32)$ heterotic) were originally thought not to contain the Standard Model, during the "duality revolution" of the 1990s it was realized that there are many more possible sources of gauge symmetry, matter, and the various interactions, such as fields localized on branes and their intersections. While the individual theories still make generic predictions, in general there is a lot of freedom to realize the Standard Model and a wide variety of additional matter sectors.

An important distinction can be made between "global" models such as heterotic string compactification and "local" models such as F-theory. In a global model, realizing chiral matter requires postulating structure on the entire extra-dimensional manifold. By contrast, in a local model, chiral matter can be realized at the intersection of branes that are contained in some arbitrarily small subregion of the manifold. This is nontrivial, because chiral matter can only be realized by brane intersections that (in a certain topological sense) span all of the extra dimensions [42]. While naively this makes local models impossible—and on simple topologies such as an n-torus they would be impossible—they are possible in more complicated geometries such as resolved orbifolds and elliptic fibrations.

Local models tend not to realize gauge unification, and in the simplest examples cannot realize the matter representations required for a GUT, such as the spinor of $SO(10)$. These two problems were more or less overcome by the development of F-theory local models [43, 44]. F-theory is also attractive in that one can more easily understand the other constructions by starting from F-theory and applying dualities than the other way around.

It was suggested in [43] that local models should be preferred because they admit a consistent decoupling limit. Essentially, this is a limit in which one takes the small subregion containing the local model to become arbitrarily small. Because observable scales (the Planck scale and the scale of matter) tend to be related to scales in the extra dimensions, it is more natural to get hierarchies in this limit. At present, the status of this argument is extremely unclear, since it is generally agreed that global models can realize hierarchies through dynamical supersymmetry breaking and otherwise. Later, we will discuss a different, cosmological argument that might favor local models.

Because of the dualities, and the existence of topology-changing transitions in string/M-theory, the usual picture is of a single "configuration space" containing all the vacua and allowing transitions (perhaps via chains of elementary transitions) between any pair of vacua. Only special cases of this picture have been worked out; for example, it has long been known that all of the simply connected Calabi–Yau 3-folds are connected by conifold transitions. More recently, "hyperconifold transitions" have been introduced that can change the fundamental group [45, 46], but it is not known whether these connect all the non-simply connected threefolds.

It is very important to complete this picture and develop concrete ways to represent and work with the totality of this configuration space. Even its most basic properties, such as any sense in which it is finite, are not really understood. Various ideas from mathematics can be helpful here; in particular, there is a theory of spaces of Riemannian manifolds in which finiteness properties can be proven, such as Gromov–Cheeger compactness. Very roughly, this says that if we place a few natural restrictions on the manifolds, such as an upper bound on the diameter (the maximum distance between any pair of points), then the space of possibilities can be covered by a finite number of finite-size balls. These restrictions can be motivated physically and lead to a very general argument that there can only be a finite number of quasirealistic string vacua [47]; however, this does not yet lead to any useful estimate of their number.

Given the topological choices of manifolds, bundles, branes, and the like, one can often use algebraic geometry to form a fairly detailed picture of a moduli space of compactifications with unbroken $\mathcal{N} = 1$ supersymmetry. Various physical constraints, of which the simplest is the absence of long-range "fifth force" corrections to general relativity, imply that the scalar fields corresponding to these moduli must gain masses. To a large extent, this so-called "moduli stabilization" problem can be solved by giving the scalars supersymmetric masses. For example, background flux in the extra dimensions can lead to a nontrivial superpotential depending on the moduli, with many supersymmetric vacua [36]. The many choices of flux also make the anthropic solution of the cosmological constant problem easy to realize [48]. Moduli stabilization also determines the distribution of vacua in the moduli space, and thus the distribution of couplings and masses in the low-energy effective theory. One can make detailed statistical analyses of this distribution, which incorporate and improve the traditional discussion of naturalness of couplings [4].

While supersymmetric effects lift many neutral scalars, it is not at all clear that it generically lifts all of them, satisfying bounds like (14.4) before taking supersymmetry breaking into account. Explicit constructions such as that of [49] are usually left with one or more light scalars, and, as we discussed earlier, one can argue that this is generic [34, 38].

Another important point that is manifest in the flux sector is what I call the "broken-symmetry paradox." Simply stated, it is that in a landscape, symmetry is heavily disfavored. One can already see this in chemistry—while the Schrödinger equation admits $SO(3)$ rotational symmetry, and this is very important for the structure of atomic and molecular orbitals, once one shifts the emphasis to studying molecules, this symmetry does not play much of a role. While a few molecules do preserve an $SO(2)$ or discrete subgroup, the resulting symmetry relations rarely have qualitatively important consequences beyond a few level degeneracies, and it is not at all true that molecules with symmetry are more abundant or favored in any way in chemical reactions.

It was shown in [50] that discrete R-symmetries are heavily disfavored in flux compactification, and the character of the argument is fairly general. Suppose we want vacua with a Z_N symmetry; then it is plausible that of the various parameters of some class of vacua including a symmetric point, order $1/N$ of them will transform trivially, and order $1/N$ will each transform in one of the $N - 1$ nontrivial representations. But, since the number of vacua is exponential in the number of parameters, symmetry is extremely disfavored. While one can imagine dynamical arguments that would favor symmetry, since these tend to operate only near the symmetric point, it is hard to see them changing the conclusion.

One virtue of this observation is that it helps explain away the gap between the many hundreds or thousands of fields of a typical string compactification (especially those with enough vacua to solve the cosmological constant problem) and the smaller number in the Standard Model, since symmetry breaking will get rid of nonabelian gauge groups and generally lift fields. But this is very different from the usual particle physics intuition.

14.5 Eternal inflation and the master vacuum

The wealth of disparate possibilities coming out of string compactification combined with the relative poverty of the data seem to force us to bring in extra structure and constraints to help solve the vacuum selection problem and test the theory. This would probably remain true even were we to discover many new particles at LHC.

A good source of extra structure is cosmology, both because there is data there and because some of the key particle physics questions (such as low-energy supersymmetry) can have cosmological consequences (such as WIMP dark matter). In addition to these more specific hints, as we discussed in Section 14.1, we have real world examples of landscapes and we know there that the dynamics that forms metastable configurations plays an absolutely essential role in preferring some configurations over others. It is entirely reasonable to expect the same here.

A very worrying point is that the dynamics of chemistry, and even big bang nucleosynthesis, is highly nonlinear and depends crucially on small energy differences. The problem of deducing abundances *ab initio*, without experimental data, is completely intractable. While this might be true of the string landscape as well, in fact the most popular scenario appears to be much simpler to analyze, since the central equations are linear.

This is the idea of eternal inflation, reviewed in [6–8] and elsewhere. There is a good deal of current work on bringing this into string theory. While I am not an expert, this seems to have two main thrusts. One is to find microscopic models of inflation or, even better, a gauge dual to inflation analogous to AdS/CFT. The other is to try to make the framework sufficiently well defined to be able to make predictions, by deriving a measure factor on the set of vacua. We will simply cite [11] for a review of the status of this field and move to discussing the concrete prescription we already quoted in Section 14.1 [13] which we call the "master vacuum" prescription:

- The measure factor is overwhelmingly dominated by the longest-lived metastable de Sitter vacuum. For other vacua, it is given by the tunneling rate from this "master" vacuum, which to a good approximation is that of the single fastest chain of tunneling events.

Once we have convinced ourselves of this, evidently the next order of business is to find the master vacuum. For some measure prescriptions, this would be an absolutely hopeless task. For example, suppose we needed to find the metastable de Sitter vacuum with the smallest positive cosmological constant. By arguments from computational complexity theory [51], this problem is intractable, even for a computer the size of the universe!

The problem of finding the longest-lived vacuum in this prescription could be much easier. A large and probably dominant factor controlling the tunneling rate out of a metastable vacuum is the scale of supersymmetry breaking [52, 53]. The intuitive reason is simply that supersymmetric vacua are generally stable, by BPS arguments. Thus, a reasonable guess is that the master vacuum is some flux sector in a vacuum with the smallest Λ_{SUSY}. The actual positive cosmological constant is less important, both because this factor cancels out of tunneling rates in the analysis of the measure factor and because there are so many choices in the flux sector available to adjust it. The relation to Λ_{SUSY} also makes it very plausible that the master vacuum is *not* anthropically allowed.

The question of how to get small Λ_{SUSY} deserves detailed study, but it is a very reasonable guess that this will be achieved by taking the topology of the extra dimensions to be as complicated as possible, and, even more specifically, by an extra-dimensional manifold with the largest possible Euler number χ. Of course it is intuitively reasonable that complexity allows for more possibilities and thus more extreme parameter values, but there is a more specific argument, which we will now explain.

The first observation is that Λ_{SUSY} is a sum of positive terms (the sum in quadrature of D- and F-breaking terms) and thus cannot receive cancellations, so one is simply trying to make the individual D- and F-terms small. If we imagine doing this by dynamical supersymmetry breaking driven by an exponentially small nonperturbative effect, then the problem is to realize a supersymmetry-breaking gauge theory with the smallest possible coupling $g^2 N$ at the fundamental scale. This coupling is determined by moduli stabilization, and is typically related to ratios of coefficients in the effective potential. These coefficients can be geometric (intersection numbers, numbers of curves, etc.) or set by quantized fluxes. To obtain a small gauge coupling, we want these coefficients to be large.

In both cases, the typical size of the coefficients is controlled by the topology of the extra dimensions. For example, the maximum value of a flux is determined by a tadpole or topological constraint, which for F-theory on a Calabi–Yau 4-fold is

$$\eta_{ij} N^i N^j + N_{D3} = \frac{1}{24}\chi. \tag{14.8}$$

Here the N^i are integrally quantized values of the 4-form flux, η_{ij} is a symmetric unimodular intersection form, and N_{D3} is the number of D3-branes sitting at points in the extra dimensions. The fluxes N^i are maximized by taking χ large and N_{D3} small, allowing large ratios of fluxes. Although the other geometric quantities are much more complicated to discuss, it is reasonable to expect similar relations.

Thus, we might look for the master vacuum as an F-theory compactification on the fourfold with maximal χ, which (as far as I know) is the hypersurface in weighted projective space given in [54] with $\chi = 24 \cdot 75852$. This compactification also allows a very large enhanced gauge group with rank 60 740, including 1276 E_8 factors [55].

With this large number of cycles, the number of similar vacua obtained by varying fluxes and other choices should be so large (10^{10000} or even more), that the nearby vacua that solve the cosmological constant problem will be similar, answering the question of predictivity raised in Section 14.1. But the complexity of this compactification suggests that it might not be easy to find the precise moduli and fluxes leading to the master vacuum. Before doing this, we need to refine the measure factor prescription, for the following reason. As stated, it assumes there is a unique longest-lived vacuum. Now, it is true that supersymmetry breaking will generate a potential on the moduli space so that de Sitter vacua will be isolated, but with this very small $\Lambda_{\rm SUSY}$ these potential barriers will be incredibly small. At the very least, one expects the tunneling rates to other vacua on (what was) the moduli space to be large. It might be a better approximation to regard the "master vacuum" as a distribution on this moduli space given by a simple probability measure, perhaps uniform or perhaps a vacuum counting measure as in [4].

The interesting tunneling events, toward anthropically allowed vacua, would be those that increase the scale of supersymmetry breaking. One might imagine that supersymmetry breaking will be associated with a single matter sector[5] (i.e., a minimal set S of gauge groups such that no matter is charged under both a group in S and a group not in S) and that these tunneling events will affect only this sector. But since the masses of charged matter depend on moduli, in parts of the moduli space where additional matter becomes light, one could get tunneling events that affect other sectors as well. We will suggest a more intuitive picture of this dynamics in Section 14.6.

Much is unclear about this picture. One very basic assumption is that we can think of the cosmological dynamics using a $(4 + k)$-dimensional split, although of course spacetime can be much more complicated. Better justification of this point would require a better understanding of inflation in string compactification. If this can only be realized as granting such a split (as appears at present to be the case), then this would be a justification; if not, not. Another question is that since there are supersymmetric transitions between compactifications with different topology, one should not even take for granted that the master vacuum is concentrated on a single topology, although this seems plausible because such transitions change the fluxes and tadpole conditions [57].

14.6   From hyperchemistry to phenomenology

Granting that the dynamics of eternal inflation and the master vacuum are an important part of the vacuum selection problem, it would be very useful to develop an intuitive picture of this dynamics. Let us suggest such a picture based on the assumptions stated above.

The starting point is to think of the various structures that lead to the gauge–matter sectors relevant for low-energy physics—groups of cycles and/or intersecting branes—as objects that can move in the extra dimensions. The idea is that we are trying to describe a distribution on a pseudo-moduli space of nearly supersymmetric vacua, and the moduli correspond to sizes of cycles, positions of branes, and the like. Of course, the background space in which they move will not be Euclidean or indeed any fixed geometry, and a really good picture must also take into account this geometrical

---

[5] A recent paper on such sectors is [56].

freedom. But, with this in mind, a picture of objects moving in a fixed six-dimensional space can be our initial picture.[6]

Next, the most important dynamical effect that could influence the tunneling rates is the possibility that as the moduli vary, new light fields come down in mass, perhaps coupling what were previously disjoint matter sectors. In the brane picture, this will happen when groups of branes come close together. Again, in the most general case, this can happen in other ways, such as by varying Wilson lines, but let us start with the simplest case to picture.

The dynamics is thus one of structured objects (groups of cycles and intersecting branes) moving about in the extra dimensions, and perhaps interacting when they come near each other—a sort of chemistry of the extra dimensions. By analogy with the familiar word "hyperspace," we might call this "hyperchemistry." As in chemistry, while the structures and their possible interactions are largely governed by symmetry (here the representation theory of supersymmetry), questions of stability and rates are more complicated to determine—although hopefully not intractable.

The basic objects or molecules of hyperchemistry are "clusters" of branes and cycles that intersect topologically. These translate into chiral gauge theories in the low-energy effective theory. Two groups of branes and cycles that do not intersect topologically are in different clusters; these can interact gravitationally, at long range, or by having vector-like matter become light, at short range.

Although the nature and distribution of the clusters is not known in four dimensions, it has recently been determined for F-theory compactifications to six dimensions with eight supercharges [58]. It turns out that the minimal clusters give rise to certain preferred gauge theories with matter that cannot be Higgsed, for example $SU(2) \times SO(7) \times SU(2)$ with half-hypermultiplets in the $(2, 8, 1) \oplus (1, 8, 2)$, or E_8 with no matter. Thus, a Calabi–Yau with many cycles will give rise to a low-energy theory with many clusters. A similar picture (though with different clusters) is expected to be true for compactifications to four dimensions as well.[7]

As a simple picture of the dynamics, we can imagine the clusters moving around in the extra dimensions, occasionally undergoing transitions (tunneling events) that change their inner structure. Thus, we have a fixed set of chiral gauge theories, loosely coupled to each other through bulk gravitational interactions. Occasionally, two clusters will collide, leading to vector-like matter becoming light. This enables further transitions such as Higgs–Coulomb or the more complicated extremal transitions in the literature.

To some extent, the details of the extra-dimensional bulk geometry would not be central to this picture—one could get away with knowing the relative distances and orientations between each pair of clusters. Our previous simplifying assumption that the clusters are moving in a fixed extradimensional geometry would imply many constraints on these parameters, which to some extent would be relaxed by

---

[6] Although F-theory postulates a 4-fold, i.e., an eight-real-dimensional space, two of these dimensions are a mathematical device used to represent a varying dilaton–axion field. The actual extra dimensions are six-dimensional.

[7] D. Morrison, private communication.

allowing the extra dimensional geometry to vary as well. In this way, our picture could accommodate all of the relevant configurations.

Granting this picture, how might the master vacuum tunnel to an anthropically allowed vacuum? Now, the Standard Model is a chiral gauge theory, and we know various ways to make it up out of branes and cycles—in other words, as a cluster. It is a cluster of moderate complexity, which within F-theory can be obtained by resolving singularities of a sort that appear naturally in 4-folds. Thus, it is natural to imagine that such clusters are already present in the master vacuum. On the other hand, the master vacuum has an extremely small supersymmetry-breaking scale, probably due to dynamics in a single cluster, with no reason to have large couplings to the Standard Model cluster.

Thus, the simplest dynamics that could create an anthropically allowed vacuum involves two steps: the supersymmetry-breaking cluster is modified to produce a larger scale of supersymmetry breaking, and its interactions with the Standard Model cluster are enhanced to produce the observed supersymmetry breaking. The first step is the one that should answer questions about the underlying scale Λ_{SUSY} of supersymmetry breaking, while the second will determine its mediation to the observable sector.

Regarding the first, it is reasonable to expect some high-scale vacua stabilized by tuned structure in the potential as in [38], with number growing as $\Lambda_{\mathrm{SUSY}}^{12}$ for reasons explained there. The number of these compared with low-cale vacua with Λ_{SUSY} exponentially small is not yet clear. However, granting that the master vacuum must be one with extremely small Λ_{SUSY}, it is already a low-scale vacuum, and thus the transition of the first step can easily be one that produces a low-scale vacuum, perhaps by varying a single flux, and thus the gauge coupling appearing in the exponential. Even if high-scale vacua can also be produced in comparable numbers, their disadvantage in solving the hierarchy problem will remain. A possible loophole would be if the mediation to the Standard Model were somehow suppressed—which seems unlikely as we argue shortly.

As for the origin of the Standard Model, these pictures suggest that it would be realized by a single matter sector in a localized region of the extra dimensions—in other words a local model. This is not because it must make sense in the decoupling limit, but rather because this is the most likely way for it to be produced by cosmological dynamics. Furthermore, there is no reason that the supersymmetry-breaking sector must be near the Standard Model sector or share matter with it. This suggests that supersymmetry breaking is generically mediated by supergravity interactions.

The generic estimate for scalar masses in supergravity mediation is $M_0 \sim F/M_{\mathrm{Plancks}}$. This might be smaller if the two sectors were "far apart" in the extra dimensions, but there is no known dynamics that would favor this. As we discussed in Section 14.2, other proposals for how this could be smaller such as sequestering are not presently believed to be generic in string theory. On the other hand, it is possible for the supersymmetry-breaking cluster and the Standard Model cluster to approach very closely so that the mediation is larger. In fact, they must be closer than the string scale, and thus (from brane model intuition) they will be coupled by vector-like matter, leading to a gauge-mediation scenario. While this is possible, since it is continuously connected to the gravitational-mediation scenario, distinguished only by varying moduli, it requires additional tuning compared with gravitational mediation.

The upshot is that gravitational mediation with $M_0 \sim F/M_{\text{Plancks}}$ seems favored, unless there is some reason that more of the alternative models satisfy the anthropic constraints. This question deserves close examination by those more expert in the field than myself, but I know of no major advantage in this regard. Indeed, one might expect gauge mediation to lead to small $M_{3/2}$ and a cosmological moduli problem. The picture also suggests that the F-terms are of the type giving rise to small gaugino masses, since they arise in a hidden matter sector.

We now recall the beyond the Standard Model part of our argument. This was to compare what seem to be the two likeliest candidate solutions of the hierarchy problem, namely, the natural supersymmetric scenario and the scenario with $\Lambda_{\text{SUSY}} \sim 30\text{--}100\,\text{TeV}$ and then an additional fine tuning. The claim is then that the additional 10^{-5} or so of fine tuning gained by naturalness is more than lost by the difficulty of solving the cosmological moduli problem, as well as meeting the other anthropic constraints, which are much stronger in the far more complicated natural supersymmetric theories. While this claim is hard to argue in the absence of any knowledge about higher-energy physics, if we believe we know the right class of theories to look at on top-down grounds, we can argue it. The class of extensions of the Standard Model that can be realized as local models in string/M-theory, interacting with a supersymmetry-breaking sector, is probably narrow enough to allow evaluating the bottom-up argument and making it quantitative. As it happens, for the question of whether we will see gauginos at LHC, it makes a great difference whether we expect $\Lambda_{\text{SUSY}} \sim 30\,\text{TeV}$ or $100\,\text{TeV}$ and whether F-terms couple to observable gauge couplings, and it would be great if the arguments could reach that level of detail.

To summarize the overall picture at this point, it is that we have three sources of information about how string/M-theory could describe our universe. Traditional particle phenomenology and astroparticle physics are of course bottom-up and motivate model building within broad frameworks such as quantum field theory and effective Lagrangians. Another source is top-down, the study of compactifications and their predictions for "physics" broadly construed. The results can be summarized in effective Lagrangians, tunneling rates between vacua and the like, and statistical summaries of this information for large sets of vacua. This is a "mathematical" definition of the landscape, which could in principle be developed *ab initio*, accepting only the most minimal real world input. Finally, there is the dynamics of early cosmology, by which the various vacua constructed in the top-down approach are created. This subject is still in its infancy—although we have pictures such as eternal inflation that might work, the details are not yet well understood, and there are variations and competing pictures yet to be explored. Simplified pictures such as hyperchemistry could help us to think physically about this dynamics.

Unless the data improve dramatically, it seems to us that all three sources must be combined to make real predictions from string/M-theory. One must understand the set of vacua, or at least those near the master vacuum. One must understand the dynamics of early cosmology and presumably tunneling rates between vacua. In general, these problems will have little or nothing to do with either Standard Model or beyond the Standard Model physics, because the relevant dynamics is at completely different energy and time scales. The other part is anthropic, but, given the vagueness and difficulty of working with the anthropic principle, it is probably better to simply call it "bottom-up" and require that we match some or all of the data to hand. The main difference with the existing paradigm in phenomenology is that we can use the top-down and early cosmology information to make a well-motivated definition of naturalness, so that if reproducing the data requires postulating an unnatural vacuum, then we have evidence against the theory. All this is a long-range project, but I think we are at the point where we can begin to work on it.

Acknowledgments

I thank Bobby Acharya, Raphael Bousso, Frederik Denef, Michael Dine, Dave Morrison, Gordy Kane, Patrick Meade, Gary Shiu, Steve Shenker, and Lenny Susskind for discussions and comments on the manuscript. This research was supported in part by DOE grant DE-FG02-92ER40697.

References

[1] T. Banks, M. Dine, and M. R. Douglas, "Time varying alpha and particle physics," Phys. Rev. Lett. **88**, 131301 (2002) [arXiv:hep-ph/0112059].

[2] N. Arkani-Hamed, L. Motl, A. Nicolis, and C. Vafa, "The string landscape, black holes and gravity as the weakest force," JHEP **0706**, 060 (2007) [arXiv:hep-th/0601001].

[3] V. Kumar and W. Taylor, "String universality in six dimensions," arXiv:0906.0987 [hep-th].

[4] M. R. Douglas and S. Kachru, "Flux compactification," Rev. Mod. Phys. **79**, 733 (2007) [arXiv:hep-th/0610102].

[5] M. R. Douglas, "Understanding the landscape," arXiv:hep-th/0602266.

[6] A. H. Guth, "Eternal inflation and its implications," J. Phys. **A40**, 6811 (2007) [hep-th/0702178 [hep-th]].

[7] A. D. Linde, "The inflationary multiverse," in B. Carr (ed.): "Universe or multiverse," pp.127–149, Cambridge University Press, Cambridge (2009).

[8] A. Vilenkin, "The Principle of Mediocrity," arXiv:1108.4990 [hep-th].

[9] L. Susskind, "Is eternal inflation past-eternal? And what if it is?," arXiv:1205.0589 [hep-th].

[10] A. Vilenkin, "Global structure of the multiverse and the measure problem," arXiv:1301.0121 [hep-th].

[11] B. Freivogel, "Making predictions in the multiverse," Class. Quant. Grav. **28**, 204007 (2011) [arXiv:1105.0244 [hep-th]].

[12] D. Harlow, S. H. Shenker, D. Stanford, and L. Susskind, "Tree-like structure of eternal inflation: a solvable model," Phys. Rev. **D85**, 063516 (2012) [arXiv:1110.0496 [hep-th]].

[13] D. Schwartz-Perlov and A. Vilenkin, "Probabilities in the Bousso–Polchinski multiverse," JCAP **0606**, 010 (2006) [hep-th/0601162].

[14] R. Bousso and R. Harnik, "The entropic landscape," Phys. Rev. **D82**, 123523 (2010) [arXiv:1001.1155 [hep-th]].

[15] R. Harnik, G. D. Kribs, and G. Perez, "A Universe without weak interactions," Phys. Rev. **D74**, 035006 (2006) [arXiv:hep-ph/0604027].

[16] S. Akula, B. Altunkaynak, D. Feldman, P. Nath, and G. Peim, "Higgs boson mass predictions in SUGRA unification, recent LHC-7 results, and dark matter," arXiv:1112.3645 [hep-ph].

[17] H. Baer, V. Barger, and A. Mustafayev, "Implications of a 125 GeV Higgs scalar for LHC SUSY and neutralino dark matter searches," arXiv:1112.3017 [hep-ph].

[18] L. J. Hall, D. Pinner, and J. T. Ruderman, "A natural SUSY Higgs near 126 GeV," arXiv:1112.2703 [hep-ph].

[19] N. Arkani-Hamed, talk at the 29th Jerusalem Winter School; <http://www.youtube.com/watch?v=QfSTvGMT41o>.

[20] B. S. Acharya, G. Kane, and P. Kumar, "Compactified string theories—generic predictions for particle physics," arXiv:1204.2795 [hep-ph].

[21] R. Barbieri, "Electroweak symmetry breaking as of 2003: on the way to the large hadron collider," arXiv:hep-ph/0312253.

[22] C. Brust, A. Katz, S. Lawrence, and R. Sundrum, "SUSY, the Third Generation and the LHC," arXiv:1110.6670 [hep-ph].

[23] L. Randall and R. Sundrum, "Out of this world supersymmetry breaking," Nucl. Phys. **B557**, 79 (1999) [arXiv:hep-th/9810155].

[24] M. Berg, D. Marsh, L. McAllister, and E. Pajer, "Sequestering in string compactifications," JHEP **1106**, 134 (2011) [arXiv:1012.1858 [hep-th]].

[25] J. L. Feng, K. T. Matchev, and T. Moroi, "Focus points and naturalness in supersymmetry," Phys. Rev. **D61**, 075005 (2000) [arXiv:hep-ph/9909334].

[26] D. Feldman, G. Kane, E. Kuflik, and R. Lu, "A new (string motivated) approach to the little hierarchy problem," Phys. Lett. **704B**, 56 (2011) [arXiv:1105.3765 [hep-ph]].

[27] N. Arkani-Hamed and S. Dimopoulos, "Supersymmetric unification without low energy supersymmetry and signatures for fine-tuning at the LHC," JHEP **0506**, 073 (2005) [arXiv:hep-th/0405159].

[28] N. Arkani-Hamed, S. Dimopoulos, G. F. Giudice, and A. Romanino, "Aspects of split supersymmetry," Nucl. Phys. **B709**, 3 (2005) [arXiv:hep-ph/0409232].

[29] J. A. Bagger, T. Moroi, and E. Poppitz, "Anomaly mediation in supergravity theories," JHEP **0004**, 009 (2000) [arXiv:hep-th/9911029].

[30] G. F. Giudice, M. A. Luty, H. Murayama, and R. Rattazzi, "Gaugino mass without singlets," JHEP **9812**, 027 (1998) [arXiv:hep-ph/9810442].

[31] G. D. Coughlan, W. Fischler, E. W. Kolb, S. Raby, and G. G. Ross, "Cosmological problems for the Polonyi potential," Phys. Lett. **B131**, 59 (1983).

[32] T. Banks, D. B. Kaplan, and A. E. Nelson, "Cosmological implications of dynamical supersymmetry breaking," Phys. Rev. **D49**, 779 (1994) [arXiv:hep-ph/9308292].

[33] B. de Carlos, J. A. Casas, F. Quevedo, and E. Roulet, "Model independent properties and cosmological implications of the dilaton and moduli sectors of 4-d strings," Phys. Lett. **B318**, 447 (1993) [arXiv:hep-ph/9308325].

[34] B. S. Acharya, G. Kane, and E. Kuflik, "String theories with moduli stabilization imply non-thermal cosmological history, and particular dark matter," arXiv:1006.3272 [hep-ph].

[35] J. R. Ellis, J. E. Kim, and D. V. Nanopoulos, "Cosmological gravitino regeneration and decay," Phys. Lett. **145B**, 181 (1984).

[36] S. B. Giddings, S. Kachru, and J. Polchinski, "Hierarchies from fluxes in string compactifications," Phys. Rev. **D66**, 106006 (2002) [hep-th/0105097].

[37] B. S. Acharya, P. Kumar, K. Bobkov, G. Kane, J. Shao, and S. Watson, "Non-thermal dark matter and the moduli problem in string frameworks," JHEP **0806**, 064 (2008) [arXiv:0804.0863 [hep-ph]].

[38] F. Denef and M. R. Douglas, "Distributions of nonsupersymmetric flux vacua," JHEP **0503**, 061 (2005) [arXiv:hep-th/0411183].

[39] M. R. Douglas, "Statistical analysis of the supersymmetry breaking scale," arXiv:hep-th/0405279.

[40] L. Susskind, "Supersymmetry breaking in the anthropic landscape," in M. "Shifman, A. Vainshtein, and J. Wheeler (eds.): a From Fields to Strings, Vol. 3," pp.1745–1749, World Scientific, Singapore (2005) [arXiv:hep-th/0405189].

[41] D. Marsh, L. McAllister, and T. Wrase, "The wasteland of random supergravities," arXiv:1112.3034 [hep-th].

[42] M. Berkooz, M. R. Douglas, and R. G. Leigh, "Branes intersecting at angles," Nucl. Phys. **B480**, 265 (1996) [hep-th/9606139].

[43] C. Beasley, J. J. Heckman, and C. Vafa, "GUTs and exceptional branes in F-theory—I," JHEP **0901**, 058 (2009) [arXiv:0802.3391 [hep-th]].

[44] R. Donagi and M. Wijnholt, "Model building with F-theory," arXiv:0802.2969 [hep-th].

[45] R. Davies, "Quotients of the conifold in compact Calabi–Yau threefolds, and new topological transitions," Adv. Theor. Math. Phys. **14**, 965 (2010) [arXiv:0911.0708 [hep-th]].

[46] R. Davies, "Hyperconifold transitions, mirror symmetry, and string theory," Nucl. Phys. **B850**, 214 (2011) [arXiv:1102.1428 [hep-th]].

[47] B. S. Acharya and M. R. Douglas, "A finite landscape?," arXiv:hep-th/0606212.

[48] R. Bousso and J. Polchinski, "Quantization of four form fluxes and dynamical neutralization of the cosmological constant," JHEP **0006**, 006 (2000) [arXiv:hep-th/0004134].

[49] S. Kachru, R. Kallosh, A. D. Linde, and S. P. Trivedi, "De Sitter vacua in string theory," Phys. Rev. **D68**, 046005 (2003) [arXiv:hep-th/0301240].

[50] M. Dine and Z. Sun, "R symmetries in the landscape," JHEP **0601**, 129 (2006) [arXiv:hep-th/0506246].

[51] F. Denef and M. R. Douglas, "Computational complexity of the landscape. I.," Ann. Phys. (NY) **322**, 1096 (2007) [arXiv:hep-th/0602072].

[52] A. Ceresole, G. Dall'Agata, A. Giryavets, R. Kallosh, and A. D. Linde, "Domain walls, near-BPS bubbles, and probabilities in the landscape," Phys. Rev. **D74**, 086010 (2006) [arXiv:hep-th/0605266].

[53] M. Dine, G. Festuccia, and A. Morisse, "The fate of nearly supersymmetric vacua," JHEP **0909**, 013 (2009) [arXiv:0901.1169 [hep-th]].

[54] A. Klemm, B. Lian, S. S. Roan, and S. -T. Yau, "Calabi–Yau fourfolds for M theory and F theory compactifications," Nucl. Phys. **B518**, 515 (1998) [arXiv:hep-th/9701023].

[55] P. Candelas, E. Perevalov, and G. Rajesh, "Toric geometry and enhanced gauge symmetry of F theory / heterotic vacua," Nucl. Phys. **B507**, 445 (1997) [arXiv:hep-th/9704097].

[56] D. Simic, "Metastable vacua in warped throats at non-isolated singularities," JHEP **1104**, 017 (2011) [arXiv:1009.3034 [hep-th]].

[57] S. Kachru, J. Pearson, and H. L. Verlinde, "Brane/flux annihilation and the string dual of a nonsupersymmetric field theory," JHEP **0206**, 021 (2002) [arXiv:hep-th/0112197].

[58] D. R. Morrison and W. Taylor, "Classifying bases for 6D F-theory models," arXiv:1201.1943 [hep-th].

15

The description of $\mathcal{N} = 1$, $d = 4$ supergravity using twisted supersymmetric fields

Laurent BAULIEU

Theory Division CERN Geneva, Switzerland, and
Laboratoire de Physique Théorique et Hautes Energies,
Sorbonnes Universités – Université Pierre et Marie Curie,
Paris, France

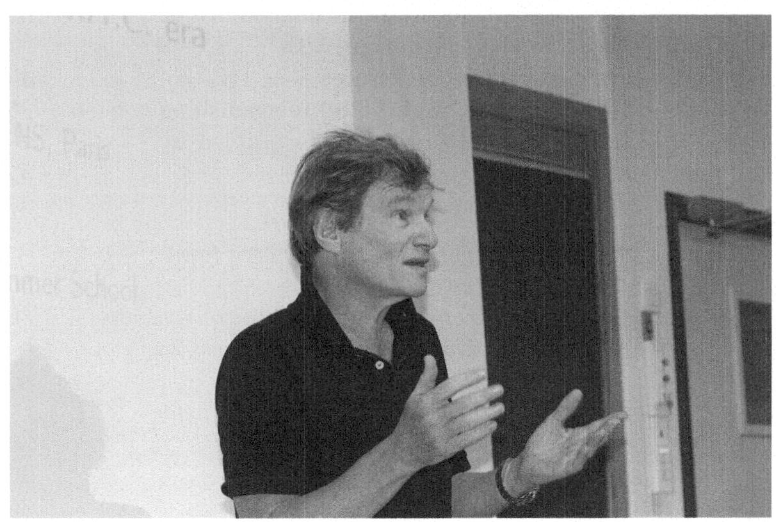

Theoretical Physics to Face the Challenge of LHC. Edited by L. Baulieu, K. Benakli, M. R. Douglas,
B. Mansoulié, E. Rabinovici, and L. F. Cugliandolo. © Oxford University Press 2015.
Published in 2015 by Oxford University Press.

Chapter Contents

This chapter shows how one can extend the method of twisted supersymmetric fields for describing global supersymmetry, as used in the context of topological field theories, to the case of local supersymmetry. As an example, the case of $\mathcal{N} = 1$ Euclidean supergravity on a 4-manifold with an almost complex structure is considered, with its couplings to scale and vector multiplets.

15.1   Introduction

Twisting is an important tool in the study of supersymmetric theories and has provided important new insights. It fundamentally means that one supercharge is singled out and used as the primary symmetry of the theory. The twist often allows for a splitting in the set of supersymmetric generators, which can be very useful. In some cases, one can find a subset of the generators that is sufficient to constrain the Lagrangian to be invariant under the full supersymmetry, while it admits off-shell closed field representations.

The first examples used nontrivial R-symmetries associated with extended supersymmetries to retain full Lorentz invariance. However, it has proved useful to consider the twist of $\mathcal{N} = 1$ theories, even if this means that only part of the Lorentz symmetry is explicitly realized: a $Spin(7)$ or $U(4)$ symmetry in dimension eight, a G_2 symmetry in dimension seven.

Here we consider the case of the simplest four-dimensional supergravity, to illustrate the formalism of twisted symmetry in curved space. We work with a Euclidean signature, which allows us to retain a $U(2)$ subgroup of the rotational symmetry. This same twist has been previously considered in the theory with only global supersymmetry [1].

In the case of the $\mathcal{N} = 1$, $d = 4$ Euclidean supergravity, only a subset of the rotational symmetry is explicitly realized after the twist, and spinors are no longer present in the theory. All fields transform as tensor products of the fundamental representation of $U(2) \subset SO(4)$. The fermionic part of the symmetry algebra consists of four fermionic twisted generators, one scalar, one vector, and one pseudoscalar. The translations are part of the supersymmetry algebra and appear, in the twisted formalism, in the anticommutator of the vector supersymmetry generators and the scalar or pseudoscalar generators. The twisted generators can be untwisted to recover the spinorial anticommuting generators of Poincaré supergravity.

The twisted superalgebra and the superalgebra of Poincaré supergravity are related in the fact that they define the same invariant action, modulo a twist. Twisted and untwisted supergravity transformation laws can be related by a linear mapping, in a way that generalizes the case of super Yang–Mills theories [1].

The construction of the twisted superalgebra is done on a 4-manifold with a Euclidean signature and an almost complex structure. In this case, the Majorana spinors can be decomposed into holomorphic and antiholomorphic forms.

Among the twisted fermionic generators, the scalar nilpotent one is of the main interest to us. It is formally similar to a BRST operator, and has an analogous interpretation as the twisted supersymmetry generator of topological Yang–Mills symmetry, two-dimensional quantum gravity or a topological string [2].

The supergravity action in a twisted form is in fact determined by the invariance under this scalar supersymmetry, with an interesting decomposition occurring for both the Einstein and Rarita–Schwinger actions. Subtle phenomena arise when one requires additional invariance under the full $SO(4)$ symmetry group.

Building the twisted superalgebra produces an interesting new framework. First, we mention that supersymmetric invariants exist as nontrivial local cocycles, a property that might be of significant importance if the twisted construction can be extended to supergravities of rank $\mathcal{N} \geq 2$. Second, the fact that invariance under the twisted scalar supersymmetry generator alone is enough to write down an action for the twisted fields might be of interest to bypass the issues raised by the lack of a system of auxiliary fields in theories such as higher-dimensional supergravities. It could be that requiring the off-shell closure of the complete Poincaré superalgebra is just too demanding. Within this approach, the super-Poincaré symmetry is not postulated, but is an emergent property once the invariance under the twisted scalar supersymmetry is imposed.

In view of these hypothetical higher-dimensional generalizations, we have computed the twisted formulation for the couplings of supergravity to scalar and vector multiplets. The results are less aesthetically pleasing than those obtained for the genuine supergravity multiplet, but their existence is a plausible four-dimensional signal that twisted formulations could also be obtained in $2n \geq 4$ dimensions, with a corresponding $U(2) \to U(n)$ generalization.

The scheme of the chapter is as follows. In Section 15.2, we recall some known facts about $\mathcal{N} = 1$, $d = 4$ supergravity in the new minimal scheme, focusing on the BRST formulation of its symmetries. In Section 15.3, we display a possible (anti-)self-dual decomposition of the supergravity action by exploring some properties of the Einstein and Rarita–Schwinger Lagrangians. In Sections 15.4 and 15.5, the twisted formalism is introduced through definitions of the twisted fields and the twisted operators corresponding to the symmetries of the supergravity action. The various curvatures needed to build the supergravity action are also displayed in twisted form. In Section 15.6, we use the so-called 1.5-order formalism to build the twisted scalar symmetry generator for all fields except the spin connection and give a primitive twisted form of the supergravity action. In Section 15.7, we explore the consequences of requiring the invariance of the action under the twisted vector symmetry, which eventually yields the complete twisted supergravity action. In Section 15.8, we compute the coupling to twisted supergravity of the twisted Wess–Zumino and vector multiplets. Finally, appendices give useful formulas.

15.2 $\mathcal{N} = 1$, $d = 4$ supergravity in the new minimal scheme

The $\mathcal{N} = 1$, $d = 4$ supergravity multiplet in the new minimal system of auxiliary fields [3] is

$$e^a, \lambda, \omega^{ab}, A, B_2. \tag{15.1}$$

Here e^a is the 1-form vielbein, the Majorana spinor $\lambda = \lambda_\mu \, dx^\mu$ is the 1-form gravitino, and ω^{ab} is the spin-connection 1-form. A and B_2 are auxiliary fields, with gauge invariances, such that the multiplet has as many bosonic and fermionic degrees of freedom both on shell and off shell, modulo the gauge invariances. The abelian 1-form gauge field $A \sim A + dc$ gauges chirality and $B_2 \sim B_2 + d\Lambda_1$, $\Lambda_1 \sim \Lambda_1 + d\Lambda_0$ is a gauge real 2-form.

The associated curvatures are

$$R^{ab} = d\omega^{ab} + \tfrac{1}{2}\left[\omega, \omega\right]^{ab},$$

$$T^a = de^a + \omega^{ab}e_b + \tfrac{i}{2}\bar{\lambda}\gamma^a\lambda,$$

$$\rho = d\lambda + \left(\tfrac{1}{2}\omega^{ab}\gamma_{ab} + A\gamma^5\right)\lambda, \tag{15.2}$$

$$G_3 = dB_2 + \tfrac{i}{2}\bar{\lambda}\gamma^a\lambda e_a,$$

$$F = dA.$$

We will often use the covariant-derivative notation $D \equiv d + \omega + A$. We use the following expression for the $\mathcal{N} = 1$ supergravity action, as in [4]:

$$I = \int_{M_4} \left(\frac{1}{4}\epsilon_{abcd}e^a \wedge e^b \wedge R^{cd}(\omega) + i\bar{\lambda} \wedge \gamma^5\gamma^a\rho(\lambda,\omega,A)\wedge e_a - 2B_2 \wedge dA + {}^*G_3 \wedge G_3\right). \tag{15.3}$$

The multiplet (15.1) is an off-shell balanced multiplet with 6 bosonic degrees of freedom defined modulo all gauge invariances, 12 fermionic ones, and 6 auxiliary ones, according to the following count:

$$e^a : \quad 6 = 16 - 6 \text{ Lorentz} - 4 \text{ reparametrizations},$$

$$\lambda : \quad 12 = 16 - 4 \text{ supersymmetries},$$

$$A : \quad 3 = 4 - 1 \text{ chiral},$$

$$B_2 : \quad 3 = 6 - 4 \text{ vector} + 1 \text{ scalar}.$$

The spin connection is not an independent field, but is fixed by the (super)covariant constraint

$$T^a(e, \lambda) = -\tfrac{1}{2}G^a_{bc}e^b e^c, \tag{15.4}$$

so that $\omega^{ab} = \omega^{ab}(e, \lambda, B_2) \equiv \omega^{ab}(e, \lambda) + \tfrac{1}{2}G^{ab}_c e^c$, where $\omega^{ab}(e, \lambda)$ is the usual spin connection seen as a function of the vielbein and gravitino. This necessary constraint expresses the fact that no first-order formalism exists for getting an off-shell closed Poincaré supersymmetry and an invariant action.

The transformation laws of the various fields under supersymmetry can be expressed using a BRST symmetry operator s, where one replaces all parameters of supergravity infinitesimal transformations by local ghost fields with opposite statistics. All ghosts transform under the BRST symmetry, in such a way that s is nilpotent. The nilpotence of s is equivalent to the off-shell closure of the system of supergravity infinitesimal transformations, as shown in [4]. This BRST symmetry can be built directly (both in the minimal and new minimal set of auxiliary fields), as outlined below.

Call ξ^μ the vector ghost for reparametrization. The other ghosts are those of local SUSY (χ), Lorentz symmetry (Ω), the chiral $U(1)$ symmetry (c), and the 2-form gauge symmetry (B_1^1). The ξ^μ-dependent part of the supergravity BRST algebra decouples by redefining

$$\hat{s} = s - L_\xi, \quad \hat{d} = d + \hat{s} + i_\phi, \tag{15.5}$$

where the vector field ϕ is a bilinear in the supersymmetry ghost χ,

$$\phi^\mu = -\frac{i}{2}\bar{\chi}\gamma^\mu\chi = s\xi^\mu - \xi^\nu\partial_\nu\xi^\mu, \tag{15.6}$$

i_V is the interior derivative on the manifold for a given vector V, and L is the Lie derivative, $L_V = i_V d + d i_V$. One has the important property

$$\hat{d} = \exp(-i_\xi)(d + s)\exp(+i_\xi), \tag{15.7}$$

which ensures that $(d+s)^2 = 0$ and $\hat{d}^2 = 0$ are equivalent, and $s^2 = 0 \Leftrightarrow \hat{s}^2 = L_\phi$. The supergravity BRST transformations can be obtained by imposing constraints on the curvatures (15.2), in a way that merely generalizes the Yang–Mills case. Using ghost unification allows for a direct check of the off-shell closure by means of the Bianchi identities. In the end, one finds the following action of the BRST operator $\hat{s}$ on the fields:

$$\hat{s}e^a = -\Omega^{ab}e_b - i\bar{\chi}\gamma^a\lambda,$$

$$\hat{s}\lambda = -D\chi - \Omega^{ab}\gamma_{ab}\lambda - c\gamma^5\lambda,$$

$$\hat{s}B_2 = -dB_1^1 - i\bar{\chi}\gamma^a\lambda e_a, \tag{15.8}$$

$$\hat{s}A = -dc - \frac{1}{2}i\bar{\chi}\gamma^5\gamma^a X_a,$$

$$\hat{s}\omega^{ab} = -(D\Omega)^{ab} - i\bar{\chi}\gamma^{[a}X^{b]},$$

where the spinor X_a is

$$X_a = \rho_{ab}e^b - \left(\frac{1}{2}G_{abc}\gamma^{bc} + \frac{1}{12}\epsilon_{abcd}G^{bcd}\gamma^5\right)\lambda. \tag{15.9}$$

The ghost transformation laws can be found in Appendix 15.A. They are such that the closure relation $s^2 = 0 \Leftrightarrow \hat{s}^2 = L_\phi$ is satisfied. The way in which the BRST symmetry transforms the supersymmetry ghost will have nontrivial consequences in the twisted formulation.

By using the twist formulas of Majorana spinors as in [1, 5–9], one could analytically continue and twist by brute force these transformations in Euclidean space. We will rather try to obtain the twisted formulation in a more straightforward way, so as to unveil and better understand the mechanisms taking place in the twisted formalism. Therefore, we now proceed to our direct construction of the twisted superalgebra, keeping in mind that both untwisted and twisted formulations can be compared at any given stage.

As we will see, all of the information about supergravity is actually contained in the twisted scalar nilpotent generator that is hidden in the Poincaré supersymmetry algebra. To reach this result, we need to separate both the Einstein and Rarita–Schwinger Lagrangians into parts depending only on the self-dual or the anti-self-dual parts of the spin connection.

15.3 Self-dual decomposition of the supergravity action

Each of the Einstein and Rarita–Schwinger Lagrangians can be naturally split into two parts: one that depends only on the self-dual components of the spin-connection and another that depends only on the anti-self-dual ones. These two parts are equal modulo suitable boundary terms. In the case of the Einstein Lagrangian, this property has already been used for other types of twisting [9].

The Einstein Lagrangian can be written as[1]

$$L_E = \frac{1}{4}\epsilon_{abcd}e^a e^b R^{cd} = \frac{1}{2}e^a e^b \left(R^+_{ab} - R^-_{ab}\right). \tag{15.10}$$

Since the $SO(4)$ Lie algebra splits into two parts, the self-dual components of the curvature $R^{\pm ab} = d\omega^{\pm ab} + \omega^{\pm a}_c \omega^{\pm cb}$ depend only on the components of the spin connection $\omega^{\pm ab}$ with the same self-duality.

In supergravity, the torsion is often taken to be $T_a = De_a + \frac{i}{2}\bar\lambda\gamma_a\lambda$, but to establish the equality between the two parts of the Einstein Lagrangian, it is simpler to also use the purely bosonic torsion $t_a \equiv De_a$, which satisfies the Bianchi identity $Dt_a = R_{ab}e^b$. Indeed, contracting this identity with e^a, we have

$$e^a Dt_a = e^a e^b(R^+_{ab} + R^-_{ab}), \tag{15.11}$$

while

$$D(e^a t_a) = t^a t_a - e^a Dt_a. \tag{15.12}$$

We then get

$$L_E = -e^a e^b R^-_{ab} + \frac{1}{2}t^a t_a - \frac{1}{2}d(e^a t_a)$$

$$= -e^a e^b R^-_{ab} - \frac{i}{2}\bar\lambda\gamma^a\lambda T_a + \frac{1}{2}T^a T_a - \frac{1}{2}d\left(e^a T_a - \frac{i}{2}e^a\bar\lambda\gamma_a\lambda\right) \tag{15.13}$$

$$= +e^a e^b R^+_{ab} + \frac{i}{2}\bar\lambda\gamma^a\lambda T_a - \frac{1}{2}T^a T_a + \frac{1}{2}d\left(e^a T_a - \frac{i}{2}e^a\bar\lambda\gamma_a\lambda\right). \tag{15.14}$$

The second line is obtained by expressing t_a in terms of T_a, remembering that $\bar\lambda\gamma^a\lambda\bar\lambda\gamma_a\lambda = 0$ when λ is a Majorana spinor.

---

[1] Our conventions for (anti-)self-dual tensors are collected in Appendix 15.B.

Since T^a is constrained to be zero or a quantity independent of the spin connection, the expressions obtained for the Einstein action depend only on the anti-self-dual part ω^{-ab} (in the case of (15.13)) or the self-dual part ω^{+ab} (for (15.14)) of the spin connection.

An analogous property holds for the Rarita–Schwinger Lagrangian. We can derive it using the decomposition of the gravitino on its chiral components (which are not independent for a Majorana spinor). Defining $\lambda = \lambda^+ + \lambda^-$ with $\lambda^\pm = \frac{1}{2}(1 \pm i\gamma^5)\lambda$, we write[2]

$$L_{RS} = i\,\bar{\lambda}\gamma^5\gamma^a\rho e_a = \bar{\lambda}^+\gamma^a\rho^- e_a - \bar{\lambda}^-\gamma^a\rho^+ e_a, \qquad (15.15)$$

using $\bar{\lambda}^\pm\gamma^a\lambda^\pm = 0$.[3] By adding a suitable total divergence, we get

$$L_{RS} = 2\bar{\lambda}^+\gamma^a\rho^- e_a - \bar{\lambda}^-\gamma^a\lambda^+ T_a + d(\bar{\lambda}^-\gamma^a\lambda^+ e_a) \qquad (15.16)$$

With anticommuting Majorana fermions, we have the identity $\bar{X}^-\gamma_a Y^+ = -\bar{Y}^+\gamma_a X^-$. Since the chiral projections commute with the generators of Lorentz transformations on spinors, we simply have $\rho^- = D(\lambda^-)$. Chiral fermions give the minimal representations of the subalgebras associated with the self-dual and anti-self-dual parts of the rotation generators, so that ρ^- depends only on the anti-self-dual part of the spin connection ω^{-ab}:

$$\rho^- = \left(d + \tfrac{1}{2}\omega^{-ab}\gamma_{ab} + iA\right)\lambda^-. \qquad (15.17)$$

The Rarita–Schwinger action can therefore be written as

$$I_{RS} = i\int \bar{\lambda}\gamma^5\gamma^a D^{(\omega)}\lambda e_a = \int 2\bar{\lambda}^+\gamma^a D^{(\omega^-)}\lambda^- e_a - \bar{\lambda}^-\gamma^a\lambda^+ T_a. \qquad (15.18)$$

We have succeeded in expressing $I_E + I_{RS}$ in a way that depends only on either the self-dual or the anti-self-dual part of the spin connection, whenever the constraint on the torsion is independent of the spin connection. This condition is necessary for the closure of the supersymmetry algebra acting on the vielbein.

15.4 Twisted supergravity variables

In order to be able to twist the theory, we must work in a Euclidean space with an almost complex structure, i.e., a map on each tangent space $J(x)$ with $J^2 = -1$, or, more explicitly, $J^\mu_\rho(x) J^\rho_\nu(x) = -\delta^\mu_\nu$.

Introducing complex coordinates $z_m, \bar{z}_{\bar{m}}$, where $m = 1, 2$, we can locally reduce the complex structure to a diagonal one, $J_m{}^n = i\delta_m{}^n$, $J_{\bar{m}}{}^{\bar{n}} = -i\delta_{\bar{m}}{}^{\bar{n}}$. Making use of a compatible metric to lower one of the indices in J, J becomes an antisymmetric tensor with $J_{m\bar{n}}$ as the only nonvanishing components.

---

[2] See Appendix 15.B for the details of our chirality conventions.

[3] Care must be taken in Minkowski space, where the conjugation changes chirality, so that, for example, $\overline{\lambda^+} = \bar{\lambda}^-$.

The tensor $J_{m\bar{n}}$ can be used instead of the metric to lower and raise indices in the tangent space, according to $X^m = -iJ^{m\bar{n}}X_{\bar{n}}$ and $X^{\bar{m}} = iJ^{\bar{m}n}X_n$. In order to keep our formulas as uncluttered as possible, we will use a notation similar to Einstein's notation for contracting antiholomorphic and holomorphic $SU(2)$ indices by means of the complex structure constant tensor, as follows:

$$X^a Y_a = g^{ab} X_a Y_b = -iJ^{m\bar{n}}(X_m Y_{\bar{n}} + X_{\bar{n}} Y_m) \equiv X_m Y_{\bar{m}} - X_{\bar{m}} Y_m. \qquad (15.19)$$

The antisymmetry of the tensor $J_{m\bar{n}}$ implies that we must be careful about the ordering of indices. It explains the minus sign appearing in the last term of (15.19).

Twisting must be done in Euclidean space, where it is known that there are no Majorana spinors. We therefore forget the Majorana condition, the effect of which can be recovered afterwards from a careful consideration of the Wick rotation [10]. We associate with the spinor $(\lambda^\alpha, \lambda_{\dot\alpha})$ the following four quantities with only holomorphic or antiholomorphic indices:

$$(\Psi_m, \Psi_{\bar{m}\bar{n}}, \Psi_0). \qquad (15.20)$$

The indices m and $\bar{m}$ take two different values and the object $\Psi_{\bar{m}\bar{n}}$ is antisymmetric in its indices, so that it only has one nonzero component.

The twisted components of a spinor (15.20) are defined from the following linear mapping, which uses Pauli matrix elements [1, 5–9]:

$$\Psi_m = \lambda^\alpha (\sigma_m)_{\alpha\dot{1}},$$

$$\Psi_{\bar{m}\bar{n}} = \bar{\lambda}_{\dot\alpha}(\bar{\sigma}_{\bar{m}\bar{n}})^{\dot\alpha}{}_{\dot{2}}, \qquad (15.21)$$

$$\Psi_0 = \bar{\lambda}_{\dot\alpha}\delta^{\dot\alpha}_{\dot{2}}.$$

In Appendix 15.C, we give the expression of the twists of $\Gamma\lambda$ as functions of the twisted components of λ for some elements Γ of the Clifford algebra.

This construction reduces the tangent space $SO(4)$ symmetry to an $SU(2) \times U(1) \subset SO(4)$ symmetry. With this change of variables, $SO(4)$-invariant expressions can be related to their twisted counterparts, which generally split into a sum of independently $U(2)$-invariant terms. For instance, the Rarita–Schwinger Lagrangian can be decomposed as follows:

$$\bar{\lambda}\gamma^5\gamma^a \rho e_a = (\Psi_0 \rho_m + \Psi_m \rho_0)e_{\bar{m}} - (2\Psi_{\bar{m}\bar{n}}\rho_n - \Psi_n \rho_{\bar{m}\bar{n}})e_m. \qquad (15.22)$$

The commuting Majorana ghost of local supersymmetry χ is twisted as follows:

$$\chi \sim (\chi_m, \chi_{\bar{m}\bar{n}}, \chi_0), \qquad (15.23)$$

and the vector field in (15.6), $\phi^\mu = -\frac{1}{2}i\bar\chi\gamma^\mu\chi = s\xi^\mu - \xi^\nu\partial_\nu\xi^\mu$, is now given by

$$\phi_m = -\chi_m\chi_0, \quad \phi_{\bar m} = -\chi_{\bar m\bar n}\chi_n. \tag{15.24}$$

When the parameter of vector supersymmetry vanishes, $\chi_m = 0$, the vector field ϕ vanishes.[4]

A consistent interpretation of the twisted supersymmetry involves only fermionic global charges. Thus, in what follows, $\chi_m, \chi_{\bar m\bar n}, \chi_0$ will be treated as constant ghosts. We will build a set of corresponding generators $\delta_{\bar m}, \delta_{mn}, \delta$ that satisfy anticommutation relations that close independently of the equations of motion (off-shell closure), but possibly modulo bosonic gauge transformations. We will consider the operation

$$Q = \chi_m\delta_{\bar m} + \chi_{\bar m\bar n}\delta_{mn} + \chi_0\delta. \tag{15.25}$$

For a vanishing gravitino field, Q is nilpotent, off-shell, and modulo bosonic gauge transformations. It turns out that the global Q invariance is a sufficiently strong condition to determine the supergravity action. In fact, it gives a Ward identity that is sufficient to control the quantum perturbative behavior of the theory generated by the Q-invariant action, once all its gauge invariances are gauge-fixed in a BRST invariant way. When the gravitino field is not zero, the closure algebra is more involved. We will see that it involves supersymmetry transformations with gravitino-field-dependent structure coefficients.

In this construction, the supergravity action is, however, fully determined by the global supersymmetry operation Q. Local supersymmetry is warranted because of the systematic construction of the charges $\delta_{\bar m}$, δ_{mn}, δ in a way that is compatible with the Bianchi identities of all field curvatures.

The four generators $(\delta, \delta_{\bar m}, \delta_{mn})$ must act on all the twisted fields of the multiplet (15.1), with the following g-grading assignments:

field	grading	field	grading
e_m	0	A	0
$e_{\bar m}$	0	B_2	0
Ψ_m	1	ω_{mn}	0
Ψ_0	-1	$\omega_{\bar m\bar n}$	0
$\Psi_{\bar m\bar n}$	-1	$\omega_{m\bar n}$	0

generators	grading
δ	1
$\delta_{\bar m}$	-1
δ_{mn}	1

---

[4] This condition means that χ is a pure spinor, and it is not surprising that it entails great simplifications in the formalism, as in [11].

The commutation properties of the various fields are always obtained by computing the sum of the form degree and the grading g of fields (for instance, e_m is an anticommuting object since the form degree is 1 and $g = 0$; Ψ_m is a commuting object since the form degree is 1 and $g = 1$; etc.). After having obtained a classical action that is invariant under the twisted nilpotent global supersymmetry Q, one must in principle check that it remains invariant under local supersymmetry by giving a coordinate dependence to $(\chi_0, \chi_m, \chi_{\bar{m}\bar{n}})$. This is in fact automatically realized, since all derivatives will appear as supercovariantized ones.

If we now generalize $(\chi_0, \chi_m, \chi_{\bar{m}\bar{n}})$ into local commuting (twisted) Faddeev–Popov ghosts, we get the operator

$$\hat{s} = \chi_0(x)\delta + \chi_m(x)\delta_{\bar{m}} + \chi_{\bar{m}\bar{n}}(x)\delta_{mn}. \tag{15.26}$$

Its action on the classical fields is the same as that of the standard BRST transformations in twisted form.

In the flat-space $\mathcal{N} = 1$ super Yang–Mills theory [1], the three nilpotent symmetry generators δ and $\delta_{\bar{p}}$ satisfy the off-shell closure anticommutation relations $\delta^2 = 0$, $\{\delta_{\bar{p}}, \delta_{\bar{q}}\} = 0$, and $\{\delta, \delta_{\bar{p}}\} = \partial_{\bar{p}}$.

The situation is more complicated in supergravity. In this case, one indeed has the property $\hat{s}^2 = L_\phi$, where the vector field ϕ has been defined in (15.24). One also has the transformation law $\hat{s}\chi \sim i_\phi\Psi$ (see Appendix 15.A), which remains true even when the supersymmetry ghosts are assumed to be constant. This implies the following supergravity generalization:

$$\delta^2 = 0, \quad \{\delta_{\bar{p}}, \delta_{\bar{q}}\} = 0,$$

$$\{\delta, \delta_{\bar{p}}\} = L_{\bar{p}} - \sum_{a=0,m,\bar{m}\bar{n}} \Psi_{\bar{p},a}\delta_{\bar{a}}. \tag{15.27}$$

These anticommutation relations hold modulo bosonic gauge transformations. The derivative $L_{\bar{p}}$ is the Lie derivative along the vector field dual to the vielbein component $e_{\bar{p}}$. In fact, the supersymmetry generators that occur in the expression for $\{\delta, \delta_{\bar{p}}\}$ occur proportionally to the components $\Psi_{\bar{p},a}$ of the gravitino field $\Psi_a \equiv \Psi_{m,a}e_{\bar{m}} - \Psi_{\bar{m},a}e_m$. One thus recognizes the expected feature of supergravity: the anticommutator $\{\delta, \delta_{\bar{p}}\}$ closes on supersymmetry generators with field-dependent coefficients, proportionally to gravitino-field components. Therefore, the anticommutator $\{\delta, \delta_{\bar{q}}\}$ is expected to involve the fourth symmetry generator δ_{pq}, whose existence can be checked afterward in the twisted method.

Once δ and $\delta_{\bar{p}}$ have been determined, the δ- and $\delta_{\bar{p}}$-invariant action turns out to be automatically invariant under a δ_{pq} symmetry. In the four-dimensional supergravity, the relations between δ_{pq} and the other generators δ and $\delta_{\bar{p}}$ are satisfied off shell.

The fermionic scalar operator δ can be extended as a globally well-defined object (provided there is a complex structure). We will focus mainly on the question of its direct construction. In fact, $\delta_{\bar{p}}$ and δ_{pq} can only be given a geometrical interpretation on a coordinate patch.

15.5 The supergravity curvatures in the $U(2) \subset SO(4)$-invariant formalism

In Section 15.3, we have shown that both the Einstein and Rarita–Schwinger actions depend only on the self-dual or anti-self-dual components of the spin connection. In $SU(2) \subset SO(4)$ notation, the self-duality condition on an antisymmetric Lorentz tensor, $F_{ab} = \frac{1}{2}\epsilon_{abcd}F^{cd}$, reads

$$F_{\bar{m}\bar{n}} = F_{mn} = 0, \qquad F_{m\bar{m}} \equiv iJ^{m\bar{n}}F_{m\bar{n}} = 0, \tag{15.28}$$

while the anti-self-duality condition $F_{ab} = -\frac{1}{2}\epsilon_{abcd}F^{cd}$ reads

$$F_{m\bar{n}} - iJ_{m\bar{n}}F_{p\bar{p}} = 0. \tag{15.29}$$

Thus, the spin connection $\omega^{ab} = \omega^{+ab} + \omega^{-ab} \equiv (\omega_{mn}, \omega_{\bar{m}\bar{n}}, \omega_{m\bar{n}})$ splits into self-dual and anti-self-dual parts,

$$\begin{aligned}
\omega^{+ab} &\sim (0, 0, \omega_{m\bar{n}} - iJ_{m\bar{n}}\omega), \\
\omega^{-ab} &\sim (\omega_{mn}, \omega_{\bar{m}\bar{n}}, iJ_{m\bar{n}}\omega),
\end{aligned} \tag{15.30}$$

respectively, where $\omega \equiv iJ_{\bar{m}n}\omega_{m\bar{n}}$.

The $SO(4)$ Lie algebra is the product of two $SU(2)$ corresponding to the self-dual and anti-self-dual generators. Therefore, the anti-self-dual part of the curvature 2-form $R^- \sim (R_{mn}, R_{\bar{m}\bar{n}}, R)$ and its Bianchi identities depend only on the anti-self-dual part of the connection ω^{-ab}:

$$\begin{aligned}
R &= d\omega + 2\omega_{mn}\omega_{\bar{m}\bar{n}}, \\
R_{mn} &= d\omega_{mn} - \omega\omega_{mn}, \\
R_{\bar{m}\bar{n}} &= d\omega_{\bar{m}\bar{n}} + \omega\omega_{\bar{m}\bar{n}}, \\
dR &= 2R_{mn}\omega_{\bar{m}\bar{n}} - 2\omega_{mn}R_{\bar{m}\bar{n}}, \\
dR_{mn} &= R_{mn}\omega - R\omega_{mn}, \\
dR_{\bar{m}\bar{n}} &= R\omega_{\bar{m}\bar{n}} - R_{\bar{m}\bar{n}}\omega.
\end{aligned} \tag{15.31}$$

The $SO(4)$ symmetry acts only as this $SU(2)$ on Ψ_0 and $\Psi_{\bar{m}\bar{n}}$, owing to chirality properties. We can thus define the $SU(2)$-covariant curvatures for Ψ_0 and $\Psi_{\bar{m}\bar{n}}$:

$$\begin{aligned}
\rho_0 &= d\Psi_0 - \left(\frac{1}{2}\omega - A\right)\Psi_0 + \omega_{mn}\Psi_{\bar{m}\bar{n}}, \\
\rho_{\bar{m}\bar{n}} &= d\Psi_{\bar{m}\bar{n}} + \left(\frac{1}{2}\omega + A\right)\Psi_{\bar{m}\bar{n}} - \omega_{\bar{m}\bar{n}}\Psi_0.
\end{aligned} \tag{15.32}$$

Their Bianchi identities are

$$\begin{aligned}
D\rho_0 &= \left(-\frac{1}{2}R + F\right)\Psi_0 + R_{mn}\Psi_{\bar{m}\bar{n}}, \\
D\rho_{\bar{m}\bar{n}} &= \left(\frac{1}{2}R + F\right)\Psi_{\bar{m}\bar{n}} - R_{\bar{m}\bar{n}}\Psi_0.
\end{aligned} \tag{15.33}$$

The curvature ρ_m of Ψ_m involves only the self-dual part of the spin connection. We can skip its definition, since it is not needed in the supergravity action.

The torsion involves both self-dual and anti-self-dual components of the spin connection:

$$
\begin{aligned}
T_m &= de_m + \omega_{mn}e_{\bar{n}} - \omega_{m\bar{n}}e_n + \Psi_m\Psi_0, \\
T_{\bar{m}} &= de_{\bar{m}} + \omega_{\bar{m}n}e_{\bar{n}} - \omega_{\bar{m}\bar{n}}e_n + \Psi_{\bar{m}\bar{n}}\Psi_n,
\end{aligned}
\tag{15.34}
$$

$$
\begin{aligned}
DT_m &= R_{mn}e_{\bar{n}} - R_{m\bar{n}}e_n + \rho_m\Psi_0 - \Psi_m\rho_0, \\
DT_{\bar{m}} &= R_{\bar{m}n}e_{\bar{n}} - R_{\bar{m}\bar{n}}e_n + \rho_{\bar{m}\bar{n}}\Psi_n - \Psi_{\bar{m}\bar{n}}\rho_n.
\end{aligned}
\tag{15.35}
$$

We now use the $SU(2)$ notation to decompose the Einstein and Rarita–Schwinger Lagrangians as sums of terms that are separately $SU(2)$-invariant, using the expressions (15.13) and (15.18):

$$
I_E = \int -\Big(Re_me_{\bar{m}} + R_{mn}e_{\bar{m}}e_{\bar{n}} + R_{\bar{m}\bar{n}}e_me_n\Big) - \Big(\Psi_m\Psi_0T_{\bar{m}} - \Psi_{\bar{m}\bar{n}}\Psi_nT_m\Big) + T_mT_{\bar{m}},
\tag{15.36}
$$

$$
I_{RS} = \int -\Big(2\rho_{\bar{m}\bar{n}}\Psi_ne_m - 2\rho_0\Psi_me_{\bar{m}}\Big) + \Big(\Psi_m\Psi_0T_{\bar{m}} - \Psi_{\bar{m}\bar{n}}\Psi_nT_m\Big).
\tag{15.37}
$$

Equations (15.36) and (15.37) are interesting. However, at first sight, they are not yet very suggestive about the existence of a twisted scalar supersymmetry.

In fact, to build the scalar supersymmetry, we depart from the method used in [4]. The so-called 1.5-order formalism, once it has been adapted to the twisted fields of supergravity, will neatly separate the various terms of the invariant actions (15.36) and (15.37).

15.6 The 1.5-order formalism with $SU(2)$-covariant curvatures

The justification for the 1.5-order formalism for supergravity is detailed in [12]. One first builds a supersymmetry that acts on all fields except the spin connection ω. The later is taken not to transform under supersymmetry in a first step.

The second-order formalism transformation law of ω is the one compatible with all Bianchi identities of the theory, including that of the Riemann curvature.

In the 1.5-order formalism, it is particularly simple to obtain the twisted scalar supersymmetry on all fields but the spin connection, by imposing consistent constraints on the ghost-dependent curvatures.

The ghost-dependent curvatures are obtained by the substitutions

$$
d \to \hat{d} = d + \chi_0\delta_{1.5} + i_\phi, \quad \Psi \to \hat{\Psi} = \Psi + \chi.
\tag{15.38}
$$

We are concerned only with the scalar supersymmetry for the moment. Thus, we only retain a constant χ_0 as the only nonvanishing component in χ. Since $\chi_m = 0$, we have $\phi_m = \phi_{\bar{m}} = 0$ and $\hat{d} = d + \chi_0 \delta_{1.5}$. The property $\hat{d}^2 = 0$ implies $\delta_{1.5}^2 = 0$ on all fields. The 1.5-order formalism constraints that are compatible with the Bianchi identities are

$$\hat{R} = R, \quad \hat{R}_{mn} = R_{mn}, \quad \hat{R}_{\bar{m}\bar{n}} = R_{\bar{m}\bar{n}}, \quad \hat{F} = F,$$
$$\hat{\rho}_0 = \rho_0, \quad \hat{\rho}_{\bar{m}\bar{n}} = \rho_{\bar{m}\bar{n}}, \quad \hat{\rho}_m = \rho_m, \tag{15.39}$$
$$\hat{G}_3 = G_3, \quad \hat{T}_m = T_m, \quad \hat{T}_{\bar{m}} = T_{\bar{m}},$$

where G_3 is the field strength of the 2-form B_2, defined in twisted form as

$$\hat{G}_3 = \hat{d}B_2 + \hat{\Psi}_m \hat{\Psi}_0 e_{\bar{m}} - \hat{\Psi}_{\bar{m}\bar{n}} \hat{\Psi}_n e_m. \tag{15.40}$$

We now use (15.38) and pick up the term with ghost number 1 in (15.39). This gives the $\delta_{1.5}$ transformation laws for all fields:

	$\delta_{1.5}$
e_m	$-\Psi_m$
$e_{\bar{m}}$	0
Ψ_m	0
Ψ_0	$\frac{1}{2}\omega - A$
$\Psi_{\bar{m}\bar{n}}$	$\omega_{\bar{m}\bar{n}}$
ω_{mn}	0
$\omega_{\bar{m}\bar{n}}$	0
ω	0
A	0
B_2	$-\Psi_m e_{\bar{m}}$

$$\tag{15.41}$$

The curvatures transform as

$$\delta_{1.5}R = 0, \qquad \delta_{1.5}R_{mn} = 0, \qquad \delta_{1.5}R_{\bar{m}\bar{n}} = 0, \qquad \delta_{1.5}F = 0,$$
$$\delta_{1.5}\rho_0 = -\frac{1}{2}R + F, \qquad \delta_{1.5}\rho_{\bar{m}\bar{n}} = -R_{\bar{m}\bar{n}}, \qquad \delta_{1.5}\rho_m = 0. \tag{15.42}$$

We can therefore build three $\delta_{1.5}$-invariant Lagrangians that respectively contain the three independent $SU(2)$-invariant pieces $R e_m e_{\bar{m}}$, $R_{mn} e_{\bar{m}} e_{\bar{n}}$, and $R_{\bar{m}\bar{n}} e_m e_n$ of the Einstein Lagrangian:

$$R_{mn} e_{\bar{m}} e_{\bar{n}},$$
$$R_{\bar{m}\bar{n}} e_m e_n + 2\rho_{\bar{m}\bar{n}} \Psi_n e_m, \tag{15.43}$$
$$R e_m e_{\bar{m}} - 2\rho_0 \Psi_m e_{\bar{m}} - 2F B_2.$$

The action

$$I = \int \alpha R_{mn} e_{\bar{m}} e_{\bar{n}} + \beta(R_{\bar{m}\bar{n}} e_m e_n + 2\rho_{\bar{m}\bar{n}} \Psi_n e_m) + \gamma(R e_m e_{\bar{m}} - 2\rho_0 \Psi_m e_{\bar{m}} - 2F B_2) \tag{15.44}$$

is thus invariant under the transformations (15.41), for all possible values of the coefficients α, β, and γ. Lorentz symmetry is obtained when $\alpha = \beta = \gamma$.

Alternatively, in a method that is closer to the we used in [4], we can directly check the invariance of the action (15.44) by computing the following quantities, using the Bianchi identities for the curvatures:

$$\hat{D}(\hat{R}_{mn}\hat{e}_{\bar{m}}\hat{e}_{\bar{n}}) = 2\hat{R}_{mn}(\hat{T}_{\bar{m}} - \hat{\Psi}_{\bar{m}\bar{p}}\hat{\Psi}_{p})\hat{e}_{\bar{n}},$$

$$\hat{D}(\hat{R}_{\bar{m}\bar{n}}\hat{e}_{m}\hat{e}_{n}) = 2\hat{R}_{\bar{m}\bar{n}}(\hat{T}_{m} - \hat{\Psi}_{m}\hat{\Psi}_{0})\hat{e}_{n},$$

$$\hat{D}(\hat{R}\hat{e}_{m}\hat{e}_{\bar{m}}) = \hat{R}(\hat{T}_{m} - \hat{\Psi}_{m}\hat{\Psi}_{0})e_{\bar{m}} - \hat{R}\hat{e}_{m}(\hat{T}_{\bar{m}} - \hat{\Psi}_{\bar{m}\bar{p}}\hat{\Psi}_{p}), \tag{15.45}$$

$$\hat{D}(\hat{\rho}_{\bar{m}\bar{n}}\hat{\Psi}_{n}\hat{e}_{m}) = \left[\left(\frac{1}{2}\hat{R} + \hat{F}\right)\hat{\Psi}_{\bar{m}\bar{n}} - \hat{R}_{\bar{m}\bar{n}}\hat{\Psi}_{0}\right]\hat{\Psi}_{n}\hat{e}_{m} + \hat{\rho}_{\bar{m}\bar{n}}\hat{\rho}_{n}\hat{e}_{m}$$
$$-\hat{\rho}_{\bar{m}\bar{n}}\hat{\Psi}_{n}(\hat{T}_{m} - \hat{\Psi}_{m}\hat{\Psi}_{0}),$$

$$\hat{D}(\hat{\rho}_{0}\hat{\Psi}_{m}\hat{e}_{\bar{m}}) = \left[\left(-\frac{1}{2}\hat{R} + \hat{F}\right)\hat{\Psi}_{0} + \hat{R}_{pq}\hat{\Psi}_{\bar{p}\bar{q}}\right]\hat{\Psi}_{m}\hat{e}_{\bar{m}} + \hat{\rho}_{0}\hat{\rho}_{m}\hat{e}_{\bar{m}} - \hat{\rho}_{0}\hat{\Psi}_{m}(\hat{T}_{\bar{m}} - \hat{\Psi}_{\bar{m}\bar{p}}\hat{\Psi}_{p}),$$

$$\hat{D}(\hat{F}\hat{B}_{2}) = \hat{F}(\hat{G}_{3} - \hat{\Psi}_{m}\hat{\Psi}_{0}\hat{e}_{\bar{m}} + \hat{\Psi}_{\bar{m}\bar{n}}\hat{\Psi}_{n}\hat{e}_{m}).$$

Taking the part with ghost number 1 of these equations and retaining only $\chi_0 \neq 0$, we obtain the $\delta_{1.5}$ transformations of the various terms in the action:

$$\delta_{1.5}(R_{mn}e_{\bar{m}}e_{\bar{n}}) = 0,$$

$$\delta_{1.5}(R_{\bar{m}\bar{n}}e_{m}e_{n}) = -2R_{\bar{m}\bar{n}}\Psi_{m}e_{n},$$

$$\delta_{1.5}(Re_{m}e_{\bar{m}}) = -R\Psi_{m}e_{\bar{m}}, \tag{15.46}$$

$$\delta_{1.5}(\rho_{\bar{m}\bar{n}}\Psi_{n}e_{m}) = -R_{\bar{m}\bar{n}}\Psi_{n}e_{m},$$

$$\delta_{1.5}(\rho_{0}\Psi_{m}e_{\bar{m}}) = \left(-\tfrac{1}{2}R + F\right)\Psi_{m}e_{\bar{m}},$$

$$\delta_{1.5}(FB_{2}) = -F\Psi_{m}e_{\bar{m}},$$

which ensure that $\delta_{1.5}(I) = 0$.

The formulas (15.45) are actually quite useful to directly compute the action of the vector supersymmetry $\delta_{\bar{p}}^{1.5}$, by generalizing to the case where $\chi_p \neq 0$. Using a ghost expansion as for the scalar symmetry, we get

$$\delta_{\bar{p}}^{1.5}(R_{mn}e_{\bar{m}}e_{\bar{n}}) = 2R_{mn}\Psi_{\bar{m}\bar{p}}e_{\bar{n}},$$

$$\delta_{\bar{p}}^{1.5}(R_{\bar{m}\bar{n}}e_{m}e_{n}) = 2R_{\bar{p}\bar{n}}\Psi_{0}e_{n},$$

$$\delta_{\bar{p}}^{1.5}(Re_{m}e_{\bar{m}}) = -R\Psi_{0}e_{\bar{p}} + Re_{m}\Psi_{\bar{m}\bar{p}}, \tag{15.47}$$

$$\delta_{\bar{p}}^{1.5}((\rho_{\bar{m}\bar{n}}\Psi_{n}e_{m}) = \left[-\left(\frac{1}{2}R + F\right)\Psi_{\bar{m}\bar{p}} + R_{\bar{m}\bar{p}}\Psi_{0}\right]e_{m},$$

$$\delta_{\bar{p}}^{1.5}(\rho_{0}\Psi_{m}e_{\bar{m}}) = \left[\left(-\frac{1}{2}R + F\right)\Psi_{0} + R_{mn}\Psi_{\bar{m}\bar{n}}\right]e_{\bar{p}},$$

$$\delta_{\bar{p}}^{1.5}(FB_{2}) = -F(\Psi_{0}e_{\bar{p}} + \Psi_{\bar{m}\bar{p}}e_{m}).$$

We find that $\delta_{\bar{p}}^{1.5}$ is another symmetry of the complete action, provided that $\alpha = \beta = \gamma$, in which case the $SU(2)$ symmetry is enlarged to $SO(4)$.

However, we must be careful in the interpretation of this vector symmetry, since it cannot be obtained by twisting the supersymmetry generators $(Q^\alpha, Q_{\dot\alpha})$. Indeed, $\delta_{1.5}$ and $\delta_{\bar{p}}^{1.5}$ do not have the right anticommutation relations, since $\{\delta_{1.5}, \sigma_{\bar{p}}^{1.5}\}\Psi = 0$, in contradiction with the twisted supersymmetry algebra (15.27). In fact the 1.5-order formalism, which is useful to determine the invariant action, does not properly define the supersymmetry generators. We must determine the ω transformations consistent with the constraints, which appear as equations of motion in the 1.5-order formalism.

With the invariant action (15.44), the equations of motion of the anti-self-dual spin connection give $12 = 3 \times 4$ equations that can be solved algebraically to determine the 12 components of the three 1-forms ω_{mn}, $\omega_{\bar{m}\bar{n}}$, and ω, as functions of e and Ψ. The precise values then depend on the parameters α, β, and γ.

We can then compute the $\delta_{1.5}$ transformations of these functions through the chain rule to obtain the transformations of ω_{mn}, $\omega_{\bar{m}\bar{n}}$, and ω. Since $\delta_{1.5}$ is nilpotent on e and Ψ, this procedure gives a nilpotent transformation in the second-order formalism, where $\omega_{mn}, \omega_{\bar{m}\bar{n}}$, and ω are not independent fields.

The case of interest is for the rotationally invariant action (15.44), which has $\alpha = \beta = \gamma$. In this case, the spin-connection equations of motion give

$$\frac{\delta}{\delta\omega}I(e, \Psi, B_2, \omega) = e_m T_{\bar{m}}^{(\omega^-)} = 0,$$

$$\frac{\delta}{\delta\omega_{mn}}I(e, \Psi, B_2, \omega) = e_{[\bar{m}} T_{\bar{n}]}^{(\omega^-)} = 0, \qquad (15.48)$$

$$\frac{\delta}{\delta\omega_{\bar{m}\bar{n}}}I(e, \Psi, B_2, \omega) = e_{[m} T_{n]}^{(\omega^-)} = 0.$$

Here $T^{(\omega^-)}$ is a function only of ω^-:

$$T_m^{(\omega^-)} = de_m + \omega_{mn}e_{\bar{n}} + \Psi_m \Psi_0,$$

$$T_{\bar{m}}^{(\omega^-)} = de_{\bar{m}} - \omega_{\bar{m}\bar{n}}e_n + \Psi_{\bar{m}\bar{n}}\Psi_n.$$

These 12 equations fix the 12 components of the anti-self-dual part of the spin connection, $\omega = \omega(e, \Psi)$, $\omega_{mn} = \omega_{mn}(e, \Psi)$, and $\omega_{\bar{m}\bar{n}} = \omega_{\bar{m}\bar{n}}(e, \Psi)$, as functions of the vielbein and the twisted gravitino. These components are the anti-self-dual parts of the complete spin connection that satisfy the constraint $T_m = T_{\bar{m}} = 0$,

As a consequence of the chain rule, $\omega(e, \Psi)$, $\omega_{mn}(e, \Psi)$, and $\omega_{\bar{m}\bar{n}}(e, \Psi)$ transform under supersymmetry, and the 1.5-order formalism guarantees that

$$I = -\int R_{mn}e_{\bar{m}}e_{\bar{n}} + (R_{\bar{m}\bar{n}}e_m e_n + 2\rho_{\bar{m}\bar{n}}\Psi_n e_m) + (Re_m e_{\bar{m}} - 2\rho_0\Psi_m e_{\bar{m}} - 2FB_2) \quad (15.49)$$

is still supersymmetric.

To avoid the heavy calculations from the chain rule, we can use the formalism used in [4] and determine modified horizontality conditions for the field strengths $\hat{R}$

and $\hat{F}$ at ghost numbers 1 and 2, such that the Bianchi identities are satisfied and the constraints are invariant. The invariance of the constraints is equivalent to the satisfaction of the chain rule. We define

$$\hat{R} = R + R^{(1)} + R^{(2)}, \tag{15.50}$$
$$\hat{F} = F + F^{(1)} + F^{(2)}, \tag{15.51}$$

while keeping

$$\hat{T} = T,$$
$$\hat{\rho} = \rho, \tag{15.52}$$
$$\hat{G}_3 = G_3.$$

The ghost-number-2 part of the Bianchi identity on the torsion $\hat{T}$ ensures that when $\chi_m = 0$, $R^{(2)} = F^{(2)} = 0$. The condition $\hat{G}_3 = G_3$ implies $\delta B_2 = -\Psi_m e_{\bar{m}}$, and

$$\hat{\rho}_0 = (d+s)\hat{\Psi}_0 - \left(\frac{1}{2}\hat{\omega} - \hat{A}\right)\hat{\Psi}_0 + \hat{\omega}_{mn}\hat{\Psi}_{\bar{m}\bar{n}} = \rho_0,$$
$$\hat{\rho}_{\bar{m}\bar{n}} = (d+s)\hat{\Psi}_{\bar{m}\bar{n}} + \left(\frac{1}{2}\hat{\omega} + \hat{A}\right)\hat{\Psi}_{\bar{m}\bar{n}} - \hat{\omega}_{\bar{m}\bar{n}}\hat{\Psi}_0 = \rho_{\bar{m}\bar{n}}, \tag{15.53}$$

together with their respective Bianchi identities, imply

$$R^{(1)} = 2F^{(1)},$$
$$R^{(1)}_{\bar{m}\bar{n}} = 0. \tag{15.54}$$

Finally, the part with ghost number 1 of the Bianchi identity on $\hat{T}$, (15.34), implies

$$R^{(1)}_{mn} = -\frac{1}{2}\left(\rho_{p[n,m]}e_{\bar{p}} + \rho_{\bar{p}[n,m]}e_p\right),$$
$$R^{(1)} = \left(\rho_{\bar{p}\bar{m},m}e_p + \rho_{p\bar{m},m}e_{\bar{p}}\right). \tag{15.55}$$

These values of R^1 and F^1 determine the transformation laws of ω and A, so that the second-order scalar supersymmetry transformations that leave invariant the action (15.49) are

	1δ (with $\delta^2 = 0$)
e_m	$-\Psi_m$
$e_{\bar{m}}$	0
Ψ_m	0
Ψ_0	$\frac{1}{2}\omega - A$
$\Psi_{\bar{m}\bar{n}}$	$\omega_{\bar{m}\bar{n}}$
ω_{mn}	$-\frac{1}{2}\left(\rho_{p[n,m]}e_{\bar{p}} + \rho_{\bar{p}[n,m]}e_p\right)$
$\omega_{\bar{m}\bar{n}}$	0
ω	$\rho_{\bar{p}\bar{m},m}e_p + \rho_{p\bar{m},m}e_{\bar{p}}$
A	$\frac{1}{2}\left(\rho_{\bar{p}\bar{m},m}e_p + \rho_{p\bar{m},m}e_{\bar{p}}\right)$
B_2	$-\Psi_m e_{\bar{m}}$

$$\tag{15.56}$$

We have used a notation where ρ_{mn}, $\rho_{\bar{m}\bar{n}}$, and $\rho_{m\bar{n}}$ are the components of the 2-form ρ on the vielbein basis, i.e., $\rho = \frac{1}{2}\left(\rho_{mn}e_{\bar{m}}e_{\bar{n}} + \rho_{\bar{m}\bar{n}}e_m e_n + \rho_{m\bar{n}}e_m e_{\bar{n}}\right)$. The indices to the right of the comma refer to the twisted spinor indices 0, m or $\bar{m}\bar{n}$.

15.7   Vector supersymmetry and nonvanishing torsion

There is no vector supersymmetry $\delta_{\bar{p}}$ for the action (15.49) that can satisfy the off-shell closure relation $\{\delta, \delta_{\bar{p}}\} = L_{\bar{p}} - \Psi_{\bar{p},a}\delta_{\bar{a}}$. Indeed, suppose that such a symmetry existed. The off-shell closure means $\hat{d}^2 = (d + \chi_0\delta + \chi_p\delta_{\bar{p}} + i_\phi)^2 = 0$, with $\phi_m = -\chi_m\chi_0 \neq 0$. Thus, the Bianchi identity,

$$\hat{d}G_3 = -\hat{\Psi}_m\hat{\rho}_0\hat{e}_{\bar{m}} + \hat{\rho}_m\hat{\Psi}_0\hat{e}_{\bar{m}} + \hat{\Psi}_m\hat{\Psi}_0\hat{T}_{\bar{m}} - \hat{\rho}_{\bar{m}\bar{n}}\hat{\Psi}_n\hat{e}_m + \hat{\Psi}_{\bar{m}\bar{n}}\hat{\rho}_n\hat{e}_m - \hat{\Psi}_{\bar{m}\bar{n}}\hat{\Psi}_n\hat{T}_m, \quad (15.57)$$

has a nontrivial ghost-number-2 part, which is

$$i_\phi G_3 = \chi_m\chi_0 T_{\bar{m}}. \quad (15.58)$$

Therefore, the torsion cannot be taken identically equal to zero, which implies that the Lagrangian found in Section 15.6 must be modified by terms that have an off-shell relevance. To remain in the context of a Lorentz-invariant action, we use the following constraints on the torsion, which generalize (15.58):

$$T_m = de_m + \omega_{mn}e_{\bar{n}} - \omega_{m\bar{n}}e_n + \Psi_m\Psi_0 = \frac{1}{2}\left(G_{m\bar{p}\bar{q}}e_p e_q - G_{mp\bar{q}}e_{\bar{p}}e_q\right),$$
$$T_{\bar{m}} = de_{\bar{m}} + \omega_{\bar{m}n}e_{\bar{n}} - \omega_{\bar{m}\bar{n}}e_n + \Psi_{\bar{m}\bar{n}}\Psi_n = \frac{1}{2}\left(G_{\bar{m}pq}e_{\bar{p}}e_{\bar{q}} - G_{\bar{m}\bar{p}q}e_p e_{\bar{q}}\right). \quad (15.59)$$

The value of the spin connection is therefore changed, and the distortion on the horizontality condition (15.50) becomes

$$R^{(1)}_{mn} = -\frac{1}{2}\left(\rho_{p[n,m]}e_{\bar{p}} + \rho_{\bar{p}[n,m]}e_p + G_{mn\bar{p}}\Psi_p\right),$$
$$R^{(1)} = \rho_{\bar{p}\bar{m},m}e_p + \rho_{p\bar{m},m}e_{\bar{p}} + G_{m\bar{p}\bar{m}}\Psi_p. \quad (15.60)$$

The scalar supersymmetry transformations are now

<table>
<tr><td></td><td>δ (with $\delta^2 = 0$)</td></tr>
<tr><td>e_m</td><td>$-\Psi_m$</td></tr>
<tr><td>$e_{\bar{m}}$</td><td>0</td></tr>
<tr><td>Ψ_m</td><td>0</td></tr>
<tr><td>Ψ_0</td><td>$\frac{1}{2}\omega - A$</td></tr>
<tr><td>$\Psi_{\bar{m}\bar{n}}$</td><td>$\omega_{\bar{m}\bar{n}}$</td></tr>
<tr><td>ω_{mn}</td><td>$-\frac{1}{2}\left(\rho_{p[n,m]}e_{\bar{p}} + \rho_{\bar{p}[n,m]}e_p + G_{mn\bar{p}}\Psi_p\right)$</td></tr>
<tr><td>$\omega_{\bar{m}\bar{n}}$</td><td>0</td></tr>
<tr><td>ω</td><td>$\rho_{\bar{p}\bar{m},m}e_p + \rho_{p\bar{m},m}e_{\bar{p}} + G_{m\bar{p}\bar{m}}\Psi_p$</td></tr>
<tr><td>A</td><td>$\frac{1}{2}\left(\rho_{\bar{p}\bar{m},m}e_p + \rho_{p\bar{m},m}e_{\bar{p}} + G_{m\bar{p}\bar{m}}\Psi_p\right)$</td></tr>
<tr><td>B_2</td><td>$-\Psi_m e_{\bar{m}}$</td></tr>
</table>

$$(15.61)$$

With $T \neq 0$, the variation of the action found in Section 15.6 involves new terms proportional to $T\delta\omega$, with must be compensated by the variation of new terms quadratic in G.

We have

$$\delta G_{mp\bar{q}} = \rho_{\bar{q}p,m} - G_{mp\bar{r}}\Psi_{\bar{q},r} - 2G_{m\bar{r}\bar{q}}\Psi_{p,r},$$

$$\delta G_{mp\bar{q}} = \rho_{\bar{p}\bar{q},m} - 2G_{m\bar{r}\bar{q}}\Psi_{\bar{p},r}, \tag{15.62}$$

$$\delta e = -\frac{1}{2}\epsilon_{\bar{p}\bar{n}rs}\Psi_{p}e_{n}e_{\bar{r}}e_{\bar{s}},$$

$$\delta(^{*}G_{3}G_{3}) = -eG_{\bar{m}pq}\left(G_{r\bar{p}\bar{q}}\Psi_{\bar{r},m} + 2G_{m\bar{r}\bar{q}}\Psi_{\bar{p},r}\right) \tag{15.63}$$

Here $^{*}G_{3}$ denotes the Hodge dual of G_{3} and e is the volume form built from $(e_{m}, e_{\bar{m}})$.

From the relation (15.58) between the torsion and the 3-form G_{3}, we have

$$T_{m}T_{\bar{m}} + {}^{*}G_{3}G_{3} = -\frac{1}{4}\left(G_{m\bar{p}\bar{q}}G_{\bar{m}\bar{r}s}e_{p}e_{q}e_{r}e_{\bar{s}} + G_{mp\bar{q}}G_{\bar{m}rs}e_{\bar{p}}e_{q}e_{\bar{r}}e_{\bar{s}}\right). \tag{15.64}$$

We thus add the term $T_{m}T_{\bar{m}} + {}^{*}G_{3}G_{3}$ to the action (15.49), which cancels the effect of the variations of the spin connection given in (15.61) under the δ symmetry. The resulting invariant action is

$$I_{\text{tot}} = -\int R_{mn}e_{\bar{m}}e_{\bar{n}} + (R_{\bar{m}\bar{n}}e_{m}e_{n} + 2\rho_{\bar{m}\bar{n}}\Psi_{n}e_{m}) + (Re_{m}e_{\bar{m}} - 2\rho_{0}\Psi_{m}e_{\bar{m}} - 2FB_{2})$$

$$-T_{m}T_{\bar{m}} - {}^{*}G_{3}G_{3}. \tag{15.65}$$

Using (15.36) and (15.37), this action can be written as

$$I_{\text{tot}} = \int L_{E} + L_{RS} + 2FB_{2} + {}^{*}G_{3}G_{3} \tag{15.66}$$

This is nothing more that the complete supergravity action of (15.3).

This action is also invariant under $\delta_{\bar{p}}$ and δ_{pq}, since it is equivalent to the one determined to be invariant under the complete untwisted BRST symmetry operator in [4]. The transformations under all twisted supersymmetry generators of the fields are

	δ	$\delta_{\bar{p}}$	δ_{pq}
e_{m}	$-\Psi_{m}$	$iJ_{m\bar{p}}\Psi_{0}$	0
$e_{\bar{m}}$	0	$\Psi_{\bar{p}\bar{m}}$	$-2iJ_{\bar{m}[p}\Psi_{q]}$
Ψ_{m}	0	$iJ_{\bar{p}m}\left(\frac{1}{2}\omega - A\right) + \omega_{\bar{p}m}$	0
Ψ_{0}	$\frac{1}{2}\omega - A$	0	$-\omega_{pq}$
$\Psi_{\bar{m}\bar{n}}$	$\omega_{\bar{m}\bar{n}}$	0	$2J_{\bar{m}[p\|}J_{\bar{n}\|q]}\left(\frac{1}{2}\omega + A\right)$
ω_{mn}	$X_{[m,n]}$	$-\frac{1}{2}iJ_{m\bar{p}}\left(\rho_{\bar{q}n,0}e_{q} + \rho_{qn,0}e_{\bar{q}}\right) - \frac{1}{2}G_{mn\bar{p}}\Psi_{0}$	0
$\omega_{\bar{m}\bar{n}}$	0	$-\frac{1}{2}\left(\rho_{\bar{q}\bar{n},\bar{m}\bar{p}}e_{q} + \rho_{q\bar{n},\bar{m}\bar{p}}e_{\bar{q}} + G_{\bar{m}\bar{n}q}\Psi_{\bar{p}\bar{q}}\right)$	$-iJ_{\bar{m}[p}X_{\bar{n},\|q]}$
$\omega_{m\bar{n}}$	$2X_{m,\bar{n}}$	$\frac{1}{2}iJ_{m\bar{p}}\left(\rho_{\bar{q}\bar{n},0}e_{q} + \rho_{q\bar{n},0}e_{\bar{q}}\right) + \frac{1}{2}\left(G_{m\bar{p}\bar{n}}\Psi_{0} - G_{mq\bar{n}}\Psi_{\bar{p}\bar{q}}\right)$	0
A	$X_{m,\bar{m}}$	$\frac{1}{2}\left(\rho_{\bar{q}\bar{p},0}e_{q} + \rho_{q\bar{p},0}e_{\bar{q}} - G_{m\bar{p}\bar{m}}\Psi_{0} + G_{mq\bar{m}}\Psi_{\bar{p}\bar{q}}\right)$	$X_{p,q}$
B_{2}	$-\Psi_{m}e_{\bar{m}}$	$-\Psi_{0}e_{\bar{p}} - \Psi_{\bar{p}\bar{m}}e_{m}$	$-2\Psi_{[p}e_{q]}$

with the twisted X spinor in (15.9) defined as

$$X_{m,n} = -\frac{1}{2}\left(\rho_{pn,m}e_{\bar{p}} + \rho_{\bar{p}n,m}e_p + G_{mn\bar{p}}\Psi_p\right). \tag{15.67}$$

Since these transformations are obtained directly from the Bianchi identities and the modified horizontality conditions for field strengths, the three anticommutation relations (15.27) hold true.[5]

15.8   Matter and vector multiplets coupled to supergravity

In this section, we will compute both the scalar and vector symmetries acting on the matter fields, so we will retain $(\chi_0, \chi_p) \neq 0$ when we expand the curvature equations in ghost number. The invariant actions for both multiplets can be expressed as δ-exact terms, in a way that generalizes the flat-space case [1].

15.8.1   The Wess–Zumino multiplet

The Wess–Zumino matter multiplet is (P, σ, H), where P is a complex scalar field, σ a Majorana spinor (higgsino), and H a complex auxiliary field, twisted into $(\phi, \bar{\phi}, \sigma_0, \sigma_{\bar{m}}, \sigma_{mn}, B_{\bar{m}\bar{n}}, B_{mn})$. The various field strengths are

$$\begin{aligned}
\hat{P} &= \hat{D}\phi + \hat{\Psi}_m\sigma_{\bar{m}}, \\
\hat{\bar{P}} &= \hat{D}\bar{\phi} - \hat{\Psi}_0\sigma_0 - \hat{\Psi}_{\bar{m}\bar{n}}\sigma_{mn}, \\
\hat{\Sigma}_0 &= \hat{D}\sigma_0 + B_{mn}\hat{\Psi}_{\bar{m}\bar{n}}, \\
\hat{\Sigma}_{\bar{m}} &= \hat{D}\sigma_{\bar{m}} - B_{\bar{m}\bar{n}}\hat{\Psi}_n, \\
\hat{\Sigma}_{mn} &= \hat{D}\sigma_{mn} + B_{mn}\hat{\Psi}_0, \\
\hat{H}_{mn} &= \hat{D}B_{mn}, \\
\hat{H}_{\bar{m}\bar{n}} &= \hat{D}B_{\bar{m}\bar{n}},
\end{aligned} \tag{15.68}$$

with the covariant derivative D explicitly defined as

$$\begin{aligned}
\hat{D}\phi &= \hat{d}\phi + w\hat{A}\phi, \\
\hat{D}\bar{\phi} &= \hat{d}\bar{\phi} - w\hat{A}\bar{\phi}, \\
\hat{D}\sigma_0 &= \hat{d}\sigma_0 + \left(\frac{1}{2}\hat{\omega} - w'\hat{A}\right)\sigma_0 + \hat{\omega}_{\bar{m}\bar{n}}\sigma_{mn}, \\
\hat{D}\sigma_{\bar{m}} &= \hat{d}\sigma_{\bar{m}} + \left(\frac{1}{2}\hat{\omega} + w'\hat{A}\right)\sigma_{\bar{m}} - \hat{\omega}_{\bar{m}n}\sigma_{\bar{n}}, \\
\hat{D}\sigma_{mn} &= \hat{d}\sigma_{mn} - \left(\frac{1}{2}\hat{\omega} + w'\hat{A}\right)\sigma_{mn} - \hat{\omega}_{mn}\sigma_0, \\
\hat{D}B_{mn} &= \hat{d}B_{mn} - w''\hat{A}B_{mn}, \\
\hat{D}B_{\bar{m}\bar{n}} &= \hat{d}B_{\bar{m}\bar{n}} + w''\hat{A}B_{\bar{m}\bar{n}}.
\end{aligned} \tag{15.69}$$

---

[5] The explicit verification is nontrivial, since it relies on the expression of the spin connection, expressed as a solution of (15.59).

To have Bianchi identities, we must have $w' = w + 1$ and $w'' = w + 2$. We obtain

$$\hat{D}\hat{P} = w\hat{F}\phi + \hat{\rho}_m\sigma_{\bar{m}} - \hat{\Psi}_m\hat{\Sigma}_{\bar{m}},$$

$$\hat{D}\hat{\bar{P}} = -w\hat{F}\bar{\phi} - \hat{\rho}_0\sigma_0 - \hat{\rho}_{\bar{m}\bar{n}}\sigma_{mn} + \hat{\Psi}_0\hat{\Sigma}_0 + \hat{\Psi}_{\bar{m}\bar{n}}\hat{\Sigma}_{mn},$$

$$\hat{D}\hat{\Sigma}_0 = \left[\frac{1}{2}\hat{R} - (w+1)\hat{F}\right]\sigma_0 + \hat{R}_{\bar{m}\bar{n}}\sigma_{mn} + \hat{H}_{mn}\hat{\Psi}_{\bar{m}\bar{n}} + B_{mn}\hat{\rho}_{\bar{m}\bar{n}},$$

$$\hat{D}\hat{\Sigma}_{\bar{m}} = \left[\frac{1}{2}\hat{R} + (w+1)\hat{F}\right]\sigma_{\bar{m}} - \hat{R}_{\bar{m}n}\sigma_{\bar{n}} - \hat{H}_{\bar{m}\bar{n}}\hat{\Psi}_n - B_{\bar{m}\bar{n}}\hat{\rho}_n, \qquad (15.70)$$

$$\hat{D}\hat{\Sigma}_{mn} = \left[-\frac{1}{2}\hat{R} - (w+1)\hat{F}\right]\sigma_{mn} - \hat{R}_{mn}\sigma_0 + \hat{H}_{mn}\hat{\Psi}_0 + B_{mn}\hat{\rho}_0,$$

$$\hat{D}\hat{H}_{mn} = -(w+2)\hat{F}B_{mn},$$

$$\hat{D}\hat{H}_{\bar{m}\bar{n}} = (w+2)\hat{F}B_{\bar{m}\bar{n}}.$$

The distorted horizontality conditions that are compatible with the Bianchi identities and warrant off-shell closure are as follows:

$$\hat{P} = P,$$

$$\hat{\bar{P}} = \bar{P},$$

$$\hat{\Sigma}_0 = \Sigma_0 + \hat{\Psi}_p\left(\bar{P}_{\bar{p}} - \frac{1}{2}wG_{m\bar{p}\bar{m}}\bar{\phi}\right),$$

$$\hat{\Sigma}_{\bar{m}} = \Sigma_{\bar{m}} - \hat{\Psi}_0\left(P_{\bar{m}} + \frac{1}{2}wG_{p\bar{m}\bar{p}}\phi\right), \qquad (15.71)$$

$$\hat{\Sigma}_{mn} = \Sigma_{mn} + \hat{\Psi}_{[m}\left(\bar{P}_{n]} - \frac{1}{2}wG_{n]q\bar{q}}\bar{\phi}\right),$$

$$\hat{H}_{mn} = H_{mn} + \hat{\Psi}_p(\Sigma_{\bar{p},mn} + S_{\bar{p},mn}) - i\hat{\Psi}_p J_{\bar{p}[m}(\Sigma_{n],0} + S_{n],0}),$$

$$\hat{H}_{\bar{m}\bar{n}} = H_{\bar{m}\bar{n}} - 2\hat{\Psi}_0(\Sigma_{[\bar{m},\bar{n}]} + S_{[\bar{m},\bar{n}]}),$$

where

$$S_{\bar{p},mn} - iJ_{\bar{p}[m}S_{n],0} = 2iwG_{q\bar{r}\bar{q}}J_{\bar{p}[m}\Psi_{n],r}\bar{\phi} - i\frac{1}{2}wJ_{\bar{p}[m}G_{n]q\bar{p}}\Psi_{\bar{q},p}\bar{\phi} + i\frac{1}{2}wJ_{\bar{p}[m}G_{n]q\bar{q}}\sigma_0$$

$$-\frac{1}{2}(w+2)G_{\bar{q}q\bar{p}}\sigma_{mn} + G_{m\bar{p}n}\sigma_0,$$

$$S_{[\bar{m},\bar{n}]} = \left(P_{[\bar{m}} - \frac{1}{2}wG_{q\bar{q}[\bar{m}}\right)\Psi_{\bar{n}],0} + \left(P_q - \frac{1}{2}wG_{rq\bar{r}}\right)\Psi_{[\bar{m},\bar{n}]\bar{q}} - G_{q\bar{q}[\bar{m}}\sigma_{\bar{n}]}$$

$$-G_{\bar{m}\bar{n}p}\sigma_{\bar{p}} + \frac{1}{2}w\rho_{\bar{m}\bar{n},0}\phi - \frac{1}{2}w\rho_{q\bar{q},\bar{m}\bar{n}}\phi.$$

The ghost-number-1 parts of these equations give the scalar and vector transformations of the fields:

$$\delta\phi = 0, \qquad\qquad \delta_{\bar{p}}\phi = -\delta_{\bar{p}},$$

$$\delta\bar{\phi} = \delta_0, \qquad\qquad \delta_{\bar{p}}\bar{\phi} = 0,$$

$$\delta\sigma_0 = 0, \qquad\qquad \delta_{\bar{p}}\sigma_0 = \bar{P}_{\bar{p}} - \frac{1}{2}wG_{m\bar{p}\bar{m}}\bar{\phi},$$

$$\delta\sigma_{\bar{m}} = -P_{\bar{m}} - \frac{1}{2}wG_{pm\bar{p}}\phi, \qquad \delta_{\bar{p}}\sigma_{\bar{m}} = B_{\bar{p}\bar{m}}, \qquad\qquad (15.72)$$

$$\delta\sigma_{mn} = -B_{mn}, \qquad\qquad \delta_{\bar{p}}\sigma_{mn} = i\left(\bar{P}_{[m|} - \frac{1}{2}wG_{q\bar{q}[m|}\bar{\phi}\right)J_{n]\bar{p}},$$

$$\delta B_{mn} = 0, \qquad\qquad \delta_{\bar{p}}B_{mn} = (\Sigma_{\bar{p},mn} + S_{\bar{p},mn}) - iJ_{\bar{p}[m}(\Sigma_{n],0} + S_{n],0}),$$

$$\delta B_{\bar{m}\bar{n}} = -2(\Sigma_{[\bar{m},\bar{n}]} + S_{[\bar{m},\bar{n}]}), \quad \delta_{\bar{p}}B_{\bar{m}\bar{n}} = 0.$$

The anticommutation relations (15.27) can be explicitly verified for all fields, in a much easier way than for the supergravity multiplet (see Appendix 15.D).

15.8.2   The vector multiplet

The twisted vector multiplet is $(B, \xi_m, \xi_{\bar{m}\bar{n}}, \xi_0, h)$, with B a $U(1)$ gauge field, $(\xi_m, \xi_{\bar{m}\bar{n}}, \xi_0)$ its twisted Majorana supersymmetric partner, and h a real auxiliary field. The field strengths are

$$\hat{\mathcal{F}} = \hat{d}B - (\hat{\Psi}_0\xi_m + \hat{\Psi}_m\xi_0)e_{\bar{m}} - (\hat{\Psi}_p\xi_{\bar{m}\bar{p}} + \hat{\Psi}_{\bar{m}\bar{p}}\xi_p)e_m,$$

$$\hat{\Xi}_0 = \hat{D}\xi_0 - h\hat{\Psi}_0,$$

$$\hat{\Xi}_m = \hat{D}\xi_m + h\hat{\Psi}_m, \qquad\qquad (15.73)$$

$$\hat{\Xi}_{\bar{m}\bar{n}} = \hat{D}\xi_{\bar{m}\bar{n}} - h\hat{\Psi}_{\bar{m}\bar{n}},$$

$$\hat{\mathcal{H}} = \hat{d}h,$$

where $\hat{D}$ is given by $\hat{D}\xi_0 = \hat{d}\xi_0 - \frac{1}{2}\hat{\omega}\xi_0 + \hat{A}\xi_0 + \hat{\omega}_{mn}\xi_{\bar{m}\bar{n}}$, etc. The Bianchi identities for these field strengths are

$$\hat{d}\hat{\mathcal{F}} = (\hat{\Psi}_0\hat{\Xi}_m + \hat{\Psi}_m\hat{\Xi}_0 - \hat{\rho}_0\xi_m - \hat{\rho}_m\xi_0)\hat{e}_{\bar{m}} + (\hat{\Psi}_p\hat{\Xi}_{\bar{m}\bar{p}} + \hat{\Psi}_{\bar{m}\bar{p}}\hat{\Xi}_p - \hat{\rho}_p\xi_{\bar{m}\bar{p}} - \hat{\rho}_{\bar{m}\bar{p}}\xi_p)\hat{e}_m$$

$$+ (\hat{\Psi}_m\xi_0 + \hat{\Psi}_0\xi_m)\hat{T}_{\bar{m}} + (\hat{\Psi}_{\bar{m}\bar{p}}\xi_p + \hat{\Psi}_p\xi_{\bar{m}\bar{p}})\hat{T}_m,$$

$$\hat{D}\hat{\Xi}_0 = \left(-\frac{1}{2}\hat{R} + \hat{F}\right)\xi_0 + \hat{R}_{mn}\xi_{\bar{m}\bar{n}} - \hat{\mathcal{H}}\hat{\Psi}_0 - h\hat{\rho}_0, \qquad\qquad (15.74)$$

$$\hat{D}\hat{\Xi}_m = -\left(\frac{1}{2}\hat{R} + \hat{F}\right)\xi_m - \hat{R}_{\bar{p}m}\xi_p + \hat{\mathcal{H}}\hat{\Psi}_m + h\hat{\rho}_m,$$

$$\hat{D}\hat{\Xi}_{\bar{m}\bar{n}} = \left(\frac{1}{2}\hat{R} + \hat{F}\right)\xi_{\bar{m}\bar{n}} - \hat{R}_{\bar{m}\bar{n}}\xi_0 - \hat{\mathcal{H}}\hat{\Psi}_{\bar{m}\bar{n}} - h\hat{\rho}_{\bar{m}\bar{n}},$$

$$\hat{d}\hat{\mathcal{H}} = 0.$$

The supersymmetry is defined by the constraints

$$\hat{\mathcal{F}} = \mathcal{F},$$
$$\hat{\Xi}_0 = \Xi_0 + \mathcal{F}_{mn}\hat{\Psi}_{\bar{m}\bar{n}},$$
$$\hat{\Xi}_m = \Xi_m - \mathcal{F}_{\bar{p}m}\hat{\Psi}_p, \tag{15.75}$$
$$\hat{\Xi}_{\bar{m}\bar{n}} = \Xi_{\bar{m}\bar{n}} + \mathcal{F}_{\bar{m}\bar{n}}\hat{\Psi}_0,$$
$$\hat{\mathcal{H}} = \mathcal{H} + \hat{\Psi}_p(\Xi_{\bar{p},0} + G_{m\bar{p}n}\xi_{\bar{m}\bar{n}}),$$

which give

$$\begin{aligned}
\delta B &= \xi_m e_{\bar{m}}, & \delta_{\bar{p}} B &= \xi_0 e_{\bar{p}} + \xi_{\bar{m}\bar{p}} e_m, \\
\delta \xi_0 &= h, & \delta_{\bar{p}} \xi_0 &= 0, \\
\delta \xi_m &= 0, & \delta_{\bar{p}} \xi_m &= \mathcal{F}_{\bar{p}m} - i J_{\bar{p}m} h, \\
\delta \xi_{\bar{m}\bar{n}} &= \mathcal{F}_{\bar{m}\bar{n}}, & \delta_{\bar{p}} \xi_{\bar{m}\bar{n}} &= 0, \\
\delta h &= 0, & \delta_{\bar{p}} h &= \Xi_{\bar{p},0} + G_{m\bar{p}n}\xi_{\bar{m}\bar{n}}.
\end{aligned} \tag{15.76}$$

The algebra closure relations (15.27) are satisfied by all fields (see Appendix 15.D).

15.9 Conclusions and outlook

The supergravity action, within the new minimal auxiliary field structure, is basically completely determined by a single (twisted) scalar supersymmetry generator, which is nilpotent and quite analogous to the one encountered in the twisted super Yang–Mills theory. By requiring the existence of a vector supersymmetry generator that anticommutes consistently with the scalar one, we find a set of generators that can be identified as the twisted version of the ordinary super-Poincaré generators. The fourth symmetry δ_{mn} occurs for free, and allows us to untwist the system into the ordinary formulation.

There is an underlying localization around gravitational instantons that seems of interest in this construction. The construction can be extended to the twisted formulation of the Wess–Zumino and vector multiplets coupled to the supergravity multiplet. Generalizations to higher-dimensional supergravities could be of interest, and an analogous twist could be used to split the Poincaré symmetry of, for example, $d = 10$ supergravity into smaller and (hopefully) simpler sectors.

Appendix A: The BSRT symmetry from horizontality conditions

The supergravity transformations can be expressed as BRST transformations, in a way that merely generalizes the Yang–Mills case (ghost unification, horizontality equations for the curvatures, etc.) [4]. Denote the BRST operator of the supergravity transformation by s and its ghost by ξ. The other ghosts are those of local SUSY (χ), Lorentz symmetry (Ω), the chiral $U(1)$ symmetry (c), and the 2-form gauge symmetry (B_1^1). We get the usual transformation laws of classical fields by changing the ghosts into local parameters, with the opposite statistics. Their off-shell closure property is equivalent to the nilpotency of the graded differential operator s. The difficult part of the supergravity BRST symmetry is its dependence on the supersymmetry ghost χ. The reparametrization invariance can be absorbed by redefining $\hat{s}$ as $\hat{s} = s - L_\xi$, with $s\xi^\mu = \xi^\nu \partial_\nu \xi^\mu + \frac{1}{2}\bar{\chi}\gamma^\mu\chi$. With this property, the off-shell closure relation $s^2 = 0$ is equivalent to $\hat{s}^2 = L_{\bar{\chi}\gamma^\mu\chi}$. Reparametrization invariance is decoupled by the operation $\exp(-i_\xi)$, when classical and ghost fields are unified into graded sums, a property that was found for the study of gravitational anomalies but turns out to be very useful for the construction of supergravity BRST symmetries. For the $\mathcal{N} = 1$, $d = 4$ supergravity in the new minimal scheme, the action of the operator $\hat{s}$ is as follows:

$$\hat{s}e^a = -\Omega^{ab}e_b - i\bar{\chi}\gamma^a\lambda,$$

$$\hat{s}\lambda = -D\chi - \Omega^{ab}\gamma_{ab}\lambda - c\gamma^5\lambda,$$

$$\hat{s}B_2 = -dB_1^1 - i\hat{\chi}\gamma^a\lambda e_a, \qquad (15.\text{A}.1)$$

$$\hat{s}A = -dc - \frac{1}{2}i\bar{\chi}\gamma^5\gamma^a X_a,$$

$$\hat{s}\omega^{ab} = -(D\Omega)^{ab} - i\bar{\chi}\gamma^{[a}X^{b]},$$

where the spinor X_a is $X_a = \rho_{ab}e^b - (\frac{1}{2}G_{abc}\gamma^{bc} + \frac{1}{12}\epsilon_{abcd}G^{bcd}\gamma^5)\lambda$. X_a vanishes when we use the equations of motion of the gravitino and of the (propagating) auxiliary fields. The property $s^2 = 0$, equivalent to $\hat{s}^2 = L_{\bar{\chi}\gamma^\mu\chi}$, is warranted by the ghost transformation laws [4]. At the root of these equations, is a unification between classical fields and ghosts [4], which is analogous to the one that occurs when analyzing anomalies by descent equations. In fact, everything boils down to computing constraints on the curvatures, which satisfy the following Bianchi identities:

$$\hat{T}^a \equiv \hat{d}e^a + (\omega + \Omega)^{ab}e_b + \frac{1}{2}i(\bar{\lambda} + \bar{\chi})\gamma^a(\lambda + \chi) = -\frac{1}{2}G^a_{bc}e^b e^c,$$

$$\hat{\rho} \equiv \hat{d}(\lambda + \chi) + (\omega + \Omega + A + c)(\lambda + \chi) = \frac{1}{2}\rho_{ab}e^a e^b,$$

$$\hat{G}_3 \equiv \hat{d}(B_2 + B_1^1 + B_0^2) + \frac{1}{2}i(\bar{\lambda} + \bar{\chi})\gamma^a(\lambda + \chi)e^a = \frac{1}{6}G_{abc}e^a e^b e^c, \quad (15.\text{A}.2)$$

$$\hat{R}^{ab} \equiv \hat{d}(\omega + \Omega) + (\omega + \Omega)^2 = R^{ab} - i\bar{\chi}\gamma^{[a}X^{b]} - \frac{1}{4}i\bar{\chi}\gamma^c\chi G^{ab}_c,$$

$$\hat{F} \equiv \hat{d}(A + c) = F - \frac{1}{2}i\bar{\chi}\gamma^5\gamma^a X_a - \frac{1}{24}i\bar{\chi}\gamma^a\chi\epsilon_{abcd}G^{bcd}.$$

By expansion at ghost number 1, we find the transformation laws in (15.8) and at ghost number 2 those of the ghosts:

$$\hat{s}\chi = -i_\phi\lambda - \Omega\chi - c\chi,$$

$$\hat{s}c = -i_\phi A - \frac{1}{24}i\bar{\chi}\gamma^a\chi\epsilon_{abcd}G^{bcd},$$

$$\hat{s}B_1^1 = -i_\phi B - dB_0^2 - \frac{1}{2}i\bar{\chi}\gamma^a\chi e_a, \qquad (15.\text{A}.3)$$

$$\hat{s}B^2 = -i_\phi B_1^1,$$

$$\hat{s}\Omega^{ab} = -i_\phi\omega^{ab} - \frac{1}{2}i[\Omega, \Omega]^{ab} - \frac{1}{2}i\bar{\chi}\gamma^c\chi G^{ab}_c.$$

Appendix B: Tensor and chirality conventions

The normalization of the completely antisymmetric four-index symbol with tangent-space indices is

$$\epsilon_{0123} = 1. \tag{15.B.1}$$

Once twisted, this is taken to be

$$\epsilon_{1\bar{1}2\bar{2}} = 1. \tag{15.B.2}$$

The dual of an antisymmetric Lorentz tensor is

$$\tilde{F}_{ab} = \frac{1}{2}\epsilon_{abcd}F^{cd}. \tag{15.B.3}$$

The self-dual and anti-self-dual parts of F_{ab} are

$$F^{\pm}_{ab} = \frac{1}{2}(F_{ab} \pm \tilde{F}_{ab}). \tag{15.B.4}$$

We take γ_5 such that $(\gamma_5)^2 = -1$ and define the chiral projections

$$\begin{aligned}
\lambda^{\pm} &= \frac{1 \pm i\gamma_5}{2}\lambda, \\
\bar{\lambda}^{\pm} &= \bar{\lambda}\frac{1 \pm i\gamma_5}{2},
\end{aligned} \tag{15.B.5}$$

in order to have $\lambda = \lambda^+ + \lambda^-$ and $\bar{\lambda} = \bar{\lambda}^+ + \bar{\lambda}^-$. Then, we have the useful identity

$$\bar{\lambda}^+\gamma^a\lambda^+ = \bar{\lambda}^+\gamma_5\gamma^a\gamma_5\lambda^+ = -i\bar{\lambda}^+\gamma^a(-i)\lambda^+ = -\bar{\lambda}^+\gamma^a\lambda^+ = 0, \tag{15.B.6}$$

and similarly $\bar{\lambda}^-\gamma^a\lambda^- = 0$. Finally, once in twisted form, the chiral projections of spinor separate its various components according to

$$\begin{aligned}
\lambda^+ &\sim (0, \Psi_p, 0), \\
\lambda^- &\sim (\Psi_0, 0, \Psi_{\bar{m}\bar{n}}).
\end{aligned}$$

Appendix C: The action of γ matrices on twisted spinors

The action of a γ matrix on a twisted spinor with components $(\Psi_0, \Psi_m, \Psi_{\bar{m}\bar{n}})$ is defined as follows:

	0	$\bar{p}$	pq
$\gamma_m\Psi$	$i\Psi_m$	$-J_{m\bar{p}}\Psi_0$	0
$\gamma_{\bar{m}}\Psi$	0	$i\Psi_{\bar{m}\bar{p}}$	$2J_{\bar{m}[p}\Psi_{q]}$

$$\tag{15.C.1}$$

Similarly, the action of a γ matrix on a twisted spinor with components $(\sigma_0, \sigma_{\bar{m}}, \sigma_{mn})$, such as that appearing in the Wess–Zumino muliplet, is

		0	p	$\bar{p}\bar{q}$
$\gamma_m \sigma$		0	$i\sigma_{mp}$	$-J_{m[\bar{p}}\sigma_{\bar{q}]}$
$\gamma_{\bar{m}} \sigma$		$i\sigma_{\bar{m}}$	$-J_{p\bar{m}}\sigma_0$	0

$$(15.\text{C}.2)$$

These conventions allow us to retrieve the Clifford algebra for the twisted γ matrices:

$$\{\gamma_m, \gamma_n\} = 0,$$
$$\{\gamma_{\bar{m}}, \gamma_{\bar{n}}\} = 0,$$
$$\{\gamma_m, \gamma_{\bar{n}}\} = -iJ_{m\bar{n}} \equiv g_{m\bar{n}}.$$

We also define the γ_{ab} matrices in twisted form as

$$\gamma_{m\bar{n}} = \gamma_m \gamma_{\bar{n}} - \gamma_{\bar{n}} \gamma_m,$$
$$\gamma_{mn} = \gamma_m \gamma_n - \gamma_n \gamma_m,$$
$$\gamma_{\bar{m}\bar{n}} = \gamma_{\bar{m}} \gamma_{\bar{n}} - \gamma_{\bar{n}} \gamma_{\bar{m}},$$

which act on the two kinds of twisted spinors according to the following tables

		0	p	$\bar{p}\bar{q}$
$\gamma_{mn} \Psi$		0	0	$-2J_{m[\bar{p}}J_{\bar{q}]n} \Psi_0$
$\gamma_{\bar{m}\bar{n}} \Psi$		$2\Psi_{\bar{m}\bar{n}}$	0	0
$\gamma_{m\bar{n}} \Psi$		$iJ_{m\bar{n}}\Psi_0$	$2iJ_{p\bar{n}}\Psi_m - iJ_{m\bar{n}}\Psi_p$	$-iJ_{m\bar{n}}\Psi_{\bar{p}\bar{q}}$

$$(15.\text{C}.3)$$

		0	$\bar{p}$	pq
$\gamma_{mn}\sigma$		$2\sigma_{mn}$	0	0
$\gamma_{\bar{m}\bar{n}}\sigma$		0	0	$-2J_{\bar{m}[p}J_{q]\bar{n}}\sigma_0$
$\gamma_{m\bar{n}}\sigma$		$-iJ_{m\bar{n}}\sigma_0$	$-\frac{3i}{2}J_{m\bar{p}}\sigma_{\bar{n}} + \frac{i}{2}J_{m\bar{n}}\sigma_{\bar{p}}$	$iJ_{m\bar{n}}\sigma_{pq}$

$$(15.\text{C}.4)$$

Appendix D: Algebra closure on the fields of matter and vector multiplets

In this appendix, we give some examples of the anticommutation relations (15.27) on some matter fields of the Wess–Zumino and vector multiplets.

Starting with the ϕ and $\bar{\phi}$ fields of the Wess–Zumino multiplet, we need their transformation laws under the pseudoscalar symmetry in order to check (15.27). These are obtained in the same way as the scalar and vector symmetry transformation laws, namely, by isolating the part of ghost number 1 in the horizontality conditions on $\hat{P} = P$ and $\hat{\bar{P}} = \bar{P}$ and keeping $\chi_{mn} \neq 0$. This yields

$$\delta_{mn}\phi = 0, \qquad \delta_{mn}\bar{\phi} = \sigma_{mn}. \qquad (15.\text{D}.1)$$

The transformation laws in (15.72) allow us to compute straightforwardly

$$\delta^2 \phi = 0,$$
$$\{\delta_{\bar{p}}, \delta_{\bar{q}}\}\phi = -(B_{\bar{p}\bar{q}} + B_{\bar{q}\bar{p}}) = 0, \tag{15.D.2}$$
$$\{\delta, \delta_{\bar{p}}\}\phi = \left(P_{\bar{p}} + \frac{1}{2}wG_{m\bar{p}\bar{m}}\phi\right)$$
$$= \partial_{\bar{p}}\phi + \left(wA_{\bar{p}} + \frac{1}{2}wG_{m\bar{p}m}\right)\phi + \Psi_{\bar{p},m}\sigma_{\bar{m}}$$
$$= \partial_{\bar{p}}\phi + \delta^{\text{gauge}}(A, G)\phi - \sum_{a=0,m,\bar{m}\bar{n}} \Psi_{\bar{p},a}\delta_{\bar{a}}\phi.$$

where the last equality is a consequence of (15.72) and (15.D.1).

Similarly, for $\bar{\phi}$,

$$\delta^2 \bar{\phi} = \delta\sigma_0 = 0,$$
$$\{\delta_{\bar{p}}, \delta_{\bar{q}}\}\bar{\phi} = 0, \tag{15.D.3}$$
$$\{\delta, \delta_{\bar{p}}\}\bar{\phi} = \left(\bar{P}_{\bar{p}} - \frac{1}{2}wG_{m\bar{p}\bar{m}}\bar{\phi}\right)$$
$$= \partial_{\bar{p}}\bar{\phi} - \left(wA_{\bar{p}} + \frac{1}{2}wG_{m\bar{p}\bar{m}}\right)\bar{\phi} - (\Psi_{\bar{p},0}\sigma_0 + \Psi_{\bar{p},\bar{m}\bar{n}}\sigma_{mn})$$
$$= \partial_{\bar{p}}\bar{\phi} + \delta^{\text{gauge}}(A, G)\bar{\phi} - \sum_{a=0,m,\bar{m}\bar{n}} \Psi_{\bar{p},a}\delta_{\bar{a}}\bar{\phi},$$

again using (15.72) and (15.D.1) for the last equality.

Turning to the B field of the vector multiplet, the horizontality condition on its field strength $\hat{\mathcal{F}} = \mathcal{F}$ allows us to compute

$$\delta_{mn} B = \xi_n e_m, \tag{15.D.4}$$

and the transformation laws (15.76) of the vector multiplet fields yield

$$\delta^2 B = \delta(\xi_m e_{\bar{m}}) = 0,$$
$$\{\delta_{\bar{p}}, \delta_{\bar{q}}\}B = \xi_0 \Psi_{\bar{p}\bar{q}} + \xi_{\bar{p}\bar{q}}\Psi_0 + \xi_0 \Psi_{\bar{q}\bar{p}} + \xi_{\bar{q}\bar{p}}\Psi_0 = 0, \tag{15.D.5}$$
$$\{\delta, \delta_{\bar{p}}\}B = he_{\bar{p}} + \mathcal{F}_{\bar{m}\bar{p}}e_m - \xi_{\bar{m}\bar{p}}\Psi_m + \mathcal{F}_{\bar{p}m}e_{\bar{m}} - iJ_{\bar{p}m}he_{\bar{m}} + \xi_m \Psi_{\bar{p}\bar{m}}$$
$$= \mathcal{F}_{\bar{p}m}e_{\bar{m}} - \mathcal{F}_{\bar{p}\bar{m}}e_m - \xi_{\bar{m}\bar{p}}\Psi_m + \xi_m \Psi_{\bar{p}\bar{m}}$$
$$= \partial_{\bar{p}}B - (\Psi_{\bar{p},0}\xi_m + \Psi_{\bar{p},m}\xi_0)\,e_{\bar{m}} - (\Psi_{\bar{p},q}\xi_{\bar{m}\bar{q}} + \Psi_{\bar{p},\bar{m}\bar{q}}\xi_q)\,e_m$$
$$= \partial_{\bar{p}}B - \sum_{a=0,m,\bar{m}\bar{n}} \Psi_{\bar{p},a}\delta_{\bar{a}}B,$$

where, for the last equality, we have used the B transformations given by (15.76) and (15.D.4).

Acknowledgments

I thank my collaborators M. Bellon and S. Reys, with whom I worked out the construction.

References

[1] L. Baulieu and G. Bossard, *Reconstruction of $N = 1$ supersymmetry from topological symmetry*, Phys. Lett. **B632** (2006) 138 [arXiv:hep-th/0507004]; L. Baulieu, *SU(5)-invariant decomposition of ten-dimensional Yang–Mills supersymmetry*, Phys. Lett. **B69** (2011) 63 [arXiv:1009.3893[hep-th]].

[2] L. Baulieu and I. M. Singer, *The topological sigma model*, Commun. Math. Phys. **125** (1989) 227; L. Baulieu and I. M. Singer, *Conformally invariant gauge fixed actions for 2-D topological gravity*, Commun. Math. Phys. **135** (1991) 253; L. Baulieu and I. M. Singer, *Topological Yang–Mills symmetry*, Nucl. Phys. Proc. Suppl. **5B** (1988) 12; L. Baulieu, H. Kanno and I. M. Singer, *Special quantum field theories in eight-dimensions and other dimensions*, Commun. Math. Phys. **194** (1998) 149 [arXiv:hep-th/9704167].

[3] M. S. Sohnius and P. C. West, *An alternative minimal off-shell version of $N = 1$ Supergravity*, Phys. Lett. **B105** (1981) 353; *The tensor calculus and matter coupling of the alternative minimal auxiliary field formulation of $N = 1$ supergravity*, Nucl. Phys. **B198** (1982) 493; A. Galperin, V. Ogievetsky and E. Sokatchev, *On matter couplings in $N = 1$ supergravities*, Nucl. Phys. **B252** (1985) 435.

[4] L. Baulieu and M. P. Bellon, *p-forms and supergravity: gauge symmetries in curved space*, Nucl. Phys. **B266** (1986) 75.

[5] A. Johansen, *Twisting of $N = 1$ SUSY gauge theories and heterotic topological theories*, Int. J. Mod. Phys. **A10** (1995) 4325 [arXiv:hep-th/9403017].

[6] E. Witten, *Supersymmetric Yang–Mills theory on a four manifold*, J. Math. Phys. **35** (1994) 5101 [arXiv:hep-th/9403195].

[7] A. D. Popov, *Holomorphic analogs of topological gauge theories*, Phys. Lett. **B473** (2000) 65 [arXiv:hep-th/9909135]; T. A. Ivanova and A. D. Popov, *Dressing symmetries of holomorphic BF theories*, J. Math. Phys. **41** (2000) 2604 [arXiv:hep-th/0002120].

[8] C. Hofman and J. -S. Park, *Cohomological Yang–Mills theories on Kähler 3 folds*, Nucl. Phys. **B600** (2001) 133 [arXiv:hep-th/0010103]; J.-S. Park, *$N = 2$ topological Yang–Mills theory on compact Kähler surfaces*, Commun. Math. Phys. **163** (1994) 113 [arXiv:hep-th/9304060]; J. -S. Park, *Holomorphic Yang–Mills theory on compact Kähler manifolds*, Nucl. Phys. **B423** (1994) 559 [arXiv:hep-th/9305095].

[9] L. Baulieu and A. Tanzini, *Topological symmetry of forms, $N = 1$ supersymmetry and S-duality on special manifolds*, J. Geom. Phys. **56** (2006) 2379 [arXiv:hep-th/0412014].

[10] H. Nicolai, *A possible constructive approach to (super Φ^3) in four-dimensions. 1. Euclidean formulation of the model*, Nucl. Phys. **B140** (1978) 294.

[11] N. Berkovits, *Perturbative Super-Yang–Mills from the Topological $AdS_{(5)} \times S^5$ sigma model*, JHEP **0809** (2008) 088 [arXiv:0806.1960 [hep-th]].

[12] P. Van Nieuwenhuizen, *Supergravity*, Phys. Rep. **68** (1981) 189.

16
AdS crunches, CFT falls, and cosmological complexity

José Luis BARBÓN[1] and Eliezer RABINOVICI[2]

[1]Institute de Física Teórica IFT UAM-CSIC,
Universidad Antónoma de Madrid,
Cantoblanco, Madrid, Spain

[2]Racah Institute of Physics,
The Hebrew University,
Jerusalem, Israel

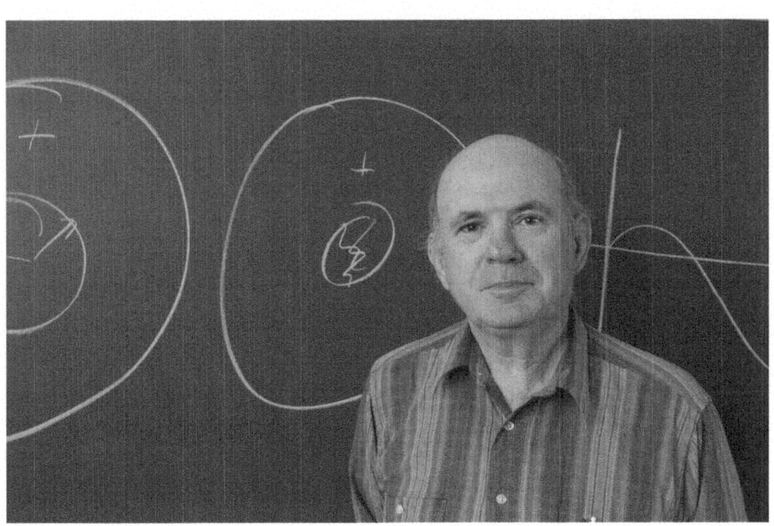

Theoretical Physics to Face the Challenge of LHC. Edited by L. Baulieu, K. Benakli, M. R. Douglas, B. Mansoulié, E. Rabinovici, and L. F. Cugliandolo. © Oxford University Press 2015. Published in 2015 by Oxford University Press.

Chapter Contents

We discuss aspects of the holographic description of crunching AdS cosmologies. We argue that crunching FRW models with hyperbolic spatial sections are dual to semi-classical condensates in deformed de Sitter CFTs. De Sitter-invariant condensates with a sharply defined energy scale are induced by effective negative-definite relevant or marginal operators, which may or may not destabilize the CFT. We find this result by explicitly constructing a 'complementarity map' for this model, given by a conformal transformation of the de Sitter CFT into a static time-frame, which reveals the crunch as an infinite potential-energy fall in finite time. We show that, quite generically, the crunch is associated with a finite-mass black hole if the de Sitter $O(d,1)$ invariance is an accidental IR symmetry, broken down to $U(1) \times O(d)$ in the UV. Any such regularization cuts off the eternity of de Sitter spacetime. Equivalently, the dimension of the Hilbert space propagating into the crunch is finite only when de Sitter is not eternal.

16.1   Introduction

The resolution of cosmological singularities has been a permanent fixture in the 'to do' list of string theory since its quantum gravitational interpretation was launched. Successful singularity resolutions by various instances of 'stringy geometry' always apply to timelike singularities that may be regarded as 'impurities' in space. These singularities are resolved by a refinement in the quantum description of the impurity, often by identifying additional light degrees of freedom supported at the singularity locus.*

Spacelike singularities looking like *bangs* and *crunches* in General Relativity have so far resisted close scrutiny. At the most naive level, they represent a challenge to the very notion of Hamiltonian time evolution. In the case of spacelike singularities censored by black hole horizons, they posed a famous historic challenge to S-matrix unitarity. The advent of notions such as black hole complementarity, holography, and the anti-de Sitter/conformal field theory (AdS/CFT) correspondence have resulted in a conceptual framework in which black hole singularities should be resolved by a refinement of the hole's quantum description, albeit nonperturbative and highly nonlocal in this case.

On general grounds, any problem that can be successfully embedded into an AdS/CFT environment should admit an honest Hamiltonian answer. In this sense, the occurrence of crunches in the interior of AdS black holes poses no serious threat to the CFT Hamiltonian description. The black hole and everything inside is described by a finite-dimensional subspace of the full Hilbert space, and thus the crunch must be 'deconstructed' within this class of states, even if the details of such a deconstruction remain largely unknown.

Potentially more serious is the situation where a crunch engulfs a globally defined, asymptotically AdS spacetime, for then the whole CFT Hilbert space seems destined for the crunch. Such a radical situation occurs in the future development

Journal of High Energy Physics, 'AdS crunches, SFT falls and cosmological complemetarity', April 2011, 2011:44, by José L.F. Barbón & Eliezer Rabinovici © SISSA 2011. With kind permission of Springer Science+Business Media.

of Coleman–de Luccia (CdL) bubbles nucleated inside a false AdS vacuum [1]. The interior of the bubble contains a crunching cosmology that eventually engulfs the whole AdS spacetime, right up to the boundary, not to mention the complicated pattern of multibubble nucleation and collision. This poses a 'clear and present danger' for the CFT Hamiltonian picture.

In this chapter, we discuss various aspects of this conundrum. We first review the construction of highly symmetric bubble-like backgrounds with a crunchy destiny and AdS asymptotic behavior. These backgrounds include the CdL single-bubble configurations, but can be much more general, and are characterized by an exact $O(d, 1)$ symmetry. On the dual holographic side, this symmetry can be realized by specifying the CFT states as living on an eternal d-dimensional de Sitter (dS) spacetime.

A central observation in this chapter is the identification of a simple 'complementarity map' that relates the formulation of the CFT in de Sitter spacetime to another description appropriate for an 'observer' who falls into the crunch in finite time. The large amount of symmetry determines this map to be a conformal transformation to the same CFT defined on a static Einstein spacetime. Using results from [2], we argue that the crunching states are seen in this frame as infinite negative-energy falls, their precise nature depending on whether the condensate was stable or unstable in the de Sitter-frame description. We discuss the implications of this statement for the interpretation in terms of a 'cosmological complementarity' using in particular a regularization that strictly reverts the model into a standard case of black hole complementarity [3].

16.2   AdS crunches and their dS duals

In this section, we review the basic issues arising in the construction of CFT duals of AdS crunching cosmologies. We begin with a description of the relevant geometries and subsequently introduce the corresponding dual CFT structures. Many details of relevance to these constructions can be found in [4–9].

16.2.1   The crunches

We shall refer to 'AdS crunches' as a particular class of Friedmann–Robertson–Walker (FRW) cosmologies with $O(d, 1)$-invariant spatial sections (i.e., d-hyperboloids $\mathbf{H}^d$),

$$ds^2_{\mathrm{FRW}} = -dt^2 + G(\mathrm{t})\, ds^2_{\mathbf{H}^d}. \tag{16.2.1}$$

The profile function $G(\mathrm{t})$ solves Einstein's equations with negative cosmological constant and a generic $O(d, 1)$-invariant matter distribution modeled by a set of fields $\varphi(\mathrm{t})$ depending only on the FRW time coordinate t. In general, for smooth initial conditions at some fixed time $\mathrm{t} = \mathrm{t}_0$, this spacetime has curvature singularities both in the future (crunch) and the past (bang). If the matter contribution is small, the metric is close to an exact AdS_{d+1} in FRW parametrization, corresponding to $G(t) = \sin^2 t$, at least for a long time. In the pure AdS case, the points $\mathrm{t} = 0, \pi$ are only coordinate singularities signaling the Killing horizons associated with the hyperbolic sections becoming null at this locus.

The behavior of the FRW patch in pure AdS suggests that a crunching cosmology of type (16.2.1) could be given initial smooth data by matching across a zero of the function $G(t)$, tuned with a locally static matter distribution. This is precisely the case if the FRW cosmology is regarded as the interior of an expanding bubble, in a generalization of the classic work by Coleman and de Luccia [1]. It is convenient to parametrize such backgrounds in terms of the Euclidean versions with $O(d+1)$ isometries. Let us consider the metric

$$ds^2_{\text{ball}} = d\rho^2 + F(\rho)\, d\Omega_d^2, \tag{16.2.2}$$

satisfying the field equations with an $O(d+1)$-symmetric matter distribution $\varphi(\rho)$. We term it the 'ball' on account of its $O(d+1)$ symmetry, even if it may be noncompact in general. Smoothness at the center of the ball requires $F(\rho) \approx \rho^2$ and $\varphi(\rho) \approx \varphi_0 + \frac{1}{2}\varphi_0'\rho^2$ as $\rho \to 0$.

Writing $d\Omega_d^2 = d\theta^2 + \cos^2\theta\, d\Omega_{d-1}^2$, we generate a Lorentz-signature metric with $O(d, 1)$ symmetry by the analytic continuation $\theta = i\tau$. We call this metric the 'bubble':

$$ds^2_{\text{bubble}} = d\rho^2 + F(\rho)\left(-d\tau^2 + \cosh^2\tau\, d\Omega_{d-1}^2\right) = d\rho^2 + F(\rho)\, ds^2_{\text{dS}_d}, \tag{16.2.3}$$

where the group $O(d, 1)$ acts on global de Sitter sections dS_d. By construction, the matter fields are de Sitter-invariant functions $\varphi(\rho)$, so all features of the metric and matter fields expand like a de Sitter spacetime, i.e., we have a generalized notion of an 'expanding bubble'. This bubble background is time-symmetric around $\tau = 0$, where it can be formally matched to the Euclidean $O(d+1)$-invariant 'ball'. Therefore, we may interpret this construction as a time-symmetric cosmology with bang and crunch, or as a crunching cosmology that evolves from a particular initial condition obtained from some quantum-cosmological tunneling event, *à la* Hartle–Hawking [10].

At $\rho = 0$ the dS_d sections become null and they may be further extended as the nearly null $\mathbf{H}^d$ sections of the FRW patch. By mimicking the pure AdS case, we can achieve this matching by the coordinate redefinition $\rho = it$ and $y = \tau + i\pi/2$:

$$ds^2_{\text{FRW}} = -dt^2 + G(t)\left(dy^2 + \sinh^2 y\, d\Omega_{d-1}^2\right) = -dt^2 + G(t)\, ds^2_{\mathbf{H}^d}, \tag{16.2.4}$$

where the smooth matching requires $G(t) \approx t^2 \approx -F(it)$ near $t = 0$. For the rest of the fields, $\varphi(\rho)$ continues to an $O(1, d)$-invariant function $\varphi(t)$ with small-t behavior $\varphi(t) \approx \varphi_0 - \frac{1}{2}\varphi_0'' t^2$. Hence, the result is an FRW model with negative spatial curvature (16.2.1), which eventually crunches, barring fine-tuning.

16.2.2 The duals

We now restrict further the form of the ball metric to asymptote AdS, $F(\rho) \to \sinh^2\rho$ as $\rho \to \infty$. Using the Euclidean AdS/CFT rules [11], this background describes a certain large-N master field for a perturbed dual CFT on the Euclidean d-sphere $\mathbf{S}^d$:

$$\int_{\mathbf{S}^d} \mathcal{L}_{\text{QFT}} = \int_{\mathbf{S}^d} \mathcal{L}_{\text{CFT}} + \sum_{\mathcal{O}} \int_{\mathbf{S}^d} \frac{g_{\mathcal{O}}}{(\Lambda_{\mathcal{O}})^{\Delta_{\mathcal{O}}-d}}\, \mathcal{O}, \tag{16.2.5}$$

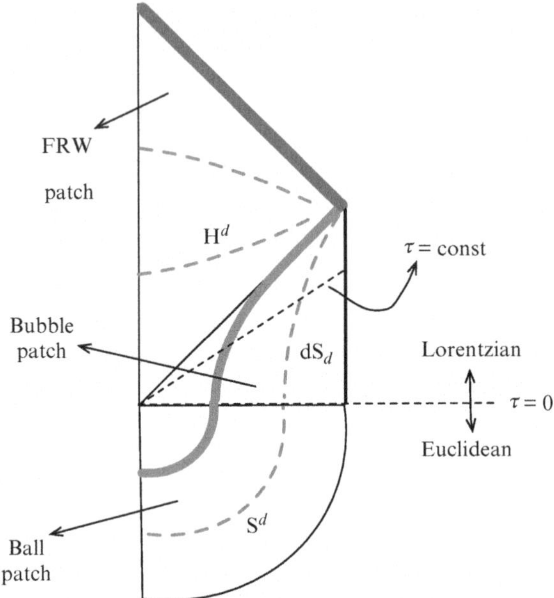

Fig. 16.1 Schematic diagram showing the analytic construction of the crunching FRW spacetime, with $\mathbf{H}^d$ spatial sections, matching to the 'bubble' patch with dS_d timelike sections, and finally the Euclidean 'ball' background, with $\mathbf{S}^d$ sections. The Euclidean piece is $O(d+1)$-invariant, whereas the Lorentz-signature piece is $O(d,1)$-invariant. The gray line signals the radius $\rho = \rho_{\mathcal{O}} \sim \log \Lambda_{\mathcal{O}}$, where the metric begins with differ significantly from the asymptotic AdS form. Equivalently, it is associated with the energy scale $\Lambda_{\mathcal{O}}$ in the dual QFT.

where $\Delta_{\mathcal{O}}$ is the conformal dimension of the perturbing operator, and the dimensionless source terms $g_{\mathcal{O}}$ are determined by the boundary values of the different fields $\varphi_{\mathcal{O}}$ according to the rule

$$g_{\mathcal{O}} = \lim_{\rho \to \infty} \left(e^{-\rho} \Lambda_{\mathcal{O}} \right)^{\Delta_{\mathcal{O}} - d} \varphi_{\mathcal{O}}(\rho), \tag{16.2.6}$$

with $\Delta_{\mathcal{O}}$ the conformal dimension of the operator $\mathcal{O}$ and $\Lambda_{\mathcal{O}}$ the energy scale set by the operator perturbation. All bulk dimensions are measured in units of the asymptotic AdS radius of curvature, and all CFT length dimensions are measured in units of the $\mathbf{S}^d$ radius.

For the case considered here, with $O(d+1)$ symmetry, the $g_{\mathcal{O}}$ are actually constant on $\mathbf{S}^d$ and therefore represent couplings rather than sources. Consistency at the level of the field equations requires that only the couplings associated with relevant or marginal operators may be nonvanishing, since otherwise the backreaction would destroy the assumed AdS asymptotic behavior of the metric. This condition can actually be extended to include also marginal operators, i.e., we have $g_{\mathcal{O}} = 0$ for $\Delta_{\mathcal{O}} \geq d$ with no loss of generality, since a marginal perturbation can be conventionally folded into the definition of $\mathcal{L}_{\mathrm{CFT}}$.

Using the UV/IR correspondence, scales $\Lambda_{\mathcal{O}} \gg 1$ are associated with characteristic geometric features at radii $\rho_{\mathcal{O}} \sim \log \Lambda_{\mathcal{O}}$, and thus we may speak of the radial development of the gravity solution as depicting a certain renormalization group flow. If the theory has no other large dimensionless parameters, we may encounter a number of different qualitative scenarios according to the overall geometrical features of the solution:

1. The flow may become singular inside the ball at a radius of order $\rho_{\mathcal{O}}$. In some cases, the singularity admits a geometric resolution, for example by a vanishing cycle in an additional compact factor of the spacetime, producing a 'confining hole' at the center of the ball. The Lorentzian versions of such models would define confining gauge theories on de Sitter, examples of which can be found in [8] and references therein. Irrespectively of an eventual resolution of the singularity, any such background that does not reach smoothly $\rho = 0$ cannot be Wick-rotated into an FRW patch and thus does not provide crunch models.

2. A flow with $\Lambda_{\mathcal{O}} \gg 1$ may evolve into an approximate IR fixed point at the origin of the ball, thus depicting a flow between a UV fixed point CFT_{+} and an IR fixed point CFT_{-}. This corresponds to a 'thin-walled bubble' of AdS_{-} inside AdS_{+} with radius $\bar{\rho} \sim \log \Lambda_{\mathcal{O}}$, so that the bulk fields at the $\rho = 0$ origin of the ball come close to a local minimum of the supergravity potential with $m_{\varphi}^{2}(\mathrm{AdS}_{-}) > 0$.

3. The flow below the threshold $\Lambda_{\mathcal{O}}$ may continue without approaching an IR fixed point or a gap before it reaches $\rho = 0$. In this case, we have roughly a bubble with 'thick walls', whose interior differs significantly from AdS, but may still define $O(d,1)$-invariant crunches by the procedure outlined above, provided the background is smooth at the origin.[1] An interesting case of a 'thick-walled' bubble is the situation with $\Lambda_{\mathcal{O}} \ll 1$, where the deformation is so small compared with the scale of the $\mathbf{S}^{d}$ sphere that the 'bubble' is but a small 'hump' around $\rho = 0$ (cf. the appendix of [9]). A well-studied class of solutions of this form can be found in [4], using a truncated four-dimensional supergravity model with one scalar field close to a local BF-stable [12] maximum of the potential, $-d^{2}/4 < m_{\varphi}^{2}(\mathrm{AdS}_{+}) \leq 0$. The resulting solutions are constructed in global coordinates and admit two dual state interpretations in a CFT that is deformed by either marginal (cf. [4]) or relevant (cf. [9]) operators, depending on the choice of standard or alternative quantization for the bulk scalar. The physics of the two interpretations is very different, since the marginal deformation was found to trigger an instability of the CFT on dS_{d} or on $\mathbf{S}^{d}$, whereas the relevant case is believed to be locally stable.

In all previous cases, smoothness of metric and fields implies that, generically, relevant and/or marginal operators are turned on at the UV fixed point. However, in

---

[1] The so-called 'thin-wall' approximation refers to the idealization in which the bubble's shell is regarded as having zero thickness. In this chapter, we will refer to a 'thin-walled bubble' whenever the interior contains an approximate AdS_{-} metric, and a 'thick-walled bubble' corresponds to a bubble with no recognizable AdS metric in its interior. This terminology is meant to give a qualitative description of the bubble, rather than a strict implementation of the 'thin-wall approximation'.

special situations, we may have 'flows' that are normalizable at the boundary, so that no operators, relevant or marginal, are turned on. For example, any smooth flow that starts at the boundary from a local minimum of the supergravity potential, $m_\varphi^2(\text{AdS}_+) > 0$, must necessarily be a normalizable deformation of pure AdS, because any amount of non-normalizable deformation backreacts strongly at $\rho = \infty$ and destroys the AdS asymptotic behavior. These normalizable flows are the CdL bounces, which break the conformal symmetry spontaneously, and thus come in continuous families (moduli spaces) associated with bulk translations of the $O(d+1)$-invariant solution. In addition, there are dilute limits with (at least) approximate multibubble solutions.

In our conventions, we regard a marginal coupling as part of the unperturbed CFT. Therefore, any non-normalizable master field that induces a marginal operator in the CFT Lagrangian may be regarded as a normalizable master field of the deformed CFT. This means that flows associated with marginal operators can be conventionally treated as CdL-type backgrounds. The defining feature of the CdL instantons is their normalizable nature at the outer boundary, irrespective of their detailed structure in the interior; i.e., we may have CdL instantons realized as 'bubbles of nothing' [13], as nongeometric impurities, or as smooth bubble-like backgrounds. It is the last class that allows us to study crunches in their real-time development, although they only have a putative 'true vacuum' inside for the case of thin walls (see [14] for a tour around the various pitfalls of the theory of CdL tunneling).

The Wick rotation of any of these Euclidean 'ball metrics' (i.e., master fields) into the bubble spacetime defines a large-N *state* in the same QFT formulated on the Wick rotation of the $\mathbf{S}^d$ slices, i.e., the de Sitter slices. We have the real-time QFT on dS_d with action

$$\int_{\text{dS}_d} \mathcal{L}_{\text{QFT}} = \int_{\text{dS}_d} \mathcal{L}_{\text{CFT}} - \sum_{\mathcal{O}_{\text{relevant}}} \int_{\text{dS}_d} \frac{g_{\mathcal{O}}}{(\Lambda_{\mathcal{O}})^{\Delta_{\mathcal{O}}-d}} \mathcal{O}. \qquad (16.2.7)$$

Geometrical features at radii $\rho_{\mathcal{O}} \sim \log \Lambda_{\mathcal{O}} \gg 1$ correspond to fixed energy scales for the QFT on de Sitter spacetime, measured in units of the Hubble constant of dS_d. For instance, we may have a confining theory in de Sitter space, which corresponds in the bulk to an expanding a 'bubble of nothing' (in this case associated with a non-normalizable deformation of asymptotic AdS). A case of more interest for the purpose of discussing crunches is the state obtained by Wick rotation of the 'domain wall flow', which defines a state looking like the vacuum of a CFT_+ in the UV and as the vacuum of a CFT_- in the IR. In the bulk, we simply see a thin-walled bubble of AdS_- expanding exponentially into the external AdS_+.

In this last situation, there is an alternative CFT representation of the bubble interior, in terms of the IR CFT fixed point: we just write the same expression as in (16.2.7), replacing the UV CFT_+ by the IR CFT_-,

$$\int_{\text{dS}_d} \mathcal{L}_{\text{QFT}_-} = \int_{\text{dS}_d} \mathcal{L}_{\text{CFT}_-} - \sum_{\mathcal{O}_{\text{irrelevant}}} \int_{\text{dS}_d} \frac{g_{\mathcal{O}}}{(\Lambda_{\mathcal{O}})^{\Delta_{\mathcal{O}}-d}} \mathcal{O}, \qquad (16.2.8)$$

and restricting the sum over perturbing operators to the infinite tower of *irrelevant* operators, according to the operator content of the CFT$_-$ fixed point (cf. [9]). This gives an approximate Wilsonian description of the bubble's interior with UV cutoff $\Lambda_\mathcal{O}$, after the bubble's wall and whatever lies outside have been 'integrated out'. In particular, the bubble could be sitting inside an asymptotic $(d+1)$-dimensional de Sitter or Minkowski spacetime, and the IR description would be very similar, provided the AdS$_-$ fixed point exists. Thus, universality of the Wilsonian flow around an IR fixed point explains the fact that all nearly AdS crunching FRW cosmologies look roughly the same, irrespective of the initial conditions. The downside of this Wilsonian description is that details of the UV completion are hidden in the properties of the full tower of irrelevant operators in (16.2.8).

The crunch singularities of the FRW patch start at the boundary and 'propagate inwards' into the bulk. Therefore, the crunch makes its first appearance in the deep-UV regime of the dual QFT, and its properties are potentially very sensitive to the details of the UV completion.

16.3   Facing the CFT crunch time is complementary

The Lagrangian (16.2.7) gives a seemingly well-defined holographic representation of the bubble patch, i.e., a de Sitter-invariant state of a deformed CFT in de Sitter spacetime. The Lagrangian (16.2.8) gives also a well-defined, albeit *approximate*, description of the bubble quantum mechanics in the case that an approximate AdS$_-$ interior exists. Both of these 'CFT-on-dS' pictures have a causal patch in the bulk that leaves out the crunch, since it happens 'after' the end of de Sitter time $\tau = \infty$. On the other hand, the $\tau = 0$ surface of the bubble patch is a valid Cauchy surface for the complete crunching manifold in the bulk. This means that the $\tau = 0$ state of the theory (16.2.7) *does* contain all the relevant information to probe the crunch. In order to expose this information, we need a 'complementarity transformation' which in this case is essentially determined by the symmetries of the problem.

To find the complementarity map, notice that an 'infalling' observer is characterized by meeting the crunch in finite time. In standard black hole states, only sufficiently IR probes have the chance to fall into the black hole (i.e., thermalize) and become eligible 'to meet the crunch'. This is actually a complication for the problem of finding the complementarity map in the QFT, since it entangles it with the renormalization group. In the case of the AdS cosmological crunches, however, the singularity is visible from the boundary, and thus it can be probed by arbitrarily UV states of the theory. So one strategy is to simply find a time variable in the boundary that, unlike de Sitter time, sees the crunch coming in finite time.

Any dS$_d$ slice at constant ρ corresponds to an accelerating, asymptotically null trajectory that hits the AdS$_+$ boundary in finite static time. This suggests that we should use static AdS time in order to describe states in such a way that they 'fall' into the crunch in finite time (i.e., infalling observers). Static time is defined as the time coordinate t adapted to the asymptotic timelike Killing vector $\partial/\partial t$ in AdS$_+$. This Killing vector exists with a good approximation in the 'exterior' of the bubble wall trajectory. Hence, we may parametrize the near-boundary metric of the deformed AdS in a neighborhood of $t = \tau = 0$ as

$$ds^2_{\text{bubble}} \approx -dt^2 \left(1 + r^2\right) + \frac{dr^2}{1 + r^2} + r^2 \, d\Omega^2_{d-1}. \tag{16.3.1}$$

This metric defines states looking in the UV like the vacuum of a CFT on the Einstein space $\mathbf{E}_d = \mathbf{R} \times \mathbf{S}^{d-1}$. Let the metric on the Einstein space be given by $ds^2_{\text{E}} = -dt^2 + d\Omega^2_{d-1}$, which is conformally related to the dS_d metric as

$$ds^2_{\text{dS}} = \Omega^2(t) \, ds^2_{\text{E}} \,, \qquad \Omega(t) = \cosh \tau = \frac{1}{\cos t}, \tag{16.3.2}$$

where $t = \int \Omega^{-1}(\tau) \, d\tau = 2 \tan^{-1}\left[\tanh(\tau/2)\right]$. The conformal transformation thus defined maps the 'eternity' of de Sitter time into a finite interval of Einstein time, and therefore the associated Hamiltonian 'meets' the crunch in finite t time. The extension beyond the interval $-\pi/2 < t < \pi/2$ is not guaranteed, however, since the conformal transformation is singular at $t = \pm t_\star = \pm\pi/2$, the Weyl function $\Omega(t)$ having a simple pole there. Nevertheless, the transformation is a well-defined symmetry in the domain of definition of $\Omega(t)$, and we may study the physical behavior of the theory at the edges.[2]

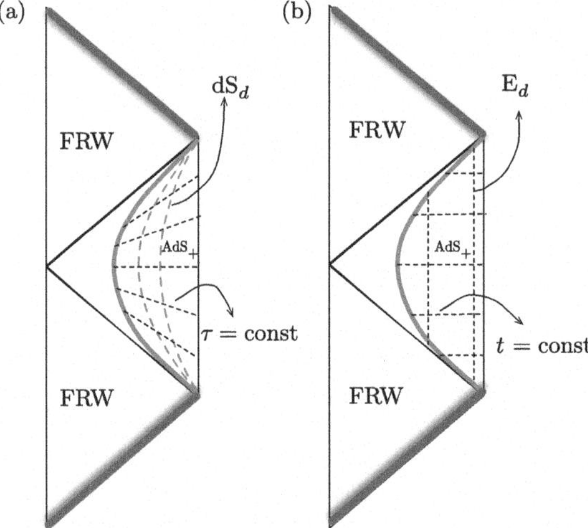

Fig. 16.2 The AdS$_+$ region of the bubble patch, coordinated along the $O(d, 1)$-invariant dS-frame (a) and the $U(1) \times O(d)$-invariant E-frame (b). The crunch and its corresponding bang by time-reversal symmetry are separated by an infinite amount of dS-frame time τ. In E-frame time, their time separation is finite, $\Delta t = \pi$.

---

[2] Conformal maps interpreted as 'complementarity transformations' appear in [15], under a slightly different guise.

16.3.1 Crashing the CFT by irresponsible driving

We can now rewrite the model (16.2.7) in the Einstein (E)-frame by acting with the conformal transformation (16.3.2). Since a given operator transforms as $\mathcal{O} \rightarrow \Omega(t)^{-\Delta_\mathcal{O}} \mathcal{O}$ we find that the model (16.2.7) at *fixed* values of the couplings $g_\mathcal{O}$ can be equivalently rewritten on the Einstein manifold as[3]

$$\int_{\mathrm{E}_d} \mathcal{L}_{\mathrm{QFT}} = \int_{\mathrm{E}_d} \mathcal{L}_{\mathrm{CFT}} - \sum_{\mathcal{O}_{\mathrm{relevant}}} \int_{\mathrm{E}_d} J_\mathcal{O}(t)\, \mathcal{O}, \qquad (16.3.3)$$

where

$$J_\mathcal{O}(t) = \frac{g_\mathcal{O}}{(\Lambda_\mathcal{O}(t))^{\Delta_\mathcal{O} - d}}, \qquad \Lambda_\mathcal{O}(t) = \Omega(t)\, \Lambda_\mathcal{O}. \qquad (16.3.4)$$

If only marginal operators are turned on, this transformation is a symmetry of the deformed CFT, and the E-frame Lagrangian has no explicit time dependence. On the other hand, each relevant operator that is turned on at the UV fixed point CFT_+ breaks the conformal symmetry, and that is reflected in the E-frame theory as an explicit time-dependent 'driving' term proportional to $J_\mathcal{O}(t)\mathcal{O}$. Notice that $\Omega(t)$ diverges as $t \rightarrow t_\star$, and, since $d - \Delta_\mathcal{O} > 0$ for a relevant operator, the E-frame driving term $J_\mathcal{O}(t)$ 'blows up' in finite time. This conclusion holds for any $O(d, 1)$-invariant and *relevant* perturbation of the de Sitter field theory (such time-dependent deformations were invoked in [16, 17] to avert the occurrence of multibubble solutions). So far, this analysis leaves out the case of CdL bubbles, which include the case of an exactly marginal deformation, and will be studied in Section 16.3.2.

We now argue that the value of the relevant deformation, for example whether $g_\mathcal{O}$ may be 'sufficiently positive' or 'sufficiently negative' does have a bearing on the physical interpretation in terms of a crunching cosmology. We shall give two heuristic arguments in this section, and another one in Section 16.3.2, showing that crunching backgrounds are associated with CFT deformations contributing a sufficiently *negative* potential energy.

In order to gain some intuition about such relevant driving terms, we can look at a simple model of a *classical* conformal field theory with similar physical phenomena to those described here. Consider the $O(N)$ sigma model defined on a four-dimensional de Sitter space of unit Hubble constant, and perturbed by a mass operator

$$\int_{\mathrm{dS}_4} \mathcal{L}_{\vec{\phi}} = - \int_{\mathrm{dS}_4} \left(\frac{1}{2} \partial_\mu \vec{\phi} \cdot \partial^\mu \vec{\phi} + \vec{\phi}^2 + g_4 \left(\vec{\phi}^2 \right)^2 + g_2 \Lambda^2 \vec{\phi}^2 \right), \qquad (16.3.5)$$

where we set $\Lambda \gg 1$ in order to be able to neglect the Hubble contribution to the mass and let $g_4 > 0$ ensure the global stability of the model. The mass operator $\vec{\phi}^2$ is relevant but nonleading for large values of $\vec{\phi}$. For a positive-definite mass perturbation, $g_2 > 0$,

---

[3] In this discussion, we neglect the effect of conformal anomalies, a subject of great interest for future work.

the theory acquires a mass gap of order Λ and has a trivial IR limit. For a negative-definite mass perturbation, $g_2 < 0$, the minimum of the potential is found at the vacuum condensate $|\vec{\phi}|_{\rm vac} \propto \Lambda$, and its low-lying excitations are the familiar Goldstone bosons with $N - 1$ degrees of freedom, the slow de Sitter expansion introducing just small thermal corrections to these vacuum states.[4] Thus, this simple model with $\Lambda \gg 1$ allows us to emulate two scenarios of the classification in Section 16.2.2. Namely, it gives an example of scenario (1) for $g_2 > 0$ (a gapped phase), and a dS-invariant domain-wall flow, or scenario (2), for $g_2 < 0$.

When written in the E-frame variables, this theory has Lagrangian

$$\int_{{\rm E}_4} \mathcal{L}_{\vec{\phi}} = - \int_{{\rm E}_4} \left(\frac{1}{2} \partial_\mu \vec{\phi} \cdot \partial^\mu \vec{\phi} + \frac{1}{2} \vec{\phi}^{\,2} + g_4 \left(\vec{\phi}^{\,2} \right)^2 + g_2 \Lambda^2(t) \vec{\phi}^{\,2} \right), \qquad (16.3.6)$$

where now the field theory lives on a static 3-sphere but the mass operator is time-dependent, with a scale $\Lambda(t) = \Lambda\,\Omega(t)$ diverging at $t = t_\star$.

For $g_2 > 0$, i.e., with no condensate in the dS description, the theory (16.3.6) exhibits an increasing gap that eventually decouples all states from the static-sphere vacuum. On the other hand, for $g_2 < 0$, the growing tachyonic perturbation sends the typical field values of the symmetry-breaking ground state to infinity, with ever increasing kinetic energy and (negative) potential energy. Given the stationary 'condensate' field configuration in the dS theory, $\vec{\phi}_{\rm vac}$, with $\partial_\tau \vec{\phi}_{\rm vac} = 0$, the corresponding solution in the E-frame theory is $\Omega(t)\vec{\phi}_{\rm vac}$, which diverges as $t \to \pm\pi/2$.

This suggests that any *coherent* quantum state that is peaked around some nonzero dS-invariant configuration in the dS theory will be mapped in the E-frame theory to a time-dependent coherent state whose support in field space is transferred to large field values. We shall refer to this transfer of 'power' in coherent states from the IR to the UV as the 'CFT fall'.

Note that this happens in the E-frame formalism (16.3.6) as a result of the driving term being negative-definite, even if the system is stable at any finite value of the time variable. On the other hand, in the de Sitter variables (16.3.5), we are simply describing a certain stationary state looking like a thermal excitation of the stable symmetry-breaking vacuum. Essentially the same physics is obtained in any model in which the formation of a condensate is controlled by the sign of a relevant operator, with a less-relevant one (not necessarily marginal) protecting the UV stability.

This example suggests that a positive-energy driving term, which is large in Hubble units, should be associated with an ever-increasing mass gap, dual to the expanding 'confinement bubble of nothing' in the bulk. Conversely, a state with nontrivial IR content, such as one having soft degrees of freedom of an infrared $\rm CFT_-$, should be associated with driving operators $J_{\mathcal{O}}(t)\,\mathcal{O}$ with a negative contribution to the potential energy.

In our qualitative discussion of the $O(N)$ model, we have chosen the case $\Lambda \gg 1$ to emphasize a phase structure with either a clear mass gap or a clear bosonic condensate

---

[4] The negative energy density at the $g_2 < 0$ vacuum does not mean that we lose de Sitter, since gravity is not dynamical, i.e., Newton's constant is zero in the CFT.

as a ground state, in a way that is visible in the classical approximation. For $g_2\Lambda^2$ of the order of the Hubble scale squared, or smaller, the question of whether there is a condensate or a gap depends on the nature of the quantum corrections in the de Sitter background. For weakly coupled field theories, we do not expect a vacuum condensate to survive the thermal de Sitter bombardment for $\Lambda < 1$, so that the critical value of the mass coupling g_2^* separating gapped phases from condensates (perhaps metastable or even unstable ones) should be strictly *negative* and $\mathcal{O}(1)$. On the other hand, for the purposes of studying holographic duals of crunches, we are interested in semiclassical states arising as large-N master fields, and here large-N effects might allow for small-field condensates surviving the dS thermal bath, corresponding to a *positive* critical value of the mass deformation, $g_2^* > 0$, in our toy example.

For the particular case of the $O(N)$ model on de Sitter, the value of g_2^* at large N is an interesting question that deserves further study (cf. [18]). For a CFT admitting a large-N gravity dual, we can get this information from the gravity solution. Consider, for example, a model like that described in the appendix of [9]. Here we have a flow that is 'stopped' by the finite-size effects of $\mathbf{S}^d$ before it goes nonlinear; i.e., we have $\Lambda_{\mathcal{O}} \ll 1$ or scenario (3) of Section 16.2.2. If the gravity solution turns on a relevant boundary operator, the field $\varphi(\rho)$ starts at the boundary of the ball at a local (BF-stable) AdS$_+$ maximum of the bulk potential, which we denote conventionally $\varphi_+ = 0$. If the smooth $\varphi(\rho)$ solution stays small throughout the 'ball', $\varphi(\rho = 0)$ remains close to the value of φ at the maximum, and it makes no difference in which direction we perturb away from $\varphi_+ = 0$ (see Fig. 16.3).

If we now gradually increase $\Lambda_{\mathcal{O}}$ past the inverse size of the sphere $\mathbf{S}^d$, the gravity solution becomes nonlinear before reaching $\rho = 0$ and, in a potential with two extrema, such as that depicted in Fig. 16.3, it *does* make a difference in which direction we flow away from $\varphi_+ = 0$. In particular, flowing to negative values of φ, we enter the basin of attraction of an AdS$_-$ minimum, so that, if the initial conditions and the detailed form of the potential are just right, we may have a domain-wall solution with $\Lambda_{\mathcal{O}} \gg 1$. Conversely, flowing to positive φ, the scalar field will run away and the solution will eventually develop a singularity. Since resolved 'confining holes' are seen in the $(d + 1)$-dimensional gravity theory as singularities, this is a typical case of a gapped phase.

In summary, for $\Lambda_{\mathcal{O}} \gg 1$, we recover the phenomenology of the $O(N)$ model with *large* Λ, suggesting that this is a generic situation; namely, large, positive-definite, relevant deformations lead to gapped phases, whereas large, negative-definite, relevant deformations lead to condensates. It is only the latter that can be used to investigate crunches.

The supergravity picture also indicates that 'small', $\Lambda_{\mathcal{O}} \ll 1$, flows of relevant operators on $\mathbf{S}^d$ do generate small, stable condensates on the dS-CFT, which can be used as holographic duals of crunches [9]. The gravity solution ensures that this condensate exists independently of the sign of the microscopic coupling, provided the flow is sufficiently weak throughout the ball. While the large $\Lambda_{\mathcal{O}}$ condensates are visible in a weakly coupled description of the dS-CFT, the small $\Lambda_{\mathcal{O}}$ condensates arise as a peculiar property of strongly coupled dS-CFTs admitting gravity duals.

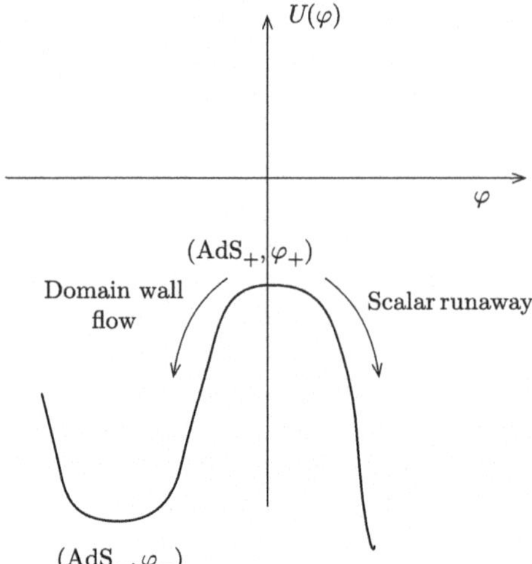

Fig. 16.3 A generic bulk potential with two extrema has inequivalent flows for the two directions of φ, provided these flows enter the nonlinear regime. The arrows indicate the inward evolution of the bulk scalar field $\varphi(\rho)$, starting from an initial value $\varphi_+ = 0$ at the boundary of the ball. In the figure, the direction of negative fields may lead to smooth domain wall flow, whereas the direction of positive fields leads to scalar runaway, which generally produces singularities in the $(d+1)$-dimensional gravity description.

We shall return once more to these issues in Section 16.4, aided by a phenomenological effective action, allowing us to map out the different scenarios of Section 16.2.2.

16.3.2   The CdL falls

Our interpretation of crunches as CFT falls can be made considerably sharper in the case that we describe the bubble in the strict thin-wall approximation. In this setup, the Euclidean background consists of an AdS_- ball of finite radius $\bar{\rho}$, surrounded by an exact AdS_+ metric. The physical parameters of the background are summarized by a charge q, controlling the jump in the AdS cosmological constant when entering the bubble, and a tension parameter σ for the thin shell. The condition for the Lorentzian bubble to expand is that $0 < \sigma < q$. The same problem for a planar domain wall would yield a static solution at any value of $\bar{\rho}$ in the case $\sigma = q$. For this reason, we refer to the condition $\sigma \geq |q|$ as a 'BPS bound', despite the fact that supersymmetry does not feature explicitly in our analysis. With this terminology, we say that only shells violating the BPS bound correspond to ever-expanding bubbles.

Since AdS_+ remains strictly unperturbed outside the bubble, this approximation describes the bubbles as normalizable states, i.e., as CdL bubbles. Therefore, the dynamics of such bubble is determined by a marginal operator in the CFT_+ fixed point.

It was shown in [2] that this operator can be captured given the thin-wall dynamical data, i.e., the tension σ and charge q of the effective brane building the bubble's shell.

The dynamics of thin-walled vacuum bubbles, defined in terms of junction conditions [19, 20], can be summarized in the effective brane action (cf. [2])

$$I = -\sigma \, \mathrm{Vol\,[shell]} + d \cdot q \cdot \mathrm{Vol\,[bubble]}, \qquad (16.3.7)$$

where the first term is of Nambu–Goto type and the second term, proportional to the volume of the bubble, is of Wess–Zumino type.

A general brane configuration can be parametrized by a collective radial field $\rho(x)$, where x coordinates the conformal boundary spacetime, where the CFT is defined. Using then the results of [21] and [2], we can find the derivative expansion of (16.3.7) after a convenient field redefinition from $\rho(x)$ to a canonically normalized field $\phi(x)$. The leading terms for smooth and large bubbles are

$$\mathcal{L}_{\mathrm{eff}}[\phi] = -\frac{1}{2}(\partial\phi)^2 - \frac{d-2}{8(d-1)}\mathcal{R}_d\,\phi^2 - \lambda\,\phi^{2d/(d-2)} + \mathcal{O}\left(\phi^{2(d-4)/(d-2)}, \partial^4\right), \quad (16.3.8)$$

where we recognize the conformal mass coupling to the background curvature and the classical marginal interaction of a conformal scalar field in d dimensions, with coupling

$$\lambda = \left(\frac{d-2}{2}\right)^{2d/(d-2)} \sigma^{2d/(d-2)}\left(1 - \frac{q}{\sigma}\right). \qquad (16.3.9)$$

Note that, precisely for the BPS-violating case corresponding to expanding bubbles, $0 < \sigma < q$, we have $\lambda < 0$ and an *unbounded* negative potential energy fall. Hence, we confirm that the crunch at $t = t_\star$ corresponds to the fall down a conformally invariant cliff that was lurking in the CFT Hamiltonian.

A crucial check of this effective Lagrangian is the successful matching of dilute instanton-gas measures, computed in the bulk CdL description, with those corresponding to the Fubini instantons [22] of (16.3.8) (cf. [2]; see also [23]). This matching is perfect for the instanton action, at the quantitative level, in the limit $\sigma \to q - 0$.

The Lagrangian (16.3.8) gives an asymptotic expansion for large $\rho(x)$, which corresponds to large $\phi(x)$ for $d \geq 2$ and to small $\phi(x)$ for $d = 1$. The precise expression in (16.3.8) is only valid for $d \neq 2$, the $d = 2$ case being special because of the occurrence of Liouville interactions. We should emphasize at this point that (16.3.8) is not of course the full CFT Lagrangian. Rather, it is the effective Lagrangian of a particular set of configurations with the bulk geometrical interpretation of expanding shells. In models with a detailed microscopic definition, such as those based on maximally supersymmetric Yang–Mills theory, the thin shells can be associated with particular branes, such as spherical D3-branes in the $\mathrm{AdS}_5 \times \mathbf{S}^5$ model with a double-trace deformation studied in [24]. In these cases, the system can gradually jump among $\mathcal{O}(N)$ supergravity vacua by ejecting D3-branes. A similar model with different details is the same theory defined on a compact hyperboloid (cf. [15, 25]).

As expected, we find that the CFT supporting a CdL bubble does have an absolutely unstable direction at large values of the collective field ϕ. Since this unstable operator is found to be marginal, it is conformally invariant and thus *also visible* in the dS-frame CFT. The large-bubble action of this dS-CFT sector is obtained by writing (16.3.8) on dS_d:

$$\int_{\mathrm{dS}_d} \mathcal{L}_{\mathrm{eff}}[\phi] = -\int_{\mathrm{dS}_d} \left(\frac{1}{2}(\partial\phi)^2 + \frac{d(d-2)}{8}\phi^2 + \lambda\,\phi^{2d/(d-2)} + \dots \right), \qquad (16.3.10)$$

where we have used $\mathcal{R}_d = d(d-1)$ for dS_d. The dS-invariant solution corresponding to the thin-walled CdL bubble is $\phi_{\mathrm{bubble}} = \bar{\phi}$ with

$$\bar{\phi} = \left(\frac{(d-2)^2}{8|\lambda|} \right)^{(d-2)/4},$$

the constant field configuration at the maximum of the potential. This homogeneous field configuration coincides of course with the $O(d+1)$-invariant Euclidean solution, a local maximum of the Euclidean action, demonstrating explicitly its 'bounce' character (i.e., the existence of one negative fluctuation eigenmode.)

The theory in E-frame variables is

$$\int_{\mathrm{E}_d} \mathcal{L}_{\mathrm{eff}}[\tilde{\phi}] = -\int_{\mathrm{E}_d} \left(\frac{1}{2}(\partial\tilde{\phi})^2 + \frac{(d-2)^2}{8}\tilde{\phi}^2 + \lambda\tilde{\phi}^{\,2d/(d-2)} + \dots \right), \qquad (16.3.11)$$

with the E-frame field related to the dS-frame field through $\tilde{\phi} = \Omega(t)^{(d-2)/2}\,\phi$. Notice that the curvature mass is different from that of the dS_d theory, because now $\mathcal{R}_d = (d-1)(d-2)$. This slight difference in the potential means that the dS-invariant bubble solution is not seen at the maximum of the E-frame potential, but rather corresponds to the time-dependent zero-energy trajectory

$$\tilde{\phi}_{\mathrm{bubble}}(t) = \Omega(t)^{(d-2)/2}\,\bar{\phi} \,,$$

so that now $\bar{\phi}$ is the time-symmetric $t = 0$ turning point of the 'CFT-fall', or the nucleation point if we think of the real-time bubble as emerging from a pure AdS_+ background by a spontaneous tunneling process [2]. It is clear that any such CdL bubble can be nucleated anywhere inside AdS_+, so that any classical solution of (16.3.10) is metastable to further nucleation of Fubini bubbles, including the $O(d,1)$-invariant configuration $\phi = \bar{\phi}$ that we have hitherto considered (cf. [2, 16]).

In general, unstable operators can be expected to be marginal only in an approximate sense. In the absence of extra degrees of freedom, the $\lambda\phi^{2d/(d-2)}$ theory is not exactly conformally invariant, since λ renormalizes logarithmically.[5] Take for example the well-known case of $d = 4$, where negative λ is asymptotically free, leading to the corrected potential

$$\lambda\phi^4 \rightarrow \lambda(\phi)\phi^4 = -\frac{\phi^4}{\log(\phi/\Lambda_{\mathrm{IR}})}\,, \qquad (16.3.12)$$

---

[5] This is true both in perturbation theory and in the bulk picture when λ is associated with a double-trace operator [26].

where Λ_{IR} is the RG-invariant strong-coupling scale in the IR. Hence, under quantum corrections, the fall is not exactly conformal, the instantons are not exactly defined as normalizable solutions, and they exist only in an approximate sense. The corrected background is actually marginally relevant, and we are back to the discussion in Section 16.2, where the driving source is given by the term (16.3.12) with a time-dependent IR Landau pole[6] $\Lambda_{\phi^4}(t) = \Lambda_{\mathrm{IR}}\Omega(t)$. Incidentally, this argument gives additional evidence supporting our prior interpretation of driven crunches as associated with negative energy falls, at least for the case of marginally relevant operators, whose effects can be approximated by those of a marginal operator.

16.4   Attempt at a 'thin-thesis'

Given that a marginally relevant operator can produce effects qualitatively similar to those of an exactly marginal operator, it is of interest to pursue the dynamical description of more general bubbles in terms of effective Lagrangians of the type (16.3.10) and (16.3.11). In particular, let us consider bubbles in the generic situation where there are relevant operators turned on in the dual dS-CFT. If the bubbles are thin-walled, i.e., an approximate AdS$_-$ patch is visible in the interior, we can expect the global dynamics of the bubble to be well described by a single collective field $\phi(x)$, of the type introduced in Section 16.3.2. Even for thick bubbles, we may expect the qualitative energetics to be accounted for by a collective field controlling the overall size and shape of a large and smooth bubble. After integrating out the remaining degrees of freedom of the full dS-CFT, we can write down a phenomenological Landau–Ginzburg model for ϕ whose leading operators, in a large-ϕ and long-distance expansion, are completely determined by conformal symmetry:

$$\int_{\mathrm{dS}_d} \mathcal{L}_{\mathrm{eff}}[\phi] = -\int_{\mathrm{dS}_d} \left(\frac{1}{2}(\partial\phi)^2 + \frac{d(d-2)}{8}\,\phi^2 + \sum_{\Delta \leq d} \lambda_\Delta\,(\Lambda_\Delta)^{d-\Delta}\,\mathcal{O}_{\mathrm{eff}}^{(\Delta)}(\phi) + \dots \right),$$

$$(16.4.1)$$

where $\mathcal{O}_{\mathrm{eff}}^{(\Delta)}(\phi) = \phi^{2\Delta/(d-2)}$ is the effective operator of classical conformal dimension $\Delta \leq d$, accounting for the leading effects of any relevant or marginal operators $\mathcal{O}_\Delta$ that may be turned on at the UV fixed point CFT$_+$, as in (16.2.7). In principle, the Lagrangian (16.4.1) can be rigorously derived in the large-N limit, starting from a given supergravity background in 'the ball'. The analysis in [2], using the extreme thin-wall approximation, captures just the marginal coupling and the curvature-induced mass term. Computing systematic corrections to the extreme thin-wall approximation should yield the couplings λ_Δ of the conformal symmetry-breaking operators with $\Delta < d$.

The marginal coupling λ_d controls the extreme UV behavior, at large values of the collective field ϕ, and thus it must be positive if the undeformed CFT$_+$ is to

---

[6] The time-dependent IR Landau pole $\Lambda_{\phi^4}(t)$ eventually becomes larger than unity at times $|t_s - t_\star| \sim (\Lambda_{\mathrm{IR}})^{-1}$; i.e., slightly before the crunch, the E-frame description becomes nonperturbative on the scale of the $\mathbf{S}^{d-1}$ sphere.

be absolutely stable. The example of Section 16.3, corresponding to CdL bubbles in the thin-wall approximation, had $\lambda_d = \lambda < 0$, leaving a globally unstable direction. By allowing logarithmic effective operators as in (16.3.12), we can also use the model to discuss marginally relevant falls (cf. [24]). Nongeneric CFTs may have $\lambda_d = 0$, like, for instance, $\mathcal{N} = 4$ Super Yang–Mills projected along the Coulomb branch. In that situation, the global stability depends on the leading less-relevant operator.

Despite the similarity to (16.3.5) and its obvious generalizations, it is important to notice that the model (16.4.1) has a very different status. While (16.3.5) is a microscopic (UV) definition of a toy deformed CFT, we have to think of (16.4.1) as a large-N effective Lagrangian for the single collective mode $\phi(x)$. Therefore, the classical approximation to (16.4.1) describes all large-N quantum dynamics of the underlying CFT, for the particular case of states looking like bulk bubbles. Notice also that the effective couplings λ_Δ appearing in (16.4.1) are functions of the microscopic couplings $g_\mathcal{O}$ featuring in (16.2.7) or the toy model (16.3.5). However, they are related by a priori complicated dynamics, and no simple relation exists between, say, the sign of a given effective coupling λ_Δ and the analogous microscopic coupling g_Δ, except perhaps when these couplings are sufficiently large, and we have a configuration that is well-approximated by a thin-walled bubble.

The essential qualitative behavior can be illustrated by a simplified case with a single relevant operator inducing a scale Λ, and a single marginal operator of coupling λ:

$$\int_{\mathrm{dS}_d} \mathcal{L}_{\mathrm{eff}}[\phi] = -\int_{\mathrm{dS}_d} \left(\frac{1}{2}(\partial\phi)^2 + \frac{d(d-2)}{8}\,\phi^2 + \lambda\,\phi^{\,2d/(d-2)} \right.$$
$$\left. + \lambda_\Delta\,\Lambda^{d-\Delta}\,\phi^{\,2\Delta/(d-2)} + \dots \right). \tag{16.4.2}$$

We choose $\lambda > 0$ to ensure global stability of the CFT$_+$ fixed point, and we assume that neither λ nor $|\lambda_\Delta|$ is parametrically large, so that the only energy hierarchy in the system is controlled by the scale Λ.

dS-invariant bubbles or, equivalently, large-N dS-invariant states in the dS theory are described in this approximation as extrema of the effective potential in (16.4.2). For $\lambda_\Delta \geq 0$, the only dS-invariant solution is the dS vacuum, with no scalar condensate $\bar\phi = 0$. Nontrivial condensates require $\lambda_\Delta < 0$, corresponding to a negative-definite, relevant perturbation in the *effective* theory. In this situation, there are still different scenarios depending on the value of Δ and the strength of the relevant perturbation, compared with the Hubble scale. For very relevant perturbations, $\Delta < d - 2$, the only nonzero bubble solutions occur in the weak-perturbation regime, $\Lambda \ll 1$, where we find a local minimum determining a small dS-invariant bubble $\bar\phi_- \sim \Lambda^\alpha \ll 1$, with

$$\alpha \equiv \frac{(d-2)(d-\Delta)}{2(d-2-\Delta)}.$$

This type of stable dS condensate is reminiscent of scenario (3) in the classification of Section 16.2.2; i.e., it is qualitatively similar to the case studied in the appendix of [9], where the condensate is so small that it is stabilized by the positive curvature-induced mass of dS. We remind the reader that while this condensate requires a negative-definite effective coupling $\lambda_\Delta < 0$, this could be compatible with a small range of positive values of the microscopic relevant coupling g_Δ (cf. the discussion in Section 16.3.1).

On the other hand, for less relevant operators, $d > \Delta > d - 2$, it is the strong-perturbation limit, $\Lambda \gg 1$, that yields interesting solutions. We have a stable minimum at $\bar{\phi}_- \sim \Lambda^{(d-2)/2}$ and a local *maximum* near the origin, $\bar{\phi}_+ \sim \Lambda^\alpha \ll 1$.

Finally, for $\Delta = d - 2$, both the small-Λ minimum and the large-Λ maximum degenerate to $\bar{\phi} = 0$ in this crude approximation, whereas the large-Λ stable minimum is present at $\bar{\phi}_- \sim \Lambda^{(d-2)/2}$.

Any dS-invariant solution at a minimum of (16.4.2) is a stable background modeling a crunch with a well-defined status as a stationary state in the dS-CFT. For $\Lambda \gg 1$, we have the domain-wall scenario (2), in the classification of Section 16.2.2. For $\Lambda \ll 1$, we have seen that we can parametrize a model of type (3) in the same list.

The situation is different for the dS-invariant states at a local maximum of the (16.4.2) potential, such as $\bar{\phi}_+ \sim \Lambda^\alpha$ for less relevant operator perturbations. At the purely classical level, this state is interpreted as a bulk CdL bubble. Thus, this is an example of a normalizable perturbation of a bulk background with relevant operators turned on at the boundary. The dynamical implications are entirely similar to the previous discussion of CdL bubbles associated with marginal operators; i.e., any such small-field condensate will degrade by further uncontrolled bubble nucleations and collisions.

Unlike the case of the absolutely unstable dS theories of Section, 16.3, there is now a finite amount of potential energy available in the dS-frame potential, since the dS theory is absolutely stable for $\lambda > 0$.[7] This means that the condensate-free dS vacuum decays in this theory toward a 'superheated' dS_d state—at least when probed on distance scales smaller than the Hubble length (above the Hubble length, thermalization of the scalar field fluctuations will not be as effective). The reheating temperature is of order $\Lambda \gg 1$, much larger than the starting dS temperature. Remarkably, there are bulk descriptions of superheated dS_d spaces precisely for the static patch, in terms of bulk hyperbolic black holes (see [8] and references therein for a recent discussion of these holographic duals in their de Sitter incarnation).

16.4.1 Going down your own way

To any classical solution $\phi_{cl}(x)$ of (16.4.2), we can associate a classical solution $\tilde{\phi}_{cl}(x) = \Omega(t)^{(d-2)/2}\,\phi_{cl}(x)$ of the 'driven' E-frame theory

---

[7] A similar model was proposed in [2] using a negative-definite marginally relevant operator to introduce the local instability, and an exactly marginal operator of the type studied in [27] to stabilize the system.

$$\int_{E_d} \mathcal{L}_{\text{eff}}[\tilde{\phi}] = -\int_{E_d} \left(\frac{1}{2}(\partial\tilde{\phi})^2 + \frac{(d-2)^2}{8}\tilde{\phi}^2 + \lambda\tilde{\phi}^{\,2d/(d-2)} \right. \tag{16.4.3}$$
$$\left. + \lambda_\Delta \Lambda(t)^{d-\Delta}\tilde{\phi}^{\,2\Delta/(d-2)} + \dots \right),$$

where $\Lambda(t) = \Omega(t)\Lambda$ is the by now familiar time-dependent scale that effects the 'driving'. This theory has a time-dependent potential with a growing gap at the origin for $\lambda_\Delta > 0$ and a negative well becoming infinitely deep in finite time for any $\lambda_\Delta < 0$.

The E-frame description of a nontrivial dS-invariant state $\phi_{\text{bubble}} = \bar{\phi} \neq 0$ is a time-dependent bubble field $\tilde{\phi}_{\text{bubble}}(x) = \Omega(t)^{(d-2)/2}\bar{\phi}$ exercising what we call the 'CFT fall', i.e. it goes to infinity in time $\pi/2$ from its $t = 0$ turning point at $\bar{\phi}$, having started at infinity at $t = -\pi/2$.

While the kinetic energy of this field in the E-frame diverges as $t \to t_\star$, its E-frame potential energy density also diverges to *negative values*. Even the value at the turning point $t = 0$ has a nonpositive energy density, because the positive mass term in (16.4.3) is smaller than the dS-frame mass term by an amount $\frac{1}{4}(d-2)\bar{\phi}^2$.

The E-frame fall of a stable dS-invariant state looks quite different from that of a CdL-like state. In the case of a configuration sitting at a minimum of the dS potential, its E-frame or 'infalling' representation involves a rolling field that is 'gently held' by the simultaneous fall of the E-frame potential well (cf. Fig. 16.4). It is interesting to ask if this E-frame field configuration sits at the instantaneous minimum of the time-dependent E-frame potential, or if rather it 'rolls' to some extent, relative to the overall fall of the potential itself. The answer is that the $\tilde{\phi}_{\text{bubble}}(t)$ configuration is slightly shifted from the instantaneous minimum of the driven potential, the displacement becoming smaller as time goes by. This is again a consequence of the slight mismatch

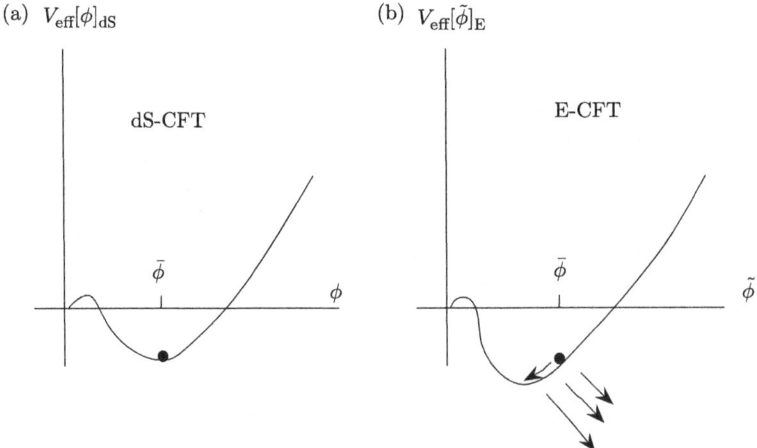

Fig. 16.4 Picture a stable fall. In (a), the dS-invariant state, $\phi_{\text{bubble}} = \bar{\phi}$, is pictured as the locally stable black dot in the dS-frame. In (b), the E-frame state $\tilde{\phi}_{\text{bubble}}(t)$ executes a combined motion: there is a slow roll down the E-frame potential, starting at $\bar{\phi}$ at $t = 0$ and approaching the minimum, while simultaneously the whole potential well falls down to infinity as $t \to t_\star$.

of curvature-induced masses, i.e., the factor of $d(d-2)$ versus $(d-2)^2$ between (16.4.2) and (16.4.3), an entirely analogous effect to the more dramatic case of the marginal fall discussed in Section 16.3, where the potential did not acquire time dependence in the E-frame, but the field configuration did. We can explicitly illustrate the effect in the case of a large ($\Lambda \gg 1$) four-dimensional mass deformation, $\Delta = 2$ and $d = 4$. We find

$$\bar{\phi} = \left(\frac{\Lambda^2 - 1}{2\lambda}\right)^{1/2}$$

for the dS-frame solution. The E-frame field is

$$\tilde{\phi}_{\text{bubble}}(t) = \Omega(t)\,\bar{\phi}\,,$$

while the instantaneous minimum sits at

$$\tilde{\phi}_{\min}(t) = \left(\frac{\Omega^2(t)\Lambda^2 - 1/2}{2\lambda}\right)^{1/2}.$$

Hence, $\tilde{\phi}_{\text{bubble}}(t)$ is slightly larger than $\tilde{\phi}_{\min}(t)$, the mismatch approaching zero as $t \to t_\star$, and being maximal at $t = 0$.

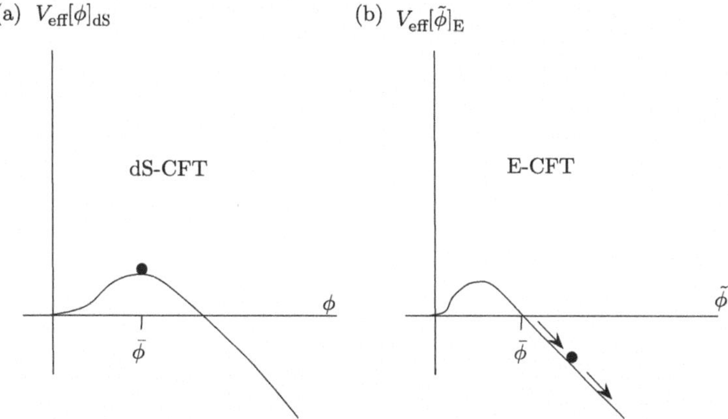

Fig. 16.5 Picture of a CdL fall. The stationary state $\phi_{\text{bubble}} = \bar{\phi}$ of the dS-frame CFT sits at a local maximum (black dot in (a)). In the E-frame CFT (b), we have a time-dependent falling state $\tilde{\phi}_{\text{bubble}}(t)$. The potential changes slightly, so that the 'sphaleron' point $\bar{\phi}$ of the dS-frame is mapped to the turning point of the E-frame configuration. If the negative slope is controlled by a marginal operator, the E-frame potential is time-independent. If the slope is controlled by a relevant operator, there is typically a receding minimum further down the potential, which may be reached by the moving dot only at the crunch time $t = t_\star$.

The stated qualitative differences between the CdL-type falls and the 'stable' falls refer to the behavior of classical dS-invariant configurations at the extrema of the dS-CFT potential. We may also consider perturbations around these extrema, of the form $\phi(\tau, \Omega_\alpha) = \bar{\phi} + \delta\phi(\tau, \Omega_\alpha)$, where Ω_α parametrizes $\mathbf{S}^{d-1}$. At the linearized level, $\delta\phi$ solves a conformally invariant Klein–Gordon equation on dS, with long-time asymptotic behavior

$$\delta\phi(\tau, \Omega_\alpha) \sim \exp(\gamma_\pm \tau) , \qquad \gamma_\pm = \frac{1-d}{2}\left(1 \mp \sqrt{1 - \frac{4m^2}{(d-1)^2}}\right),$$

where m is the effective mass of the linearized field $\delta\phi$. Here we see crucial differences between the stable and unstable dS-invariant vacua. Stable vacua have $m^2 > 0$ and $\mathrm{Re}(\gamma_\pm) < 0$, leading to decaying perturbations in the dS-frame. After transformation to the E-frame, the harmonic fluctuations are still suppressed relative to the zero mode in the $t \to t_\star$ limit. In particular, the gradient energy never dominates over the kinetic energy of the field zero mode. This means that the crunch is quite homogeneous, except for possible nonlinearities generated at an intermediate time scale.

On the other hand, for the case of CdL solutions, $m^2 < 0$ and $\mathrm{Re}(\gamma_+) > 0$, so that there is an unstable solution leading to the growth of harmonic perturbations on the $\mathbf{S}^{d-1}$ sphere. This leads to a rapid dominance of the energy by the spatial gradient terms. Over at the E-frame, the gradient modes get excited in the fall and dominate the energy density, a case of 'tachyonic preheating' (see [28] for a review). A recent detailed analysis of such processes for a CdL fall can be found in [29].

These simple considerations regarding nonhomogeneous configurations show that while crunches associated with stable CFT falls 'have no hair', in the sense that the homogenous solution is linearly stable as $t \to t_\star$, crunches associated wtih CdL falls are quite 'hairy', even at the level of single-bubble dynamics.

16.4.2   Rules of engagement?

We finish this section with some general considerations on the overall physics picture implied by the effective Landau–Ginzburg approach.

One would like to identify definite field-theoretical hallmarks for the crunch, and we have highlighted several candidates, none of which is perfect, but each of which manifested an important aspect of the crunching phenomenon. An indication in the E-frame was an infinite energy fall, which came in essentially two flavors.

In one class of 'CFT fall' the E-frame potential is itself time-dependent but stable for any time before the crunch. The value of the potential at its minimum is negative and becomes more and more negative as the time approaches the crunch time. The field has an expectation value that shifts to the UV—that is, to larger and larger values. A potential in the dS-frame that is negative at its minimum and that has a next-to-leading operator with a large negative coupling would be mapped to the desired form in the E-frame.

The other type of potential is one that is unbounded for any time in both Einstein and de Sitter frames. It may be more palatable to accept that the crunches associated with the stabilized potentials can exist in a theory of gravity, even if those associated with the second type of potentials are classically well defined for a finite time interval.[8]

These scenarios are particularly clear-cut when the energy scale associated with the condensate is much larger than the Hubble scale. This corresponds in the bulk with a thin-walled bubble of large size compared with the AdS radius of curvature. In this case, it is natural to expect that the sign of the effective coupling $\lambda_{\mathcal{O}}$ is correlated with the sign of the microscopic coupling $g_{\mathcal{O}}$, so that a large and negative value of $g_{\mathcal{O}}(\Lambda_{\mathcal{O}})^{d-\Delta_{\mathcal{O}}}$ is expected to be a hallmark for the crunch in the microscopic specification of the CFT. Conversely, a large and positive $g_{\mathcal{O}}(\Lambda_{\mathcal{O}})^{d-\Delta_{\mathcal{O}}}$ would be a hallmark of a gapped theory with no crunch in its bulk version.

When the energy scale associated with the condensate is not large in Hubble units, the geometrical picture becomes murkier. If the slightly negative operator is sufficiently relevant, we have found small condensates with thin walls in the Landau–Ginzburg model, mimicking the expected behavior of supergravity solutions with bubbles that are very small in units of the AdS curvature radius. Such supergravity solutions are, strictly speaking, outside the realm of the thin-wall approximation, and therefore reducing the number of effective fields to one single collective mode becomes questionable. Yet it is in such circumstances that a crunch can be reliably identified in the bulk within a valid linear approximation of the supergravity equations. This linearity implies that there cannot be a strict correlation between the signs of $\lambda_{\mathcal{O}}$ and $g_{\mathcal{O}}$ in these cases.

All examples of crunches considered in this chapter seem to conform to a general rule, namely one needs a large-N worth of *massless* degrees of freedom at the Hubble scale, coexisting with a semiclassical condensate, which itself could be large or small in Hubble units. Expectation values of collective fields measuring the condensate may then serve as 'order parameters' for the existence of the crunch. The gapless character of the condensates seems to be essential. Semiclassical condensates exist in gapped theories, such as gluon condensates in a confining AdS/CFT model, and yet such theories provide unambiguous crunching models only when the confining scale is small in Hubble units, so that the glueballs still look essentially massless at the Hubble scale.

16.5 Falling on your sword

In this section, we introduce a regularized version of the single-bubble crunching dynamics that simply makes the fall finite, further elaborating on the discussion in [2, 4]. We will see that the result is a conventional black hole final state, thus adding support to our complementarity interpretation of the map between Einstein and de Sitter frames.

From the point of view of the CFT in E-time frame, the crunch is associated with a finite-time fall, down an infinite cliff of negative potential energy. The geometry codifies

---

[8] Beyond the $N = \infty$ limit, which corresponds to the classical approximation to (16.3.11), the fate of the CdL-fall model depends on poorly understood multibubble dynamics [16, 20]. Even at the level of the $1/N$ expansion, the quantum evolution of a single bubble suffers from ambiguities on time scales arbitrarily close to $t = 0$ (D. Marolf, unpublished).

a state in the QFT that is transferring support to UV modes, with all the characteristic energy scales diverging proportionally to $\Omega(t)$. The infinite character of the fall is a consequence of the $O(d,1)$ symmetry of the state, since any dS-invariant configuration $\phi_{\text{bubble}} = \bar{\phi}$, with constant $\bar{\phi}$, is mapped to a configuration whose time dependence is just dictated by the blowing-up Weyl factor $\Omega(t)$. Hence, any regularization of the fall must break dS symmetry close to the boundary. In the dS-time frame, this means breaking the eternal character of de Sitter spacetime.

When the crunch is a result of an explicit driving term, the breaking of the $O(d,1)$ symmetry must be prescribed by hand, simply declaring that the driving source $J_{\mathcal{O}}(t)$ stops growing before the pole at $t = t_\star$. If we stop the bubble as some fixed radius in the E-frame metric, $r_{\max} = \Lambda_{\text{E}}$, the state breaks the $O(d,1)$ symmetry to an $U(1) \times O(d)$ symmetry, which is the global symmetry of the CFT on the Einstein manifold. In dS-frame variables, the stopping of the bubble is equivalent to terminating the 'eternity' of de Sitter, with a limiting time

$$\tau_{\max} \sim \log(\Lambda_{\text{E}}/\Lambda_{\mathcal{O}}).$$

The long-time evolution in the E-frame will take the system to a generic state with the unbroken $U(1) \times O(d)$ symmetry. If the potential energy released is large enough, those states look like a locally thermal state in the QFT, or a black hole in the bulk description.

We may estimate the energy and entropy of this final black hole in the following way. Since the driving operator $\mathcal{O}$ has dimension $\Delta_{\mathcal{O}}$, the expectation value at long times in the E-frame is of order $\langle \mathcal{O} \rangle \sim N_{\text{eff}} (\Lambda_{\text{E}})^{\Delta_{\mathcal{O}}}$, where N_{eff} is the central charge of the CFT, or number of effective field species in the UV limit. Therefore, the amount of potential energy released is of order

$$\langle H_{\text{driving}} \rangle \sim \frac{g_{\mathcal{O}}}{(\Lambda_{\text{E}})^{\Delta_{\mathcal{O}}-d}} \, N_{\text{eff}} \, (\Lambda_{\text{E}})^{\Delta_{\mathcal{O}}} \sim g_{\mathcal{O}} \, N_{\text{eff}} \, (\Lambda_{\text{E}})^d.$$

If all this energy is eventually thermalized in the E-frame QFT, it will take the form $N_{\text{eff}} (T_{\text{eff}})^d$, which gives an effective 'reheating' temperature

$$T_{\text{eff}} \sim (g_{\mathcal{O}})^{1/d} \, \Lambda_{\text{E}} \; .$$

If $T_{\text{eff}} \gg 1$, the bulk representation of this state will be a large AdS black hole of entropy

$$S_{\text{BH}} \sim N_{\text{eff}} (T_{\text{eff}})^{d-1} \sim N_{\text{eff}} \, (g_{\mathcal{O}})^{(d-1)/d} \, (\Lambda_{\text{E}})^{d-1}, \tag{16.5.1}$$

where all quantities are normalized dimensionally to the unit size of the E-frame sphere. Since $g_{\mathcal{O}} < \mathcal{O}(1)$ as part of the Wilsonian convention in defining the effective energy scales, we find that the entropy of the resulting black hole is always bounded by the maximal information capacity of the E-frame QFT, defined with a Wilsonian cutoff at scale Λ_{E}:

$$S_{\text{BH}} < S_{\max}(\Lambda_{\text{E}}). \tag{16.5.2}$$

In the case of CdL bubbles, or spontaneous decay, the same arguments apply, except that now the $O(d,1)$ symmetry is broken to $U(1) \times O(d)$ by postulating a stabilization potential in the E-frame Hamltonian H_{CFT} at field values of order $\phi_{\mathrm{max}} \sim \Lambda_{\mathrm{E}}$. For the situation studied in Section 16.4, in the thin-wall approximation, the estimates about the properties of the final state apply with $g_{\mathcal{O}} \sim |\lambda| \ll 1$ and N_{eff} the fraction of degrees of freedom carried by the bubble's shell, so that the information-theoretic bound (16.5.2) is far from saturated. In general, the details of the approach to the typical thermalized state are much more involved here, since due attention must be paid to multibubble collisions that occur within the $O(d,1)$-invariant region, $r < \Lambda_{\mathrm{E}}$.

The fundamental aspect of the regularization is to regard the $O(d+1)$ group (or its Lorentzian counterpart) as an accidental symmetry emerging below a scale Λ_{E}. Above this scale, the symmetry of the state is only the $U(1) \times O(d)$ group of the

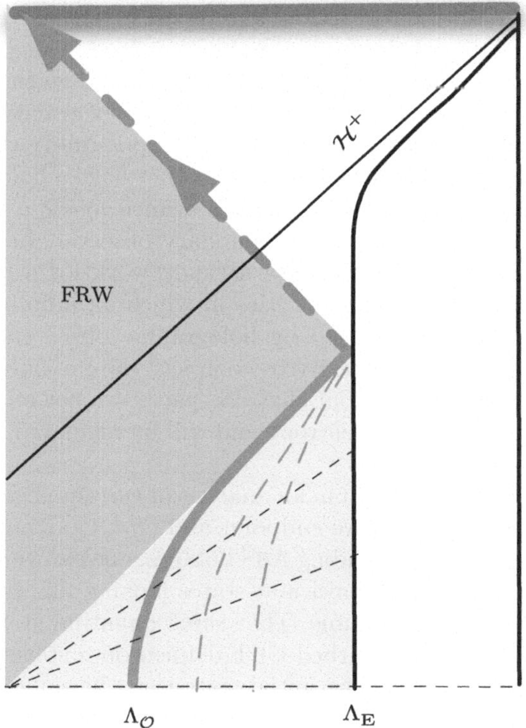

Fig. 16.6 Causal diagram of the regularized crunch model. The shaded region is the part of the bulk with approximate $O(d,1)$ symmetry. The bubble patch is shown by light shading and the FRW patch by dark shading. The unshaded part is the bulk region realizing the UV symmetry group $U(1) \times O(d)$. The ingoing flux of energy from the bubble collision at the UV wall bounds the FRW region and forms the final black hole. As $\Lambda_{\mathrm{E}} \to \infty$, this bolt of energy diverges, as does the black hole size, producing the FRW crunch.

Einstein space. Going back to the original problem posed by (16.2.1), the resolution of the crunch by a UV breaking of the $O(d, 1)$ symmetry puts the finger of blame on the large isometry of the FRW model on noncompact spatial sections. If this symmetry is broken to $U(1) \times O(d)$ outside a compact set, the crunch is tamed in the sense that it resides inside a black hole. However, it would be wrong to claim that the crunch inside the black hole is the precise regularization of the cosmological crunch of (16.2.1). A glance at the causal diagram in Fig. 16.6 shows that the cosmological crunch is associated with the boundary of the region with $O(d, 1)$ symmetry, i.e., the null surface produced by the 'backflow' from the collision of the bubble with the UV wall. Inside the final black hole event horizon, this surface coincides with the apparent horizon of the black hole.

16.6 Conclusions

Singularities have been encountered time and again in physics. In most cases, they marked the limits of validity of the approximation involved. The drive to discover what lies beyond the approximation originated from the knowledge that these singularities are not present in the phenomena described. In the study of gravity, a new way emerged to understand such singularities: one considered the possibility that they are cloaked by horizons. This was actually realized in systems that have a holographic description. The finite entropy that could be absorbed by a crunch inside a black hole in AdS is captured in principle by the holographic boundary observer. In this paper, we have shown explicitly how such a complementarity may work for a class of cosmological crunches. We see that even such singularities in which an infinite amount of entropy flows into the crunch can be decoded by holographic observers, provided they are prepared to wait for a de Sitter eternity to complete the measurement. We have also shown that if in some way it turns out that dS spaces are not eternal [30], then these singularities will involve only finite entropy and will be regulated, as crunches in black holes are, by the system itself.

We have distilled these lessons from an analysis of certain negative-curvature FRW backgrounds with a crunching future endpoint and $O(d, 1)$ symmetry. By embedding these FRW cosmologies inside expanding AdS bubbles, one can view these backgrounds as the evolution of certain $O(d, 1)$-invariant states looking like Bose condensates of a perturbed CFT on de Sitter spacetime. The *same* quantum state can be codified in the Hilbert space of *another* perturbed CFT defined on a static Einstein spacetime. This alternative representation of the initial state uses the same basic CFT, but now perturbed by time-dependent couplings. These two descriptions of the initial state are related by a conformal transformation that we interpret as a 'complementarity map' in the sense in which this term is used in discussions of black hole information theory.

For those dS-invariant states whose bulk development has a crunch, and the condensate has a sharply defined energy scale, we argue that the E-frame (infalling) description consists of an infinite negative-energy fall, where the quantum state coherently shifts its support to the UV under the action of an unbounded Hamiltonian, either through an explicit time-dependent driving term or through an unbounded potential. We view this behavior, which we term the 'CFT fall', as the CFT landmark of a crunch. When transformed back into the dS-frame picture, the $O(d,1)$-invariant state is seen as a large-N master field for a dS-CFT perturbed by *sufficiently* negative-definite relevant or marginal operators.

As a peculiarity of the large-N limit, we can have semiclassical condensates that are very small compared with the Hubble scale. In this case, the form of the gravity solution shows similar qualitative behavior, although it is not possible to sharply trace the 'crunchy' character to the sign of the microscopic coupling. Still, if an effective Landau–Ginzburg description should exist in terms of a single collective field, it is expected to follow the general picture above.

The $O(d,1)$-invariant condensates that harbor crunches in their bulk description fall into two broad classes, depending on whether they are stable or unstable states in the deformed dS-CFT. In the first case, they give self-consistent holographic models for the crunch. In the second case, corresponding to bulk backgrounds with the interpretation of CdL bubbles, the dynamics is heavily corrected by finite-N effects involving multibubble nucleation and collisions, and even the quantum $1/N$ corrections pose a consistency challenge.

We have also investigated an explicit regularization of the CFT fall, introducing a hard UV wall with the manifest $U(1) \times O(d)$ symmetry of the E-frame theory. The $O(d,1)$ symmetry is then regarded as an accidental IR symmetry. Since the CFT fall transfers the support of the state to the UV, the reduced symmetry of the wall determines the long-time dynamics of the system, so that it approaches the generic state with $U(1) \times O(d)$ symmetry, i.e., a locally thermalized state, or a black hole in bulk parlance. Within this interpretation, the FRW crunch is regularized as the null 'backflow' of debris from the collision of the CFT state with the UV wall. Upon removal of the UV wall, it is the diverging energy of this back flow that produces the crunch. As a byproduct, this regularization establishes a direct relation between finiteness of the black hole entropy and the non-eternal character of the de Sitter state. At the same time, it shows that our 'cosmological complementarity map' can be regarded as a limit of the more standard, and yet more mysterious, black hole complementarity map.

Looking at our results in the large, it is tempting to promote the scenario depicted here to the rank of a general rule, namely, that the quantum description of spacelike singularities is always going to involve Hamiltonian 'falls', most likely of the 'stable' type, which seem well defined enough. This would apply strictly to the case in which an infinite-dimensional Hilbert space can 'fall into' a crunch or 'come from' a bang. For finite-entropy crunches/bangs, one expects any continuous-time Hamiltonian description to be at best approximate (cf. [31]).

At this point, we may ask: Who is afraid of singular Hamiltonians? The 'infalling' Hamiltonians described here act for a finite time and therefore *must* be singular. From the holographic point of view, it makes no sense to go beyond the crunch, and thus there is no need for the Hamiltonian description to be regular at $t = t_\star$. In any case, the examples discussed in this chapter show vividly how an infinite fall propagated by an unbounded Hamiltonian can be a valid 'history' of a completely regular state.

We have one state and two noncommuting operator algebras that measure it. In one operator algebra, described as a de Sitter-CFT, the 'history' is that of a stationary state, whereas in the other operator algebra, characterized as a driven Einstein-CFT, we have a singular Hamiltonian for a finite time. They are completely equivalent for the interval $-t_\star < t < t_\star$, and that is all we need, because there is nothing before the bang, and nothing after the crunch, just as there is nothing left outside the eternity of de Sitter.

Acknowledgments

We are indebted to T. Banks, R. Brustein, J. Martínez–Magán, and S. Shenker for useful discussions. We thank the Galileo Galilei Institute for hospitality. E. Rabinovici wishes to thank Stanford University for hospitality. The work of J. L. F. Barbón was partially supported by MEC and FEDER under a grant FPA2009-07908, the Spanish Consolider-Ingenio 2010 Programme CPAN (CSD2007-00042), and Comunidad Autónoma de Madrid under grant HEPHACOS S2009/ESP-1473. The work of E. Rabinovici was partially supported by the Humbodlt Foundation, a DIP grant H-52, the American–Israeli Bi-National Science Foundation, and the Israel Science Foundation Center of Excellence.

References

[1] S. R. Coleman and F. De Luccia, "Gravitational effects on and of vacuum decay," Phys. Rev. **D21**, 3305 (1980). L. F. Abbott and S. R. Coleman, "The collapse of an anti-de Sitter bubble," Nucl. Phys. **B259**, 170 (1985).

[2] J. L. F. Barbón and E. Rabinovici, "Holography of AdS vacuum bubbles," JHEP **1004**, 123 (2010) [arXiv:1003.4966 [hep-th]].

[3] L. Susskind, L. Thorlacius and J. Uglum, "The stretched horizon and black hole complementarity," Phys. Rev. **D48**, 3743 (1993) [arXiv:hep-th/9306069].

[4] T. Hertog and G. T. Horowitz, "Holographic description of AdS cosmologies," JHEP **0504**, 005 (2005) [arXiv:hep-th/0503071]. T. Hertog and G. T. Horowitz, "Towards a big crunch dual," JHEP **0407**, 073 (2004) [arXiv:hep-th/0406134].

[5] S. Elitzur, A. Giveon, M. Porrati, and E. Rabinovici, "Multitrace deformations of vector and adjoint theories and their holographic duals," JHEP **0602**, 006 (2006) [arXiv:hep-th/0511061]; Nucl. Phys. Proc. Suppl. **171**, 231 (2007).

[6] B. Craps, T. Hertog, and N. Turok, "Quantum resolution of cosmological singularities using AdS/CFT," arXiv:0712.4180 [hep-th]. N. Turok, B. Craps, and T. Hertog, "From Big Crunch to Big Bang with AdS/CFT," arXiv:0711.1824 [hep-th].

[7] S. Hawking, J. M. Maldacena, and A. Strominger, "DeSitter entropy, quantum entanglement and AdS/CFT," JHEP **0105**, 001 (2001) [arXiv:hep-th/0002145]. A. Buchel and A. A. Tseytlin, "Curved space resolution of singularity of fractional D3-branes on conifold," Phys. Rev. **D65**, 085019 (2002) [arXiv:hep-th/0111017]. A. Buchel, P. Langfelder, and J. Walcher, "Does the tachyon matter?" Ann. Phys. (NY) **302**, 78 (2002) [arXiv:hep-th/0207235]. A. Buchel, "Gauge/gravity

correspondence in accelerating universe," Phys. Rev. **D65**, 125015 (2002) [arXiv:hep-th/0203041]. A. Buchel, P. Langfelder, and J. Walcher, "On time-dependent backgrounds in supergravity and string theory," Phys. Rev. **D67**, 024011 (2003) [arXiv:hep-th/0207214]. T. Hirayama, "A holographic dual of CFT with flavor on de Sitter space," JHEP **0606**, 013 (2006) [arXiv:hep-th/0602258]. M. Alishahiha, A. Karch, E. Silverstein, and D. Tong, "The dS/dS correspondence," AIP Conf. Proc. **743**, 393 (2005) [arXiv:hep-th/0407125]. A. Buchel, "Inflation on the resolved warped deformed conifold," Phys. Rev. **D74**, 046009 (2006) [arXiv:hep-th/0601013]. O. Aharony, M. Fabinger, G. T. Horowitz, and E. Silverstein, "Clean time-dependent string backgrounds from bubble baths," JHEP **0207**, 007 (2002) [arXiv:hep-th/0204158]. V. Balasubramanian and S. F. Ross, "The dual of nothing," Phys. Rev. **D66**, 086002 (2002) [arXiv:hep-th/0205290]. S. F. Ross and G. Titchener, "Time-dependent spacetimes in AdS/CFT: bubble and black hole," JHEP **0502**, 021 (2005) [arXiv:hep-th/0411128]. R. G. Cai, "Constant curvature black hole and dual field theory," Phys. Lett. **B544**, 176 (2002) [arXiv:hep-th/0206223]. V. Balasubramanian, K. Larjo, and J. Simon, "Much ado about nothing," Class. Quant. Grav. **22**, 4149 (2005) [arXiv:hep-th/0502111]. J. He and M. Rozali, "On bubbles of nothing in AdS/CFT," JHEP **0709**, 089 (2007) [arXiv:hep-th/0703220]. J. A. Hutasoit, S. P. Kumar, and J. Rafferty, "Real time response on dS_3: the topological AdS black hole and the bubble," JHEP **0904**, 063 (2009) [arXiv:0902.1658 [hep-th]].

 [8] D. Marolf, M. Rangamani, and M. Van Raamsdonk, "Holographic models of de Sitter QFTs," arXiv:1007.3996 [hep-th].

 [9] J. Maldacena, "Vacuum decay into anti de Sitter space," arXiv:1012.0274 [hep-th].

[10] J. B. Hartle and S. W. Hawking, "Wave function of the universe," Phys. Rev. **D28**, 2960 (1983).

[11] J. M. Maldacena, "The large N limit of superconformal field theories and supergravity," Adv. Theor. Math. Phys. **2**, 231 (1998) [Int. J. Theor. Phys. **38**, 1113 (1999)] [arXiv:hep-th/9711200]. S. S. Gubser, I. R. Klebanov, and A. M. Polyakov, "Gauge theory correlators from non-critical string theory," Phys. Lett. **B428**, 105 (1998) [arXiv:hep-th/9802109]. E. Witten, "Anti-de Sitter space and holography," Adv. Theor. Math. Phys. **2**, 253 (1998) [arXiv:hep-th/9802150].

[12] P. Breitenlohner and D. Z. Freedman, "Stability in gauged extended supergravity," Ann. Phys. (NY) **144**, 249 (1982). P. Breitenlohner and D. Z. Freedman, "Positive energy In anti-de Sitter backgrounds and gauged extended supergravity," Phys. Lett. **B115**, 197 (1982).

[13] E. Witten, "Instability of the Kaluza–Klein vacuum," Nucl. Phys. **B195**, 481 (1982).

[14] T. Banks, "Heretics of the false vacuum: gravitational effects on and of vacuum decay. II," arXiv:hep-th/0211160. T. Banks, "Landskepticism or why effective potentials don't count string models," arXiv:hep-th/0412129. T. Banks, "TASI Lectures on Holographic Space-Time, SUSY and Gravitational Effective Field Theory," arXiv:1007.4001 [hep-th].

[15] G. Horowitz, A. Lawrence, and E. Silverstein, "Insightful D-branes," JHEP **0907**, 057 (2009) [arXiv:0904.3922 [hep-th]].

[16] D. Harlow, "Metastability in anti de Sitter space," arXiv:1003.5909 [hep-th].

[17] D. Harlow and L. Susskind, "Crunches, hats, and a conjecture," arXiv:1012.5302 [hep-th].

[18] V. Asnin, E. Rabinovici, and M. Smolkin, "On rolling, tunneling and decaying in some large N vector models," JHEP **0908**, 001 (2009) [arXiv:0905.3526 [hep-th]].

[19] W. Israel, "Singular hypersurfaces and thin shells in general relativity," Nuovo Cim. (Ser. 10) **B44**, 1 (1966) [Erratum **B48**, 463].

[20] S. K. Blau, E. I. Guendelman, and A. H. Guth, "The dynamics of false vacuum bubbles," Phys. Rev. **D35**, 1747 (1987). G. L. Alberghi, D. A. Lowe, and M. Trodden, "Charged false vacuum bubbles and the AdS/CFT correspondence," JHEP **9907**, 020 (1999) [arXiv:hep-th/9906047]. B. Freivogel, V. E. Hubeny, A. Maloney, R. C. Myers, M. Rangamani, and S. Shenker, "Inflation in AdS/CFT," JHEP **0603**, 007 (2006) [arXiv:hep-th/0510046].

[21] N. Seiberg and E. Witten, "The D1/D5 system and singular CFT," JHEP **9904**, 017 (1999) [arXiv:hep-th/9903224].

[22] S. Fubini, "A new approach to conformal invariant field theories," Nuovo Cim. **A34**, 521 (1976).

[23] S. de Haro and A. C. Petkou, "Instantons and conformal holography," JHEP **0612**, 076 (2006) [arXiv:hep-th/0606276]. S. de Haro, I. Papadimitriou, and A. C. Petkou, "Conformally coupled scalars, instantons and vacuum instability in AdS_4," Phys. Rev. Lett. **98**, 231601 (2007) [arXiv:hep-th/0611315]. I. Papadimitriou, "Multi-trace deformations in AdS/CFT: exploring the vacuum structure of the deformed CFT," JHEP **0705**, 075 (2007) [arXiv:hep-th/0703152].

[24] A. Bernamonti and B. Craps, "D-brane potentials from multi-trace deformations in AdS/CFT," JHEP **0908**, 112 (2009) [arXiv:0907.0889 [hep-th]].

[25] J. L. F. Barbón and J. Martínez-Magán, "Spontaneous fragmentation of topological black holes," JHEP **1008**, 031 (2010) [arXiv:1005.4439 [hep-th]].

[26] E. Witten, "Multi-trace operators, boundary conditions, and AdS/CFT correspondence," arXiv:hep-th/0112258. M. Berkooz, A. Sever, and A. Shomer, "Double-trace deformations, boundary conditions and spacetime singularities," JHEP **0205**, 034 (2002) [arXiv:hep-th/0112264].

[27] O. Aharony, B. Kol, and S. Yankielowicz, "On exactly marginal deformations of $N = 4$ SYM and type IIB supergravity on $AdS_5 \times S^5$," JHEP **0206**, 039 (2002) [arXiv:hep-th/0205090].

[28] L. Kofman, "Tachyonic preheating," arXiv:hep-ph/0107280.

[29] L. Battarra and T. Hertog, "Particle production near an AdS crunch," JHEP **1012**, 017 (2010) [arXiv:1009.0992 [hep-th]].

[30] A. M. Polyakov, "Decay of vacuum energy," Nucl. Phys. **B834**, 316 (2010) [arXiv:0912.5503 [hep-th]].

[31] T. Banks and W. Fischler, "Space-like singularities and thermalization," arXiv:hep-th/0606260. T. Banks, "Pedagogical notes on black holes, de Sitter space, and bifurcated horizons," arXiv:1007.4003 [hep-th].

High-energy collisions of particles, strings, and branes

Gabriele VENEZIANO

Collège de France, Paris, France, and
Theory Division CERN, Geneva, Switzerland

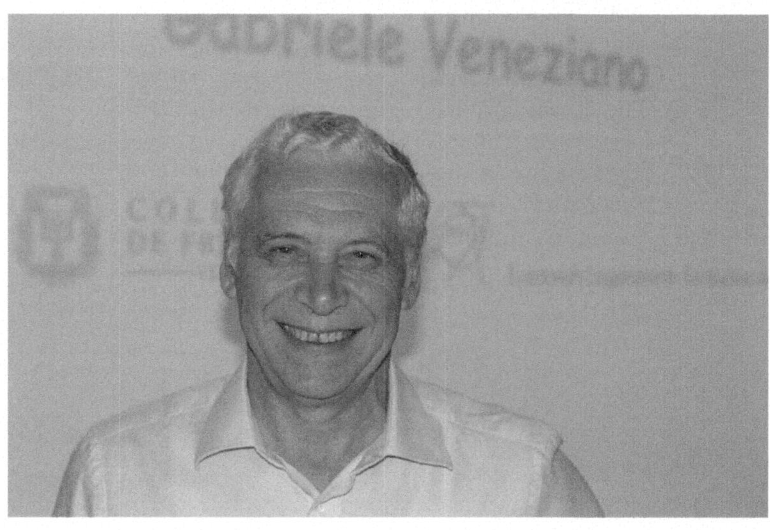

Theoretical Physics to Face the Challenge of LHC. Edited by L. Baulieu, K. Benakli, M. R. Douglas, B. Mansoulié, E. Rabinovici, and L. F. Cugliandolo. © Oxford University Press 2015. Published in 2015 by Oxford University Press.

Chapter Contents

We summarize some 25 years of work on the transplanckian-energy collisions of particles, strings, and branes, seen as a theoretical laboratory for understanding how gravity and quantum mechanics can be consistently combined in string theory. The ultimate aim of the exercise is to understand whether and how a consistent quantization of gravity can solve some long-standing paradoxes, such as the apparent loss of information in the production and decay of black holes at a semiclassical level.

Considerable progress has been made in understanding the emergence of General Relativity expectations and in evaluating several kinds of quantum string corrections to them in the weak-gravity regime while keeping unitarity manifest. While some progress has also been made in the strong-gravity/gravitational collapse domain, full control of how unitarity works in that regime is still lacking.

17.1 Motivations and outline

Progress in fundamental physics has often been based on stepping up in energy, either experimentally or through theoretical (gedanken) experiments. The realization, for instance, that a theory of the weak interactions based on fundamental massive vector particles would violate unitarity at very (and at the time unrealistically) high energies was one of the ingredients that led eventually to the idea of spontaneous symmetry breaking and to the present electroweak standard model.

When dealing with candidate theories of quantum gravity, the need for very (unrealistically?) high energies is even more obvious. Indeed, while classical gravity—or classical string theory—has no intrinsic energy scale, quantum and string gravity do: the Planck mass M_P and the string mass scale M_s, respectively. Both are presumably too high for real experiments, except for those that presumably occurred naturally in the early universe.

In this chapter, we will use very high (i.e. transplanckian) energy to expose in a clear way some of the deep conceptual problems that seem to emerge when one tries to combine the basic principles of General Relativity with those of Quantum Mechanics, the two great revolutions that took place in physics about a century ago.

The issue of a possible loss of information/quantum coherence in processes where a black hole is produced and then evaporates has been the subject of much debate since Hawking's observation [1] that black holes should emit an exactly thermal spectrum of light particles, known as Hawking radiation. Progress coming from string theory, in particular on the microscopic understanding of black hole entropy [2] and on the AdS/CFT correspondence [3], have lent strong support [4] to the "no-information-loss" camp. In spite of these developments, several issues still remain unclear. One would like to understand, for instance, how exactly information is retrieved and what this implies on the properties of the *pure* final state that a given *pure* initial state generates through its unitary evolution.

There is a second, less fundamental but phenomenologically interesting, reason for studying high-energy collisions. Models have been proposed [5] in which gravity, being sensitive to some "large" extra dimensions of space, becomes strong at an effective energy scale M_D that is much smaller than the "phenomenological" four-dimensional

Planck energy $M_P \sim 10^{19}$ GeV. Assuming M_D to be not too far from the few TeV scale, a variety of interesting strong-gravity signals could be expected [6] when the LHC turns on.

We will start by recalling briefly some well-known results on gravitational collapse criteria in classical General Relativity (CGR). When naively applied to our collision problem, they lead naturally to a two-dimensional "phase diagram" with a "phase transition" curve separating a "dispersion" region from a "collapse" one. Furthermore, the dispersion region can be divided into two subregions depending on the relative sizes of the impact parameter b and the string length l_s. These two subregions will then be discussed, in succession, and an explicitly unitary ansatz for the S-matrix will be presented.

We will then present the first serious attempt to move into the collapse region of parameter space. Here success is much more limited, in particular in what concerns control of inelastic unitarity. Finally, we will turn our attention to a supposedly simpler problem, that of the high-energy scattering of a light closed string off a stack of D-branes, describe analogies and differences with respect to the previous problem, and present the progress made so far. We shall conclude with a brief summary and outlook.

17.2   Gravitational collapse criteria: a brief review

There are many analytic as well as numerical CGR results on whether some given initial data should lead to gravitational collapse or to a completely dispersed final state. The two phases would be typically separated by a critical hypersurface in the parameter space of the initial states. The problem has some amusing analogies with the physics of phase transitions in statistical systems. In fact, the approach to criticality resembles that of phase transitions (the order of the transition and critical exponents can be defined by analogy).

For pure gravity, in a classic work, Christodoulou and Klainerman [7] have found a finite-measure parameter-space region bordering Minkowski spacetime and lying on the dispersion side of the critical surface. In the case of spherical symmetry, regions on the collapse side have been found, analytically by Christodoulou [8] and numerically by Choptuik and collaborators [9].

In the absence of any special symmetry, Christodoulou [10] has identified another collapse-bound region. It is characterized by a lower bound on incoming energy per unit advanced time holding uniformly over the full solid angle. More precisely, denote by $\mu(v, \theta, \phi)$ the incoming (null) energy per unit advanced time v and solid angle $d\Omega$ entering the system during a "short" interval $\delta \equiv \delta v$. Then, if

$$M(\theta, \phi, \delta) \equiv \int_0^\delta dv\, \mu(v, \theta, \phi) > \frac{k}{8\pi}, \qquad (17.2.1)$$

a closed trapped surface (CTS) forms with a Schwarzschild radius $R_S > k - O(\delta) > 0$.

Unfortunately, such a beautiful criterion is not useful for two-body collisions, the energy being concentrated in two narrow back-to-back cones, but the general idea of the method still applies. This consists in the identification of a CTS at a certain point in the system's evolution. It should be stressed that such criteria can only be of the sufficiency type. Identification of a CTS guarantees collapse, whereas the opposite situation does not lead to any firm conclusion, since it can be the result of one's inability to follow the evolution of the system for sufficiently long times.

Examples of criteria that can be established in the case of two-body collisions are as follows:

- Point-particle collisions:
  - $b = 0$: For a head-on collision of pointlike massless particles, Penrose [11] has argued that there is a lower bound on the fraction of the incoming energy that goes into forming a black hole:

$$M_{\mathrm{BH}} > E/\sqrt{2} \sim 0.71\sqrt{s}\,. \tag{17.2.2}$$

  - $b \neq 0$: Eardley and Giddings [12] have generalized the above result to a collision at a generic impact parameter b. One example in $D = 4$ is

$$\left(\frac{R_S}{b}\right)_{\mathrm{cr}} \leq 1.25 \quad (R_S \equiv 2G\sqrt{s})\,. \tag{17.2.3}$$

- The Eardley and Giddings approach was generalized further to extended sources in [13]. One example is the central collision of two homogeneous null discs of radius L, where one finds

$$\left(\frac{R_S}{L}\right)_{\mathrm{cr}} \leq 1\,. \tag{17.2.4}$$

Finally, we should mention that Choptuik and Pretorius [14] have obtained new numerical results for a highly relativistic axisymmetric situation (their results will be compared with ours in Section 17.6).

So far, our considerations have been purely classical. What happens when we go from the classical to the quantum problem? We can certainly prepare pure initial states that correspond, roughly, to the classical data by specifying the centre-of-mass energy $\sqrt{s}$ of the collision and, instead of the impact parameter, the total angular momentum $J \sim bE$. We can then ask several interesting questions:

- Does a unitary S-matrix (evolution operator) always describe the evolution of the system?
- If so, does such an S-matrix develop singularities as one approaches a critical (parameter-space) surface?
- If so, what happens in its vicinity? Does the nature of the final state change as one goes through it?
- Is there a relation between the classical and quantum critical surfaces?
- What happens to the final state deep inside the collapse region? Does it resemble at all Hawking's thermal spectrum for each initial pure state?

All these questions are obviously related to the information paradox/puzzle.

As already mentioned, there can be more phenomenological motivations for studying transplanckian-energy (TPE) collisions, i.e. finding signatures of string/quantum gravity at the LHC. This is in principle possible in Kaluza–Klein models with large extra dimensions, in brane-world scenarios, and in general if the true quantum gravity scale can be lowered to the TeV scale. However, even in the most optimistic situation, the LHC will be quite marginal for producing black holes, let alone semiclassical ones. The question then is this:

- Can there be some precursors of BH behaviour even below the expected black hole-production threshold?

Perhaps surprisingly, the answer will turn out to be positive.

TPE string collisions represent a perfect theoretical laboratory for studying these questions within a framework that claims to be a fully consistent quantum theory of gravity. We can hardly imagine a simpler pure initial state that could lead to black hole formation and whose unitary evolution we would like to understand/follow. TPE is obviously need in order to have a chance of forming (and studying) a semiclassical black hole, i.e. one with $R_S \gg l_P$. As it turns out, TPE also simplifies the theoretical analysis by allowing the use of some semiclassical approximation.

17.3   The expected phase diagram

Collisions of light particles at superplanckian energies ($E = \sqrt{s} \gg M_D$) have received considerable attention since the late 1980s. While in [15, 16] the focus was on $D = 4$ collisions in the field theory limit, two groups have carried out the analysis within superstring theory, possibly allowing for a number of "large" extra dimensions. In the approach due to Gross, Mende, and Ooguri (GMO) [17], one starts from a genus-by-genus analysis of fixed-angle scattering, and then attempts an all-genus resummation. In the work by Amati, Ciafaloni, and myself (ACV) [18–20], one starts from an all-order eikonal description of small-angle scattering and then attempts to push the results towards larger and larger angles. In the approach by Fabbrichesi et al. [21], one relates, at arbitrary scattering angle, the semiclassical S-matrix to a boundary term and tries to estimate it in terms of classical solutions.

The picture that has emerged (see e.g. [22] for some reviews) is best explained by working in impact parameter ($b = 2J/E$) space, rather than in scattering angle (θ) or momentum transfer. We can thus represent the various regimes of superplanckian collisions by appealing to an (E, b) plane or, equivalently but more conveniently, to an (R_S, b) plane, where[1]

$$R_S(E) \sim (G_D E)^{1/(D-3)} \tag{17.3.1}$$

is the Schwarzschild radius associated with the centre-of-mass energy E. Since both coordinates in this plane are lengths, we can also mark on its axes two (process-independent) lengths: the Planck length l_D and the string length l_s. We shall use the following definitions:

---

[1] We shall denote by G_D the D-dimensional Newton constant and simply by G the four-dimensional one.

$$l_s = \sqrt{2\alpha'\hbar} = M_s^{-1}, \quad G_D = l_D^{D-2} = M_D^{2-D}, \tag{17.3.2}$$

where α' is the open-string Regge-slope parameter (equal to twice that of the closed string). We will assume string theory to be (very) weakly coupled:

$$l_s = (g_s)^{-2/(D-2)} l_D \gg l_D, \quad \text{i.e.} \, M_D = M_s(g_s)^{-2/(D-2)} \gg M_s, \tag{17.3.3}$$

where g_s is the string coupling constant. We shall keep g_s (and hence $l_D/l_s = M_s/M_D$) fixed and very small.

By definition of transplanckian energy, $R_S > l_D$. Since we also restrict ourselves to $b > l_D$, a small square near the origin is not considered. The rest of the diagram is divided essentially into three regions (see Fig. 17.1):

- The first region, characterized by $b > \max(l_s, R_S)$, is the easiest to analyse and corresponds to small-angle quasi-elastic scattering.
- The second region, $R_S > \max(b, l_s)$, is the most difficult: this is where we expect black hole formation to show up. Unfortunately, in spite of much effort (see e.g. [20, 21, 23]), not much progress has been achieved in the way of going through the $b = R_S > l_s$ boundary of Fig. 17.1.
- Finally, the third region $(b, R_S < l_s)$, whose very existence depends on working in a string theory framework, has provided some very interesting insight [19] into how string effects may modify classical and quantum gravity expectations once the string scale is approached. The reason why progress could be made by ACV in this regime, unlike in the previous one, is that string-size effects intervene *before* large classical corrections make the problem intractable as $b \to R_S$. The physical reason for this is that string-size effects prevent the formation of a putative black

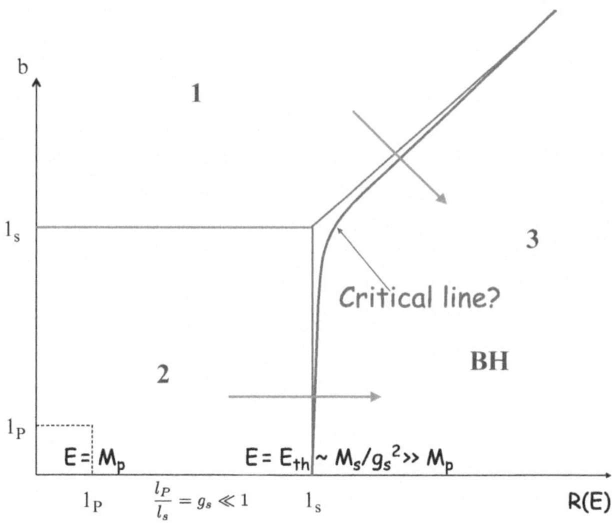

Fig. 17.1 Phase diagram of transplanckian scattering showing three different kinematic regions and two different paths towards the regime of large black hole production. Here $l_P = l_D$.

hole whose radius would be smaller than l_s. Instead, it is found [19] that a maximal deflection angle $\theta_{\max} \sim (R_S/l_s)^{D-3}$ is reached at an impact parameter of order l_s (for which the colliding strings graze each other). If one considers scattering at angles larger than such $\theta_{\max}$, one finds (see, e.g., [22]) an exponential suppression of the cross section, in very good agreement with the results obtained by GMO [17] through their very different approach. This region merges into the previous one at $R_S \sim l_s$, corresponding to the expected energy threshold for black hole production at $E = E_{\rm th} \sim g_s^{-2} M_s$, in agreement with the so-called correspondence [24, 25] between black holes and fundamental strings.

17.4　The small-angle regime: deflection angle and tidal excitation

General arguments, as well as explicit calculations, suggest the following form for the elastic S-matrix at TPE:

$$S(E,b) \sim \exp\left(i\frac{A_{cl}}{\hbar}\right) \equiv e^{2i\delta(E,M,b)},$$

$$\delta(E,M,b) = \frac{G_D s}{\hbar}\frac{b^{4-D}}{\Omega_{D-4}}\left[1 + O\left(\left(\frac{R_S}{b}\right)^{2(D-3)}\right) + O\left(\frac{\lambda_s^2}{b^2}\right) + O\left(\frac{\lambda_P^{D-2}}{b^{D-2}}\right) + \cdots\right],$$

$$R_S^{D-3} = \frac{16\pi G_D \sqrt{s}}{(D-2)\Omega_{D-1}}, \quad \Omega_d \equiv \frac{2\pi^{d/2}}{\Gamma(d/2)}. \tag{17.4.1}$$

Here we have written explicitly the leading term at large b, followed by "corrections" that are controlled either by the ratio l_s/b (so-called string corrections) or by the ratio R_S/b (so-called classical corrections), while corrections proportional to the Planck length are systematically ignored for the reasons already mentioned. The first kind of corrections will be discussed here; the second kind will be discussed in Section 17.6.

Note, however, that both kinds of corrections may become relevant even when the corresponding ratio is still very small. The reason is that, unlike the leading term, corrections are not necessarily real. Whenever they contain an imaginary part, the resulting damping of the elastic S-matrix becomes important as soon as the overall quantity in the exponent (including the large pre-factor) becomes of order one.

17.4.1　The point-particle limit at large b

This regime can be described by resumming the leading-eikonal field theoretical diagrams (crossed ladders included). This restores elastic unitarity since the large partial-wave amplitude, by exponentiation, becomes a harmless rapidly varying phase. This fact can actually be used to justify a saddle-point approximation when we transform back the S-matrix from impact parameter to (centre-of-mass) scattering angle (or momentum transfer q) space.

The position of the saddle point is given by

$$b_s^{D-3} = \frac{8\pi G_D \sqrt{s}}{\theta\,\Omega_{D-2}} \sim \frac{R_S^{D-3}}{\theta}, \tag{17.4.2}$$

and can be seen as the generalization of Einstein's deflection formula for ultrarelativistic collisions and extended to arbitrary D. It corresponds precisely to the relation between impact parameter and deflection angle in the (Aichelburg–Sexl) metric [26] generated by a relativistic point-particle of energy E. Note that this effective metric is not put in by hand: it is an "emergent" semiclassical metric generating the expected deflection.

We conclude the discussion of this regime with the following important remark: high-q_T is not necessarily short-distance in high-energy gravitational scattering! Indeed, as can be seen from (17.4.2), at fixed θ, larger E probes larger b. The reason is simple: because of the eikonal exponentiation, $G_D s b^{4-D}/\hbar$ also gives the average/dominant loop number. The total momentum transfer $q \sim \theta E$ is thus shared among $O(s \sim E^2)$ exchanged gravitons to give

$$q_{\text{ind}} \sim \frac{\hbar q b^{D-4}}{G_D s} \sim \frac{\hbar\theta}{b}(R/b)^{3-D} \sim \frac{\hbar}{b_s}, \tag{17.4.3}$$

thus recovering the uncertainly-principle relation and the conclusion that the process is soft, even at large q, provided that b is sufficiently large.

17.4.2 String corrections at large b

Even at large b, graviton exchange can excite one or both strings. The physical reason [27] is that a string moving in a nontrivial metric feels tidal forces as a result of its finite size. A simple argument gives the critical impact parameter b_t below which this tidal excitation phenomenon kicks in (in agreement with what was found by direct calculation by ACV!). It is indeed parametrically larger than l_s:

$$b_t \sim \left(\frac{G_D s l_s^2}{\hbar}\right)^{1/(D-2)}. \tag{17.4.4}$$

These effects are neatly captured, at the leading eikonal level, by replacing the impact parameter b by a shifted impact parameter, displayed by each string's position operator (stripped of its zero modes) evaluated at $\tau = 0$ (equal to the collision time) and averaged over σ. This leads to a unitary operator eikonal formula for the S-matrix:

$$S(E,b) \to \hat{S}(E,b) = \exp[2i\langle\delta(E, b - X_u + X_d)\rangle], \tag{17.4.5}$$

where

$$\langle\delta(E, b - X_u + X_d)\rangle \equiv \frac{1}{4\pi^2} \int_0^{2\pi} d\sigma_u \int_0^{2\pi} d\sigma_d\, :\delta\left(b + \hat{X}_d(\sigma_d, 0) - \hat{X}_u(\sigma_u, 0)\right): \tag{17.4.6}$$

Several quantities can be computed from this general formula—for instance the mass distribution of the excited strings. One finds [18] that such a distribution grows roughly like the density of string states (i.e. exponentially) up to a certain maximal excitation mass ($M_{\max} \sim G_D s l_s b^{2-D}$) and then sharply cuts off.

Also, in order to conserve probability, the cross section for each exclusive process (including the elastic one) is exponentially damped. For instance,

$$\sigma_{\rm el} \sim \exp(-G_D s \lambda_s^2 b^{2-D}). \tag{17.4.7}$$

In other words, the whole process of tidal excitations produces a sort of statistical (though nonthermal) ensemble of final states, while strictly maintaining quantum coherence.

17.5 The string-gravity regime: a precocious black hole behaviour?

Because of (good old Dolen–Horn–Schmit) duality, even single-graviton exchange does not give a real scattering amplitude. The imaginary part is due to formation of closed strings in the s-channel. Since the imaginary part of the tree amplitude lacks the Coulomb singularity, it is exponentially damped at large impact parameter. This is why this contribution is irrelevant in region I but important in region III.

The average number of closed strings produced is given by the average number of cut gravi-reggeons according to the AGK cutting rules [28] (see [29] for details). This is still given by the eikonal phase, but this time by its imaginary part:

$$\langle N_{\rm CGR}\rangle = 4\,{\rm Im}\,\delta = \frac{G_D s l_s^2}{(Y\lambda_s)^{D-2}} = O\left(\frac{s}{M_*^2}\right), \tag{17.5.1}$$

where $M_* \sim M_s/g_s \sim \sqrt{M_s M_{\rm th}}$ will turn out to play an important role in the following. Note that M_* coincides, up to numerical factors, with the mass of D0-branes (see e.g. [30]), possibly just as a coincidence.

If we forbid particle production, we are again penalized by an exponential factor. For instance, the elastic cross section is damped as

$$\sigma_{\rm el} \sim \exp(-8\,{\rm Im}\,\delta) = \exp\left[-\frac{G_D s l_s^2}{(Y l_s)^{D-2}}\right]. \tag{17.5.2}$$

Amusingly, such a suppression (which coincides with (17.4.7) at $b \sim l_s$) resembles a statistical factor $\exp(-S_{\rm bh})$, where $S_{\rm bh}$ is the Bekenstein–Hawking entropy of a black hole of mass $\sqrt{s}$. Such a suppression is known to appear in the elastic amplitude for the scattering of a particle off a classical black hole when the impact parameter goes below that of classical capture (see e.g. [31]). For $D = 4$ the agreement holds up to a numerical factor, while for $D > 4$ the functional dependence is different. For any value of D, however, agreement with a black-hole-type suppression holds (up to factors $O(1)$) as one approaches $E_{\rm th}$.

Let us now look instead at the typical final state that roughly saturates the cross section. The total energy will be shared among N_{CGR} CGRs, giving an average energy per CGR:

$$\langle E \rangle_{\text{CGR}} = \frac{\sqrt{s}}{\langle N_{\text{CGR}} \rangle} \sim \frac{M_*^2}{\sqrt{s}}. \tag{17.5.3}$$

The average energy of the final states thus *decreases* as the energy is *increased* within our window. This is quite unlike what one is accustomed to in particle physics, but is similar to what we expect in black hole physics! Once more, for $D = 4$ the functional dependence on $\sqrt{s}$ of $\langle E \rangle_{\text{CGR}}$ follows that of a thermal spectrum with a Hawking temperature $T_H \sim \hbar/R_S$, while for $D > 4$ the functional dependence is different. For all values of D, however, agreement (up to factors $O(1)$) with Hawking temperature expectations occurs at E_{th}. An "antiscaling" behaviour, corresponding to

$$\langle E \rangle_{\text{CGR}} \sqrt{s} = M_*^2 = M_s^2 g_s^{-2}, \tag{17.5.4}$$

holds [32] for any D in the energy window $M_* < E < E_{\text{th}} = g_s^{-2} M_s$.

An interesting signature even below the actual threshold of black hole production!

17.6 The strong-gravity regime: towards the large-angle/collapse phase?

We shall now address the more difficult question of how to deal with what we called classical corrections, those characterized by the expansion parameter $(R/b)^{2(D-3)}$ and which become important when the scattering angle becomes $O(1)$. It was understood quite early on [20] that these corrections are associated with (the resummation of) a particular class of diagrams, those in which the gravitons exchanged between the two fast-moving particles only interact (if at all) at tree level. It is of course not unexpected that classical corrections are related to tree diagrams, but in our context we have to be precise about the meaning of a "tree diagram". In the following discussion, we shall limit ourselves to the point-particle limit and to $D = 4$. While the second limitation looks easy to dispose of (actually, some of the infrared problems we shall encounter disappear for $D > 4$), the first limitation is hard to circumvent. Ideally, one would like to find, for the classical corrections, a simple recipe, like that of (17.4.5), for taking the string-size corrections into account. No such a generalization has been found so far.

Standard reasoning strongly suggests that the sum of all (connected and disconnected once the external lines are removed) diagrams simply gives the exponential of the connected diagrams, the latter therefore being directly related to the phase of the semiclassical S-matrix. Power counting confirms this assumption. If n gravitons are exchanged and interact with a connected tree, we find

$$A_{\text{cl}}(E, b) \sim G^{2n-1} s^n \sim G s R^{2(n-1)} \to G s (R/b)^{2(n-1)}, \tag{17.6.1}$$

which is the expected scaling for $D = 4$.

Summing tree diagrams should amount to solving a classical field theory, and the question therefore is: Which is the effective field theory describing transplanckian scattering? There is actually a good candidate for it: the effective action proposed long ago by Lipatov [33]. Unfortunately, this is still too complicated to attempt any kind of (analytic or numerical) solution.

In [23], ACV proposed a simplified version of Lipatov's action in which the longitudinal dynamics is frozen and factored out. One is then left with a much more manageable $D = 2$ effective action (corresponding to the coordinates transverse to the collision axis) containing four fields: the $++$ and $--$ components of the metric, sourced by the energy–momentum tensor of the two fast particles, together with a complex field ϕ representing the two physical polarizations of physical gravitons. In $D = 4$, one polarization is affected by infrared divergences, which in principle can be cured by considering infrared-safe observables, but will be actually neglected for the sake of simplicity. Thus, the complex scalar field gets replaced by a real one, for a total of three real fields. The action, for whose explicit form we refer to [23], contains up to four derivatives but is otherwise nice looking. Its equations of motion are rather simple and admit a perturbative expansion in our "small" parameter R_S/b.

The semiclassical approximation amounts to solving the equations of motion and to computing the classical action on the solution after imposing suitable boundary, reality, and regularity conditions on it [23]. The resulting problem is still too hard for analytic study, but can be dealt with numerically. In an impressive paper, Marchesini and Onofri [34] managed to solve directly the resulting partial differential equations (PDEs) by fast Fourier transform methods and concluded that real, regular solutions only exist if

$$b > b_c \sim 2.28 R_S \,, \tag{17.6.2}$$

to be compared with the CTS lower bound of [12] $b_c > 0.80 R_S$. Thus the "ACV value" for b_c is a factor 2.85 or so above the CTS lower bound by Eardley and Giddings.

For an analytic approach, we have to turn to an even simpler problem: axisymmetric beam–beam collisions [23, 35]. The data in this case lie in two functions, $R_1(r), R_2(r)$, that correspond to the gravitational radii associated with the centre-of-mass energy in each beam below a distance r from the symmetry axis. This is a simpler, yet rich, problem, for several reasons:

- The sources contain several parameters, and we can look for critical surfaces in their multidimensional space.
- The CTS criterion is simple (see below).
- Numerical results are coming in (see e.g. [14]).
- The "bad" infrared-singular polarization is not produced.
- Last but not least: PDEs become ODEs.

Here we give a short account of the main results obtained in this problem [35]:

- *ACV versus CTS criterion—some general results:*

1. The criterion for the existence of a CTS in the case of axisymmetric beam–beam collisions reads as follows [13]: if there exists an r_c such that

$$R_1(r_c)R_2(r_c) = r_c^2\,, \tag{17.6.3}$$

then we can construct a CTS, and therefore a black hole must form. In [35], the following theorem was proved:
   - *Whenever the Kohlprath–Veneziano criterion (17.6.3) holds, the ACV field equations do not admit regular real solutions.*
   Thus the CTS criterion implies the one based on the ACV equations, but not necessarily the other way around!
2. At the opposite end, a sufficient criterion for the existence ACV can be given:[2] if the inequality

$$\frac{R_1(r)R_2(r)}{R^2} \leq \frac{4r^4}{(3R^2 + 2r^2)^2}\left[1 - \frac{R^2}{2r^2}\log\left(1 + \frac{2r^2}{3R^2}\right)\right]^2 \tag{17.6.4}$$

   holds at all r, then the ACV equations admit regular, real solutions.
- *Three particular examples:*
   1. Particle scattering off a ring-shaped beam with all the energy concentrated at $r = b$ (thus $R_2(r) = R\,\theta(r - b)$). This case can be dealt with analytically, since it leads to a simple cubic equation that has real solutions if and only if

$$b^2 > \frac{3\sqrt{3}}{2}R_S^2 \equiv b_c^2\,. \tag{17.6.5}$$

   Thus we find $(b/R_S)_c \sim 1.61$, to be compared with the CTS prediction [13] $(b/R_S)_c \geq 1$.
   The following two examples can be solved numerically with Mathematica:
   2. The collision of two homogeneous beams of radius L. One finds

$$\left(\frac{R_S}{L}\right)_c \sim 0.47, \quad \text{while} \quad \left(\frac{R_S}{L}\right)_c^{\text{CTS}} < 1.0\,. \tag{17.6.6}$$

   3. Two beams having a Gaussian profile of width L. Here our L_c turns out to be a factor of about 2.70 above the CTS lower bound.

In conclusion, while the ACV-based results are never in contradiction—and even in qualitative agreement with—those based on the CTS criterion, there is typically a factor of 2–3 discrepancy between them. This could be due either to our rough approximations or to the CTS criteria being too loose (or to a combination of both).

An amusing coincidence appears to point in this latter direction. In an interesting paper, Choptuik and Pretorius [14] analysed a "similar" situation numerically (the relativistic central collision of two solitons of fixed mass and transverse size). They found black hole formation to occur at a critical Lorentz boost parameter γ_c (i.e.

---

[2] P.-L. Lions, private communication.

basically R_c) that is a factor 2–3 below the naive CTS value (but still in the relativistic regime where a connection to our process is possibly justified).

The conclusions that can be drawn on string–string collisions in the strong-gravity regime can be summarized by saying that the above results are encouraging (even better than one could have expected), but also that real control over the different approximations is lacking, in particular on the freezing of longitudinal dynamics. This is probably at the origin of some puzzles we find[3] in connection with gravitational radiation at $b \gg R$. It seems that the fraction of incoming energy getting lost in gravitational radiation becomes $O(1)$ already in the small-angle regime. Unfortunately, this is a regime in which there appears to be no reliable general relativistic calculation.

An even bigger problem is an apparent violation of unitarity in this regime. Since the solution is no longer real below b_c, a new elastic-unitarity deficit appears, which, unlike the previous ones (related to the opening of identified inelastic channels), has no simple physical interpretation.[4] Recent work [36] suggests that, perhaps, one should not use regular complex solutions below b_c, but rather stick to the reality of the solution, abandoning the constraint of regularity at $r = 0$. As a consequence, the action computed on the solution blows up (because of the above singularity) for $b < b_c$ and one would have to invoke short-distance (string?) corrections in order to restore unitarity, something not totally unreasonable, after all.

17.7   High-energy string–brane collisions: an easier problem?

In order to make some progress on the small-b regime, we have recently turned our attention to a hopefully easier problem: the high-energy collision of a light closed string off a stack of D_p-branes [37]. The brane configuration was chosen to be the simplest possible: N infinitely extended parallel branes spanning $p + 1$ directions inside the ambient $(9 + 1)$-dimensional spacetime.

By playing with the residual $(p+1)$-dimensional Lorentz invariance, we can always go to a frame in which the closed string moves in a hyperplane perpendicular to the brane system and impinges on it, carrying an energy E, at an impact parameter b. The brane system conserves energy, but can absorb a transverse momentum q. Let us start with some general comments:

As in the case of string–string collisions, we are not assuming any metric: calculations are done in flat spacetime (the N Dp-branes being introduced via the boundary state formalism [38]). There are, also in this case, three relevant scales in the problem:

- the impact parameter b related to the (orbital) angular momentum $J = bE$ of the incoming string, with $J >> \hbar$ (justifying a semiclassical treatment);
- the scale R_p of the (expected) emerging geometry (see below);
- the string length l_s.

---

[3] M. Ciafaloni and G. Veneziano, unpublished.

[4] Taking it as an indication of black hole formation would seem too good to be true!

These three lengthscales lead to a phase diagram resembling that of Fig. 17.1, but with the collapse region replaced by one of capture of the closed string by the brane system. Since the stack of D-branes is infinitely heavy, we expect the emergent metric to be well described by the classical metric produced by the branes themselves. This is known to be given by

$$ds^2 = \frac{1}{\sqrt{H(r)}}\left(\eta_{\alpha\beta}\,dx^\alpha\,dx^\beta\right) + \sqrt{H(r)}(\delta_{ij}\,dx^i\,dx^j), \qquad (17.7.1)$$

where the indices $\alpha, \beta, \ldots$ run along the Dp-brane worldvolume, the indices $i, j, \ldots$ indicate the transverse directions, $r^2 = \delta_{ij}x^i x^j$, and

$$H(r) = 1 + \left(\frac{R_p}{r}\right)^{7-p}, \qquad R_p^{7-p} = \frac{g_s N(\sqrt{2}\pi l_s)^{7-p}}{(7-p)\Omega_{9-p}}. \qquad (17.7.2)$$

Note that the ratio R_p/l_s can be tuned by varying $g_s N$ (with $g_s \ll 1$, $N \gg 1$).

At very high energy, gravity, in the form of graviton exchange, dominates. Yet we can neglect closed string loops below an $E_{\max}$ that goes to infinity with N. This problem is expected to be easier than the two-particle/string collisions problem. This is because the closed string, though very energetic, still acts as a probe of the geometry induced by the infinitely extended (hence infinitely heavy) brane system. We therefore expect a negligible backreaction on the geometry.

At the disc (tree) and annulus (one-loop) level, an effective classical brane geometry emerges from the calculation under the reasonable assumption that the exponentiation persists at higher loop level. This is seen, again, through the classical deflection formulae that are satisfied at the saddle point of the b-integral. Furthermore, unlike in the case of string–string scattering, the agreement with general relativistic expectations can be checked explicitly at next-to-leading order in the deflection angle, and an extension to all orders appears to be within reach. Indeed, a nontrivial calculation of a subleading term in the annulus diagram gives the following next-to-leading expression for the deflection angle:

$$\Theta_p = \sqrt{\pi}\left[\frac{\Gamma\left((8-p)/2\right)}{\Gamma\left((7-p)/2\right)}\left(\frac{R_p}{b}\right)^{7-p} + \frac{1}{2}\frac{\Gamma\left((15-2p)/2\right)}{\Gamma\left(6-p\right)}\left(\frac{R_p}{b}\right)^{2(7-p)} + \cdots\right],$$
$$(17.7.3)$$

in agreement with the expansion of the exact (though somewhat implicit) classical expression.

Tidal effects can also be computed, and they turn out to be in complete agreement with what one would obtain (to leading order in R_p/b and $(l_s/b)^2$) by quantizing the string in the D-brane metric. Indeed, one can justify, at high energy and leading order in $(l_s/b)^2$, a "Penrose pp-wave limit" for the D-brane metric and then study the nonlinear σ-model describing string fluctuations in that background. Amusingly, at this order the result is the same as the one we described for a string moving in the Aichelburg–Sexl metric—something that can be understood in terms of a Lorentz contraction of the metric along the direction of the incoming energetic string.

Once more, these effects become relevant below a critical impact parameter b_t that is parametrically larger than the string scale:

$$b_t^{8-p} = \frac{\pi}{2}\alpha'\sqrt{\pi s}(7-p)\frac{\Gamma\left((8-p)/2\right)}{\Gamma\left((7-p)/2\right)}R_p^{7-p}\,. \qquad (17.7.4)$$

The tidal excitation spectrum has been double-checked by considering the tree-level exclusive process [39] and the full microscopic understanding of the allowed transition is being clarified [40].

It is also interesting to look at the imaginary part of the tree-level diagram in analogy with what we have already discussed for string–string collisions. In both cases, closed strings (corresponding to a reggeized graviton) are exchanged in the t-channel. However, in this latter case, the imaginary part is due to formation of heavy *open* strings in the s-channel. As one goes to impact parameters smaller than l_s, this imaginary part becomes very relevant and should damp the elastic process in favour of copious production of many open strings living on the branes. Going to higher and higher energies, the average number of these open strings produced goes up so fast that the average mass of each open string produced will eventually go to zero. It is tempting to assume that the dynamics of these massless open strings will be described by a conformal field theory living on the branes. For $p = 3$, where the metric near the boundary is AdS_5, we may hope to make contact with the famous ADS/CFT correspondence [3] within a truly S-matrix approach.

17.8 Summary and outlook

I hope to have passed the message that transplanckian energy collisions in flat spacetime are an ideal theoretical laboratory for studying several conceptual issues (cf. the information puzzle) arising from interplay of quantum mechanics and gravity within a fully consistent framework. Highlighting the main achievements so far:

- At sufficiently large distances, we have been able to reproduce classical expectations (gravitational deflection, tidal effects) and extend them to the case of extended objects within a unitarity-preserving semiclassical description;
- When string-size effects dominate, we found no evidence for black hole formation (again in agreement with classical expectations), but, instead, a rapid increase in the multiplicity and a corresponding softening of the final state resembling a smooth transition to a Hawking-evaporation-like regime.
- In the regime of strong gravitational fields, our successes are still limited. Amusingly, a drastic approximation of the dynamics appears to reproduce at a semiquantitative level expectations based on CTS collapse criteria.
- No firm conclusion can be drawn on this regime without more work. Some features of the present approach may not survive a more complete treatment (e.g. on longitudinal dynamics, which was frozen in the present approach). Many issues remain to be settled (in particular the saturation of unitarity), possibly because of our drastic approximations.

- A general pattern seems to emerge whereby, at the quantum level, the transition between the dispersive and collapse phases is smoothed out by quantum mechanics. As some critical value of the impact parameter is approached, the nature of the final state changes smoothly from that characteristic of a dispersive state to one reminiscent of Hawking radiation (very high multiplicity and very low energies).
- Transplanckian-energy string collisions off a stack of D-branes seem to offer a new tool to study all these issues within an easier setup. We have already seen how classical expectations from an effective metric are reproduced both through deflection formulae and from tidal excitations at leading and next-to-leading order. Generalization to higher (all) orders looks within reach.
- Extension to the classical-capture regime should be possible, and will allow an understanding of how quantum coherence is preserved through the production of a coherent multi-open-string state living on the branes.
- In the case of D3-branes, we hope that this gedanken experiment will shed some new light on the AdS/CFT correspondence within an S-matrix framework.

Acknowledgments

I wish to thank the organizers of the beautiful Les Houches Summer School for the invitation and for the gentle pressure they exercised to have my lectures written up.

References

[1] S. W. Hawking, *Nature* **248** (1974) 30; *Commun. Math. Phys.* **43** (1975) 199.
[2] A. Strominger and C. Vafa, *Phys. Lett.* **B379** (1996) 99; for a review, see J. R. David, G. Mandal, and S.R. Wadia, *Phys. Rep.* **369** (2002) 549.
[3] J. M. Maldacena, *Adv. Theor. Math. Phys.* **2** (1998) 231; S. S. Gubser, I. R. Klebanov, and A. M. Polyakov, *Phys. Lett.* **B428** (1998) 105; E. Witten, *Adv. Theor. Math. Phys.* **2** (1998) 253.
[4] J.M. Maldacena, *JHEP* **0304** (2003) 021; J. L. F. Barbon and E. Rabinovici, *JHEP* **0311** (2003) 047.
[5] I. Antoniadis, *Phys. Lett.* **B246** (1990) 377; N. Arkani-Hamed, S. Dimopoulos, and G. Dvali, *Phys. Lett.* **B429** (1998) 263; L. Randall and R. Sundrum, *Phys. Rev. Lett.* **83** (1999) 3370 and 4690.
[6] S. Dimopoulos and G. Landsberg, *Phys. Rev. Lett.* **87** (2001) 161602; S. B. Giddings and S. Thomas, *Phys. Rev.* **D65** (2002) 056010; G. F. Giudice, R. Rattazzi, and J. D. Wells, *Nucl. Phys.* **B630** (2002) 293.
[7] D. Christodoulou and S. Klainerman, *The Global Nonlinear Stability of the Minkowski Space*, Princeton University Press, Princeton, NJ (1993).
[8] D. Christodoulou, *Commun. Pure Appl. Math.* **44** (1991), 287; *Commun. Math. Phys.* **109** (1987) 613.
[9] M. W. Choptuik, *Phys. Rev. Lett.* **70** (1993) 9. For a review, see C. Gundlach, *Phys. Rep.* **376** (2003) 339.

[10] D. Christodoulou, arXiv: 0805.3880 [gr-qc].

[11] R. Penrose, unpublished (1974).

[12] D. M. Eardley and S. B. Giddings, *Phys. Rev.* **D66** (2002) 044011; H. Yoshino and Y. Nambu, *Phys. Rev.* **D67** (2003) 024009; S. B. Giddings and V. S. Rychkov, *Phys. Rev.* **D70** (2004) 104026.

[13] E. Kohlprath and G. Veneziano, *JHEP* **0206** (2002) 057.

[14] M. W. Choptuik and F. Pretorius, *Phys. Rev. Lett.* **104** (2010) 111101.

[15] G. 't Hooft, *Phys. Lett.* **B198** (1987) 61.

[16] I. J. Muzinich and M. Soldate, *Phys. Rev.* **D37** (1988) 359.

[17] D. J. Gross and P. F. Mende, *Phys. Lett.* **B197** (1987) 129; *Nucl. Phys.* **B303** (1988) 407; P.F. Mende and H. Ooguri, *Nucl. Phys.* **B339** (1990) 641.

[18] D. Amati, M. Ciafaloni, and G. Veneziano, *Phys. Lett.* **B197** (1987) 81; *Int. J. Mod. Phys.* **A3** (1988) 1615.

[19] D. Amati, M. Ciafaloni, and G. Veneziano, *Phys. Lett.* **B216** (1989) 41; G. Veneziano, in *Proc. Superstrings 89, Texas A&M University, 1989*, eds. R. Arnowitt et al. (World Scientific, Singapore, 1990), p. 86.

[20] D. Amati, M. Ciafaloni, and G. Veneziano, *Nucl. Phys.* **B347** (1990) 550 and **B403** (1993) 707.

[21] M. Fabbrichesi, R. Pettorino, G. Veneziano, and G.A. Vilkovisky, *Nucl. Phys.* **B419** (1994) 147.

[22] G. Veneziano in *Proc. Pascos Conference, Northeastern University, Boston, 1990*, eds. P. Nath and S. Rencroft (World Scientific, Singapore, 1990), p. 486; in *Proc. 2nd Paris Cosmology Colloquium, Paris, 1994*, eds. H. J. de Vega and N. Sanchez (World Scientific, Singapore, 1995), p. 322.

[23] D. Amati, M. Ciafaloni, and G. Veneziano, *JHEP* **0802** (2008) 049.

[24] G. Veneziano, *Europhys. Lett.* **2** (1986) 133; in *Proc. Meeting on Hot Hadronic Matter: Theory and Experiments, Divonne, June 1994*, eds. J. Letessier, H. Gutbrod, and J. Rafelsky (Plenum Press, New York, 1995), p. 63; L. Susskind, "Some speculations about black hole entropy in string theory", hep-th/9309145; E. Halyo, A. Rajaraman, and L. Susskind, *Phys. Lett.* **B392** (1997) 319; E.Halyo, B. Kol, A. Rajaraman, and L. Susskind, *Phys. Lett.* **B401** (1997) 15.

[25] G. T. Horowitz and J. Polchinski, *Phys. Rev.* **D55** (1997) 6189 and **D57** (1998) 2557; T. Damour and G. Veneziano, *Nucl. Phys.* **B568** (2000) 93.

[26] P. C. Aichelburg and R. U. Sexl, *Gen. Rel. Grav.* **2** (1971) 303; see e.g. [13] for its generalization.

[27] S. B. Giddings, *Phys. Rev.* **D74** (2006) 106005.

[28] V. A. Abramovskij, V.N. Gribov, and O.V. Kancheli, *Sov. J. Nucl. Phys.* **18** (1974) 308.

[29] G. Veneziano, JHEP **0411** (2004) 001.

[30] J. Polchinski, *String Theory*, Vol. II (Cambridge University Press, Cambridge, 1998).

[31] N. Sanchez, *Phys. Rev.* **D18** (1978) 1030 and 1798.

[32] G. Veneziano, *JHEP* **0411** (2004) 001.

[33] L.N. Lipatov, *Nucl. Phys.* **B365** (1991) 614.

[34] G. Marchesini and E. Onofri, *JHEP* **0806** (2008) 104.

[35] G. Veneziano and J. Wosiek, *JHEP* **0809** (2008) 023 and 024.

[36] M. Ciafaloni and D. Colferai, *JHEP* **0811** (2008) 047; *JHEP* **0912** (2009) 062.

[37] G. D'Appollonio, P. Di Vecchia, R. Russo, and G. Veneziano, *JHEP* **1011** (2010) 100.

[38] P. Di Vecchia and A. Liccardo, in *M-Theory and Quantum Geometry*, eds. L. Thorlacius and T. Jonsson (Kluwer, Dordrecht, 2000), p. 1 [arXiv:hep-th/9912161].

[39] W. Black and C. Monni, *Nucl. Phys.* **B859** (2012) 299; M. Bianchi and P. Teresi, JHEP **1201** (2012) 161.

[40] G. D'Appollonio, P. Di Vecchia, R. Russo, and G. Veneziano, JHEP **1311** (2013) 126.

The manufacturer's authorised representative in the EU for product
safety is Oxford University Press España S.A. of El Parque Empresarial
San Fernando de Henares, Avenida de Castilla, 2 - 28830 Madrid
(www.oup.es/en or product.safety@oup.com). OUP España S.A. also acts
as importer into Spain of products made by the manufacturer.
Printed and bound by CPI Group (UK) Ltd, Croydon, CR0 4YY

06/07/2026

02157624-0001